THIRD EDITION

ESSENTIALS OF SPORTS
PERFORMANCE TRAINING

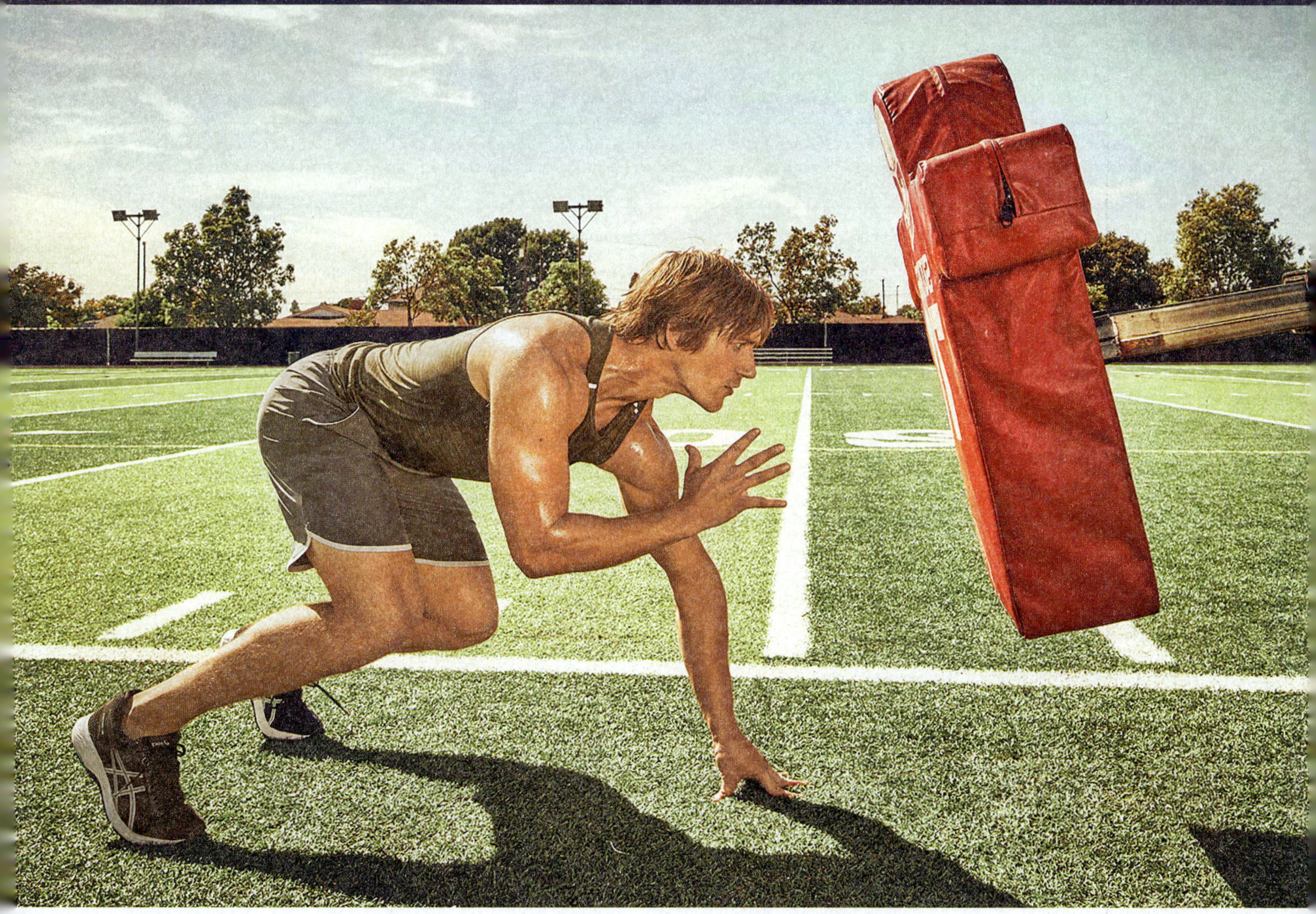

EDITORS

Kyle Stull, DHSc, MS, LMT, CSCS, NASM-CPT, CES, PES
Brian G. Sutton, EdD, MS, MA, CSCS, CES, PES

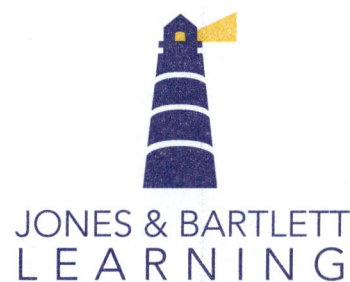

JONES & BARTLETT
LEARNING

World Headquarters
Jones & Bartlett Learning
25 Mall Road
Burlington, MA 01803
978-443-5000
info@jblearning.com
www.jblearning.com

National Academy of Sports Medicine
355 E. Germann Road
Suite 201
Gilbert, AZ 85297
800-460-6276

Jones & Bartlett Learning books and products are available through most bookstores and online booksellers. To contact Jones & Bartlett Learning directly, call 800-832-0034, fax 978-443-8000, or visit our website, www.jblearning.com.

Substantial discounts on bulk quantities of Jones & Bartlett Learning publications are available to corporations, professional associations, and other qualified organizations. For details and specific discount information, contact the special sales department at Jones & Bartlett Learning via the above contact information or send an email to specialsales@jblearning.com.

Production Credits

Senior Director, Content Production and Delivery: Christine Emerton
Director, Product Management: Matthew Kane
Product Manager: Whitney Fekete
Manager, Content Management: Tiffany Sliter
Content Manager: Summer Ibrahim
Manager, Intellectual Properties and Content Production: Kristen Rogers
Content Production Manager: Jennifer Risden and Madelene Nieman
Senior Digital Project Specialist: Colleen Lamy

Senior Director of Supply Chain: Ed Schneider
Procurement Manager: Wendy Kilborn
Composition: S4Carlisle Publishing Services
Cover & Text Design: NASM
Media Development Editor: Faith Brosnan
Rights Specialist: Robin Silverman
Cover Image: © NASM
Printing and Binding: Lakeside Book Company

Library of Congress Cataloging-in-Publication Data
Names: National Academy of Sports Medicine, issuing body. | Stull, Kyle, 1980- editor.
Title: Essentials of sport performance training / [edited by] Kyle Stull.
Other titles: NASM's essentials of sports performance training
Description: Third edition. | Burlington, MA : Jones & Bartlett Learning, 2026. | Revised edition of: NASM's essentials of sports performance training. | Includes bibliographical references and index.
Identifiers: LCCN 2024013414 | ISBN 9781284281767 (hardcover)
Subjects: LCSH: Physical education and training.
Classification: LCC GV341 .N286 2026 | DDC 613.7/11--dc23/eng/20240417
LC record available at https://lccn.loc.gov/2024013414

6048

Printed in the United States of America
28 27 26 25 24   10 9 8 7 6 5 4 3 2 1

CONTENTS

SECTION 1: COACHING AND SPORTS PSYCHOLOGY   1

01   INTRODUCTION TO THE PERFORMANCE TRAINING PROFESSION   3

02   COACHING AND INTERPERSONAL COMMUNICATION SKILLS   19

SECTION 3: ASSESSMENTS, TESTING, AND MONITORING   203

FOREWORD

Congratulations on taking this step to set yourself apart in the competitive sports performance training industry. Thank you for entrusting us to provide the education and tools to improve your skill set and enhance the services you provide to your athletes. Applying the knowledge and skills presented in this course will give you the information, insight, and inspiration needed to help athletes of all levels achieve peak performance.

NASM is the world leader in fitness certification, continuing education, and professional development for health and fitness professionals and sports performance coaches. Our evidence-based approach to creating practical strategies has created what many consider the current standard in professional education in the health and fitness industry.

Scientific research and techniques continue to evolve—and as a result, you must remain on the cutting edge to be competitive. Designed exclusively by NASM, the Optimum Performance Training® (OPT™) Model is the industry's first evidence-based training system founded on the scientific rationale of human movement science. Now, more than ever, a Sports Performance Coach must fully understand all components of exercise programming. The OPT Model is your solution. Using this model, you can successfully train any athlete toward any goal.

This new edition of *NASM Essentials of Sports Performance Training* has been updated with the current evidence, strategies, and training techniques designed to equip Sports Performance Coaches with the necessary skills to optimize the athletic development of their athletes.

Welcome to the team, and we look forward to helping you influence the future of athletic development.

Sincerely,
The National Academy of Sports Medicine

NEW TO THIS EDITION

Based on feedback from past students and sports performance professionals, the Third Edition includes several updates compared to the previous edition.

1. **Additional Chapters.** This textbook includes new chapters, expanding the textbook from 16 to 23 chapters. These additional topics will assist in creating a more well-rounded Sports Performance Coach.
2. **Updated Chapter Content.** All of the topics in this textbook have been updated to include new information and updated research provided and reviewed by the industry's most well-respected sports performance professionals.
3. **Glossary of Terms.** We have updated our glossary to include many terms and definitions.

The Third Edition comes with a variety of new educational features, including the following:

- New illustrations that bring principles and concepts to life
- Updated tables that summarize additional information not included in the body of the text
- New anatomical images that clearly identify important structures of the human body
- Text boxes that discuss relevant research and expanded content
- Updated photos that show proper execution of exercises

CONTRIBUTORS

EDITORS

Kyle Stull
DHSc, MS, LMT, CSCS, NASM-CPT,
CES, PES

Brian Sutton
EdD, MS, MA, CSCS, CES, PES

PEER REVIEW AND DEVELOPMENTAL EDITING

Tony Ambler-Wright
MS, BCTMB, LMT, CPSS, CSCS,
NASM-CES, PES, CSNC

Wendy Batts
MS, NMT, NASM-CPT, CES, PES

David Behm
PhD

Scott W. Cheatham
PhD, DPT, ATC, NASM-CPT,
CES, PES

Brad Dieter
PhD, MS

Michael Elliott
MS, NASM-CPT, CES, PES

Lauren Hyser
USAW-L2, CrossFit-L2, ESC-L2, PN1

Joel Jamieson
CSCS, NSCA-CPT, USAW

Morey Kolber
PhD, PT, OCS

Ken Miller
MS, NASM-CPT, CES, PES

Theresa Miyashita
PhD, MA, ATC, NASM-CES, PES

Aaron Nelson
MS, ATC, NASM-CES

Rick Richey
DHSc, MS, LMT

Justin Russ
CSCS, RSCC, NASM-PES, USAW,
USA Track and Field-L1

Kyle Stull
DHSc, MS, LMT, CSCS, NASM-CPT,
CES, PES

Brian Sutton
EdD, MS, MA, CSCS, CES, PES

Julius Thomas
MS, CSNS

AUTHORS

Bryan Burnstein
MS, AT-Ret, CSCS, USAW-ASPC,
NASM-CES/PES/FNS

Scott W. Cheatham
PhD, DPT, ATC, NASM-CPT,
CES, PES

Rodney Corn
MS, PES, CES, PTA Global-CPT

Adam Feit
PhD, CSCS*D, SCCC, PES

Mary Kate Feit
PhD, CSCS, SCCC

Rick Howard
DSc, CSCS*D, RSCC*E, FNSCA

Scott Howell
PhD, CSCS, CPT

Matt Jordan
PhD, CSCS

Jordan M. Joy
PhD, CSCS*D, CISSN

Justin Kilian
PhD

Joseph G. Kenn III
MA, CSCS, RSCC*E, SCCC,
MSCC, PN1

William J. Kraemer
PhD, CSCS*D, FACSM, FNSCA

Kerry Martin
PhD

Tony Moreno
PhD, CSCS*D

Brian T. Oddi
PhD, PES, CSS

Ben Reuter
PhD, CSCS*D, ATC

Tony Ricci
EdD MS, FISSN, CSCS, PES,
CES, CNS

Rick Richey
DHSc, MS, LMT, CES, PES

Alan Russell
MS, LAT, ATC, PES, CES

Tim Sharpe
DACM, MS

Brian Sutton
EdD, MS, MA, CSCS, CES, PES

Dan van Zandt
MS, CSCS

Nick Winkelman
PhD

PRODUCT TEAM

Casey DeJong – Senior Instructional
Designer

Ian Montel – Product Manager

Andrew Payne – Instructional
Designer

Melissa Schimmel – Project Manager

Kyle Stull – Content Development
Manager

SPECIAL THANKS

- Nurture Digital
- Reflection Software
- NASM Marketing
  Creative Team

SECTION 1

COACHING AND SPORTS PSYCHOLOGY

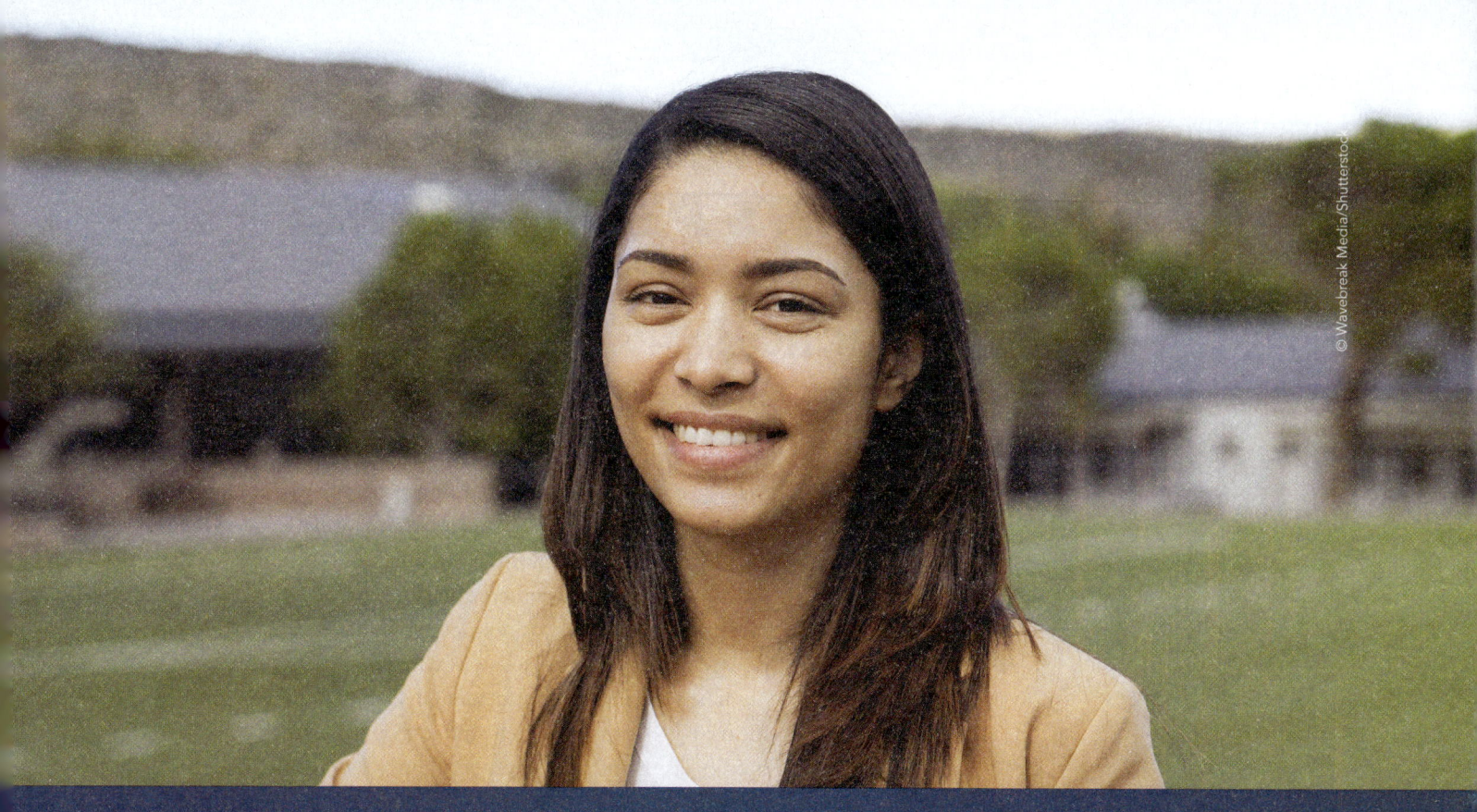

INTRODUCTION TO THE PERFORMANCE TRAINING PROFESSION

CHAPTER ONE

LEARNING OBJECTIVES

Upon completion of this chapter, the Sports Performance Coach will be able to:

- **Differentiate** sports performance training from traditional personal training and generalized exercise instruction.

- **Understand** the roles of the various members of the Integrated Sports Performance Team.

- **Identify** scope of practice, ethical and professional behaviors, and referral strategies.

- **Identify** the different types of clients who make up the athlete spectrum.

LESSON 1: AN INTRODUCTION TO SPORTS PERFORMANCE COACHING

INTRODUCTION

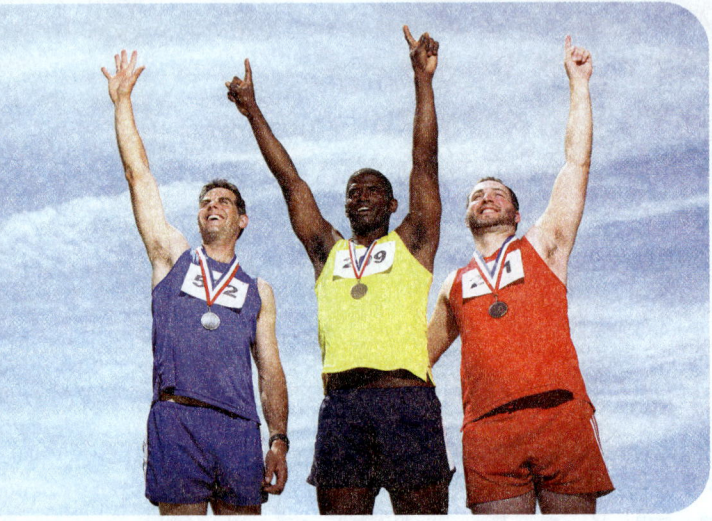

© Hurst Photo/Shutterstock

Even in the time of the ancient Olympics, high-performance elements were a part of athletic preparation. The ancient Greeks trained within macro- and micro-training cycles and used specialized tactical preparation, specialized equipment, psychological preparation, and proper recovery to prepare for the Olympic Games. Additionally, athletes were supported by coaches, doctors, physiotherapists, and massage therapists, much as they are today (Smith & Smolianov, 2020). Although research examining the science behind sports performance has taken place since the ancient Greek era, it was not until the mid-1970s that research shifted from assessing resistance training as the primary method of improving athleticism to more detailed physical performance capabilities for those seeking athletic elitism and the ideals surrounding the holistic approach to training.

As athletes progress toward elite status in their sport, organizational expectations and societal pressures increase. For some athletes, these increases have led to burnout, poor mental health, and risk-taking behaviors (Lindgren & Barker-Ruchti, 2017; Rice et al., 2016). In turn, the field of sports science has recognized the need for a holistic approach to athlete development.

> ### ✔ CHECK IT OUT
>
> Boyd Epley was the University of Nebraska's first full-time strength and conditioning coach. He was hired in 1969 and shortly thereafter helped found the National Strength and Conditioning Association, bringing together the first group of like-minded professionals. This was a pivotal moment in the industry and began a paradigm shift in collegiate athletics (Shurley & Todd, 2012).

HOLISTIC APPROACH →

Considers the personal, emotional, cultural, academic, athletic, and social identity of the athlete, as well as nutrition, sleep, and recovery, and how these elements influence the athlete's performance.

A **holistic approach** considers the personal, emotional, cultural, academic, athletic, and social identity of the athlete, as well as nutrition, sleep, and recovery, and how these elements influence the athlete's performance (Egan, 2019; Lindgren & Barker-Ruchti, 2017; Mujika et al., 2018) (**Figure 1.1**). By emphasizing a good balance of performance enhancement, results, and health and well-being, the Sports Performance Coach can focus on the athlete as a whole (**Figure 1.2**) and train the individual athlete's developmental needs as the means to the end.

Today's Sports Performance Coach uses a holistic approach while working as an integral member of the Integrated Sports Performance Team to assist athletes of varying

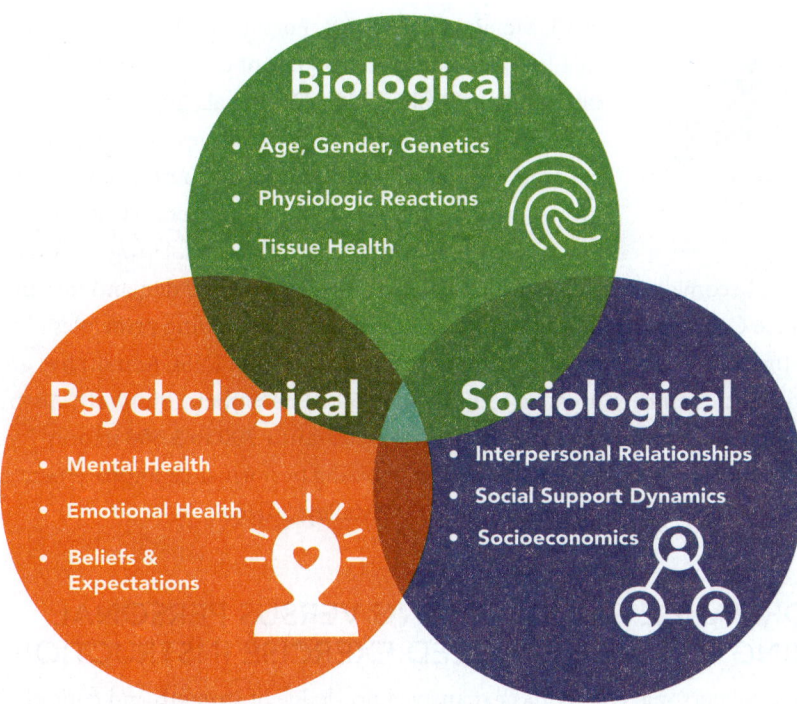

FIGURE 1.1 Holistic Approach

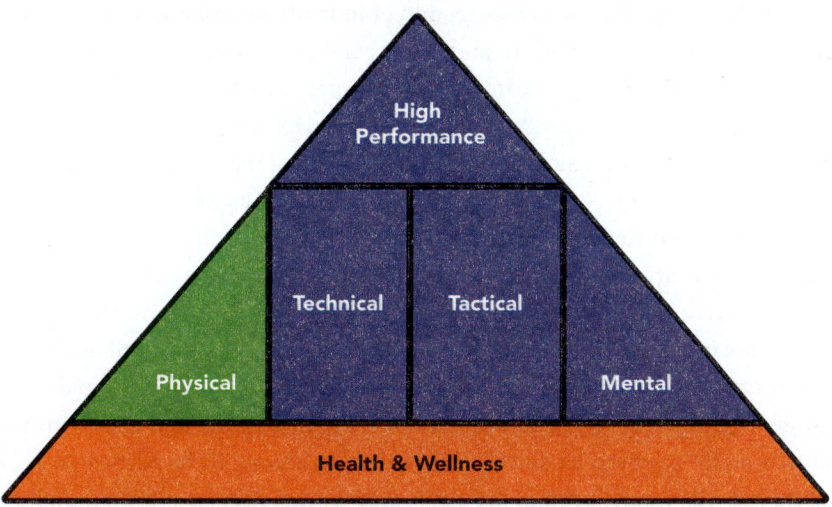

FIGURE 1.2 Holistic Athlete Development

skills and abilities in reaching their goals. In the United States, the Bureau of Labor Statistics (n.d.) projects that the number of people employed in occupations in sports is expected to grow much faster than average through 2030. This course is designed to help meet the needs of this growing industry by ensuring that the Sports Performance Coach learns what it means to fill that role and how to use an athlete-centric approach to optimize athletic development.

PARTICIPATION IN SPORTS

Increasing evidence shows that participating in sports has benefits above the physical effects, including improved mental and social health, improved social interaction and self-esteem, fewer depressive symptoms, and reduced stress (Eime et al., 2013; Jenkin et al.,

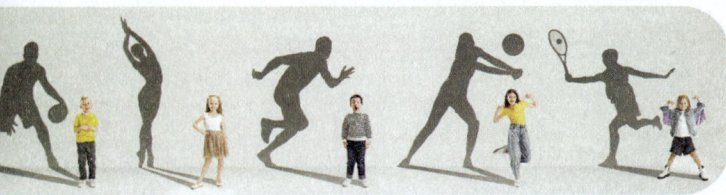

2018; Moeijes et al., 2018). Further, research has demonstrated that the academic performance of children and adolescents is linked to physical activity (Dyer et al., 2017).

As participation in sports continues to climb, competition becomes greater, and the demand for performance training grows stronger. As recent as the 20th century, strength training was viewed as harmful for some sports. However, as new research has become available, a shift has occurred, increasing the demand for Sports Performance Coaches with in-depth knowledge of strength training principles. As an example, the National Strength and Conditioning Association (NSCA, n.d.) has grown from an original membership of 76 to more than 60,000 members. Similarly, Australian Strength and Conditioning memberships increased from 1,300 to 3,500 in only 7 years because many coaches and athletes began recognizing performance improvement and injury reduction benefits from such training (O'Malley, 2016).

PERFORMANCE CONDITIONING VERSUS PERSONAL TRAINING AND GENERALIZED EXERCISE INSTRUCTION

The traditional personal trainer has expansive knowledge of strength and conditioning principles and enters the workforce either by starting a private fitness business or by delivering personal or group training sessions at public gyms. Working with a personal trainer is appropriate for the wide cross section of individuals looking to increase their physical activity, optimize their health and fitness, and even compete in recreational competitions. For individuals and teams looking to maximize performance and compete at the highest levels, however, working with a Sports Performance Coach is necessary. Performance conditioning requires advanced knowledge of the scientific principles of human anatomy, physiology, kinesiology, and biomechanics, as well as the practitioner's ability to apply this knowledge in a dynamic high-performance environment.

Personal trainers are integral members of the fitness community and work with a client's medical team to develop the most appropriate exercise program. However, fitness professionals are often not considered members of the individual's overall healthcare team, which can lead to them working in silos toward their client's fitness goals. While fitness professionals often build a referral network of other health and fitness providers, the onus falls on the client to facilitate communication among these parties. In a personal trainer–client relationship, the client must either disclose information between practitioners or initiate the communication and give consent for discussion. This often differs for a Sports Performance Coach, who acts as part of an interdisciplinary team where athlete-centered communication is central. Athletes as part of a team provide consent to allow the interdisciplinary performance team to collaborate to support their individual readiness, safety, and health.

To ensure optimal and safe outcomes regardless of the level of activity, training programs must be scientifically based and match the level of participation. General fitness programs are often designed to fit around the space, equipment, and time constraints of the client. It is common for an average client to allocate only a short window of time each week for such a program and to train in the same location with the same equipment. Average clients have common goals, with weight loss being one of the most desired changes.

By comparison, serious athletes have more performance-based goals and fewer body composition goals. In addition, reaching performance-based goals may require specialized equipment and programming that fits a unique schedule. Some athletes have several weeks or even several months of an off-season to recover and correct muscle imbalances before they begin training for the next season. Others might need to fit recovery, corrective exercise, and increasing strength and power into a relatively short window of time. Accordingly, the Sports Performance Coach must have in-depth knowledge of different periodization models and be able to structure a training program into specific phases to create the best opportunity for maximal performance during the competitive season or a specific event. These training programs prepare the athlete for the repetitive and often unpredictable demands of specific positions within sports.

Sports Performance Coaches recognize that athletic movements are functional and must be trained in a more complex and dynamic environment to achieve optimal neuromuscular efficiency and performance. They must design training programs that incorporate the entire **human movement system (HMS)** through all planes of motion, integrating flexibility, core, balance, plyometric, resistance, metabolic energy system, sport-specific training, and speed, agility, and quickness (SAQ) training into the program (McGill & Montel, 2019).

ADDRESSING THE GAP

When pursuing a career in sports training, it is important to understand the gap between the information and education available. Traditional strength and conditioning certifications are often promoted as the "gold standard" in sports performance education. Although this knowledge is certainly valuable, modern sports performance training goes beyond traditional strength and conditioning programming.

Sports participation continues to grow, leading to increased competition and greater demand for high-level performance training of athletes. The Sports Performance Coach must go beyond understanding assessment protocols, principles of programming and periodization, and various strength training systems, by also understanding how to connect and effectively communicate with athletes.

Sports Performance Coaches can increase the demand for their services by taking the following steps:

- Learning *how* to coach
- Developing interpersonal communication skills
- Exploring performance psychology and its role in sports
- Having working knowledge of rest and recovery strategies
- Understanding how to train for injury prevention

> ### HUMAN → MOVEMENT SYSTEM (HMS)
>
> The muscular, skeletal, and nervous systems; also known as the kinetic chain.

📋 COACH'S CORNER

While the Sports Performance Coach should not promote themselves as a sports psychologist, understanding some of the underlying tenets of the mind can play a vital role in performance development.

NASM's Sports Performance Enhancement Specialization addresses these gaps by providing the learner with the most scientifically accurate information, allowing for continued growth and advancement of the industry.

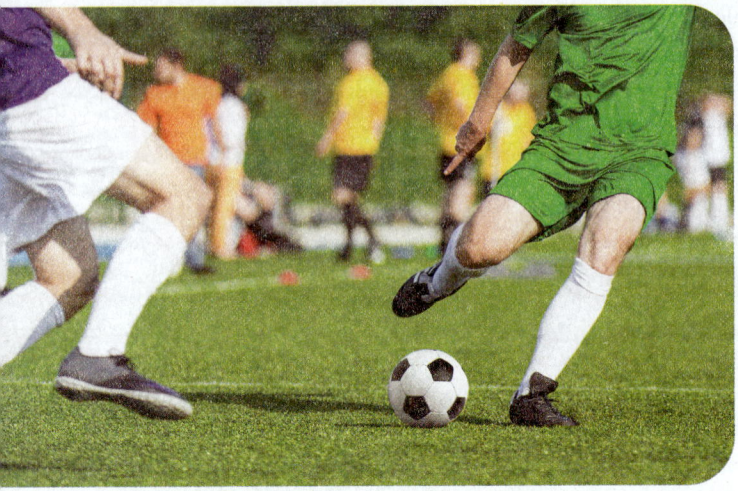

© Matimix/Shutterstock

THE ATHLETE SPECTRUM

The term *athlete* comes from the Greek word *athlos*, which means "achievement," and is often associated with someone who competes in events that require physical strength, speed, endurance, and sport-specific skills and who performs at an elite level within their chosen sport (Araújo & Scharhag, 2016; Laquale, 2009). However, the modern-day use of this term has expanded to include more than professional or semi-professional status. Its scope includes recreational athletes, youth and adolescent athletes, senior athletes, competitive amateur athletes, and collegiate, semi-professional, and professional status athletes. Within this expanding demographic, the Sports Performance Coach must understand the needs of athletes across the entire spectrum.

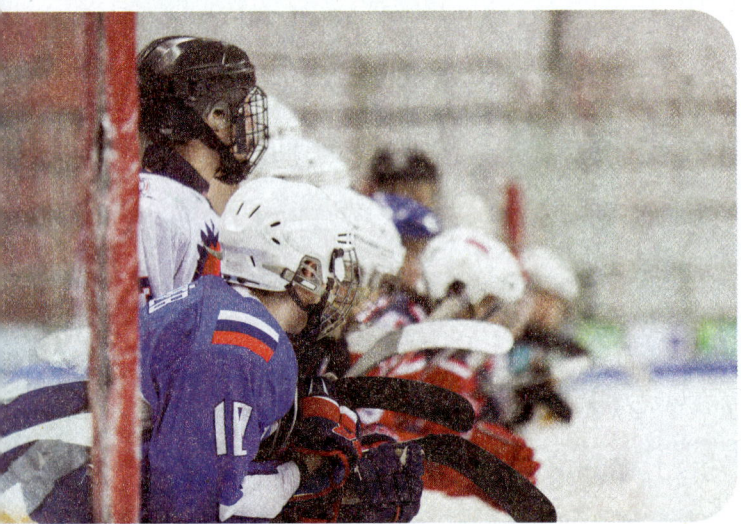

© Pavel L Photo and Video/Shutterstock

RECREATIONAL ATHLETES AND WEEKEND WARRIORS

Recreational athletes participate in sports to be social, stay physically active, and have fun (Laquale, 2009). A weekend warrior is an individual who does not train regularly or who trains extremely hard for a very short time leading up to an event. The recreational athlete and the weekend warrior typically do not train properly for their sport or activity. Recreational athletes might participate in organized athletic competitions, and they train at a lower intensity than individuals who seek to be competitive. Both the weekend warrior and recreational athlete are at a higher risk for injury secondary to their lack of training or inefficient training, and they often do not train under the guidance of an appropriately educated Sports Performance Coach.

COMPETITIVE ATHLETE SPECTRUM

The competitive athlete spectrum ranges from well-trained athletes who compete on a regular basis without any financial gain to collegiate athletes, and those who make careers out of their skill as professional athletes, such as Olympians and individuals who receive financial compensation for their performance. Sports experts continue to debate the classifications of amateur versus professional athlete status, and it is not the job of the Sports Performance Coach to delineate where the athlete falls within this spectrum.

However, it is important to understand that differences exist, and the Sports Performance Coach must consider the complexity of physical and mental demands when designing a program for the various types of athletes. Such training must be goal oriented and sport specific and must utilize an appropriate periodized training system within a holistic athlete development program. **Periodized** training is best described as a planned approach to training that divides complex training programs into smaller, more distinct, and more manageable phases (Hornsby et al., 2020). The training program needs to provide sufficient training stimuli to allow an athlete to progress toward the next level of competition while also increasing durability and longevity.

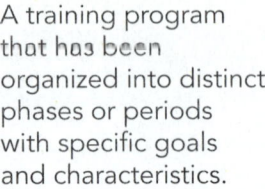

PERIODIZED →

A training program that has been organized into distinct phases or periods with specific goals and characteristics.

YOUTH AND ADOLESCENT CLIENTS

Recent research shows that almost 60% of U.S. children and adolescents ages 6 to 17 years participate in organized sports (Hyde et al., 2020). Many of these young athletes compete in multiple sports; however, sports specialization is common at young ages, depending on the sport. The Sports Performance Coach must understand that youth and adolescent athletes are not miniature adults. The goal when working with children is to motivate them to enjoy athletics and to encourage physical activity throughout adulthood. Unfortunately, competitive athletic programs and sport specialization frequently result in burnout among young athletes.

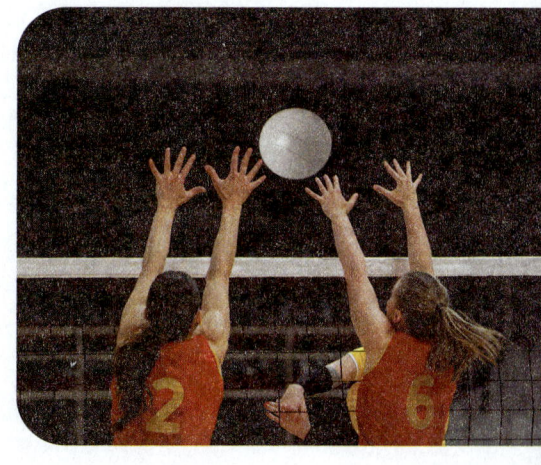

© Sportoakimirka/Shutterstock

Training programs for young athletes must focus on general athleticism while keeping it fun and building a desire to remain active. Research shows that young athletes grow into active adults. In one long-term study, individuals who participated in sports between the ages of 9 and 18 were five to six times more likely to be active into adulthood (Telama et al., 2006). In some cases, participating in youth sports just once a week led to a higher chance of being active adults. Without question, regular physical activity early in life can translate into a healthier future. The chances of youth athletes continuing on to become collegiate and professional athletes is slim, however. The National Collegiate Athletic Association (NCAA, n.d.) reports that only 7% of the 7 million high school athletes progress to collegiate athletics; of that group, only 2% become professional athletes. Therefore, the focus should be on developing healthy athletes who love being physically active rather than getting young athletes to a professional status.

LESSON 2: MAXIMIZING TEAM SUCCESS: THE ROLE OF INTEGRATED SPORTS PERFORMANCE TEAMS

THE INTEGRATED SPORTS PERFORMANCE TEAM

Sport is one of North America's leading industries, generating nearly $500 billion in revenues annually. Spectators spend almost $18 billion each year attending sporting events, with another $10 billion going toward event-day purchases and incidentals (Kim & Trail, 2010; Smith & Smolianov, 2020). In terms of the desire for spectators to attend sporting events, team performance is a large motivator or constraint: If a team has a winning record, attendance numbers increase; conversely, attendance numbers trend downward if a team has a losing record. Further, teams that advance to playoffs and championships generate even greater revenues. Thus, a team's performance directly impacts the amount of revenue generated by the parent organization (Smith & Smolianov, 2020), and having athletes perform at their highest capabilities is important to ensure good team outcomes.

To win, athletes need to be ready to perform, be in peak condition, and be available for the coaches to implement a strategic game plan. Over the past decade, there has been a shift in how professional teams and elite sports organizations approach the care and management of athletes—because athletes who suffer from injuries and lack of conditioning are no longer assets to their teams. To provide the optimal environment for athletes to be successful, sports teams use an athlete-centered model (**Figure 1.3**), ultimately building a support system whose focus is the care and development of each athlete.

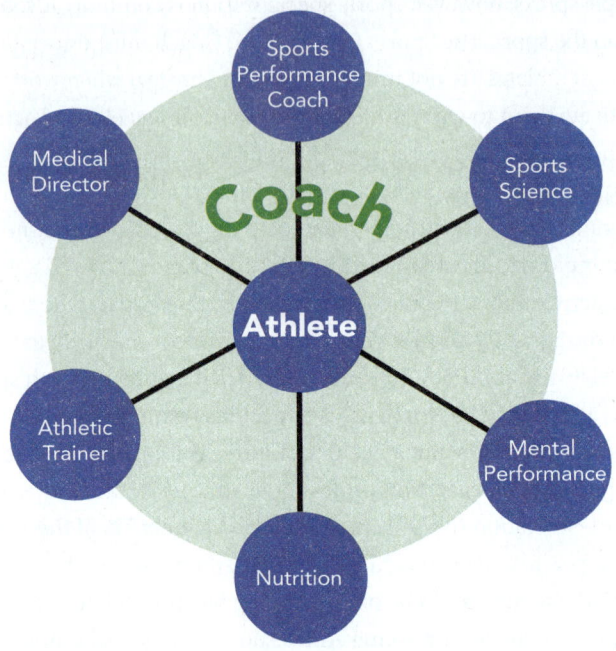

FIGURE 1.3 Athlete-Centered Model

Providing appropriate support for an athlete requires a multidisciplinary approach in which practitioners and coaches draw on knowledge from various disciplines, such as sport-specific coaching, performance medicine, and performance conditioning. A more cohesive and effective approach is working within an **Integrated Sports Performance Team** that collaborates to analyze, synthesize, and harmonize links between the disciplines to create a coordinated and coherent whole-team approach (Choi & Pak, 2006). Effective communication among members of the Integrated Sports Performance Team is critical to its success.

The Integrated Sports Performance Team supports the health and well-being of the athlete, keeping the athlete on the field of play and maximizing their athletic performance. The Integrated Sports Performance Team includes the following members:

- The athlete
- Performance director
- Sports coaches
- Sports Performance Coaches
- Athletic trainers
- Physical therapists
- Sports physicians
- Registered dieticians or nutrition specialists
- Licensed massage therapists
- Sports psychologists or mental performance coaches

Many athletes like to be involved in the management of their own performance, especially when it comes to objective measures to improve performance. Therefore, it is important that the Integrated Sports Performance Team create an environment where the athlete is supported and nurtured to develop some autonomy.

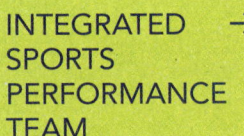

INTEGRATED SPORTS PERFORMANCE TEAM

Analyzes, synthesizes, and harmonizes links between the disciplines to create a coordinated and coherent whole-team approach.

PERFORMANCE DIRECTOR

As teams move away from a multidisciplinary structure and embrace the concept of an interdisciplinary functioning performance unit, a new role has emerged: the performance director. The role of the performance director is to create an environment for success through collaboration with other team members (Sotiriadou & De Bosscher, 2013) (**Figure 1.4**). This individual must have strong management, organizational, and communication skills to effectively lead and manage the team and to align with other stakeholders across the organization. Additionally, a performance director needs extensive knowledge of elite-level programs, coaching, and athletes. They must have a high level of self-motivation, effective time management skills, and a strong work ethic (Smith & Smolianov, 2020). Individuals in this role have, at a minimum, a bachelor's degree in sport administration, physiology, kinesiology, or equivalent experience and typically five or more years in high performance or a related field. As this role continues to adapt to changing demands, more organizations are looking for an individual with a graduate-level degree and increased work-related experience.

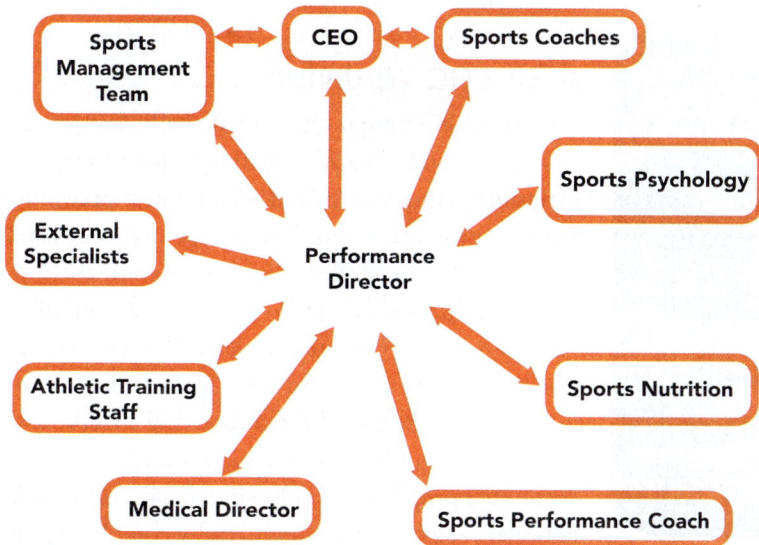

FIGURE 1.4 Performance Director Role

SPORTS COACHES

Typically, the sports coach is the most influential member of the Integrated Sports Performance Team for the athlete. Sports coaches can vary by sport but generally include the head coach, assistant coaches, and various position-specific coaches. The athlete understands that the coach ultimately determines the athlete's path to success (i.e., playing time and exposure). A good head coach is an expert in the tactical and strategic methods needed to get the best performance out of the athlete. Additionally, the head coach must be able to recruit talented athletes and put together a cohesive and competent coaching staff. This coaching staff is then responsible for ensuring a safe and effective environment for competition.

Although a traditional educational route is not required for an individual to become a sports coach, standards, competencies, and certification requirements, which can vary among countries and sports, may be established for this role. For example, Canada and Australia have national coaching certifications, whereas other countries, such as the United States, leave certification requirements up to the individual sport's governing body.

SPORTS PERFORMANCE COACH

Experienced strength and conditioning coaches who understand the demands of elite performance and know how to effectively communicate with athletes are well suited to take on the role of the Sports Performance Coach. The Sports Performance Coach must be able to understand and apply foundational principles of sports nutrition, sports psychology, athletic training, organizational management, coaching, and motivation to a wide spectrum of athletes. Additionally, they must be able to assess and design programs for the elite athlete. Although specific certifications and education vary depending on the job level and employer, most high-level Sports Performance Coaches have a bachelor's degree (graduate-level degree preferred) in sports science, exercise science, kinesiology, or a related field of study along with a recognized certification.

© Matimix/Shutterstock

ATHLETIC TRAINERS

Athletic trainers are multi-skilled healthcare practitioners who can provide a variety of athletic-based services, including primary care, injury and illness prevention, wellness promotion and education, emergency care, examination and clinical diagnosis, therapeutic intervention, and rehabilitation of injuries and medical conditions. According to the National Athletic Trainers' Association, the minimum entry point into the athletic training profession is a bachelor's degree. After completing a Commission on Accreditation of Athletic Training Education (CAATE)–accredited program of study, students become eligible for national certification by successfully completing the Board of Certification (BOC) examination and filing for their respective state licensure. Currently, athletic trainers are licensed or otherwise regulated in 49 states and the District of Columbia.

© Alexander Lukatskiy/Shutterstock

PHYSICAL THERAPIST

As part of the Integrated Sports Performance Team, physical therapists work with the athletic trainer (or are sometimes dual-credentialed as an athletic trainer) to properly evaluate and treat athletes' injuries and provide prevention strategies. Physical therapists must complete a graduate level of education (most have earned a doctoral degree), pass a nationally recognized certification examination, and become licensed in the state in which they practice. Some professional athletic teams and leagues employ athletic trainers and physical therapists to perform distinct roles.

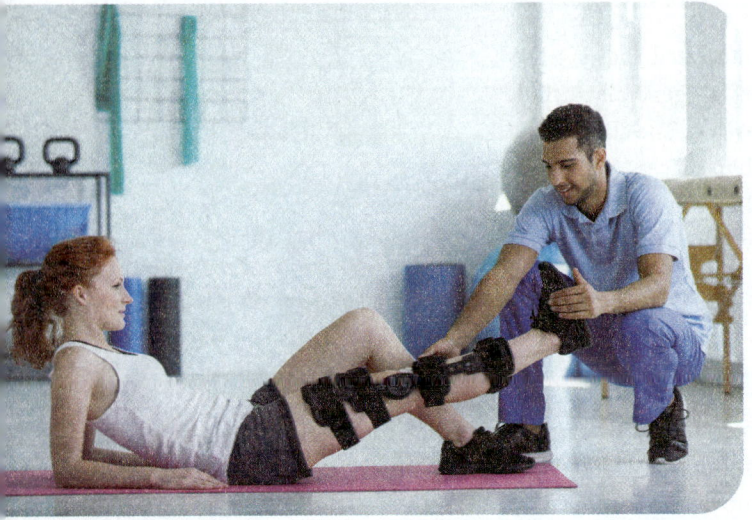

© Ground Picture/Shutterstock

SPORTS PHYSICIANS

Depending on the level of competition, sports physicians might be directly employed by the organization. Most often, these individuals are community physicians who have demonstrated excellence in their profession and understand the dynamics of high-level athleticism. Teams often collaborate with multiple sports physicians in various specialties ranging from general health to orthopedic medicine. Having a physician with a specialization in sports medicine available is important when a team needs to make decisions about an athlete's playing status and, in particular, about their return to play following an injury. A physician unfamiliar with the demands of sport may clear an athlete for return based solely on physiological healing. However, that athlete might not be functionally ready to return, thus increasing the risk of reinjury. Having a sports physician as part of the Integrated Sports Performance Team mitigates these types of issues.

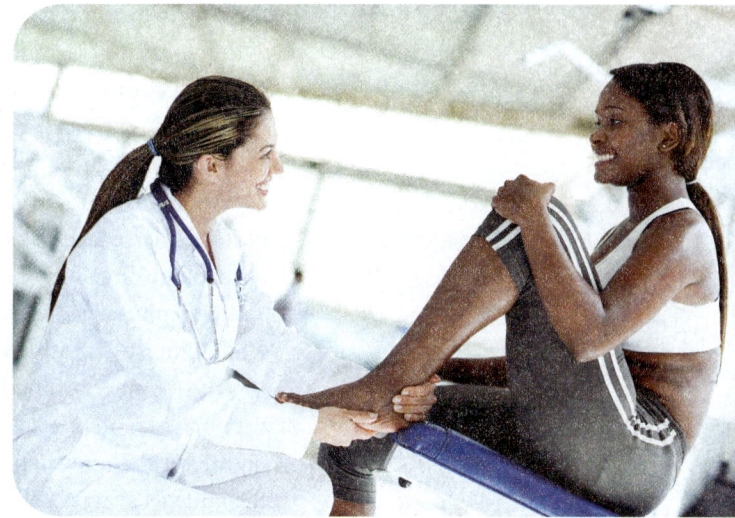

© ESB Professional/Shutterstock

BOARD-CERTIFIED SPECIALIST IN SPORTS DIETETICS

Proper fueling and hydration are vitally important pieces of the performance puzzle. The strategies implemented by a board-certified specialist in sports dietetics (CSSD) include educating athletes on the proper nutrition to get the most out of workouts and to achieve faster recovery times, weight management, injury rehabilitation, and pain alleviation. Most sports dieticians have a strong background working with male and female athletes.

Many athletes rely on supplements to enhance performance and maintain health. Further, it is highly recommended that athletes seek out the sports dietician's advice and recommendations on proper supplement use (Maughan et al., 2018). To help athletes make safe decisions, the sports dietician must have detailed knowledge of dietary and supplement dosing recommendations and regulations in sports.

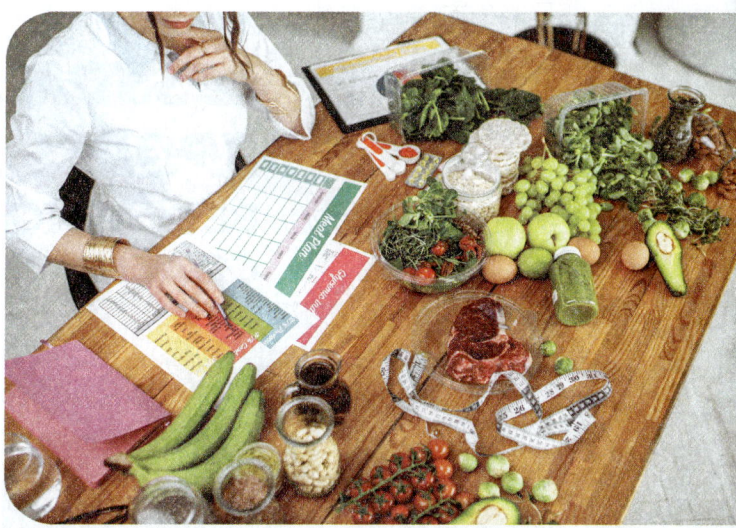

© RossHelen/Shutterstock

LICENSED MASSAGE THERAPIST

Licensed massage therapists (LMTs) complement the work of the athletic trainer and physical therapist in providing enhanced mobility and recovery tactics to reduce the risk of injury. LMTs must complete formal education and meet the requirements set by their specific state for licensure. While not required, additional training in sports-specific massage may be beneficial.

SPORTS PSYCHOLOGIST AND MENTAL PERFORMANCE COACH

An often overlooked component of athlete preparedness is mental training and support. Many individuals in this role have received a doctoral degree in psychology and additional

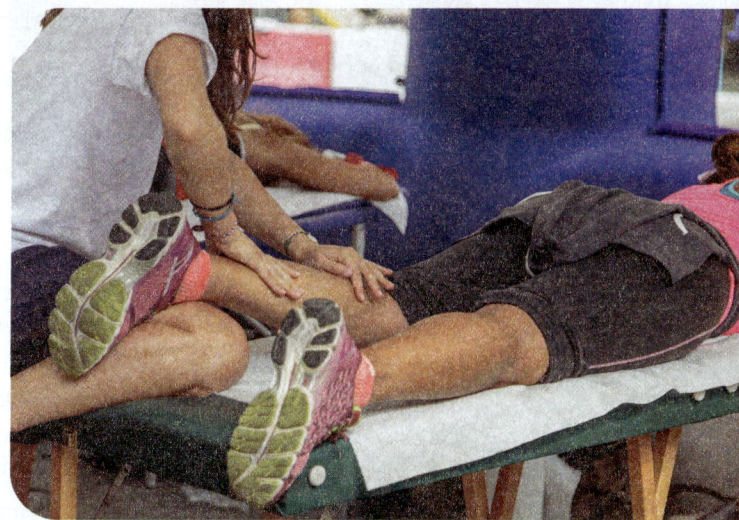

© Giorgio Rossi/Shutterstock

training to become sports psychologists. While sports psychologists are trained to deal with mental illness, much of this field focuses on understanding people's performance, mental processes, and well-being in sports settings (Meijen, 2019). A sports psychologist's role includes helping athletes to manage anxiety, use mental strategies to build motivation and self-confidence, develop mental toughness, and increase concentration.

Another role focusing on mental training is the mental performance coach. A mental performance coach or consultant must also have a graduate degree in a field related to psychology or sports science, but a doctoral degree or state licensure is not required. Thus, a mental performance coach may have specific limitations on their practice, but can still be vital in improving athletes' mental performance.

The members of the Integrated Sports Performance Team must work together to support each other as well as to support the athlete. The integration aspect of this team highlights the importance of communication among members, which is crucial to the athlete's success. When there are gaps in communication or alignment among the performance team, mistakes can lead to injury or the athlete not being properly prepared. Both outcomes can lead to loss of trust.

LESSON 3: BECOMING A SPORTS PERFORMANCE COACH
BECOMING A SPORTS PERFORMANCE COACH

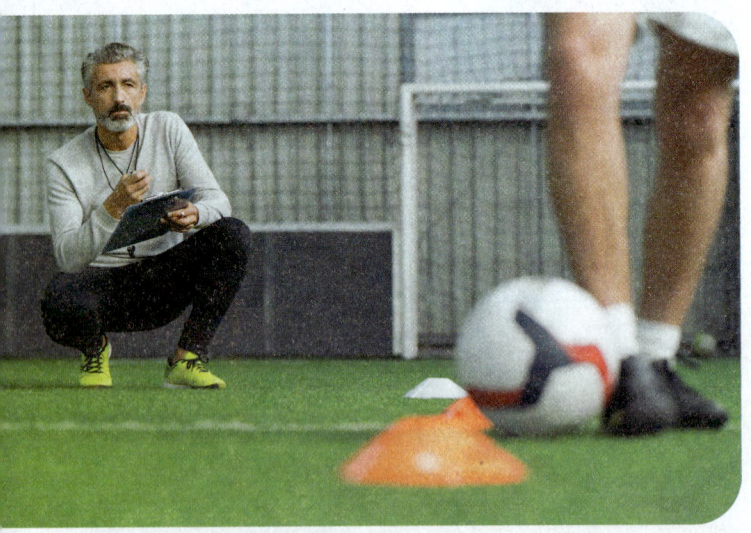
© ALPA PROD/Shutterstock

Many Sports Performance Coaches develop the dedication and desire to help other athletes after being athletes themselves (Lynch & Mallett, 2006; Miller et al., 1996; Sarı & Soyer, 2010; Schinke et al., 1995). However, being a former athlete is not a requirement for becoming an effective Sports Performance Coach. Great coaches, above all, exhibit the desire to help others succeed. They are often on the same level as great leaders in both sports and business.

Once the passion to work with athletes exists, becoming a great coach requires education. Some certifications and jobs in the sports performance field require a bachelor's degree in a related field of study, such as sports science, exercise science, kinesiology, health, or life sciences. University degrees offer many advantages, such as the advanced study of topics essential to performance training, exposure to a variety of disciplines, and opportunities for practical experience.

However, formal degrees are not a hard-and-fast requirement. There are no national or state licensure requirements to become a Sports Performance Coach, although employers are more likely to hire individuals who have a credible certification. Certifications are earned when an individual meets a professional organization's requirements to sit for a certification examination, granting them the right to use the organization's credentials upon receiving a passing score. Licensure focuses on meeting a set of regulations from a state or national government agency. Further, positions in the sports science realm require varying levels of experience, specialized training, educational background, and additional certifications. When hiring for these roles, employers examine their organizational needs, and the requirements are often based on that population's athletic status and desired outcomes.

A Sports Performance Coach can work in many different venues, so it is helpful to seek out internship opportunities and find a mentor who can provide guidance on career goals. It is common for professional teams to recruit candidates for paid internships through industry job boards. Additionally, as the field of sports performance continues to evolve, it is crucial that Sports Performance Coaches take advantage of learning opportunities, such as workshops and conferences, for career advancement. Opportunities also exist in elite-level sports, collegiate sports at varying levels, high school and youth sports, and clubs or studios. Another opportunity is to work as a private or individual Sports Performance Coach. This trend is becoming more common across professional and elite-level athletics because of the one-on-one attention an athlete receives.

Regardless of the venue, the Sports Performance Coach has a responsibility to individual athletes, the athletic team and affiliated organization, the Integrated Sports Performance Team and, if the athlete is a minor, the parents. The Sports Performance Coach must also recognize that beyond the advancement of the athlete, they serve in a role that can impact the profession and the sport in which they work.

SCOPE OF PRACTICE AND ETHICAL PRACTICES

Because the Sports Performance Coach's scope of practice includes athletes at all levels of competition, the Sports Performance Coach needs to understand how the various physical, mental, and emotional loads impact an athlete's training and development for their age and physical maturity. It is a part of the job to push the athlete out of their comfort zone without intentionally harming the athlete by going beyond one's base of knowledge.

> **⚠ CRITICAL**
>
> The Sports Performance Coach is not a therapist and has an obligation to understand when it is appropriate for an athlete to be referred for physical or mental services. For example, an athlete who complains of pain needs to be referred to the athletic trainer or sports physician for an evaluation. Similarly, an athlete who consistently complains of a lack of energy or is in a poor mood should be referred to the sports dietician to discuss proper fueling and hydration or to the mental performance consultant for further support.

The Integrated Sports Performance Team aims to keep the athlete in the game. The safety of the athlete in regard to proper training, injury prevention, and proper rehabilitation must always remain at the forefront. The Sports Performance Coach has an ethical obligation to remain within their scope of practice and must understand how to integrate the knowledge from other Integrated Sports Performance Team members to maintain athlete safety and contribute to the return of the athlete post injury.

PLAYER SAFETY AND THE RETURN-TO-PLAY PROCESS

The Sports Performance Coach is an integral part of the return-to-play process for injured athletes. During the early phases of rehabilitation, the medical team will take the most active role in leading the care plan. As the athlete progresses, the medical staff continues to coordinate the plan, and the Sports Performance Coach becomes much more involved in the day-to-day delivery of the plan, as the program progresses toward functional, sports-specific activities. Throughout this process, communication with the doctors and family (if applicable) is streamlined through the medical team.

INAPPROPRIATE CONDUCT

The Sports Performance Coach must not participate in any inappropriate conduct, such as sexual harassment or discrimination, or knowingly instruct an athlete to participate in inappropriate training, including the use of banned substances. Sports Performance Coaches need to remain up-to-date on regulations regarding performance enhancers, including any relevant position statements from the World Anti-Doping Agency (WADA) and the specific sport's governing body (e.g., NCAA, National Football League, National Basketball Association, National Hockey League, Major League Baseball). Athletes with questions on these topics, including about new supplements they are thinking of taking, should be referred to a qualified sports dietician. Furthermore, every Sports Performance Coach needs to know the code of ethics associated with their specific work environment.

SUMMARY

A career in high-performance sports is exciting and challenging. Understanding the educational and training demands of the career path in which the Sports Performance Coach chooses to practice is important. As an integral member of the Integrated Sports Performance Team, the Sports Performance Coach works closely with the athlete to achieve optimal performance and to advance to the next level of athleticism. By collaborating with other sport-minded professionals, the Sports Performance Coach can have a large impact on the athlete, the outcome of a competition, and the longevity of the athlete's career.

KEY TAKEAWAYS

- The athlete spectrum: The Sports Performance Coach works with a variety of athletes, including semi-professional and professional, collegiate, recreational, youth, adolescent, and senior athletes. For this reason, the Sports Performance Coach must have knowledge of foundational sports performance research across the entire athletic spectrum.
- Integrated Sports Performance Team: The sports performance industry is one of the largest industries in North America, generating nearly $500 billion annually. Today, sports team owners, managers, and coaching staff are demanding that athletes be better, faster, and stronger. Winning requires that athletes be ready to perform and available when needed. In the past decade, athlete health care and performance management have begun to shift to an athlete-centered model, providing athletes with multidisciplinary support.

- Becoming a Sports Performance Coach: Sports Performance Coaches often have a background as athletes, but excelling as a performance coach also requires an understanding of sports science, exercise science, kinesiology, and anatomy and physiology. After becoming a Sports Performance Coach, opportunities exist across the entire athletic spectrum. Regardless of their place of employment, the Sports Performance Coach has a responsibility to the individual athlete, the team, and the affiliated organization.

REFERENCES

Araújo, C. G., & Scharhag, J. (2016). Athlete: A working definition for medical and health sciences research. *Scandinavian Journal of Medicine & Science in Sports, 26*(1), 4–7.

Bureau of Labor Statistics, U.S. Department of Labor. (n.d.). *Occupational outlook handbook: Athletes and sports competitors.* https://www.bls.gov/ooh/entertainment-and-sports/athletes-and-sports-competitors.htm

Choi, B. C. K., & Pak, A. W. (2006). Multidisciplinarity, interdisciplinarity and transdisciplinarity in health research, services, education and policy: 1. Definitions, objectives, and evidence of effectiveness. *Clinical & Investigative Medicine 2006; 29*(6), 351–364.

Dyer, A. M., Kristjansson, A. L., Mann, M. J., Smith, M. L., & Allegrante, J. P. (2017). Sport participation and academic achievement: A longitudinal study. *American Journal of Health Behavior, 41*(2), 179–185. https://doi.org/10.5993/AJHB.41.2.9

Egan, K. P. (2019). Supporting mental health and well-being among student-athletes. *Clinics in Sports Medicine, 38*(4), 537–544.

Eime, R. M., Young, J. A., Harvey, J. T., Charity, M. J., & Payne, W. R. (2013). A systematic review of the psychological and social benefits of participation in sport for children and adolescents: Informing development of a conceptual model of health through sport. *International Journal of Behavioral Nutrition and Physical Activity, 10*(1), 98. https://doi.org/10.1186/1479-5868-10-98

Hornsby, W. G., Fry, A. C., Haff, G. G., & Stone, M. H. (2020). Addressing the confusion within periodization research. *Journal of Functional Morphology and Kinesiology, 5*(3), 68. https://doi.org/10.3390/jfmk5030068

Hyde, E. T., Omura, J. D., Fulton, J. E., Lee, S. M., Piercy, K. L., & Carlson, S. A. (2020). Disparities in youth sports participation in the U.S., 2017–2018. *American Journal of Preventive Medicine, 59*(5), e207–e210. https://doi.org/10.1016/j.amepre.2020.05.011

Jenkin, C. R., Eime, R. M., Westerbeek, H., & van Uffelen, J. G. Z. (2018). Sport for adults aged 50+ years: Participation benefits and barriers. *Journal of Aging and Physical Activity, 26*(3), 363–371. https://doi.org/10.1123/japa.2017-0092

Kim, Y. K., & Trail, G. (2010). Constraints and motivators: A new model to explain sport consumer behavior. *Journal of Sport Management, 24*(2), 190–210.

Laquale, K. (2009). Nutritional needs of the recreational athlete. *Athletic Therapy Today, 14*(1), 12–15.

Lindgren, E. C., & Barker-Ruchti, N. (2017). Balancing performance-based expectations with a holistic perspective on coaching: A qualitative study of Swedish women's national football team coaches' practice experiences. *International Journal of Qualitative Studies on Health and Well-being, 12*(1). 13538580. https://doi.org/10.1080/17482631.2017.1358580

Lynch, M., & Mallett, C. (2006). Becoming a successful high-performance track and field coach. *Modern Athlete and Coach, 44*, 15–20.

Maughan, R. J., Burke, L. M., Dvorak, J., Larson-Meyer, D. E., Peeling, P., Phillips, S. M., Rawson, E. S., Walsh, N. P., Garthe, I., Geyer, H., Meeusen, R., van Loon, L. J. C., Shirreffs, S. M., Spriet, L. L., Stuart, M., Vernec, A., Currell, K., Ali, V. M., Budgett, R. G., … Engebretsen, L. (2018). IOC consensus statement: Dietary supplements and the high-performance athlete. *British Journal of Sports Medicine, 52*(7), 439–455. https://doi.org/10.1136/bjsports-2018-099027

McGill, E. A., & Montel, I. (Eds.). (2019). *Essentials of sports performance training.* Jones & Bartlett Learning.

Meijen, C. (Ed.). (2019). *Endurance performance in sport: Psychological theory and interventions.* Routledge.

Miller, P. S., Bloom, G. A., & Salmela, J. H. (1996). The roots of success: From athletic leaders to expert coaches. *Coaches Report. 2*(2), 18–20.

Moeijes, J., van Busschbach, J. T., Bosscher, R. J., & Twisk, J. W. R. (2018). Sports participation and psychosocial health: A longitudinal observational study in children. *BMC Public Health, 18*(1), 702. https://doi.org/10.1186/s12889-018-5624-1

Mujika, I., Halson, S., Burke, L. M., Balagué, G., & Farrow, D. (2018). An integrated, multifactorial approach to periodization for optimal performance in individual and team sports. *International Journal of Sports Physiology and Performance, 13*(5), 538–561. https://doi.org/10.1123/ijspp.2018-0093

National Collegiate Athletic Association. (n.d.). *NCAA* [Fact sheet]. https://www.nsca.com/contentassets /873d10c7f5c0470d8f8cf666fda84445/nsca-fact-sheet_final.pdf

National Strength and Conditioning Association. (n.d.). *Who is the NSCA?* https://www.nsca.com/about-us /about-us/

O'Malley, L. (2016, March 31). *Women in strength and conditioning.* Wintec. https://www.wintec.ac.nz/the-coach /blog/women-in-strength-and-conditioning

Rice, S. M., Purcell, R., De Silva, S., Mawren, D., McGorry, P. D., & Parker, A. G. (2016). The mental health of elite athletes: A narrative systematic review. *Sports Medicine, 46*(9), 1333–1353. https://doi.org/10.1007 /s40279-016-0492-2

Sarı, İ., & Soyer, F. (2010). The scope, development and the characteristics of expertise in sports coaching context. *Journal of Human Sciences, 7*(2), 1173–1185. https://www.j-humansciences.com/ojs/index.php/IJHS/article /view/1463

Schinke, R. J., Bloom, G. A., & Salmela, J. H. (1995). The career stages of elite Canadian basketball coaches. *Avante,* 1, 48–62.

Shurley, J. P., & Todd, J. S. (2012). The strength of Nebraska: Boyd Epley, Husker Power, and the formation of the strength coaching profession. *Journal of Strength and Conditioning Research, 26*(12), 3177–3188.

Smith, J., & Smolianov, P. (2020). The high-performance management model: From Olympic and professional to university sport in the United States. *Sport Journal, 41*(2). https://thesportjournal.org/article/the-high -performance-management-model-from-olympic-and-professional-to-university-sport-in-the-united -states/#

Sotiriadou, P., & De Bosscher, V. (Eds.). (2013). *Managing high-performance sport.* Routledge.

Telama, R., Yang, X., Hirvensalo, M., & Raitakari, O. (2006). Participation in organized youth sport as a predictor of adult physical activity: A 21-year longitudinal study. *Pediatric Exercise Science, 18*(1), 76–88. https:// doi.org/10.1123/pes.18.1.76

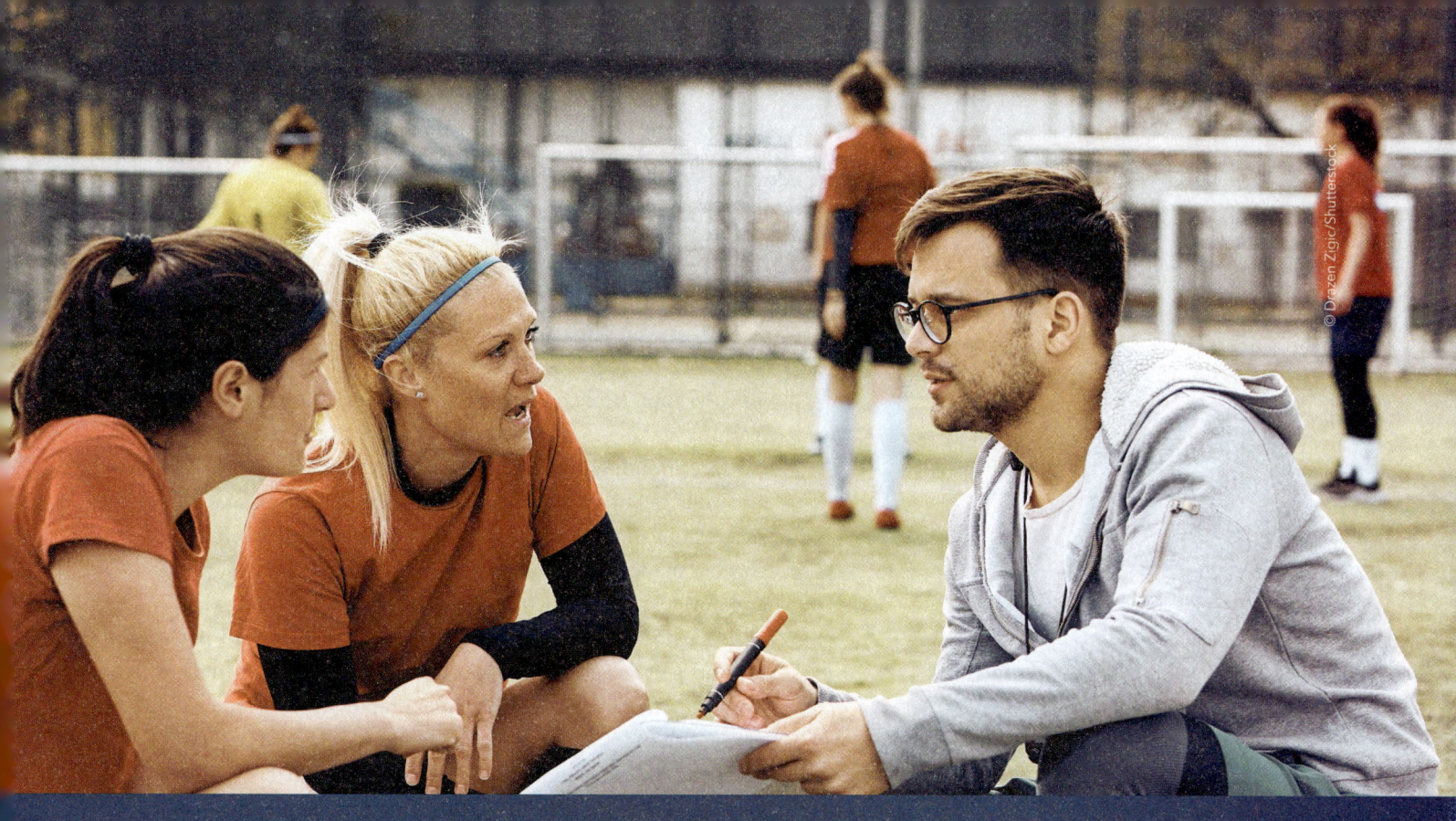

COACHING AND INTERPERSONAL COMMUNICATION SKILLS

CHAPTER TWO

LEARNING OBJECTIVES

Upon completion of this chapter, the Sports Performance Coach will be able to:

- **Define** elements of effective communication.
- **Identify** factors that optimize interpersonal communication.
- **Discuss** elements of effective coaching delivery and optimal session planning.
- **Describe** characteristics of an effective coaching style.
- **Differentiate** internal cueing from external cueing for skill acquisition.

LESSON 1: COACHING KNOWLEDGE AND COMMUNICATION

INTRODUCTION

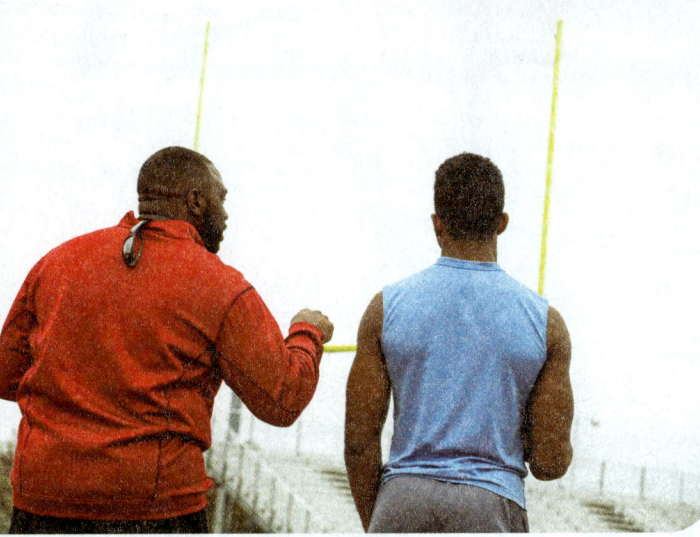

© Pixelheadphoto digitalskillet/Shutterstock

To enter into the field of coaching is to enter the world of learning and development. Coaches know that it takes work—hard, continuous, purposeful work—to change behavior and build better habits. This is as true for a nutrition coach as it is for a strength coach. But even the most purposeful coaches may not always apply their knowledge about learning and development to their own craft, and coaches rarely seek coaching for themselves.

The act of coaching is as much a skill as the movements it is meant to influence. Just as movement represents a complex web of muscles and joints that work together to achieve a desired outcome, coaching comprises a complex web of behaviors that help the athlete achieve those ends. One can easily argue that coaches need coaching and guidance just as much as the athletes they support. Coaches need someone to help make the invisible behaviors, like communication, visible. Only after a behavior becomes visible can it be defined, assessed, and modified.

The mission of this chapter is to define and outline the collection of behaviors that have the greatest impact on athlete learning and development. This chapter provides a foundational set of tools to help coaches normalize the continuous improvement of their behavior. This journey begins with the most basic question: What is a coach?

THE COACH

Originally, a coach was a physical vehicle that took people from where they were to where they wanted to be (similar to a car to an average person). Because the core function of a coach is to help people get where they are going, it is unsurprising that "coach" has become the adopted title of those responsible for developing others within a given industry.

From life coaches to business coaches, and from sports coaches to performance coaches, the word **coach** is now used to describe people who are responsible for guiding others to where they want to be. Regardless of the discipline, a coach guides the individual along the winding path toward their goals. It is important to recognize that the coach cannot walk the path for the person; they can only show them the way.

No matter how well the coach knows the path and how many times they have traveled it themselves, if they do not know how to reveal the path to another person through word or demonstration, they will be unsuccessful in their pursuits. To illustrate, consider the following interaction between a performance coach and an athlete.

> Coach: "Today we're going to progress you from the goblet squat to the back squat."
> Athlete: "Sounds good, coach!"
> Coach: "Okay, to begin, I will demonstrate the movement and talk you through the technique. First, I want you to get under the bar, stand up, step back, and widen your stance shoulder-width apart. I then want you to focus on keeping your chest

COACH →

A person who is responsible for guiding others from where they are to where they want to be.

up, elbows down, and core tight. Once you feel set,
I want you to push your hips down and back, squatting
as low as you can while keeping your knees straight
and your chest up. I then want you to focus on standing
straight up, pushing your hips up and forward, and
squeezing your glutes at the top."

Athlete: "Okay, I'll give it a shot."

Watching the athlete perform the squat, the coach can
see they are hesitant and notices that they are struggling
to control their core, hips, and knees despite the coach's
detailed instructions.

Coach: "Talk to me about what you were feeling during the
squat."

Athlete: "I'm not really sure, I was just squatting."

Coach: "Okay, but what were you focusing on during the squat?
Did you remember to focus on everything I told you?"

Athlete: "Kind of. I didn't know exactly what to focus on."

Coach: "No worries, totally normal. On this next set, focus on keeping your chest up,
knees aligned, and sit back like you're sitting in a chair. Just remember to be strong
as you stand up and drive your hips forward. You've got this!"

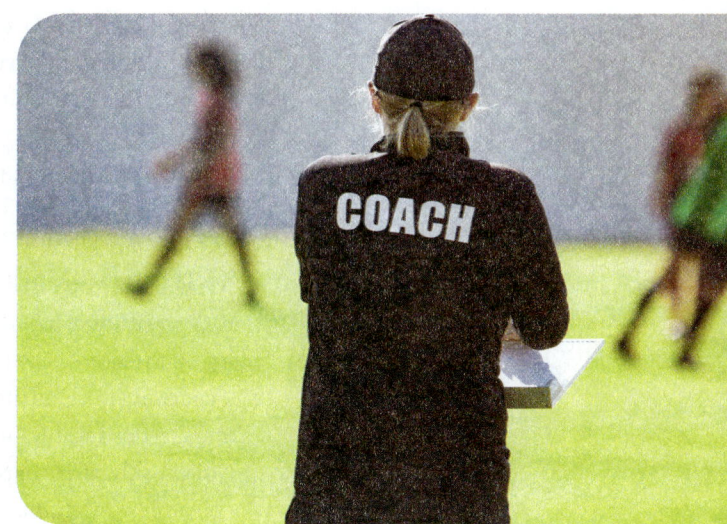

© Chalermpon Poungpeth/Shutterstock

Over the next few weeks, the coach continued using the same coaching language,
emphasizing detailed technical points. Although the athlete made progress, it was
inconsistent and impermanent. Despite the athlete's visible frustration at times, the coach
asked them to continue focusing on the same technical points and encouraged the athlete
to stick with the process.

This kind of interaction between coach and athlete is all too common. In fact, many
would praise this coach for their detailed knowledge of the squat pattern and clear
articulation of its technical points. But knowledge of the squat alone may not help the
athlete to learn. While technical knowledge is important, it is only as valuable as a coach's
ability to translate it into a form that the athlete can absorb and apply to themselves. Put
metaphorically, a coach with a lot of knowledge but no way of communicating it is like
someone with a fortune sealed in a keyless chest. Knowledge and information are useless
when there is no way to access it.

COACHING FORMS OF KNOWLEDGE: THE WHAT AND HOW

Famed University of California, Los Angeles (UCLA) basketball
coach John Wooden is often credited with saying, "You haven't
coached until they've learned." Wooden's words remind us
that coaching is about learning. Learning is a permanent change
to a movement or skill that can be expressed without reminders,
feedback, or prompts from a coach. Put simply, learning is
about the athlete's ability to own change. From this perspective,
one could argue that the athlete's coach from the story fell short
of the criteria on which all coaching is evaluated.

Clearly, the coach in the story knew what to coach.
However, the athlete's inability to convert the coach's words
into an improved squat pattern suggests that something was

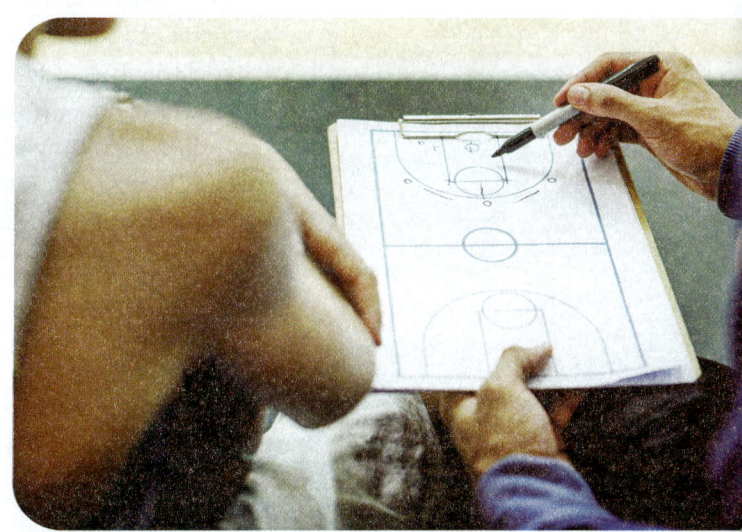

© Rawpixel.com/Shutterstock

impeding progress. One explanation for the athlete's slow progress is that they did not have the physical ability to perform the squat, meaning they did not have the mobility, stability, or strength needed to squat effectively.

If this is the case, the coach needs to develop these qualities in parallel to the squatting pattern, recognizing that the athlete's improvement will be directly related to upgrading the underlying qualities. Put simply, no amount of verbal instruction, good or bad, will make a difference if the barrier to improvement is physical. In the words of sprint coach Stu McMillan, "You can't fix a [physical] problem with a technical cue." However, if the athlete's squatting barrier is not a physical one, two possible explanations are left, both falling on the side of the coach. The coach has either identified the wrong technical error (e.g., coaching knee position when the problem resides in the hips) or identified the correct technical error but is failing to communicate it to the athlete (i.e., no learning takes place).

Collectively, these explanations provide a blueprint that can help coaches pinpoint why an athlete might not be learning. Likewise, this blueprint highlights the forms of knowledge that coaches must develop to minimize coaching missteps.

📋 COACH'S CORNER

The first form of knowledge a coach must seek to develop is their *knowledge of what* to coach. This includes an understanding of anatomy, physiology, biomechanics, and program design. This type of knowledge is central to building goal-specific programs and understanding the biomechanics of the movements being coached. In large part, someone's knowledge of what is theoretical and exists independent of the athlete it is meant to influence.

The second form of knowledge is the *knowledge of how* to coach to translate this information into a language the athlete can understand and apply. This form of knowledge is dependent on the athlete, while the coach figures out how to communicate a technical change (e.g., the balance of flexion in the knees versus hips during the descent of a back squat) in a way that the athlete can understand and apply to their own movement.

Traditionally, knowledge of *what* to coach has been emphasized within degree programs and certifications, leaving coaches to figure out *how* to coach on their own. This is a problem: If a coach is unaware of the difference between the knowledge of what and knowledge of how, they are less likely to seek the latter and more likely to confuse it with the former. For example, coaches often fail to make a distinction between the language used to describe a movement biomechanically and the language used to coach it. For many, describing a movement biomechanically becomes the same as coaching it. We do not mean to suggest that biomechanical knowledge and the communication of it is not important—it certainly is. However, when it is unaccompanied by the communication tools designed to support athlete understanding, enjoyment, and learning, both coach and athlete will fall short.

To illustrate, consider the following upgraded interaction between the same coach and athlete from earlier.

Coach: "You've made some really good progress on the goblet squat over the last few weeks. How do you feel about progressing to the back squat?"

Athlete: "Really good, coach!"

Coach: "Great! Before we get into the back squat, let's go through some of your focus points from the goblet squat."

Athlete: "Athletic stance. Sit behind the bell. Be proud."

Coach: "Exactly! Okay, the only difference with the back squat is the setup—everything else is virtually the same. Before we get going, let me give you a quick demonstration on the setup. First, step under the bar and grab it as if to bend it over your back; second, stand up and step back; third, take a wide stance like the goblet squat."

The coach continues by demonstrating three repetitions, emphasizing the cues "sit behind the bar" at the bottom and "be proud—stand proud" at the top.

Coach: "Still got it! Okay, your turn, what are you going to focus on?"

Athlete: "Sitting back and staying proud!"

Coach: (While demonstrating one final repetition) "That's right, sit back behind the bar like you're sitting on a tiny stool. Let's go!"

Over the next three sets of back squats, the coach mainly observed, asking the athlete about the general feeling of the movement and focal points. Both were happy about a positive first day of back squatting, successfully transferring learnings from the goblet squat to the back squat.

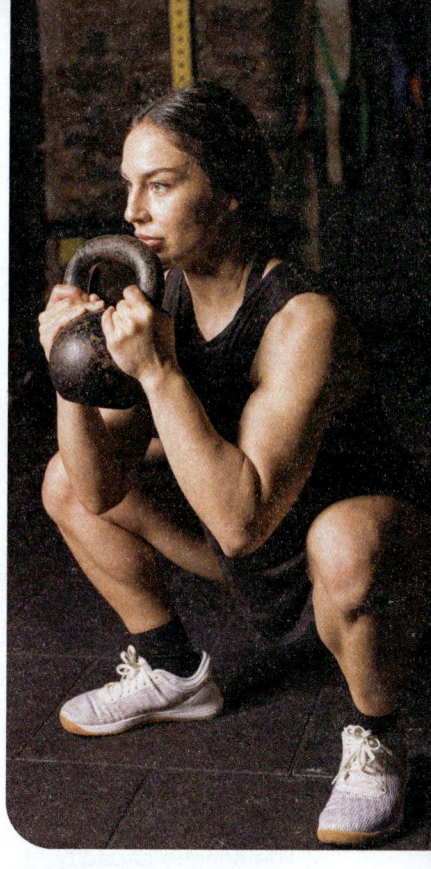

© Berkomaster/Shutterstock

In comparing the interactions in the two stories, reflect on the similarities and the differences in terms of knowledge of *what* and *how* is useful. In both cases, it's clear that the coach understands the biomechanics of the squat pattern—a reflection of their knowledge of what to coach. A key difference is the amount of biomechanical information offered to the athlete. Specifically, in the first story, the coach verbalizes technical reminders for the setup, downward phase, and upward phase of the squat. In contrast, the coach in the second story provides only technical information about the setup, leveraging demonstration and the athlete's familiarity with the goblet squat to convey the movement pattern itself. In this case, the coach provides the athlete with the minimal viable information needed to perform the squat efficiently and effectively.

By minimizing the information the athlete has to mentally process, the coach reduces the risk of confusion, misdirected focus, and overthinking—a reflection of the coach's knowledge of how to coach. Further, the second coach actively involves the athlete in creating the major focus point to guide the movement pattern. By facilitating a simple, singular focus, the coach and athlete are clear on how the movement is performed (e.g., "like you are *sitting on a tiny stool*" or "as if you were *standing proud*").

These singular coaching cues guide the whole movement using visually rich language that is easy to act out. Moreover, each cue implies how the whole body works to achieve the desired movement goal, minimizing the need to think about each body part independently (Wulf et al., 2001). In the second story, the coach uses language like the conductor of an orchestra, emphasizing one focus to coordinate a symphony of joints. In contrast, in the first story, the coach instructs the athlete to think about a multitude of joints and limbs while simultaneously trying to use them. This is analogous to thinking about the legs while walking or focusing on the hand instead of the glass it is reaching for. Ultimately, knowledge of what to coach focuses on the parts, while knowledge of how to coach focuses on the whole.

While the other chapters in this text are rightly dedicated to the *knowledge of what* to coach, this chapter is wholly focused on the *knowledge of how* to coach. The following lessons take an athlete-centered approach, outlining the strategies a coach needs to get the right information off the program and into the person. The central purpose of this chapter is to help the coach learn how to share the right information at the right time and in the right way to drive an enjoyable experience that supports athlete learning. As part of this approach, every strategy must be judged by its capacity to stimulate movement learning, empowering the athlete to leave each session better than when they came in—by owning the change.

In addition, this chapter focuses on interpersonal communication and movement communication. **Interpersonal communication (IC)** focuses on the coach's capacity to connect with the athlete, build buy-in, and create a motivationally rich environment that the athlete enjoys being a part of. Put simply, IC is about the person-to-person connection that is the fabric of successful relationships. **Movement communication (MC)** focuses on the coach's capacity to use language to generate movement learning.

LESSON 2: LEARNING NEW MOVEMENTS

INFLUENCING MOVEMENT

The core function of a Sports Performance Coach is to positively influence **movement learning**. This includes moving with improved coordination, speed, strength, and other movement-related goals. The key question is how a coach influences an athlete's movement. To answer this question, it is necessary to consider where movement comes from.

One might say that the impetus for movement begins in the brain, flows through the nervous system, and triggers a series of muscle contractions that act on the skeletal system to produce motion. This certainly explains how motion is created, but does so independent of the context shaping it. Only through context can the contents of a movement be fully understood and coached (Newell, 1986).

For example, the hand changes shape to meet the glass it intends to grip. Likewise, the legs coordinate their actions differently based on the type of terrain they are moving over. Watch someone walk up a set of stairs versus down a rocky hill, and you will see two different movement patterns despite the same goal of getting from Point A to Point B. In both cases, the hand and legs successfully complete the task without additional thought from the person to which they are attached. The person provides the intention—grab this or go there—and the body complies by producing a movement pattern suitable for achieving the desired goal. These examples demonstrate that movement always exists in the space between the perceiver (athlete) and the perceived (environment). We do not move in a vacuum void of a physical context. Movement always requires both the intentions of the athlete and the environment in which those intentions are played out. As such, it is the responsibility of the coach to learn the subtle art of influencing rather than interrupting the movement space between athlete and environment.

With an understanding of where movement comes from, a coach is now ready to inquire about how best to influence it. The first thing to recognize is that movement does not require a coach. People move and learn to move all the time without coaches. Children typically learn to sit, crawl, stand, walk, run, and roll without coaching. Even if the child wanted to take the advice of an encouraging parent, they would struggle to do so if they are in a preverbal state. Even into adulthood, people might take up golfing, tennis, surfing, or snowboarding, and they can successfully do so without any coaching. However, in each case, a person reaches a level of competency and then sees their progress stall.

While the level of performance one can achieve without coaching is individualized, everyone plateaus at some point. It is at this point that a person either resigns themselves to this level of ability or finds a coach. A coach is needed to get beyond "good enough" and push the person toward their potential. This good-enough phenomenon comes from the fact that humans are movement generalists.

Being a movement generalist means that humans can perform diverse movement skills at a very average level. Compared to the rest of the animal kingdom, humans are not the best sprinters, climbers, swimmers, or lifters. But despite this, humans can perform *all* of these movements with far greater ease than any one animal that is the best in any particular area. Nevertheless, humans need help to get beyond their natural movement learning set point; this is where coaches come in. That said, coaches should respect an athlete's affinity for learning movement organically. When studying movement in its natural form, coaches should recognize when to influence the movement and when to be influenced by it.

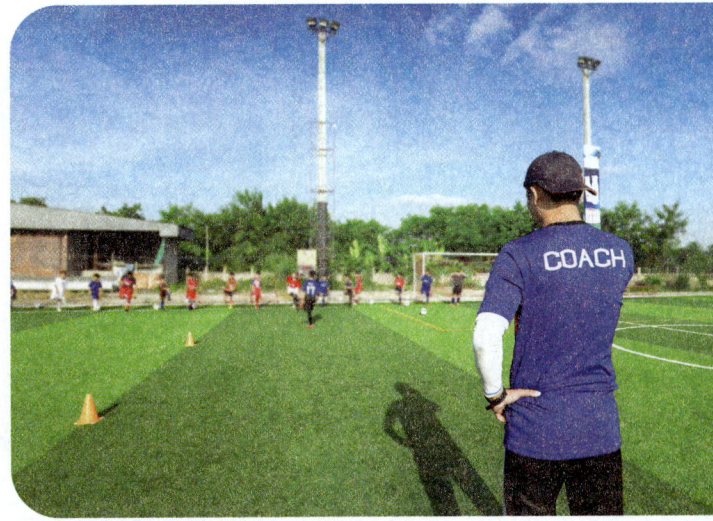
© Red mango/Shutterstock

This last point is best understood through a key coaching principle: *Watch it before you coach it*. This means that the coach watches the athlete move before they coach them on how to move. Many coaches commit the error of making a long speech on the nuances of a movement before ever watching the athlete perform it. Coaches certainly want to explain the goal of the movement, provide a demonstration, and cover safety information. However, providing too many details will interfere with the athlete's natural capacity to pursue a movement goal within a given environmental context (Liao & Masters, 2001). Moreover, when observing a prematurely coached movement, it is difficult to know which errors are the athlete's and which are the result of the coach's untimely instruction. By watching a movement in its natural form, the coach can identify and prioritize the aspect of the movement that, if modified, will help the athlete improve their performance. From here, the coach identifies the best coaching strategy for that athlete regarding the specific movement error they are trying to overcome.

VERBAL AND NONVERBAL COACHING

With a clear understanding of when to step in and when to step back, a coach can consider the tools at their disposal for positively influencing an athlete's movement. There are two primary ways to influence a movement: verbally or nonverbally (**Figure 2.1**). As movement is the product of athlete plus environment, it's unsurprising that the verbal strategy targets the athlete and the way they focus on the environment, whereas the nonverbal strategy targets the environment and the way it naturally captures the athlete's focus.

Verbal coaching strategies—also known as top-down strategies because they start with the athlete and move toward the environment—represent spoken communications meant to influence movement learning. The goal of verbal coaching strategies is to help the athlete craft a mental focus that optimizes how they perform a given movement.

In contrast, **nonverbal coaching** strategies—also known as bottom-up strategies because they start in the environment and move toward the athlete—represent the aspects of the environment that are influenced by the coach and designed to drive

VERBAL COACHING →

Spoken communications meant to influence movement learning.

NONVERBAL COACHING →

The aspects of the environment that are influenced by the coach and designed to drive athlete adaptation and learning.

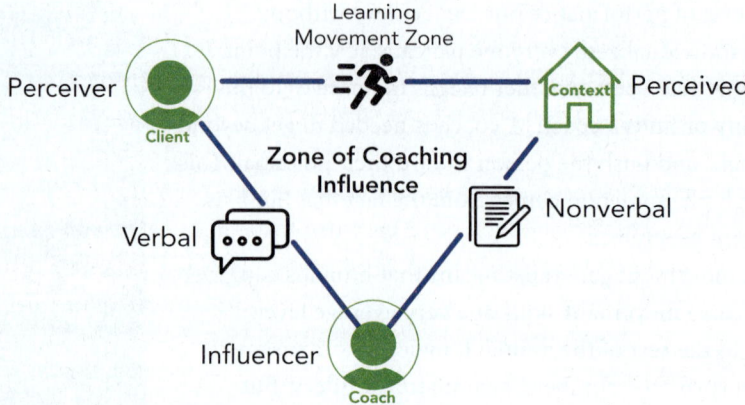

FIGURE 2.1 Movement Influence Model (Adapted from Winkelman, 2021)

Data from Winkelman, N. (2021). The language of coaching: The art and science of teaching movement. Champaign, IL: Human Kinetics

athlete adaptation and learning. They include the physical space the athlete trains in, the program they follow, and the specifics of their exercises. Both verbal and nonverbal strategies are always present—the athlete is always focusing on something, and there is always something to focus on. It's a matter of whether a coach can tap into the respective strategies to nudge understanding and learning.

Consider the back squat from the previous coaching stories to demonstrate how these strategies work. In both stories, the coaches used the verbal path to influence the movement. Independent of which coach did it best, both were using words to shape the athlete's focus with the intention of improving the back squat. It is possible, however, that the coaches could have used a nonverbal strategy to stimulate the same movement changes. To illustrate this, consider a final interaction between the same coach and athlete.

> Coach: "You made really good progress on the back squat during our last session. The depth and control of the movement looked great."
>
> Athlete: "Thanks, coach! I thought it felt pretty good for my first time doing it."
>
> Coach: "There was one aspect of the movement we said we'd focus on today."
>
> Athlete: "Oh yeah, my knees—they're kind of wobbly. I think you called them my headlights."
>
> Coach: "Yes! Nice memory. Just like a car, we want to keep those headlights pointed where?"
>
> Athlete: "Forward!"
>
> Coach: "Right again. To help with this, I want you to step into this blue mini-band and pull it just above your knees."
>
> The athlete steps into the mini-band.
>
> Coach: "Perfect. Now, before we get under the bar, I want you to set your athletic stance and perform a few bodyweight squats."
>
> The coach observes as the athlete performs five bodyweight squats with the mini-band just above their knees.
>
> Coach: "Okay. How did it feel? What did you notice?"
>
> Athlete: "I could definitely feel the tension around my knees and hips. I actually felt like I had greater control despite the resistance."
>
> Coach: "That's the goal. Let's get under the bar and see how you do."

In this story, the coach introduced a physical **constraint**. A constraint can be understood as something that eliminates or restricts certain actions. In this case, a piece of equipment provided a nonverbal change to the environment that naturally influenced how the athlete moved. The coach used a mini-band around the knees to target the athlete's control of knee position. Ironically, the mini-band accentuated the error, pulling the knees inward, even though the coach wants the athlete's knees to point forward, like headlights.

However, this accentuation of the error provided the athlete with increased sensory information about their knees, making it easier to naturally find the right body position. Just as someone can't scratch an itch they can't feel, a person can't change a movement error they don't notice. As such, nearly all nonverbal constraints are meant to increase the athlete's natural awareness of a movement error, increasing the odds that they can self-correct.

The question remains: Which is superior, verbal or nonverbal coaching strategies? In general, there is no single best way—the best way is the one that works for the athlete. That said, one could argue that nonverbal coaching strategies are a more natural way to influence movement patterns because they deal directly with the environment.

Moreover, nonverbal coaching strategies decrease the odds that a coach will put forth a counterproductive idea that either encourages an athlete to focus on the wrong thing or disrupts the natural flow of movement execution with overthinking. Despite the organic nature of nonverbal coaching strategies, however, they have significant limitations. First, coaches still need to communicate with the athlete on an interpersonal level and provide a basic level of instruction for the movement. As such, coaches should have a blueprint for how to best deploy these communication strategies. Moreover, there is no guarantee that the physical constraint will generate the desired movement. Some athletes are more sensitive to these environmental nudges than others. Coaches, in turn, need to be able to synthesize a coaching cue that guides the athlete's focus toward the desired movement change. In all cases, the coach is shaping the way the athlete pays attention, getting them to focus on the right things, in the right way, at the right time. In the end, if the right focus is generated, the right movement can emerge, independent of how the focus was triggered.

> ## ✔ CHECK IT OUT
>
> **Learning-supportive coaching** covers both verbal and nonverbal strategies, and each type of strategy has a breadth and depth that cannot be covered in a single chapter. With a clear understanding of what a coach is and the ways the coach influences movement, the stage is set to construct a blueprint for effective coaching communication.

CONSTRAINT →

Something that eliminates certain possibilities for action.

LEARNING-SUPPORTIVE COACHING →

A type of coaching that includes both verbal and nonverbal strategies.

THE COMMUNICATION BLUEPRINT

While coaches frequently communicate with athletes, the communication used in the training session has the greatest impact on those athletes' experience and learning. Thus, a training session provides a natural canvas on which to map the communication strategies underpinning a developed knowledge of how to coach.

It is helpful to think of a training session as a story with a beginning, a middle, and an end.

> Beginning: Acts as a preview of the session, foreshadowing what can be expected.
> Middle: The physical actioning of those expectations, guided by the dialogue between athlete and coach.
> End: The review of the session, revealing lessons learned.

Although certain communication strategies are unique to each part of the story, they always fall into either the interpersonal communication (IC) strand (i.e., person-focused) or the movement communication (MC) strand (i.e., movement-focused). As outlined in the communication blueprint (**Figure 2.2**), the communication strands form a DNA-like double helix featuring a natural alternation between person-focused dialogue (e.g., "How did you do on your exams?") and movement-focused dialogue (e.g., "On this next repetition, let's focus on …"). These two forms of communication are inextricably linked and depend on each other to optimize the athlete's experience and learning.

RAPPORT BUILDING →

A coach's ongoing process of getting to know an athlete.

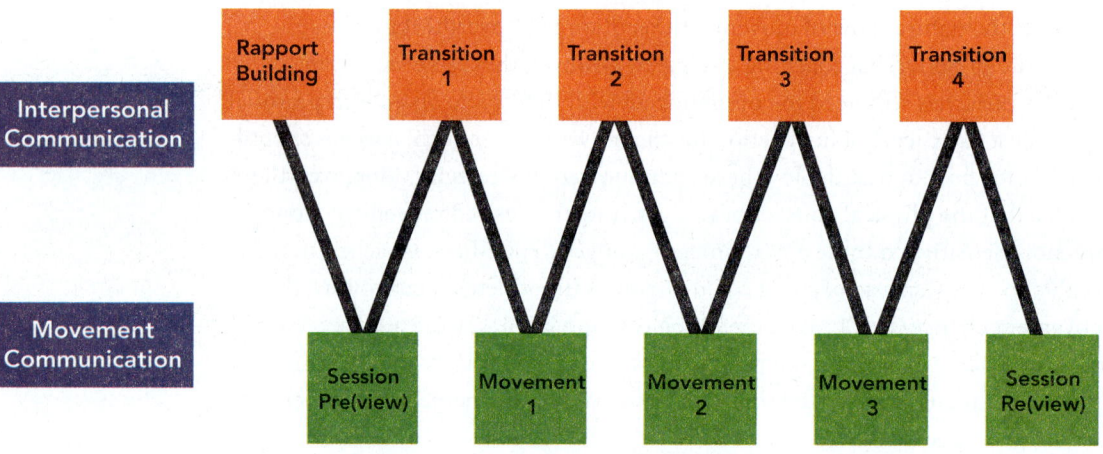

FIGURE 2.2 The Communication Blueprint

Data from Winkelman, N. (2021). The language of coaching: The art and science of teaching movement. Champaign, IL: Human Kinetics

Within the communication blueprint, the *beginning* is characterized by two communication strategies: rapport building and the session preview. Coaches start by building rapport with the athlete, followed by previewing the training session. This follows social convention and meets the expectation that an athlete is a person first and a player second. **Rapport building** invites the coach to check in, see how the athlete is doing, and ask any relevant life- or sport-related questions. In the simplest of terms, it is the ongoing process of getting to know the athlete. This check-in signals to the athlete that the coach cares about them as a person while providing the coach with relevant information that might influence the training session (e.g., the athlete didn't get much sleep because they were studying for an exam).

Rapport building, which might take seconds to minutes, is followed by the session preview. The **session preview** is the business end of the conversation that outlines *what* will happen during the session, *why* it will happen in terms of the athlete's goals, and *how* it will happen.

SESSION PREVIEW →

The business end of the conversation that outlines what, why, and how.

In this story, the coach introduced a physical **constraint**. A constraint can be understood as something that eliminates or restricts certain actions. In this case, a piece of equipment provided a nonverbal change to the environment that naturally influenced how the athlete moved. The coach used a mini-band around the knees to target the athlete's control of knee position. Ironically, the mini-band accentuated the error, pulling the knees inward, even though the coach wants the athlete's knees to point forward, like headlights.

However, this accentuation of the error provided the athlete with increased sensory information about their knees, making it easier to naturally find the right body position. Just as someone can't scratch an itch they can't feel, a person can't change a movement error they don't notice. As such, nearly all nonverbal constraints are meant to increase the athlete's natural awareness of a movement error, increasing the odds that they can self-correct.

The question remains: Which is superior, verbal or nonverbal coaching strategies? In general, there is no single best way—the best way is the one that works for the athlete. That said, one could argue that nonverbal coaching strategies are a more natural way to influence movement patterns because they deal directly with the environment.

Moreover, nonverbal coaching strategies decrease the odds that a coach will put forth a counterproductive idea that either encourages an athlete to focus on the wrong thing or disrupts the natural flow of movement execution with overthinking. Despite the organic nature of nonverbal coaching strategies, however, they have significant limitations. First, coaches still need to communicate with the athlete on an interpersonal level and provide a basic level of instruction for the movement. As such, coaches should have a blueprint for how to best deploy these communication strategies. Moreover, there is no guarantee that the physical constraint will generate the desired movement. Some athletes are more sensitive to these environmental nudges than others. Coaches, in turn, need to be able to synthesize a coaching cue that guides the athlete's focus toward the desired movement change. In all cases, the coach is shaping the way the athlete pays attention, getting them to focus on the right things, in the right way, at the right time. In the end, if the right focus is generated, the right movement can emerge, independent of how the focus was triggered.

CONSTRAINT →

Something that eliminates certain possibilities for action.

✔ CHECK IT OUT

Learning-supportive coaching covers both verbal and nonverbal strategies, and each type of strategy has a breadth and depth that cannot be covered in a single chapter. With a clear understanding of what a coach is and the ways the coach influences movement, the stage is set to construct a blueprint for effective coaching communication.

LEARNING-SUPPORTIVE COACHING →

A type of coaching that includes both verbal and nonverbal strategies.

THE COMMUNICATION BLUEPRINT

While coaches frequently communicate with athletes, the communication used in the training session has the greatest impact on those athletes' experience and learning. Thus, a training session provides a natural canvas on which to map the communication strategies underpinning a developed knowledge of how to coach.

It is helpful to think of a training session as a story with a beginning, a middle, and an end.

> Beginning: Acts as a preview of the session, foreshadowing what can be expected.
> Middle: The physical actioning of those expectations, guided by the dialogue between athlete and coach.
> End: The review of the session, revealing lessons learned.

Although certain communication strategies are unique to each part of the story, they always fall into either the interpersonal communication (IC) strand (i.e., person-focused) or the movement communication (MC) strand (i.e., movement-focused). As outlined in the communication blueprint (**Figure 2.2**), the communication strands form a DNA-like double helix featuring a natural alternation between person-focused dialogue (e.g., "How did you do on your exams?") and movement-focused dialogue (e.g., "On this next repetition, let's focus on …"). These two forms of communication are inextricably linked and depend on each other to optimize the athlete's experience and learning.

Spontaneous Communication Skills

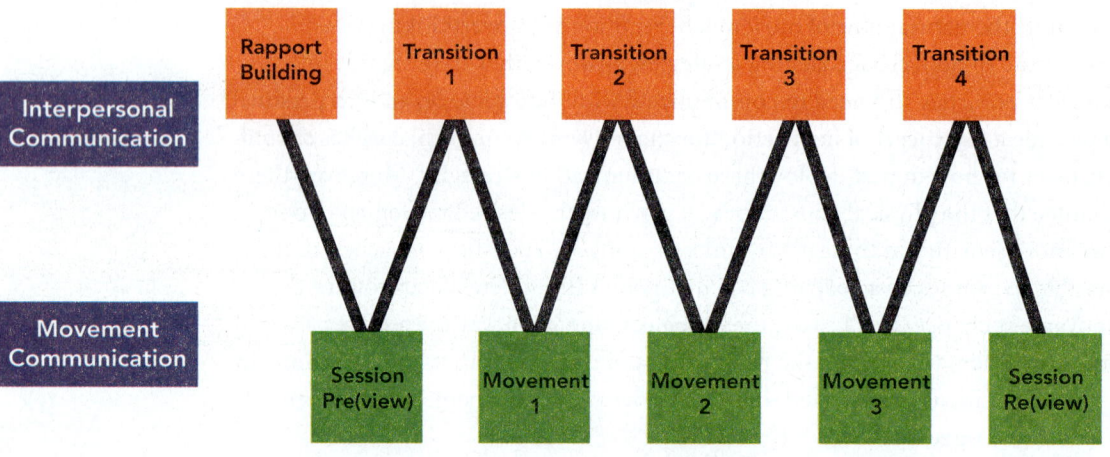

Coaching Communication Loop

FIGURE 2.2 The Communication Blueprint

Data from Winkelman, N. (2021). The language of coaching: The art and science of teaching movement. Champaign, IL: Human Kinetics

Within the communication blueprint, the *beginning* is characterized by two communication strategies: rapport building and the session preview. Coaches start by building rapport with the athlete, followed by previewing the training session. This follows social convention and meets the expectation that an athlete is a person first and a player second. **Rapport building** invites the coach to check in, see how the athlete is doing, and ask any relevant life- or sport-related questions. In the simplest of terms, it is the ongoing process of getting to know the athlete. This check-in signals to the athlete that the coach cares about them as a person while providing the coach with relevant information that might influence the training session (e.g., the athlete didn't get much sleep because they were studying for an exam).

Rapport building, which might take seconds to minutes, is followed by the session preview. The **session preview** is the business end of the conversation that outlines *what* will happen during the session, *why* it will happen in terms of the athlete's goals, and *how* it will happen.

To illustrate the session preview in action, consider the following example of a coach taking a soccer team through a linear speed session.

The What
Coach: "Team, building on our speed session from last week, we will continue to focus on our acceleration or short speed over 10 yards. Can anyone tell us why this is so critical to our sport?"

The Why
Athlete: "Because most possessions are won or lost over a short distance of sprinting."
Coach: "Exactly! So just like last week, we'll go through our prep drills, wall drills, resisted sprints, and finish off with our free sprint races."

The How
Coach: "Before we get started, I want you to find a partner and take 60 seconds, 30 seconds each, to discuss your key focus and objective for this session. Each of you knows what you need to work on, so discuss this with your partner and explain your focus to get 1% better today."

There is a natural flow covering what the athletes will do, why they are doing it, and how to complete it. The best session preview is a dialogue rather than a monologue because it allows the coach to involve the athlete in the learning journey, connecting one session to the next. Like rapport building, the session preview might take seconds to minutes based on the athlete, the type of training session, and how familiar the athlete is with the session content.

When training is under way, the coach sets their sights on facilitating the session and coaching movement. Session facilitation is composed of drill organization, time management, and the transition from one drill or exercise to the next. Good session facilitation ensures the coach has

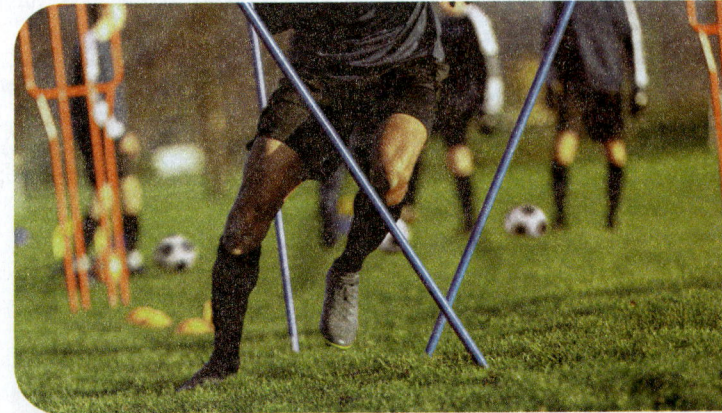
© Matimix/Shutterstock

time to effectively coach each movement. This middle portion of the communication blueprint still has a natural ebb and flow between IC and MC. To demonstrate, consider the following interaction between the coach and one of the soccer players in the speed session.

Coach: "Okay, team, take 90 seconds' recovery. Stride out, stretch out, or grab a shot of water. Let's make sure we're doing something to get our body right for this last sprint. How have those last few sprints felt?

Athlete: "Okay, I guess. I'm just feeling a little distracted with exams coming up."

Coach: "Totally get it. I remember how challenging it was to play sports in college while studying for exams. It's not for everyone, but here you are getting it done!"

Athlete: "Yeah (laughing), I guess you're right."

Coach: "So here we are with one rep to go. What do you think we can focus on to ace this last sprint?"

Athlete: "I really liked that steep hill analogy you mentioned earlier."

Coach: "Perfect. Imagine that steep hill is just in front of you. From the first step you have to push like heck to explode up it—let's get it!"

An interaction like this is likely to take less than a minute, but it has a far-reaching impact on the quality of the coach–athlete relationship and the desired movement outcome:

1. The coach signals that they see the athlete by approaching them individually during the break.
2. By asking how the athlete feels, the coach invites the athlete to share off-the-field information that might be relevant.
3. The coach signals understanding, empathizing with the athlete and sharing a common experience.
4. With the athlete feeling seen and heard, there is space to draw attention back to the task, getting the most out of the final sprint.

📋 COACH'S CORNER

When a coach takes a person-centered approach and blends IC and MC, it creates an environment that allows an athlete to thrive. When an athlete feels understood as a person, it enables the athlete to become who they want to be as a player within their sport.

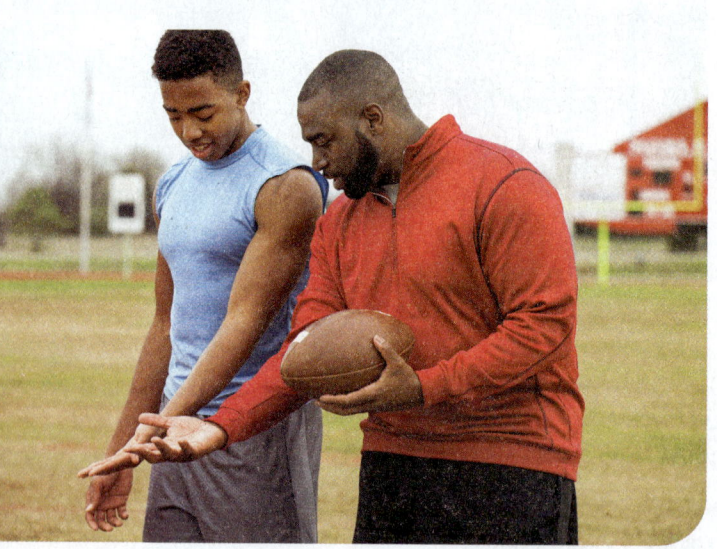

© Pixelheadphoto digitalskillet/Shutterstock

The middle portion of the communication blueprint has a looping quality, as there is a natural opportunity to engage the athlete before, during, and after each rep or set of each exercise or drill. The coaching communication loop is central to effective coaching because it is where the most information is shared and the greatest dialogue is had.

Finally, the coach arrives at the *end* of the training session and the communication blueprint. Like the beginning, the end summarizes what has occurred and what learnings can go forward. During the session review, the coach focuses on the key progress points and the remaining opportunities for improvement. While this can be done in many ways, one of the simplest is known as the 2 + 2 method. In this method, the coach offers or invites the athlete to share the top two positives from the session and the top two opportunities for improvement. To demonstrate this session review, consider this final interaction between the coach and the soccer players within the speed session.

Coach: "That's a wrap. Bring it in. Great session, everyone. I thought the overall effort and intensity you brought was top class. However, your voices are the ones that matter. Let's go through our 2 + 2. Who wants to share the top positives from today?"

Athlete: "I thought we really got after the sprints at the end. Everyone looked smoother in their acceleration the last week. I know I definitely felt better."

Coach: "Absolutely. We've been using that analogy of sprinting up a steep hill, and it appears that we are seeing improved knee drive, which gives the sense of speed and smoothness. What else went well today?"

Athlete: "I think we're really coming together as a team and doing a good job encouraging and coaching each other."

Coach: "1,000%! The chat from the group, the words of encouragement, and even your cues to one another are phenomenal. Let's keep driving these behaviors as we move forward. Okay, what are our opportunities for growth?"

Athlete: "I think we need to start the session with better intensity and remember that if we're meant to sprint 10 yards, we sprint 12. I still feel like we're hitting the brakes too early."

Coach: "Anyone disagree or see it differently? No? Okay, let's build on those points in our next session—start hard and finish hard."

The session review is a mixture of person-centered and movement-centered points. Although a coach might decide to be the sole voice providing the feedback, it is also wise to include the athlete when appropriate, as it is ultimately their learning journey. The more involved the athlete is, the greater their sense of ownership and drive to succeed will be. Hidden in every person's intuition is the knowledge that they are more likely to commit to the path they choose rather than the one chosen for them. In the end, coaches must see the session review as a way to memorialize learning and generate the content for the next session preview.

 COACH'S CORNER

With the communication blueprint outlined, coaches are ready to consider the strategies they can use to bring it to life and adapt it to the individuals they support. The one constant in coaching is that what works for one does not work for all. As such, coaches benefit from developing the skills and behaviors underpinning an agile coaching style.

LESSON 3: COACHING MOVEMENT

MOVEMENT COMMUNICATION

Between the two forms of communication outlined, interpersonal and movement, movement communication is more straightforward. A coach knows how the athlete needs to move, which movements the athlete needs to perform, and which aspects of those movements need improvement. In the same way that a session can be planned and programmed, coaches can apply a similar system to how they will coach it. Traditionally, periodization models provided the foundation to build programs that achieved a desired physical adaptation. Here, an analogous approach is used to help coaches plan sessions in terms of how they will coach them, while still recognizing that this planning requires some level of in-session flexibility. This system is known as the coaching communication loop.

COACHING COMMUNICATION LOOP

The **coaching communication loop (CCL)** is a five-step model used to coach movement within the middle portion of the communication blueprint (Winkelman, 2021).

COACHING COMMUNICATION LOOP (CCL) →

The five-step model used to coach movement within the middle portion of the communication blueprint.

CCL is a naturalistic communication model born out of the observation necessary to communicate before, during, and after a movement is performed. This model provides a communication structure that stabilizes communication behaviors, increasing the odds that the coach is as consistent in their approach to coaching as they are in their programming.

The five steps of the CCL model are described in the following subsections. The description of each step is followed by an example conversation between a coach and an athlete learning to bench press that demonstrates this step of the CCL.

STEP 1: DESCRIBE IT

Describe means the same thing as *instruct*. When describing a movement, the coach provides the minimal information required for the athlete to clearly understand and complete the movement safely. When describing a movement, a coach typically wants to share three types of information. The first is basic information pertaining to the movement itself. This includes a basic technical description of what needs to happen. The second is information pertaining to performing the movement safely. This is of particular importance when an athlete is, for example, using a barbell or if the movement requires another person. The third is information that boosts the athlete's perceived competency or psychological readiness. For example, recall the second story about the back squat. In that story, the coach described the back squat in terms of its similarity with the goblet squat. Because the athlete was competent in the goblet squat, this reference carried their confidence over while mapping relevant cues from one movement to the next.

> Coach: "I know that you did the bench press in your high school program, but I would love to take you through our approach to coaching it at Bulldog State. How does that sound?"
>
> Athlete: "Great, coach!"
>
> Coach: "Right on. Okay, the first thing is the setup. Like the foundation of a house, we want it to be strong and stable. So, lay down on the bench. Keep your feet flat on the ground and bring them back until you feel a little tension in your legs, and then set your grip. We always use a spotter, so we'll hand off the bar on '1-2-3' and you say, 'My bar.' After you have the bar, you bring it straight down, tap your chest, fire it back up, rinse and repeat. Any questions?"
>
> Athlete: "No. That is very similar to how we did it back at school."
>
> Coach: "Yeah, I know your old strength coaches. They are top-class and have been to a few of the seminars we have run in the past. But enough talk, let me get under the bar and give you a quick demonstration."

STEP 2: DEMONSTRATE IT

Although describing a movement is important, most agree that a demonstration is non-negotiable. Ask an athlete whether they'd prefer a description or a demonstration, and most will choose the latter. This is because humans have mirror neurons that allow them to embody the movement they're watching as if performing it themselves. In essence, the brain circuits used to perform the movement are the same ones that fire up when someone watches another person perform it (Cohro-Mcrino et al., 2006). This further supports why minimizing verbal information is so important, as much of it is redundant to what the athlete sees in a quality demonstration. A description and demonstration work together to provide the athlete with the complete picture and relevant knowledge about the picture, increasing the likelihood of success.

The coach sits on the bench, briefly highlighting each step in the setup. The coach then proceeds to unrack the bar, showing each phase of the bench press with cue words.

Coach: "Load, hold, explode."

STEP 3: CUE IT

Both athletes and coaches occasionally find themselves saying, "I know WHAT to do, I just don't know HOW to do it." This sense, which one can have in any aspect of life, points to the realization that knowing *what* doesn't imply knowing *how*. It suggests why many great coaches can't do what they say, and great athletes can't explain what they do. Coaches must identify coaching language that can be translated into more than words and thoughts. Coaches must find a flavor of coaching language that is easily converted into images, sensations, and actions. This is the purpose of the coaching cue. The coaching cue provides the athlete with a singular focus that guides the way they move, much like an address in a GPS guides where someone drives. In the same way a person trusts the GPS to provide optimized directions, a coach can trust the athlete's body to deliver optimized movement. In both cases, it comes down to getting the cue right.

There is a specific type of coaching language that is easily converted into physical movement. This type of language creates the coaching cue, ensuring that the last thing the athlete hears and focuses on helps them arrive at the desired destination.

Coach: "Any questions?"
Athlete: "Nope, let's get after it!"
Coach: "I like it. One question for you: How will your spotter know to let go of the bar?"
Athlete: "My bar!"
Coach: "Perfect. Now for this first round, let's use our mantra 'Load, hold, explode.' I'll say it aloud to help you get your pacing."

STEP 4: DO IT

By now, the athlete's knowledge of what to do and how to do it can be brought into focus with a singular cue. With the singular focus cue guiding the movement, the athlete is ready to physically perform the movement. Only through physical practice does learning take place. The coaching language that preceded the movement is designed to optimize the learning experience, not replace it.

From a communication perspective, coaches should rarely speak while the athlete moves. In most cases, asking an athlete to think about a coach's words while moving disrupts the movement. Unless a coach is cueing rhythm, as in "push-push-push" during an acceleration sprint or "pop-one-two-pop" during a skip, where the words act like a metronome, a coach should speak minimally during movement. Principally, the slower the movement is, the easier it is to get away with parallel coaching. However, coaches are strictly cautioned to weigh the pros and cons of coaching while the athlete moves. The line between influence and interruption is very thin.

The athlete gets under the bar and sets up. After saying, "My bar," the coach lets them have it. As promised, the coach provides a long "loooad" and "hooold," and a short "explode" to help the athlete with timing.

Athlete: "My bar!"
Coach: "Loooooad. Hooooold. Explode!"

After watching the athlete's first set, the coach notices they have good control on the way down but need a bit more speed on the way up, given the short "explode" cue.

STEP 5: DEBRIEF IT

When the athlete completes the rep or set, there is a natural opportunity to review what happened and identify further improvements. In this context, debriefing is synonymous with providing feedback. The goal of the debriefing is to identify whether the focus cue positively influenced the movement and therefore needs to be *repeated*; the meaning behind the focus cue was correct, but the cue itself needs to be *refined*; or the focus cue has either lost its potency after having been used for too long or had a negative impact on the movement and therefore needs to be *retired* for that athlete and that specific movement.

It is important that the debriefing takes the form of a dialogue as opposed to a monologue. While the coach is able to objectively determine the impact of the focus cue on the movement itself, only the athlete can share if they focused on the cue, they understood the cue, or the cue gave them the right feeling or sensation while performing the movement. With a new pair of sneakers, a person doesn't know if they like them until they try them on. It is the same for coaching cues: Sometimes an athlete needs to try a few cues before finding the one that feels best.

> Athlete: "Wow, that is a lot slower than I normally bench press."
> Coach: "Don't you know it. Long and slow makes the muscle grow! Outside of getting used to this new speed, how did this first set feel?"
> Athlete: "Pretty good, I just felt a little sluggish when I went to push the bar."
> Coach: "That's exactly what I saw. How about we shorten that hold at the bottom, make it more of a controlled tap. Then, as you go to push, I want you to focus on accelerating the bar through the ceiling—just remember to hold on!"
> Athlete: "Sounds good—let's bring the roof down."
> Coach: "Now we're talking."

With an understanding of the five-step CCL model, coaches can consider how to deploy this tool in practice (**Figure 2.3**). The CCL consists of a long loop and a short loop.

Coaching Communication Loop

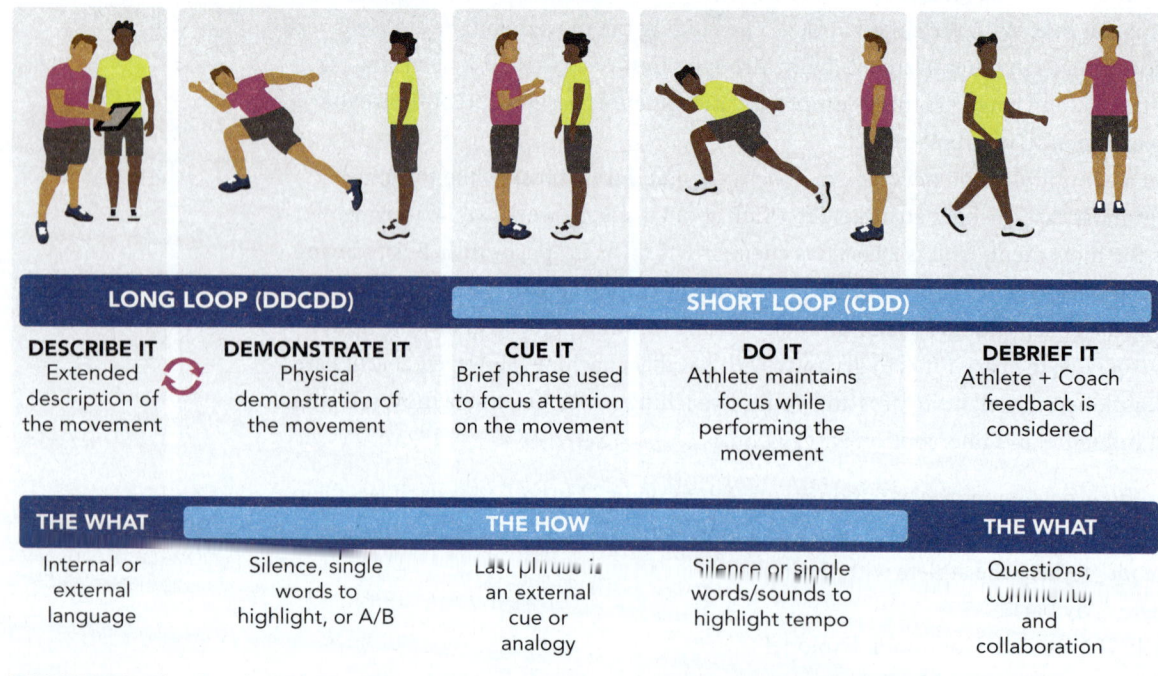

LONG LOOP (DDCDD)		SHORT LOOP (CDD)		
DESCRIBE IT Extended description of the movement	**DEMONSTRATE IT** Physical demonstration of the movement	**CUE IT** Brief phrase used to focus attention on the movement	**DO IT** Athlete maintains focus while performing the movement	**DEBRIEF IT** Athlete + Coach feedback is considered

THE WHAT	THE HOW			THE WHAT
Internal or external language	Silence, single words to highlight, or A/B	Last phrase is an external cue or analogy	Silence or single words/sounds to highlight tempo	Questions, comments, and collaboration

FIGURE 2.3 The Coaching Communication Loop

Reproduced with permission from Winkelman, N. (2021). The language of coaching: The art and science of teaching movement. Champaign, IL: Human Kinetics.

The long loop, which includes all five steps of the CCL model, is used when teaching a movement for the first time or providing an athlete with a refresher. Logically, after the athlete hears the initial description and has a clear picture through demonstration, there is no reason to continue repeating those first two steps. Thus, the short loop, which includes just the last three steps of the model, is used to coach a movement the athlete is already familiar with. If the coach is coaching, there is a need to Cue it, so that the athlete can Do it, and so the athlete and coach can Debrief it.

The story presented here outlines the CCL model and all five steps of the long loop, and each step has evident flexibility. Notably, as the coach continues working with the athlete, they pivot to the short loop, focusing on the Cue, Do, and Debrief portions. Many of the interpersonal communication elements show up throughout the CCL model. Although movement communication is the goal, the coach's interpersonal communication skills forge the path to get there. But the intended destination of the coach and athlete leads straight back to the cue and the focus that helps unlock the next level of progress in the athlete's movement learning journey.

CREATING CUES

The cue is the last thing a coach says to an athlete before they move, so this communication shapes the athlete's focus during the actual movement. The challenge for a coach is identifying the language that informs rather than interferes with movement performance. Coaches have the added challenge of observing the athlete from a bird's-eye view but creating focus cues that easily translate to a first-person perspective. From a practical standpoint, coaches are trying to create cues that make actionable sense from the athlete's perspective and help them optimize their movement in relation to the immediate physical environment.

INTERNAL AND EXTERNAL CUEING

Coaches might be surprised to know that an entire field of study examines the impact of coaching cues on performance and learning—the study of attentional focus. Championed by Dr. Gabriele Wulf, this field now features more than 20 years of research and more than 200 papers written on the topic.

Coaching cues and an athlete's focus exist on a continuum comparable to the zoom lens on a camera. When zoomed in, the athlete is focused on the movement of their body, which is known as an internal focus. An **internal focus** is triggered by any cue that encourages the athlete to focus on moving a joint (e.g., "flex your hip"), limb (e.g., "lift your leg"), or muscle (e.g., "squeeze your glute"). As suggested by this term, the athlete is encouraged to think about their body while simultaneously moving their body.

In contrast, when zoomed out, the athlete is focused on the impact their movement has on the physical environment, which is known as an external focus. An **external focus** is triggered by any cue that encourages the athlete to focus on the movement outcome (e.g., "jump as high as you can") or the environmental impact needed to achieve that outcome (e.g., "explode off the ground to jump as high as you can"). An external focus is so named because it is external to the body; thus, the body is implied rather than the explicit focus. Put simply, an internal focus prioritizes the micro while the external focus prioritizes the macro.

INTERNAL FOCUS →
When an athlete focuses on specific body movements or sensations while performing a skill.

EXTERNAL FOCUS →
When an athlete directs attention toward external factors in the environment, focusing on the intention of the movement outcome.

To further illustrate the difference between an internal and external focus, three examples are provided here:

Upward Phase of a Barbell Romanian Deadlift (RDL)
Internal focus: Focus on driving your hips forward.
External focus: Focus on driving the bar up toward the ceiling.

Upward Phase of a Wide Grip Pull-Up
Internal focus: Focus on squeezing your shoulder blades together.
External focus: Focus on pulling the bar toward the ground.

Outward Phase of Broad Jump
Internal focus: Focus on rapidly extending your hips.
External focus: Focus on rapidly pushing the ground away.

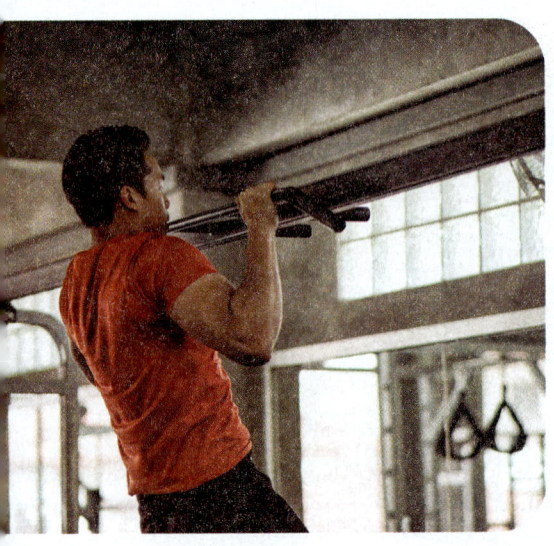

© Blanscape/Shutterstock

What role does each cue play in the athlete's movement learning journey? The coach must reflect on the three cueing examples to move closer to the answer to this question. Putting themselves in the shoes of the athlete, the coach needs to consider which cue is preferred to maximize movement performance and learning. For example, for the barbell RDL, which cue best supports the weight lifted, speed of movement, and technical quality? For the wide grip pull-up, which cue supports the reps completed and range of motion? For the broad jump, which cue generates the farthest jump? The curious coach is encouraged to test and physically try these different cues while performing the outlined movements.

When given the option, athletes and coaches consistently prefer external cues (Winkelman et al., 2021). First, in purely practical terms, an external focus directly connects the athlete to the environment through their movement. As such, an external focus strengthens the existing link between perceiver and perceived, and it translates well to the first-person perspective as the athlete is holding the bar, pulling the bar, and pushing off the ground. An internal focus, by contrast, asks the athlete to retreat into the body, inadvertently breaking the bond between athlete and environment.

Moreover, an internal focus implies that the part is greater than the whole. For example, the broad jump involves every joint and muscle in the body, but the internal focus asks the athlete to focus solely on their hips. In contrast, the external focus invites the whole body to work together to push the ground away.

Both intuition and research point toward the superiority of an external focus. Review of numerous studies—across strength (Halperin et al., 2016), power (Vance et al., 2004), endurance (Marchant et al., 2011), and efficiency (Lohse et al., 2011); across lifting (Schutts et al., 2017), sprinting (Winkelman et al., 2017), jumping (Porter et al., 2013), and agility (Porter et al., 2010); and across experience level (Wulf & Su, 2007), physical ability level (Beck et al., 2018), and sport (Wulf et al., 2002)—reveals that performance and learning are consistently better when adopting an external focus of attention. This does not mean that people do not get better with an internal focus: They do, just not at the same rate or to the same degree as when under the guidance of an external focus (Wulf, 2013). When the evidence is combined with natural intuition, there is a strong case that coaches should prioritize the use of external cues for the cueing portion of the CCL.

However, internal language is still important when learning. Internal language is central to both the Describe and Debrief portions of the CCL. It allows the coach and the athlete to discuss the movement biomechanically and outline what happens during the motion. This is particularly important for highly technical movements, such as pitching a baseball, and for aesthetic sports that are subjectively scored, such as dance, gymnastics, and diving. Without a way to talk about what the body is doing, there is little basis for understanding what the external focus cue is trying to achieve. This is especially true if a coach is trying to use video analysis with an athlete. Hence, many coaches use a hybrid cue that combines an internal description with an external focus.

The critical move is to ensure that the external cue is the last thing the athlete hears, clearly delineating the role of the internal language (the *what*) and the external focus (the *how*). There is room for all forms of coaching language, as long as coaches organize their words regarding the desired outcome. This skill requires coaches to recognize that internal language elevates an athlete's knowledge of what to do, whereas external language elevates their knowledge of how to do it. Both forms of knowledge are valuable, but the latter is what athletes are ultimately judged by. For example, at no time does an athlete take a written exam on sprinting: The exam is sprinting. Coaches are cautioned not to confuse their desire to explain a movement with what is necessary for the athlete to perform it.

When they use the CCL in its long and short forms, coaches have a repeatable process for saying the right things at the right time. The CCL model allows for significant flexibility within each step, catering to the athlete's needs.

📋 COACH'S CORNER

To see how separation of the internal focus and external focus might occur, with the external cue being presented last, consider the following examples:

Push Phase of Sprint Acceleration
"On your next sprint, we need to focus on getting more *hip and knee extension* [internal focus]. To achieve this, I want you to focus on *pushing the ground away* [external focus]."

Downward Phase of Single-Leg Romanian Deadlift
"As you lower, we want to focus on keeping your *body long from head to heel*, while *flexing through your hip* [internal focus], creating a T at the bottom of the motion. To achieve this, I want you to focus on pushing the bottom of your shoe toward the wall behind you—put your footprint on the wall [external cue]."

LESSON 4: SENDING AND RECEIVING THE INTENDED MESSAGE
INTERPERSONAL COMMUNICATION

Interpersonal communication (IC) is more spontaneous than movement communication (MC). Coaches use IC strategies in a flexible way to get the most out of their MC. To recognize that coaches do not go around yelling out cues in isolation is to recognize that

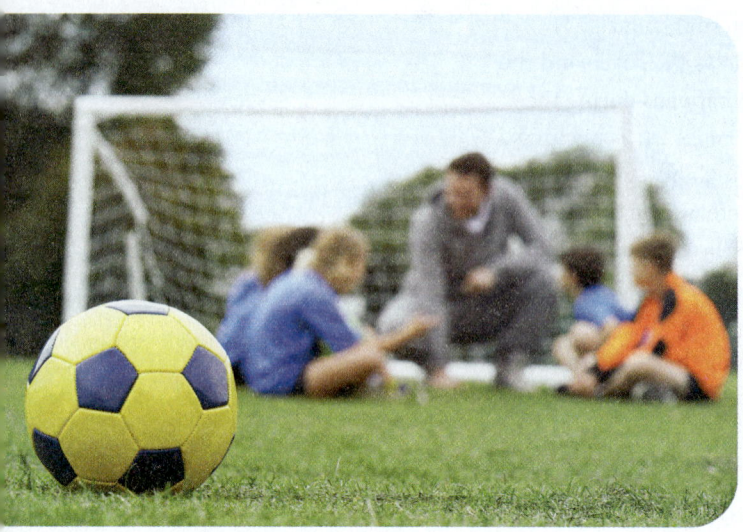

© SpeedKingz/Shutterstock

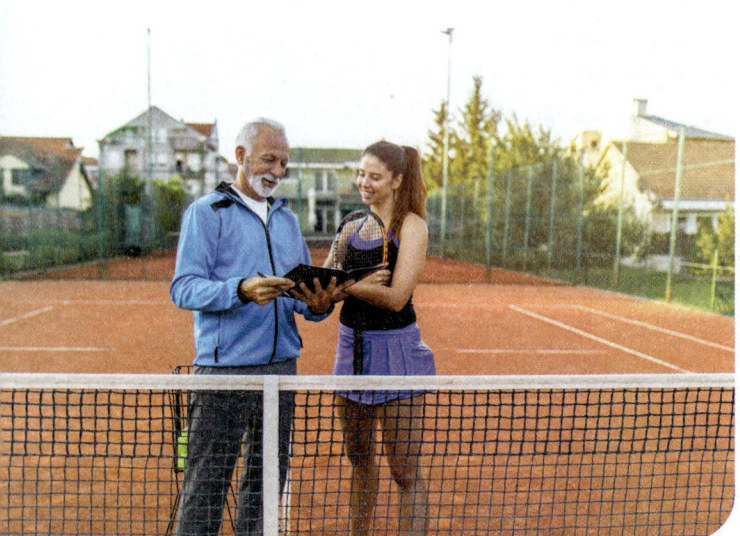

© Hedgehog94/Shutterstock

there are IC valleys that lead to the MC peaks. IC is how the coach communicates how to move. It is the collection of the small interactions that a coach and athlete have on their way to the right cue and that elusive "aha" moment. It is the questions, stories, moments of connection, shared understanding, and overcoming of differences that make two people want to engage with each other. Without IC, the best MC falls short.

By chance or by choice, coaches adopt a speaking pattern known as their communication style. If they do not engage in reflection or do not receive feedback, coaches can struggle to understand their style and its impact on athletes. For example, when an athlete's behavior comes into question, the athlete commonly shoulders the blame. Coaches state that the athlete does not understand or is not applying themselves. Rarely do coaches ask if an athlete's poor understanding is due to a lack of communication. Similarly, the athlete who does not appear to apply themselves may be responding poorly to the negative speech pattern the coach uses as motivation. The coach is a physical variable within the athlete's learning journey and needs to be reviewed just as a training program is reviewed (Mallett, 2005).

COMMUNICATION STYLE

Whereas MC targets the language needed to help the athlete learn to move better, IC creates the conditions for that learning. For example, if an athlete were asked to describe their coach, their response would characterize the coach's IC style.

If enough athletes were asked to describe their coach, it would become clear that coaches operate on a communication continuum, characterized by a controlling style at one end and an autonomy-supportive style at the other (Mageau & Vallerand, 2003). To demonstrate these styles, consider the following coach–athlete interactions.

COACH–ATHLETE INTERACTION 1

Coach: "You're late again. This is unacceptable and unfair to your teammates who are here on time. Come talk to me after training."

Athlete: "Sorry, coach."

Coach: "Okay, everyone, the program is up on the screen with your main lift loads. Let's get on the platforms and start warming up for our hang cleans."

The coach paces up and down the room, eyeing each athlete as they progressively increase their loads on the hang clean.

Coach: "Cut the chat. I want you focused on what you're doing. The season is just around the corner and these lifts have never been more important."

The coach starts targeting specific athletes, yelling out coaching cues from a central position in the room.

Coach: "Catch that bar with a proud chest. Explode through that bar. Get your hips back. That's it, that's what we're looking for."

The coach continues like this throughout the session, maintaining a central position and calling out cues and commands over the pumping music.

Coach: "Team, I thought we did a good job after a slow start. We need to relish every opportunity to get under the bar and get better. Our first game is in three weeks, and we need to be ready on and off the field. Get to class and I'll see you first thing tomorrow. Right?"

Athlete: "Yes, coach!"

COACH–ATHLETE INTERACTION 2

Athlete: "Sorry I'm late, coach."

The coach nods, giving the athlete time to join the team.

Coach: "Good morning, everyone, how are we feeling?"

Team: "Good coach!" "Great coach!"

The team laughs in approval.

Coach: "That's good. We have a big day in front of us. Another opportunity to get better with the season just around the corner! Okay, take a moment and have a look at the screen. Your main lifts and loads are outlined. Are there any questions?"

Athlete: "Coach, if our hang clean is at the standard, can we start pulling from the ground?"

Coach: "Great question. Yes, that is fine. Just make sure I get my eyes on your last few sets."

Coach: "Any other questions? Okay, if not, just grab me if anything pops up throughout the session."

As the team disperses to their lifting platforms, the coach walks with the athlete who arrived late.

Coach: "Is everything all right? That was the second time you were late this week, which is unlike you."

Athlete: "Yeah, I'm really sorry, I haven't been sleeping very well. I'm dealing with some family stuff."

Coach: "Is there anything I can do? You can also speak with someone in player support."

Athlete: "Thanks, coach. No, I think I'm okay, everything should be sorted by next week."

Coach: "Well, you let me know if you need any help."

Athlete: "I will, and I won't be late again. Thank you!"

As the athlete finds their platform, the coach starts to move through the room, stopping briefly to say a few words to each athlete.

Coach: "Loving that bar speed, keep it up. You're dropping under that bar so much faster, nice work. That's it, keep snapping those elbows forward."

Athlete: "Coach, can you have a look at my next set?"

Coach: "Sure thing, let's have a look."

The athlete proceeds to perform a set of power cleans, pulling from the floor as discussed during the session preview.

Coach: "How'd it feel pulling from the ground? What did you notice—good or bad?"

Athlete: "I kind of felt my hips shoot up. It was like I lost all my tension when I started to pull the bar from the ground."

Coach: "What do you think you can focus on to reclaim that tension and connection with the bar?"

Athlete: "Pulling the bar harder?"

Coach: "I like it. Yes, let's focus on pulling the bar. One way to think of this is like you are pulling yourself into the ground, giving you the sensation of bending the bar.

So on your last set here, let's pull ourselves into the ground and bring that tension through the pull."

Athlete: "Perfect, thanks coach!"

The coach continues like this, having similar micro-coaching conversations throughout the session, still maintaining a global presence and calling out messages of encouragement and session flow as needed.

These coach–athlete interactions demonstrate how noticeably different communication styles can facilitate the same training session. One style is not principally better, but individuals generally prefer one style over the other. Putting themselves in the role of the athlete, coaches can more easily consider which style they would have preferred as an athlete and compare that to their current coaching style. Although some coaches feel they use a more controlling style, as outlined in the first interaction, others feel more autonomy-supportive, like the coach in the second interaction. Still others see themselves as somewhere in the middle, wavering between the two styles. Principal differences exist between the two styles, and the preference of each style appears to be context specific.

CONTROLLING STYLE

The **controlling style** is best defined as a monologue-heavy approach to communication. This style is characterized by statements and commands rather than questions and conversation.

A coach who uses this style comes across as direct and to the point. They speak with certainty and seek to tell the athlete what they expect and whether they achieved it. Although this style is often labeled as being authoritative or autocratic, the negative framing is misleading and obscures the utility of this coaching style when used for the right reasons in certain situations.

For example, consider a coach working with a high school athlete for the first time. If this athlete has no experience lifting weights, the coach initially defaults to a controlling style. This style is preferred for two reasons. First, there is a legitimate safety risk when lifting weights. As such, the coach must be clear and direct so the athlete is not put at risk. Second, when the athlete has no experience lifting weights, the nature of the relationship requires that the coach does more of the talking and teaching early on, giving the athlete time to accumulate knowledge of what to do and how to do it.

The controlling style gets a bad reputation because coaches overuse it. The coach might continue to use a controlling style long after the athlete has accumulated a significant understanding of their body, movement, training, and what works for them. When the controlling style is taken too far, it can undermine the athlete's autonomy, leading to demotivation and ambivalence. In essence, an athlete is told what to do and is given no voice in their learning journey. This behavior can dissociate the athlete from their results and the effort required to achieve them, because the athlete cannot see the connection between their influence on the process and the outcome. In contrast, when an athlete feels involved in relevant features of their learning journey, they see the connection between effort and outcome. With a sense of self-control and the responsibility that comes with it, athletes develop a more intrinsically directed motivation resulting in greater focus, effort, and, ultimately, a better result (Mageau & Vallerand, 2003).

CONTROLLING → STYLE

A monologue-heavy approach to communication.

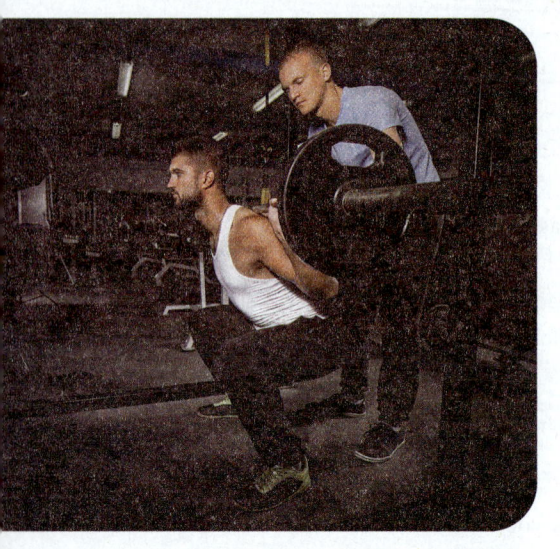

© Bokan/Shutterstock

When considering this coaching style, be mindful that some athletes do not experience the controlling style as controlling. Some athletes feel that having a coach who exclusively tells them what to do allows them to focus their energy on execution. These athletes make a conscious choice to be in the presence of the controlling-style coach and accept their guidance. When considered in a social context, the controlling style signals that the coach knows what they are talking about and that they are an expert. For many, this status engenders trust, confidence, and peace of mind. Thus, the controlling style has a role in every coach–athlete journey. It is up to the coach to identify when it is best to use this interaction style versus pivot to a more autonomy-supportive style based on their understanding of the athlete.

AUTONOMY-SUPPORTIVE STYLE

The **autonomy-supportive style** is defined as a dialogue-driven approach to communication. This style is characterized by questions and conversation rather than statements and commands. A coach using this style values the input from the athlete and recognizes the importance of athlete autonomy. While the coach is clear about the expected outcomes and the process needed to get there, they recognize that each athlete travels an individual path. This style is associated with the understanding that what works for one does not work for all. Thus, the autonomy-supportive coach realizes that the only way to unlock the individual's potential is to involve them in the journey.

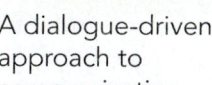

AUTONOMY-SUPPORTIVE STYLE →

A dialogue-driven approach to communication.

Adopting an autonomy-supportive style of communication does not mean that the athlete is given the keys to the kingdom and asked to write and coach their own program on day one. Taking such an extreme stance may, in fact, undermine the athlete's autonomy, as the athlete's decision to work with a coach who can guide them was an expression of autonomous behavior. At every stage of the athlete's journey, there is an unspoken expectation that the coach will provide insight and direction when the athlete needs it. The following example demonstrates a betrayal of this expectation, and how autonomy can be misused.

> Coach: "I am going to demonstrate the power clean and then I want you to give it a try."
> Athlete: "Sounds good."
> The coach demonstrates the movement three times, providing no instruction on setup or execution.
> Coach: "Okay, your turn. Let's see you go through three repetitions, taking your time between each rep."
> Athlete: "So, you want me to just do what you did?"
> Coach: "Yes, exactly, I want to see how you perform the movement."
> The athlete approaches the bar. A bit confused, they ask the coach about the right way to set up and catch the bar. After three somewhat awkward repetitions, the coach and athlete debrief.
> Coach: "So, how did those reps feel?"
> Athlete: "Good, I guess. I am not really sure what I am doing."
> Coach: "That is normal. I want you to explore the movement until you find a comfortable way of performing it. What do you think you can focus on to get a bit better on your next set?"

Athlete: "I'm not really sure. What do you think I should focus on?"

Coach: "Let's do a few more sets, and we will find the focus and technique that works for you."

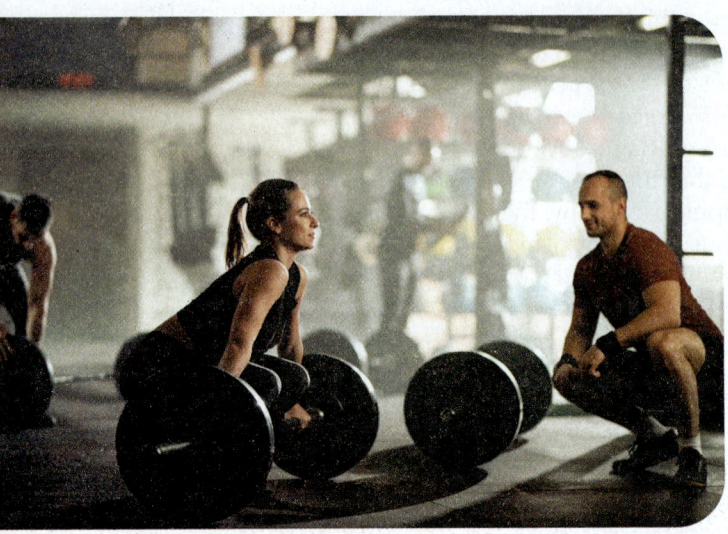

© Drazen Zigic/Shutterstock

Athlete autonomy is beneficial and associated with more intrinsic motivation and may result in a higher level of effort and better overall performance (Amorose & Anderson-Butcher, 2007). However, it is not a fix-all. The previous example demonstrates the flaw in that thought process. When a coach gives an athlete autonomy in a situation where they do not want it, they unintentionally take it away.

At this point, a coach needs to recognize that the uniform application of a single coaching style is unlikely to result in the desired outcome for either the coach or the athlete. Instead, it is more appropriate to think of these styles as modes of coaching whereby a coach switches between modes within and across sessions as the athlete and the context require it. To illustrate this fluid use of communication modes, consider this version of the previous coaching interaction.

Coach: "Hey, am I right in saying this is the first time you've done the full power clean?"

Athlete: "Yes. I've done the hang clean a few times, but I've never been coached."

Coach: "No worries, we'll make sure we change that. To start, I'm going to walk you through the setup and give you a few pointers on how to execute the movement."
The coach briefly explains the setup and demonstrates three repetitions, highlighting key pointers along the way.

Coach: "Your turn. I want you to run through the setup three times and then have a go at three full repetitions. Take your time and feel free to ask questions along the way."
The athlete proceeds as outlined by the coach. They stop to ask a few questions, but comfortably work through the repetitions.

Coach: "Okay, first things first: Did you feel comfortable in the setup?"

Athlete: "Yes. Getting close and pulling myself into the ground really seemed to help. I did have one question on how wide my hands should be."

Coach: "You want your hands to be just outside your legs, but not so far that you feel like you have to slouch. Okay, second part: How did the movement feel? Connected or disconnected, smooth or choppy, explosive or slow?"

Athlete: "It felt good, pretty smooth overall."

Coach: "That's good. Can I share one observation with you?"

Athlete: "Please."

Coach: "Once the bar clears your knees, you really want to accelerate it toward the ceiling. To get the feeling of this, I find athletes respond really well to either moving with the same intention as a vertical jump or with the sense of stealing or ripping the bar away from the ground. Do either of those cues resonate with you?"

Athlete: "I really like stealing the bar from the ground. I can feel how that will help with my speed."

Coach: "Great, let's give this a go."

This example demonstrates how control and autonomy can coexist. Throughout the story, the coach involves the athlete at relevant moments, providing direct instruction where it makes sense. Notably, the most important bit of autonomy came at the end, when the coach provided controlled choice. Here the coach controls what the athlete focuses on but does so in a way that the athlete is involved. This involvement helps the coach because the athlete's choice helps the coach understand what words work best for them. While this A/B choice might not seem like a lot, a large body of work shows that simple choices significantly improve movement learning compared to coaching environments that do not use controlled choice (Sanli et al., 2013).

Both the controlling and autonomy-supportive communication modes are critical to a coach's interpersonal skillset. Generally, a coach starts with a more controlling style, unlocking autonomy as the athlete earns the right to it. However, strategic autonomy, like controlled choice, can and should be used early in the training process. It helps the coach identify what makes sense to the athlete and gives the athlete ownership of the process. Finally, whether they operate in controlling or autonomy-supportive mode, coaches face the challenge of getting to know each athlete. This builds rapport and provides the coach with the information needed to coach the athlete.

For example, imagine a coach working with an athlete on sprinting. The coach struggles to get the athlete to gradually rise as they go from acceleration to maximal speed. The coach then remembers the athlete telling them their mother was a fighter pilot. This prompts the coach to offer the analogy, "As you are sprinting, gradually rise like a jet taking off." The athlete's eyes widen with familiarity, and the cue does the trick. As this example illustrates, knowing the athlete makes it easier to coach and guide them down a familiar path. To unlock this knowledge, a coach needs only two tools: the ability to ask questions and to listen without judgment.

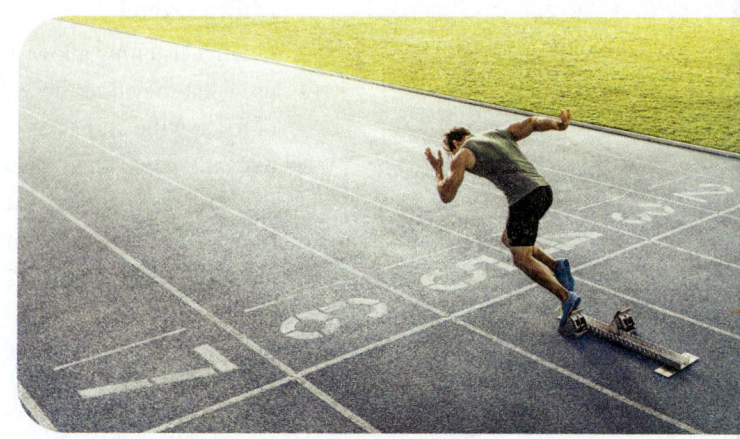
© Jacob Lund/Shutterstock

ASKING AND LISTENING

Coaches and athletes only speak or listen in each communication style or mode. Although speaking is certainly important, a coach's listening quality is the defining difference between the good and the great. Only when a coach listens can they access the athlete's language, experience, and perspective. This information forms the core of who the athlete is, which opens up a few opportunities for the coach.

First, how people use language, including slang, is regional and generational: An athlete uses the language from where and when they grew up. Because language is how people describe and codify the world around them, a coach's use of an athlete's language helps with understanding. Second, getting to know the athlete provides the coach with access to their life experiences. An athlete's life experiences provide the coach with reference material that they can use to help the athlete understand new concepts. By making analogies, a coach can use familiar concepts to teach unfamiliar ones. Finally, listening is required to gain insight into an athlete's perspective. This is particularly important during the Debrief step of the CCL, where the coach wants to access the athlete's experience using the focus cue. Moreover, if a coach continues to use coaching cues that are not working, they need to get the athlete's perspective on which focus works best.

In all cases, listening is the main skill deployed by the coach. Specifically, coaches need to employ **active listening** to intently focus on what is said rather than making judgments or preplanned responses while the athlete is speaking (Treasure, 2017). If a coach

ACTIVE →
LISTENING

Intently focusing on what is said rather than making judgments or preplanned responses while the athlete is still speaking.

summons a response before the athlete is done talking, they interfere with their ability to hear what the athlete is saying.

Moreover, it is easy to tell active listening from passive listening. When someone is in the presence of an active listener, they feel they have that person's full attention, often receive questions, and are always given the space to finish what they have to say. Further, when in the presence of an active listener, a person is more likely to speak because they feel heard. A coach who masters active listening is more likely to have athletes who feel comfortable communicating, questioning, and sharing the information that the coach requires to make them better.

While effective listening is the goal, a coach must have something to listen to. As such, the athlete must be invited to share or feel comfortable doing so voluntarily. Leaning on this logic, the following strategies can help coaches get the most out of their asking and listening skills.

MIRRORING

If active listening allows the coach to access the athlete's life locker, **mirroring** helps them use what they find there. Notably, a coach should try to learn how to speak *athlete* instead of forcing the athlete to learn how to speak *coach*. This means the coach can mirror the relevant words and phrases the athlete organically shares in regular daily conversations. Without being forced, the coach wants to find natural situations where they can replace their language with the athlete's.

This verbal mirroring can also be prompted more explicitly. For example, after offering an athlete a cue, a great way to identify if they understand its meaning is to prompt them with one of the following:

- "What are you going to focus on?"
- "What does this cue mean to you?"
- "Put this cue into your own words."

The coach must listen closely to how the athlete responds to the prompt. To illustrate, consider how this coach uses the second prompt.

Coach: "On your next set of goblet squats, I want you to focus on <u>sitting behind the kettlebell</u>. So, what does that cue mean to you?"
Athlete: "You want me to <u>push</u> my hips <u>back</u> as I <u>squat down to the floor</u>."
Coach: "Exactly, focus on <u>pushing back</u> as you <u>squat down to the floor</u>."

Here is a perfect example of mirroring an athlete's words. The coach offers the cue, "focus on sitting behind the kettlebell." The athlete interprets that cue as "push my hips back as I squat down to the floor." The coach then refines the cue, editing out "hips back" and mirroring the athlete's language: "Exactly, focus on pushing back as you squat down to the floor." This is a simple and effective strategy to get the cues from the athlete's words, lowering their barrier to understanding.

CONTROLLED CHOICE

Another way to involve the athlete is by giving them a **controlled choice** over the coaching cue (Wulf & Lewthwaite, 2016). While the coach curates the choices, the athlete gets to choose the cue that makes the most sense to them. This provides the coach with further access to the athlete's language preferences and understanding of the movement.

Here are some example prompts the coach can use to trigger the choice:

- "Which of the following cues do you prefer?"
- "Which of the following cues makes the most sense to you?"
- "Which of the following cues will help you achieve X—technical change?"

The coach should listen closely to which choice the athlete makes. To illustrate this, consider the following example of a coach using the third prompt.

Coach: "As you are sprinting, we need to get a bit more hip flexion. Which of the following cues do you feel help you get more knee drive: (a) drive your knees toward the finish, (b) drive out like you're sprinting up a steep set of stairs, or (c) drive your knees forward as if to shatter a pane of glass."

Athlete: "I think all of those could help, but I really like C."

Coach: "C it is—drive your knees forward as if to shatter a pane of glass."

As the example illustrates, the use of controlled choice actively involves the athlete, providing the coach with an opportunity to listen and understand their perspective. This inevitably stimulates conversation that helps the athlete and coach find shared meaning.

CUE CREATION

The final strategy is the ultimate form of athlete autonomy and coach listening. Specifically, after a coach feels an athlete has reached the point where they understand the movement well enough, they can give them more control of the **cue creation** process.

In this case, the coach lays out the technical error that must be corrected and gives the athlete the first shot at identifying a suitable cue. For example, in the case of a single-leg RDL, a coach might say, "What do you think you can focus on to stay long from head to heel during the downward portion of the RDL?" In the case of a vertical jump, a coach might say, "What do you think you can focus on to get more vertical power during your vertical jump?" Sometimes the athlete identifies a brilliant cue. At other times, a conversation ensues. Either way, the coach and athlete work to co-create a custom cue built from the words in the athlete's language locker. The method provides the coach and athlete with insights that bring them closer to shared meaning.

> **CUE CREATION →**
>
> A process in which the coach provides the technical error that needs to be corrected and gives the athlete the first opportunity to identify a suitable cue.

SUMMARY

A coach takes others from where they are to where they want to be. This chapter first discussed the forms of knowledge that coaches must pursue—knowledge of what to coach and how to coach it. Coaches typically receive more formal development in the former, leaving the development of the latter up to chance.

Recognizing that movement exists in the space between athlete and environment is key to influencing movement. Coaches are not necessary for movement learning to occur, but they are required for movement learning to be optimized. There are two primary ways to influence a movement—verbal coaching and nonverbal programming. Both forms of influence are valuable when used in the right way and at the right time.

The communication blueprint is a model that outlines the way interpersonal and movement communication show up within a training session. Like a story, the communication blueprint has a beginning, a middle, and an end, replete with distinct communication strategies the coach can use to get the most out of the athlete. Movement communication can be facilitated by the coaching communication loop (CCL). The five-step CCL model is used to organize coaching language so that coaches say the right things at the right time to optimize athlete learning. This guides the coach toward a deeper discussion of the coaching cue, the last thing the athlete hears before they move. While the coaching cue is responsible for establishing the athlete's focus while they move, the coach can learn the best language to generate focus for that specific athlete. Internal language maps to an athlete's understanding of what to do, and external language maps to their understanding of how to do it. Both forms of communication are necessary, but coaches need to prioritize the use of external language when cueing.

Interpersonal communication is the soil in which movement communication thrives. By choosing the most appropriate place on the communication continuum flanked by controlling and autonomy-supportive behaviors, coaches can learn nuanced ways to build a healthy coach–athlete relationship. The basic skills of speaking and listening are required for interpersonal communication. Coaches are encouraged to think about the importance of listening, recognizing that it is the only time they are accessing the athlete's language, experiences, and perspective. This information informs the coach how best to individualize the coaching experience to meet the athlete's unique needs. Mirroring, controlled choice, and cue co-creation are another set of strategies that can help coaches involve the athlete in their learning journey.

Pursuit of the craft of coaching is a lifelong journey with no finish line. This proposition is exciting for anyone who values the path more than the destination. Although this path provides great joy, it also presents great challenges. The strategies are the tools coaches can apply to overcome these barriers. Coaches must recognize that they are much like their athletes—always learning, making mistakes, and overcoming. To this end, coaches need to give themselves the space to grow, be patient, and look up occasionally to see how far they have come. By engaging in self-awareness and self-care, a coach is far more likely to build an environment that encourages an athlete to do the same.

KEY TAKEAWAYS

- Influencing movement: The primary purpose of a performance coach is to improve movement by enhancing coordination, speed, and strength. Coaches should engage in both verbal and nonverbal communication when working with athletes. Verbal communication targets the athlete and the way they focus on the environment; nonverbal communication targets the environment and the way it captures the athlete's focus.
- Communication blueprint: Communication must include a natural alternation between person-focused dialogue and movement-focused dialogue. These two interact to optimize the athlete's experience and learning.
- Movement communication: The five steps of the coaching communication loop (CCL) are (a) describe it, (b) demonstrate it, (c) cue it, (d) do it, and (e) debrief it. CCL is a natural communication model that focuses on the communication necessary before, during, and after a movement is performed.
- Interpersonal communication: Interpersonal communication is how the coach communicates to the athlete how to move. It is more spontaneous than movement communication, where the coach is encouraged to be flexible, integrating several different strategies. The most common interpersonal communication styles used in coaching are controlling and autonomy-supportive style.

REFERENCES

Amorose, A. J., & Anderson-Butcher, D. (2007). Autonomy-supportive coaching and self-determined motivation in high school and college athletes: A test of self-determination theory. *Psychology of Sport and Exercise, 8*(5), 654–670.

Beck, E. N., Intzandt, B. N., & Almeida, Q. J. (2018). Can dual task walking improve in Parkinson's disease after external focus of attention exercise? A single blind randomized controlled trial. *Neurorehabilitation and Neural Repair, 32*(1), 18–33.

Calvo-Merino, B., Grèzes, J., Glaser, D. E., Passingham, R. E., & Haggard, P. (2006). Seeing or doing? Influence of visual and motor familiarity in action observation. *Current Biology, 16*(19), 1905–1910.

Halperin, I., Williams, K. J., Martin, D. T., & Chapman, D. W. (2016). The effects of attentional focusing instructions on force production during the isometric mid-thigh pull. *Journal of Strength & Conditioning Research, 30*(4), 919–923.

Liao, C.-M., & Masters, R. S. (2001). Analogy learning: A means to implicit motor learning. *Journal of Sports Sciences, 19*(5), 307–319.

Lohse, K. R., Sherwood, D. E., & Healy, A. F. (2011). Neuromuscular effects of shifting the focus of attention in a simple force production task. *Journal of Motor Behavior, 43*(2), 173–184.

Mageau, G. A., & Vallerand, R. J. (2003). The coach–athlete relationship: A motivational model. *Journal of Sports Sciences, 21*(11), 883–904.

Mallett, C. J. (2005). Self-determination theory: A case study of evidence-based coaching. *Sport Psychologist, 19*(4), 417–429.

Marchant, D. C., Greig, M., Bullough, J., & Hitchen, D. (2011). Instructions to adopt an external focus enhance muscular endurance. *Research Quarterly for Exercise and Sport, 82*(3), 466–473.

Newell, K. (1986). Constraints on the development of coordination. In M. G. Wade & H. T. A. Whiting (Eds.), *Motor development in children: Aspects of coordination and control* (pp. 341–360). Martinus Nihjoff, Dordect.

Porter, J. M., Anton, P. M., Wikoff, N. M., & Ostrowski, J. B. (2013). Instructing skilled athletes to focus their attention externally at greater distances enhances jumping performance. *Journal of Strength & Conditioning Research, 27*(8), 2073–2078.

Porter, J. M., Nolan, R. P., Ostrowski, E. J., & Wulf, G. (2010). Directing attention externally enhances agility performance: A qualitative and quantitative analysis of the efficacy of using verbal instructions to focus attention. *Frontiers in Psychology, 1*(216), 1–7.

Sanli, E. A., Patterson, J. T., Bray, S. R., & Lee, T. D. (2013). Understanding self-controlled motor learning protocols through the self-determination theory. *Frontiers in Psychology, 3*, 611.

Schutts, K. S., Wu, W. F. W., Vidal, A. D., Hiegel, J., & Becker, J. (2017). Does focus of attention improve snatch lift kinematics? *Journal of Strength & Conditioning Research, 31*(10), 2758–2764.

Treasure, J. (2017). *How to be heard: Secrets for powerful speaking and listening.* Mango Publishing.

Vance, J., Wulf, G., Tollner, T., McNevin, N., & Mercer, J. (2004). EMG activity as a function of the performer's focus of attention. *Journal of Motor Behavior, 36*(4), 450–459.

Winkelman, N. (2021). *The language of coaching: The art and science of teaching movement.* Human Kinetics.

Winkelman, N., Clark, K., Razon, S., Jarmuz, A., & Whale, A. (2021). *Sport-imagery ability and preference for attentional cueing in motor skills instruction.* Unpublished research.

Winkelman, N., Clark, K. P., & Ryan, L. J. (2017). Experience level influences the effect of attentional focus on sprint performance. *Human Movement Science, 52*, 84–95.

Wulf, G. (2013). Attentional focus and motor learning: A review of 15 years. *International Review of Sport and Exercise Psychology, 6*(1), 77–104.

Wulf, G., & Lewthwaite, R. (2016). Optimizing performance through intrinsic motivation and attention for learning: The OPTIMAL theory of motor learning. *Psychonomic Bulletin & Review, 23*(5), 1382–1414.

Wulf, G., McConnel, N., Gartner, M., & Schwarz, A. (2002). Enhancing the learning of sport skills through external-focus feedback. *Journal of Motor Behavior, 34*(2), 171–182.

Wulf, G., McNevin, N., & Shea, C. H. (2001). The automaticity of complex motor skill learning as a function of attentional focus. *Quarterly Journal of Experimental Psychology, 54*(4), 1143–1154.

Wulf, G., & Su, J. (2007). An external focus of attention enhances golf shot accuracy in beginners and experts. *Research Quarterly for Exercise and Sport, 78*(4), 384–389.

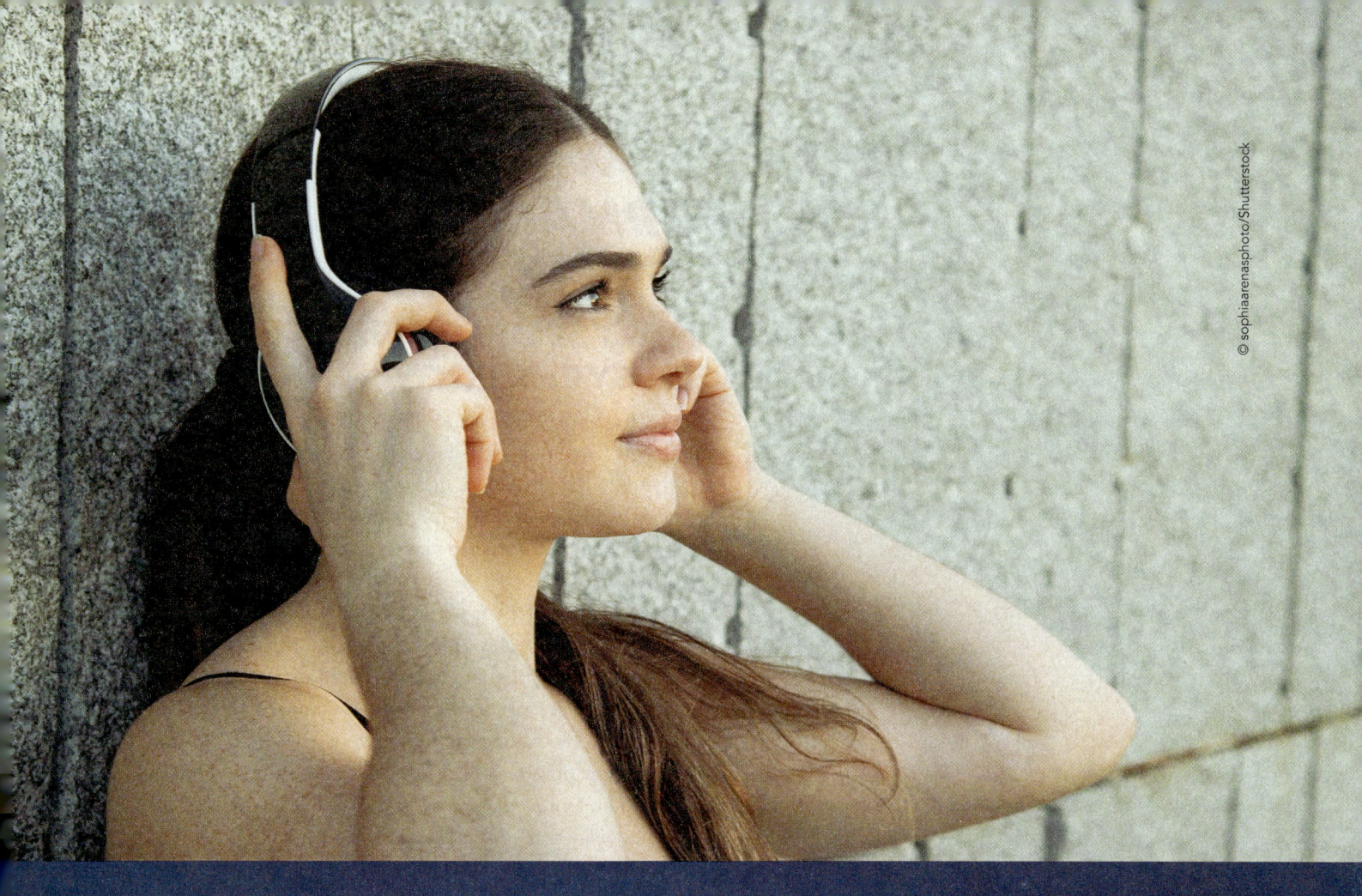

PSYCHOLOGY IN SPORTS PERFORMANCE

CHAPTER THREE

LEARNING OBJECTIVES

Upon completion of this chapter, the Sports Performance Coach will be able to:

- **Define** sports psychology.
- **Define** internal motivation and its relationship to athletic success.
- **Explain** the role of mental skills training in improving sports performance.
- **Identify** the relationship between mental readiness and return to sport after injury.
- **Identify** mental skills training methods to optimize athletic performance.

LESSON 1: SPORTS AND PERFORMANCE PSYCHOLOGY THEORY

INTRODUCTION TO SPORTS AND PERFORMANCE PSYCHOLOGY

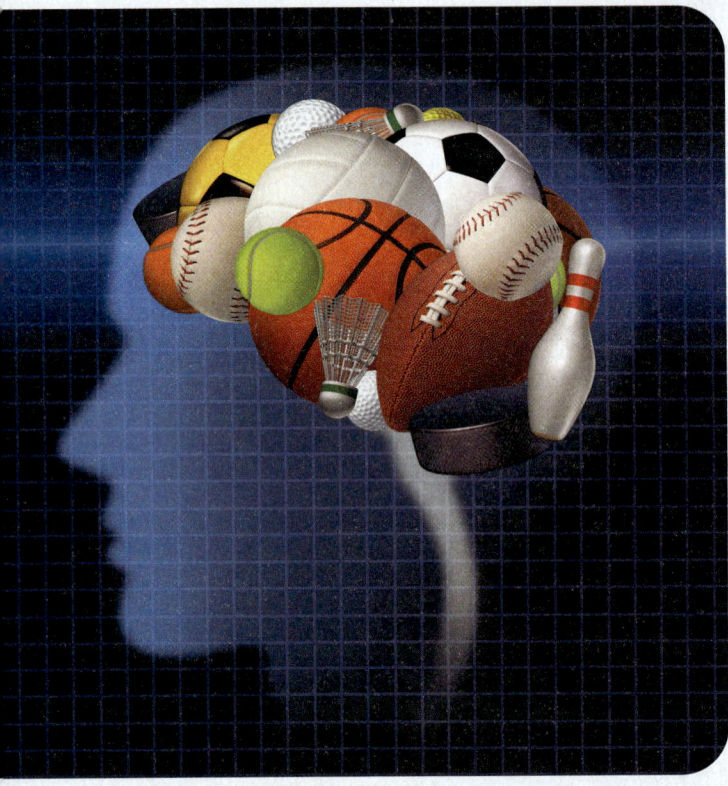

© Lightspring/Shutterstock

Athletes know that their minds play an integral role in physical performance. Yankees catcher Yogi Berra once said that 90% of the game is mental, and the other half is physical. While his numbers might not add up, the message is clear: Mental performance plays a significant role in sports performance.

It is well known that thoughts affect physiology. *What* and *how* athletes think creates a physiological state that either limits or optimizes their ability to perform. For example, an athlete suffering from excessive anxiety before a competition may experience overactivation of their nervous system (also known as sympathetic dominance), leading to an inability to diffuse tension and maintain optimal focus. Excessive anxiety and worry can delay reaction time and impair the ability to monitor and judge situations correctly (Bali, 2015).

Consider an Olympic athlete training for four years for an event, and then having anxiety be the factor that limits their performance—not their athletic ability. These kinds of situations are a primary reason that the field of **sports psychology** is experiencing rapid growth and acceptance from the scientific and sports communities.

SPORTS PSYCHOLOGY →

The study of performance, mental processes, and well-being of people in sporting settings while considering psychological theory and methods.

✔ CHECK IT OUT

Sports psychology traces its roots back to the ancient Olympic Games, but modern studies of sports psychology date to roughly 1880 (Kornspan, 2012). Coleman Griffith began working at the University of Illinois in 1915 and is often touted as the father of sports psychology in North America. Griffith authored the books *Psychology of Coaching* in 1926 and *Psychology of Athletics* in 1928. While Griffith worked in the United States, Avkentsy Puni of the Soviet Union published theories on psychological preparation for competition, optimal emotional arousal, and self-regulation, which were considered groundbreaking and beyond what was being studied in North America at that time (Gould & Weinberg, 2015).

Sports and performance psychology continues to evolve. As part of this evolution, other fields, including clinical psychology, physical education, and kinesiology, influence the discipline. Sociocultural factors, such as the growth of Olympic sports, professional sports, Title IX, television contracts, and social media, also inform the path taken by sports and performance psychology. The scientific community and those involved in sports training know that preparing an athlete's mind for success is imperative in reaching performance excellence.

The primary objective of sports and performance psychology is to help athletes achieve and consistently replicate performance excellence. **Performance excellence** can be defined as the consistent on-demand execution of a learned skill. One common way of describing this excellence is as a *flow* state. Mihaly Csikszentmihalyi (1990), who originally introduced flow theory in the 1970s, later described it as a state of consciousness where someone is wholly absorbed into what they are doing to the exclusion of all other thoughts and emotions. This has also been described as being in the *zone*. No matter what it is called, this experience is related to an optimal mental and physical state that inspires peak performance (Biasutti, 2017).

> **PERFORMANCE→ EXCELLENCE**
>
> The consistent on-demand execution of a learned skill.

> 👍 **HELPFUL HINT**
>
> According to Csikszentmihalyi, flow occurs when challenges and skills are in balance; it is then that an individual achieves an optimal psychological state. The total focus that occurs in flow fosters a positive experience in which individuals move their experience from average to optimal. Although flow often leads to positive outcomes, the essence of this state is complete engagement in the present. Essentially, performance excellence leads to flow, and flow leads to performance excellence.

A consistent factor emerging from stories of flow is that it is experienced when individuals push themselves beyond their current abilities but believe they can succeed (Biasutti, 2017). This perspective draws attention to Bandura's **theory of self-efficacy**. Self-efficacy is an individual's belief in their capacity to execute the skills necessary to produce a specific performance outcome (Bandura, 1994). In sports, much of this theory is rooted in an athlete's confidence.

The Sports Performance Coach is at the forefront in this era, where the athlete's mind is trained with as much attention and planning as the athlete's muscles, heart, and lungs. In this exciting progression in sports performance, the Sports Performance Coach plays a complementary role in advancing the athlete's mindset by approaching their role in the following ways:

> **THEORY OF → SELF-EFFICACY**
>
> An individual's belief regarding their own capability to produce performances that lead to anticipated outcomes.

- Collaborate with sports and performance psychologists and mental performance consultants.
- Understand the mental qualities that help athletes achieve performance excellence.
- Stress the importance of mental performance training and share basic mental skills training strategies with athletes.
- Create a positive and supportive training environment for athletes to maximize their abilities and enjoy the sporting experience.
- Establish effective communication methods with athletes.

SPORTS AND PERFORMANCE PSYCHOLOGY DEFINED

Sports and performance psychology can be defined in numerous ways. Some definitions focus on the act of sports psychology, whereas others stress what the sports psychologist implements. Without a clear definition for the field, identifying specific training models and the services and scope of the practice is a challenge.

Meijen (2019) defined sports psychology as understanding people's performance, mental processes, and well-being in sporting settings while considering psychological theory and methods. Meijen's definition should be part of the Sports Performance Coach's understanding of this field because it addresses the athlete's well-being.

> ✔ **CHECK IT OUT**
>
> Several definitions of sports psychology include exercise, which might blur the definitions and scope of the disciplines. The study of sports psychology and exercise psychology are often coupled.

Table 3.1 offers common definitions of sports psychology. Note that each source offers a slightly different interpretation. Independent of these differences, the Sports Performance Coach must understand the principles underlying an athlete's mental performance and ability to achieve performance excellence, as well as their enjoyment of the experience.

TABLE 3.1 Common Definitions of Sports Psychology

Source	Definition
Division 47 of the American Psychological Association (n.d.)	Sports psychology is the scientific study of the psychological factors that are associated with participation and performance in sports, exercise, and other types of physical activity.
European Federation of Sport Psychology (1996)	Sports psychology is concerned with the psychological foundations, processes, and consequences of the psychological regulation of sports-related activities of one or several persons acting as the subject(s) of the activity.
Meijen (2019)	Sports psychology is about understanding people's performance, mental processes, and well-being in sporting settings, considering psychological theory and methods.
Gill and Williams (2008)	Sports psychology is the scientific study and application of human behavior in a sports and exercise environment.

Debate also continues regarding what the field should be called. Hays (2006) described performance psychology as helping people learn how to perform better and more consistently in endeavors where excellence counts. This definition accurately characterizes the context of athletics and sports psychology. As a result, the field is embracing the label of *sports and performance psychology*, and several universities now offer academic programs under the same name.

As yet, this evolving field does not enjoy the same nomenclature standards, time-honored principles, and defined scope of practice that other sports science disciplines have. It is also facing challenges because of its rapid growth and acceptance as a valuable discipline. For the Sports Performance Coach, this evolution emphasizes the need to understand mental performance and educate athletes about mental skills training.

🤖 GETTING TECHNICAL

As the field of sports and performance psychology gains acceptance as a credible science, two central questions remain:

- Who might practice as a sports psychologist?
- What does sports psychology entail?

Both questions have no clear answers, and various governing bodies and career disciplines within the field continue to vigorously debate these issues.

Today, a licensed sports psychologist holds a PsyD or PhD in psychology and frequently performs a multidisciplinary role in managing and advancing athletic performance. These doctors diagnose mental health disorders such as depression and anxiety and provide psychotherapy interventions for treatment.

Sports psychologists often counsel athletes in a clinical setting, including helping athletes manage mood and anxiety. They also work on advancing mental skills strategies, such as restoring or building motivation, mental toughness, goal planning, concentration, and self-confidence.

While the laws regarding the scope of practice vary from state to state, qualified professionals can provide mental skills training to enhance athletic performance without holding a degree or licensure in psychology. Individuals holding a master's degree in sports psychology or an approved field, and who have 400 hours of experiential hours in counseling, can sit for the Certified Mental Performance Consultant (CMPC) exam offered by the Association for Applied Sports Psychology. Those holding the CMPC certification can provide mental skills training and are called mental performance consultants or cognitive performance specialists.

SPORTS AND PERFORMANCE PSYCHOLOGY THEORIES

There are a host of theories in sports and performance psychology, and as the field continues to grow and thrive, new theories continue to arise. Many theories for achieving sports performance excellence are adopted and refined from the field of psychology.

Theories in sports and performance psychology are centered on the mental qualities associated with performance excellence. Providing an in-depth discussion and comparison of these theories is beyond the scope of this chapter and the responsibility of the Sports Performance Coach. However, having foundational knowledge of the recognized theories can help the coach understand potential mental and physical barriers that may impact the athlete's performance and well-being.

ORIENTATIONS

Theories fall under various categorizations, including behavioral, personality, and performance excellence, such as building confidence, motivation, and resiliency.

ORIENTATIONS →

The theoretical framework and basis from which sports and performance psychologists obtain information on the mental qualities of an athlete.

No one theory fits best for any athlete. Instead, most athletes perform better through the integration of several theories.

Orientations form the theoretical framework from which sports and performance psychologists obtain information on the mental qualities of an athlete. It is helpful for the Sports Performance Coach to know these orientations but to develop their own framework to ascertain information from their athletes.

> ⚠ **CRITICAL**
>
> The sports psychologist and mental performance consultant gains insight into an athlete's behaviors through all orientations, and so might the Sports Performance Coach. But, above all, observing, listening, communicating, and monitoring information that athletes provide through actions, thoughts, and discussions is the foundation of any orientation.
>
> Adhering to this framework allows the Sports Performance Coach to better understand an athlete's mental qualities or needs. This helps the coach create a positive training environment and an atmosphere in which the athlete can achieve performance excellence.

PSYCHOPHYSIOLOGICAL ORIENTATION

PSYCHO-
PHYSIOLOGICAL →
ORIENTATION

The study of behavior during sport to gain insight into an athlete's physiology and brain.

The **psychophysiological orientation** studies behaviors performed during a sport to help a coach gain insight into an athlete's physiology and mental state (Gould & Weinberg, 2015). This orientation seeks to control physiology as a method for advancing performance excellence. These measurements are best accomplished by assessing heart rate, heart rate variability (HRV), brain waves, autonomic nervous system readiness, and muscle activation. Neurofeedback and biofeedback also provide insight into physiological markers.

Because of the equipment needed to obtain the physiological measurements, this approach might seem impractical for the Sports Performance Coach. However, portable and affordable devices can accurately measure physiological qualities, giving the Sports Performance Coach insight into an athlete's heart rate, HRV, and other physical factors. As a result, the Sports Performance Coach can observe an athlete's physiological response and recommend mental skills strategies, including relaxation strategies during periods of high anxiety and hyperarousal. For example, the Sports Performance Coach can advise rhythmic breathing to an archer who needs to reduce their anxiety, relax their body, and lower their heart rate.

It is important for the Sports Performance Coach to understand that regulating physiological qualities helps an athlete achieve their optimal performance.

SOCIAL PSYCHOLOGICAL ORIENTATION

SOCIAL →
PSYCHOLOGICAL
ORIENTATION

The belief that behavior in sport is determined by a complex interaction between environment and the athlete's personal biological make up.

Sports psychologists and mental performance consultants who emphasize the **social psychological orientation** view sport behavior as a complex interaction between the environment and the athlete's biology. For example, a swimmer may have an adverse reaction when performing in front of large crowds. If the Sports Performance Coach observes this relationship, they may invite a few participants to watch the athlete practice, gradually increasing the size of the audience. Over time, the athlete will adapt, learning to maintain focus on the task rather than the crowd. The heart of social psychological orientation is knowing the athlete and which situations hinder versus help their performance.

COGNITIVE BEHAVIORAL ORIENTATION

The **cognitive behavioral orientation** focuses on an athlete's thoughts and the interpretation of those thoughts and their abilities as determinants of behavior. This orientation also sees the environment as a factor, but it centers on cognition as the primary influencer (Gould & Weinberg, 2015). As such, sports psychologists and mental performance consultants aim to help athletes stop or reframe negative thoughts and reconstruct cognition into positive thoughts and self-talk.

For example, a hockey goalie who gave up a goal to bring the game to a tie must now reframe any thoughts about failing to block the next shot. The cognitive processing and self-talk that stop negative thoughts must be constructed well in advance of competition and practiced with frequency—attempting to do so only during competition won't yield the desired results. The Sports Performance Coach can also assist with this orientation by observing athletes' thoughts and behaviors during practice and creating a positive training environment that fosters mental qualities such as self-efficacy, motivation, and confidence.

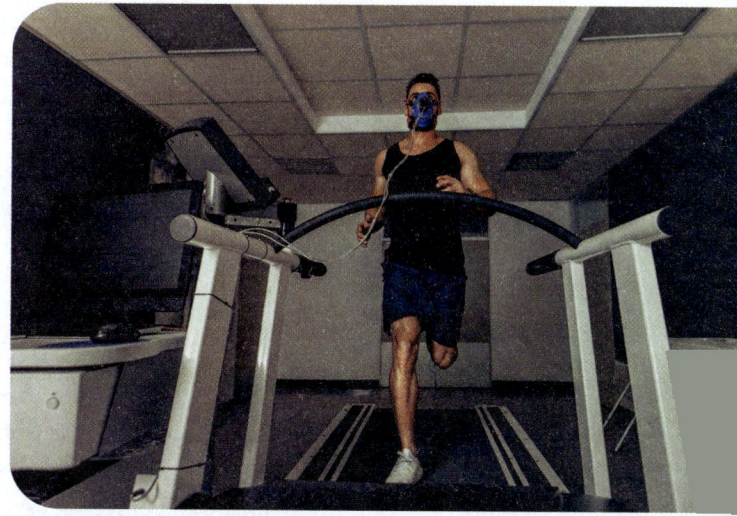
© Jacob Lund/Shutterstock

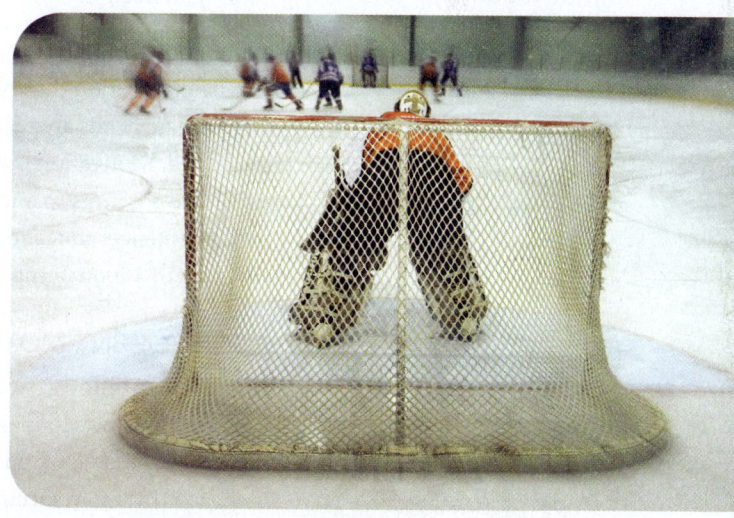
© DmitrijsDmitrijevs/Shutterstock

FOUNDATIONAL THEORIES IN SPORTS AND PERFORMANCE PSYCHOLOGY

Performance theories are often coupled with mental qualities that positively impact performance (Kingston & Wilson, 2008). Mental skills that are foundational for performance excellence include the following:

- Motivation
- Goal setting
- Confidence
- Arousal management
- Mental toughness
- Resiliency

Being aware of these theories adds value to the Sports Performance Coach's services to athletes.

THEORY OF SELF-EFFICACY

As noted earlier, the theory of self-efficacy focuses on an individual's belief in their ability to produce performances that lead to anticipated outcomes. In this theory, Bandura (1994) linked the qualities of confidence and expectations. In essence, when athletes demonstrate high levels of self-efficacy, they are more likely to believe that they have the capacity to achieve a task, whether the circumstances are optimal or challenging. Although self-efficacy and motivation are two separate concepts, they are closely connected. Bandura

> **COGNITIVE BEHAVIORAL ORIENTATION** →
>
> The psychophysiological orientation that focuses on an athlete's cognition and thoughts as determinants of their behavior.

proposed that self-efficacy is also the determinant of motivation. In other words, self-efficacy affects how much effort and focus someone puts into achieving goals and how resilient they are when faced with challenges.

A key focus of sports and performance psychology is the association between self-efficacy and performance. Research findings consistently support the notion that self-efficacy has a positive relationship on performance. Indeed, when physical abilities and skills are equal, athletes with higher self-efficacy outperform those with lower self-efficacy (Moritz et al., 2000).

SELF-DETERMINATION THEORY

Self-determination theory centers on creating and sustaining motivation (Deci & Ryan, 1985) and is one of the more widely accepted theories in sports and performance psychology. This theory suggests that people are motivated to grow and change by three innate and universal psychological needs:

- Competence
- Connection
- Autonomy

Self-determination theory proposes that people become self-determined when these three innate needs are fulfilled. In the sports arena, if these needs are met, an athlete stays motivated. Motivation serves as the core of performance excellence and is the driving force an athlete commits to and practices to master their sport. By understanding athletes' needs for competence, concentration, and autonomy, the Sports Performance Coach can create and sustain a motivating training environment for those athletes.

ACHIEVEMENT MOTIVATION THEORY

Achievement motivation theory was first introduced in 1953 and has since evolved to refer to a person's efforts to master a task, achieve excellence, overcome obstacles, perform better than others, and take pride in exercising talent (Kingston & Wilson, 2008). Heckhausen and Maher (2013) more succinctly defined achievement motivation theory as a person's capability to strive for excellence where the execution of that activity can either succeed or fail.

As in many other theories, motivation is a central tenet of achievement motivation theory. Motivation is consistently evolving and undulating with each athlete. The Sports Performance Coach must be aware of this variability and observe all motivational factors for athletes. Some athletes are motivated by process and competence; others are motivated by comparing their abilities to others and finding their purpose through winning.

MENTAL FITNESS MODEL

The **Mental FITness model** identifies Focus, Inspiration, and Trust as the critical components for conceptualizing and facilitating performance excellence (Aoyagi et al., 2017). This model emphasizes athletes focusing their minds, trusting their training, allowing their bodies to perform, and finding purpose in their performance. The athletes' purpose must be inspiring and fulfilling for their souls. The Mental FITness model also contends that focus and inspiration are foundational for achieving performance excellence.

The Mental FITness model suggests that determining an athlete's core values and connecting those values with purpose and meaning is essential to achieving performance excellence. It also suggests trusting the athlete's ability to let go of conscious control to allow for automatic responses when learning motor skills. The model emphasizes an external focus, so the Sports Performance Coach may use an autonomy-supportive

---

SELF-DETERMINATION THEORY →

The belief that one can create and sustain motivation.

ACHIEVEMENT MOTIVATION THEORY →

A person's efforts to master a task, achieve excellence, overcome obstacles, perform better than others, and take pride in exercising talent.

MENTAL FITNESS MODEL →

A model that identifies focus, inspiration, and trust as critical ingredients for conceptualizing and facilitating performance excellence.

coaching style to help athletes identify individual purpose and meaning. The Mental FITness model goes beyond the efforts of physical training, skill acquisition, and mental skills application by linking performance to purpose, meaning, and satisfaction.

P.A.C.E. SPORTS PSYCHOLOGY MODEL

The **P.A.C.E. sports psychology model**, developed by Cohen (2012), focuses on Perception, Activation, Concentration, and Execution. This model emphasizes these four qualities as vital for achieving performance excellence. Additionally, the model serves as a framework for measuring and augmenting these qualities (**Table 3.2**).

TABLE 3.2   P.A.C.E. Sports Psychology Model

Quality	Definition
Perception	The thoughts, feelings, imagery, and self-talk an athlete has about their technical and psychological skills, performance environment, and goals.
Activation	The optimal level of arousal that leads to success. Performance limitations happen at a less than or greater than optimal level. Determining the optimal level takes collaboration between the athlete and the coach. The Sports Performance Coach can refer to Hanin's (1997) individual zone of optimal functioning (IZOF) to identify an athlete's ideal level of arousal.
Concentration	The ability to exert deliberate mental effort toward what is most important in any given situation (Moran, 2012). The model suggests attending to the most relevant information, discarding potential distractions, and coordinating simultaneous actions. There is an emphasis on coaches creating an environment where athletes can learn to regulate concentration and decide what to focus on at the correct time.
Execution	The ability to perform motor skills automatically, leaving time, room, and energy for a greater focus on concentration.

> ⚠ **CRITICAL**
>
> It is not within the scope of practice of the Sports Performance Coach to focus exclusively on the four qualities of the P.A.C.E. sports psychology model. However, sharing the importance of the qualities with athletes can prove highly valuable.

SPORTS CONFIDENCE THEORY

Sports confidence theory is a sport-specific theory of confidence that focuses on the belief or degree of certainty an athlete has about their ability to be successful in sport (Vealey, 1986). This theory measures two factors:

1. **State sports confidence (SC state):** Situational confidence that wavers and might be skill-specific. SC state can be developed through learning and practice. For

P.A.C.E. SPORTS→ PSYCHOLOGY MODEL

A mental fitness model that emphasizes the qualities of perception, activation, concentration, and execution as vital to performance excellence.

SPORTS → CONFIDENCE THEORY

The belief or degree of certainty individuals possess about their ability to be successful in sport.

STATE SPORTS → CONFIDENCE (SC STATE)

Situational confidence that wavers and is usually skill-specific.

example, a basketball player might have great self-confidence in their accuracy of shooting from the three-point range but struggle at sinking free throws from the foul line.

2. **Trait sports confidence (SC trait)**: Global confidence that remains consistent across skills or sports. It is generally considered a natural part of an individual's demeanor. SC trait has benefits but also poses challenges to improving abilities if an athlete is too confident. For example, a basketball player might be confident in shooting from the three-point range, and that confidence transfers to all skills within the sport.

**TRAIT SPORTS →
CONFIDENCE
(SC TRAIT)**

Global confidence consistent with an athlete's personality.

To help athletes achieve confidence in sports, Vealey suggested the strategies outlined in **Table 3.3**. Vealey contended that it is vital for an individual to build mastery of an important skill because it builds confidence in their ability to achieve other skills and, in turn, builds confidence across their participation in sports. The theory rests largely on boosting the SC state. The Sports Performance Coach needs to be cognizant of Vealey's strategies and integrate them into their training philosophy and style.

TABLE 3.3 Strategies for Achieving Confidence in Sports

Strategy	Defining Characteristics
Mastery of skill	The athlete feels they have acquired skill mastery and perceives that they have made progress.
Styling	The athlete's confidence increases when they demonstrate high performance in several important skills.
Physical and mental preparation	The athlete's confidence increases when they feel adequately prepared for competition/performance.
Social reinforcement	The athlete has increased confidence when they receive praise and approval from significant others, particularly from teammates.
Effective leadership	Leadership promotes confidence in team members.
Environmental comfort	Athletes who lack self-confidence are best helped when they are coached under optimal conditions (e.g., coaching an athlete who lacks confidence without others observing).

GOAL-SETTING THEORY

**GOAL-SETTING →
THEORY**

The effects of setting goals on subsequent performance.

Goal-setting theory suggests that an athlete is motivated by working toward an objective goal, which in turn improves performance. Individuals who set specific and challenging goals perform better than those who set general, easy-to-reach goals (Locke & Latham, 2002). These goals are generally objective and focus on attaining proficiency on a task, usually within a specified time frame (Locke & Latham, 2002). Goal-setting theory encourages athletes to focus on skill mastery rather than a specific performance outcome, such as winning a competition.

Locke and Latham suggested five principles are important in goal setting:

1. Clarity
2. Challenge
3. Commitment
4. Feedback
5. Task complexity

Goal setting is universally accepted as an integral component for achieving success and reaching performance excellence.

LESSON 2: MOTIVATION
MOTIVATION AS THE DRIVING FORCE FOR SUCCESS

In sports and performance psychology, no word is utilized or emphasized more than *motivation*. **Motivation** is a fundamental quality needed to achieve performance excellence. Mastering any skill takes grueling hours of practice, working through discomfort, training with minor injuries, and sacrificing time with family and friends. Motivation also guides other peripheral preparations necessary for performance excellence, such as sound dietary practices, proper hydration, and adequate sleep and recovery.

Most theories centered on motivation attempt to explain, measure, and develop it. Deci and Ryan (1985) describe motivation as a drive that maintains, directs, and channels behavior over time. The most crucial element in this definition is *channeling behaviors over time* because motivation is a fleeting quality.

Discussing the factors that foster or hinder motivation is beyond the scope of this chapter and the requirements for the Sports Performance Coach. However, an understanding of self-determination theory and the principles of intrinsic and extrinsic motivation offers a sound foundation of knowledge for the Sports Performance Coach.

MOTIVATION →

The direction and intensity of one's effort.

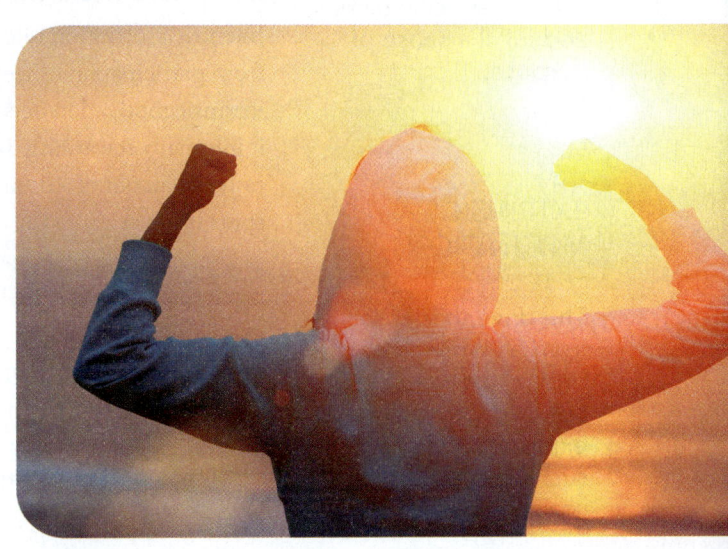

© Dirima/Shutterstock

SELF-DETERMINATION THEORY

Self-determination theory states that people are motivated to grow and change by three innate and universal psychological needs. Specifically, individuals become self-determined when their needs for competence, connection, and autonomy are fulfilled.

- *Competence* refers to the need to experience one's behaviors as enacted—the sense that the person is mastering their skill and has done a good job.
- *Connection* refers to the importance of interaction, the experience of caring for others, and having purposeful interactions and relationships.
- *Autonomy* refers to the experience of acting from choice rather than feeling pressured to act. Considered a fundamental psychological need, autonomy predicts well-being, and in the case of an athlete, a continued focus and sense of enjoyment while engaging in their sport.

The Sports Performance Coach must be aware of these needs and understand their significance to athletes. Knowing the needs highlighted in self-determination theory helps the Sports Performance Coach consider the relevant forces of motivation for athletes and helps them use the proper listening, observational, and communication skills to foster motivation.

> **📋 COACH'S CORNER**
>
> Sports Performance Coaches can advance their coaching abilities by understanding the central needs of competence, connection, and autonomy as fundamental qualities for long-term motivation.

INTRINSIC MOTIVATION →

The drive that arises from an individual's inner desires to achieve specific tasks and fulfill a sense of purpose.

EXTRINSIC MOTIVATION →

The drive that arises from an individual's desire to engage in behavior to obtain external rewards, such as titles, money, praise, or fame.

TYPES OF MOTIVATION

Psychologists who study motivation have detailed its contributing factors and the approaches and theories that explain it. In many fields, including sports psychology, motivation is categorized as either **intrinsic motivation** or **extrinsic motivation**.

INTRINSIC MOTIVATION

Intrinsic motivation refers to doing an activity for the pleasure and satisfaction derived from participation (Sheehan et al., 2018). The most self-determined form of motivation, intrinsic motivation occurs when an individual engages in a behavior because they find it internally rewarding. In essence, the individual performs the activity for its own sake rather than out of a desire to obtain external rewards. For athletes, participation in the sport is the reward (Lee et al., 2012).

For example, a woman starting her journey in Brazilian Jiu-Jitsu might have long-term aspirations of achieving her black belt. However, if she is internally motivated, the primary reasons she participates might be her love of the art, the process of learning and mastering new skills, and the joy of embracing new challenges.

The essence of intrinsic motivation is that the person must take pleasure in the processes involved in improving existing skills and applying new skills in their sport. If they don't find the sport pleasurable, they are less likely to engage in the hours, weeks, months, and years of practice necessary to master skills and achieve performance excellence.

EXTRINSIC MOTIVATION

Extrinsic motivation differs from intrinsic motivation in that an athlete participates in activities to attain an outcome tied to a reward rather than out of the joy of participation or a sense of purpose. Extrinsic rewards might come in the form of praise, fame, titles, or money. Although extrinsic motivation is often viewed negatively, it has many positive effects.

For example, a student might not enjoy a specific subject. However, they understand that studying hard and getting good grades makes them more likely to get into the college of their choice. In elite sports, extrinsic rewards can be a significant motivating factor. For example, a professional athlete may put extra effort in during the last year of their contract so that they can potentially sign a larger contract the following year. Further, it is rare for any athlete to reach elite status without at least some desire for extrinsic rewards. Similarly, youth athletes have high extrinsic motivation: Praise and rewards can, in turn, help foster greater enjoyment of sports participation at a young age.

However, athletes with only extrinsic motivation are less likely to persist in the face of challenges or defeat and may put in less effort if the expected outcome is not achieved (Sheehan et al., 2018). Therefore, the Sports Performance Coach should consider strategies to help foster internal motivation and increase athlete competence.

APPROACHES TO MOTIVATION

Motivation is a multidimensional and complex concept. Having some knowledge of where motivation originates may help the Sports Performance Coach understand why it may waver and be fleeting with some athletes. Sport psychologists suggest there are three general views of where motivation originates:

- Trait-centered view
- Situation-centered view
- Interactional view

The **trait-centered view** (also called the participant-centered view) asserts that motivation is a product of an individual's personal characteristics—the athlete's personality determines whether they are motivated. In essence, the trait-centered view assumes an individual is born motivated. An athlete's personality can also explain their lack of motivation. Although genetic contributions play a role in an athlete's motivation, the trait-centered view discounts the impact of coaching and positive reinforcement.

The **situation-centered view** contends that motivation is determined by the given situation. According to this view, motivation is influenced by external, situational factors rather than internal traits. For example, if an athlete receives negative reinforcement from a coach and feels inept in their abilities in contrast to their peers, they might lose motivation to participate and may even permanently shun the sport. In essence, the situational-centered view suggests that the environment dictates motivation.

The **interactional view** contends that motivation results from the interaction of participant factors (i.e., trait-centered) and situational factors (i.e., situation-centered) (Gould & Weinberg, 2015). **Figure 3.1** depicts how the trait-centered view and situation-centered view cooperate and blend into the interactional approach.

Interactional View of Motivation

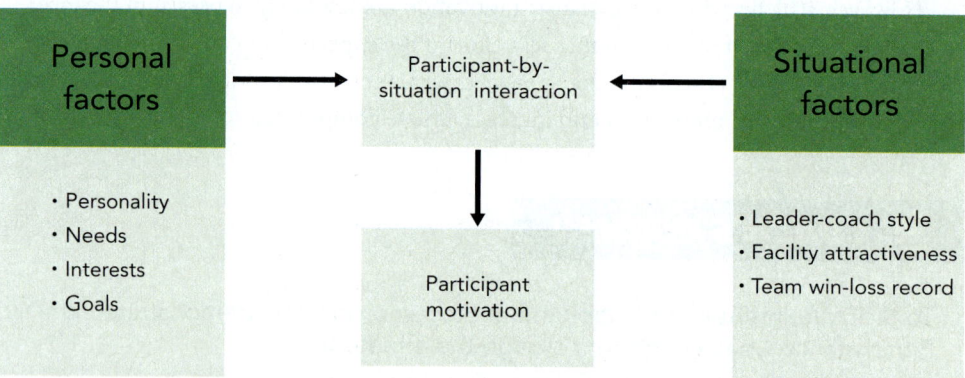

FIGURE 3.1 Interactional View of Motivation

Reproduced with permission from Gould, D. & Weinberg, R., 2015. Foundations of sport and exercise psychology (6th ed.). Human Kinetics.

📋 COACH'S CORNER

The interactional view of motivation may be considered the most rational view because it is multidimensional. However, coaches and trainers often neglect to consider that an athlete's motivation is impacted by a multitude of factors outside of the sport itself, such as family, friends, and culture. The Sports Performance Coach must understand all motivation orientations to gain insight into the multidimensional nature of motivation and increase their ability to cultivate athletes' mental skills.

LESSON 3: MENTAL SKILLS AND PERFORMANCE

MENTAL SKILLS TRAINING

Coaches and athletes often attempt to correct performance limitations through additional physical practice and may not pay as much attention to improving mental performance. Mastering mental performance is no different from mastering physical performance, in that both require consistent practice and focused attention. For example, a trainer might instruct a boxer to relax, breathe, and focus between rounds. However, if they have not practiced relaxation and breathing techniques or developed an effective imagery practice, then they will not be able to employ relaxation strategies and will not know what, precisely, to *focus* on. Therefore, athletes must develop these skills beforehand.

Mental skills training (MST) helps athletes process their thoughts and actions in the manner most apt to improve mental and physical performance. MST refers to the systematic and consistent practice of specific mental and psychological skills to enhance performance, increase enjoyment, and achieve greater self-satisfaction (Gould & Weinberg, 2015).

MST includes techniques and exercises designed to improve skills such as goal setting, visualization, positive self-talk, stress management, concentration, mindfulness, and establishing routines. It is often used in sports, performance arts, and other high-pressure settings, but can be beneficial in many other areas, such as education and business. This section defines the qualities and skills an athlete must practice to reach performance excellence. The Sports Performance Coach can support athletes and assist in developing a well-designed MST program only when they understand these qualities.

> **MENTAL SKILLS →
> TRAINING (MST)**
>
> A systematic approach to developing specific mental and psychological skills to enhance performance, increase enjoyment, and achieve greater self-satisfaction.

MENTAL SKILLS TRAINING QUALITIES AND SKILLS

Mental skills training is composed of distinct qualities and skills. The following framework for MST includes key qualities that are essential for developing effective mental MST programs and helping athletes and other performers improve their mental game.

SET SPECIFIC AND CHALLENGING GOALS

Goal setting is perhaps the most important aspect of an MST program. As is necessary to accomplish any task in a timely manner, goals should be prioritized when developing mental skills. Goal setting is simply the process of developing a plan to accomplish something. The plan focuses on the necessary actions to achieve an object or aim. Goals need to be specific, challenging but achievable, and measurable (objective) as opposed to general. Further, effective goals are written and recorded.

MST can help athletes set and achieve goals by teaching them how to break the overall goal into smaller, more manageable steps. In sports and performance psychology, goals are categorized into one of three types: outcome, performance, or process (Gould & Weinberg, 2015) (**Table 3.4**). Although some goals may receive more attention than others, athletes must focus on all three types of goals.

> **GOAL SETTING →**
>
> The process of developing a plan to accomplish something.

SMART Goals

Numerous theories are associated with developing goals in sports, but SMART goals remain a practical approach for the Sports Performance Coach and athletes. The acronym

TABLE 3.4 Sports and Performance Psychology Goal Categories

Category	Definition	Example
Outcome goals	Focus on a given result	An athlete finishes first in the 400-meter hurdles race or winning a tennis match. These goals are not achieved in isolation because one's competitor might be formidable and they might win the events.
Performance goals	Focus on achieving a specific criterion or performance measure independently of other competitors	The athlete focuses on running their best time in the mile or by beating their score from the last round of golf on a given course. The focus is not on beating another opponent, but rather on optimizing one's personal performance.
Process goals	Focus on a specific skillset that contributes to long-term success in a sport	A soccer player concentrates on keeping the opposite arm of the kicking leg farther from the body while striking. These goals build confidence as the athlete achieves small steps toward improving performance.

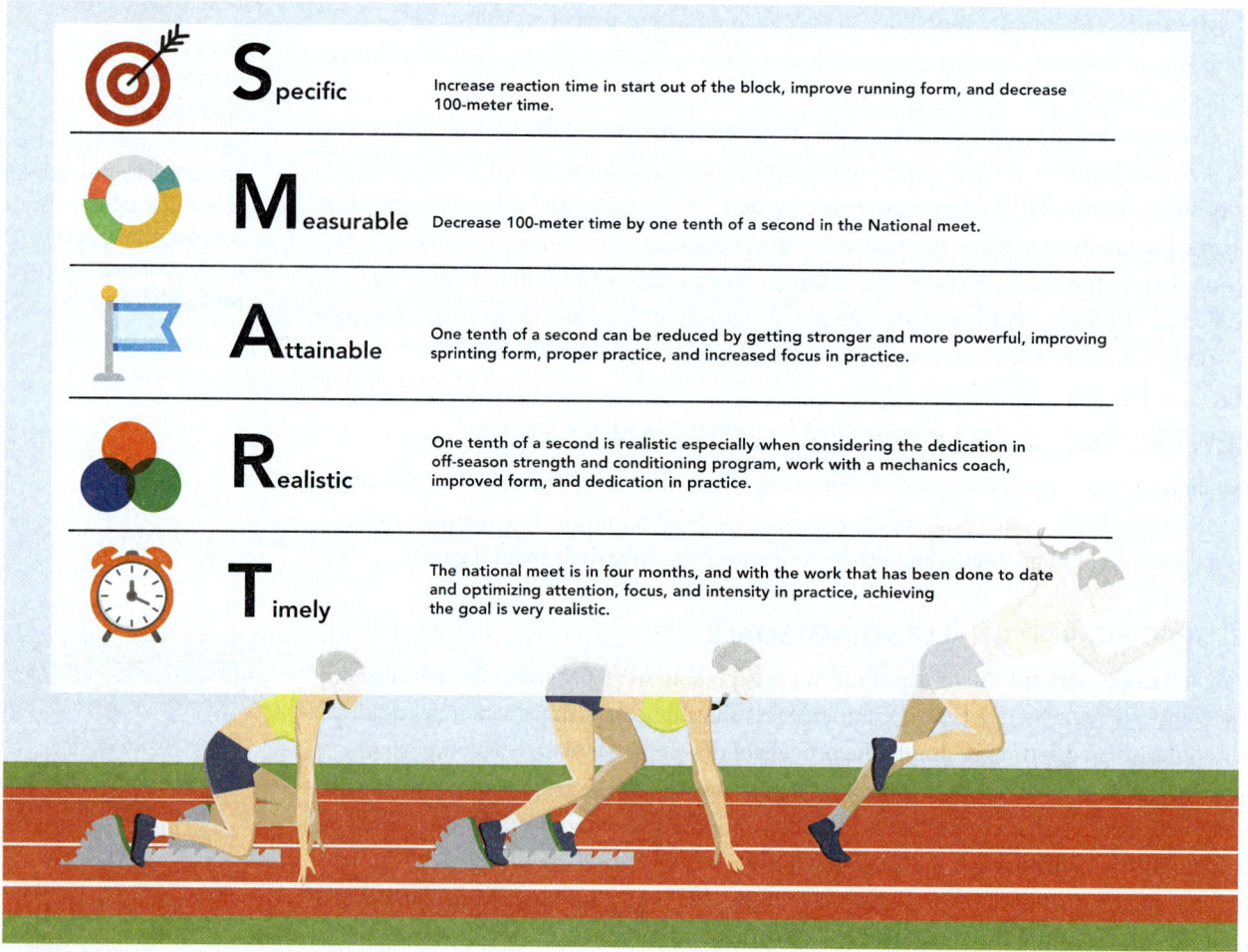

FIGURE 3.2 SMART Goals Example

SMART stands for Specific, Measurable, Attainable, Realistic, and Timely. **Figure 3.2** is an example of a long-term goal framework developed with a Sports Performance Coach and a track and field athlete.

A comprehensive goals strategy generally includes more details, but the example in Figure 3.2 shows how the framework is applied. Goal setting is a vital piece of MST because it plays an integral role in building confidence, arousal, and resiliency. The Sports Performance Coach must ensure that SMART goals are clearly written, and it's a good idea for the athlete to journal their progress and accomplishments toward both their short- and long-term goals.

STRIVE TO MAINTAIN SELF-CONFIDENCE

Self-confidence refers to an athlete's belief in their ability to successfully perform a task or achieve a goal. When athletes have high levels of self-confidence, they are more likely to perform at their best, take on challenges, and persist in the face of setbacks. Confidence and self-efficacy, as described by Bandura (1977) and Vealey (1986), is the ultimate goal that a sports psychologist or mental performance consultant hopes to achieve with their athletes. Confidence impacts concentration, attention, effort, emotions, and other skills. MST can help athletes build self-confidence by setting goals, practicing positive self-talk, and developing positive coping strategies.

Sport and performance psychology views self-confidence as a trainable skill. The Sports Performance Coach can build this skill through basic yet effective methods (Gould & Weinberg, 2015):

- *Focus on performance accomplishments.* Develop short-term goals that an athlete can achieve and build on. Journaling is an effective tool: Athletes should track their progress, essentially building a résumé of achievements they can see and reflect on.
- *Think confidently.* Emphasize instruction and motivational cues during practice and competition. Have athletes reflect on their previous accomplishments to foster confidence in their ability to master future skills and challenges.
- *Create a goal map.* A goal map is an individualized plan for an athlete that consists of process goals and defined strategies for attaining them. Goal maps also include methods, such as a rubric, for measuring performance in relation to goals.
- *Prepare physically.* Develop well-designed programs that help an athlete reach elite physical conditioning and diminish the effects of fatigue. Research reveals perceived associations between physical and mental fatigue and changes in behavior can decrease motivation and enthusiasm (Russell et al., 2019). Other changes associated with fatigue include altered concentration and reduced attention to detail. Adding performance limitations due to a controllable factor, such as physical conditioning, is easy to remedy.

PRACTICE IMAGERY AND VISUALIZATION

Imagery and visualization, also known as mental rehearsal, mental practice, or mental warm-up, is a form of simulation in which a person creates a multisensory experience (tactile, visual, auditory, or olfactory) through stored information and memory. Imagery techniques can be classified into two types: cognitive-specific and cognitive-general.

Cognitive-specific imagery involves recreating specific movements or actions involved in a skill or task. This type of imagery is task-specific and involves visualizing the movements, sensations, and outcomes associated with performing a particular skill. For example, a soccer player might use cognitive-specific imagery to visualize themselves dribbling past an opponent or taking a successful penalty kick.

Cognitive-general imagery involves imagining more general scenarios or situations related to a sport or activity. This type of imagery is not specific to a particular task or skill, but rather involves visualizing the overall experience of performing the sport. For example, a hockey player might imagine a positive experience in competition, such as scoring an overtime goal in a playoff game.

SELF-CONFIDENCE

The belief that one can successfully perform a task or achieve a goal.

IMAGERY →

A form of simulation in which a person creates a multisensory experience, such as tactile, visual, auditory, or olfactory, through stored memory and information.

COGNITIVE-SPECIFIC IMAGERY

A form of imagery that involves the specific movements or actions used in a particular skill or task.

COGNITIVE-GENERAL IMAGERY

A form of imagery that involves the overall experience of the performance.

Imagery is divided into internal and external forms. With **internal imagery**, an athlete executes a skill from their vantage point: They see, feel, and hear what they would while applying the skill live. This can help athletes improve kinesthetic awareness, or the sense of how their body moves and feels during a skill or task, and help fine-tune techniques through mental rehearsal.

External imagery focuses on viewing oneself from an outside perspective, such as from the vantage point of a competitor or fan. For example, a goalkeeper in soccer might view themselves blocking a penalty kick from the vantage point of the striker. This can help athletes improve situational awareness by visualizing themselves in specific game situations and anticipating potential challenges. Further, external imagery can improve spatial awareness by visualizing the locations of teammates, opponents, and other elements of the game environment.

Evidence continues to support imagery as a method for learning and advancing motor skills, as well as improving the mental qualities required for performance excellence (Gould & Weinberg, 2015). Imagery is a tough skill to measure in other people, but athletes can improve the vividness of their skills with time.

PETTLEP

An effective motor imagery practice should incorporate as many senses as an athlete can activate. One model that serves as a popular framework to help athletes develop and refine mental skills is PETTLEP (Holmes & Collins, 2001). PETTLEP stands for:

- Physical
- Environment
- Task
- Timing
- Learning
- Emotion
- Perspective

Figure 3.3 depicts the seven components of PETTLEP, including what each refers to when applying imagery. The components of PETTLEP help an athlete activate multiple senses and develop vivid images that are as close to the actual skill or competition as possible.

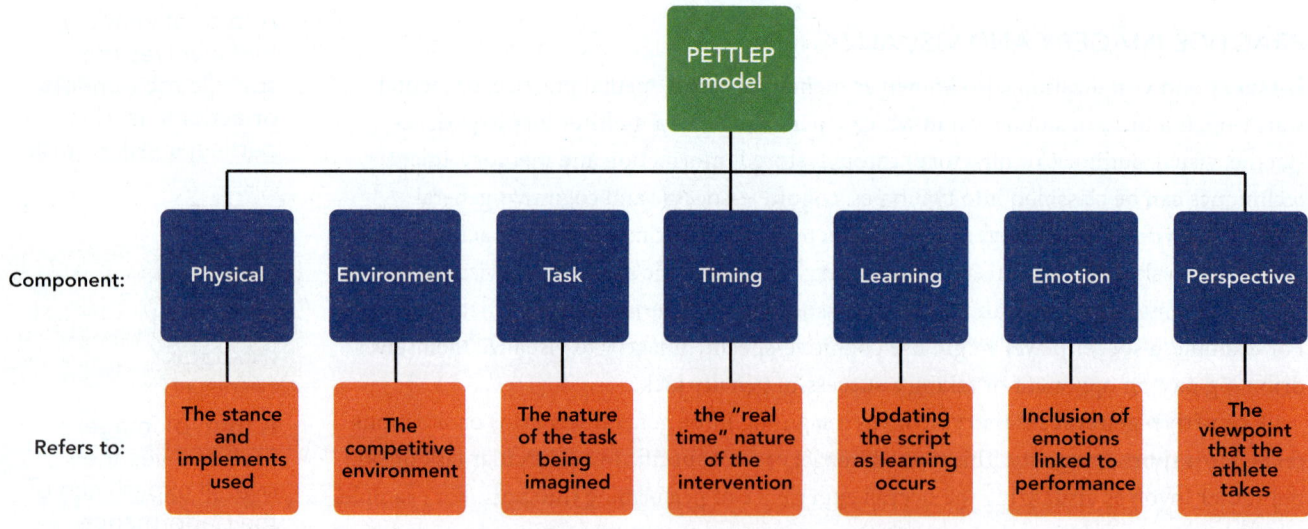

FIGURE 3.3 PETTLEP Model

Reproduced with permission from Wakefield C., & Smith, D. (2012). Perfecting practice: Applying the pettlep model of motor imagery. Journal of Sport Psychology, 3(1), 1-11.

The following example depicts a mixed martial arts athlete using PETTLEP for reducing pre-fight anxiety:

- Physical: The fighter imagines being relaxed pre-fight while having her hands wrapped. She activates the tactile vividness of sitting in the chair while having her hands wrapped by wrapping her fingers around her wrists. She then imagines standing and warming up, feeling her muscular system in the proper sequence from head to toe while striking practice pads and mitts in her warm-up.

- Environment: The fighter imagines stepping into the cage, seeing the fencing, and hearing the background and noise of the crowd. She uses positive self-talk statements while imagining that she is relaxed and prepared for the fight.

- Task: The fighter imagines her name announced. She looks across at her opponent, relaxed and confident, and focuses on her fight plan and skills.

- Timing: The fighter imagines the pre-fight events, keeping the duration of each imagined event as close as possible to the real-time duration. This imagery reduces uncertainty during competition and the fighter's anxiety associated with the unknown.

- Learning: The fighter and her coaches practice and discuss the optimal way to perform a pre-competition routine, using what she has learned during practices for future competitions.

- Emotion: As the fighter imagines the events in a relaxed state, she couples it with rhythmic breathing. This technique builds the connection from imagery to pre-competition preparation.

- Perspective: The fighter feels, hears, sees, and smells everything as she will the night of the fight, viewing herself internally and externally.

The ability to create such vivid imagery varies and improves over time with practice. However, with a basic understanding of the components needed for effective imagery, the Sports Performance Coach can guide an athlete to use this valuable mental skill.

👍 HELPFUL HINT

Athletes might use imagery as instruction or for motivation and confidence. In instructional imagery, a golfer might use all their senses to imagine the proper foot and hand positioning, correct grip, flawless backswing, and perfect follow-through while driving the golf ball off a tee. If an error is made during the imagery practice, the athlete should correct the error and repeat the sequence as needed. All too often, athletes will stop the imagery practice when errors occur. However, part of the skill is learning to handle and correct such errors.

In motivational or confidence-building imagery, a swimmer might see themselves on the podium after taking first place in the 50-meter freestyle event.

CONTINUOUSLY IMPROVE CONCENTRATION

Concentration refers to an athlete's ability to exert deliberate mental effort to focus on what is most important in any situation and to maintain that focus over time. In sports, concentration is essential for optimal performance, as it allows athletes to

CONCENTRA- →
TION

The ability to exert deliberate mental effort to focus on what is most important in any situation and maintain that focus over time.

INTERNAL FOCUS →

When an athlete focuses on specific body movements or sensations while performing a skill.

EXTERNAL FOCUS →

When an athlete directs attention toward external factors in the environment, focusing on the intention of the movement outcome.

BROAD FOCUS →

Taking in a large amount of information and processing it quickly, such as an entire field of play.

NARROW FOCUS →

Taking in specific bits of information, such as a specific area or individual.

process information quickly, make decisions, and execute their skills and strategies effectively. Gould and Weinberg (2015) contend that concentration consists of four constructs:

- Focusing on the relevant cues in the environment (selective attention)
- Maintaining that attentional focus over time
- Having awareness of the situation and performance errors
- Shifting attentional focus when necessary

Attentional Styles

Attentional (focus) styles refer to individual differences in how people attend to and process information. These styles can be broadly described as existing on a continuum ranging from **internal focus** to **external focus** and from **broad focus** to **narrow focus** (Nideffer & Sagal, 2006) (**Table 3.5**).

TABLE 3.5 Concentration and Attention Styles

	EXTERNAL	INTERNAL
Broad	*Assessing* Considering the general external environment.	*Analyzing* Reviewing general thoughts and emotions throughout a performance.
Narrow	*Acting* Focusing outward on the execution of a given skill.	*Preparing* Readying to execute a given skill (i.e., mental rehearsal).

Data from Nideffer, R. M., & Sagal, M. S. (2006). Attentional control and sport performance. In J. M. Williams (Ed.), Applied sport psychology: Personal growth to peak performance (5th ed., pp. 377-399). McGraw-Hill.

An external focus has shown to be superior in skills that rely on balance, accuracy, speed and endurance, and maximum force production (Wulf, 2013). An external focus also promotes increased performance outcomes, movement efficiency, and movement kinematics. Therefore, an external focus is generally recommended for the optimal execution of a task. One way a Sports Performance Coach could apply this concept is to instruct a track athlete to focus on a fixed point 5 yards beyond the finish line rather than on the optimal sprinting posture. Or, a quarterback could use an external focus by concentrating on where the ball is placed in the receiver's hands instead of his throwing mechanics.

In contrast, an internal focus is recommended during many aspects of MST, such as when practicing relaxation techniques and mindfulness practices (Coffey et al., 2010). Directing the focus inward helps the athlete process many mental and physical experiences.

A broad focus involves taking in a large amount of information and processing it quickly. When using a broad focus, a quarterback can survey the entire field, assess the positioning and movements of all the players on the field, and make quick decisions based on this information. This type of focus is useful when the quarterback needs to scan the field for open receivers or potential openings for a run play.

A narrow focus, in contrast, involves focusing on a specific area or player on the field. When using a narrow focus, the quarterback can concentrate on a specific receiver, for example, and analyze their movements and positioning to make a more accurate throw. This type of focus is useful when the quarterback needs to make a quick and accurate throw to a specific receiver, especially when under pressure.

Milley and Ouelette (2021) recommended the following strategies for advancing concentration and attentional focus:

- Focus on controllable factors versus uncontrollable factors.
- Simulate training; mimic competition situations.
- Perform distraction drills to teach athletes to shift attention between tasks.
- Create concentration cues that can be used to reset attention during a performance.

DEVELOP STRESS MANAGEMENT STRATEGIES

Sports and performance psychologists have theorized how hyperarousal and anxiety lead to declines in performance. Their consensus is that athletes must regulate both to achieve performance excellence.

Arousal is a blend of physiological and psychological activity in a person; it refers to the intensity dimensions of motivation at a particular moment (Wesson et al., 2000). The intensity of arousal ranges from no level of arousal (unconscious) to completely aroused, such as running full speed after a soccer ball. The inverted-U theory (**Figure 3.4**) proposes that sporting performance improves as arousal levels increase, but there is a threshold point of performance (Yerkes & Dodson, 1908). If arousal increases beyond that threshold, performance might diminish. Hyperarousal can negatively impact performance by causing athletes to become distracted, lose focus, or experience physical symptoms such as increased heart rate or tension. Although arousal does not always travel a path along an inverted-U shape, this theory suggest that under-arousal (hypoarousal) could limit performance as much as hyperarousal.

AROUSAL
The level of psychological and physiological activation that an athlete experiences.

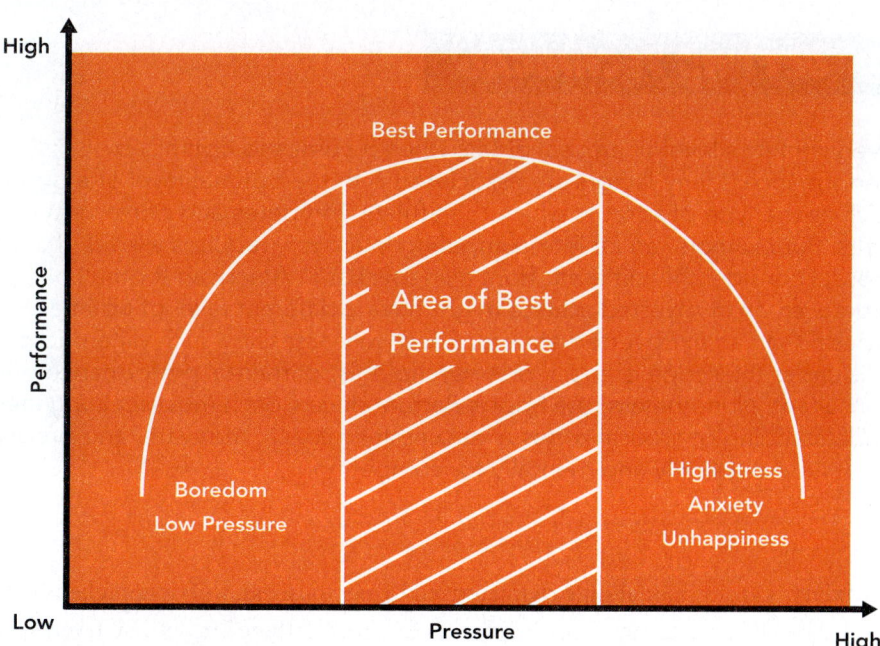

FIGURE 3.4 Inverted-U Theory

Reproduced with permission from Yerkes, R.M., & Dodson, J.D. (1908). The relation of strength of stimulus to rapidity of habit-formation. Journal of Comparative Neurology and Psychology, 18, 459–482.

The Sports Performance Coach must recognize that the optimal level of arousal is specific to each athlete. Hanin's (1997) model of the individual zone of optimal functioning (IZOF) (**Figure 3.5**) accounts for individual differences by demonstrating that each athlete has a unique level of arousal in their quest for performance excellence. The IZOF suggests that the best performance will occur when athletes are in their optimal zone, which is characterized by a balance between the level of arousal or anxiety and the skill level.

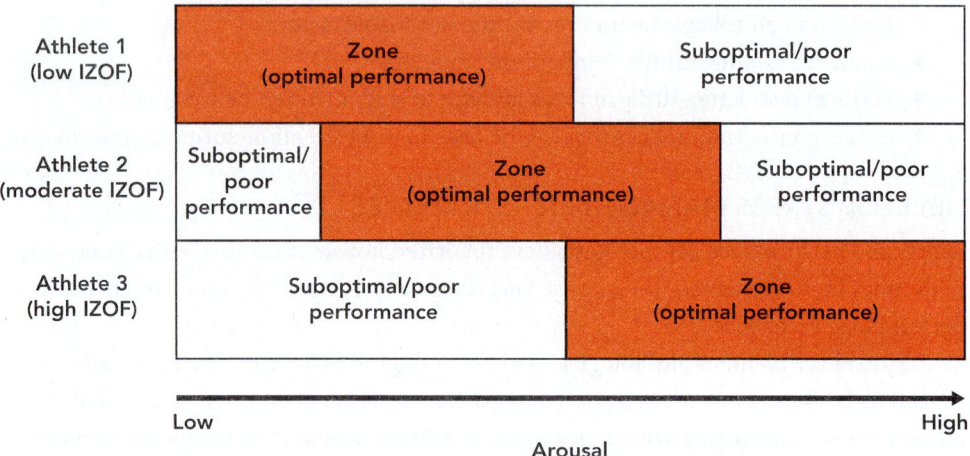

FIGURE 3.5 Hanin's Model of the Individual Zone of Optimal Functioning

Based on Hanin, Y. (1997). Emotions and athletic performance: Individual zones of optimal functioning model. European Yearbook of Sport Psychology, 37 (3), 223-232.

The inverted-U theory and IZOF models are only two theories among many that pertain to the optimal levels of arousal regarding performance excellence. To learn more, the Sports Performance Coach should continue researching other theories, such as drive theory, catastrophe theory, multidimensional theory, and reversal theory.

🤖 GETTING TECHNICAL

Every athlete's level of arousal differs when it comes to optimized performance. Many factors are associated with the optimal level of arousal, such as the type of sport in which the athlete competes and personality traits. For example, an athlete competing in archery requires a level of arousal considerably different from a linebacker in American football. Moreover, an introverted athlete might have a different level of optimal arousal than an extroverted athlete. Effectively assessing such differences falls under the scope of the sports psychologist or mental performance consultant. Nonetheless, the Sports Performance Coach must seek a general understanding of arousal zones to successfully coach, motivate, and prepare an athlete physically and mentally for competition.

ANXIETY →

An emotional state characterized by nervousness, worry, and apprehension, which is associated with activation or arousal of the body.

Anxiety is an emotional state characterized by nervousness, worry, apprehension, and arousal. Anxiety is not always negative, but, as for arousal, there are optimal levels specific to each athlete. Anxiety can positively affect performance by increasing physical arousal, resulting in increased energy, motivation, and focus and helping athletes stay more alert during competition. However, when anxiety increases beyond the optimal range, adverse effects on performance can occur. For example, high levels of anxiety can cause distraction, leading to errors and mistakes and adversely affecting an athlete's confidence.

The effects of anxiety on performance are complex and can vary depending on the individual athlete, the sport, and the level and direction of the anxiety experienced. Athletes can benefit from working with a sports psychologist or mental performance consultant to learn how to manage anxiety levels and find their optimal zone of functioning.

DEVELOP MENTAL TOUGHNESS AND ERROR MANAGEMENT SKILLS

Athletes who possess **mental toughness** are competitive, committed, and self-motivated, and can sustain concentration under high-pressure situations. Even after a setback, such as a bad pass in football or a faulted serve in tennis, they maintain a high degree of self-belief and self-efficacy (Sutton, 2021). These athletes are quick to discard setbacks and excel when conditions are less than optimal (Clough & Strycharczyk, 2015).

According to Crust and Clough (2005), mental toughness dictates how individuals deal effectively with challenges and pressure regardless of the circumstances. Additionally, athletes with mental toughness have a high internal locus of control: They believe they have control over the outcomes in their life or performance; external factors play no role.

Sports psychologists and mental performance consultants often emphasize the four C's—that is, the four components of mental toughness identified by Crust and Clough (2005):

- Control: Mentally tough athletes have the capacity to retain control even when confronted with barriers and difficult circumstances.
- Commitment: Athletes with mental toughness are not only inclined to create detailed goals, but also have the commitment to do what is necessary to achieve these goals. They deliver on their promises to themselves as well as to their teammates and coaches.
- Confidence: An athlete is unlikely to possess mental toughness without confidence. Self-confidence is the belief that one can successfully perform a desired behavior (Gould & Weinberg, 2015). With mental toughness, the athlete's confidence remains intact, even under the most challenging of situations.
- Challenge: This component comprises the extent to which an individual pushes back their boundaries, embraces change, and accepts risk. Mentally tough athletes see challenges as opportunities, not threats, and as a potential source of growth.

Error management in MST helps athletes develop a healthy and positive mindset toward errors. Athletes must be able to manage errors and setbacks effectively. Errors are a natural part of the learning process, and how athletes respond to them can significantly impact their performance and well-being. By developing a positive attitude toward errors, athletes can learn from their mistakes, adopt new strategies, and continue to improve over time.

The Sports Performance Coach can use the Sports Mental Toughness Questionnaire developed by Sheard et al. (2009) to gain insights into an athlete's mental toughness and resilience. The full questionnaire can be found in Appendix E. Higher scores indicate greater mental toughness. The scores can be used to identify areas of strength and potential areas for development in an athlete's mental toughness.

Error Management

Improving error management—the ability to overcome errors—is a learned ability closely tied to mental resiliency. The field of sports and performance psychology has developed

---

MENTAL TOUGHNESS →

The ability to cope with stress, pressure, and challenges while maintaining focus and motivation.

ERROR MANAGEMENT →

The ability to mitigate the effects of errors and to overcome them.

numerous strategies to improve error management skills with athletes. One common and effective method for amending errors is ARSE, developed by Solomon and Becker (2004). ARSE stands for Acceptance, Review, Strategize, and Execute:

- Acceptance: Acknowledge the error and accept the frustration it has caused.
- Review: Analyze the situation and determine how and why the error occurred.
- Strategize: Plan an adjustment to make the necessary corrections for the future.
- Execute: Sustain a positive mindset and prepare for the next play.

The principles of error management strategies center on teaching the athlete to acknowledge the reason for an error and then prepare mentally and physically for immediate correction. The Sports Performance Coach can share these important and effective strategies with athletes.

Mental toughness and error management are closely related when it comes to sports performance. Both are essential for athletes to achieve optimal performance, cope with stress, and overcome setbacks. The relationship between mental toughness and error management can be explained as follows:

- Mental toughness serves as a foundation for error management because it helps athletes maintain composure and deal with mistakes without being overwhelmed by negative emotions.
- Athletes who possess mental toughness understand that errors are an inevitable part of sports and can provide valuable learning opportunities.
- Mental toughness helps athletes regulate emotions and engage in positive self-talk.
- Mental toughness fosters adaptability and flexibility, allowing athletes to adjust their strategies and techniques in response to errors.
- In team sports, mental toughness contributes to psychological safety, which is a sense of trust and support among teammates encouraging athletes to take risks, communicate openly about errors, and collaborate to find solutions, leading to more effective error management.
- Mental toughness allows athletes to recover from setbacks and errors more quickly, helping them to maintain their motivation and commitment to improvement, and ultimately fostering long-term growth and better sports performance.

ESTABLISH ROUTINES

> ### ROUTINE →
>
> A sequence of relevant thoughts and actions that an athlete systematically engages in before the performance of practice or competition.

A pre-performance (readiness) **routine** is a sequence of tasks, thoughts, and actions an athlete engages in before performing a specific sport skill (Moran, 1996). Athletes need to develop pre-performance routines to get into a state of readiness in both practice and competition. Some routines may include reciting positive self-talk cues and using multisensory imagery or visualization. By establishing a consistent pattern of behavior and preparation, athletes can reduce stress and anxiety, enhance focus and concentration, and build the confidence needed to achieve performance excellence.

Readiness routines are a teachable mental skill, and coaches and athletes are well served to develop and implement them. The Sports Performance Coach plays an influential role in promoting the importance of routines with their athletes by developing and using them in training sessions.

Readiness routines should include behaviors and actions. Although these behaviors and actions are often specific to each athlete, some guidelines can help in developing routines to enhance readiness (**Table 3.6**).

TABLE 3.6 Developing Routines for Enhancing Readiness Guidelines

Guideline for Enhancing Readiness	Definition
Simplicity	Keep routines simple and include thoughts and actions that the athlete can remember effectively.
Controlled and rhythmic breathing	Rhythmic breathing prepares the athlete to execute their routine in a methodical manner and remain focused.
Positive self-talk	Develop short statements and affirmations to recite throughout the routine.
Imagery	Imagine specific skills that will be performed in competition while using positive self-talk statements.
Task-specific skills	Perform skills that will be applied during the competition.
Replicable	Routines must be easy to repeat, making them an automatic part of preparation.

The Sports Performance Coach can assist athletes to develop a readiness routine, ensure it is performed effectively, and help athletes reach performance excellence in practice and competition.

✔ **CHECK IT OUT**

A readiness routine should consist of mindful preparation with a specific purpose. It should include systematic engagement and task-relevant thoughts and actions to ensure it will translate from pre-competition into the competition.

The following strategies are recommended for developing an effective pre-practice routine:

- Understand the goal of the routine and how it relates to advancing abilities in practice and competition.
- Recognize the demands and tasks and apply purpose to the actions and thoughts toward the routine and competition.
- Develop individualized routines.
- Apply the routine in a comparable environment and of a similar duration prior to competition.
- Apply cognitive and neuromotor demands to the skills.
- Understand that routines evolve as athletes advance their level of skill.

PRACTICE POSITIVITY

Positivity is a key component of MST, as it helps athletes foster a constructive mindset and maintain emotional stability under pressure. Staying positive plays a crucial role in an athlete's success, affecting various aspects of performance, mental well-being, and long-term growth (Seligman & Csikszentmihalyi, 2000). A positive mindset can help athletes

SELF-TALK

The automatic statements and purposeful techniques athletes use to direct sport-related thinking.

POSITIVE BODY LANGUAGE →

The conscious use of nonverbal cues and gestures to communicate confidence, focus, and a winning attitude.

POSITIVE ATTITUDE →

A constructive mindset characterized by optimism, self-confidence, and resilience.

SPORTSMAN-SHIP →

A situation-specific set of behaviors involving concern and respect for rules, opponents, and officials, as well as a positive approach to sporting events.

maintain concentration, boost motivation and commitment, and recover better after errors. Ways to practice positivity can include positive self-talk, positive body language, and an overall positive attitude. As with all mental skills, positivity can be learned and refined. Therefore, athletes need to establish a positivity practice.

Self-talk refers to the automatic statements athletes use to direct their sport-related thinking. Positive self-talk is an essential skill for athletes because it helps them stay confident, focused, and motivated. MST can teach athletes how to identify and replace negative thoughts and self-talk with positive, supportive ones. However, it is important to recognize that negative self-talk will inevitably occur at times. Thus, an essential aspect of MST is learning how to quickly reframe these thoughts with positive talk.

Positive body language is the conscious use of nonverbal cues and gestures to communicate confidence, focus, and a winning attitude. In sports, body language can have a significant impact on an athlete's performance and can influence their opponents, teammates, coaches, and even the audience. Positive body language is universal. For example, in a study of blind and seeing athletes, they all displayed the same body language after winning a race (Tracy & Matsumoto, 2008). Victorious athletes raised their arms, tilted their heads, and puffed out their chests, while defeated athletes displayed slumped shoulders, head down, and narrowed chests.

A **positive attitude** can be defined as a constructive mindset characterized by optimism, self-confidence, and resilience. These characteristics allow an athlete to maintain focus, effectively manage challenges, and consistently pursue personal growth and improvement in their sport. This attitude includes embracing setbacks as learning opportunities, emphasizing strengths and achievements, and fostering a growth mindset to continually seek new challenges.

 ✔ CHECK IT OUT

Recent research in the field of psychology has significantly contributed to our understanding of how body language can impact mindset and behavior. Researchers suggest that adopting power poses can lead to increased confidence, decreased stress, and changes in neuroendocrine levels (Carney et al., 2010; Huang et al., 2011). However, according to Elkjaer et al. (2020), avoiding defeated postures, such as slumped shoulders and a narrowed chest, might be more important than the expression of victorious postures. Thus, Sports Performance Coaches must encourage athletes to avoid such postures as much as possible.

MAINTAIN SPORTSMANSHIP

The American Psychological Association (APA, n.d.) defines **sportsmanship** as situation-specific behaviors that involve concern and respect for rules, opponents, and officials, as well as a positive approach to participating in sporting events. Sportsmanship can be taught, and coaches can foster it by creating a culture and code of conduct for their athletes. While definitions of sportsmanship vary, most definitions address and include *concern* and *respect* along with the following behaviors:

- Winning and losing with character
- Shaking hands with opponents after a game

- Congratulating an excellent effort by opponents
- Demonstrating care for injured opponents
- Respecting the rules and officials
- Encouraging lesser-skilled teammates

Sportsmanship is not often considered a skill, but it is a set of behaviors that an athlete can identify, practice, and apply as much as any other mental skill.

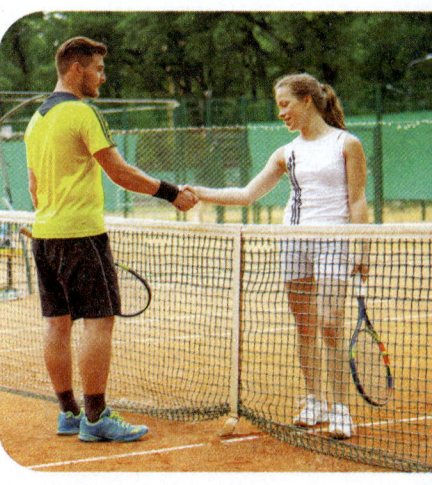

© Luckyraccoon/Shutterstock

✔ CHECK IT OUT

Team sports make up many of the world's most popular sports. Some qualities the Sports Performance Coach observes with team members exhibiting good sportsmanship include a willingness to do the following:

1. Play any role on a team.
2. Communicate.
3. Hold themselves and others accountable.
4. Develop meaningful relationships.
5. Invest themselves in the success of others.
6. Put team success before their own.

APPLYING MENTAL SKILLS TRAINING

Mental skills must be learned and practiced if they are to be effective. Just as motor skills require hours of weekly practice and months to reach elite levels of physical conditioning, the capacity for an athlete to use mental skills also requires concerted effort. Learning and applying MST effectively involves three phases: education, acquisition, and practice (Gould & Weinberg, 2015) (**Table 3.7**).

TABLE 3.7 Basic Phases of Mental Skills Training

Phase	Summary
Education	An athlete recognizes the importance of mental performance in sports and makes an effort to learn MST.
Acquisition	An athlete is introduced to MST strategies. For example, an athlete battling pre-performance anxiety might try progressive relaxation, rhythmic breathing, or positive self-talk.
Practice	After a specific MST approach has been chosen, the athlete integrates it as part of training. The athlete must practice for weeks for the approach to have a positive and lasting effect.

The most suitable role for the Sports Performance Coach in MST is to educate athletes on the importance of mental performance and make them aware of the strategies available to them. The coach can also play an assistant role in the acquisition and practice phases under the guidance of a sports psychologist or mental performance consultant. MST is the primary means through which athletes advance mental performance. In training sessions with athletes, the Sports Performance Coach can integrate readiness practices, emphasize positive self-talk strategies, and use external focus cues to help the athlete perform well and build their self-confidence.

LESSON 4: ADDITIONAL CONSIDERATIONS IN SPORTS PSYCHOLOGY

PERFORMANCE ANXIETY MANAGEMENT

Performance anxiety is a type of hyperarousal experienced before or during an event. It elicits performance-limiting effects when uncontrolled. Although uncontrolled anxiety in sports and physical activity is not the sole issue that gave rise to sports psychology, it is one of the more common and significant issues that athletes confront on a regular basis. Anxiety is a state most people have experienced inside or outside the realm of sport, and quite often, their association is a negative one.

It is important to manage anxiety in sports because the onset of anxiety before practice or during competition further increases the intensity and levels of anxiety. Anxiety can be a negative emotional state characterized by nervousness, worry, and apprehension associated with activation or arousal of the body. The two primary forms are **cognitive anxiety** (the psychological component) and **somatic** (the physiological component).

When cognitive anxiety is uncontrolled, an athlete has negative expectations about their success, negative self-talk, images of failure, worries about performance, an inability to concentrate, and disrupted attention (Bali, 2015). Likewise, when somatic anxiety is not controlled, the athlete experiences negative physical symptoms, such as nervousness, high blood pressure, dry throat, muscular tension, rapid heart rate and breathing, sweaty palms, and upset stomach. Both types of anxiety are interconnected, influencing each other and causing performance to suffer in many circumstances.

However, anxiety is not always negative, and modest levels may be beneficial as part of the pre-competitive sports experience. The Sports Performance Coach can use the Sports Anxiety Scale-2 (SAS-2) developed by Smith et al. (2006) to quickly gain insight into an athlete's anxiety level before or during a sporting event. This tool has been extensively used in research and clinical practice to monitor anxiety levels and guide MST programs. The full version of SAS-2 can be found in Appendix E.

A host of MST strategies can be applied for anxiety management. In particular, mindfulness and relaxation are two commonly used practices that a Sports Performance Coach can easily integrate into athlete programs.

MINDFULNESS FOR MANAGING PERFORMANCE ANXIETY

Mindfulness is the psychological process of bringing attention to the internal and external experiences occurring in the present and accepting the moment as it happens. The primary goal of mindfulness is to be present rather than rehashing the past or imagining the future. Accordingly, focusing on the present can decrease anxiety, helping to manage stress, improve focus, and enable performance at higher levels.

By remaining *in the moment*, an athlete diverts their focus away from anxiety triggered by past failures or fear of future disappointments. Like all skills, mindfulness requires daily practice to become efficient in applying it. An athlete can achieve mindfulness through the aggregate of other mental skills, such as rhythmic breathing, motor imagery, positive self-talk, and readiness routines.

Mindfulness in sports is represented by being fully engaged in what is presently occurring. For example, an athlete who made an error on a previous play is best served by being resilient and not dwelling on the error, and by not concerning themselves with the possibility of future failures.

STRATEGIES FOR FOSTERING MINDFULNESS

Acceptance and commitment therapy (ACT) is a type of cognitive-behavioral therapy (CBT) that does not aim to eliminate negative thoughts and emotions, but rather seeks to develop a more accepting, compassionate, and goal-directed attitude toward oneself (Hayes et al., 2012). ACT has gained a popular following in sports. It encourages athletes not to suppress and remove feelings, but to be present with them, let them flow, and then move toward valued behavior. ACT recognizes that negative thoughts and emotions will arise but teaches that the athlete has the power to redirect and reframe them into constructive actions and behaviors.

ACT can help athletes who are struggling with performance anxiety to develop a more accepting and nonjudgmental attitude toward their thoughts and emotions. By cultivating mindfulness and self-compassion, athletes can learn to manage their anxiety more effectively and focus on performance goals rather than fears. Similarly, ACT can play a beneficial role in performance by helping athletes to identify their core values and goals, take action to achieve them, and maintain a positive mindset despite failure and setbacks.

The clinical application of ACT is not within a Sports Performance Coach's scope of practice. However, the coach can share the principles of ACT with athletes as they strive to understand and implement mindfulness. ACT skills (**Figure 3.6**) have been adapted from Hayes et al. (2012) to apply to the Sports Performance Coach.

ACCEPTANCE AND COMMITMENT THERAPY (ACT) →

A psychological practice that helps individuals develop greater psychological flexibility and well-being by focusing on accepting and having a compassionate attitude toward negative thoughts and emotions and taking committed action toward achieving goals.

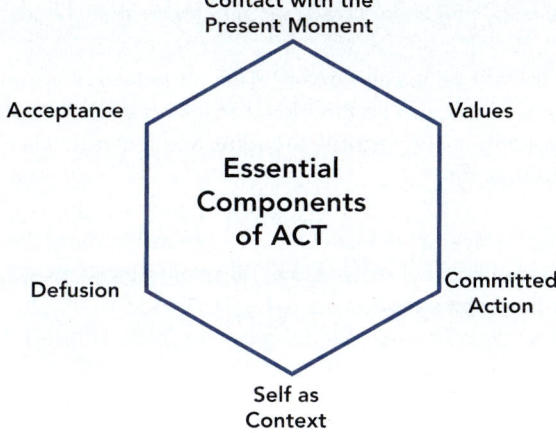

FIGURE 3.6 Essentials of ACT

MINDFULNESS–ACCEPTANCE–COMMITMENT (MAC) →

A psychological practice that combines mindfulness-based techniques with acceptance and commitment therapy to help develop greater psychological flexibility and well-being.

The psychological practice known as **mindfulness–acceptance–commitment (MAC)** combines mindfulness techniques with ACT. MAC has gained recognition and acceptance among sports psychologists in large part due to its emphasis on practicing mindfulness (Gardner & Moore, 2004). Further, MAC can be applied to a range of sports and levels of athletic ability, can be used to enhance individual and team performance, and can cover a wide range of anxiety-inducing thoughts and behaviors.

Both ACT and MAC can be effective for athletes, as both aim to help individuals develop greater psychological flexibility, resilience, and well-being. ACT primarily focuses on developing acceptance, mindfulness, and values-based action, while MAC combines these elements with additional mindfulness-based techniques. MAC may be a better choice if an athlete is specifically interested in developing mindfulness skills. **Table 3.8** describes the basic skills of ACT and suggests how Sports Performance Coaches and athletes can integrate them into their daily routines.

TABLE 3.8 Acceptance and Commitment Therapy Skills

Skill	Description
Diffusion	Stepping back and creating distance from anxious thoughts and feelings rather than trying to suppress or control them. An athlete who envisions making a mistake in an important game must recognize that the vision/thought is separate from themselves, create distance from it, imagine the feelings passing by, and then refocus attention to the present moment.
Acceptance	Allowing negative feelings to exist without attempting to suppress or stop them. Instead of struggling against, attempting to hide, or focusing on negative thoughts, an athlete might let them come and go, while acknowledging that they are a normal response to high-pressure situations. Then, the athlete can refocus attention to the present moment.
Contact with the present moment	Focusing attention on the present moment rather than getting caught up in anxious thoughts and worries about the future. An athlete can redirect focus from a negative thought to body sensations, such as breathing or muscle tension, to become more aware of their response to the anxiety. Then, the athlete can refocus on the task at hand and take action to achieve their goals.
Values	Clarifying personal values helps an individual gain a sense of purpose and meaning and stay motivated. Once values have been identified, the athlete can connect them to performance goals and use them as a source of motivation. When anxiety increases, the athlete can reframe negative thoughts or behaviors in a way that aligns with their values.
Committed action	Consistently taking action toward values and goals, even in the face of anxiety-producing thoughts and feelings. This skill is based on the idea that taking action toward something meaningful, rather than avoiding uncomfortable thoughts and feelings, will result in feelings of success and increased motivation.
Self as context	Thoughts and feelings are not necessarily facts or truths, but rather mental events that arise and pass away in the context of broader experience. By shifting focus away from identifying with or getting caught up in negative thoughts and feelings and toward attaining a broader sense of self, athletes can develop greater psychological flexibility and resilience.

RELAXATION STRATEGIES

The terms *relaxation* and *mindfulness* are often used interchangeably. However, although they are interconnected, they are actually separate practices. Many types of relaxation practices are available, such as meditation, massage, and yoga. While these should be a part of every athlete's weekly routine, athletes also need strategies that are easy to access and implement as a pre-practice or pre-competition routine. Two such relaxation strategies are **progressive relaxation** and **rhythmic breathing**. Both of these strategies, when practiced consistently, create an autonomic response that eases mental and muscular tension.

The premise behind progressive relaxation is that tension and relaxation are mutually exclusive; muscles cannot be relaxed and tense simultaneously. By regularly practicing progressive relaxation, athletes can learn to recognize the physical signs of anxiety and can use this technique to manage their symptoms, thereby helping them maintain a positive and motivated mindset. Athletes may begin by focusing on just two to four muscle groups, then slowly progress to focusing on the full body. An entire progressive relaxation session may take as little as 20 minutes.

📋 COACH'S CORNER

General steps for applying progressive relaxation:

1. Find a quiet and comfortable place.
2. Establish a relaxed breathing pattern.
3. Focus on sensations of tension followed by warmth and relaxation.
4. Begin at the toes and progress toward the head.
5. Practice regularly to build a habit and make it easier to access the technique on demand.

Rhythmic breathing is an immediate and effective method for mitigating tension and lowering anxiety. An individual's breathing rate influences their parasympathetic system, working to counter the activation of the sympathetic system or the fight-or-flight response. Rhythmic breathing promotes a sense of stability, centeredness, and relaxation (Gould & Weinberg, 2015). Many guidelines suggest that a breathing ratio of approximately 1:2, with the exhale lasting twice as long as the inhale, can trigger the body's relaxation response. Research has also substantiated the importance of breathing deeply, usually by inhaling through the nose, allowing for the expansion of the abdominal area rather than the chest, called **diaphragmatic breathing (DBR)**. This breathing method is particularly effective for reducing anxiety and stress and improving overall mental health (Fincham et al., 2023).

✔ CHECK IT OUT

Researchers examining the effects of DBR in healthy adults have found that it reduces cortisol levels and improves attention and mood (Ma et al., 2017). This type of breathing focuses on breathing deeply from the diaphragm, allowing for increased oxygen intake, and a full exhalation. With a full exhale, the individual draws their abdominal region inward to *force* as much air out of the lungs as possible. A long exhale allows for more oxygen to be taken in on the next cycle and activates the vagus nerve, which in turn activates the parasympathetic nervous system, promoting relaxation and well-being (Brown & Gerberg, 2005).

PROGRESSIVE RELAXATION

The process of diffusing muscle tension by contracting and subsequently relaxing a group of muscles, bringing awareness to the physical sensations of tension and relaxation.

RHYTHMIC BREATHING

Intentionally controlling and regulating breathing patterns to reduce stress and anxiety.

DIAPHRAGM-ATIC BREATHING (DBR) →

Breathing deeply by allowing the expansion of the abdominal area.

Rhythmic breathing is a simple and effective strategy for reducing anxiety. The most positive aspect of rhythmic breathing is that an athlete can perform it anywhere, so the Sports Performance Coach can apply this strategy with their athletes no matter the location. Moreover, because rhythmic breathing creates a relaxed state, every other mental skill is improved when coupled with rhythmic breathing.

📋 COACH'S CORNER

Steps for effective rhythmic breathing:

1. Lie in a supine position.
2. Place one hand on your abdomen, below the ribs.
3. Breathe in through your nose for 3 to 4 seconds. Focus on raising your hand with your abdomen. Aim for minimal movement in your chest.
4. Hold your breath briefly after inhalation to allow more time for oxygen to diffuse into the bloodstream.
5. Breathe out through the mouth with pursed lips for about 6 seconds. The hand on your abdomen should lower with the exhale.
6. In the initial phases of training, practice rhythmic breathing for up to 10 minutes. This duration trains the body to foster parasympathetic influence.
7. Focus on the relaxation that this breathing exercise produces. Check that your muscles and mind are relaxed.

Mindfulness and relaxation strategies optimize mood, increase awareness and focus, and reduce anxiety. Both strategies are simple in principle, but to be useful tools in reducing anxiety and fostering performance excellence, they must be applied in tandem with attention to detail and frequent practice.

INTRODUCTION TO MENTAL READINESS AFTER INJURY

An athlete's readiness to return to play, based on both their physical and mental health, falls under the discretion of medical professionals, such as a physician, physical therapist, and licensed sports psychologist. If the Sports Performance Coach is working with an athlete during injury rehabilitation or in preparation for return to play, they must collaborate with the appropriate medical professionals and work under their guidance.

The Sports Performance Coach can play an integral role by providing positive support and fostering the athlete's confidence through the rehabilitative process. Common mental challenges with athletes returning to play include:

- Anxiety over suffering a reinjury
- Increased performance anxiety
- Concern over meeting the expectations of others
- Diminished physical and mental self-efficacy
- Concerns about returning to their pre-injury performance abilities (Gould & Weinberg, 2015)

MST is effective with athletes returning to sports because it reduces negative psychological outcomes and anxiety associated with reinjury and improves coping skills (Madrigal, 2015). The Sports Performance Coach can support MST for athletes preparing to return to play. Some of the skills that are appropriate in this context include imagery, building motivation, goal setting, self-talk, and relaxation.

Imagery involves the rehearsal of motor activities without making actual movements. Athletes can use the skill without distributing mechanical and physical loads on the injured area. Physical therapists often provide the mental cues for what a patient should imagine while rehabbing.

The PETTLEP (physical, environment, task, timing, learning, emotion, and perspective) model is also used in rehabilitation settings. For example, athletes can use visualization techniques that include specific environments

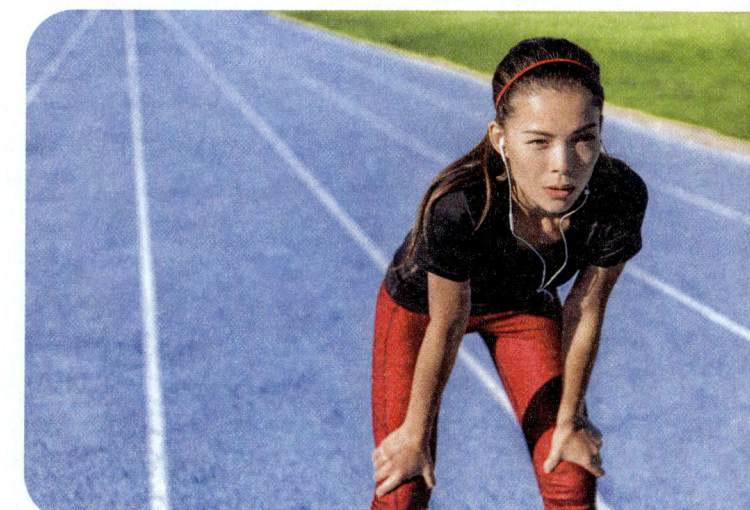
© Mariday/Shutterstock

to imagine themselves performing the physical movements required for the sport, even if they are unable to perform them physically due to their injury. By mentally rehearsing these movements, athletes can maintain their motor patterns and improve confidence and preparedness for returning to play.

Motivation plays an integral role in preparing athletes for sports after injury. Athletes who exhibit higher levels of intrinsic motivation tend to have better rehabilitation outcomes, including greater adherence to rehabilitation programs, and a greater likelihood of returning to sports after injury (Goddard et al., 2021). Although intrinsic motivation is often considered more beneficial for rehabilitation, some evidence suggests that extrinsic motivation can also play a positive role in promoting adherence to rehabilitation programs and facilitating a successful return to play. For example, individuals motivated by external factors, such as competition, tend to have higher exercise adherence and better functional outcomes than those driven solely by certain intrinsic factors (Ednie & Stibor, 2016).

However, extrinsic motivation may not be a good thing for all athletes. Some athletes with high levels of extrinsic motivation display diminished confidence, unsatisfying performance, and heightened competitive anxiety (Podlog & Eklund, 2005). The Sports Performance Coach should be able to recognize the underlying motivation drive and assist in maintaining and building an athlete's level of motivation, both intrinsic and extrinsic when necessary, albeit under the guidance of the medical professionals supervising the athlete's rehabilitative process.

Goal setting is a powerful tool for athletes returning to play after an injury. Goal setting can provide focus and direction by helping athletes set specific goals, and it increases motivation by helping athletes have a sense of purpose for their rehabilitation. Process goals, outcome goals, and rehabilitation timelines must be set and guided by a physical therapist. However, after an athlete is cleared for training, the Sports Performance Coach can collaborate with the integrated performance team to plan and map goals together.

Positive self-talk can be an effective tool in helping athletes return to play after injury by reducing anxiety, enhancing confidence, and increasing motivation (Van Raalte et al., 2020). It is particularly effective when combined with other rehabilitation techniques, such as goal setting and visualization. Clear goals and a sense of purpose are imperative when using self-talk in rehabilitation scenarios. The athlete can apply several types of self-talk through mental skills training:

- Focused self-talk: An athlete concentrates on what must be done during rehab and the assigned protocols from medical professionals.
- Instructional self-talk: An athlete ensures that exercises and rehabilitative practices are performed in a technically correct manner.
- Motivational self-talk: An athlete reminds themselves of past successes in rehab or instances in which they performed successfully during difficult training sessions, practices, or competitions.

Relaxation techniques such as breathing, progressive muscle relaxation, and meditation are useful strategies to help with emotional regulation, healing, and a timely return to play (Hooi & Wah, 2018). Aquatherapy has also gained attention as an effective tool for reducing pain, improving range of motion, and facilitating early functional progress in patients recovering from anterior cruciate ligament (ACL) reconstruction (Buckthorpe et al., 2019). Additionally, aquatic therapy can be used in combination with traditional rehabilitation methods to improve outcomes for patients undergoing ACL reconstruction. Aquatherapy may also be referred to as aqua relaxation because the warmth of the water can increase circulation and promote relaxation.

 COACH'S CORNER

A systematic review by Gledhill et al. (2017) concluded that psychological skills training, including cognitive relaxation, imagery, and goal setting, can effectively reduce injury risk, promote recovery, and enhance psychological well-being in athletes. Tailored programs delivered by qualified professionals are recommended for optimal effectiveness. Sports Performance Coaches should align their practice with the recommendations of athletes' mental health practitioners to provide comprehensive support, integrating both physical training and mental readiness.

A host of factors come into play when the medical team considers an athlete's return to play after an injury. Most of these decisions are not within the scope of the Sports Performance Coach and are made by medical personnel. Under the guidance of the medical team, however, the Sports Performance Coach can keep the athlete mentally prepared to return to high levels of competition.

SUMMARY

The sports and performance psychology field continues to enjoy rapid growth and acceptance in both the scientific and sporting communities. The licensed sports psychologist has the broadest scope of practice rights in the field, including working with athletes in clinical and applied settings. The mental performance consultant applies mental skills strategies with clients outside of a clinical setting. The Sports Performance Coach plays a collaborative role with these professionals and helps athletes set goals, build mental resiliency, reduce performance anxiety, develop pre-competition routines, and increase confidence and self-efficacy. Beyond helping athletes build strength, power, and speed, the Sports Performance Coach enhances mental performance, helps athletes find more enjoyment in sports, and guides them toward performance excellence by possessing knowledge of mental skills training.

KEY TAKEAWAYS

- Sports psychology is the understanding of performance, mental processes, and well-being in a sports setting while simultaneously considering psychological theories and methods.
- Athletes' cognition of themselves significantly influences their physiology. Anxiety can lead to muscle tension, decreased concentration, and a delay in reaction time. If not managed, these effects can limit the athlete's performance.
- Foundational theories in sports and performance psychology center on qualities associated with performance excellence. Such theories include self-determination theory, achievement motivation theory, the Mental FITness model, the P.A.C.E sports psychology model, and the sports confidence theory.
- Motivation is the drive that maintains, directs, and channels behavior over time. Motivation is multidimensional, and research indicates that intrinsic motivation and the desire for competence, connection, and autonomy are central to creating and maintaining it.
- Mental skills training (MST) is the systematic and consistent practice of mental or psychological skills to enhance performance, increase enjoyment, or achieve greater sport self-satisfaction. The Sports Performance Coach uses mental skills training to help athletes process their thoughts and actions in a manner apt to improve their mental and physical performance.
- The mental qualities and skills consistent with performance excellence include self-efficacy, confidence, motivation, arousal and anxiety, imagery, concentration, mental toughness and resiliency, positive self-talk, goal setting, and mindfulness.
- To establish automatic and immediate effects of mental skills, mental skills training requires daily practice over several weeks and months.
- Mindfulness and rhythmic breathing can help an athlete control their anxiety while also regulating the optimal level of arousal.

REFERENCES

American Psychological Association. (n.d.). *APA dictionary of psychology.* https://dictionary.apa.org/

American Psychological Association, Division 47. (n.d.). *What is sport, exercise, & performance psychology?* https://www.apadivisions.org/division-47/about/resources/what-is

Aoyagi, M., Cohen, A., Poczwardowski, A., Metzler, J., & Statler, T. (2017). Models of performance excellence: Four approaches to sport psychology consulting. *Journal of Sport Psychology in Action, 9*(2), 94–10. https://doi.org/10.1080/21520704.2017.1355861

Bali, A. (2015). Psychological factors affecting sports performance. *International Journal of Physical Education, Sports and Health, 1*(6), 92–95.

Bandura, A. (1977). Self-efficacy: Toward a unifying theory of behavioral change. *Psychological Review, 84,* 191–215.

Bandura, A. (1994). Self-efficacy. In V. S. Ramachaudran (Ed.), *Encyclopedia of human behavior* (Vol. 4, pp. 71–81). Academic Press.

Biasutti, M. (2017). Flow and optimal experience. In *Reference module in neuroscience and biobehavioral psychology* (p. B9780128093245061000). Elsevier. https://doi.org/10.1016/B978-0-12-809324-5.06191-5

Brown, R. P., & Gerbarg, P. L. (2005). Sudarshan kriya yogic breathing in the treatment of stress, anxiety, and depression: Part II—clinical applications and guidelines. *Journal of Alternative and Complementary Medicine, 11*(4), 711–717. https://doi.org/10.1089/acm.2005.11.711

Buckthorpe, M., Pirotti, E., & Villa, F. D. (2019). Benefits and use of aquatic therapy during rehabilitation after ACL reconstruction: A clinical commentary. *International Journal of Sports Physical Therapy, 14*(6), 978–993.

Carney, D. R., Cuddy, A. J., & Yap, A. J. (2010). Power posing: Brief nonverbal displays affect neuroendocrine levels and risk tolerance. *Psychological Science, 21*(10), 1363–1368. https://doi.org/10.1177/0956797610383437

Clough, P., & Strycharczyk, D. (2015). *Developing mental toughness: Coaching strategies to improve performance, resilience and wellbeing* (2nd ed.). Kogan Page.

Coffey, K. A., Hartman, M., & Fredrickson, B. L. (2010). Deconstructing mindfulness and constructing mental health: Understanding mindfulness and its mechanisms of action. *Mindfulness, 1*(4), 235–253. https://doi.org/10.1007/s12671-010-0033-2

Cohen, A. (2012). The P.A.C.E. performance program: Integrating sport psychology into training programs. *Olympic Coach Magazine, 23*(3), 5–9.

Crust, L., & Clough, P. J. (2005). Relationship between mental toughness and physical endurance. *Perceptual and Motor Skills, 100*(1), 192–194.

Csikszentmihalyi, M. (1990). *Flow: The psychology of optimal experience*. Harper & Row.

Deci, E. L., & Ryan, R. M. (1985). The General Causality Orientations Scale: Self-determination in personality. *Journal of Research in Personality, 19*, 109–134.

Ednie, A. J., & Stibor, M. D. (2016). Extrinsic motivations: Relevance and significance for exercise adherence. *Journal of Physical Activity Research, 1*(1), 26–30. https://pubs.sciepub.com/jpar/1/1/6/

Elkjaer, E., Mikkelsen, M. B., Michalak, J., Mennin, D. S., & O'Toole, M. S. (2020). Expansive and contractive postures and movement: A systematic review and meta-analysis of the effect of motor displays on affective and behavioral responses. *Perspectives on Psychological Science.* https://doi.org/10.1177/1745691620919358

European Federation of Sport Psychology. (1996). Position statement of the European Federation of Sport Psychology (FEPSAC): I. Definition of sport psychology. *Sport Psychologist, 10*(3), 221–223.

Fincham, G. W., Strauss, C., Montero-Marin, J., & Cavanagh, K. (2023). Effect of breathwork on stress and mental health: A meta-analysis of randomised-controlled trials. *Scientific Reports, 13*(1), 432. https://doi.org/10.1038/s41598-022-27247-y

Gardner, F. L., & Moore, Z. E. (2004). A mindfulness–acceptance–commitment (MAC) based approach to athletic performance enhancement: Theoretical considerations. *Behavior Therapy, 35*, 707–723.

Gill, D. L., & Williams, L. (2008). *Psychological dynamics of sport and exercise* (3rd ed.). Human Kinetics.

Gledhill, A., Murray, E., & Forsdyke, D. (2017). Psychological interventions associated with injury prevention: A systematic review. *British Journal of Sports Medicine, 51*(4), 321–322. https://doi.org/10.1136/bjsports-2016-097372.97

Goddard, K., Roberts, C.-M., Byron-Daniel, J., & Woodford, L. (2021). Psychological factors involved in adherence to sport injury rehabilitation: A systematic review. *International Review of Sport and Exercise Psychology, 14*(1), 51–73. https://doi.org/10.1080/1750984X.2020.1744179

Gould, D., & Weinberg, R. (2015). *Foundations of sport and exercise psychology* (6th ed.). Human Kinetics.

Hanin, Y. L. (1997). Emotions and athletic performance: Individual zones of optimal functioning model. *European Yearbook of Sport Psychology, 1*, 29–72.

Hayes, S. C., Strosahl, K. D., & Wilson, K. G. (2012). *Acceptance and commitment therapy: The process and practice of mindful change* (2nd ed.). Guilford Press.

Hays, K. F. (2006). Being fit: The ethics of practice diversification in performance psychology. *Professional Psychology: Research and Practice, 37*(3), 223–232.

Heckhausen, H., & Maher, B. A. (2013). *The anatomy of achievement motivation*. Elsevier Science.

Holmes, P. S., & Collins, D. J. (2001). The PETTLEP approach to motor imagery: A functional equivalence model for sport psychologists. *Journal of Applied Sport Psychology, 13*(1), 60–83. https://doi.org/10.1080/10413200109339004

Hooi, L.B., & Wah, T.E. (2018). Injured athletes and a new invention of relaxation techniques. *International Research Journal of Pharmacy and Medical Sciences, 1*(4). 78–81.

Huang, L., Galinsky, A. D., Gruenfeld, D. H., & Guillory, L. E. (2011). Powerful postures versus powerful roles: Which is the proximate correlate of thought and behavior? *Psychological science, 22*(1), 95–102. https://doi.org/10.1177/0956797610391912

Kingston, K., & Wilson, K. M. (2008). The application of goal setting in sport. In S. Mellalieu & S. Hanton (Eds.), *Advances in applied sport psychology* (pp. 75–123). Routledge. https://doi.org/10.4324/9780203887073

Kornspan, A. S. (2012). History of sport and performance psychology. In S. M. Murphy (Ed.), *The Oxford handbook of sport and performance psychology* (pp. 3–23). Oxford University Press.

Lee, W., Reeve, J., Xue, Y., & Xiong, J. (2012). Neural differences between intrinsic reasons for doing versus extrinsic reasons for doing: An fMRI study. *Neuroscience Research, 73*(1), 68–72. https://doi.org/10.1016/j.neures.2012.02.010

Locke, E. A., & Latham, G. P. (2002). Building a practically useful theory of goal setting and task motivation: A 35-year odyssey. *American Psychologist, 57*(9), 705–717. https://doi.org/10.1037/0003-066X.57.9.705

Ma, X., Yue, Z. Q., Gong, Z. Q., Zhang, H., Duan, N. Y., Shi, Y. T., Wei, G. X., & Li, Y. F. (2017). The effect of diaphragmatic breathing on attention, negative affect and stress in healthy adults. *Frontiers in Psychology, 8*, 874. https://doi.org/10.3389/fpsyg.2017.00874

Madrigal, L (2015). Psychological skills for injury prevention and recovery. *Women in Sport and Physical Activity Journal.* https://doi.org/10.1123/WSPAJ.2014-0024

Meijen, C. (2019). *Endurance performance in sport: Psychological theory and interventions.* Routledge.

Milley, K. R., & Ouellette, G. P. (2021). Putting attention on the spot in coaching: Shifting to an external focus of attention with imagery techniques to improve basketball free-throw shooting performance. *Frontiers in Psychology, 12.* 645676. https://doi.org/10.3389/fpsyg.2021.645676

Moran, A. (1996). *The psychology of concentration in sport performance: A cognitive approach.* Psychology Press.

Moran, A. (2012). Concentration: Attention and performance. In S. M. Murphy (Ed.), *The Oxford handbook of sport and performance psychology* (pp. 117–130). Oxford University Press. https://doi.org/10.1093/oxfordhb/9780199731763.013.0006

Moritz, S. E., Feltz, D. L., Fahrbach, K. R., & Mack, D. E. (2000). The relation of self-efficacy measures to sport performance: A meta-analytic review. *Research Quarterly for Exercise and Sport, 71*, 280–294.

Nideffer, R. M., & Sagal, M. S. (2006). Attentional control and sport performance. In J. M. Williams (Ed.), *Applied sport psychology: Personal growth to peak performance* (5th ed., pp. 377–399). McGraw-Hill.

Podlog, L., & Eklund, R. C. (2005). Return to sport after serious injury: A retrospective examination of motivation and psychological outcomes. *Journal of Sport Rehabilitation, 14*(1), 20–34. https://doi.org/10.1123/jsr.14.1.20

Russell, S., Jenkins, D., Rynne, S., Halson, S. L., & Kelly, V. (2019). What is mental fatigue in elite sport? Perceptions from athletes and staff. *European Journal of Sport Science, 19*(10), 1367–1376. https://doi.org/10.1080/17461391.2019.1618397

Seligman, M. E. P., & Csikszentmihalyi, M. (2000). Positive psychology: An introduction. *American Psychologist, 55*(1), 5–14. https://doi.org/10.1037/0003-066X.55.1.5

Sheard, M., Golby, J., & van Wersch, A. (2009). Progress toward construct validation of the Sports Mental Toughness Questionnaire (SMTQ). *European Journal of Psychological Assessment, 25*, 186–193. http://doi.org/10.1027/1015-5759.25.3.186

Sheehan, R. B., Herring, M. P., & Campbell, M. J. (2018). Associations between motivation and mental health in sport: A test of the hierarchical model of intrinsic and extrinsic motivation. *Frontiers in Psychology, 9*, 707. http://doi.org/10.3389/fpsyg.2018.00707

Smith, R. E., Smoll, F. L., Cumming, S. P., & Grossbard, J. R. (2006). Measurement of multidimensional sport performance anxiety in children and adults: The Sport Anxiety Scale-2. *Journal of Sport & Exercise Psychology, 28*, 479–501.

Solomon, G., & Becker, A. (2004). *Focused for fastpitch.* Human Kinetics.

Sutton, J. (2021). *What is sports psychology? 9 scientific theories and examples.* https://positivepsychology.com/sports-psychology/

Tracy, J. L., & Matsumoto, D. (2008). The spontaneous expression of pride and shame: Evidence for biologically innate nonverbal displays. *PNAS Journal, 105*(33), 11655–11660. https://doi.org/10.1073/pnas.0802686105

Van Raalte, J. L., Brewer, B. W., Rivera, P. M., & Petitpas, A. J. (2020). The effectiveness of self-talk for athletic injury rehabilitation: A systematic review. *Journal of Sport Rehabilitation, 29*(3), 352–359.

Vealey, R. (1986). Conceptualization of sport confidence and competitive presentation: Preliminary investigation and instrument development. *Journal of Sport Psychology, 8*, 221–246.

Wesson, K., Wiggins, N., Thompson, G., & Hartigan, S. (2000). *Sport and PE* (2nd ed.). Hodder & Stoughton Educational.

Wulf, G. (2013). Attentional focus and motor learning: A review of 15 years. *International Review of Sport and Exercise Psychology, 6*(1), 77–104. https://doi.org/10.1080/1750984X.2012.723728

Yerkes, R. M., & Dodson, J. D. (1908). The relation of strength of stimulus to rapidity of habit-formation. *Journal of Comparative Neurology and Psychology, 18*(5), 459–482.

SECTION 2

INTRODUCTION TO SPORTS SCIENCE

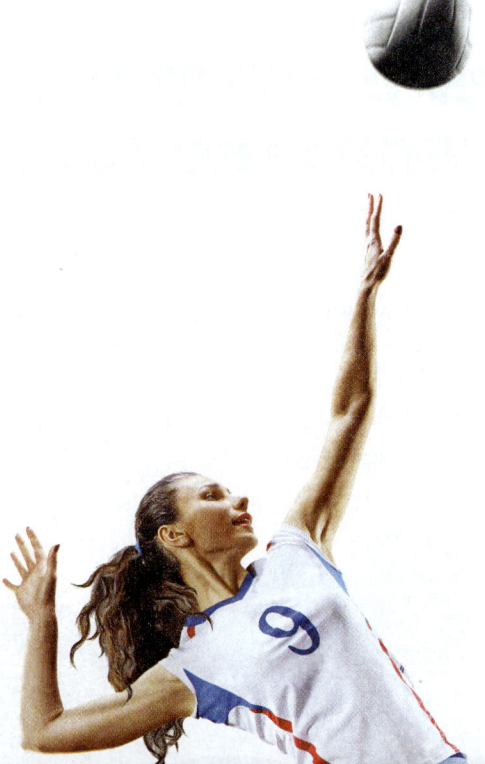
© Eugene Onischenko/Shutterstock

INTRODUCTION TO SPORTS PERFORMANCE TRAINING

CHAPTER FOUR

LEARNING OBJECTIVES

Upon completion of this chapter, the Sports Performance Coach will be able to:

- **Describe** the scientific principles of training.
- **Identify** integrated training principles.
- **Explain** the benefits of integrated training for sports performance.
- **Discuss** NASM's Optimum Performance Training™ Model as a foundation for implementing integrated training.

LESSON 1: INTRODUCTION TO INTEGRATED TRAINING

INTRODUCTION

The Sports Performance Coach plans a progressive and systematic approach toward developing the necessary attributes for an athlete's peak athletic performance. This type of training is based on the interrelationships of exercise science, kinesiology, exercise physiology, neuromechanics, biomechanics, and human movement science, as well as clinical and application-oriented professions such as strength and conditioning, athletic training, and physical therapy (**Figure 4.1**).

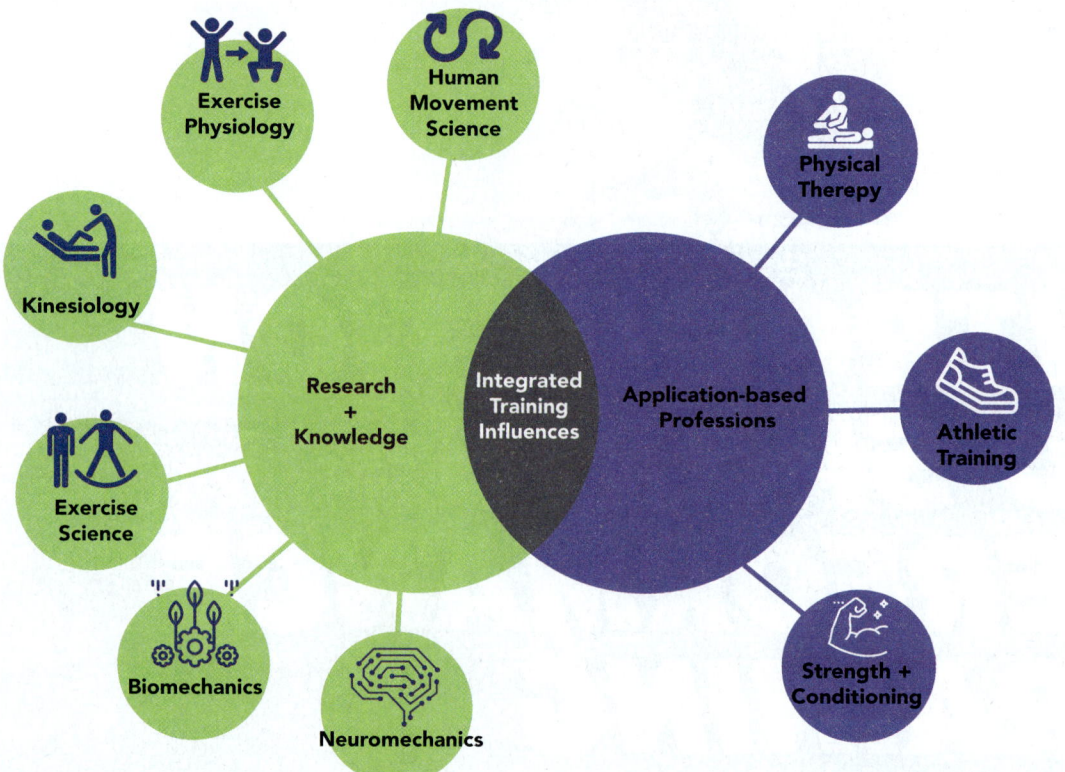

FIGURE 4.1 Integrated Training Influences

A well-rounded approach is critical to ensure that exercise program development, administration, and evaluation address each athlete's complex and comprehensive needs. Exercises designed to improve performance date back to earlier civilizations of the Chinese dynasties. Their methods to improve muscular strength were documented, indicating they focused on maintaining the preparedness of military soldiers (Kraemer et al., 2017). However, it wasn't until the 1970s that research further defined the effectiveness of planned, progressive training methods, which incorporated many aspects of athletic performance and human movement science. Interestingly, this line of research downplayed the role of force production alone and fueled debates over traditional (e.g., isolated, single-plane, artificially supported bodyweight) versus functional (e.g., multiplanar, multisensory, multimodal, posture variations) approaches to exercise and program development.

Traditional strength and conditioning programs focus on absolute or maximal strength gain in isolated muscles—chiefly the prime movers in the body—throughout single planes of motion. Examples of common traditional exercises include barbell squats, deadlifts, bench presses, overhead presses, leg extensions, and leg curls. Many of these exercises are performed with the athlete's body weight artificially supported, such as on a bench (**Figure 4.2**).

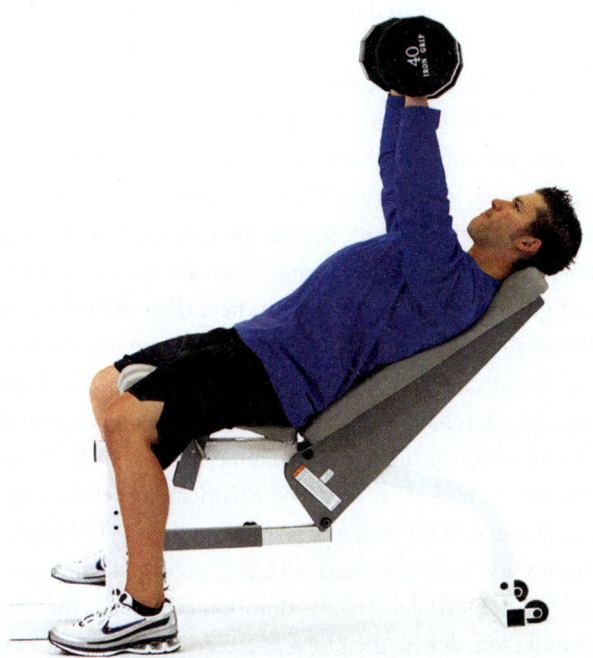

FIGURE 4.2 Bodyweight Artificially Supported During Incline Dumbbell Press

Although these exercises develop useful elements of performance, the Sports Performance Coach needs to take a broader look at overall athletic function. Integrated training evolved through a multidisciplinary approach to physical training. In the 1970s, researchers sought the best methods to produce muscular endurance, strength, hypertrophy, power, and speed. During that time, another body of knowledge was developing centered on the study of pain. Janda and Lewit, two neurologists and physical therapists from Czechoslovakia, studied the role of independent muscles in the context of interdependent multi-joint movement. They observed how muscles in healthy individuals functioned together to allow movement through all planes of motion and how these muscles were subgrouped according to the body's motion (Janda, 1978; Lewit, 1994). A group of primarily Australian researchers eventually determined that muscle activation of the trunk and deep abdominal stabilizers preceded movement of the limbs in athletes without back pain (Comerford & Mottram, 2001; Hodges & Richardson, 1996; Mayhew et al., 1983; O'Sullivan et al., 1998; Richardson et al., 2002; Sahrmann, 1992).

This "feedforward" firing sequence was found to be absent or delayed in athletes with a history of low back pain, establishing a connection between neuromuscular activity, pain, and function (Hodges & Richardson, 1997). These ideas quickly advanced to connect the altered function of hip muscles following ankle injury (Beckman & Buchanan, 1995; Bullock-Saxon, 1994) and its concomitant relationship to knee pain (Frederickson et al., 2000; Hewett et al., 1996; Padua et al., 2012a) and back pain (Cibulka et al., 1998; Hides et al., 1994; O'Sullivan et al., 1997; Sahrmann, 1992).

The proposed solutions to restore neuromuscular activity patterns centered on improving lumbo-pelvic-hip complex stability. The neuromuscular approach popularized in Australia involved performing a "drawing in" maneuver before any trunk or limb movement (Hodges et al., 1996; Richardson et al., 2002). Researchers in Sweden (Bergmark, 1989) and Canada (McGill & Cholewicki, 2001) utilized a bracing approach, also called "hollowing." From a structural engineering perspective, these researchers viewed the spine as an unstable stack of bone that could be stabilized only through correct tensioning of the muscles that connected not only spinal segment to segment, but also spine to extremity—similar to the support wires in a suspension bridge.

Human movement is a collaborative effort involving joint complexes, muscle groups, and central nervous system (CNS) control (Janda, 1978; Panjabi, 1992a; Sahrmann, 1992). If a movement task presents a problem, the CNS provides the solution through the recruitment of specific muscle fibers and the coordination of multi-joint motion. Sometimes these solutions are effective; at other times, they are not. For example, athletes who learn motor patterns through trial and error, poor training techniques, and repetition have altered movement quality that may negatively affect their athletic performance (Richardson & Jull, 1995). Over time, it became clear that there was a strong relationship between the stability of the lumbo-pelvic-hip complex (Barr et al., 2005; Barr et al., 2007; Comerford & Mottram, 2001), rehabilitation (Nadler, Malanga, Feinberg, et al., 2002; Panjabi, 1992b; Sahrmann, 1992), athletic performance (Hewett et al., 1996; Hides et al., 1994), musculoskeletal injury (Hewett et al., 1999; Mandelbaum et al., 2005; McGill, 2001; Myer et al., 2002; Nyland et al., 2002), and injury-risk reduction (Boling et al., 2009).

In 2000, American physical therapist Michael Clark presented the Optimum Performance Training™ (OPT) Model. This landmark method was the first to integrate multidisciplinary research from across the globe and blend performance-enhancement outcomes with an injury-prevention focus. The comprehensive OPT Model aims to improve all components of human movement through a progressive and systematic approach to developing function.

Function in athletics represents multiplanar movements that involve acceleration, deceleration, and stabilization during sports actions (Clark, 2000). Peak athletic function is best developed through an integrated training approach. **Integrated training** is a comprehensive approach that attempts to improve all components necessary for an athlete to perform at the highest level of competition with an injury risk mitigation focus. This is best achieved through the development of functional strength and neuromuscular efficiency.

Functional strength is the ability of the neuromuscular system to efficiently produce force, reduce force, and dynamically stabilize multiple joint segments during athletic tasks (Edgerton et al., 1996; Panjabi, 1992a, 1992b; Sahrmann, 2011). Functional athletic activities occur in multiple planes of motion and require acceleration, deceleration, and dynamic stabilization (Clark, 2000; Ford et al., 2003; Frederickson et al., 2000; Ireland et al., 2003; McClay & Manal, 1999; Nyland et al., 2002; Powers, 2003).

Neuromuscular efficiency is the ability of the CNS to allow agonists, antagonists, synergists, stabilizers, and **neutralizers** (muscles that counteract unwanted actions of other muscles) to work interdependently during dynamic athletic activities (Edgerton et al., 1996; Enoka, 2002; Neumann, 2017; Sahrmann, 2011).

Muscles improve strength (i.e., force production) capacity with adequate overload. However, the Sports Performance Coach must determine if this new level of muscle strength suffices to function adequately in the multisensory, neuromuscular environment required for many athletic tasks. Strength alone is insufficient to develop all the attributes (DiStefano et al., 2013) required to implement the athletic task within preferred biomechanical postures (Hewett & Bates, 2017). Therefore, the Sports Performance Coach must aim to provide a comprehensive approach that improves all biomotor abilities (flexibility, endurance, strength, coordination, speed) and their derived qualities (mobility, stability, balance, agility, power) to optimize performance and lower associated injury risks (Boling et al., 2009; Clark, 2000; Hewett & Bates, 2017; Padua & Marshall, 2006).

This comprehensive approach signals a paradigm shift in physical training and conditioning toward optimizing the entire human movement system (HMS) through all planes of motion. To achieve these outcomes, the Sports Performance Coach must develop and deliver training programs that integrate proven training principles and components in a systematic, progressive, and planned manner. As a result of such programs, athletes should be able to move more effectively, perform better, and recover faster.

📋 COACH'S CORNER

All muscles function in all planes of motion at all times, although their specificity is determined by the exercise and joint position. At different joint angles, muscles demonstrate different qualities (Neumann, 2010). For example, during the barbell squat exercise, the gluteus medius and adductor muscle group work in the frontal plane, along with the internal and external oblique muscles in the transverse plane, as *neutralizers* to prevent undesired movements and to allow efficient movement in the desired sagittal plane direction.

LESSON 2: FUNDAMENTAL CONCEPTS OF SPORTS TRAINING
THE SCIENTIFIC PRINCIPLES OF TRAINING

Developing an integrated training program might appear to be an arduous and complex task. Integrated training programs are rooted in scientific principles of training, which provide the background and context for which the programs are created.

GENERAL ADAPTATION AND FITNESS–FATIGUE MODELS

The Sports Performance Coach's comprehensive, sport-specific training program must account for many variables. From the most fundamental perspective, a training program is a collection of individual training sessions. Each training session introduces various stimuli to deliver the desired physiologic responses. These training stimuli have an impact on the athlete's performance. Performance tends to be reduced immediately after a training session and may stay reduced for a few days.

Following the initial reduction in performance, there is a rebound, such that performance improves. These observations are partly explained by the body's predictable responses to stress (general adaptation syndrome) and the relationship between fitness and fatigue (fitness–fatigue model). These

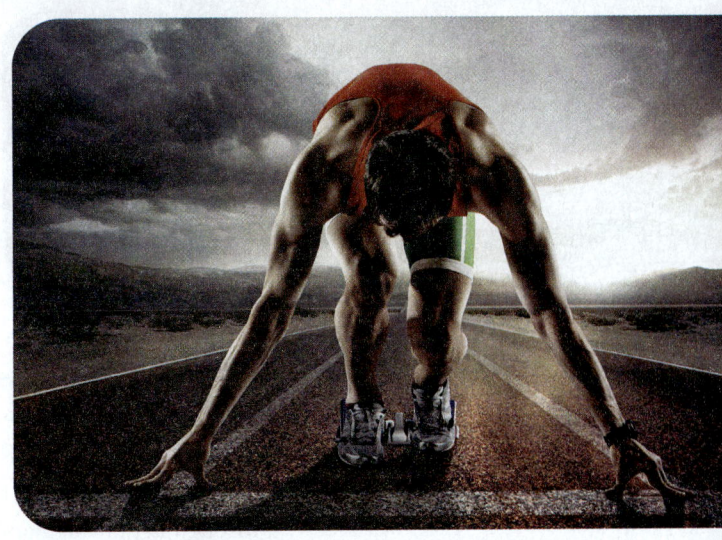

© Rocksweeper/Shutterstock

models are helpful for analyzing the effects of training and recovery on athletic performance.

GENERAL ADAPTATION SYNDROME

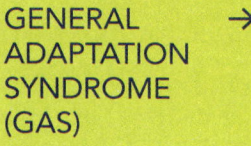

Maintaining the dynamic balance between training stimuli and adequate rest, recovery, and regeneration is a constant challenge for practitioners. To develop progressive training programs that deliver the desired physiologic adaptations, the Sports Performance Coach needs to consider the body's natural response to stress and the process used to restore its physiologic balance. The body's natural balance, called **homeostasis**, must be altered to produce the desired physiologic adaptation (Cunanan et al., 2018; Selye, 1976). The disturbance of homeostasis by tissue overload produces an initial decline in performance (i.e., fatigue), which is then followed by a supercompensation effect wherein performance increases (Cunanan et al., 2018).

To describe the body's predictable reaction to stress, Hans Selye introduced the notion of the **general adaptation syndrome (GAS)** in 1936. Although his theory was not specific to physical training, it evolved into a practical model of training planning in which progressive training loads are alternated with appropriate recovery periods (Cunanan et al., 2018). Adaptation to stress follows a predictable pattern that includes three stages of response (Selye, 1976):

- Alarm
- Resistance development
- Exhaustion

Alarm

The alarm stage is the body's initial reaction to a stressor. This stage is generally considered a negative reaction to stress, but it allows for the activation of protective processes within

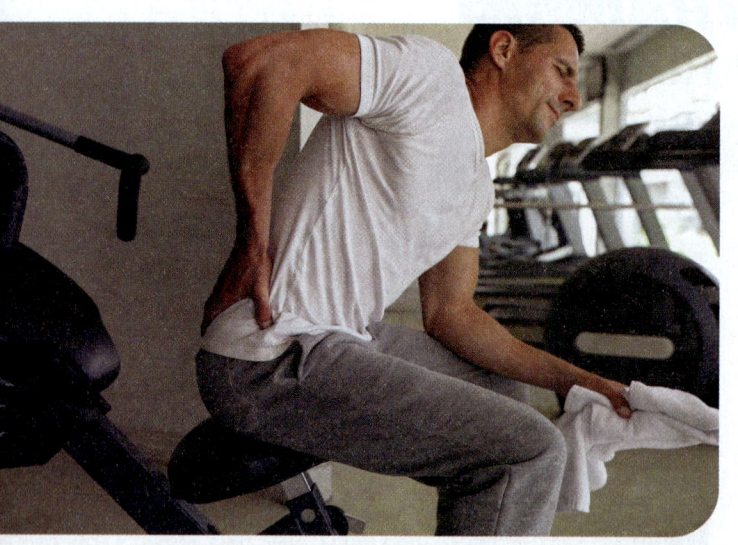

the body. For example, when an athlete begins resistance training, their body is subjected to the stress of increased amounts of force on the bones, joints, muscles, connective tissues, and nervous system. This stress creates a need for increased oxygen and blood supply to the right areas of the body and increased neural recruitment to the muscles. Initially, the athlete's body is very inefficient at responding to the demands placed upon it; thus, it increases its ability to meet new demands (Cunanan et al., 2018; Selye, 1976).

Consider the typical response to an unaccustomed exercise or a sudden increase in a training program. The new work is performed, and over the next two or three days, the muscles exhibit classic delayed-onset muscle soreness (DOMS). During this period of DOMS, any attempt at replicating or advancing the soreness-inducing exercise is limited by the factors contributing to the soreness.

© Albina Gavrilovic/Shutterstock

Resistance Development

The second stage is called resistance development. During this stage, the body increases its functional capacity as it adapts to the stressor, assuming it is repeated. After repeated training sessions, the HMS increases its capability to efficiently recruit muscle fibers through neural adaptations such as improved rate coding and synchronicity, and it distributes oxygen and blood to the proper areas in the body through improved vascularization and metabolic efficiency. After adaptation, the athlete requires further stress to produce a new response and a higher level of performance (Cunanan et al., 2018; Selye, 1976).

Manipulating the amount of weight an athlete uses is one of many ways to increase stress on the body. When introducing a new exercise to a conditioned individual, the intensity gradually increases after the residual effects of DOMS subside. The athlete's performance continues to improve until a new level of homeostasis is reached; the athlete can maintain this level with adequate training. Applying a variety of training stresses is advantageous, and allowing the body to acclimate to the demands imposed by each exercise so as to demonstrate improvement and progress is known as **supercompensation**.

Exhaustion

The final stage is called exhaustion. Prolonged stress or stress that exceeds the athlete's adaptive potential produces distress. Too much stress on the system leads to performance detriments because of injury or staleness (Cunanan et al., 2018; Selye, 1976). However, the stressors induced by training are only one of the multiple types of stress to which the athlete must respond. Additional stressors include emotional, psychological, social, and biological factors. The culmination of multiple stress inputs can lead to exhaustion.

An athlete in the exhaustion stage can suffer from a variety of issues that reduce performance, such as:

- Stress fractures
- **Muscle strain**
- Joint and muscle pain
- Emotional fatigue
- Altered sleep patterns

Training must be cycled through stages that increase the stress placed on the HMS and allow for sufficient rest and recuperation. A continued increase in resistance with the intention of stressing the muscles of the body to produce a size or strength change can lead to injury of the muscle, joint, or connective tissue.

The muscle, connective, and nervous tissues have different potentials to adapt to stress. Thus, training programs must provide a variety of intensities and stresses to optimize the adaptation of each kind of tissue for the best possible results (Clark, 2000).

🤖 GETTING TECHNICAL

Optimal tissue development is dependent on adequate stress and recovery. Due to their individual biology, athletes' body tissues will respond differently to stress, which affects their rate of adaptation. Poor blood supply to connective tissues (such as bone, ligaments, tendons, and cartilage) delays nutritional delivery, leading to variable remodeling rates when compared to muscle tissue (Kannus, 2000; McArdle, 2010; Neumann, 2017).

FITNESS–FATIGUE MODEL

Expanding on the GAS model, which identifies the initial performance deficit that occurs immediately following exercise (Chiu & Barnes, 2003), the **fitness–fatigue model** explains how different stressors produce different physiological responses (Bannister, 1991).

SUPERCOM-PENSATION →

Allowing the body to acclimate to the demands imposed by each exercise to demonstrate improvement and progress.

MUSCLE STRAIN →

Trauma to the muscle tissue, most commonly occurring at the musculoskeletal junction.

FITNESS–FATIGUE MODEL →

A framework in which an individual's performance at any given time is determined by the balance between their level of fitness and their level of fatigue.

For example, resistance training produces different physiological adaptations than prolonged cardiorespiratory training, which is defined largely by fatigue.

Fatigue occurs when working muscles (peripheral fatigue) are altered through cellular function and metabolite accumulation or at higher levels of the CNS (central fatigue). In this model, *fitness* refers to adaptations inside the CNS and the muscle–tendon–joint complex that contribute to improved performance. In other words, fitness represents the positive effects of exercise, whereas fatigue represents the adverse effects. By this definition, *performance* is the sum of these factors. The fitness–fatigue model is not a replacement for the GAS model but rather a more accurate representation of the stimulus–response relationships and a more detailed explanation of how performance improves over time.

For example, assume a progressive training program increases an athlete's maximal vertical jump. The GAS model identifies an improvement in jump performance, whereas the fitness–fatigue model (**Figure 4.3**) looks at the performance attributes required to increase jump height, such as motor unit recruitment, rate of force production, joint stability, range of motion, muscle strength, athlete motivation, rest, and recovery (Chiu & Barnes, 2003).

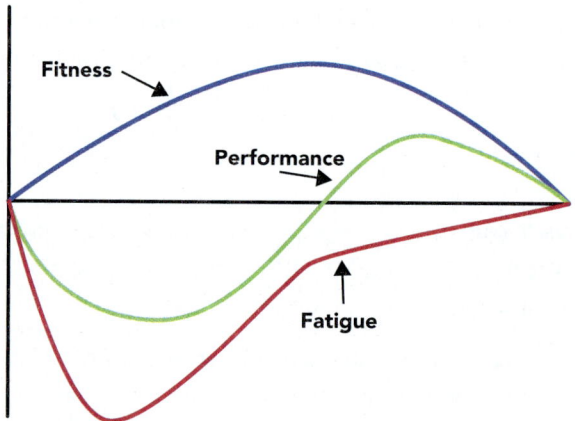

FIGURE 4.3 Fitness–Fatigue Model

Data from Chiu, L. Z. F & Barnes, J. L. (2003). The fitness-fatigue model revisited: Implications for planning short- and long-term training. *Strength & Conditioning Journal, 25*(6), 42–51.

PRINCIPLE OF SPECIFICITY

PRINCIPLE OF SPECIFICITY →

The adaptive response of specific recruitment of muscles and its associated adaptation to a sport-specific task or training activity. Also known as the SAID (specific adaptation to imposed demands) principle.

The **principle of specificity** is often referred to as the SAID (specific adaptation to imposed demands) principle. This principle states that the body undergoes specific adaptations to the type of demand placed on it. For example, if an athlete trains by lifting heavy weights, the primary adaptations support higher levels of maximal strength. If an athlete trains by lifting lighter weights for many repetitions, the primary adaptations support higher levels of local muscle endurance. This simple concept implies that the athlete gets what they train for. However, the SAID principle is often used out of context and can be misleading because different tissues in the body respond to different stimuli intended to achieve specific goals.

The body must progress through stages of adaptation to ensure all the necessary tissues are developed properly to meet the desired goal. For example, connective tissue adapts more slowly than muscle, and it must be strong for muscles to generate high levels of tension. Therefore, if a coach places a training emphasis on muscular hypertrophy and strength first, then the absence of prior training that allows the connective tissue to increase its strength increases the risk of injury.

Type I muscle fibers, which are important for postural stabilization, function differently than type II muscle fibers. To train with higher intensities, an athlete must use proper postural stabilization. Both types of fibers need to be trained specifically to prepare them to support higher levels of training. This is the primary purpose behind the three main outcomes of training within the OPT Model.

> ⚠ **CRITICAL**
>
> The SAID principle must be used appropriately within the context of the OPT Model, which progresses the program through a series of logical steps. Do not use the SAID principle as justification to skip progressions through the model, as this can lead to potential injury and athletic breakdown.

The degree of adaptation during training is directly related to the program's mechanical, neuromuscular, and metabolic specificity (Kraemer & Ratamess, 2000; Tan, 1999). In other words, the more specifically the Sports Performance Coach manipulates the exercise routine to meet the actual goal, the greater the specific carryover the training program has on that goal.

Mechanical specificity refers to the weight and movements required of the body (Behm, 1995; Rutherford et al., 1986). For example, for athletes to develop endurance in their legs, they must use light weights over many repetitions of leg exercises. For athletes to develop maximal strength in their chest, they must use heavy weights during chest-related exercises.

Neuromuscular specificity refers to the speed of contraction and exercise selection (Hakkinen, 1994; McEvoy & Newton, 1991). For example, for an athlete to develop higher levels of power in the legs, they must use low weight at high velocity of contraction in a plyometric manner, such as in plyometric training (**Figure 4.4**).

| **MECHANICAL SPECIFICITY** → |
| The weight and movements required of the body. |

| **NEURO-MUSCULAR SPECIFICITY** → |
| The speed of contraction and exercise selection. |

| **INTER-MUSCULAR COORDINATION** → |
| The ability of the neuromuscular system to allow all muscles to work together with proper activation and timing between them. |

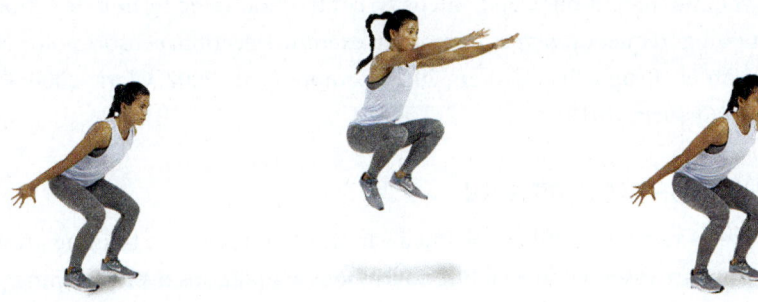

FIGURE 4.4 Training for Power

Nyland et al. (2014) examined muscle activation and coordination patterns through electromyography (EMG) measurements during a kicking motion following progressive resistance training. The testing group demonstrated a change to earlier muscle activation, earlier peak ground reaction force, and improved kick quickness. These results suggest that resistance training influences **intermuscular coordination**, which aids in improving sports skills. Thus, resistance training directly enhances speed, agility, and quickness and reinforces the importance of each part of integrated training for overall athletic development (Hakkinen et al., 1985). To develop higher levels of stability while pulling, an athlete needs to perform back exercises using controlled, unstable exercises at slower speeds, such as a single-leg cable row (Behm, 1995; Sale, 1988) (**Figure 4.5**).

METABOLIC →
SPECIFICITY

The metabolic route needed to supply energy for a specific exercise accounting for intensity and duration.

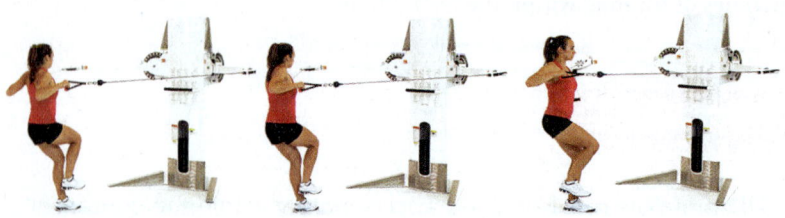

FIGURE 4.5 Training for Stability

Overall strength development is velocity-dependent (Janusevicius et al., 2017) and reflects neuromuscular factors of antagonistic muscles. For example, heavy resistance training causes greater increases in strength at slower speeds than at fast speeds. Faster movement training develops greater improvements in strength at faster speeds.

Metabolic specificity refers to the metabolic route needed to supply energy quickly for a specific exercise. To develop endurance, training should include prolonged bouts of exercise with minimal rest periods between sets that produce energy through the aerobic pathways. To develop maximal strength or power, training should include longer rest periods, so that the intensity of each bout of exercise remains high. Energy is supplied through the anaerobic pathways (Parra et al., 2000; Viru & Viru, 2000).

PRINCIPLE OF →
PROGRESSIVE
OVERLOAD

Increasing the intensity or volume of exercise programs using a systematic and gradual approach.

PRINCIPLE OF PROGRESSIVE OVERLOAD

The **principle of progressive overload** focuses on providing the appropriate training stimulus to elicit the optimal physical, physiological, and performance adaptations. A tissue adapts to a stimulus: Thus, the tissue needs the overload or it will not adapt. A well-designed resistance training program imposes continued demands that force progressive adaptations (Kraemer & Ratamess, 2004). The HMS responds to the imposed demands incurred during training (SAID principle); this can occur through manipulation of training volume (repetitions, sets), intensity, contraction velocity, muscle actions, rest intervals, training frequency, planes of motion, exercise selection, sensorimotor challenges, and exercise order (Brughelli & Cronin, 2007; Campos et al., 2002; Clark, 2000; Fleck & Kraemer, 1997; Issurin, 2010).

PRINCIPLE OF →
VARIATION

Variation in training programs is necessary to stimulate new adaptations.

PRINCIPLE OF VARIATION

The **principle of variation** utilizes planned variations in resistance training programs. These variations are essential to enabling continuous adaptations over a training period while preventing injury. Notably, periodized resistance training programs lead to superior physical, physiological, and performance improvements compared to nonperiodized training programs (DiStefano et al., 2013; Fleck & Kraemer, 1997; Issurin, 2010; Marx et al., 2001; Rhea, Ball, et al., 2002). Moreover, specific combinations of volume and intensity produce specific training adaptations. A high training volume equates to cellular or hypertrophic changes, whereas high intensity equates to neural adaptations. A planned training program that incorporates progressive and systematic variation (multiplanar, multisensory) produces long-term, consistent adaptations to movement efficiency, tissue load tolerance, and reduced risk of overtraining and injury (Clark, 2000; Franchi et al., 2017; Issurin, 2010; Rhea, Alvar, et al., 2002; Rhea et al., 2003; Rhea, Ball, et al., 2002).

PRINCIPLE →
OF INDIVIDUAL-
IZATION

Individuals have unique physical characteristics, fitness levels, goals, and preferences that should be taken into account when designing and implementing training programs.

PRINCIPLE OF INDIVIDUALIZATION

The Sports Performance Coach must also consider the **principle of individualization** when designing exercise programs. This principle suggests that the athlete's age, general medical history, injury history, training background, work capacity, recoverability, structural integrity, psychological readiness, training needs or goals, and sport will affect the training plan. Each athlete responds to a program tailored to address their specific needs or goals (Fleck & Kraemer, 1997; Issurin, 2010; Judge et al., 2003; Kraemer & Ratamess, 2004; Tan, 1999). A generic programming strategy based on the particular sport and a desired physiologic adaptation might not adequately address an individual's specific needs based on their training and health history (Padua et al., 2012b; Zhang et al., 2018).

PRINCIPLE OF TRANSFER EFFECT

The **principle of transfer effect** states that training of one skill can transfer to the performance of a different skill. Ultimately, developing performance-enhancing qualities through planned training programs is beneficial only if applying these qualities improves athletic performance. This principle can be applied within individual sports or to specific sports movements. According to the SAID principle, the more specific the training, the greater the likelihood that training gains will transfer to performance (Loturco et al., 2014; Rhea et al., 2008; Wilson et al., 1996). For example:

- A single-leg squat might enhance sprint performance more than swimming.
- Jump rope exercises might improve agility and dynamic foot control for a tennis player but may have little impact on serve velocity.

Researchers report that the performance of slow, heavily loaded strength training enhances maximal strength but not the rate of force production (Campos et al., 2002; Kanehisa & Miyashita, 1983). Conversely, plyometric training increases the rate of force production with minimal effect on maximal strength (Campos et al., 2002; Ewing et al., 1990; Hakkinen et al., 1985; Loturco et al., 2014; Rhea et al., 2008).

PRINCIPLE OF INTERFERENCE EFFECT

Many sports and sporting movements require muscular size, endurance, strength, power, and speed. Therefore, planned conditioning programs that strive to improve these physical attributes are essential. Performance programs that simultaneously combine resistance training to develop muscle hypertrophy, strength, and power with aerobic exercise to develop endurance are called **concurrent training**.

Concurrent training, relative to resistance training alone, negatively impacts muscular hypertrophy, strength, and power (Fyfe et al., 2014; Hickson, 1980; Kraemer et al., 1995; Wilson et al., 2012), but improves short- and long-duration endurance activities (Fyfe et al., 2014; Wilson et al., 2012). Research indicates that endurance exercise might interfere with the metabolic effects of exercise (sustained fatigue, substrate shortage) and compromise cellular remodeling activated by the resistance exercise (Fyfe et al., 2014). This interference in the development of some physical attributes is known as the **principle of interference effect**. The exact mechanism by which this interference effect occurs is not fully understood, but is likely multifactorial because training is so highly individualized. Some athletes experience deficits in strength performance after concurrent training, whereas others demonstrate gains (Karavirta et al., 2011; Wilson et al., 2012), including those participating in endurance-based activities such as marathons or

---

PRINCIPLE OF TRANSFER EFFECT →

Training or practice of one skill can have a positive effect on the performance of another related skill.

CONCURRENT TRAINING →

Simultaneous use of two or more training modalities for improving more than one biomotor ability, with the aim of improving sports performance at the training session or micro-cycle level.

PRINCIPLE OF INTERFERENCE EFFECT →

The impairment or blunting of a desired training effect because of the application of a conflicting training stimulus.

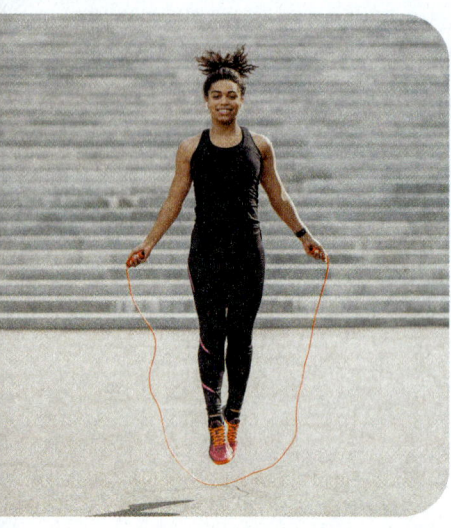
© Prostock-studio/Shutterstock

triathlons (Fei et al., 2020), and especially those who engage in higher-intensity resistance training (Fei et al., 2020).

Table 4.1 provides tips that the Sports Performance Coach can employ with an athlete to optimize performance and minimize interference (Blagrove, 2014; Fyfe et al., 2014; Hickson, 1980; Karavirta et al., 2011; Wilson et al., 2012).

TABLE 4.1 Recommendations for Optimizing Performance While Minimizing Interference

Separate endurance and resistance training by 6 hours (performing endurance training first) to optimize the timing window of protein synthesis. Resistance training sessions should be separated by 24 hours.
Decrease activities that involve running prior to resistance training. Running can have a high interference effect because it is a highly specialized skill that involves a complex combination of neuromuscular, cardiovascular, and metabolic adaptations.
Utilize a split-body resistance training routine to allow for greater focus on specific muscle groups and movements, which can improve neuromuscular coordination, strength, and hypertrophy without negatively affecting other muscle groups or movements.
If strength-based outcomes are the priority, reduce the frequency of endurance training to three or fewer sessions per week. The intensity per session can be increased.

🤖 GETTING TECHNICAL

In a six-week study of recreational endurance runners, Fei et al. (2020) found that a concurrent training approach that combined endurance running with either concurrent complex training (strength and power) or higher-intensity strength training improved maximal oxygen uptake (VO_2 max), eccentric and concentric leg strength, vertical jumping power, and running economy. In this study, the athletes performed resistance training elements twice weekly and their usual running activities four to six days per week. These data demonstrate that concurrent training with higher-intensity resistance loads might minimize the interference effects (Fei et al., 2020).

PRINCIPLE OF → REVERSIBILITY

Benefits of training are not permanent and can be lost if training is discontinued or reduced in frequency, intensity, or duration.

PRINCIPLE OF REVERSIBILITY

Modern training methods focus on developing biomotor abilities (i.e., strength, muscle size, power, neuromuscular control) that increase athletic performance. These attributes of enhanced fitness do not persist indefinitely, however (Chiu & Barnes, 2003; Terzis et al., 2008). The training stimulus must be periodically altered; otherwise, a detraining effect will occur. This phenomenon of detraining is widely known as the "use it or lose it" principle and was formerly called the **principle of reversibility**. When the training stimulus is terminated, the stimulus that continually alters the body's homeostasis also ends. In turn, the body adapts to accommodate this lesser state of physiologic performance and achieves a new homeostasis through muscle atrophy and metabolic downregulation (Andersen et al., 2005; Chiu & Barnes, 2003).

Some evidence shows that when load progression is reduced, adaptations gained from chronic exercise diminish at a slower rate than those achieved rapidly (Mujika & Padilla, 2001b; Romer & McConnell, 2003; Terzis et al., 2008). This rate of predictable decline can be slowed by implementing planned active-recovery training periods (Issurin, 2010; McArdle, 2010). Each training adaptation has certain residual training effects and a predictable timeline for their decline.

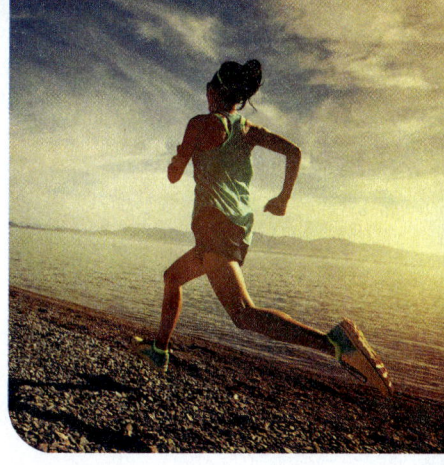

© Lzf/Shutterstock

> ### ⚠ CRITICAL
>
> To achieve optimal performance, an athlete must train their biomotor qualities in the correct order (e.g., stabilization and endurance, then strength, then power) (Clark, 2000; Issurin, 2010). This sequencing can be useful when planning short- and long-term training (Clark, 2000; Gibala & McGee, 2008; Mujika & Padilla, 2001a, 2001b).

LESSON 3: GUIDELINES FOR SPORTS PERFORMANCE TRAINING
INTEGRATED PERFORMANCE TRAINING TENETS

Effective athletic performance enhancement training programs involve much more than manipulated training loads. Considering that nearly all athletic endeavors require a rate of force production and reduction in multiple planes of motion and in response to an unpredictable environment, the Sports Performance Coach must focus on the following tenets of training.

TRAINING IN ALL PLANES OF MOTION

Athletic actions occur in all three planes of motion: sagittal, frontal, and transverse (Ford et al., 2003; Kipp et al., 2011; McClay & Manal, 1999; Nyland et al., 2002; Powers, 2003) (**Figure 4.6**). Individual muscles also function in all three planes to provide dynamic joint control (Neumann, 2017). However, many athletic injuries occur in the frontal and transverse planes (Beckman & Buchanan, 1995; Bell et al., 2012; Boling et al., 2009; Bullock-Saxon, 1994; Chappell & Limpisvasti, 2008; Di Stasi, 2013; Ford et al., 2003; Frederickson et al., 2000; Hewett & Bates, 2017; Ireland et al., 2003).

Traditional strength and conditioning exercises often focus on the sagittal plane (e.g., squat, close-grip row, lunge, deadlift, etc.), primarily emphasizing concentric force production. An athletic activity might appear to predominantly occur in one plane (e.g., sprinting in the sagittal plane), but an athlete must control movements in the other two planes of motion to perform effectively (Franchi et al., 2017; Frederickson et al., 2000; Hewett & Bates, 2017; Ireland et al., 2003). Training only in the sagittal plane does not

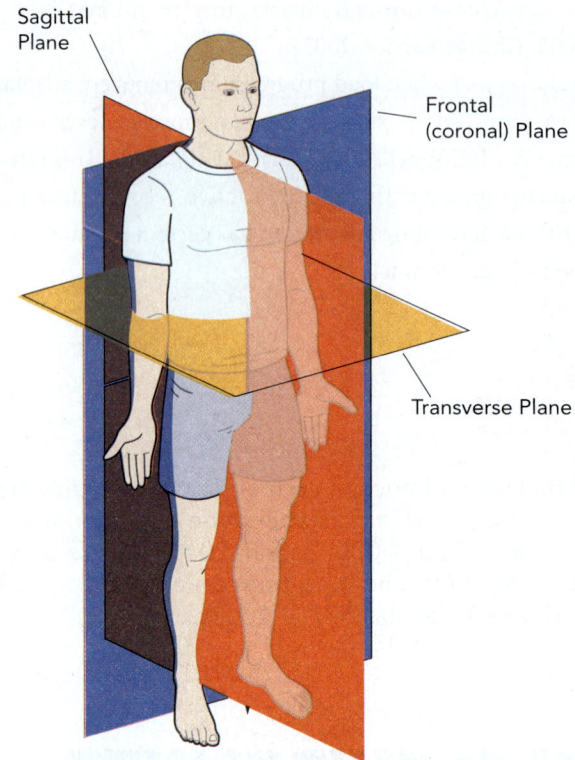

FIGURE 4.6 Planes of Motion

effectively prepare the athlete's muscles dominant in the frontal and transverse planes (Boling et al., 2009; Frederickson et al., 2000), nor does it affect the co-contractions required to perform efficiently at varying levels of speed (Clark, 2000; Janusevicius et al., 2017; Macrum et al., 2012; Rhea et al., 2009). Thus, this kind of single-plane training elevates injury risks (Boling et al., 2009).

✔ CHECK IT OUT

As an illustration of dominance in one plane with controlled movements in the other two planes, consider the action of sprinting. Sprinting is the culmination of powerful extension of the hip, knee, and ankle in the sagittal plane; counter-rotation of the hips and shoulders in the transverse plane; and controlled and resisted hip adduction in the frontal plane. Collectively, these actions result in unilateral sagittal plane movement.

Efficient movement in the intended direction requires efforts to buffer the unwanted effects of movements in the other two planes. It is important to realize that movement occurs in all three planes of motion at every joint. When sprinting, the goal is not to eliminate movements in the frontal and transverse planes, but rather to minimize overaccentuated movement and lessen the detracting impacts of the desired movement in the sagittal plane.

POSTURE

The summation of the positions that all joints of the body are in at any given time.

TRAINING WITH OPTIMAL POSTURE

Posture is a dynamic controlling quality, altering the neural input to the acting musculature (Wilson et al., 1996). Therefore, the optimal alignment of each segment of the HMS is a cornerstone of any functional sports performance program. If one component of the HMS is out of alignment, other components have to compensate for it (Gomes-Neto et al., 2017; Knox et al., 2017; Park et al., 2021; Pourheidary et al., 2019; Sueki, 2013), decreasing neuromuscular efficiency and increasing the chance of injury (Beckman & Buchanan, 1995; Bullock-Saxon, 1994; Padua et al., 2012a).

> ⚠ **CRITICAL**
>
> Allowing an athlete to perform exercises with poor lumbar posture can result in muscle imbalances (Hodges et al., 1996) and injury (Cibulka et al., 1998; Hodges et al., 1996; McGill et al., 2009; O'Sullivan et al., 1998; Richardson et al., 2002).

Poor posture during training can lead to muscle imbalances, joint dysfunctions, and impairment of movement (McGill, 2004; Padua et al., 2012b; Sahrmann, 2011). Training with proper posture ensures optimal results and decreases the risk of developing muscle imbalances, joint dysfunctions, and tissue overload (Comerford & Mottram, 2001; Huxel Bliven & Anderson, 2013; McKeon et al., 2008; Wilson et al., 1996). Poor training posture also includes poor exercise technique. For example, during the barbell squat, some athletes have a predisposition to adopt a wide-foot stance combined with a toe-out lateral rotation posture. This stance, which increases the base of support and allows for greater control of postural sway (Lorenzetti et al., 2018), also pre-shortens the piriformis and increases activation of the biceps femoris and lateral gastrocnemius (Clark, 2000). Although the athlete's overall performance is temporarily improved when measured by total

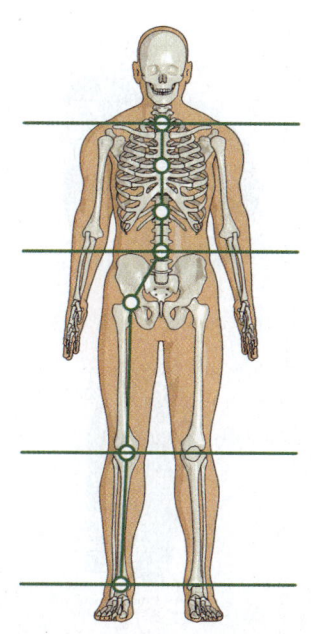 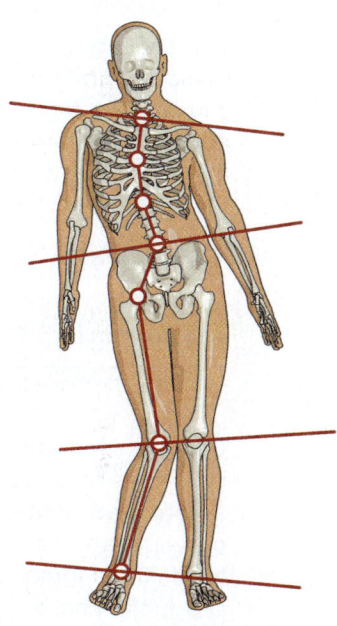

© SKYKIDKID/Shutterstock

resistance moved, this positioning negatively affects joint structures (Clark, 2000; Han et al., 2013; Lorenzetti et al., 2018; Nyland et al., 2002) and facilitates altered movement patterns (Boling et al., 2009; Eckard et al., 2018; Ford et al., 2003; Hewett et al., 2005; Powers, 2003) that elevate injury risks (Hewett & Bates, 2017; Hewett et al., 2005). Although a slight toe-out position and wide stance can be valuable for competitive weightlifting, a neutral hip position with the feet facing forward is recommended during most training (Han et al., 2013; Hewett & Bates, 2017; Lorenzetti et al., 2018). A functional, integrated training program that involves the entire HMS ensures that an athlete maintains structural integrity while performing exercises correctly and with proper postural control (Cobb et al., 2014; McGill et al., 2009).

TRAINING FOR OPTIMAL MUSCLE BALANCE

Muscles function optimally from an ideal predetermined length or an optimal **length–tension relationship** (Neumann, 2017). An athlete's length–tension relationship is altered when a muscle is stimulated at a length less than or greater than this optimal

> **LENGTH–TENSION RELATIONSHIP** →
>
> The resting length of a muscle and the tension the muscle can produce at this resting length.

length, altering the body's **force–couple relationships** and joint kinematics (Janda, 1978; Panjabi, 1992a; Sahrmann, 2011). Subtle changes in posture, pattern overload, injury, and decreased neuromuscular efficiency can alter the resting length of a muscle (Medeiros & Lima, 2017), which can then lead to muscle imbalances (Gilchrist et al., 2008; Medeiros & Martini, 2018). Muscle overactivity, adaptive muscle shortening, or both can cause **altered reciprocal inhibition** and **synergistic dominance** (Barr et al., 2005; Barr et al., 2007; Frederickson et al., 2000; Hides et al., 1994; Hungerford et al., 2003; Janda, 1978). Altered reciprocal inhibition decreases force production by the prime mover and leads to compensation by the synergists (Janda, 1978; Nyland et al., 2002). Synergistic dominance leads to altered movement patterns and decreased neuromuscular control (Hungerford et al., 2003; Janda, 1978; Nyland et al., 2002). The Sports Performance Coach must plan and execute all sports performance programs to develop optimal muscle balance (Freitas et al., 2018), thereby ensuring that athletes maintain the structural integrity of the entire HMS through its optimal range of motion (**Figure 4.7**).

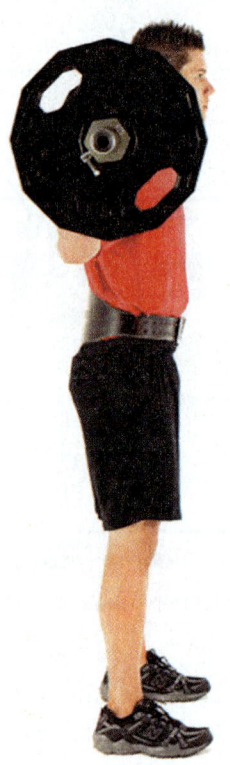
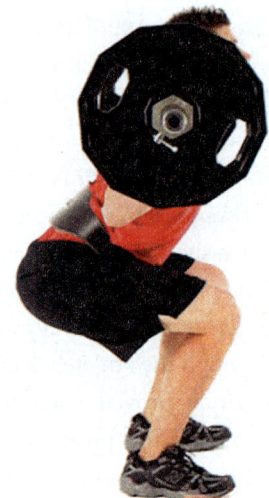

FIGURE 4.7 Training with Proper Technique

TRAINING FOR OPTIMAL MUSCLE FUNCTION

Muscles function eccentrically, isometrically, and concentrically in all three planes of motion (Janda, 1978; Neumann, 2010, 2017; Sahrmann, 2011). All movements are complex events orchestrated by the CNS. The CNS executes preprogrammed patterns of movements that are modified in response to gravity, ground reaction forces, and momentum. For example, the CNS allows the gluteus maximus to work *eccentrically* to decelerate hip flexion, internal rotation, adduction, and tibial internal rotation; *isometrically* to stabilize the sacroiliac joint; and *concentrically* to extend and externally rotate the hip (Janda, 1978; Neumann, 2010, 2017; Sahrmann, 2011). The typical way to strengthen the gluteus maximus is to have the athlete perform sagittal plane hip flexion and extension exercises (e.g., squats, lunges, step-ups) with little attention to transverse-plane eccentric function or the stabilization capacity of the gluteus maximus. It is important to remember that muscles have anatomic individuality but lack functional individuality (Neumann, 2010, 2017; Sahrmann, 2011).

To efficiently and effectively prepare athletes for optimal performance and injury prevention, an integrated sports performance training program must include the following elements:

- Focus on multiplanar training while activating the entire spectrum of muscle contraction (eccentric, isometric, and concentric) through the optimal range of motion
- Incorporate multiple modalities (free weights, dumbbells, cables, machines, tubing, medicine balls)
- Include flexibility, core, balance, plyometrics, speed, agility, quickness, integrated resistance training, and sports-specific conditioning (Clark, 2000; Gilchrist et al., 2008; Palmer et al., 2015; Wiggins et al., 2016; Willardson, 2004)

> ### ✔ CHECK IT OUT
>
> Because a muscle's action is dependent on the body's position and the muscle's interaction with gravity and the ground, the CNS recruits an appropriate, coordinated muscle response in preparation for the movement task (Kita et al., 2019; Maniar et al., 2018; Sueki et al., 2013). A seemingly simple task, such as reaching for a door handle, requires complex coordination of trunk and hip stabilizers: the forward motion of the arm and hand toward the door handle and the grip motion with fine motor control of the hand and fingers.

SYSTEMATIC AND PROGRESSIVE TRAINING

Many traditional strength and conditioning programs focus on isolated, uniplanar exercises to maximize absolute strength gains and hypertrophy. However, the HMS evolved using all three planes of motion as an interdependent unit, and the CNS naturally optimizes the selection of muscle synergies to perform integrated movement patterns (Ford et al., 2003; Herman et al., 2012; Ireland et al., 2003; Lee et al., 2001; McClay & Manal, 1999; Sahrmann, 2011). As a result, isolated training does little to improve overall athletic performance. In contrast, training that exploits integrated, functional movement patterns targets synergistic muscles to regulate isometric, concentric, and eccentric force while dynamically stabilizing the entire HMS in all three planes of motion.

This type of training maximizes motor unit recruitment and facilitates a greater overall training response (Thompson et al., 2007; Vera-Garcia et al., 2000). The athlete who applies an integrated, functional approach to training develops high levels of dynamic flexibility, core strength, neuromuscular control, power, speed, agility, quickness, and functional strength (Caraffa et al., 1996; Hewett et al., 1996; Hewett et al., 1999; Luebbers, 2003). In addition, an athlete could develop similar, or even greater, levels of hypertrophy following improved motor unit recruitment. The primary goals of a sports performance training program are to prevent injury and increase athletic performance measures, including flexibility, core, balance, power, speed, agility, quickness, strength,

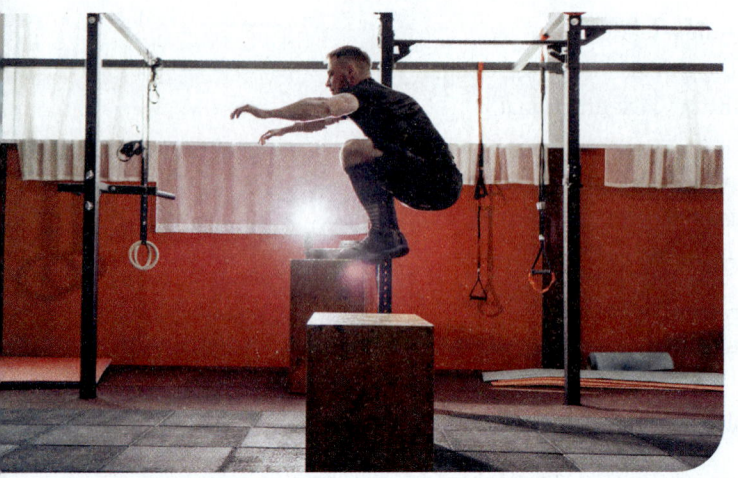
© Mirage_studio/Shutterstock

and sport-specific cardiovascular efficiency. The Sports Performance Coach can use various methods to stimulate these improvements in athletes. By integrating each training component into the training plan, the coach offers athletes the best route to improved performance.

When designing an integrated performance program, the Sports Performance Coach must perform a comprehensive sports performance assessment, using data to evaluate the demands of a given sport. Above all, the program must be safe. Choosing the components of a sports performance program requires careful selection of exercises that meet the specific criteria for the particular athlete.

Exercises in a sports performance training plan must be progressive, be proprioceptively challenging, stress multiple planes of motion, integrate multiple joints when possible, challenge the entire contraction velocity spectrum (slow, fast, explosive), and be as sport-specific as possible. The Sports Performance Coach needs to follow a progressive, systematic, functional continuum to allow optimal performance adaptations. The following key concepts are necessary for proper exercise progression:

- Slow to fast
- Simple to complex
- Familiar to unfamiliar
- Low force to high force
- Eyes open to eyes closed
- Static to dynamic
- Correct execution of increased repetitions, sets, and intensity

With such an approach, athletes can develop optimal levels of functional strength and dynamic stabilization. Neural adaptations become the focus of the program instead of striving for absolute strength gains. Increasing the proprioceptive demands in a multisensory environment (e.g., stability ball, foam pad, balance disc, wobble board) is an important concept in athletic development. The Sports Performance Coach must also emphasize quality before quantity of training and seek to manage the sensory information stimulating the athlete's CNS. If athletes train with poor technique and neuromuscular control, they may develop poor motor patterns and stabilization. Therefore, an athlete's program must focus on the functional continuum.

 COACH'S CORNER

To determine if a program is functional, answer the following questions:

- Is it progressive?
- Is it systematic?
- Is it sport-specific?
- Is it integrated?
- Is it proprioceptively challenging?
- Is it based on functional anatomy and evidence-based practices?

UTILIZATION OF THE STRETCH–SHORTENING CYCLE

Many sports that require sprinting, cutting, jumping, and throwing rely heavily on integrating an athlete's speed, strength, and power (Adams et al., 1992; Baker, 1996; Gehri et al., 1998; Hewett et al., 1996; Luebbers et al., 2003; Rumpf et al., 2013). Therefore, explosive force and force reduction are vital factors in athletic performance.

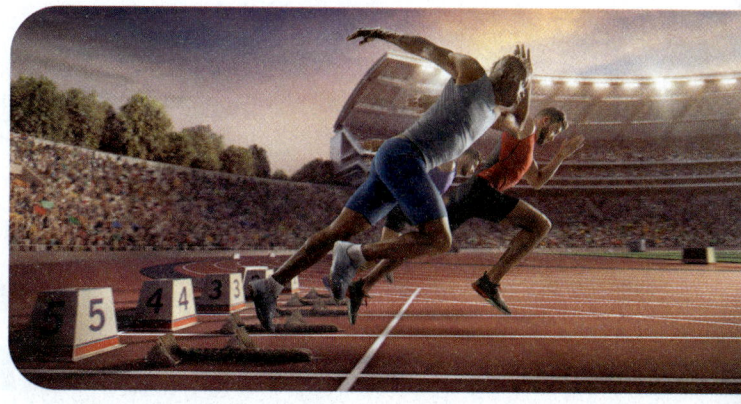

© Alex Kravtsov/Shutterstock

Specific exercises increase power output and explosiveness and train muscles to do more work in less time (Holcomb et al., 1996; Luebbers et al., 2003; Wilson et al., 1993; Wilson et al., 1996). This increase in power occurs when an athlete utilizes the **stretch–shortening cycle**—that is, the transition of an activated muscle from an eccentric contraction (deceleration) to a rapid, concentric contraction (acceleration) (Bosco et al., 1981; Bosco et al., 1982; Chmielewski et al., 2005; Rassier & Herzog, 2005; Turner & Jeffreys, 2010).

The rapid eccentric contraction creates a stretch reflex, storing potential energy used to produce a concentric contraction more forceful than would otherwise be generated by the resting muscle (Luebbers et al., 2003; Potteiger et al., 1999). The shorter the amount of time between the eccentric and concentric contractions means the greater amount of potential energy is stored and becomes available for more concentric force production (Bosco et al., 1981; Bosco et al., 1982; Chmielewski et al., 2005; Clutch et al., 1983; Hewett et al., 1996; Wagner & Kocak, 1987). Stabilization strength, core strength, and neuromuscular efficiency help to control the time between the eccentric and concentric contractions (Clark, 2000). When an athlete optimizes eccentric strength, neuromuscular efficiency, and stabilization strength, they realize greater concentric force production (Chimera et al., 2004; Hewett et al., 1996; Hewett et al., 1999; Luebbers et al., 2003; Sherry & Best, 2004). Thus, exercises that accentuate the stretch–shortening cycle are valuable in an athlete's overall development (Caraffa et al., 1996; Chimera et al., 2004; Frederickson et al., 2000; Hewett et al., 1996; Hewett et al., 1999; Junge et al., 2002; Luebbers et al., 2003; Paterno et al., 2004).

> ### STRETCH– SHORTENING CYCLE →
>
> A muscle reflex referred to as the myotatic or stretch reflex that imparts the ability to store and release elastic energy of the tendons.

ASSESSMENT-BASED TRAINING

Movement impairments at slow, controlled speeds do not improve when loads are increased (Bagherian et al., 2018; van Melick et al., 2019). Therefore, the Sports Performance Coach should use validated assessments to evaluate movement quality before advancing a training program. Failing to assess movement quality can impose training stress that exceeds the athlete's tissue (muscle, ligament, bone) tolerance, resulting in musculoskeletal injury (Bagherian et al., 2018). Muscle and joint imbalances are related to poor movement quality and affect strength (Bell et al., 2008; DiStefano et al., 2013; Stanley et al., 2019), range of motion (Bell et al., 2012; Macrum et al., 2012; Mauntel et al., 2013), and movement efficiency (Macrum et al., 2012; Mauntel et al., 2014). These factors combine to increase injury risk (Eckard et al., 2018; Kollock et al., 2016; Rabin et al., 2014).

After identifying the attributes of poor movement, the Sports Performance Coach must utilize an evidence-based approach to improve the athlete's movement quality. Muscle imbalances can lead to reciprocal inhibition, synergistic dominance, and altered movement patterns. In contrast, a targeted and individualized approach to corrective exercise will increase muscle activation and improve overall muscle efficiency (Bagherian et al., 2018; Bell et al., 2012; Frederickson et al., 2000; Hewett et al., 2005; Sullivan et al.,

2013; Verrelst et al., 2013). One of the purest forms of performance enhancement seeks to eliminate factors that limit athletic performance. To do so, the Sports Performance Coach can emphasize exercise techniques that promote efficient biomechanical movement patterns. For example, the ball bridge and single-leg squat exercises provide the optimal neuromuscular activation patterns to eventually improve posture in a barbell squat.

LESSON 4: ELEMENTS OF COMPREHENSIVE TRAINING
INTEGRATED TRAINING COMPONENTS

The Sports Performance Coach must take a broad, multivariate approach to match all the training and competition demands of athletic performance. Diligently developing the integral components of a comprehensive training program can help athletes improve their performance and reduce their risk of injury. Although deficiencies identified from movement quality assessments can indicate a need to highlight one component more than others, a complete integrated training program includes the following elements:

- Flexibility training
- Core training
- Balance training
- Plyometric training
- Speed, agility, and quickness training
- Resistance training
- Energy systems development

FLEXIBILITY TRAINING

Muscle imbalances and poor flexibility decrease performance and increase the risk of injury (Baxter et al., 2017; Cibulka et al., 1998; Knapik et al., 1991; Nadler, Malanga, Bartoli, et al., 2002; Nadler, Malanga, Feinberg, et al., 2002; Sherry & Best, 2004; Witvrouw et al., 2003). Working on the complete flexibility continuum (i.e., static, active, and dynamic stretching) is an effective technique for improving range of motion (ROM) (Baxter et al., 2017; Behm et al., 2014; Blackburn et al., 2004; Davis et al., 2005; Hanten et al., 2000; Kokkonen et al., 2007; Shrier, 2004; Winters et al., 2004). Therefore, the Sports Performance Coach should include all forms of flexibility training in a comprehensive training program to develop optimal functional ROM and neuromuscular efficiency (Bell-Jenie et al., 2016; Brooks & Cressey, 2013). The most effective programs utilize a chronic approach to stretching to optimize joint ROM, reduce stiffness, and decrease stretch-induced pain (Freitas et al., 2018; Medeiros & Lima, 2017; Medeiros & Martini, 2018; Riley & Van Dyke, 2012). Static stretching, followed by dynamic movements that require active muscular contraction and multi-segment coordination, allows an athlete to develop neuromuscular control (Riley & Van Dyke, 2012).

However, improvements made to tissue extensibility will revert to pretraining levels if the athlete discontinues flexibility

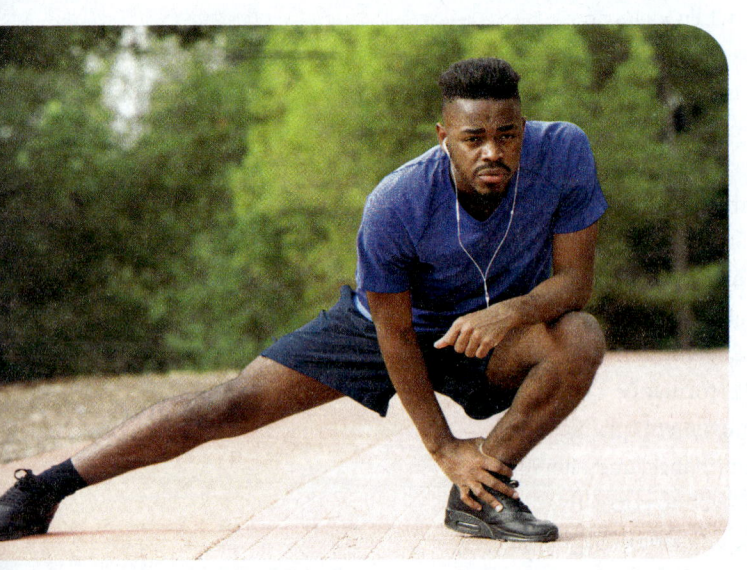

training (Padua et al., 2012b). Therefore, an athlete must perform passive stretching daily—the principle of reversibility kicks in after 24 hours (Riley & Van Dyke, 2012). In addition to enhancing mobility, flexibility training improves muscular contractions and functional movement tasks (Medeiros & Lima, 2017).

CORE TRAINING

Core training is the foundation on which a progressive sports performance training program is built. Unfortunately, many athletes develop the strength, power, and endurance in their prime movers but neglect to develop adequate neuromuscular control, strength, power, and endurance in their core (Afyon, 2014; Barr et al., 2005; Barr et al., 2007; Heiderscheit & Sherry, 2007; Hodges & Richardson, 1997; Hungerford et al., 2003; McGill, 2001; McGill & Cholewicki, 2001; Richardson et al., 2002; Taskin, 2016; Yapici, 2016). Core training is a systematic and progressive approach to developing muscle balance, neuromuscular efficiency, strength, power, and endurance in an athlete's core musculature (Abdelraouf & Abdel-Aziem, 2016; Barr et al., 2007; Clark, 2000; Heiderscheit & Sherry, 2007; Wilson et al., 2006). An athlete's core must function optimally to harness the strength and power of the prime movers (Bagherian et al., 2017; Huxel Bliven & Anderson, 2013; McGill, 2004; Skundric et al., 2021). A stable, strong, and reactively efficient core must be the cornerstone of all integrated sports performance and injury prevention programs (Barr et al., 2007; Heiderscheit & Sherry, 2007; Peate et al., 2007).

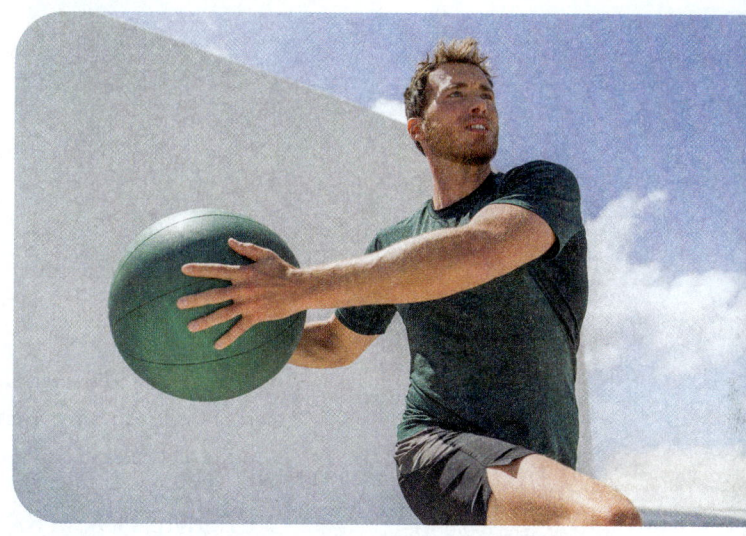
© Maridav/Shutterstock

BALANCE TRAINING

Balance training is a systematic and progressive training process designed to develop neuromuscular efficiency (Hewett & Bates, 2017). This form of training in a proprioceptively enriched environment (e.g., standing on a half foam roll, foam pad, or balance disc) stimulates neuromuscular adaptations, leading to improved intermuscular and intramuscular coordination; that is, it recruits the right muscles to work at the right time with the right amount of force for the desired outcome (Behm et al., 2015; Caldemeyer et al., 2020; Comerford & Mottram, 2001; Cruz-Dias et al., 2015; Hewett & Bates, 2017). **Intramuscular coordination** comprises the ability of the CNS to improve motor unit recruitment, **rate coding**, and synchronization within an individual muscle. In contrast, intermuscular coordination is the ability of the entire HMS and each muscular subsystem to work interdependently to improve movement efficiency. Improved intramuscular and intermuscular efficiency yields greater recruitment of the agonist musculature and less inhibition from the antagonist musculature, resulting in greater force production (Baker, 1996; Bruhn et al., 2004; Cosio-Lima et al., 2003; Gebel et al., 2018; Hahn et al., 1998; Lesinski et al., 2015; Myer et al., 2006; Yaggie & Campbell, 2006), preferred movement patterns (Olson et al., 2011; Padua et al., 2012b), and injury prevention (Caraffa et al., 1996; Chimera et al., 2004; Frederickson et al., 2000; Gebel et al., 2018; Hewett et al., 1996; Junge et al., 2002; Kovacs et al., 2014; Mandelbaum et al., 2005; Paterno et al., 2004; Schiftan et al., 2014).

Athletes who invoke high levels of neuromuscular control during the performance of common athletic tasks tend to demonstrate smaller magnitudes of frontal and transverse

INTRA-MUSCULAR COORDINATION →

The ability of the neuromuscular system to allow optimal levels of motor unit recruitment and synchronization within a muscle.

RATE CODING →

The speed of the neurological message sent by the brain to the motor units it desires to activate.

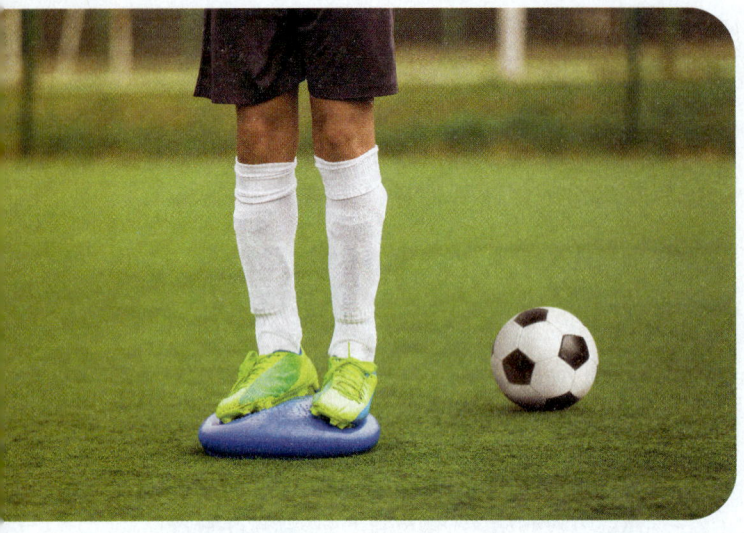
© Matimix/Shutterstock

plane compensations during movements that dominate the sagittal plane as well as decreased tensile loading of the anterior cruciate ligament (ACL) (Hewett & Bates, 2017). Exercise technique is critical to delivering consistent, desired outcomes.

Neuromuscular training improves overall multi-segmental joint biomechanics (e.g., reduced knee valgus moments, improved control and coordination of hip internal and external rotation), which lowers injury risk. These neuromuscular improvements also lead to enhanced performance (increased strength, jumping performance, reaction time, and speed) (Chappell & Limpisvasti, 2008; Hewett & Bates, 2017; Myer et al., 2006). Such training involves more than simple balancing-type exercises. Specifically, activating the hip musculature works to maintain the body's center of mass over a dynamically changing base of support (Clark, 2000). Poor neuromuscular control leads to early and excessive movement of the trunk and deviations from the center of mass, thereby extending the moment arm acting on the lower-extremity joints, and leading to excessive frontal plane loading of the knee (Di Stasi et al., 2013).

PLYOMETRIC TRAINING

Enhanced athletic performance is related to the **rate of force production** (Luebbers et al., 2003) regulated by the CNS. The demands of training should occur at the same speeds encountered during functional activities (Chmielewski et al., 2005), so that the system learns how rapidly force production is required (Devita & Skelly, 1992). Thus, the HMS moves only within a defined range of speeds set by the CNS (Chmielewski et al., 2005). Most human movement involves the stretch–shortening cycle, in which deceleration (stretch) transitions to acceleration (shortening). The HMS must react quickly following an eccentric contraction to produce a concentric contraction and impart the necessary force and acceleration in the proper direction (Chimera et al., 2004). Plyometric training overloads the stretch–shortening cycle (e.g., box jumps, squat jumps, hops) to enhance neuromuscular efficiency and the rate of force production and reduce neuromuscular inhibition by stimulating the proprioceptive mechanisms and elastic properties of the HMS (Adiguzel & Günay, 2016; Bedoya et al., 2015; Chimera et al., 2004; Hermassi et al., 2014; Hopper et al., 2017).

Reactive training is effectively an extension of the balance-training continuum, with the addition of a focus on the rate of force production and force reduction. Here, the emphasis is on progressive plyometric training and landing efficiency. The end objective is improved multi-segmental joint control as kinetic forces are distributed across joints through active connective tissues (muscles, tendons) and are less likely to be absorbed by more passive, stabilizing tissues (ligaments, cartilage) (Clark, 2000; Hewett & Bates, 2017; Padua et al., 2012a, 2012b).

Muscle force production plays a crucial role in overall performance and is often measured in terms of muscular strength. Although it is certainly important, muscular strength is just one element of functional performance. Other factors, such as flexibility, joint mobility, endurance, stability, neuromuscular efficiency, speed and agility, power, and multiplanar movement quality, are also critical elements of functional performance (DiStefano et al., 2013; Palmer et al., 2015). All of these elements work together to allow the athlete to produce force, dynamically stabilize multiple joint segments, and reduce

RATE OF FORCE PRODUCTION →

Ability of the muscles to exert maximal force output in a minimal amount of time; also known as rate of force development.

forces efficiently in all planes of motion under varying load conditions (Clark, 2000).

SPEED, AGILITY, AND QUICKNESS TRAINING

Human movement occurs in all planes of motion at varying speeds in response to multiple stimuli. The ability to change speed and direction and react appropriately to all stimuli often makes the difference between injury and safety and success or failure (Nadler, Malanga, Bartoli, et al., 2002; Nadler, Malanga, Feinberg, et al., 2002; Padua & Marshall, 2006; Paul et al., 2016). An athlete can improve speed, change of direction, and reaction time through proper training strategies (Mills & Taunton, 2003; Rhea et al., 2009). Collectively, these strategies are known as speed, agility, and quickness training. Each of these abilities is an independent quality, yet all are related and dependent on the other to optimize human function.

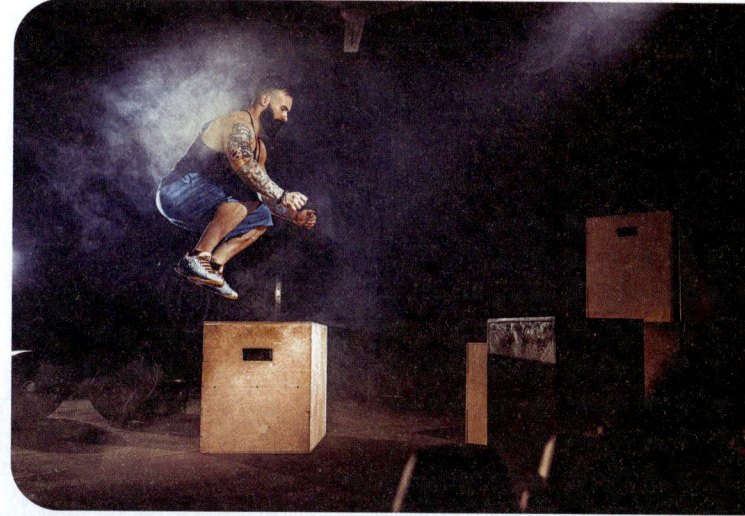

© SOK Studio/Shutterstock

RESISTANCE TRAINING

It is important for the Sports Performance Coach to support athletes' continued performance efforts and levels in a safe manner. Muscular fitness is important for both athletic performance and injury prevention (Harries et al., 2012; Peterson et al., 2004). It is expressed in various forms, including maximal strength, relative strength, strength endurance, speed strength, stabilization strength, and functional strength (Bird et al., 2005; Clark, 2000; Kraemer & Ratamess, 2004; Peterson et al., 2004). Resistance training—a general term that refers to exercise requiring the individual to exert force against a resistance—is a superior modality for increasing muscle strength, local muscular endurance, power, hypertrophy, and motor performance.

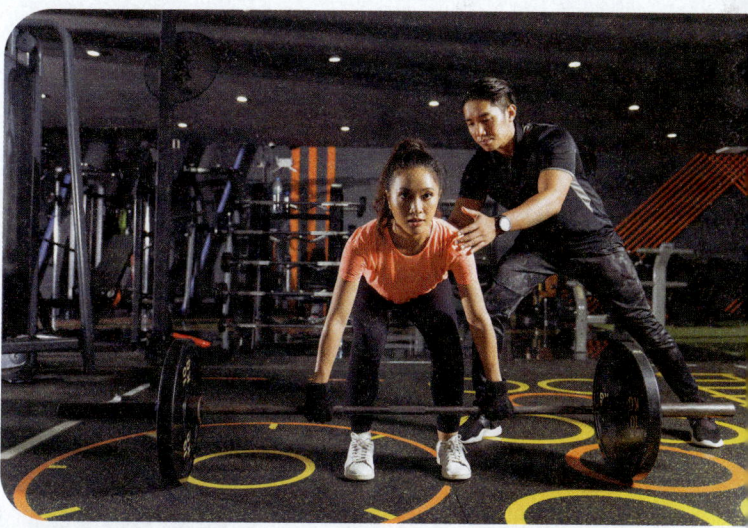

© TORWAISTUDIO/Shutterstock

Resistance training promotes improvements in all of these areas among athletes (Harries et al., 2012; Peterson et al., 2004) and is used to support optimal development and performance (Peterson et al., 2005; Rhea et al., 2009). Strength training can be sensitive to the speed of movement or exercise. Heavy resistance training causes greater strength development at slow speeds than at fast speeds, whereas faster movement training causes greater gains in strength at faster speeds (Janusevicius et al., 2017). Resistance training improves an athlete's ability to exert force, but by itself it does not alter lower-extremity movement patterns (DiStefano et al., 2013; Herman et al., 2008). Therefore, the Sports Performance Coach who is creating resistance training programs must incorporate integrated training principles to develop a comprehensive performance program that ensures each athlete achieves optimal performance and reduces their risk of injury.

ENERGY SYSTEMS DEVELOPMENT

Among the various components composing an athlete's total physical fitness program, metabolic energy system training is perhaps the most studied, misunderstood, and underrated. Energy system efficiency is the foundation for the development of overall fitness and athletic performance (Davis et al., 2005; Plews et al., 2013). Increases in efficiency, regardless of primary energy system reliance, improve training readiness and athletic performance (Davis et al., 2005; Plews et al., 2013). High-intensity interval training accelerates the metabolic changes, such as increased muscle oxidative capacity, typically seen with traditional high-volume endurance training (Gibala & McGee, 2008). While Sports Performance Coaches must be creative in designing metabolic energy system conditioning programs, athletes must know how to start a safe program that improves endurance while avoiding overtraining and minimizing their risk for injury (**Table 4.2**).

TABLE 4.2 Metabolic Energy System Conditioning Training

	Immediate Energy System (Phosphagen)	Anaerobic (Glycolytic)	Aerobic (Oxidative)
Intensity	90%–100%	30%–75%	20%–30%
Duration	5–10 seconds	1–3 minutes	>3 minutes
Work–rest ratio	1:5–1:20	1:2–1:4	0–1:3
Fuel source	Adenosine triphosphate (ATP) in muscle cells	Glycogen	Glycogen and fatty acids
Sport example	Short distance sprints	Intermittent bursts in soccer or basketball	Long-distance running

LESSON 5 : OPTIMUM PERFORMANCE TRAINING
INTRODUCTION TO THE OPTIMUM PERFORMANCE TRAINING MODEL

> **PHASE POTENTIATION** →
>
> The adaptations gained in one training phase enhance adaptations in future training phases, such that the order in which training phases are implemented assumes great importance.

The Optimum Performance Training (OPT) Model is a process of programming that systematically progresses any athlete toward any performance goal. This method is a phase potentiation model. **Phase potentiation** occurs when adaptations in one training phase enhance adaptations in future training phases; therefore, the order in which training phases are implemented is important. The OPT Model is built on a foundation of stabilization training principles (**Figure 4.8**). With the acquisition of proper levels of stabilization, an athlete can then progress into the strength level of the training model.

Program design models that include a multisensory, multimodal approach improve movement quality and performance outcomes in athlete populations, particularly when training time reaches 45 minutes in duration (DiStefano et al., 2013). That achievement indicates that even those with good movement quality can still improve multiplanar movement efficiency. As the athlete obtains ample strength, they progress into the power level of the training model.

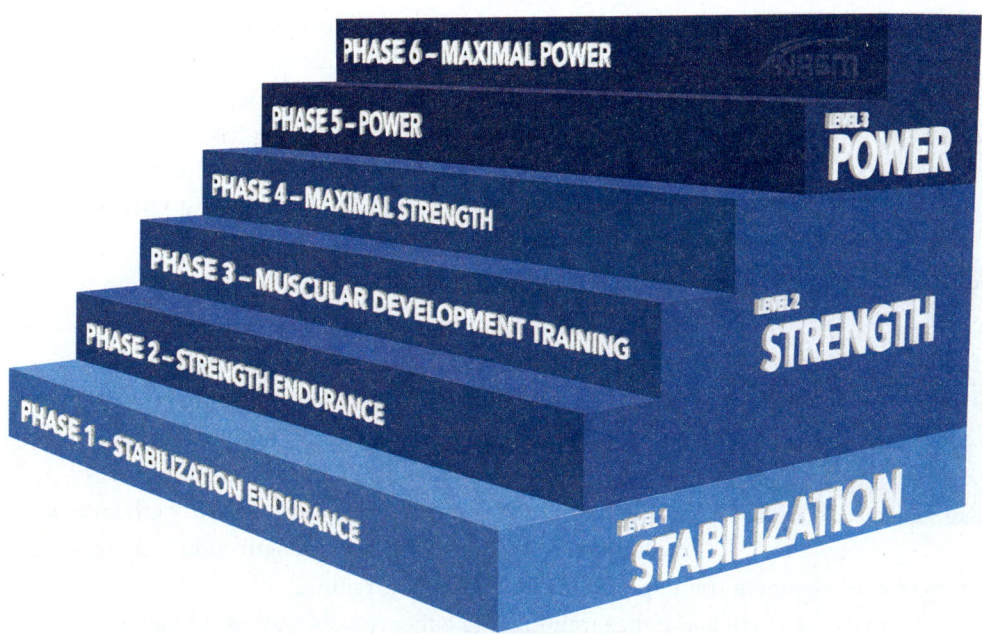

FIGURE 4.8 The OPT Model

SCIENTIFIC RATIONALE FOR THE OPT MODEL

The OPT Model is divided into stabilization, strength, and power levels. Each level is built upon and dependent on the prior level. Within each level, there are specific phases of training that an athlete progresses through:

- Phase 1: stabilization endurance training
- Phase 2: strength endurance training
- Phase 3: muscular development training
- Phase 4: maximal strength training
- Phase 5: power training
- Phase 6: maximal power training

The Sports Performance Coach must understand the scientific rationale behind each phase to properly use the OPT Model.

STABILIZATION → STRENGTH

The ability of the stabilizing muscles to provide dynamic joint stabilization and postural equilibrium during functional activities.

STABILIZATION LEVEL

The stabilization level consists of one training phase: stabilization endurance training. The main focus of this phase is to increase **stabilization strength** and develop optimal communication between the athlete's nervous and muscular systems.

The progression for the stabilization level is proprioceptively based. This means difficulty is increased by introducing more challenges to the balance and stabilization systems of the body versus simply increasing the load (Behm & Colado, 2013).

An athlete must do stabilization training before advancing into the strength and power phases of the OPT Model, as research shows that inefficient stabilization leads to altered force production in muscles, stress at the joints,

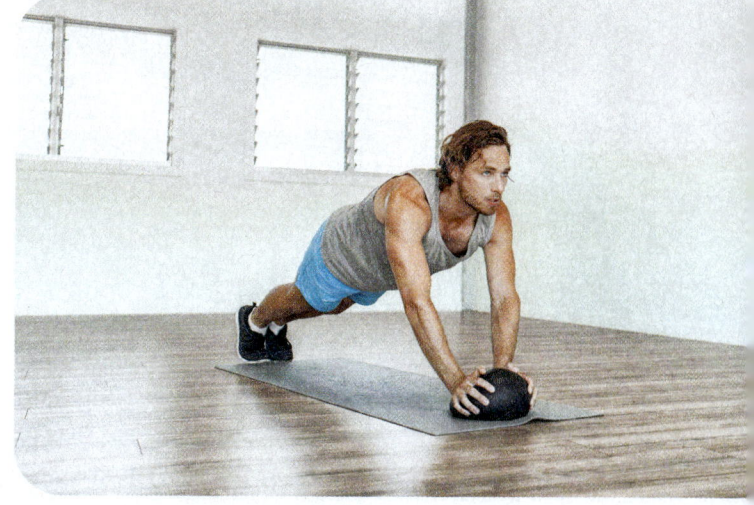

© Maridav/Shutterstock

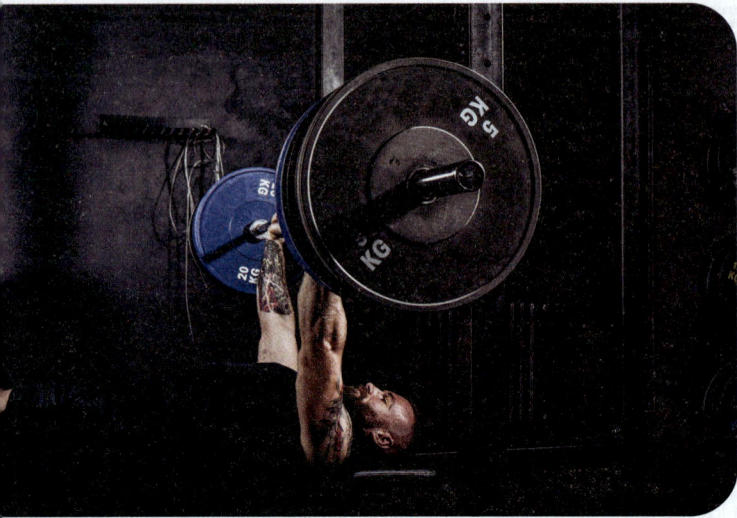

© Srdjan Randjelovic/Shutterstock

tissue overload, and injury (Edgerton et al., 1996; McGill, 2001; O'Sullivan et al., 1997; O'Sullivan et al., 1998). This level prepares the athlete's body for more demanding exercise by improving movement quality, increasing flexibility and muscle extensibility, and increasing the joint and postural stabilization mechanisms (Bagherian et al., 2018; Behm et al., 2015).

STRENGTH LEVEL

The strength level of training follows the successful completion of the stabilization level. The emphasis in this level is to enhance stabilization strength while increasing prime mover strength. This is also the level of training an athlete progresses to if their goal is muscular development (hypertrophy) or maximal strength (lifting heavy loads). The strength level of training consists of three phases: strength endurance training, muscular development training, and maximal strength training.

The goal of strength endurance training is to enhance stabilization, strength, and endurance while increasing prime mover strength. These two adaptations are accomplished by performing two exercises in a **superset** manner with similar joint dynamics. One exercise is traditional and performed in a stable environment (e.g., bench press), and the other is an integrated exercise performed in a less stable environment (e.g., suspension trainer push-up). The underlying premise is to work the prime movers predominantly with the first exercise to elicit prime mover strength. Then, by immediately following with an exercise that challenges the stabilizers, an athlete enhances their neuromuscular and postural stabilization endurance and dynamic joint stabilization (Ebben, 2002).

Other phases of the strength level are muscular development training for muscle growth and maximal strength training to increase maximal prime mover strength.

> ### SUPERSET →
>
> Two exercises performed back-to-back in rapid succession with minimal to no rest.

POWER LEVEL

The power level of the OPT Model emphasizes the development of speed and power. The speed and power with which athletes produce muscular actions determine successful performance in most sports. This level of training is necessary to enhance the speed spectrum that the athlete's body is allowed to operate within. The neuromuscular system dictates the speed with which muscles exert force. Therefore, the body can move only within a set range of speed determined by the nervous system (Devita & Skelly, 1992; Voight & Draovitch, 1991). This range is achieved through two phases of training: power training and maximal power training. The premise behind power training is the execution of a more traditional strength exercise (e.g., barbell squat) in a superset with a plyometric power exercise of similar joint dynamics (e.g., squat jumps). These exercises enhance prime mover strength while also improving the rate of force production. Maximal power training is the next progression for an athlete to produce maximal acceleration and rate of force production. This training phase is typically reserved for high-level athletes who require maximal levels of power.

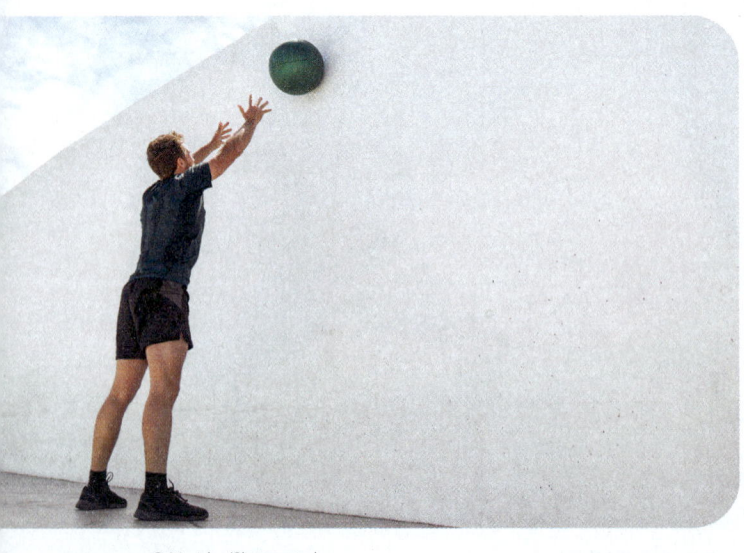

© Maridav/Shutterstock

SUMMARY

Although improvements in strength, power, and speed are often highlighted in athlete development, programming for today's athletes must also address factors such as appropriate forms of flexibility, increasing stabilization strength and endurance, and training in a multiplanar environment. All of these forms of training are specifically designed to follow the physiological principles of the HMS and to provide a systematic progression in training while minimizing injury and maximizing the athlete's results.

Although the scientific support for strength training from a traditional sense continues to evolve, it is imperative to maintain a systematic and progressive focus on all the other elements of success in sports actions. In contrast, functional activities are multiplanar movements that require acceleration, deceleration, and dynamic stabilization. The barbell squat, for example, demonstrates the "function" of passive hip flexion and active hip extension—though this does not imply that traditional exercises do not have a significant role in an integrated training approach. Every exercise supports the development of a primary physiologic outcome (e.g., stabilization, endurance, strength, power, speed). The knowledge base for appropriate program design and manipulation of training variables continues to expand as new findings, replication of old concepts, and new visions with the latest technologies emerge, and it should fuel the Sports Performance Coach's ongoing education and interest in this approach.

KEY TAKEAWAYS

- Integrated training programs are rooted in scientific principles of training, which provide the background and context for program development.
- A comprehensive sport-specific program must account for basic training principles, as well as overtraining and fatigue.
- Sport-specific training principles must consider the principles of specificity, progressive overload, variation, individualization, transfer effect, interference effect, and reversibility.
- Integrated sports performance training enhances an athlete's ability to rapidly produce force, reduce force, and stabilize joints in all planes of motion in an unpredictable environment.
- Integrated training programs focus on training in planes of motion, with optimal posture, in a progressive and systematic fashion and based on the results of assessments.
- The OPT Model is a programming process that systematically progresses any athlete to any performance goal using phase potentiation. Phase potentiation occurs when adaptations in one training phase enhance adaptations in future training phases. Thus, this model emphasizes the order in which the training phases are implemented.
- The OPT Model utilizes a sequence of training phases that progress athletes from stabilization to strength and finally to power.

REFERENCES

Abdelraouf, O. R., & Abdel-aziem, A. A. (2016). The relationship between core nonspecific low back pain. *International Journal of Sports Physical Therapy, 11*(3), 337–344.

Adams, K., O'Shea, J. P., O'Shea, K. L., & Climstein, M. (1992). The effect of six weeks of squat, plyometric and squat-plyometric training on power production. *Journal of Applied Sport Sciences, 6,* 36–41.

Adiguzel, N. S., & Günay, M. (2016). The effect of eight weeks plyometric training on anaerobic power, counter movement jumping and isokinetic strength in 15–18 years basketball players. *International Journal of Environmental and Science Education, 11*(10), 3241–3250.

Afyon, Y. A. (2014). Effect of core training on 16 year-old soccer players. *Educational Research and Reviews, 9*(23), 1275–1279.

Andersen, L. L., Andersen, J. L., Magnusson, S. P., & Aagaard, P. (2005). Neuromuscular adaptations to detraining following resistance training in previously untrained subjects. *European Journal of Applied Physiology, 93*(5), 511–518. https://doi.org/10.1007/s00421-004-1297-9

Bagherian, S., Ghasempoor, K., Rahnama, N., & Wikstrom, E. A. (2017). The effect of core stability training on functional movements in college athletes. *Journal of Sports Rehabilitation, 28*(5), 444–449.

Bagherian, S., Rahnama, N., Wikstrom, E. A., Clark, M. A., & Rostami, F. (2018). Characterizing lower extremity movement scores before and after fatigue in collegiate athletes with chronic ankle instability. *International Journal of Athletic Therapy Trainers, 23,* 27–32.

Baker, D. (1996). Improving vertical jump performance through general, special, and specific strength training: A brief review. *Journal of Strength & Conditioning Research, 10,* 131–136.

Bannister. W. (1991). Modeling elite athletic performance. In J. D. MacDougall, H. A. Wenger, & H. J. Green (Eds.), *Physiological testing of the high-performance athlete* (pp. 403–424). Human Kinetics.

Barr, K. P., Griggs, M., & Cadby, T. (2005). Lumbar stabilization: Core concepts and current literature, part 1. *American Journal of Physical Medicine & Rehabilitation, 84,* 473–480.

Barr, K. P., Griggs, M., & Cadby, T. (2007). Lumbar stabilization: Core concepts and current literature, part 2. *American Journal of Physical Medicine & Rehabilitation, 86,* 72–80.

Baxter, C., McNaughton, L. R., Sparks, A., Norton L., & Bentley, D. (2017). Impact of stretching on the performance and injury risk of long-distance runners. *Research in Sports Medicine, 25*(1), 78–91.

Beckman, S. M., & Buchanan, T. S. (1995). Ankle inversion injury and hypermobility: Effect on hip and ankle muscle electromyography onset latency. *Archives of Physical Medicine and Rehabilitation, 76,* 1138–1143.

Bedoya, A. A., Miltenberger, M. R., & Lopez, R. M. (2015). Plyometric training effects on athletic performance in youth soccer athletes: A systematic review. *Journal of Strength & Conditioning Research, 29*(8), 2351–2361.

Behm, D. G. (1995). Neuromuscular implications and applications of resistance training. *Journal of Strength & Conditioning Research, 9,* 264–274.

Behm, D. G., Bambury, A., Cahill, F., & Power, K. (2014). Effect of acute static stretching on force, balance, reaction time, and movement time. *Medicine & Science in Sports & Exercise, 36,* 1397–1402.

Behm, D. G., & Colado, J. C. (2013). Instability resistance training across the exercise continuum. *Sports Health, 5*(6), 500–503.

Behm, D. G., Muehlbauer, T., Kibele, A., & Granacher, U. (2015). Effects of strength training using unstable surfaces on strength, power and balance performance across the lifespan: A systematic review and meta-analysis. *Sports Medicine, 45,* 1645–1669.

Bell, D. R., Padua, D. A., & Clark, M. A. (2008). Muscle strength and flexibility characteristics of people displaying excessive medial knee displacement. *Archives of Physical Medicine and Rehabilitation, 89*(7), 1323–1328.

Bell, D. R., Vesci, B. J., DiStefano, L. J., Guskiewicz, K. M., Hirth, C. J., & Padua, D. A. (2012). Muscle activity and flexibility in individuals with medial knee displacement during the overhead squat. *Athletic Training and Sports Health Care, 4*(3), 117–125.

Bell-Jenie, T., Olivier, B., Wood, W., Rogers, S., Green, A., & McKinon, W. (2016). The association between loss of ankle dorsiflexion range of movement, and hip abduction and internal rotation during a step down test. *Manual Therapy, 21,* 256–261.

Bergmark, A. (1989). Stability of the lumbar spine: A study in mechanical engineering. *Acta Orthopaedica Scandinivia, Supplementa, 230,* 1–54.

Bird, S. P., Tarpenning, K. M., & Marino, F. E. (2005). Designing resistance training programs to enhance muscular fitness: A review of the acute program variables. *Sports Medicine, 35,* 841–851.

Blackburn, J. T., Padua, D. A., Riemann, B. L., & Guskiewicz, K. M. (2004). The relationships between active extensibility, and passive and active stiffness of the knee flexors. *Journal of Electromyography and Kinesiology, 14,* 683–691.

Blagrove, R. (2014). Minimising the interference effect during programmes of concurrent strength and endurance training. Part 2: Programming recommendations. *Professional Body for Strength and Conditioning, 32,* 15–22.

Boling, M. C., Padua, D. A., Marshall, S. W., Guskiewicz, K., Pyne, S., & Beutler, A. (2009). A prospective investigation of biomechanical risk factors for patellofemoral pain syndrome: The Joint Undertaking to Monitor and Prevent ACL Injury (JUMP-ACL) cohort. *American Journal of Sports Medicine, 37*(11), 2108–2116.

Bosco, C., Komi, P. V., & Ito, A. (1981). Prestretch potentiation of human skeletal muscle during ballistic movement. *Acta Orthopaedica Scandinivia, 111,* 135–140.

Bosco, C., Viitasalo, J. T., Komi, P. V., & Luhtanen, P. (1982). Combined effect of elastic energy and myoelectrical potentiation during stretch-shortening cycle exercise. *Acta Orthopaedica Scandinivia, 114,* 557–565.

Brooks, T., & Cressey, E. (2013). Mobility training of the young athlete. *Strength & Conditioning Journal, 35*(3), 27–33.

Brughelli, M., & Cronin, J. (2007). Altering the length–tension relationship with eccentric exercise: Implications for performance and injury. *Sports Medicine, 37*(9), 807–826.

Bruhn, S., Kullmann, N., & Gollhofer, A. (2004). The effects of a sensorimotor training and a strength training on postural stabilisation, maximum isometric contraction, and jump performance. *International Journal of Sports Medicine, 25*, 56–60.

Bullock-Saxon, J. E. (1994). Local sensation changes and altered hip muscle function following severe ankle sprain. *Physical Therapy, 74*, 17–28.

Caldemeyer, L. E., Brown, S. M., & Mulcahey, M. K. (2020). Neuromuscular training for the prevention of ankle sprains in female athletes: A systematic review. *Physician and Sportsmedicine, 48*(4), 363–369.

Campos, G. E., Luecke, T. J., & Wendeln, H. K. (2002). Muscular adaptations in response to three different resistance-training regimens: Specificity of repetition maximum training zones. *European Journal of Applied Physiology, 88*, 50–60.

Caraffa, A., Cerulli, G., Projetti, M., Aisa, G., & Rizzo, A. (1996). Prevention of anterior cruciate ligament injuries in soccer: A prospective controlled study of proprioceptive training. *Knee Surgery, Sports Traumatology, Arthroscopy, 4*, 19–21.

Chappell, J. D., & Limpisvasti, O. (2008). Effect of a neuromuscular training program on the kinetics and kinematics of jumping tasks. *American Journal of Sports Medicine, 36*(6), 1081–1086.

Chimera, N. J., Swanik, K. A., Swanik, C. B., & Straub, S. J. (2004). Effects of plyometric training on muscle-activation strategies and performance in female athletes. *Journal of Athletic Training, 39*, 24–31.

Chiu, L. Z. F., & Barnes, J. L. (2003). The fitness–fatigue model revisited: Implications for planning short- and long-term training. *Strength & Conditioning Journal, 25*(6), 42–51.

Chmielewski, T. L., Hurd, W. J., Rudolph, K. S., Axe, M. J., & Snyder-Mackler, L. (2005). Perturbation training improves knee kinematics and reduces muscle co-contraction after complete unilateral anterior cruciate ligament rupture. *Physical Therapy, 85*, 740–749.

Cibulka, M. T., Sinacore, D. R., Cromer, G. S., & Delitto, A. (1998). Unilateral hip rotation range of motion asymmetry in patients with sacroiliac joint regional pain. *Spine, 23*, 1009–1015.

Clark, M. A. (2000). *Integrated training for the new millennium.* National Academy of Sports Medicine.

Clutch, D., Wilton, M., McGown, C., & Bryce, G. R. (1983). The effect of depth jumps and weight training on leg strength and vertical jump. *Research Quarterly for Exercise and Sport, 54*, 5–10.

Cobb, S. C., Bazett-Jones, D. M., Joshi, M. N., Earl-Boehm, J. E., & James, C. R. (2014). The relationship among foot posture, core and lower extremity muscle function, and postural stability. *Journal of Athletic Training, 49*(2), 173–180.

Comerford, M. J., & Mottram, S. L. (2001). Movement and stability dysfunction: Contemporary developments. *Manual Therapy, 6*(1), 15–26.

Cosio-Lima, L. M., Reynolds, K. L., Winter, C., Paolone, V., & Jones, M. T. (2003). Effects of physio-ball and conventional floor exercises on early phase adaptations in back and abdominal core stability and balance in women. *Journal of Strength & Conditioning Research, 17*, 721–725.

Cruz-Dias, D., Lomas-Vega, R., Osuna-Perez, M. C., Contreras, F. H., & Martinez-Azmat, A. (2015). Effect of 6 weeks of balance training on chronic ankle instability in athletes: A randomized controlled trial. *International Journal of Sports Medicine, 36*(9), 754–760.

Cunanan, A. J., DeWeese, B. H., Wagle, J. P., Carroll, K. M., Sausaman, R., Hornsby, W. G., Haff, G. G., Triplett, N. T., Pierce, K. C., & Stone, M. H. (2018). The general adaptation syndrome: A foundation for the concept of periodization. *Sports Medicine, 48*, 787–797.

Davis, D. S., Ashby, P. E., McCale, K. L., McQuain, J. A., & Wine, J. M. (2005). The effectiveness of 3 stretching techniques on hamstring flexibility using consistent stretching parameters. *Journal of Strength & Conditioning Research, 19*, 27–32.

Devita, P., & Skelly, W. A. (1992). Effect of landing stiffness on joint kinetics and energetics in the lower extremity. *Medicine & Science in Sports & Exercise, 24*, 108–115.

Di Stasi, S., Myer, G. D., & Hewett, T. E. (2013). Neuromuscular training to target deficits associated with second anterior cruciate ligament injury. *Journal of Orthopaedic & Sports Physical Therapy, 43*(11), 772–792, A1–A11.

DiStefano, L. J., DiStefano, M. J., Frank, B. S., Clark, M. A., & Padua, D. A. (2013). Comparison of integrated and isolated training on performance measures and neuromuscular control. *Journal of Strength & Conditioning Research, 27*(4), 1083–1090.

Ebben, W. P. (2002). Complex training: A brief review. *Journal of Sports Science and Medicine, 1*, 42–46.

Eckard, T., Padua, D., Mauntel, T., Frank, B., Pietrosimone, L., Begalle, R., Goto, S., Clark, M., & Kucera, K. (2018). Association between double-leg squat and single-leg squat performance and injury incidence among incoming NCAA Division I athletes: A prospective cohort study. *Physical Therapy in Sport, 34*, 192–200.

Edgerton, V. R., Wolf, S. L., Levendowski, D. J., & Roy, R. R. (1996). Theoretical basis for patterning EMG amplitudes to assess muscle dysfunction. *Medicine & Science in Sports & Exercise, 28*, 744–751.

Enoka, R. M. (2002). *Neuromechanics of human movement* (3rd ed.). Human Kinetics.

Ewing, J. L., Wolfe, D. R., Rogers, M. A., Admundson, M. L., & Stull, G. A. (1990). Effects of velocity of isokinetic training on strength, power, and quadriceps muscle fibre characteristics. *European Journal of Applied Physiology, 61*, 159–162.

Fei, L., Nassis, G. P., Shi, Y., Han, G., Zhang, X., Gao, B., & Ding, H. (2020). Concurrent complex and endurance training for recreational marathon runners: Effects on neuromuscular and running performance. *European Journal of Sport Science, 21*(9), 1243–1253.

Fleck, S. J., & Kraemer, W. J. (1997). *Designing resistance training programs* (2nd ed.). Human Kinetics.

Ford, K. R., Myer, G. D., & Hewett, T. E. (2003). Valgus knee motion during landing in high school female and male basketball players. *Medicine & Science in Sports & Exercise, 35*, 1745–1750.

Franchi, M. V., Reeves, N. D., & Narici, M. V. (2017). Skeletal muscle remodeling in response to eccentric vs. concentric loading: Morphological, molecular, and metabolic adaptations. *Frontiers in Physiology, 8*, 447.

Frederickson, M., Cookingham, C. L., Chaudhari, A. M., Dowdell, B. C., Oestreicher, N., & Sahrmann, S. A. (2000). Hip abductor weakness in distance runners with iliotibial band syndrome. *Clinical Journal of Sports Medicine, 10*, 169–175.

Freitas, S. R., Mendes, B., Le Sant, G., Andrade, R. J., Nordez, A., & Milanovic, Z. (2018). Can chronic stretching change the muscle-tendon mechanical properties? A review. *Scandinavian Journal of Medicine & Science in Sports, 28*, 794–806.

Fyfe, J. J., Bishop, D. J., & Stepto, N. K. (2014). Interference between concurrent resistance and endurance exercise: Molecular bases and the role of individual training variables. *Sports Medicine.* https://doi.org /10.1007/s40279-014-0162-1

Gebel, A., Lesinski, M., Behm, D. G., & Granacher, U. (2018). Effect and dose–response relationship of balance training on balance performance in youth: A systematic review and meta-analysis. *Sports Medicine, 48*, 2067–2089.

Gehri, D. J., Ricard, M. D., Kleiner, D. M., & Kirkendall, D. T. (1998). A comparison of plyometric training techniques for improving vertical jump ability and energy production. *Journal of Strength & Conditioning Research, 12*, 85–89.

Gibala, M. J., & McGee, S. L. (2008). Metabolic adaptations to short-term high-intensity interval training: A little pain for a lot of gain? *Exercise and Sport Sciences Reviews, 36*(2), 58–63.

Gilchrist, J., Mandelbaum, B. R., Melancon, H., Ryan, G. W., Silvers, H. J., Griffin, L. Y., Watanabe, D. S., Dick, R. W., & Dvorak, J. (2008). A randomized controlled trial to prevent noncontact anterior cruciate ligament injury in female collegiate soccer players. *American Journal of Sports Medicine, 36*, 1476–1483.

Gomes-Neto, M., Lopes, J. M., Conceicao, C. S., Araujo, A., Brasiliero, A., Sousa, C., Carvalho, V. O., & Arcanjo, F. L. (2017). Stabilization exercise compared to general exercises or manual therapy for the management of low back pain: A systematic review and meta-analysis. *Physical Therapy in Sports, 23*, 136–142.

Hahn, S., Stanforth, D., Stanforth, P. R., & Philips, A. (1998). A 10-week training study comparing resist-a-ball and traditional trunk training. *Medicine & Science in Sports & Exercise, 30*, S199.

Hakkinen, K. (1994). Neuromuscular adaptation during strength training, aging, detraining and immobilization. *Critical Reviews in Physical and Rehabilitation Medicine, 6*, 161–198.

Hakkinen, K., Komi, P. V., & Alen, M. (1985). Effect of explosive type strength training on isometric force- and relaxation-time, electromyographic and muscle fibre characteristics of leg extensor muscles. *Acta Physiologica Scandinavica, 125*, 587–600.

Han, S., Ge, S., Liu, H., & Liu, R. (2013). Alterations in three-dimensional knee kinematics and kinetics during neutral, squeeze and outward squat. *Journal of Human Kinetics, 39*, 59–66. https://pubmed.ncbi.nlm.nih.gov /24511341/

Hanten, W. P., Olson, S. L., Butts, N. L., & Nowicki, A. L. (2000). Effectiveness of a home program of ischemic pressure followed by sustained stretch for treatment of myofascial trigger points. *Physical Therapy, 80*, 997–1003.

Harries, S. K., Lubans, D. R., & Calliste, R. (2012). Resistance training to improve power and sports performance in adolescent athletes: A systematic review and meta-analysis. *Journal of Science and Medicine in Sport, 15*, 532–540.

Heiderscheit, B., & Sherry, M. (2007). What effect do core strength and stability have on injury prevention? In D. MacAuley & T. Best (Eds.), *Evidence-based sports medicine* (2nd ed., pp. 59–72). Blackwell.

Herman, D. C., Weinhold, P. S., Guskiewicz, K. M., Garrett, W. E., Yu, B., & Padua, D. A. (2008). The effects of strength training on the lower extremity biomechanics of female recreational athletes during a stop–jump task. *American Journal of Sports Medicine, 36*(4), 733–740.

Herman, K., Barton, C., Malliaras, P., & Morrissey, D. (2012). The effectiveness of neuromuscular warm-up strategies, that require no additional equipment, for preventing lower limb injuries during sports participation: a systematic review. *BMC Medicine, 10,* 75.

Hermassi, S., Gabbett, T. J., Chelly, M. S., & Chamari, K. (2014). Effects of a short-term in-season plyometric training program on repeated-sprint ability, leg power, and jump performance of elite handball players. *International Journal of Sports Science & Coaching, 9*(5), 1205–1216.

Hewett, T. E., & Bates, N. A. (2017). Preventive biomechanics: A paradigm shift with translational approach to injury prevention. *American Journal of Sports Medicine, 45*(11), 2654–2664.

Hewett, T. E., Lindenfeld, T. N., Riccobene, J. V., & Noyes, F. R. (1999). The effect of neuromuscular training on the incidence of knee injury in female athletes: A prospective study. *American Journal of Sports Medicine, 27,* 699–706.

Hewett, T. E., Myer, G. D., Ford, K. R., Heidt, R. S., Colosimo, A. J., McLean, S. G., van den Bogert, A. J., Paterno, M. V., & Succop, P. (2005). Biomechanical measures of neuromuscular control and valgus loading of the knee predict anterior cruciate ligament injury risk in female athletes: A prospective study. *American Journal of Sports Medicine, 33*(4), 492–501.

Hewett, T. E., Stroupe, A. L., Nance, T. A., & Noyes, F. R. (1996). Plyometric training in female athletes: Decreased impact forces and increased hamstring torques. *American Journal of Sports Medicine, 24,* 765–773.

Hickson, R. C. (1980). Interference of strength development by simultaneously training for strength and endurance. *European Journal of Applied Physiology and Occupational Physiology, 45*(2), 255–263.

Hides, J. A., Stokes, M. J., Saide, M., Jull, G. A., & Cooper, D. H. (1994). Evidence of lumbar multifidus muscle wasting ipsilateral to symptoms in patients with acute/subacute low back pain. *Spine, 19,* 165–172.

Hodges, P. W., & Richardson, C. A. (1996). Inefficient muscular stabilization of the lumbar spine associated with low back pain: A motor control evaluation of transversus abdominis. *Spine, 21,* 2640–2650.

Hodges, P. W., & Richardson, C. A. (1997). Contraction of the abdominal muscles associated with movement of the lower limb. *Physical Therapy, 77,* 132–142.

Hodges, P. W., Richardson, C., & Jull, G. (1996). Evaluation of the relationship between laboratory and clinical tests of transversus abdominis function. *Physiotherapy Research International, 1,* 30–40.

Holcomb, W. R., Lander, J. E., Rutland, R. M., & Wilson, G. D. (1996). The effectiveness of a modified plyometric program on power and the vertical jump. *Journal of Strength & Conditioning Research, 10,* 89–92.

Hopper, A., Haff, E. E., Barley, O. R., Joyce, C., Lloyd, R. S., & Haff, G. G. (2017). Neuromuscular training improves movement competency and physical performance measures in 11–13-year-old female netball athletes. *Journal of Strength & Conditioning Research, 31*(5), 1165–1177.

Hungerford, B. P., Gilleard, W. P., & Hodges, P. P. (2003). Evidence of altered lumbopelvic muscle recruitment in the presence of sacroiliac joint pain. *Spine, 28,* 1593–600.

Huxel Bliven, K. C., & Anderson, B. E. (2013). Core stability training for injury prevention. *Sports Health, 5*(6), 514–522.

Ireland, M. L., Willson, J. D., Ballantyne, B. T., & Davis, I. M. (2003). Hip strength in females with and without patellofemoral pain. *Journal of Orthopaedic & Sports Physical Therapy, 33,* 671–676.

Issurin, V. B. (2010). New horizons for the methodology and physiology of training periodization. *Sports Medicine, 40*(3), 189–206.

Janda, V. (1978). *Muscles, central nervous system regulation, and back problems.* Plenum Press.

Janusevicius, D., Snieckus, A., Skurvydas, A., Silinskas, V., Trinkunas, E., Cadeau, J. A., & Kamandulis, S. (2017). Effects of high velocity elastic band versus heavy resistance training on hamstring strength, activation, and sprint running performance. *Journal of Sports Science and Medicine, 16,* 239–246.

Judge, L. W., Moreau, C., & Burke, J. R. (2003). Neural adaptations with sport-specific resistance training in highly skilled athletes. *Journal of Sports Science, 21,* 419–427.

Junge, A., Rosch, D., Peterson, L., Graf-Baumann, T., & Dvorak, J. (2002). Prevention of soccer injuries: A prospective intervention study in youth amateur players. *American Journal of Sports Medicine, 30,* 652–659.

Kanehisa, H., & Miyashita, M. (1983). Specificity of velocity in strength training. *European Journal of Applied Physiology, 52,* 104–106.

Kannus, P. (2000). Structure of the tendon connective tissue. *Scandinavian Journal of Medicine & Science in Sports, 10*(6), 312–320.

Karavirta, L., Hakkinen, K., Kauhanen, A., Arija-Blazquez, A., Sillanpaa, E., Rinkinen, N., & Hakkinen, A. (2011). Individual responses to combined endurance and strength training in older adults. *Medicine & Science in Sports & Exercise, 43,* 484–490.

Kipp, K., McLean, S. G., & Palmieri-Smith, R. M. (2011). Patterns of hip-flexion motion predict frontal and transverse plane knee torques during a single leg land and cut maneuver. *Clinical Biomechanics, 25*(5), 504–508.

Kita, K., Osu, R., Hosoda, C., Honda, M., Hanakawa, T., & Izawa, J. (2019). Neuroanatomical basis of individuality in muscle tuning function: Neural correlates of muscle tuning. *Frontiers in Behavioral Neuroscience, 13*, 28. https://doi.org/10.3389/fnbeh.2019.00028

Knapik, J. J., Bauman, C. L., Jones, B. H., Harris, J. M., & Vaughan, L. (1991). Preseason strength and flexibility imbalances associated with athletic injuries in female collegiate athletes. *American Journal of Sports Medicine, 19*, 76–81.

Knox, M. F., Chipchase, L. S., Schabrun, S. M., & Marshall, P. W. M. (2017). Improved compensatory postural adjustments of the deep abdominals following exercise in people with chronic low back pain. *Journal of Electromyography and Kinesiology, 37*, 117–124.

Kokkonen, J., Nelson, A. G., Eldredge, C., & Winchester, J. B. (2007). Chronic static stretching improves exercise performance. *Medicine & Science in Sports & Exercise, 39*, 1825–1831.

Kollock, R. O., Andrews, C., Johnston, A., Elliott, T., Wilson, A. E., Games, K. E., & Sefton, J. M. (2016). A meta-analysis to determine if lower extremity muscle strengthening should be included in military knee overuse injury prevention programs. *Journal of Athletic Training, 51*(11), 919–926.

Kovacs, E. J., Birmingham, T. B., Forwell, L., & Litchfield, R. B. (2014). Effect of training on postural control in figure skaters: A randomized controlled trial of neuromuscular versus basic off-ice training programs. *Clinical Journal of Sport Medicine, 14*, 215–224.

Kraemer, W. J., Patton, J. F., Gordon, S. E., Harman, E., Deschenes, M., Reynolds, K., Newton, R., Triplett, N., & Dziados, J. (1995). Compatibility of high-intensity strength and endurance training on hormonal and skeletal muscle adaptations. *Journal of Applied Physiology, 78*(3), 976–989.

Kraemer, W. J., & Ratamess, N. A. (2000). Physiology of resistance training. *Orthopedic Clinics of North America, 9*, 467–513.

Kraemer, W. J., & Ratamess, N. A. (2004). Fundamentals of resistance training: Progression and exercise prescription. *Medicine & Science in Sports & Exercise, 36*, 674–678.

Kraemer, W. J., Ratamess, N. A., Flanagan, S. D., Shurley, J. P., Todd, J. S., & Todd, T. C. (2017). Understanding the science of resistance training: An evolutionary perspective. *Sports Medicine, 47*, 2415–2435.

Lee, T. Q., Yang, B. Y., Sandusky, M. D., & McMahon, P. J. (2001). The effects of tibial rotation on the patellofemoral joint: Assessment of the changes in in situ strain in the peripatellar retinaculum and the patellofemoral contact pressures and areas. *Journal of Rehabilitation Research and Development, 38*, 463–469.

Lesinski, M., Hortobágyi, T., Muehlbauer, T., Gollhofer, A., & Granacher U. (2015). Dose–response relationships of balance training in healthy young adults: A systematic review and meta-analysis. *Sports Medicine, 45*(4), 557–576.

Lewit, K. (1994). The functional approach. *Journal of Orthopedic Medicine, 16*(3), 73–74.

Lorenzetti, S., Ostermann, M., Zeidler, F., Zimmer, P., Jentsch, L., List, R., Taylor, W. R., & Schellenberg, F. (2018). How to squat? Effects of various stance widths, foot placement angles and level of experience on knee, hip and trunk motion and loading. *BMC Sports Science, Medicine, and Rehabilitation, 10*, 14. https://doi.org/10.1186/s13102-018-0103-7

Loturco, I., Tricoli, V., Roschel, H., Nakamura, F. Y., Cavinato Cal Abad, C., Kobal, R., Gil, S., & Gonzalez-Badillo, J. J. (2014). Transference of traditional versus complex strength and power training to sprint performance. *Journal of Human Kinetics, 41*, 265–273.

Luebbers, P. E., Potteiger, J. A., Hulver, M. W., Thyfault, J. P., Carper, M. J., & Lockwood, R. H. (2003). Effects of plyometric training and recovery on vertical jump performance and anaerobic power. *Journal of Strength Conditioning Research, 17*, 704–709.

Macrum, E., Bell, D. R., Boling, M., Lewek, M., & Padua, D. (2012). Effect of limiting ankle-dorsiflexion on lower extremity kinematics and muscle-activation patterns during a squat. *Journal of Sport Rehabilitation, 21*, 144–150.

Mandelbaum, B. R., Silvers, H. J., Watanabe, D. S., Knarr, J. F., Thomas, S. D., & Griffin, L. Y. (2005). Effectiveness of a neuromuscular and proprioceptive training program in preventing the incidence of ACL injuries in female athletes: A 2-year follow-up. *American Journal of Sports Medicine, 33*, 1003–1010.

Maniar, N., Schache, A. G., Sritharan, P., & Opar, D. A. (2018). Non-knee-spanning muscles contribute to tibiofemoral shear as well as valgus and rotational joint reaction moments during unanticipated sidestep cutting. *Scientific Reports, 8*, 2501. https://doi.org/10.1038/s41598-017-19098-9

Marx, J. O., Ratamess, N. A., Nindl, B. C., Gotschalk, L. A., Volek, J. S., & Dohi, K. (2001). Low-volume circuit versus high-volume periodized resistance training in women. *Medicine & Science in Sports & Exercise, 33*, 635–643.

Mauntel, T. C., Beagle, R. L., Cram, T. R., Frank, B. S., Hirth, C. J., Blackburn, T., & Padua, D. A. (2013). The effect of lower extremity muscle activation and passive range of motion on a single leg squat performance. *Journal of Strength & Conditioning Research, 27*(7), 1813–1823.

Mauntel, T. C., Frank, B. F., Begalle, R. L., Blackburn, J. T., & Padua, D. A. (2014). Kinematic differences between those with and without medial knee displacement during a single-leg squat. *Journal of Applied Biomechanics, 30,* 707–712.

Mayhew, T. P., Norton, B. J., & Sahrmann, S. A. (1983). Electromyographic study of the relationship between hamstring and abdominal muscles during a unilateral straight leg raise. *Physical Therapy, 63*(11), 1769–1773.

McArdle, W. D., Katch, F. I., & Katch, V. L. (Eds.). (2010). *Exercise physiology: Nutrition, energy, and human performance* (7th ed.). Lippincott Williams & Wilkins.

McClay, I., & Manal, K. (1999). Three-dimensional kinetic analysis of running: Significance of secondary planes of motion. *Medicine & Science in Sports & Exercise, 31,* 1629–1637.

McEvoy, K. P., & Newton, R. U. (1991). Baseball throwing speed and base running speed: The effects of ballistic resistance training. *Journal of Strength & Conditioning Research, 12,* 216–221.

McGill, S. A. (2004). *Ultimate back fitness and performance.* Wabuno Publishers.

McGill, S. A., Karpowicz, A., Fenwick, C. M. J., & Brown S. H. M. (2009). Exercises for the torso performed in a standing posture: Spine and hip motion and motor patterns and spine load. *Journal of Strength & Conditioning Research, 23*(2), 455–464.

McGill, S. M. (2001). Low back stability: From formal description to issues for performance and rehabilitation. *Exercise and Sport Sciences Reviews, 29,* 26–31.

McGill, S. M., & Cholewicki, J. (2001). Biomechanical basis for stability: An explanation to enhance clinical utility. *Journal of Orthopaedic & Sports Physical Therapy, 31,* 96–100.

McKeon, P. O., Ingersoll, C. D., Kerrigan, D. C., Saliba, E., Bennett, B. C., & Hertel, J. (2008). Balance training improves function and postural control in those with chronic ankle instability. *Medicine & Science in Sports & Exercise, 40*(10), 1810–1819.

Medeiros, D. M., & Lima, C. S. (2017). Influence of chronic stretching on muscle performance: Systematic review. *Human Movement Science, 54,* 220–229.

Medeiros, D. M., & Martini, T. F. (2018). Chronic effect of different types of stretching on ankle dorsiflexion range of motion: Systematic review and meta-analysis. *The Foot, 34,* 28–35.

Mills, J., & Taunton, J. E. (2003). The effect of spinal stabilization training on spinal mobility, vertical jump, agility, and balance. *Medicine & Science in Sports & Exercise, 35,* S323.

Mujika, I., & Padilla, S. (2001a). Cardiorespiratory and metabolic characteristics of detraining in humans. *Medicine & Science in Sports & Exercise, 33,* 413–421.

Mujika, I., & Padilla, S. (2001b). Muscular characteristics of detraining in humans. *Medicine & Science in Sports & Exercise, 33*(8), 1297–1303.

Myer, G. D., Ford, K. R., & Hewett, T. E. (2002). A comparison of medial knee motion in basketball players when performing a basketball rebound. *Medicine & Science in Sports & Exercise, 34*(5), S247.

Myer, G. D., Ford, K. R., McLean, S. G., & Hewett, T. E. (2006). The effects of plyometric versus dynamic stabilization and balance training on lower extremity biomechanics. *American Journal of Sports Medicine, 34*(3), 445–455.

Nadler, S. F., Malanga, G. A., Bartoli, L. A., Feinberg, J. H., Prybicien, M., & Deprince, M. (2002). Hip muscle imbalance and low back pain in athletes: Influence of core strengthening. *Medicine & Science in Sports & Exercise, 34,* 9–16.

Nadler, S. F., Malanga, G. A., Feinberg, J. H., Rubanni, M., Moley, P., & Foye, P. (2002). Functional performance deficits in athletes with previous lower extremity injury. *Clinical Journal of Sports Medicine, 12,* 73–78.

Neumann, D. A. (2010). Kinesiology of the hip: A focus on muscular actions. *Journal of Orthopaedic & Sports Physical Therapy, 40*(2), 82–94.

Neumann, D. (2017). *Kinesiology of the musculoskeletal system: Foundations for physical rehabilitation* (3rd ed.). Elsevier Health Sciences.

Nyland, J., Love, M., Burden, R., Krupp, R., & Caborn, D. N. (2014). Progressive resistance, whole body long-axis rotational training improves kicking motion motor performance. *Physical Therapy in Sport, 15*(1), 26–32.

Nyland, J., Smith, S., Beickman, K., Armsey, T., & Caborn, D. N. (2002). Frontal plane knee angle affects dynamic postural control strategy during unilateral stance. *Medicine & Science in Sports & Exercise, 34,* 1150–1157.

Olson, T. J., Chebny, C., Willson, J. D., Kernozek, T. W., & Straker, J. S. (2011). Comparison of 2D and 3D kinematic changes during a single leg step down following neuromuscular training. *Physical Therapy in Sport, 12*(2), 93–99.

O'Sullivan, P. B., Phyty, G. D., Twomey, L. T., & Allison, G. T. (1997). Evaluation of specific stabilizing exercise in the treatment of chronic low back pain with radiologic diagnosis of spondylolysis or spondylolisthesis. *Spine, 22,* 2959–2967.

O'Sullivan, P. B., Twomey, L., & Allison, G. T. (1998). Altered abdominal muscle recruitment in patients with chronic back pain following a specific exercise intervention. *Journal of Orthopaedic & Sports Physical Therapy, 27,* 114–124.

Padua, D. A., Bell, D. R., & Clark, M. A. (2012a). Neuromuscular characteristics of individuals displaying excessive medial knee displacement. *Journal of Athletic Training, 47*(5), 525–536.

Padua, D. A., DiStefano, L. J., Marshall, S. W., Beutler, A. I., de la Motte, S. J., & DiStefano, M. J. (2012b). Retention of movement pattern changes following a lower extremity injury prevention program is affected by program duration. *American Journal of Sports Medicine, 40,* 300–306.

Padua, D. A., & Marshall, S. W. (2006). Evidence supporting ACL-injury-prevention exercise programs: A review of the literature. *Athletic Therapy Today, 11,* 11–23.

Palmer, T., Uhl, T. L., Howell, D., Hewett, T. E., Viele, K., & Mattacola, C. G. (2015). Sport-specific training targeting the proximal segments and throwing velocity in collegiate throwing athletes. *Journal of Athletic Training, 50*(6), 567–577.

Panjabi, M. M. (1992a). The stabilizing system of the spine. Part I. Function, dysfunction, adaptation, and enhancement. *Journal of Spinal Disorders & Techniques, 5*(4), 383–389; discussion 397.

Panjabi, M. M. (1992b). The stabilizing system of the spine. Part II. Neutral zone and instability hypothesis. *Journal of Spinal Disorders & Techniques, 5*(4), 390–396; discussion 397.

Park, J. H., Shin, J. H., Lee, H., Roh, J., & Park, H. S. (2021). Alterations in intermuscular coordination underlying isokinetic exercise after a stroke and their implications on neurorehabilitation. *Journal of NeuroEngineering and Rehabilitation, 18,* 110. https://doi.org/10.1186/s12984-021-00900-9

Parra, J., Cadefau, J. A., Rodas, G., & Amigo, N. (2000). The distribution of rest periods affects performance and adaptations of energy metabolism induced by high-intensity training in human muscle. *Acta Physiologica Scandinavica, 169,* 157–165.

Paterno, M. V., Myer, G. D., Ford, K. R., & Hewett, T. E. (2004). Neuromuscular training improves single-limb stability in young female athletes. *Journal of Orthopaedic & Sports Physical Therapy, 34,* 305–316.

Paul, D. J., Gabett, T., & Nassis G. (2016). Agility in team sports: Testing, training and factors affecting performance. *Sports Medicine, 46*(3), 421–442.

Peate, W. F., Bates, G., Lunda, K., Francis, S., & Bellamy, K. (2007). Core strength: A new model for injury prediction and prevention. *Journal of Occupational Medicine and Toxicology, 2,* 3. https://doi.org/10.1186/1745-6673-2-3

Peterson, M. D., Rhea, M. R., & Alvar, B. A. (2004). Maximizing strength development in athletes: A meta-analysis to determine the dose–response relationship. *Journal of Strength & Conditioning Research, 18*(2), 377–382.

Peterson, M. D., Rhea, M. R., & Alvar, B. A. (2005). Applications of the dose–response for muscular strength development: A review of meta-analytic efficacy and reliability for designing training prescription. *Journal of Strength & Conditioning Research, 19*(4), 950–958.

Plews, D. J., Laursen, P. B., Stanley, J., Kilding, A. E., & Buchheit, M. (2013). Training adaptation and heart rate variability in elite endurance athletes: Opening the door to effective monitoring. *Sports Medicine, 43*(9), 773–781.

Potteiger, J. A., Lockwood, R. H., & Haub MD. (1999). Muscle power and fiber characteristics in human skeletal muscle. *Journal of Strength & Conditioning Research, 13,* 275–279.

Pourheidary, S., Sheikhhoseini, R., & Babakhani, F. (2019). The electromyographic feedback and feedforward activity of selected lower extremity muscles during toe-in landing in female athletes. *Physical Treatments, 9*(4), 203–210.

Powers, C. M. (2003). The influence of altered lower-extremity kinematics on patellofemoral joint dysfunction: A theoretical perspective. *Journal of Orthopaedic & Sports Physical Therapy, 33,* 639–646.

Rabin, A., Kozol, Z., & Finestone, A. S. (2014). Limited ankle dorsiflexion increases the risk for mid-portion Achilles tendinopathy in infantry recruits: A prospective cohort study. *Journal of Foot and Ankle Research, 7,* 48.

Rassier, D. E., & Herzog, W. (2005). Force enhancement and relaxation rates after stretch of activated muscle fibres. *Proceedings of the Royal Society B, 272,* 475–480.

Rhea, M. R., Alvar, B. A., Ball, S. D., & Burkett, L. N. (2002). Three sets of weight training superior to 1 set with equal intensity for eliciting strength. *Journal of Strength & Conditioning Research, 16,* 525–529.

Rhea, M. R., Alvar, B. A., Burkett, L. N., & Ball, S. D. (2003). A meta-analysis to determine the dose response for strength development. *Medicine & Science in Sports & Exercise, 35,* 456–464.

Rhea, M. R., Ball, S. D., Phillips, W. T., & Burkett, L. N. (2002). A comparison of linear and daily undulating periodized programs with equated volume and intensity for strength. *Journal of Strength & Conditioning Research, 16,* 250–255.

Rhea, M. R., Kenn, J. G., & Dermody, B. M. (2009). Alterations in speed of squat movement and the use of accommodated resistance among college athletes training for power. *Journal of Strength & Conditioning Research, 23*(9), 2645–2650.

Rhea, M. R., Peterson, M. D., Oliverson, J. R., Allyon, F. N., & Potenziano, B. J. (2008). An examination of training on the VertiMax resisted jumping device for improvements in lower body power in highly trained college athletes. *Journal of Strength & Conditioning Research, 22*, 735–740.

Richardson, C. A., & Jull, G. A. (1995). Muscle control–pain control. What exercises would you prescribe? *Manual Therapy, 1*, 2–10.

Richardson, C. A., Snijders, C. J., Hides, J. A., Damen, L., Pas, M. S., & Storm, J. (2002). The relation between the transverse abdominis muscle, sacroiliac joint mechanics, and low back pain. *Spine, 27*, 399–405.

Riley, D. A., & Van Dyke, J. M. (2012). The effects of active and passive stretching on muscle length. *Physical Medicine and Rehabilitation Clinics of North America, 23*, 51–57.

Romer, L. M., & McConnell, A. K. (2003). Specificity and reversibility of inspiratory muscle training. *Medicine & Science in Sports & Exercise, 35*(2), 237–244.

Rumpf, M. C., Cronin, J. B., Oliver, J. L., & Hughes, M. G. (2013). Vertical and leg stiffness and stretch-shortening cycle changes across maturation during maximal sprint running. *Human Movement Science, 32*(4), 668–676.

Rutherford, O. M., Greig, C. A., Sargent, A. J., & Jones, D. A. (1986). Strength training and power output: Transference effects in the human quadriceps muscle. *Journal of Sports Science, 4*, 101–107.

Sahrmann, S. A. (1992). Posture and muscle imbalance: Faulty lumbo-pelvic alignment and associated musculoskeletal pain syndromes. *Orthopaedic Division Canada Physiotherapy Association, 12*, 13–20.

Sahrmann, S. (2011). *Movement system impairment syndromes of the extremities, cervical and thoracic spines.* Elsevier Health Sciences.

Sale, D. G. (1988). Neural adaptation to resistance training. *Medicine & Science in Sports & Exercise, 20*, S135–S145.

Schiftan, G. S., Ross, L. A., & Hahne, A. J. (2014). The effectiveness of proprioceptive training in preventing ankle sprains in sporting populations: A systematic review and meta-analysis. *Journal of Science, Medicine, and Sport, 18*, 238–244.

Selye, H. (1976). *The stress of life.* McGraw-Hill.

Sherry, M. A., & Best, T. M. (2004). A comparison of 2 rehabilitation programs in the treatment of acute hamstring strains. *Journal of Orthopaedic & Sports Physical Therapy, 34*, 116–125.

Shrier, I. (2004). Meta-analysis on pre-exercise stretching [Letter]. *Medicine & Science in Sports & Exercise, 36*, 1832.

Skundric, G., Vukicevic, V., & Lukic, N. (2021). Effects of core stability exercises, lumbar lordosis and low-back pain: A systematic review. *Journal of Anthropology of Sport and Physical Education, 5*(1), 17–23.

Stanley, L. E., Harkey, M., Luc-Harkey, B., Frank, B. S., Pietrosimone, B., Blackburn, T. J., & Padua, D. A. (2019). Ankle dorsiflexion displacement is associated with hip and knee kinematics in females following anterior cruciate ligament reconstruction. *Research in Sports Medicine, 27*, 21–33.

Sueki, D. G., Cleland, J. A., & Wainner, R. S. (2013). A regional interdependence model of musculoskeletal dysfunction: Research, mechanisms, and clinical implications. *Journal of Manual and Manipulative Therapy, 21*(2), 90–102.

Sullivan, K. M., Silvey, D. B. J., Button, D. C., & Behm, D. G. (2013). Roller-massager application to the hamstrings increases sit-and-reach range of motion within five to ten seconds without performance impairments. *International Journal of Sports Physical Therapy, 8*(3), 228–236.

Tan, B. (1999). Manipulating resistance training program variables to optimize maximum strength in men: A review. *Journal of Strength & Conditioning Research, 13*, 289–304.

Taskin, C. (2016). Effect of core training program on physical functional performance in female soccer players. *International Education Studies, 9*(5), 115–123.

Terzis, G., Stratakos, G., Manta, P., & Georgiadis, G. (2008). Throwing performance after resistance training and detraining. *Journal of Strength & Conditioning Research, 22*, 1198–1204.

Thompson, C. J., Cobb, K. M., & Blackwell, J. (2007). Functional training improves club head speed and functional fitness in older golfers. *Journal of Strength & Conditioning Research, 21*, 131–137.

Turner, A. N., & Jeffreys, I. (2010). The stretch-shortening cycle: Proposed mechanisms and methods for enhancement. *Strength & Conditioning Journal, 32*(4), 87–100.

van Melick, N, van Rijn, L., Nijhuis-van der Sanden, M. W. G., Hoogeboom, T. J., & van Cingel, R. E. H. (2019). Fatigue affects quality of movement more in ACL-reconstructed soccer players than in healthy players. *Knee Surgery, Sports Traumatology, Arthroscopy, 27*, 549–555.

Vera-Garcia, F. J., Grenier, S. G., & McGill, S. M. (2000). Abdominal muscle response during curl-ups on both stable and labile surfaces. *Physical Therapy, 80*, 564–569.

Verrelst, R., Willems, T., De Clerq, D., Roosen, P., Goossens, L., & Witvrouw, E. (2013). Hip muscle weakness as a risk factor for the development of exertional medial tibial pain: A prospective study. *Medicine & Science in Sports & Exercise, 45*, 196–197.

Viru, A., & Viru, M. (2000). Nature of the training response. In W. E. Garrett, Jr., & D. T. Kirkendall (Eds.), *Exercise and sport science* (pp. 67–95). Lippincott, Williams & Wilkins.

Voight, M., & Draovitch, P. (1991). Plyometrics. In M. Albert (Ed.), *Eccentric muscle training in sports and orthopedics* (pp. 45–73). Churchill Livingstone.

Wagner, D. R., & Kocak, M. S. (1997). A multivariate approach to assessing anaerobic power following a plyometric training program. *Journal of Strength & Conditioning Research, 11*, 251–255.

Wiggins, A. J., Grandhi, R. K., Schneider, D. K., Stanfield, D., Webster, K. E., & Myer, G. D. (2016). Risk of secondary injury in younger athletes after anterior cruciate ligament reconstruction: A systematic review and meta-analysis. *American Journal of Sports Medicine, 44*(7), 1861–1876.

Willardson, J. M. (2004). The effectiveness of resistance exercises performed on unstable equipment. *Strength & Conditioning Journal, 26*(5), 70–74.

Wilson, G. J., Murphy, A. J., & Walshe A. (1996). The specificity of strength training: The effect of posture. *European Journal of Applied Physiology, 73*, 346–352.

Wilson, G. J., Newton, R. U., Murphy, A. J., & Humphries, B. J. (1993). The optimal training load for the development of dynamic athletic performance. *Medicine & Science in Sports & Exercise, 25*, 1279–1286.

Wilson, J. D., Ireland, M. L., & Davis, I. (2006). Core strength and lower extremity alignment during single leg squats. *Medicine & Science in Sports & Exercise, 38*, 945–952.

Wilson, J. M., Marin, P. J., Rhea, M. R., Wilson, S. W. C., Loenneke, J. P., & Anderson, J. C. (2012). Concurrent training: A meta-analysis examining interference of aerobic and resistance exercise. *Journal of Strength & Conditioning Research, 26*(8), 2293–2307.

Winters, M. V., Blake, C. G., Trost, J. S., Marcello-Brinker, T. B., Lowe, L. M., & Garber, M. B. (2004). Passive versus active stretching of hip flexor muscles in subjects with limited hip extension: A randomized clinical trial. *Physical Therapy, 84*, 800–807.

Witvrouw, E., Danneels, L., Asselman, P., D'Have, T., & Cambier, D. (2003). Muscle flexibility as a risk factor for developing muscle injuries in male professional soccer players: A prospective study. *American Journal of Sports Medicine, 31*, 41–46.

Yaggie, J. A., & Campbell, B. M. (2006). Effects of balance training on selected skills. *Journal of Strength & Conditioning Research, 20*, 422–428.

Yapici, A. (2016). Investigation of the effects of teaching core exercises on young soccer players. *International Journal of Environmental Science Education, 11*(16), 9410–9421.

Zhang, X., Xia, R., Dai, B., Sun, X., & Fu, W. (2018). Effects of exercise-induced fatigue on lower extremity joint mechanics, stiffness, and energy absorption during landings. *Journal of Sports Science and Medicine, 17*, 640–649.

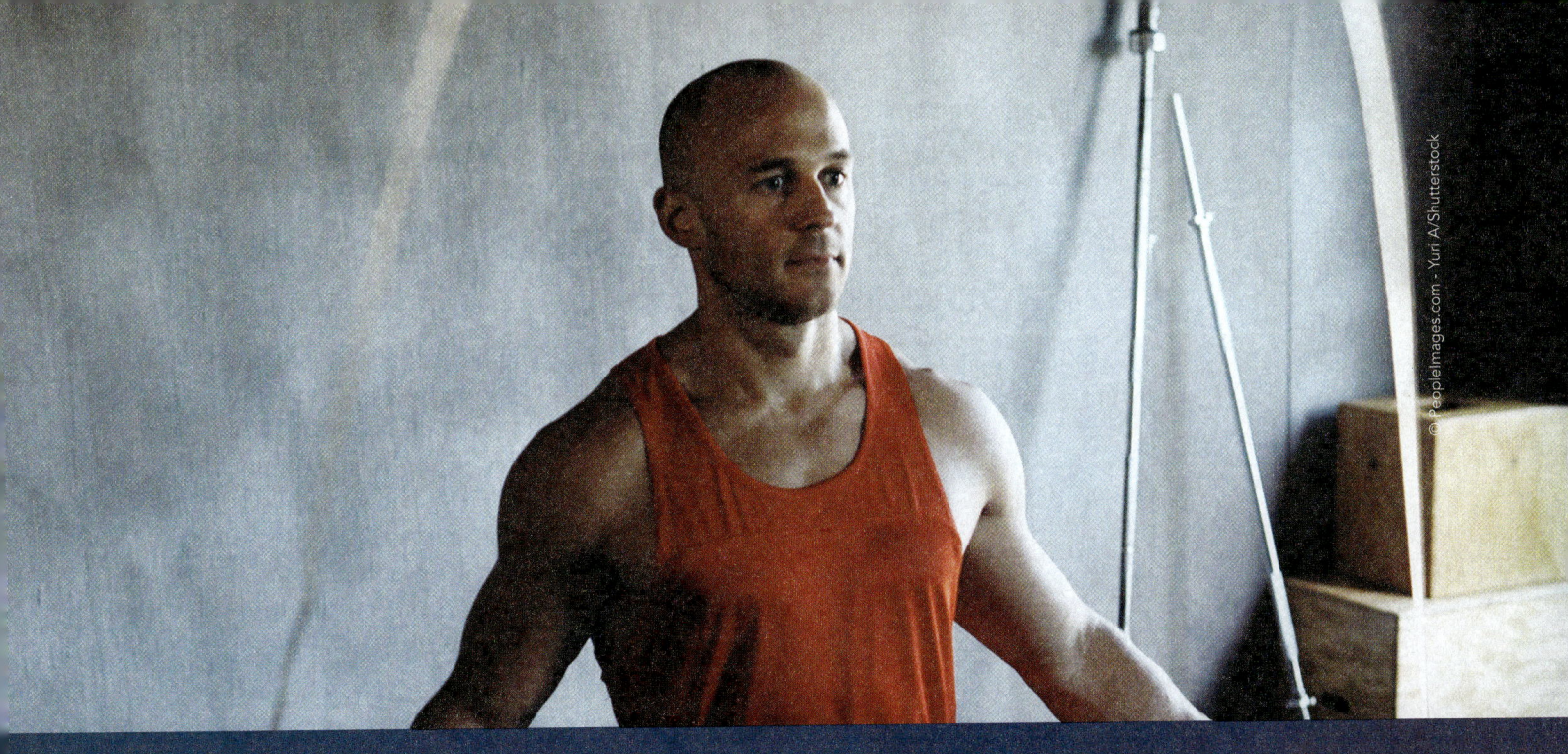

PHYSIOLOGICAL ADAPTATIONS TO SPORTS PERFORMANCE TRAINING

CHAPTER FIVE

LEARNING OBJECTIVES

Upon completion of this chapter, the Sports Performance Coach will be able to:

- **Identify** the fundamental adaptive changes in the body with exercise training that provides the basis for sports performance.

- **Explain** the roles that physiological adaptations play in athlete health and sports performance training and optimization.

- **Describe** the fundamental difference in the primary training targets for cardio endurance and resistance training workout programs.

- **Explain** key physiological adaptations (cardiovascular, endocrine, neuro-musculoskeletal) as they relate to resistance and cardio endurance training.

LESSON 1: INTRODUCTION TO PHYSIOLOGICAL ADAPTATIONS

INTRODUCTION

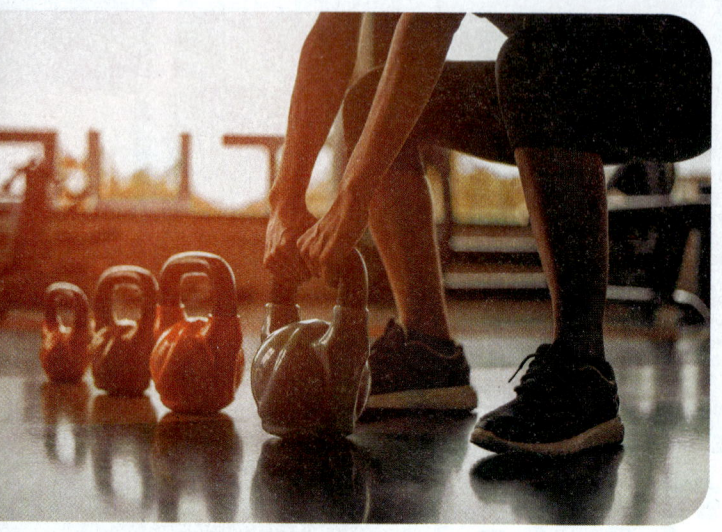

© Day Of Victory Studio/Shutterstock

The human body is consistently exposed to different stimuli. Physical exercise is one stimulus resulting in changes in structure and function, leading to sports performance and health improvements. These changes, called **adaptations**, are specific to many factors that are created by components of the program design, such as training intensity (i.e., percentage of maximum effort), frequency (i.e., number of days per week or sessions per day), and volume (i.e., amount of total work) of training. The Sports Performance Coach must understand the fundamental adaptive changes that take place in the body as a result of physical training, as this knowledge provides the basis of sports performance.

Adaptations in the different **physiological systems** are related to the targeted programs specific to training goals. The adaptive changes that occur with exercise training in men and women are essentially the same for the targeted goals of **cardiorespiratory fitness** and **neuromuscular efficiency**. However, a few notable differences may impact training of men versus women. For example, compared to women, men typically have higher testosterone levels, resulting in higher muscle mass, thicker bones, and less body fat (Blair, 2007). Each sport has different physiological demands for optimal performance, and the training programs implemented are specific to these sports' needs (Kraemer et al., 2021). However, the training for a sport always influences specific adaptive changes in each system depending on the workout.

ADAPTATION

A change by which an organism becomes better matched to its environment.

PHYSIO-LOGICAL SYSTEM →

A group of tissues that work together to perform a specific function or set of functions within the body, such as the muscular, skeletal, and nervous systems.

📋 COACH'S CORNER

The goals of performance training programs may be identical for both men and women. However, each program should be individualized, in that the frequency, intensity and load, duration, and exercise selection are specific to the athlete. Whether the athlete is male or female, the Sports Performance Coach must keep in mind the athlete's starting fitness level and desired outcomes and program proper progressions within the training program.

The underlying basis for adaptations in the human body is straightforward but might not be evident from a physiological perspective. Movements in training or competition make various external demands for specific force and power outputs to achieve the desired activity, such as running, shooting a basketball, or throwing a baseball. To understand adaptations, the Sports Performance Coach must first understand how muscle tissue is recruited to produce movement.

Movement in muscles (**Figure 5.1**) is achieved when the central nervous system (CNS) sends specific neural impulses from the motor cortex down the spinal cord and then out into the periphery. This movement stimulates muscle fibers to produce the correct amount of force and the desired movement. These muscle fibers are organized into **motor units**, which are called upon to produce the right amount of force and power. Adaptation starts when the motor units and their associated muscle fibers are activated to produce the needed force. Importantly, all other physiological systems (e.g., cardiovascular, endocrine) are then engaged to the specific level needed to support the activated motor units during and after the exercise (Duchateau & Enoka, 2011).

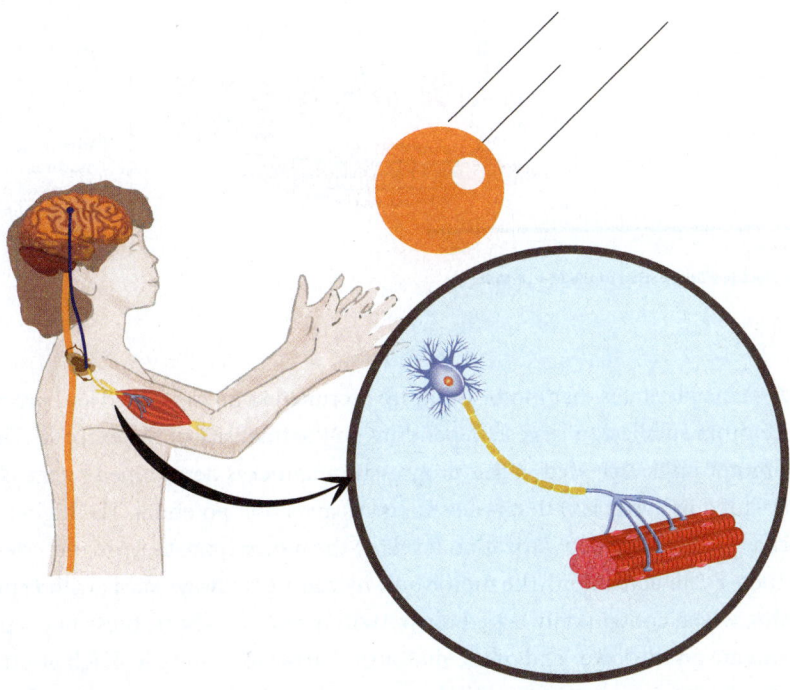

FIGURE 5.1 Neuromuscular Control

> ⚠️ **CRITICAL**
>
> Only the motor units that are stimulated will adapt to the exercise training or sport skill practice. Additionally, only the systems (e.g., endocrine, cardiovascular) needed to support the specific motor units recruited will experience adaptive changes. The magnitude of adaptation in these systems depends on the acute training variables, such as the intensity of training and the selection of exercises (i.e., how many muscles are used and in what manner).

Any physiological adaptation from exercise starts with the recruitment of a specific number and type of motor units to meet the demands for force and power. Unrecruited motor units and their associated muscle fibers do not develop beyond the level needed for normal function. Recruitment of motor units is based on the **size principle**, one of the most critical concepts in exercise and sports science (**Figure 5.2**).

CARDIO-RESPIRATORY FITNESS →

The ability of the circulatory and respiratory systems to provide the body with oxygen during activity.

NEURO-MUSCULAR EFFICIENCY →

The ability of the nervous system to recruit the correct muscles to produce force, reduce force, and dynamically stabilize the body's structure in all three planes of motion.

MOTOR UNIT →

A motor neuron and the muscle fibers it innervates or activates.

SIZE PRINCIPLE →

Motor unit recruitment occurs from smallest to largest.

The Size Principle

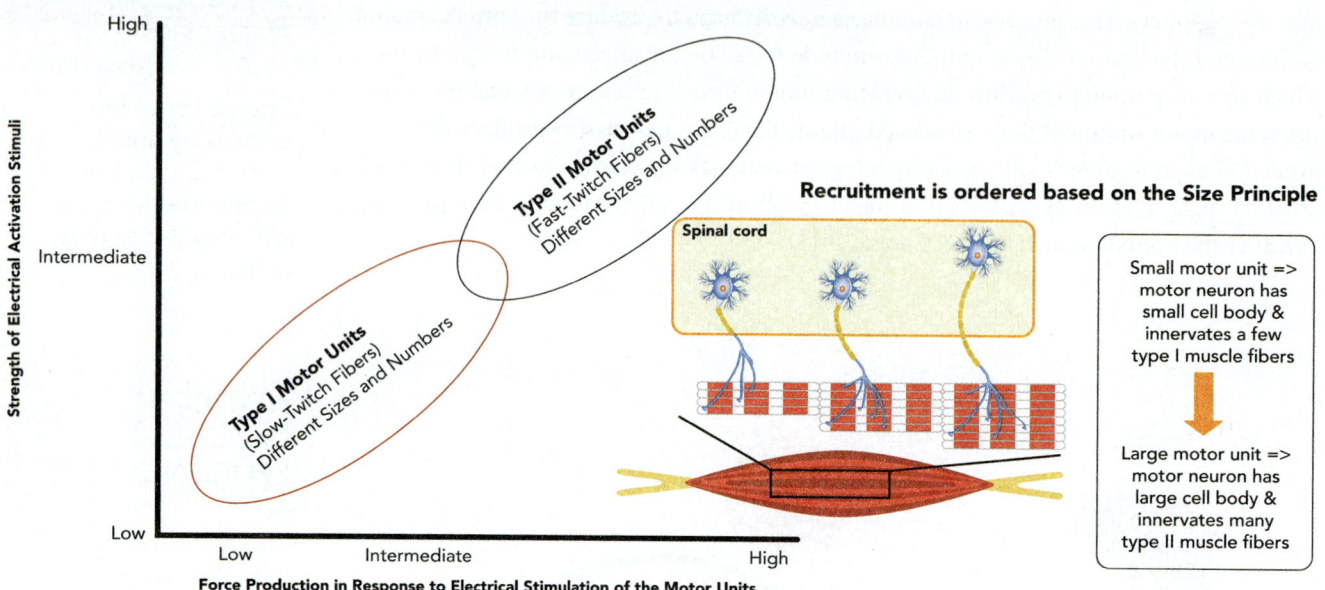

FIGURE 5.2 The Size Principle

<table>
<tr><td>

**TYPE I MOTOR →
UNIT**

An alpha motor neuron that contains only type I slow-twitch muscle fibers.

</td><td>

The size principle states that motor units are recruited in an organized and progressive order of size, from smallest to largest, depending on the intensity of the exercise. The number of motor units recruited in this progressive manner is determined by the electrical charge (measured in hertz, Hz) that is developed as an action potential. The higher the electrical charge, the more depolarization levels of the motor units that are met, resulting in greater motor unit activation. The motor unit recruitment always starts with **type I motor units**, which contain only **type I slow-twitch muscle fibers**; these fibers produce less force and are on the lower end of the motor unit array for a muscle. High electrical charges then add more motor units until the recruitment level is met and the right amount of force is achieved to produce a desired movement.

</td></tr>
</table>

TYPE I SLOW- →
**TWITCH MUSCLE
FIBER**

Muscle fibers that are small in size, generate lower amounts of force, and are more resistant to fatigue.

✔ CHECK IT OUT

The size principle was discovered over a lifetime of research by Elwood Henneman, an American neurophysiologist working at Harvard University, who studied the properties of vertebrate motor neurons. Henneman showed that whether muscle actions are concentric or eccentric, as the demands for force and power increase, more and more motor units are recruited in a progressive manner based on sizing factors (e.g., number, type, and size) to meet those demands.

**TYPE II MOTOR →
UNIT**

An alpha motor neuron that contains only type II fast-twitch muscle fibers.

How many motor units need to be recruited to reach a specific level of force to produce movement is determined by the electrical charge sent down the spinal cord from the motor cortex to all the motor units involved. This process starts with the type I motor units, which contain slow-twitch muscle fibers. The type I motor units produce less force but are always recruited first. If the electrical charge is high, then **type II motor units** containing **type II fast-twitch muscle fibers** are recruited to meet the force demands for movement. The associated adaptation to a specific sport task or training activity is based on the specific adaptation to imposed demands (SAID) principle (discussed in Chapter 4).

Finally, physiological adaptation reflects the many different physiological systems that support the active muscle in the performance of sports skills or in exercises used as part of a training program. Based on all of these factors, the Sports Performance Coach must design workouts and training programs to maximize an athlete's adaptational potential.

 **TYPE II FAST- →
TWITCH MUSCLE
FIBER**

Muscle fibers that are larger in size, generate higher amounts of force, and are faster to fatigue.

📋 COACH'S CORNER

Coaches see athletes with a natural bounce in their step, who can cut and "stop on a dime," and are naturally fast. These athletes are sometimes described as *twitchy*. This means they have a lot of type II motor units that contain fast-twitch muscle fibers that produce high levels of force, power, and speed. Although the number of type II motor units is largely genetically determined, proper training can enhance the activation efficiency and potential when needed.

BENEFITS OF SPORTS PERFORMANCE TRAINING

The most desired benefit for an athlete is an improvement in sports performance, achieved by enhancing the individual's anatomic structures and physiological functions using a systematic training approach (Kraemer et al., 2021). The effects of training programs are defined by anatomic structure and physiological system adaptations. Effective exercise programs are needed to ensure that the body responds with adaptive changes that move an athlete closer to the desired goal. Consequently, programs must address individualized training intensities, frequencies, and volumes of exercise, which allow for needed recovery and adaptations in the body's structures and physiological functions.

ATHLETE HEALTH

Sports are challenging to the health and well-being of any athlete who is striving to be the best. As competitive demands increase over an athlete's career, the challenges become even more daunting. The Sports Performance Coach must exercise care when developing sports performance programs to address the different aspects of an athlete's health, from physical to psychological (Casa et al., 2012; Chang et al., 2020; Radcliffe et al., 2018). When such training is done correctly, the benefits to an athlete after their competitive days will include optimized physical fitness and disease prevention. That is, properly designed training programs enhance the athlete's health by preventing injuries, allowing movements to be more precise and reactive, and adding to the improved functionality of physiological systems. These benefits lead to a greater potential for long-term health and resilience over an athlete's lifespan, increasing both the quality and longevity of life. Multiple components interact with an athlete's health when attempting to maximize their performance.

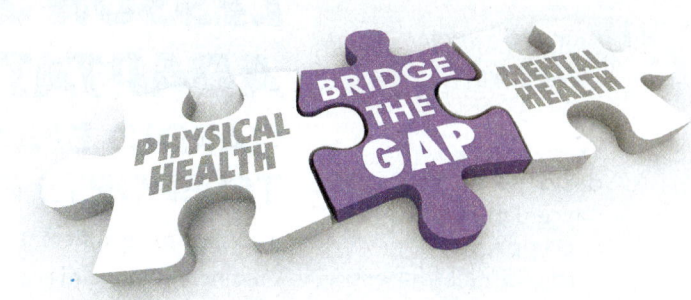

© iQoncept/Shutterstock

PERFORMANCE OPTIMIZATION

Optimizing performance requires the development of workouts and training programs that improve the body's ability to function and meet the competitive demands of a sport (Fleck & Kraemer, 2014). These processes are related to many aspects of sports performance training, including periodization of workouts, proper amounts of recovery time from workouts and competitions, sleep, proper nutrition and hydration, and developing the psychological and sociological capabilities for coping with competitive training and stress. With any training program, progressive overload with variation is vital in achieving adaptive changes (Peterson et al., 2011). **Figure 5.3** identifies various factors that can impact performance, and which a Sports Performance Coach must consider.

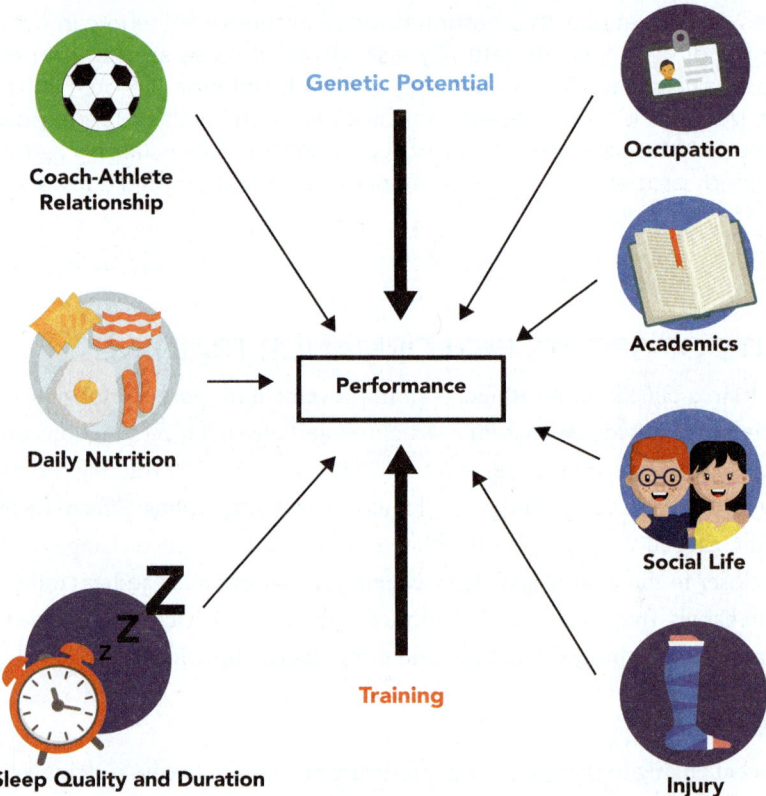

Factors that Impact Sports Performance Optimization

FIGURE 5.3: Factors That Impact Sports Performance Optimization

ENDURANCE
TRAINING →

Exercise programs designed to optimize oxygen utilization and improve cardiovascular fitness and long duration performances.

LESSON 2: CARDIO ENDURANCE ADAPTATIONS
CARDIO ENDURANCE ADAPTATIONS TO SPORTS PERFORMANCE TRAINING

There are many different forms of cardio **endurance training** and programs, which rely on different modalities and different types of equipment (Ronnestad & Mujika, 2014; Tonnessen et al., 2015). Cardio endurance training is directed toward improving the body's ability to take in and utilize oxygen for improved metabolic function and performance. This greater capability, in turn, supports the development of increased strength and power.

All athletes need various types of resistance and cardiorespiratory training to enhance their sports performance and recovery. The primary goal of a cardio endurance training program is to improve cardiorespiratory fitness, enhancing the function of the various anatomic structures and physiological functions needed to support increased endurance. It is vital for an athlete's cardiorespiratory system, which consists of the respiratory and cardiovascular systems, to adapt to improve their sports performance and support their body's increased metabolic demands. The first step is to get oxygen into the lungs, and from there into the blood, so the heart can deliver the oxygen-laden blood to the target tissues in the body.

Different modes of training impact the **cardiovascular system** and **respiratory system** to different extents based on their inherent differences as exercise modalities. Specifically, cardiovascular ("cardio") training can exist on a continuum from various types of high-intensity interval training workouts to continuous training methods (Milanovic et al., 2015).

CARDIO ENDURANCE TRAINING ADAPTATIONS

The primary purpose of the cardiorespiratory system is to deliver oxygen to the muscles and eliminate carbon dioxide, a waste product of metabolism, from the body. When a person is at rest, these functions remain somewhat constant for a given type of tissue, such as skeletal muscle. With exercise, the amount of oxygen taken out of the blood by active muscles and the amount of blood flowing through the active muscles increases substantially. As a result, the amount of oxygen delivered to the tissue increases. How well this is accomplished when exercising at the highest aerobic intensity is termed **maximum oxygen consumption**, or VO_2 max. VO_2 max is the primary measure of the multiple adaptations that take place with cardio or aerobic endurance training (Hellsten & Nyberg, 2015); this endpoint serves as the gold standard for aerobic fitness testing. The respiratory and cardiovascular systems are the two major components that are stimulated to adapt with cardio endurance training.

> ### ✔ CHECK IT OUT
>
> A common myth related to aerobic training states that running athletes must run long distances to gain improvements in maximum oxygen consumption or aerobic fitness. This is not true. In fact, long-distance road work for the anaerobic speed power athlete will only make them slower and less powerful and is a major training mistake (Wilson et al., 2012). Interval cardio sprint training can achieve the same goals of improving the anaerobic athlete's aerobic fitness to the level needed for recovery capabilities without harming speed and power (Knuttgen et al., 1973).

RESPIRATORY ADAPTATIONS

The process of respiration (**Figure 5.4**) involves the movement of air into and out of the lungs. The diffusion process in the lungs then exchanges oxygen with carbon dioxide (Dempsey et al., 1990; Romer et al., 2012). This exchange is mediated by the heart and its cardiovascular actions, which pump blood throughout the body; the blood, in turn, delivers oxygen to tissues and removes carbon dioxide from them.

CARDIO-VASCULAR SYSTEM →

The body system that transports blood to tissues of the body; includes the heart, blood vessels, and blood. Also known as the circulatory system.

RESPIRATORY SYSTEM →

The body system that brings oxygen into the lungs from breathed air while removing carbon dioxide from the lungs to the outside air; includes the airways, lungs, and respiratory muscles. Also known as the pulmonary system.

MAXIMUM OXYGEN CONSUMPTION →

(VO_2 max) The maximal amount of oxygen that the human body utilizes during sustained peak or maximal exercise.

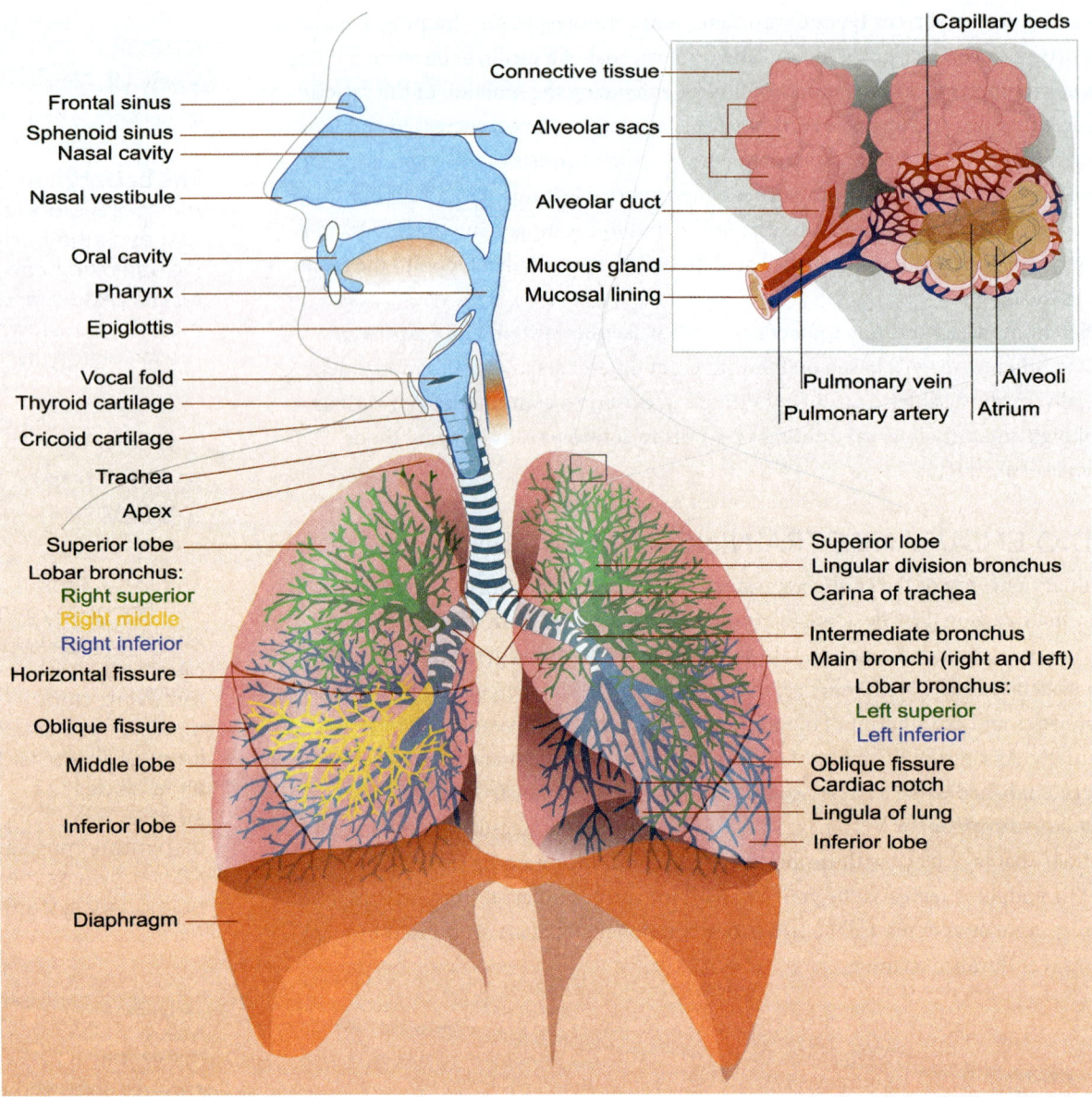

FIGURE 5.4 Component Structures of the Respiratory System

© Freepick/Shutterstock

✔ CHECK IT OUT

As exercise intensity increases, the amount of air an athlete needs to take in dramatically increases. With intense cardio endurance exercise, an athlete can increase their breathing rate from about 15 breaths per minute to more than 60 breaths per minute, taking in more than 100 liters of air per minute. Such heavy breathing creates a tremendous volume of air that needs to be moved in and out of the lungs by the respiratory muscles. In fact, research indicates that developing a ventilatory training program that mimics the specific demands of the sport can improve performance in running, cycling, swimming, and rowing (Shei, 2018).

The lungs are the major organs that capture oxygen from the air and deliver it to the blood for circulation, while taking carbon dioxide and other waste products from the blood. The respiratory system works with the cardiovascular system to provide oxygen to the body and remove carbon dioxide. Breathing is a dynamic function that relies on the inspiratory and expiratory muscles to move air into and out of the lungs (Bahensky et al., 2020). As shown in Figure 5.4, the respiratory tree (blue), the lungs, the diaphragm, and the alveoli carry out the functions of the respiratory system within the cardiorespiratory system.

With cardio training, the first adaptation enables the inspiratory and expiratory muscles to become stronger and more efficient at submaximal intensities and to tolerate higher frequencies of breathing at maximal exertion. Upper-body musculature contractions are used to accomplish proper breathing movements to get air in and out of the lungs (Aliverti, 2016). The diaphragm contracts and expands the abdominal and lower parts of the rib cage. Other muscles, including the intercostals, parasternals, scalenes, and neck muscles, act on the upper part of the pulmonary rib cage; they are engaged during both the inspiratory and expiratory processes. The expiratory muscles also include the abdominal muscles (i.e., external obliques, internal obliques, transversus abdominis, and rectus abdominis). An athlete requires coordinated contraction of the different muscle groups to breathe optimally.

📋 COACH'S CORNER

When an athlete competes intensely, abdominal conditioning is important. For example, in a basketball game or soccer match, it is apparent that the first stage of fatigue occurs in the abdominal area. This fatigue manifests as athletes bent over grasping their knees, straining to get their breath back. Given this relationship, exercise programs that strengthen and improve the endurance of the core musculature is vital to performance in sports.

The dynamics of the inspiratory and expiratory muscles function differently at rest as compared to during exercise, when increased lung volume and maximal diaphragmatic function are needed. Training programs must try to specifically address the diaphragm (Sales et al., 2016). The metabolic demands for energy, along with the changes in pH, affect both the inspiratory/expiratory muscles and the locomotive skeletal muscles. Thus, cardiorespiratory training aims to enhance the buffering of metabolic acidosis and to improve strength and endurance. The energy cost of breathing accounts for about 10% of the total oxygen consumption at higher exercise intensities (more than 90% of maximal exercise) (Kraemer et al., 2021). The ability to sustain these respiratory muscle contractions with ongoing exercise creates different levels of fatigue based on the intensity and duration of exercise stress. Therefore, cardiorespiratory fitness and adaptations are highly related to the specificity of the training program and the intensity, duration, and volume of exercise. Matching the sport's demands with the training program is vital to allow for optimal sports performance.

Men and women rely on the same respiratory system to provide oxygen to the exercising muscles, but there are some notable differences between them. First, men have larger and differently shaped lungs: Men have pyramidal-shaped lungs, whereas women's lungs are more symmetrical. Women have smaller airways leading into the lungs, making it harder for them to move air in and out of the lungs compared to men. Thus, women have to work harder at higher intensities for exercise. At peak exercise intensity, the respiratory muscles in men account for about 9% of the total body oxygen consumption compared to about 14% for women (Kraemer et al., 2021). However, women demonstrate greater endurance of the diaphragm at high-intensity exercise (greater than 90% of maximum effort) than men.

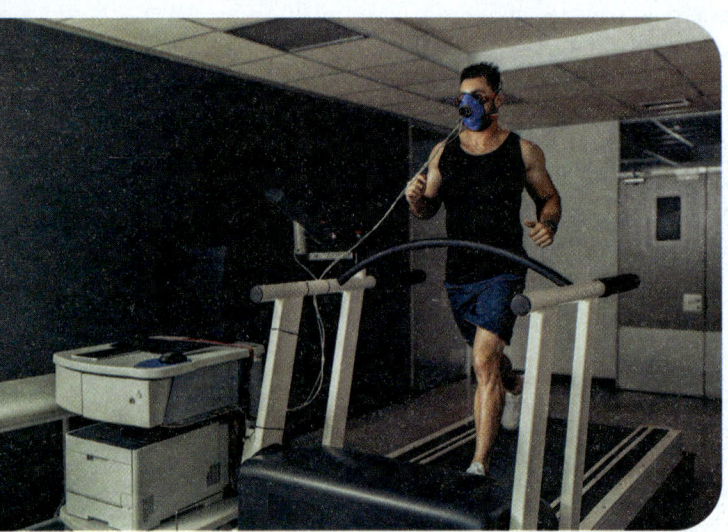

© Jacob Lund/Shutterstock

It is also essential for the respiratory muscles to assist blood flow to the active skeletal muscles needed for locomotion. Improved blood flow and capillary density is an adaptive response in all muscles, including the respiratory muscles, with training. A primary adaptation in the lungs is an increase in the number of alveoli, the functional structures in the lungs where blood flow and gas exchange occur (Romer et al., 2012).

The cost of breathing decreases during submaximal exercise, which allows more energy to be made available to the locomotive muscles. The **ventilatory equivalent** for oxygen (VE/VO_2) is also lowered, producing improvements in ventilatory efficiency. This equates to delayed fatigue in trained athletes. The effects of breathing efficiency are specific to upper- and lower-body cardio endurance training protocols. For example, when performing only arm training, athletes show improvements in VE/VO_2, but no such effects are observed when they perform only leg exercises. This makes adaptations in the VE/VO_2 specific to the upper- or lower-body modality.

VENTILATORY EQUIVALENT →

The amount of ventilation (milliliters per minute, mL/min) divided by how much oxygen is taken in (mL/min).

 COACH'S CORNER

If breathing fatigue occurs as a result of a sport that has an upper-body–predominant feature, such as water polo, it is important to include upper-body cardio training as well as typical lower-body cardio workouts in the training program.

VASCULAR-IZATION →

The process of growing blood vessels to improve oxygen and nutrient supply.

Cardio endurance exercise also increases the **vascularization** of capillaries in the lungs. This adaptation allows for greater blood flow in and out of the lungs. Oxygen uptake is enhanced due to the greater surface area in the lungs where blood can interact with the oxygen-carrying hemoglobin that passes through the pulmonary blood system. The blood in capillaries also removes carbon dioxide and other waste products from the body (Romer et al., 2012).

Other adaptations in the respiratory system associated with cardio endurance training include increased strength and endurance of the respiratory muscle fibers (**Table 5.1**). The ability to take in higher volumes of air and tolerate higher breathing rates enhances the athlete's endurance.

TABLE 5.1 Adaptations of the Respiratory System to Cardio Endurance Training

- Improved inspiratory and expiatory muscle strength and endurance
- Improved neural efficiency and signaling with better contractile coordination of respiratory muscles
- Improved toleration of pH decreases and energy demands with exercise
- Increased lung elasticity and expansion of pulmonary volumes and capacities
- Increased blood flow and number of capillaries in the inspiratory and expiratory muscles and lung tissues
- Increased number of alveoli in the lungs
- Increased lung tidal volume and lung capacity
- Decreased ventilatory oxygen demands in the inspiratory and expiratory muscles, leaving more oxygen available for use by locomotive muscles in the periphery
- Reduced energy cost of ventilation

CARDIAC ADAPTATIONS

The heart sits at the center of the cardiorespiratory system. It acts as the pump in the circulatory system, sending blood to deliver oxygen and nutrients to the cells, tissues, and organs that support exercise demands (**Figure 5.5**) (O'Leary et al., 2012). At the same time, blood returning to the heart delivers waste products that the body must dispose of, including carbon dioxide that exits the body with every exhalation. Cardio endurance training impacts this organ by supporting various structural and functional changes.

ANATOMY OF THE HEART

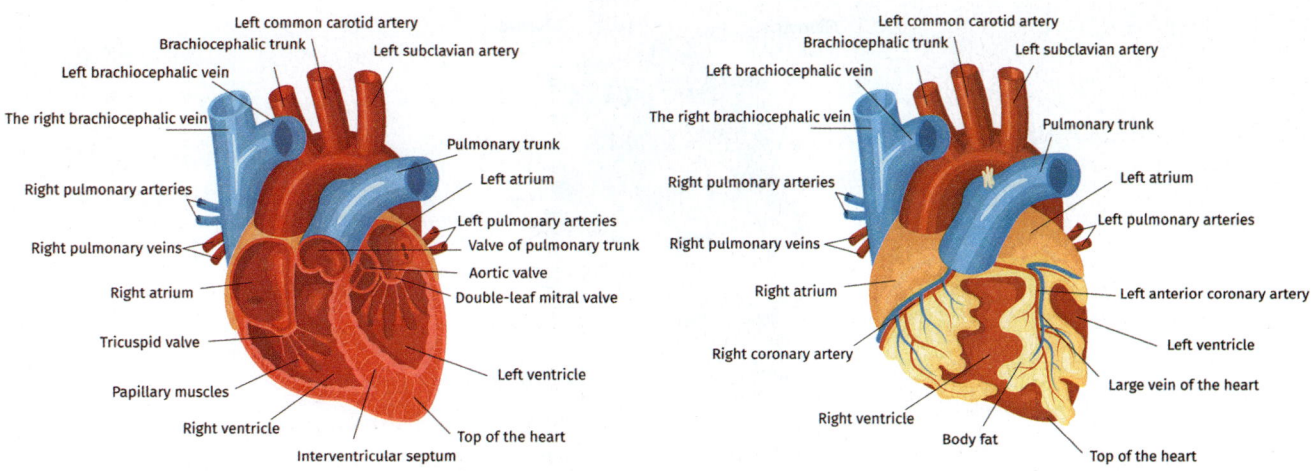

FIGURE 5.5 The Functional Blood Flow and the Heartbeat

First, cardio endurance training impacts the structure of the heart itself. Like skeletal muscle, cardiac muscle—that is, the myocardium—is capable of contraction and force production and responds to exercise stress. However, the myocardium is composed of only type I muscle fibers. The heart has a complex system that carries out its organized contraction, with the entire group of muscles in a heart chamber contracting simultaneously. This system is activated by a group of pacemaker cells, called the sinoatrial (SA) node, that cause the stimulation of the atria. The resulting neural signal is then sent to another set of cells, called the atrioventricular (AV) node, that stimulate the ventricles to contract (Moore & Brown, 2012). **Figure 5.6** illustrates the blood flow pathways and the unique unconscious activation that allows the heart chambers to contract, with the atria contracting first, followed by the ventricles. The heart rate responds to physical and psychological challenges when more blood flow is required (Moore & Brown, 2012).

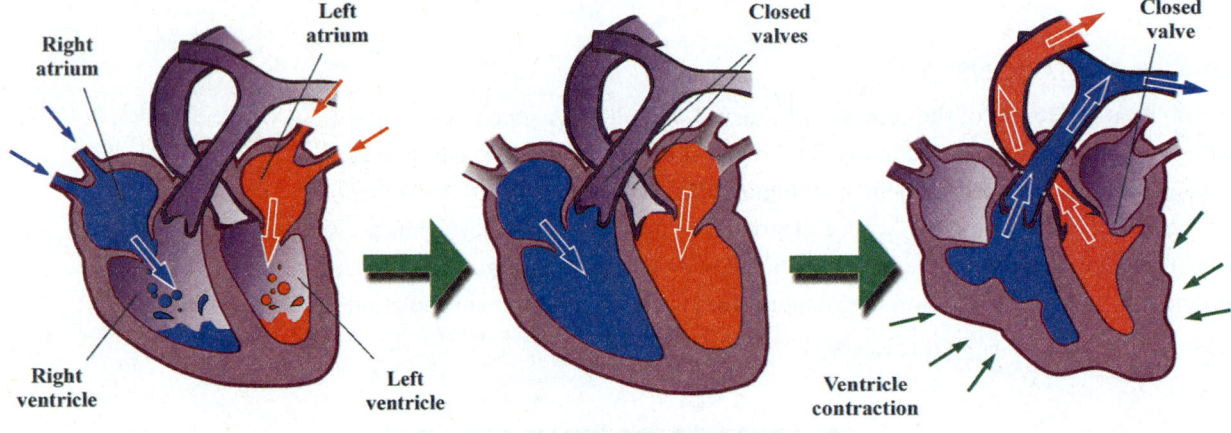

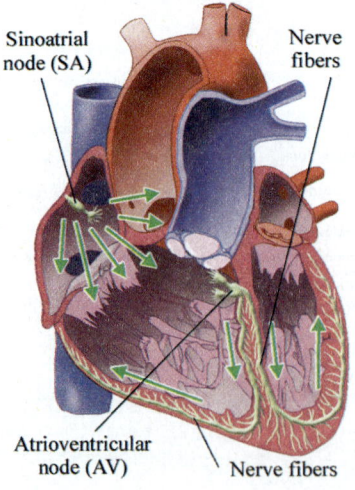

FIGURE 5.6 The Functional Blood Flow and the Heartbeat
© AmadeuBlasco/Shutterstock

The heartbeat is controlled unconsciously by the nervous system and can be visualized with an electrocardiogram (EKG). Here are some tips for understanding the diagram in Figure 5.6.

Top: Blood flow moves from the atria chambers first, sending blood to the ventricles; the ventricles then send the blood to the rest of the body. Blood in the veins (venous circulation), which comes back to the heart and is then sent to the lungs for reoxygenation, is shown in blue. The oxygenated blood pumped out to the rest of the body is shown in red.

Bottom: The activation of the heart starts with the AV node, which stimulates the atria. The neural message then goes to the SA node, which sends signals to the bottom of the ventricles to complete the heartbeat with their contraction.

With cardio training, the chambers of the heart become thicker and can produce more force to eject blood with greater velocity and pressure, which is especially important at higher exercise and competition intensities. The size and thickness of each chamber vary, with the different chambers of the heart pumping blood to different locations: The atria pump blood to the ventricle chambers; the right ventricle pumps blood to the lungs; and the left ventricle pumps blood to the rest of the body. As more work is needed to get blood to the far reaches of the body, the left ventricle increases its wall thickness through cardio training. However, this thickness does not exceed normal limits (about 13 mm), unlike with chronic hypertension pathologies. Additionally, with cardio endurance training, the volume of the left ventricular chamber increases to allow more blood to be pumped out with each beat. Because less work is needed from the right ventricle, this chamber of the heart does not experience the same increase in size.

✔ CHECK IT OUT

The fact that endurance athletes have larger hearts was first recognized at the end of the 19th century in cross-country skiers. This finding was confirmed in other endurance athletes as more advanced imaging techniques became available. An enlarged heart is considered harmless if the size falls within normal limits. In contrast, a heart enlarged beyond normal limits can be dangerous. The latter condition, called "athlete's heart syndrome," may be due to pathologies such as aortic stenosis, hypertension, ischemic heart disease, or hypertrophic obstructive cardiomyopathy.

CARDIORESPIRATORY ADAPTATIONS TO RESISTANCE TRAINING

Most resistance training programs focus on improving muscular strength and power. Resistance exercise is associated with high-pressure loads that create dramatic demands on the cardiorespiratory system and its organs. Some of the highest blood pressures recorded occur when maximal loading is achieved (MacDougall et al., 1985). Additionally, blood pressure increases with the addition of more sets with moderate to heavy loads (Fleck & Dean, 1987). The pressure changes observed far outdistance the typical pressures seen with cardio exercise, even at maximal levels of exertion. The high-pressure changes with heavy resistance exercise play protective roles by modulating the pressure levels in the abdominal, thoracic, and spinal columns to eliminate the risk of aneurysm (i.e., bulge or burst of a fluid column or structure). The increased thickness in the heart's septal wall (i.e., the wall between the chambers) reflects these dramatic pressure overloads with progressive heavy resistance exercise training (**Figure 5.7**).

Cardiorespiratory Adaptations

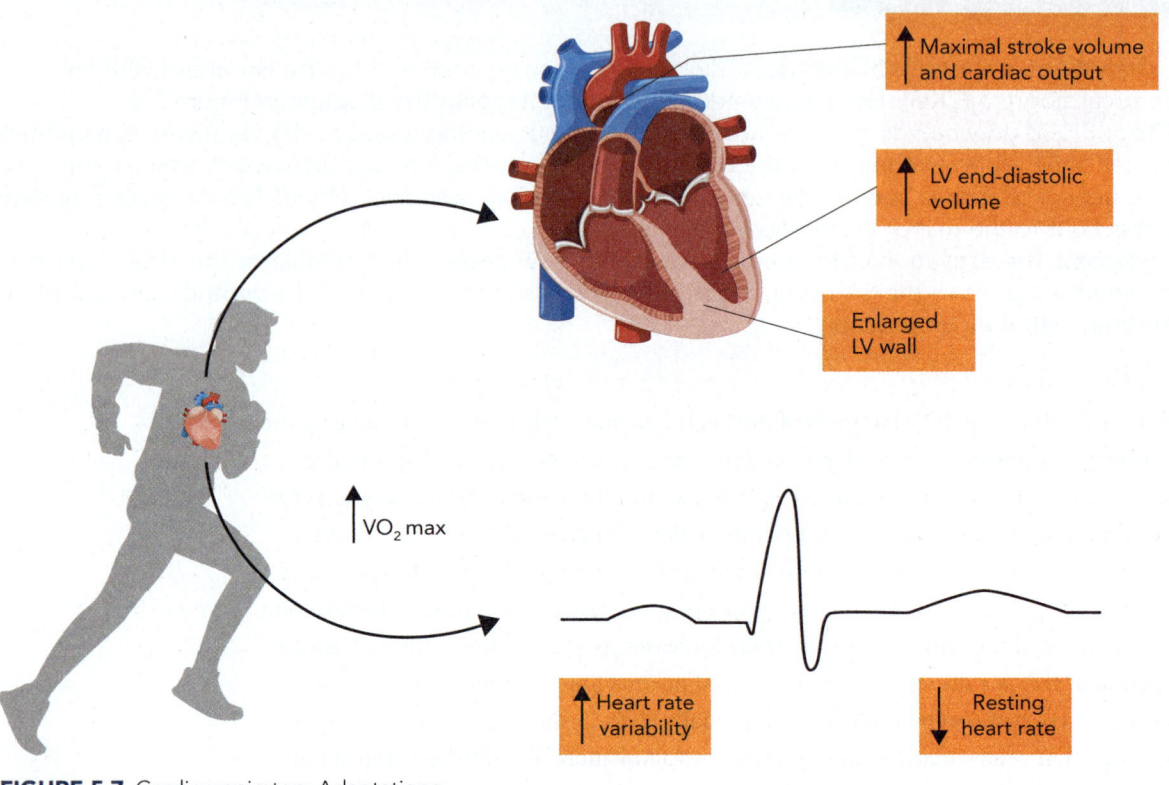

FIGURE 5.7 Cardiorespiratory Adaptations

LV: left ventricular

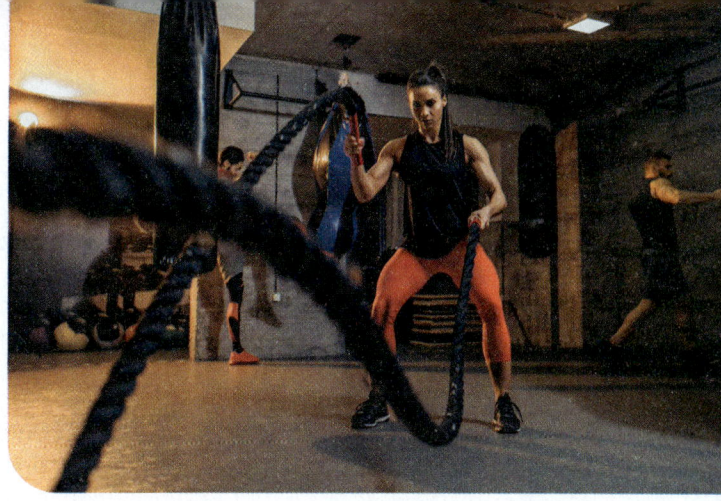
© Bbernard/Shutterstock

Some forms of resistance training, such as short-rest types of circuit weight training, improve anaerobic capacity and local muscular endurance. They accomplish this by keeping the body's normal **acid–base balance** within a tolerable range—an important effect because pH drops with intense anaerobic exercise. The pH scale ranges from 0 (strongly acidic) to 14 (strongly basic or alkaline), with the normal pH of blood being 7.40 (the normal range is 7.35–7.45). With intense exercise, blood pH can drop to 7.1, making the blood more acidic than at rest (Gordon et al., 1994).

To combat the impact of drops in pH with intense exercise, athletes can engage in training geared toward enhancing the buffering mechanisms. These buffering mechanisms neutralize hydrogen ions and reduce the decreases in pH associated with intense exercise. Such changes in pH and increases in hydrogen ion (H^+) levels are major causes of fatigue and loss of force and power in sports performance and workouts. They affect many other functions as well, including the endocrine release of growth hormones (Kraemer et al., 2021). With circuit weight training, cardiorespiratory improvements are typically observed, especially in beginners (Harber et al., 2004; Maiorana et al., 1997). Resistance training improves cardiorespiratory structures and functions very similarly to cardio training, albeit not to the same magnitude.

> **ACID–BASE BALANCE** →
>
> The balance between intake and production and elimination of hydrogen ions.

 COACH'S CORNER

When performing a resistance exercise workout with short rest periods between sets and exercises, it is vital that the athlete does not experience any symptoms of nausea, dizziness, or vomiting. These symptoms indicate an athlete is sick and are not representative of a "good workout." If such symptoms exist, stop the workout, increase the rest periods, and progress more slowly.

The lack of improvement in maximal oxygen consumption in highly fit trainees was first shown in a study by Kraemer et al. (1995). Researchers used a 4-day-a-week resistance training program in which 2 days were dedicated to strength and power, and the other 2 days were devoted to circuit-type training with supersets and bodybuilding protocols to enhance muscular endurance. However, no significant changes in the participants' maximal oxygen consumption values were noted at the end of 3 months, despite dramatic increases in their strength, power, and muscle size. The participants who did resistance and cardio endurance training improved in terms of both their strength and maximal oxygen consumption, indicating they had enhanced aerobic fitness. Ultimately, these study results emphasized the importance of training specificity in regard to the various training modalities. Although many benefits of resistance training may be observed in the cardiorespiratory system, absolute improvements in the gold standard of aerobic fitness, maximum oxygen consumption (VO_2 max), are not easily achieved once fitness levels go beyond the beginner level of sports performance fitness.

Another study raised an important point: All adaptations have windows of adaptive potential (Fleck & Kraemer, 2014). The Sports Performance Coach must pay careful attention to individualized programming for an athlete to achieve further gains in cardiorespiratory or neuromuscular efficiency variables. **Table 5.2** compares the adaptive changes that occur with cardio endurance versus resistance training programs.

TABLE 5.2 Adaptations of the Cardiac System with Cardio Endurance Training or Resistance Training

Variable	Cardio Endurance Training	Resistance Training
Right atrium wall thickness	No change	No change
Left atrium wall thickness	No change	No change
Right ventricle thickness	Small increase	No change
Left ventricle thickness	Increase	Increase
Septum wall thickness	Small increase	Increase
Right atrium chamber volume	No change	No change
Left atrium chamber volume	No change	No change
Right ventricle volume	No change	No change
Left ventricle volume	Increase	Small increase
Resting heart rate	Decrease	Small decrease
Heart rate variability	Increase	Increase
Adrenergic (adrenalin) sensitivity to stress	Decrease	Decrease
Resting diastolic blood pressure	Decrease	Variable
Resting systolic blood pressure	Decrease	Variable
Peak exercise diastolic blood pressure	Decrease	Variable
Peak exercise systolic blood pressure	Decrease	Variable

Adaptations in Cardio Training Performance

The primary variable that helps to mediate endurance performance is maximal oxygen consumption (VO_2 max) and the energy efficiency of movement at given levels of exercise intensity. The various forms of cardio training—from intervals to tempo runs to distance workouts—all attempt to improve this variable. The specificity of the modality (e.g., running versus cycle versus swimming) is also crucial for ensuring optimal endurance performance, as has been well noted by triathlon competitors. Resistance training, even when using short rest periods or circuit weight training protocols, can fall short when an athlete attempts to improve their maximal oxygen consumption. However, such training improves the efficiency of endurance performances by strengthening the peripheral musculature and reducing the stress on the heart and other central cardiorespiratory demands. Thus, including both forms of training is vital to address different targets in cardiorespiratory adaptations and their role in sports performance.

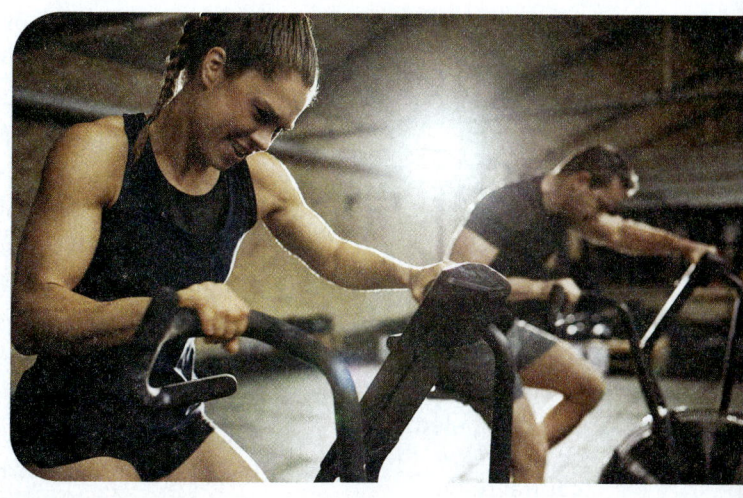

© Ground Picture/Shutterstock

LESSON 3: NEUROMUSCULAR ADAPTATIONS

NEUROMUSCULOSKELETAL ADAPTATIONS TO SPORTS PERFORMANCE TRAINING

The neuromuscular system plays an integral role in recruiting different muscles to produce movement in exercise training and sports skill performances. The performance is based on the recruitment of motor units in a progressive manner (i.e., the size principle) to meet the demands of the external resistance and the need for force and power (Duchateau & Enoka, 2011). The associated adaptations to such stimulation are related to the specificity of the training program or practice. Motor units not recruited with their associated muscle fibers show no adaptations above the everyday demands of cell function. However, as muscle fibers are recruited as a part of activated motor units, a new homeostatic function is produced. The adaptation in the neural and muscular systems occurs and is related to the training program's intensity, duration, and frequency.

ADAPTATIONS TO NERVOUS SYSTEM

The nervous system is the electrical system that controls body functions and adapts to the external environment. In essence, the nervous system controls everything in the human body. The brain and spinal cord make up the CNS. After the neuron leaves the spinal cord, it becomes part of the peripheral nervous system (PNS). Exercise training for sports performance or health results in adaptive changes in the CNS and PNS in both structure and function.

RESISTANCE TRAINING

One of the primary neural adaptations with resistance training is the reduction in inhibition and improvement of neural facilitation of muscular force. This occurs centrally in the brain and peripherally around the joints, enhancing the agonist force production and limiting the antagonist inhibition. Studies show that injury can affect brain function and inhibit peripheral force production in the lower body musculature (Flanagan et al., 2021). Additionally, injury can impact the capability of muscles to produce force. The inhibition in the nervous system often serves as a protective measure to reduce damage to the joints and muscles when they are not ready for high-force production efforts. With exercise training, this inhibition is reduced, which allows for more forceful and effective muscle actions. The primary adaptations in the nervous system involve the facilitation or inhibition of the electrical signaling of end-target organs and tissues. The activation of these peripheral targets stimulates their cellular adaptations, whether it is a myocardial heart muscle cell, a skeletal muscle cell, or an endocrine organ.

The body contains a variety of neurons of all shapes and sizes. Each neuron has a dendrite that takes information into the central body, where that information is processed. If appropriate, the information then leaves the cell body through axons to the next neuron or, in the case of muscle, to the neuromuscular junction to stimulate the muscle fibers to contract or activate. Skeletal muscle activation starts in the motor cortex of the brain. Here, the electrical stimuli to produce force are created. These electrical signals travel from the motor cortex through **alpha motor neurons**, down the spinal cord, and out to stimulate the muscle fibers that make up that motor unit (**Figure 5.8**). Repeated stimulation with a training program causes adaptations in this process.

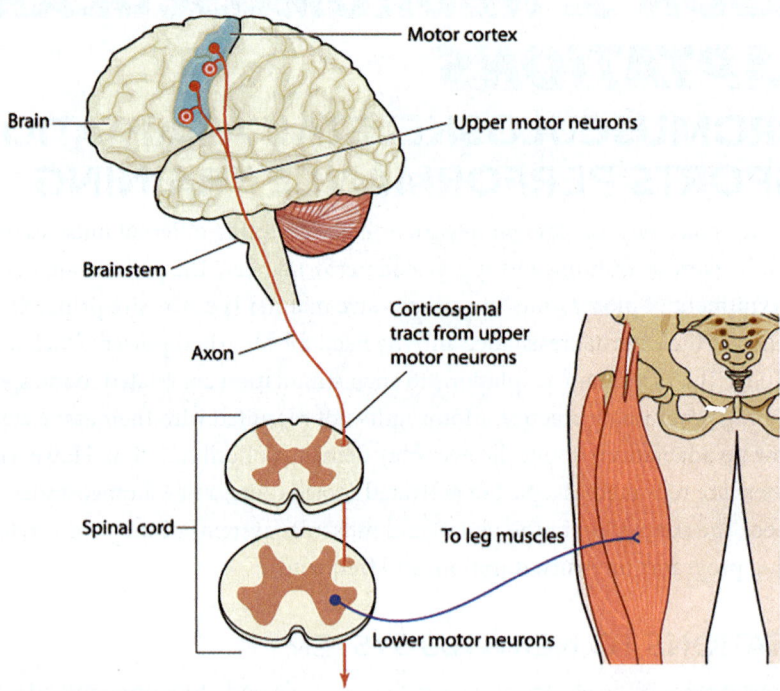

FIGURE 5.8 The Motor Unit
© Blamb/Shutterstock

✔ **CHECK IT OUT**

A motor unit activates a given set of muscle fibers to produce the force needed to meet the external force and power demands in a sports skill or a training exercise.

CARDIO TRAINING

As with resistance training, the nervous system's involvement during cardio training is specific to the activation of skeletal muscles to provide the needed force and power. Thus, the effect on the nervous system is specific to the type of workout the athlete performs. Cardiorespiratory endurance or repeated endurance capabilities represent an essential adaptive change. For athletes who do not want cardio endurance training, such as distance running, to interfere with their muscular development or power from resistance training, high-intensity interval training can be used. This training allows athletes to improve VO_2 max without decreasing speed, strength, and power. **Table 5.3** outlines the expected adaptive changes in the neuromuscular system with cardio sports performance training.

TABLE 5.3 Basic Adaptations of the Neuromuscular System to Resistance and Cardio Endurance Training

Variable responses are related to the span of resistance or cardio training programs used in different training programs.		
Variable	**Cardio Endurance Training**	**Resistance Training**
Motor unit size	Variable	Increase
Motor facilitation	Increase	Increase
Motor inhibition	Decrease	Decrease
Neurotransmitter chemicals	Variable	Increase
Type I muscle fiber size	No change or decrease	Increase
Type II muscle fiber size	No change	Increase
Intact muscle size	No change	Increase
Aerobic enzymes	Increase	Variable
Anaerobic enzymes	Variable	Increase
Mitochondria content	Increase	Variable
Capillary density per fiber	Increase	Variable
Triglyceride stores	Increase	Variable
Stored ATP	Increase	Increase
Glycogen stores	Increase	Increase
Maximal strength	No change	Increase
Local muscular endurance	Increase	Variable

CELL SIGNALING →

The process of communication between cells by biological messengers to govern cellular function.

The neuromuscular adaptations to sports performance training are the cornerstone of sports performance. An athlete's ability to produce higher muscular force is the endpoint of many different physiological adaptations that come with exercise training. The process starts with the recruitment of motor units in a workout that is part of a training program. Through this motor unit recruitment process, the nervous system begins its adaptive changes as part of the neuromuscular system. Then, the amount of muscle recruited impacts other supportive physiological systems and structures. The increases in strain and compressive forces on the connective tissues stimulate changes in density and strength. The endocrine glands are repeatedly activated to cope with stress and help in the anabolic signaling for growth and development. Thus, **cell signaling** and the adaptive changes in response to exercise training mediate the improved structure and function of the athlete.

ADAPTATIONS TO THE SKELETAL SYSTEM

The activation of muscle and the resulting movement and force production create a dramatic adaptive effect on connective tissue. **Mechanotransduction** encompasses many different processes in which cells respond to the mechanical stimuli of exercise by converting forces into molecular signaling that alters cellular mechanisms and adaptations (Herrmann et al., 2020). This process helps to explain how exercise training stimulates the many adaptive changes that occur in the body with exercise training, especially in the muscle and connective tissues and structures (Bamman et al., 2018).

⚠ **CRITICAL**

From mechanotransduction to hormonal interactions with receptors, the body's ability to adapt is based on cell signaling. Cell signaling is one of the many ways cells learn about and respond to their environment. This includes the anabolic and catabolic interactions related to exercise training and sports competition. Cells, tissues, physiological systems, and structures are all informed about and respond to the external environment of nutrition, exercise, and behaviors through cell signaling. Adaptation is related to the body's cells receiving, processing, and transmitting signals to its environment and itself. Cell signaling is a fundamental property of all cells in every living organism.

MECHANO- TRANSDUCTION →

The process by which cells convert mechanical stimuli or forces, such as pressure, tension, or stretching, into electrochemical signals that elicit specific cellular responses.

Connective tissues in the human body are sensitive to loading (Ratamess, 2022). The three common types of stress mediated by mechanotransduction are associated with the loading of connective tissue:

- *Tension* or *stress* is what an athlete feels with stretching or pulling forces on the tissues. It also occurs in tendons during muscular contractions.
- *Compression* is a stress that involves the inward pressing of the longitudinal length of the structure. For example, compression occurs in the spinal cord in a squat exercise and in the arms in an overhead military press.
- *Shear stress* occurs where forces hit tissues at oblique angles, such as during agility training. As a result of the acceleration and deceleration at different angles, this stressor on connective tissue has the greatest potential for causing injury. Indeed, one of the primary reasons sports performance training is needed is to prevent connective tissue damage from shear stress. The breakpoints of different connective tissues vary by type and stress. Connective tissue is sensitive to loading, underloading, and overtraining.

Connective tissues start at the level of the muscle fiber. They include all of the noncontractile elements in the muscle from the endomysium that covers the muscle fiber, to the perimysium that covers the fasciculus, to the epimysium that surrounds the muscle, to the noncontractile elements in the sarcomere itself with the Z-line proteins at the ends of the sarcomere, to the nebulin that keeps the actin filaments in line, to the titan that holds the myosin proteins in line and the M-line protein that holds various chemicals in place (e.g., myosin-ATPase) (**Figure 5.9**). These noncontractile proteins, called the **elastic component** of muscle, are vital for developing power in the stretch–shortening cycle. The muscle then connects to tendons, which in turn connect to bones. Additionally, ligaments connect bones together and help maintain joint alignment. A great deal of connective tissue keeps the body structures in line and gives the human body structural shape and function (Kraemer et al., 2021; Ratamess, 2022). Exercise training impacts these structures and functions.

> **ELASTIC COMPONENT** →
>
> Noncontractile proteins.

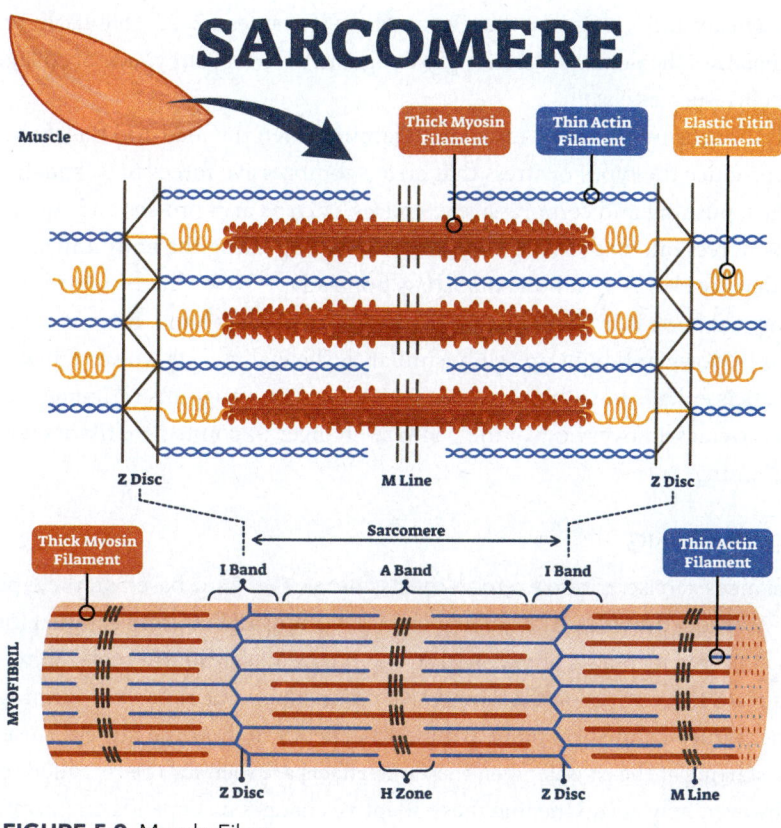

FIGURE 5.9 Muscle Fiber

© VectorMine/Shutterstock

✔ CHECK IT OUT

Muscle fibers are made up of sarcomeres that provide the contraction mechanisms of the muscle. In the fibers, actin and myosin are held in place by more connective tissues—specifically, noncontractile proteins of nebulin, titin, Z-discs, and M-lines. The connective tissues add structure to the muscle and provide the elastic component, which is important for power production in sports and training.

RESISTANCE TRAINING

The load used in a resistance exercise stimulates the motor units needed to move a specific load. The electrical charge from the nervous system runs down the line and into the muscle fibers of motor units to stimulate contraction. This produces adaptations in both the connective tissue and the muscle fibers. The noncontractile proteins (e.g., Z-discs, titan) start to increase their density (thickness) to tolerate the forces. Type I muscle fibers have naturally thicker noncontractile proteins because they are always recruited first. When athletes lift heavier loads with progressive resistance training, these connective tissues become even more dense. The connective tissue adapts with resistance training at the level of the muscle fibers.

Mechanotransduction plays a vital role in identifying the specific type of loading to which connective tissue is sensitive, especially pulling tension. The contraction of the intact muscle stimulates an increase in the proteins of the tendon, which is primarily made up of dense fibrous collagen fibers. Progressive heavy resistance training promotes increased density and strength of the tendon fibers (Ratamess, 2022). Similarly, resistance training increases the density and strength of ligaments, which are made of collagen and other proteins, such as elastin.

Finally, bone is impacted by resistance training when the load and the chosen exercises produce the types of stress that create compressive forces (e.g., squats, bench press). Thus, pushing and compressive exercises, such as arm presses and squats with a vertical compression, load on the bone structures supporting the body and are crucial for bone density changes. In bone *modeling*, bone adapts to mechanical loading; in bone *remodeling*, old bone is broken down and replaced with new bone. Bone is constantly being broken down and built up again, similar to skeletal muscle with exercise stress. This process is enhanced with proper resistance exercise programs (Ratamess, 2022). **Table 5.4** provides an overview of the primary changes in connective tissues with exercise training.

CARDIO TRAINING

Like resistance exercise, cardio exercise affects connective tissue based on the types of forces the workout provides. The loading in such training differs from external forces due to the lower percentages of maximal strength used in cardio workouts. Some cardio workouts place more stress on the connective tissues than others, such as running versus swimming. Which connective tissue is affected depends on how the muscle is used. Similarly, starting at the muscle fiber, the same effects are seen for the recruited muscle fibers. However, how far up the line these adaptive changes go depends on how many motor units are recruited. For instance, distance runners well know that high impact on hard surfaces over a long duration can result in unwanted breakdown of tissues in the entire body structure. That is why almost all endurance athletes supplement their cardio exercise with resistance training. The adaptations of the tendons, ligaments, and bone follow the same pattern of adaptation based on the different tensions and loading of the body (Table 5.4).

ADAPTATIONS TO THE MUSCULAR SYSTEM

The adaptations observed in muscles are based on the recruitment of motor units to meet the demands of sports performance and exercise training. As is the case for connective tissue, loading plays a crucial role in how the musculature adapts to the exercise and training program (Campos et al., 2002).

TABLE 5.4 Basic Adaptations of the Connective Tissues with Resistance and Cardio Endurance Training

Variable	Cardio Endurance Training	Resistance Training
Type I motor unit and muscle fiber's noncontractile proteins	Increased based on the level of loading used in the modality used	Increased, especially when heavier loads are used
Type II motor unit and muscle fiber's noncontractile fiber proteins	Few or no changes due to the lack of loading of these motor units and fibers	Increased but not to the extent of type I muscle fibers, which have naturally denser fibers made for regular use
Tendon thickness	Increased protein content but not to the same extent as with heavy loading used in resistance training	Increased protein content contributes to thicker tendons
Ligament thickness	Increased protein content but not to the same extent as with heavy loading used in resistance training	Increased protein content contributes to thicker ligaments
Collagen synthesis	Increased in loaded tendons and ligaments	Increased in loaded tendons and ligaments
Collagen breakdown	Decreased in loaded tendons and ligaments	Decreased in loaded tendons and ligaments
Number of collagen proteins	Increased in loaded tendons and ligaments	Increased in loaded tendons and ligaments
Tendon blood flow	Increased	Increased
Inflammatory markers and mediators	Decreased	Decreased
Elastic energy storage	Increased	Increased
Connective tissue strength	Increased	Increased

✔ **CHECK IT OUT**

The intact structure of skeletal muscle (**Figure 5.10**) begins at the point of tendon attachment. It then pulls out into smaller structures from bundles of fibers to the fiber itself, made up of actin and myosin, called myofibrils. Connective tissues surround each pull-out from the muscle to the muscle fiber.

SKELETAL MUSCLE

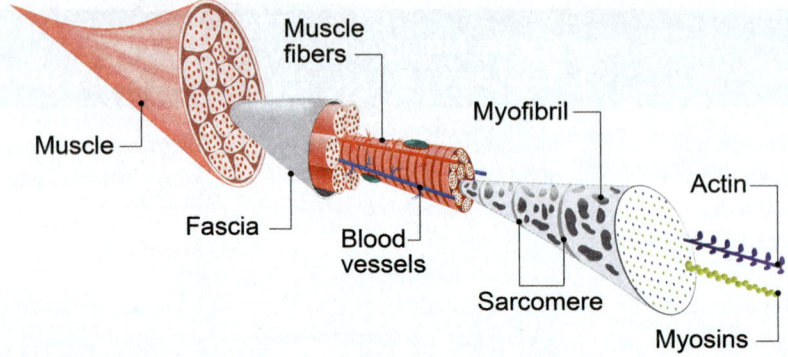

FIGURE 5.10 Skeletal Muscle
© Designua/Shutterstock

RESISTANCE TRAINING

Many types of resistance training programs are possible, spanning different configurations of the acute training variables and periodization models. However, if activated, adaptive changes start occurring in the neuromuscular system. This system includes both type I slow-twitch and type II fast-twitch muscle fibers, but not all muscles have the same complement of each motor unit type. Type I motor units with type I slow-twitch muscle fibers dominate all individuals' postural muscles (e.g., abdominal muscles). However, individuals can have different genetic complements of muscle fiber types in their locomotor muscles (e.g., thighs, calves). This allows for dramatically different sports performance potentials (e.g., sprinters versus marathon runners). The average population of human locomotor muscles ranges from 40% to 60% type I and 40% to 60% type II muscle fibers, with elite endurance or strength athletes showing either a higher slow-twitch or a higher fast-twitch fiber profile, respectively (Staron et al., 2000).

Beginning in the 1960s and continuing into the 1980s, exercise and sports scientists argued about how the phenomenon of hypertrophy occurred. Two primary questions were (1) whether this condition increased muscle fiber size or the number of muscle fibers and (2) whether the muscle broke down and then was repaired, or whether it just added protein to existing structures. By the start of the 21st century, some of these mysteries had been solved. Increased muscle fiber size, not an increased number of muscle fibers, is the primary way an intact muscle grows. Additionally, exercise stress stimulates a breakdown and repair phenomenon. First, exercise causes damage, and then a multitude of physiological signals start the recovery process to rebuild and repair the muscle, making the damaged muscle bigger and stronger (Kraemer et al., 2021).

Upon muscle breakdown, the adaptive changes that occur with skeletal muscle repair and lead to hypertrophy involve the addition of a noncontractile protein latticework and the addition of myofibrillar proteins (actin and myosin) to the outside of the fiber. The amount of sarcoplasm also increases to address the need for more fluid content created by the increased protein content; this fluid keeps all of the pressure gradients (i.e., osmotic and oncotic) in balance. Additionally, **cell swelling** occurs due to increased blood flow and energy production to the activated muscle, and temporary cell bloating occurs (Schoenfeld, 2013). This has been noted as a stimulus for muscle hypertrophy, which many lifters call the "pump" after lifting workouts. Many signaling processes (e.g., endocrine, immune) respond to the exercise stress to support the adaptive changes needed for repair and remodeling (Kraemer & Spiering, 2007). Greater hypertrophy in an intact muscle is

CELL SWELLING→

An increase in blood flow to the contracting muscle, which results in temporary cell bloating.

achieved when more motor units are recruited in a muscle. Thus, the use of progressive heavy resistance exercise training is critical. Without progressive overload, no adaptive changes will occur. The lack of an adaptive change is often called a plateau or staleness in training, but might also be due to some form of overreaching or overtraining (Fry & Kraemer, 1997). Thus, the resistance training stimulus in the workout and proper progressions are vital to promote both neural and hypertrophic neuromuscular adaptations.

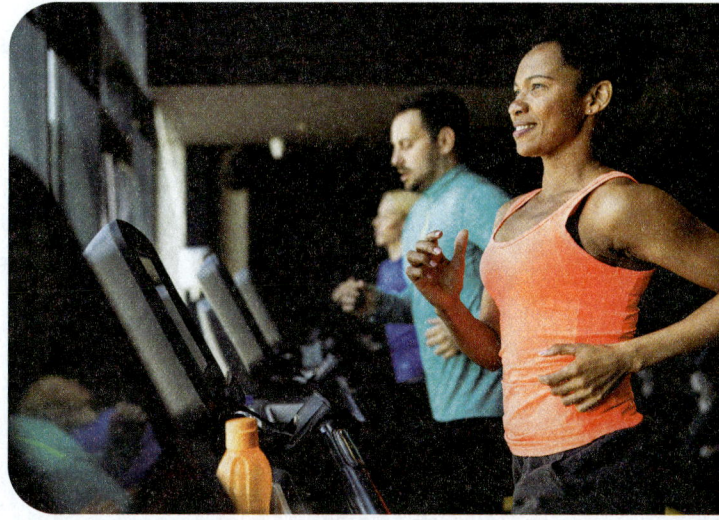

© NDAB Creativity/Shutterstock

CARDIO TRAINING

As expected from a neuromuscular perspective, the primary motor units recruited with cardio endurance exercise workouts are the type I motor units containing the type I slow-twitch muscle fibers. The cardio workout produces muscle breakdown in the recruited muscle fibers, along with the need for subsequent repair. For the most part, this repair process takes place to a greater extent in the type I muscle fibers due to the intensity of exercise when performing a typical cardio exercise workout. A similar repair and remodeling process then occurs, whether the trigger is cardio or resistance exercise. However, with routine cardio workouts, hypertrophy is limited at best due to the lower electrical charge stimulus associated with exercise stress targeting predominately low-threshold type I motor units. Cardio exercise tends to trigger remodeling and repair of the type I muscle fibers, and it is not a hypertrophy stimulus as an exercise modality. Hypertrophy is limited even with high-intensity interval training using sprints.

✔ CHECK IT OUT

When an athlete engages in high-intensity aerobic endurance training without resistance training, the type I muscle fibers get smaller (Kraemer et al., 1995). That is why elite runners use a resistance training program to maintain muscle fiber size: It does not negatively affect their endurance capacity and improves performance by increasing exercise efficiency (Bazyler et al., 2015; Hickson et al., 1980).

LESSON 4: ENDOCRINE ADAPTATIONS
ENDOCRINE ADAPTATIONS TO SPORTS PERFORMANCE TRAINING

The **endocrine system** comprises specialized glands (endocrine glands) that store and produce hormones to release into the blood when stimulated by other hormones or nerves (**Figure 5.11**) (Kraemer & Rogol, 2005). The endocrine system is complex and is involved in almost every physiological function in the body.

ENDOCRINE → SYSTEM

A group of glands that secrete chemical substances (hormones) into the blood to signal cell receptors to respond in a certain manner.

The Endocrine System

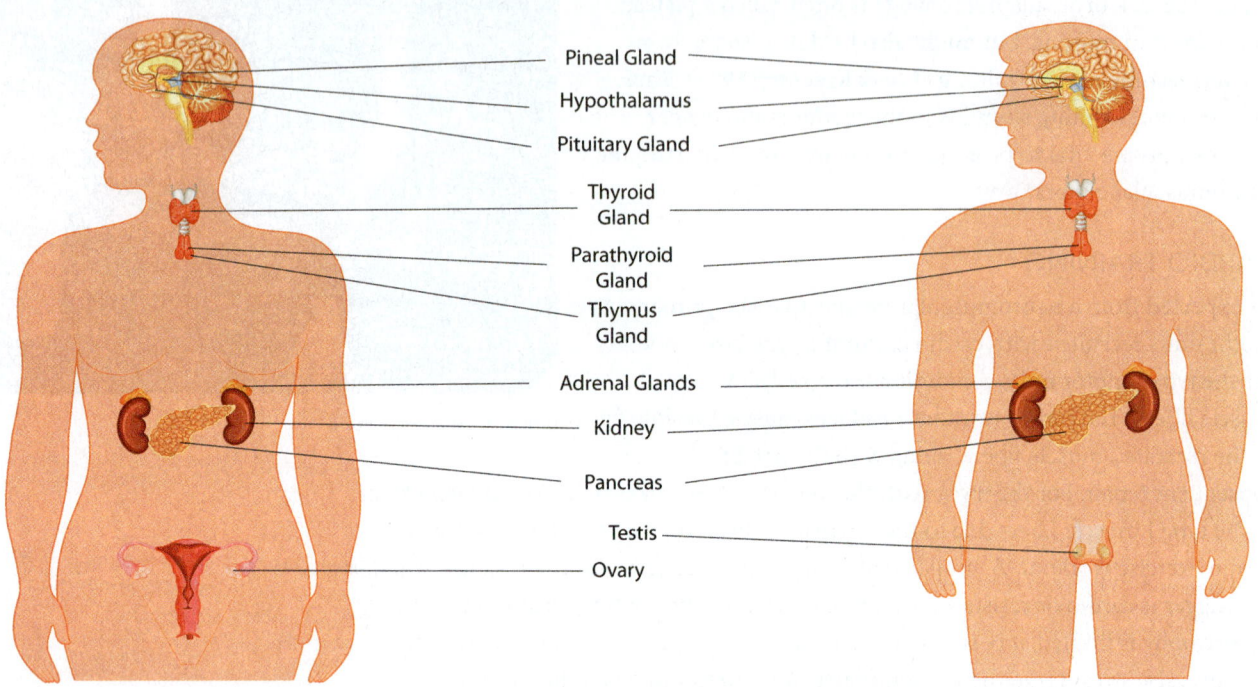

FIGURE 5.11 The Endocrine System

PARACRINE →

The action of a hormone or substance acting locally by diffusing from its source to target cells nearby.

AUTOCRINE →

An action in which a hormone or substance acts on the same cell that produced or secreted it.

MYOKINE →

A type of chemical substance released from skeletal muscle upon contraction.

In the classic endocrine function, the glands release hormones into the blood; these hormones then seek out and bind with specific receptors. Signals may be either excitatory or inhibitory in their actions. Adding to the complexity are two other forms of cell signaling created within the endocrine system. First, in **paracrine** signaling, hormones are released from cells that interact with nearby cells and their receptors, such as immune cells releasing growth hormones or thyroid hormones to affect the cells nearby to enhance growth or metabolism (Csaba, 2014). Second, in **autocrine** signaling, cells release a hormone that acts upon itself; thus, the hormone acts on the cell from which it was released.

Other substances are released in a paracrine or autocrine fashion as well. For example, **myokine** is one of the hundreds of different types of cytokines that are released by skeletal muscle cells in response to muscular contractions. **Cytokines** are small proteins (approximately 5–20 kDa) and proteoglycan peptides produced in different cells. They include chemokines, interferons, interleukins, lymphokines, and tumor necrosis factors, but are not typically hormones or growth factors (despite some terminology overlap). Additionally, cytokines released from other cell sources, such as immune cells, impact cell signaling. Such signaling interacts differently with various cells, tissues, and organs (Severinsen & Pedersen, 2020).

In skeletal muscle, the autocrine interaction involves a mechano growth factor that enhances the anabolic aspects of the muscle fiber (Goldspink, 2005; Zablocka et al., 2012). Insulin-like growth factor (IGF), mechano growth factor (MGF) (IGF 1EC), and various isoforms of IGF and MGF are important autocrine factors for repairing the muscle tissue damage that occurs with exercise (Karalaki et al., 2009; Philippou et al., 2009). IGF-I messenger RNAs (mRNAs), which encode the various isoforms of pro-IGF-I in a differential manner, regulate the responses to mechanical stress in skeletal muscle. Several studies have demonstrated that alternative splicing of IGF-I pre-mRNA gives rise to a unique peptide derived from pro-IGF-I that plays a novel role in myoblast proliferation. It is especially important for interactions not only with muscle but also with satellite cells and their differentiation to effect myoblast repair of muscle (Matheny et al., 2010). A host of cell signaling factors, both hormonal and cytokine in nature, are involved with repairing and remodeling of skeletal muscle after exercise stress.

Hormones secreted into the blood from endocrine glands can influence the body's acute coping with exercise stress and the adaptive changes associated with sports performance training (**Table 5.5**). Hormones translate information by binding to a receptor and stimulating the cell's genetic machinery; they bind only to the specific receptors they are matched with, thereby providing specificity in the endocrine response. An important concept is that for a receptor to accept and bind a hormone passing by it

CYTOKINE   →

Substances including chemokines, interferons, interleukins, lymphokines, and tumor necrosis factors, but generally not hormones or growth factors.

TABLE 5.5   Endocrine System Hormones' Basic Functions and Adaptations

Gland	Hormone Secreted	Functions
Anterior pituitary	Growth hormone (GH) Thyroid-stimulating hormone (TSH)	Tissue growth, use of fats, and protein synthesis stimulates release of insulin-like growth factors from the liver; enhanced connective tissue growth. Stimulates thyroid gland to secrete thyroid hormones T_3 and T_4.
Posterior pituitary	Antidiuretic hormone (ADH)	Uptake of water by kidneys, hydration control.
Thyroid	T_3 (triiodothyronine) and T_4 (thyroxine) Calcitonin	Vital for chemical reactions in the body; related to energy production and metabolism. Regulates levels of calcium and phosphate in the blood, opposing the action of parathyroid hormone.
Parathyroid	Parathyroid hormone (PTH)	Calcium uptake; increases calcium levels by releasing calcium from bones and increasing the amount of calcium absorbed from the small intestine; increases bone density; stimulates vitamin D_3 synthesis and metabolism.
Pancreas	Insulin and glucagon	Regulation of glucose metabolism in the body.
Adrenal cortex	Cortisol	Immune inhibition, protein breakdown, and catabolic functions.
Adrenal medulla	Catecholamines (epinephrine, norepinephrine, and dopamine)	Fight-or-flight response enhances muscular contractions, part of the stress response to exercise.
Liver	Insulin-like growth factor (IGF)	Increased protein synthesis, growth, and development of muscle and connective tissues and other cells.
Ovaries	Estrogen	Female sex characteristics, egg development, growth, and bone development.
Testes	Testosterone	Male sex characteristics, protein synthesis in all cells, and neural stimulation.

UPREGULATED →

The process whereby a receptor is made available for binding with a molecule or hormone.

DOWN-REGULATED →

The process whereby a receptor is not made available for binding with a molecule or hormone.

ANABOLIC

Metabolic process that synthesizes smaller molecules into larger units used for building and repairing tissues.

CATABOLIC

Metabolic process that breaks down molecules into smaller units used for energy.

from the circulation, it must be **upregulated**—that is, ready for interaction. If it is not upregulated, the receptor is **downregulated**—that is, it is not available for interactions with a hormone (Kraemer et al., 2021). Recruitment of skeletal muscle is one stimulus that results in the upregulation of receptors in those muscles.

Exercise, training, and the challenges of sports performances are potent stimulators of the endocrine system, which helps the body meet the demands of stress and assists in the recovery process. Yet, there is also an ongoing battle between the **anabolic** (building) and **catabolic** (breakdown) processes that are functions of the endocrine system (Kraemer et al., 2020). Optimal sports performance training can help to enhance the anabolic processes while minimizing the catabolic processes.

In both men and women, testosterone, growth hormone, and IGF are significant hormones that help to stimulate muscle fiber growth and hypertrophy (**Figure 5.12**). This process involves the hormone interacting and binding with a receptor, followed by a signal to the cell's nuclei that causes the genetic machinery to produce proteins. The catabolic hormone cortisol can interfere with this process, blocking the anabolic signaling that would otherwise lead to protein production.

Several other factors come into play and influence the endocrine system's responsiveness to stress and adaptations. For example, many people believe that reductions in hormonal levels and function inevitably occur with aging. While this statement is true to some extent, the decline is highly individualized for some hormonal systems: Not all men who are master athletes, for example, see a drop in growth hormone or testosterone (Kraemer, Kennett, et al., 2017). Nevertheless, all women do experience changes in their hormonal systems during menopause. The exercise-stimulated hormone responses might not be as great at certain phases of the lifespan, and are highly individualized for some anabolic and catabolic hormones, but still yield some positive benefits (Hakkinen et al., 2001; Izquierdo et al., 2001; Kraemer et al., 1992).

Endocrine system modulation with aging is impacted by a variety of behavioral and genetic influences, such as diet. For example, consuming a high-carbohydrate diet can lead to type 2 diabetes and obesity. Thyroid function can also be affected by aging, and monitoring of hypothyroid and hyperthyroid functions as part of an individual's annual clinical exams is crucial. In addition to exercise, lifestyle choices are vital in maintaining health and optimizing exercise training adaptations. Master athletes can benefit from sports performance training programs that enable their endocrine glands to have more robust storage and to release hormones and receptors that are responsive to those hormones' binding. Additionally, the stress of competition and everyday life typically lessens as athletes age.

ADAPTATIONS TO THE ENDOCRINE SYSTEM

In general, the adaptations of the endocrine system start with the stimulus to the gland to synthesize more hormones and then enhance its release mechanisms to secrete the hormones into the blood. Normal endocrine functions maintain balanced physiological function (homeostasis) in all the body's systems. The endocrine system is very responsive to the needs of the body, particularly the skeletal muscle, and supports the metabolic activity required for both the exercise demands and recovery processes. The endocrine system's activity starts when muscle is recruited to perform sports skills or an exercise training workout. In this process, there is both an acute response and a chronic adaptation with repetitive exposure to the stress, whether from the sport or exercise training workout.

Hormonal Influences on Growth of Fibers

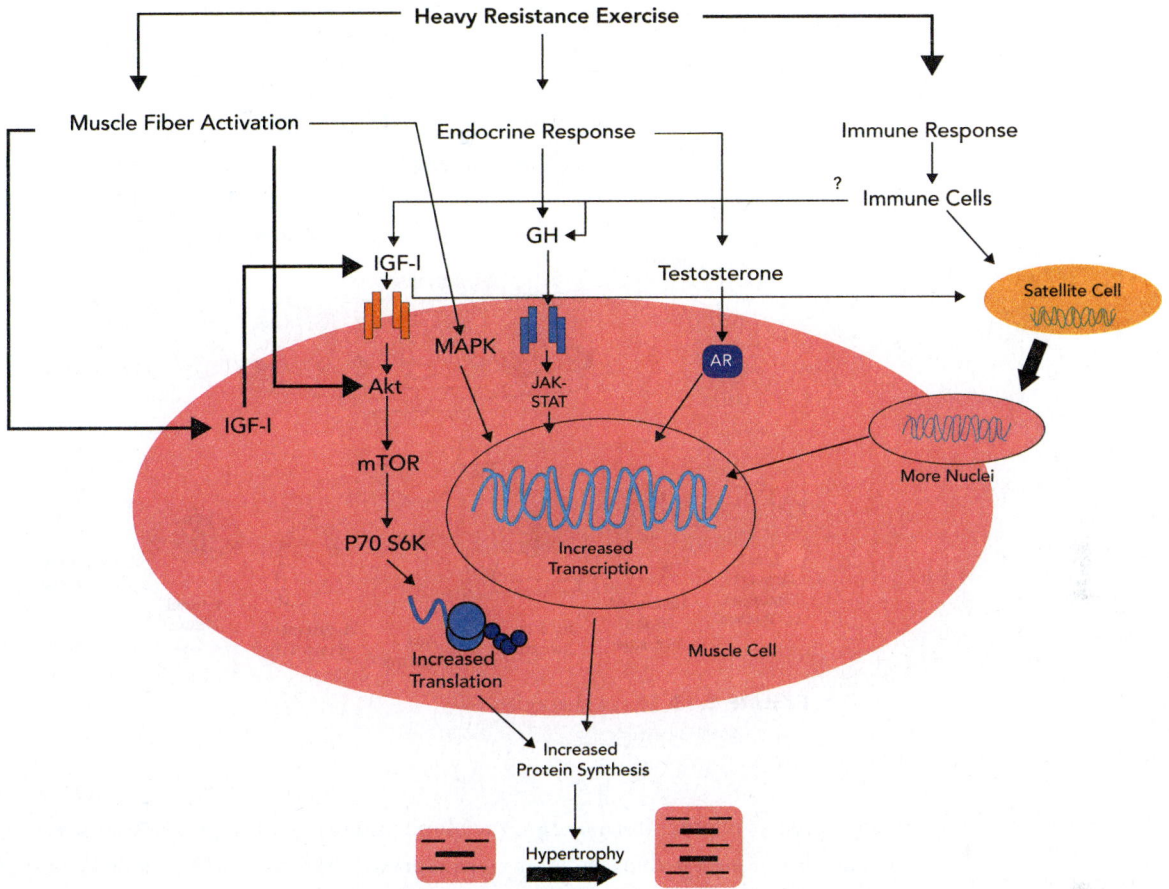

FIGURE 5.12 Endocrine Interactions That Stimulate Muscle Growth

Acutely, the endocrine responses aim to manage the demands placed on the body. Chronically, the endocrine mechanisms respond more quickly to stress and modify any overreaction. With training, the endocrine system responds more efficiently and effectively. This is accomplished with various mechanisms, including increased synthesis of hormones, increased storage capacities of hormones, improved release mechanisms, and more responsive receptors (upregulation) on the endocrine glands and target tissues. Thus, like any system, the endocrine system improves its structure and functions over time in response to exercise.

RESISTANCE TRAINING

Resistance training adaptations result from repetitive acute exposures to a given type of workout over time. Due to the number of motor units activated with typical progressive heavy resistance exercise, a host of hormones are acutely released from the glands that play different roles in the body. When high neural demands occur, the **sympatho-adrenergic-adrenal system** is activated right away. The nervous system stimulates the adrenal glands to release stress hormones and catecholamines, primarily epinephrine. These hormones help the body address the stress of exercise by enhancing muscular contractions and creating an arousal level needed for a workout.

The adrenal hormones are part of the body's fight-or-flight response (**Figure 5.13**). If the training is demanding enough (e.g., a whole-body multi-set exercise protocol),

SYMPATHO-ADRENERGIC-ADRENAL SYSTEM →

A physiological connection between the sympathetic nervous system and the adrenal medulla.

STRESS RESPONSE

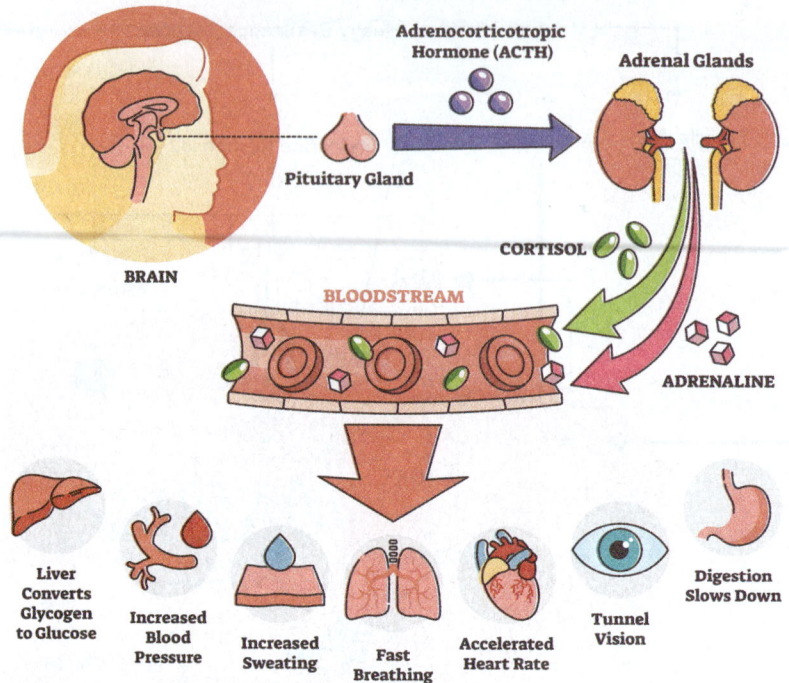

FIGURE 5.13 Stress Response
© VectorMine/Shutterstock

acute increases of other hormones in the blood also occur with the workout stress. From anabolic hormones, such as testosterone and growth hormone, to catabolic hormones, such as cortisol from the adrenal gland, increases in hormone levels occur in the recovery period to mediate the repair and remodeling of the muscles used in the training (Kraemer, Ratamess, & Nindl, 2017).

Sports performance training has always been a battle between anabolic and catabolic influences. Although the level of the catabolic hormone cortisol increases during exercise, it typically returns to the normal resting level within an hour or two. If cortisol remains elevated, which happens when recovery from a workout is not adequate, overtraining syndromes may occur. Other glands, such as the liver, pancreas, and thyroid, release hormones that help to regulate metabolism and produce the needed energy during a workout. With resistance training, the acute responses to the workout for most hormones increase. Resistance training adaptations include improved toleration of stress, especially in regard to the stress hormones. Each hormone has a specific pattern of acute responses and chronic adaptations.

CARDIO TRAINING

Cardio workouts trigger essentially the same hormonal response patterns in the blood as occur with resistance exercise. Cardio exercise recruits predominantly type I motor units with associated type I slow-twitch fibers because it typically creates lower muscular force and power needs. With higher intensities of cardio exercise, increases in the recruitment of type II motor units are observed, but not to the same extent as in progressive heavy resistance training (**Figure 5.14**).

Although the response pattern of the hormones in the blood looks similar for both an endurance workout and a resistance workout, the hormonal interactions are different.

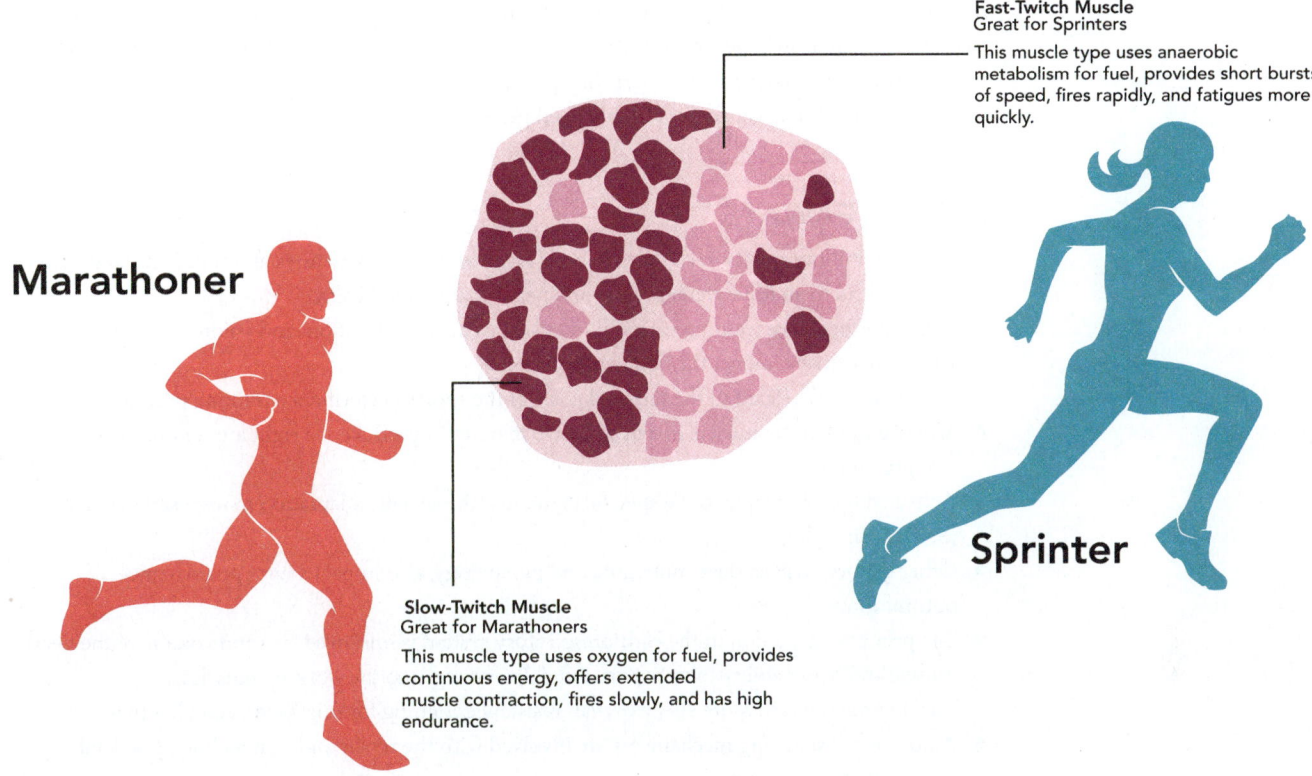

Fast-Twitch Muscle
Great for Sprinters

This muscle type uses anaerobic metabolism for fuel, provides short bursts of speed, fires rapidly, and fatigues more quickly.

Marathoner

Sprinter

Slow-Twitch Muscle
Great for Marathoners

This muscle type uses oxygen for fuel, provides continuous energy, offers extended muscle contraction, fires slowly, and has high endurance.

FIGURE 5.14 Slow-Twitch Versus Fast-Twitch Muscles

Only receptors in the muscles that are recruited to perform the activity are upregulated for increased interactions with hormones beyond resting levels. This recruitment pattern means that the type I muscle fibers predominantly interact with hormones of the endocrine system beyond normal resting homeostatic needs.

Typically, the metabolic demands are much higher for cardio training due to the higher energy needed to complete such workouts. Type I motor units are highly recruited for repetitive sports movements such as running, cycling, and swimming for long distances. Increases in the metabolic demands for energy stimulate specific endocrine glands to release hormones related to energy production and maintenance. The type I muscle fibers, which are made for long-duration exercise, need these specific hormones to help meet the muscle's energy demands and assist in the recovery process of damaged muscle. The receptors in those muscle fibers are upregulated to interact with such hormones. The type II motor units are not recruited unless an athlete participates in uphill or short sprint challenges in the workout or sports demands. The challenges to the type I motor units and their fibers imposed by cardio exercise result in training adaptations specific to these associated muscle fibers.

SUMMARY

The adaptations in the body to cardio or resistance training are specific to the types of workouts and training programs used. Muscle recruitment dictates the demands of the body's physiological structures and functions. All systems work together to enhance performance by improving each of the body's systems, including the cardiorespiratory and endocrine systems. Sports performance is enhanced by increased capabilities for utilizing oxygen with a stronger heart and an expanded respiratory system, such as occur with cardio training. Resistance training complements cardio training and results in larger muscles that produce more force and power due to enhanced motor unit activation and larger muscle fibers. In essence, sports performance training produces an athlete with greater functional capacities for enhanced performance.

KEY TAKEAWAYS

- Exercise training results in changes in both organ and tissue structures and functions, and such changes lead to an improvement in sports performance and health.
- Sports performance training varies in intensity, frequency, duration, and volume of exercise, which collectively impact the body's adaptations.
- Adaptations are related to the targeted goals of the sports performance training program.
- Motor units activate muscle in a progressive manner to produce the right amount of force (the size principle).
- Activated muscle adapts to the specific demands (the specific adaptation to imposed demands [SAID] principle).
- Other factors, such as sleep, nutrition, and psychology, also impact sports performance optimization.
- The primary adaptation in the cardiorespiratory system is improved size and volume of the heart muscle and better ability to transport and deliver oxygen to the working muscles.
- Cardio programs are more effective than resistance training for improving aerobic fitness.
- A host of cell signaling mechanisms are involved with the repair and remodeling of skeletal muscle after exercise stress.
- Resistance training increases the various connective tissues' density and resistance to injury.
- Resistance training improves the efficiency of cardio exercise.
- Resistance training reduces neural inhibition and increases the size of muscle fibers associated with the load-specific activated motor units.
- Sports performance training leads to stronger muscles, improved heart and lung functions, stronger connective tissues, and stronger muscle, all of which contribute to enhanced athlete development.

REFERENCES

Aliverti, A. (2016). The respiratory muscles during exercise. *Breathe, 12*(2), 165–168. https://doi.org/10.1183/20734735.008116

Bahensky, P., Bunc, V., Marko, D., & Malatova, R. (2020). Dynamics of ventilation parameters at different load intensities and the options to influence it by a breathing exercise. *Journal of Sports Medicine and Physical Fitness, 60*(8), 1101–1109. https://doi.org/10.23736/S0022-4707.20.10793-X

Bamman, M. M., Roberts, B. M., & Adams, G. R. (2018). Molecular regulation of exercise-induced muscle fiber hypertrophy. *Cold Spring Harbor Perspectives in Medicine, 8*(6). https://doi.org/10.1101/cshperspect.a029751

Bazyler, C. D., Abbott, H. A., Bellon, C. R., Taber, C. B., & Stone, M. H. (2015). Strength training for endurance athletes: Theory to practice. *Strength and Conditioning Journal, 37*(2), 1–12.

Blair, M. L. (2007). Sex-based differences in physiology: What should we teach in the medical curriculum? *Advances in Physiology Education, 31*(1), 23–25. https://doi.org/10.1152/advan.00118.2006

Campos, G. E., Luecke, T. J., Wendeln, H. K., Toma, K., Hagerman, F. C., Murray, T. F., Ragg, K. E., Ratamess, N. A., Kraemer, W. J., & Staron, R. S. (2002). Muscular adaptations in response to three different resistance-training regimens: Specificity of repetition maximum training zones. *European Journal of Applied Physiology, 88*(1–2), 50–60. https://doi.org/10.1007/s00421-002-0681-6

Casa, D. J., Anderson, S. A., Baker, L., Bennett, S., Bergeron, M. F., Connolly, Courson, R., Drezner, J. A., Eichner, E. R., Epley, B., Fleck, S., Franks, R., Guskiewicz, K. M., Harmon, K. G., Hoffman, J., Holschen, J. C., Jost, J., Kinniburgh, A., Klossner, D., ... Thompson, C. (2012). The inter-association task force for preventing sudden death in collegiate conditioning sessions: Best practices recommendations. *Journal of Athletic Training, 47*(4), 477–480. https://doi.org/10.4085/1062-6050-47.4.08

Chang, C. J., Putukian, M., Aerni, G., Diamond, A. B., Hong, E. S., Ingram, Y. M., Reardon, C. L., & Wolanin, A. T. (2020). Mental health issues and psychological factors in athletes: Detection, management, effect on performance, and prevention: Executive summary. *Clinical Journal of Sport Medicine, 30*(2), 91–95. https://doi.org/10.1097/JSM.0000000000000799

Csaba, G. (2014). Hormones in the immune system and their possible role: A critical review. *Acta Microbiologica et Immunologica Hungarica, 61*(3), 241–260. https://doi.org/10.1556/AMicr.61.2014.3.1

Dempsey, J. A., Johnson, B. D., & Saupe, K. W. (1990). Adaptations and limitations in the pulmonary system during exercise. *Chest, 97*(3 suppl), 81S–87S. https://doi.org/10.1378/chest.97.3_supplement.81s-a

Duchateau, J., & Enoka, R. M. (2011). Human motor unit recordings: Origins and insight into the integrated motor system. *Brain Research, 1409*, 42–61. https://doi.org/10.1016/j.brainres.2011.06.011

Flanagan, S. D., Proessl, F., Dunn-Lewis, C., Sterczala, A. J., Connaboy, C., Canino, M. C., Beethe, A. Z., Eagle, S. R., Szivak, T. K., Onate, J. A., Volek, J. S., Maresh, C. M., Kaeding, C. C., & Kraemer, W. J. (2021). Differences in brain structure and theta burst stimulation-induced plasticity implicate the corticomotor system in loss of function after musculoskeletal injury. *Journal of Neurophysiology, 125*(4), 1006–1021. https://doi.org/10.1152/jn.00689.2020

Fleck, S. J., & Dean, L. S. (1987). Resistance-training experience and the pressor response during resistance exercise. *Journal of Applied Physiology, 63*(1), 116–120. https://doi.org/10.1152/jappl.1987.63.1.116

Fleck, S. J., & Kraemer, W. J. (2014). *Designing resistance training programs* (4th ed.). Human Kinetics.

Fry, A. C., & Kraemer, W. J. (1997). Resistance exercise overtraining and overreaching. *Sports Medicine, 23*(2), 106–129. https://doi.org/10.2165/00007256-199723020-00004

Goldspink, G. (2005). Research on mechano growth factor: Its potential for optimising physical training as well as misuse in doping. *British Journal of Sports Medicine, 39*(11), 787–788. https://doi.org/10.1136/bjsm.2004.015826

Gordon, S. E., Kraemer, W. J., Vos, N. H., Lynch, J. M., & Knuttgen, H. G. (1994). Effect of acid–base balance on the growth hormone response to acute high-intensity cycle exercise. *Journal of Applied Physiology, 76*(2), 821–829. https://doi.org/10.1152/jappl.1994.76.2.821

Häkkinen, K., Pakarinen, A., Kraemer, W. J., Häkkinen, A., Valkeinen, H., & Alen, M. (2001). Selective muscle hypertrophy, changes in EMG and force, and serum hormones during strength training in older women. *Journal of Applied Physiology, 91*(2), 569–580. https://doi.org/10.1152/jappl.2001.91.2.569

Harber, M. P., Fry, A. C., Rubin, M. R., Smith, J. C., & Weiss, L. W. (2004). Skeletal muscle and hormonal adaptations to circuit weight training in untrained men. *Scandinavian Journal of Medicine & Science in Sports, 14*(3), 176–185. https://doi.org/10.1111/j.1600-0838.2003.371.x

Hellsten, Y., & Nyberg, M. (2015). Cardiovascular adaptations to exercise training. *Comprehensive Physiology, 6*(1), 1–32. https://doi.org/10.1002/cphy.c140080

Herrmann, M., Engelke, K., Ebert, R., Müller-Deubert, S., Rudert, M., Ziouti, F., Jundt, F., Felsenberg, D., & Jakob, F. (2020). Interactions between muscle and bone: Where physics meets biology. *Biomolecules, 10*(3). https://doi.org/10.3390/biom10030432

Hickson, R. C. (1980). Interference of strength development by simultaneously training for strength and endurance. *European Journal of Applied Physiology and Occupational Physiology, 45*, 255–263.

Izquierdo, M., Häkkinen, K., Ibañez, J., Garrues, M., Antón, A., Zúñiga, A., Larrión, J. L., & Gorostiaga, E. M. (2001). Effects of strength training on muscle power and serum hormones in middle-aged and older men. *Journal of Applied Physiology, 90*(4), 1497–1507. https://doi.org/10.1152/jappl.2001.90.4.1497

Karalaki, M., Fili, S., Philippou, A., & Koutsilieris, M. (2009). Muscle regeneration: Cellular and molecular events. *In Vivo, 23*(5), 779–796.

Knuttgen, H. G., Nordesjo, L. O., Ollander, B., & Saltin, B. (1973). Physical conditioning through interval training with young male adults. *Medicine & Science in Sports Exercise, 5*(4), 220–226.

Kraemer, W. J., Fleck, S. J., & Deschenes, M. R. (2021). *Exercise physiology: Integrating theory and application* (3rd ed.). Wolters Kluwer.

Kraemer, W. J., Fry, A. C., Warren, B. J., Stone, M. H., Fleck, S. J., Kearney, J. T., Conroy, B. P., Maresh, C. M., Weseman, C. A., Triplett, N. T., & Gordon, S. E. (1992). Acute hormonal responses in elite junior weightlifters. *International Journal of Sports Medicine, 13*(2), 103–109. https://doi.org/10.1055/s-2007-1021240

Kraemer, W. J., Kennett, M. J., Mastro, A. M., McCarter, R. J., Rogers, C. J., DuPont, W. H., Flanagan, S. D., Trubitt, W. J., Fragola, M. S., Post, E. M., & Hymer, W. C. (2017). Bioactive growth hormone in older men and women: It's relationship to immune markers and healthspan. *Growth Hormone & IGF Research, 34*, 45–54. https://doi.org/10.1016/j.ghir.2017.05.002

Kraemer, W. J., Patton, J. F., Gordon, S. E., Harman, E. A., Deschenes, M. R., Reynolds, K., & Dziados, J. E. (1995). Compatibility of high-intensity strength and endurance training on hormonal and skeletal muscle adaptations. *Journal of Applied Physiology, 78*(3), 976–989. https://doi.org/10.1152/jappl.1995.78.3.976

Kraemer, W. J., Ratamess, N. A., Hymer, W. C., Nindl, B. C., & Fragala, M. S. (2020). Growth hormone(s), testosterone, insulin-like growth factors, and cortisol: Roles and integration for cellular development and growth with exercise. *Frontiers in Endocrinology (Lausanne), 11*, 33. https://doi.org/10.3389/fendo.2020.00033

Kraemer, W. J., Ratamess, N. A., & Nindl, B. C. (2017). Recovery responses of testosterone, growth hormone, and IGF-1 after resistance exercise. *Journal of Applied Physiology, 122*(3), 549–558. https://doi.org/10.1152/japplphysiol.00599.2016

Kraemer, W. J., & Rogol, A. D. (Eds.). (2005). *The endocrine system in sports and exercise*. International Olympic Committee.

Kraemer, W. J., & Spiering, B. A. (2007). Skeletal muscle physiology: Plasticity and responses to exercise. *Hormone Research in Pediatrics, 66*(suppl 1), 2–16. https://doi.org/10.1159/000096617

MacDougall, J. D., Tuxen, D., Sale, D. G., Moroz, J. R., & Sutton, J. R. (1985). Arterial blood pressure response to heavy resistance exercise. *Journal of Applied Physiology, 58*(3), 785–790. https://doi.org/10.1152/jappl.1985.58.3.785

Maiorana, A. J., Briffa, T. G., Goodman, C., & Hung, J. (1997). A controlled trial of circuit weight training on aerobic capacity and myocardial oxygen demand in men after coronary artery bypass surgery. *Journal of Cardiopulmonary Rehabilitation, 17*(4), 239–247. https://doi.org/10.1097/00008483-199707000-00004

Matheny, R. W., Nindl, B. C., & Adamo, M. L. (2010). Minireview: Mechano-growth factor: A putative product of IGF-I gene expression involved in tissue repair and regeneration. *Endocrinology, 151*(3), 865–875. https://doi.org/10.1210/en.2009-1217

Milanović, Z., Sporiš, G., & Weston, M. (2015). Effectiveness of high-intensity interval training (HIT) and continuous endurance training for VO$_2$ max improvements: A systematic review and meta-analysis of controlled trials. *Sports Medicine, 45*(10), 1469–1481. https://doi.org/10.1007/s40279-015-0365-0

Moore, R. L., & Brown, D. A. (2012). The cardiovascular system: cardiac function. In P. A. Farrell, M. J. Joyner, & V. J. Caiozzo (Eds.), *ACSM's advanced exercise physiology* (2nd ed., pp. 313–331). Lippincott Williams & Wilkins.

O'Leary, D. S., Mueller, P. J., & Sala-Mercado, J. A. (2012). The cardiovascular system: Design and control. In P. A. Farrell, M. J. Joyner, & V. J. Caiozzo (Eds.), *ACSM's advanced exercise physiology* (2nd ed., pp. 297–312). Lippincott Williams & Wilkins.

Peterson, M. D., Pistilli, E., Haff, G. G., Hoffman, E. P., & Gordon, P. M. (2011). Progression of volume load and muscular adaptation during resistance exercise. *European Journal of Applied Physiology, 111*(6), 1063–1071. https://doi.org/10.1007/s00421-010-1735-9

Philippou, A., Papageorgiou, E., Bogdanis, G., Halapas, A., Sourla, A., Maridaki, M., & Koutsilieris, M. (2009). Expression of IGF-1 isoforms after exercise-induced muscle damage in humans: Characterization of the MGF E peptide actions in vitro. *In Vivo, 23*(4), 567–575.

Radcliffe, J. N., Comfort, P., & Fawcett, T. (2018). The perceived psychological responsibilities of a strength and conditioning coach. *Journal of Strength and Conditioning Research, 32*(10), 2853–2862. https://doi.org/10.1519/JSC.0000000000001656

Ratamess, N. A. (2022). *ACSM's foundations of strength and conditioning* (2nd ed.). Lippincott Williams & Wilkins.

Romer, L. M., Sheel, A. W., & Harms, C. A. (2012). The respiratory system. In P. A. Farrell, M. J. Joyner, & V. J. Caiozzo (Eds.), *ACSM's advanced exercise physiology* (2nd ed., pp. 242–296). Lippincott Williams & Wilkins.

Rønnestad, B. R., & Mujika, I. (2014). Optimizing strength training for running and cycling endurance performance: A review. *Scandinavian Journal of Medicine & Science in Sports, 24*(4), 603–612. https://doi.org/10.1111/sms.12104

Sales, A. T., Fregonezi, G. A., Ramsook, A. H., Guenette, J. A., Lima, I. N., & Reid, W. D. (2016). Respiratory muscle endurance after training in athletes and non-athletes: A systematic review and meta-analysis. *Physical Therapy in Sport, 17*, 76–86. https://doi.org/10.1016/j.ptsp.2015.08.001

Schoenfeld, B. J. (2013). Potential mechanisms for a role of metabolic stress in hypertrophic adaptations to resistance training. *Sports Medicine, 43*(3), 179–194. https://doi.org/10.1007/s40279-013-0017-1

Severinsen, M. C. K., & Pedersen, B. K. (2020). Muscle–organ crosstalk: The emerging roles of myokines. *Endocrinology Review, 41*(4), 594–609. https://doi.org/10.1210/endrev/bnaa016

Shei, R.-J. (2018). Recent advancements in our understanding of the ergogenic effect of respiratory muscle training in healthy humans: A systematic review. *Journal of Strength and Conditioning Research, 32*(9), 2665–2676. https://doi.org/10.1519/JSC.0000000000002730

Staron, R. S., Hagerman, F. C., Hikida, R. S., Murray, T. F., Hostler, D. P., Crill, M. T., & Toma, K. (2000). Fiber type composition of the vastus lateralis muscle of young men and women. *Journal of Histochemistry and Cytochemistry, 48*(5), 623–629. https://doi.org/10.1177/002215540004800506

Tønnessen, E., Svendsen, I. S., Rønnestad, B. R., Hisdal, J., Haugen, T. A., & Seiler, S. (2015). The annual training periodization of 8 world champions in orienteering. *International Journal of Sports Physiology Performance, 10*(1), 29–38. https://doi.org/10.1123/ijspp.2014-0005

Wilson, J. M., Marin, P. J., Rhea, M. R., Wilson, S. M., Loenneke, J. P., & Anderson, J. C. (2012). Concurrent training: A meta-analysis examining interference of aerobic and resistance exercises. *Journal of Strength & Conditioning Research, 26*(8), 2293–2307. https://doi.org/10.1519/JSC.0b013e31823a3e2d

Zablocka, B., Goldspink, P. H., Goldspink, G., & Górecki, D. C. (2012). Mechano-growth factor: An important cog or a loose screw in the repair machinery? *Frontiers in Endocrinology, 3*, 131. https://doi.org/10.3389/fendo.2012.00131

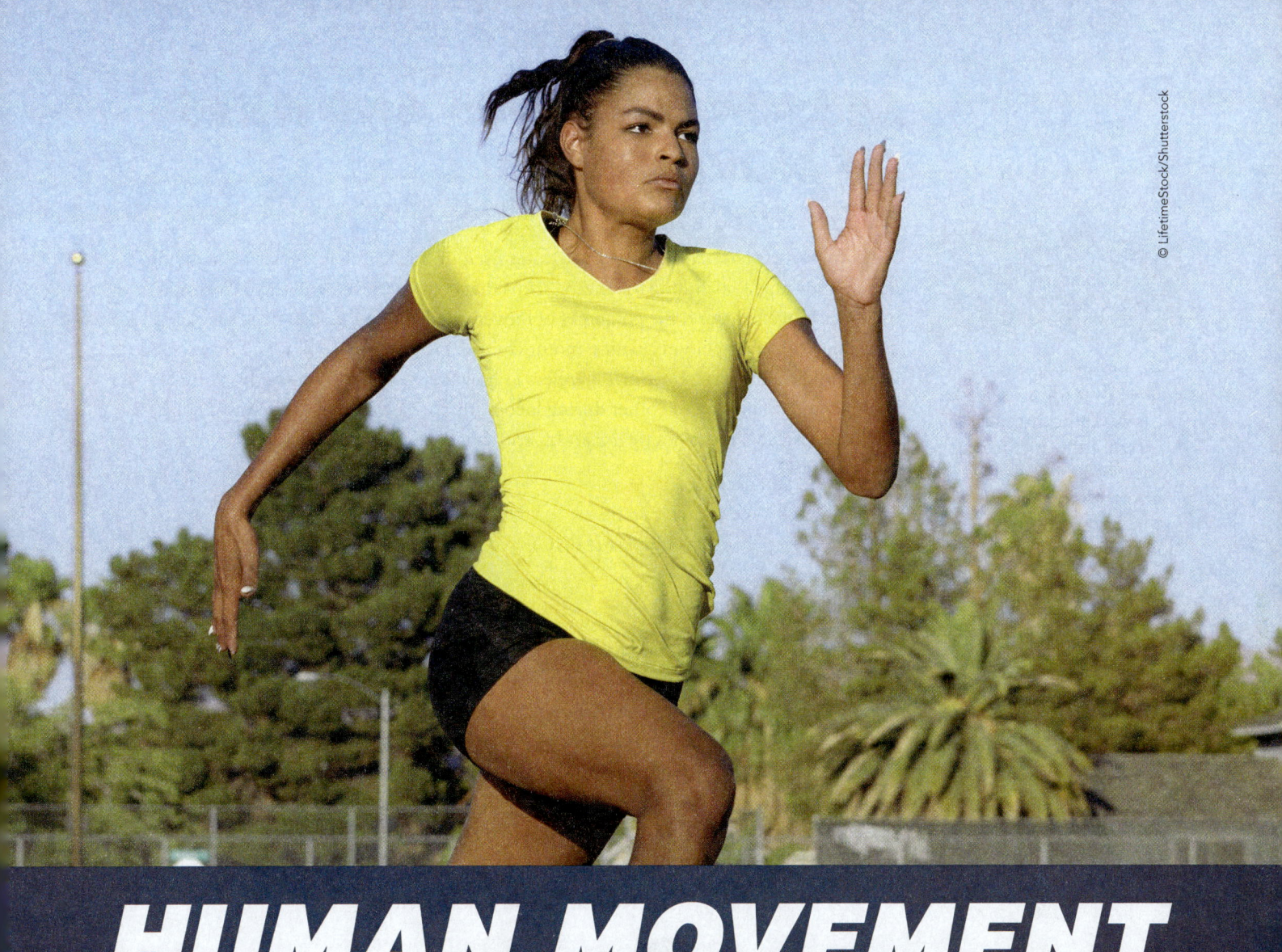

HUMAN MOVEMENT SCIENCE

CHAPTER SIX

LEARNING OBJECTIVES

Upon completion of this chapter, the Sports Performance Coach will be able to:

- **Summarize** the scientific terminology that governs exercise and movement.
- **Identify** key biomechanical concepts that define how the neuromuscular system functions.
- **Describe** motor behavior and how the neuromuscular system adapts and learns.

LESSON 1: PLANES AND AXES OF MOVEMENT

INTRODUCTION

Human movement science is a broad, interdisciplinary field that focuses on studying human movement, including the mechanisms that control movement, the factors that influence movement, and the outcomes of movement. This field draws on a range of disciplines, including biomechanics, motor control, exercise physiology, and neuroscience, among others. The term *kinetic chain* refers to how the segments of the body are linked together and influence each other during locomotion. The National Academy of Sports Medicine (NASM) identifies the major kinetic chain checkpoints as follows:

- Head and neck
- Shoulder and thoracic spine
- Lumbo-pelvic-hip complex (LPHC)
- Knees
- Foot-ankle complex

The segments of the kinetic chain allow the Sports Performance Coach to check alignment and movement compensations and make better decisions about how to program exercises for the athlete (**Figure 6.1**). Each sport, as well as different positions within the same sport, has various requirements. It is the job of the Sports Performance Coach to balance the needs and requirements of the sport with the athlete's abilities to produce, reduce, and dynamically stabilize in multiple planes, at various speeds, in a safe and coordinated fashion, which allows for optimal performance outcomes.

Kinetic Chain Checkpoints

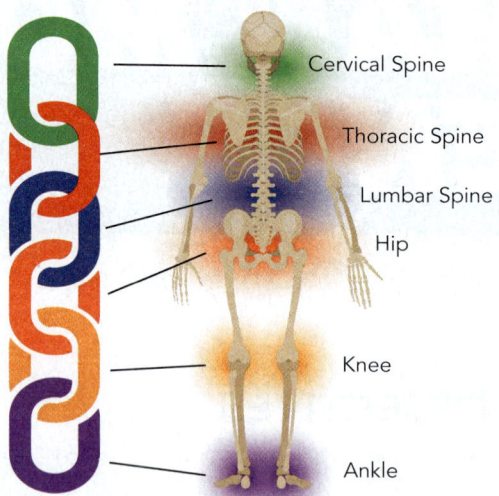

Cervical Spine
Thoracic Spine
Lumbar Spine
Hip
Knee
Ankle

FIGURE 6.1 Kinetic Chain Checkpoints

THE LANGUAGE OF HUMAN MOVEMENT SCIENCE

Human movement science has its own language. A unique set of words are used for above or below, closer or farther, near to and away from, and more in this context. To new students, it can be difficult to make sense of the reasons and rationales for using this unique jargon. However, as complexities and nuances of human movement science emerge, it is this language that makes human movement both clearer and easier to understand and describe. Each word has a specific meaning and relates to the body in a particular way. The jargon used to speak about movement provides clarity not only for the Sports Performance Coach, but also for those persons working in the exercise sciences, rehabilitative sciences, and even the medical field.

Just like learning a new language, learning the unique descriptors in the field takes practice. Becoming familiar with the terminology allows the Sports Performance Coach to incorporate these words in context while speaking, which helps to encode the terms into memory. At that point, the Sports Performance Coach can begin using these words and concepts to select well-balanced exercises as part of programming.

Although the Sports Performance Coach rarely uses these terms when speaking directly to athletes, it is integral for the Sports Performance Coach to know how to work with the athletes. Anatomic directions (**Table 6.1**) allow the Sports Performance Coach to be clear and specific about movement.

TABLE 6.1 Anatomic Directions

Directional Term	Description	Example
Superior (cranial)	Toward the head	The superior fibers of the trapezius muscle are often referred to as the upper traps.
Inferior (caudal)	Away from the head	The inferior angle of the scapula is where the latissimus dorsi attaches to the scapula.
Proximal	Toward the center of the body	The proximal attachments of the biceps brachii are on the coracoid process and supraglenoid tubercle of the scapula.
Distal	Away from the center of the body	The distal attachment of the biceps brachii is on the radial tuberosity.
Anterior	Front	During an overhead squat assessment, it is important to look at the feet and knees from an anterior view.
Posterior	Back	A posterior view during on overhead squat assessment allows the Sports Performance Coach to look for a hip shift.
Medial	Toward the midline	The medial collateral ligament is at risk during loaded knee valgus, which includes resistance training, landing, and run deceleration.
Lateral	Away from the midline	A lateral shuffle is when an athlete's body faces forward but shuffles sideways.
Superficial	Shallow, just under the skin	Subcutaneous fat is superficial fat just under the skin.
Deep	Away from the skin, farther inside the body	Visceral fat is deep fat found around organs.

(continues)

TABLE 6.1 Anatomic Directions (*continued*)

Directional Term	Description	Example
Ipsilateral	Same side	When climbing a ladder, the ipsilateral arm and leg reach up at the same time.
Contralateral	Opposite side	When running, the contralateral arm and leg move into flexion and extension.
Unilateral	On one side of the body	A unilateral dumbbell chest press increases core engagement to help stabilize the LPHC.
Bilateral	On both sides of the body	A back squat is a bilateral leg exercise designed to increase the strength of the major muscle groups of the lower body in both legs concurrently.

SAGITTAL PLANE →

An imaginary plane that divides the body into left and right.

FRONTAL PLANE →

An imaginary plane that divides the body into front and back.

TRANSVERSE PLANE →

An imaginary plane that divides the body into top and bottom.

ANATOMIC POSITION →

The position with the body erect, the arms at the sides, and the palms forward; the position of reference for anatomic nomenclature.

PLANES OF MOTION

Planes of motion are a fundamental principle for any Sports Performance Coach, trainer, or exercise specialist. As a quick refresher, there are three primary planes of motion. These planes are imaginary flat surfaces intersecting the body at 90-degree angles (**Figure 6.2**).

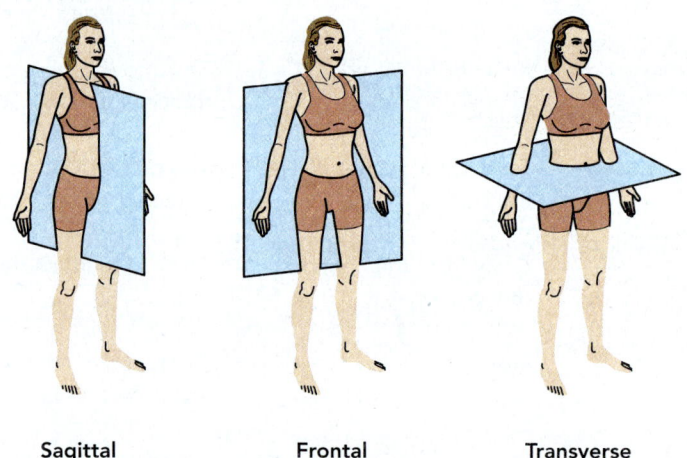

Sagittal   Frontal   Transverse

FIGURE 6.2 Anatomic Planes of the Body

The **sagittal plane** bisects the body into right and left sides; the **frontal plane** separates the body into front and back; and the **transverse plane** divides the body into top and bottom. Multiple references to planes of motion can be made when discussing movement to better clarify what these planes are and how the human movement system functions along them. However, even the strictest of movements in one plane of motion incorporates the other planes of motion, via either slighter movements or stabilization forces. That said, all movement is multiplanar and requires the human movement system (HMS) to move through and stabilize in all planes of motion.

When considering planes of motion, start in a standard position, known as the **anatomic position**, to identify the plane of motion in which movement is taking place. Planes of motion are always relative to body position. For instance, if an athlete is standing up and performing jumping jacks, they are moving in the frontal plane. If the athlete lies down to make snow angels, that movement is the same plane of motion relative to their body, even though the athlete is no longer standing.

MULTIPLANAR OR TRIPLANAR MOVEMENTS

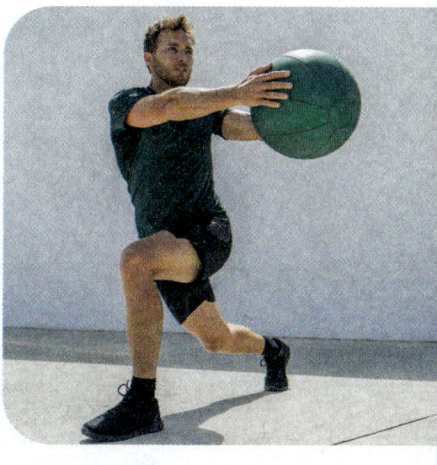

© Maridav/Shutterstock

The Sports Performance Coach must understand that movement in sports is never limited to just one plane of motion. The body continually moves in and out of all three planes of motion. Such movements are referred to as multiplanar or triplanar movements, and they indicate the dynamic nature of human movement.

For example, a first baseman lunging to the side to catch a ground ball may move in the direction of the frontal plane; however, from a lateral view, the knee and torso translate forward, and the hips backward in the sagittal plane. As the body hinges forward, rotational components emerge, creating a transverse component as well. As another example, a sprinter may travel in the sagittal plane, but they generate power for maximal speed through the counter-rotational forces of the shoulders and lower trunk. Multiple planes are moved through, allowing the human body to produce and reduce forces in all three planes while also requiring stabilization in all planes to protect and direct movement appropriately.

The Sports Performance Coach must learn about movement through the various planes and how the body works to limit degrees of freedom if the coach is to direct the athlete's body to perform within the constraints of the sport, environment, and abilities. Understanding movement and being able to identify altered or faulty movement is vital. For example, force production may be diminished if a movement is intended to be sagittal plane dominant but there is too much deviation in the frontal or transverse plane. For example, during a jump, the knees might move together in a valgus position (frontal plane adduction and transverse plane internal rotation). However, upon standing, the knees realign. The erroneous knee movement is potentially dangerous, and unnecessary movement can limit the ability to produce maximal force or speed. The same issue is seen in the running gait if the foot rotates externally (transverse plane) on the foot strike and back swing, and then realigns as the knee drives forward during the terminal swing of the leg before striking the ground again. This unnecessary deviation can overdevelop certain muscles while causing the medial hamstrings to minimize activation that is otherwise able to realign the knee joint and create less ancillary movement.

AXES OF ROTATION

Each plane of motion has an **axis of rotation** that can identify and further define the plane of motion. Axes of rotation are imaginary lines (rather than planes) that serve as the pivot point upon which the joint swivels. For instance, when an athlete is doing a bench press, if the Sports Performance Coach were to look at only the movement of the hand rather than the joint action, they might assume it is a sagittal plane movement. However, by looking at the athlete's shoulder joint and identifying the axis of rotation, the Sports Performance Coach can determine that the bench press occurs in the transverse plane (**Figure 6.3**). The axis of rotation is always perpendicular to the plane of motion.

> **AXIS OF ROTATION** →
>
> An imaginary line that runs through a joint, perpendicular to the plane of motion, serving as a pivot point upon which the bones rotate.

JOINT ACTIONS

Many movements describe the dominant plane and the direction in which the body moves when referencing the plane of motion. For instance, walking and running occur in the sagittal plane. However, the individual joints show more complexity by demonstrating multiplanar movement. For example, during walking, the hip, knee, and ankle joints will

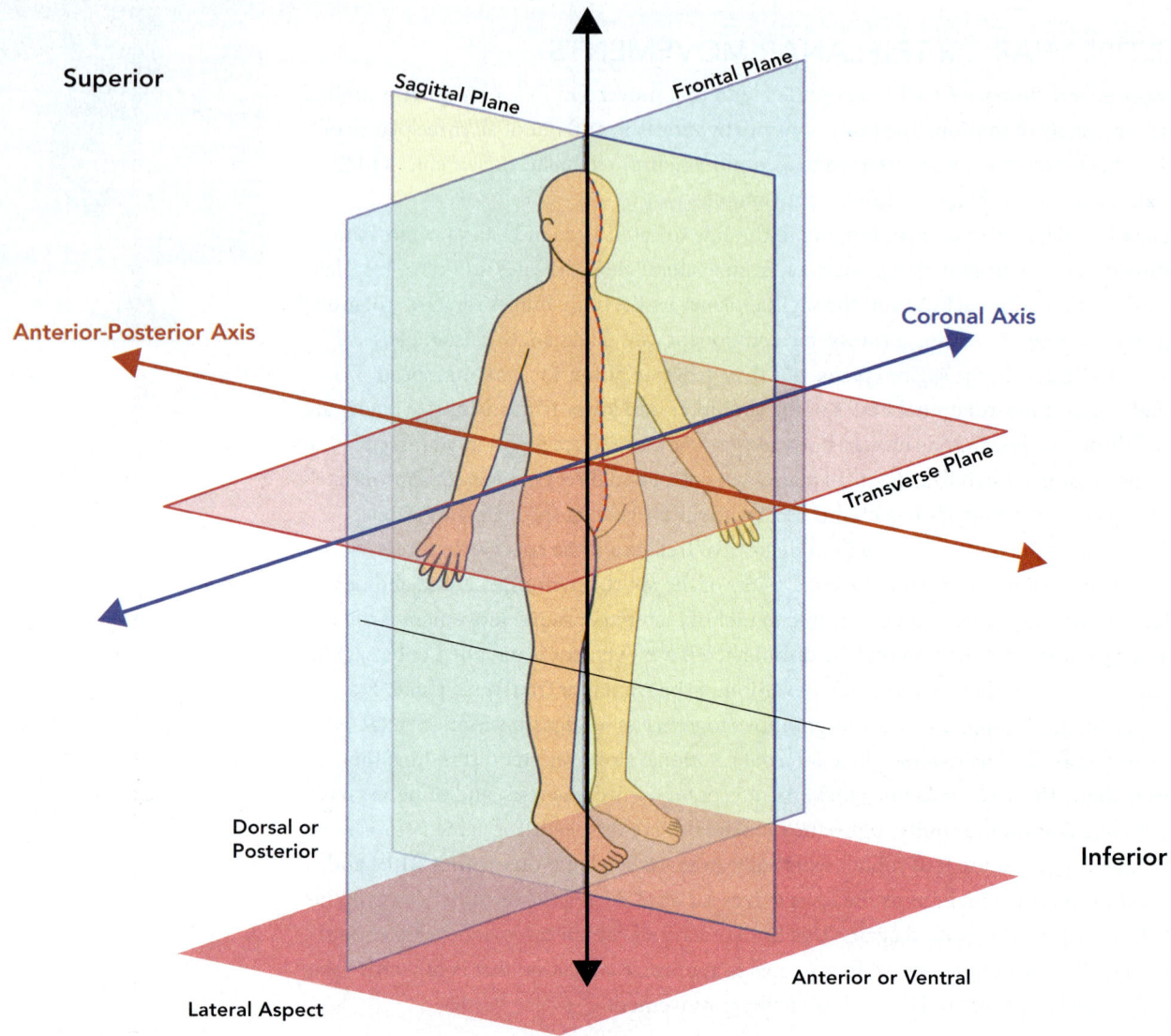

Axes of Rotation

Superior

Sagittal Plane

Frontal Plane

Anterior-Posterior Axis

Coronal Axis

Transverse Plane

Dorsal or
Posterior

Inferior

Anterior or Ventral

Lateral Aspect

FIGURE 6.3 Axes of Rotation

move in two or more planes to reduce, produce, and stabilize forces. Therefore, while the resultant movement of walking is considered sagittal plane dominant, the joint actions will include at least some movement in all planes. The Sports Performance Coach should understand joint actions to identify movement.

ANTERIOR–POSTERIOR AXIS

ANTERIOR– →
POSTERIOR AXIS

An imaginary line
that passes through a
joint from anterior to
posterior.

The **anterior–posterior axis**, also known as the sagittal axis, is an imaginary line that passes through a joint in an anterior to posterior direction. Movement about the anterior–posterior axis is in the frontal plane (**Table 6.2**). For example, this axis runs through the anterior–posterior shoulder joint, so movement around that pivot point entails abduction and adduction of the arm in the frontal plane. In a side shuffle, the hip joints move around the anterior–posterior axis, which allows the hips to move laterally in the frontal plane. Similarly, the anterior–posterior axis through the shoulder allows the arms to swing overhead in the frontal plane, as in a jumping jack or as a means to distract attention or block a shot in basketball.

TABLE 6.2   Examples of Anterior–Posterior Axis

Axis/Plane	Motion
Anterior–posterior axis/ frontal plane	**Abduction:** Movement of the appendicular skeleton away from the anatomic midline of the body.
	Adduction: Movement of the appendicular skeleton toward the anatomic midline of the body in the frontal plane.
	Lateral flexion: Occurs at the spine when the column of the spine bends to either the right or left side.
	Scapular upward rotation: Upward rotation of the scapula that occurs when the inferior angle of the scapula rotates away from the spine (laterally) and upward.
	Scapular downward rotation: Downward rotation of the scapula that occurs when the inferior angle of the scapula rotates toward the spine (medially) and downward.

MEDIOLATERAL AXIS

The **mediolateral axis**, also known as the frontal or coronal axis, is an imaginary line that passes through a joint in a medial to lateral direction, allowing movement to take place in the sagittal plane (**Table 6.3**). This axis runs through the majority of joints of long bones and is pivotal in human locomotion. You can visualize the mediolateral line as running through the big toes, ankles, knees, hips, shoulders, and elbows, allowing all these joints to flex and extend in the sagittal plane during running patterns. Although all these joints have some movement in other planes while running, the sagittal is the primary plane of motion, and the mediolateral axis is the primary pivot point.

**MEDIOLATERAL →
AXIS**

An imaginary line that passes through a joint from medial to lateral.

TABLE 6.3   Examples of Mediolateral Axis

Axis/Plane	Motion
Mediolateral axis/sagittal plane	**Flexion:** The decreasing angle of two (or more) bones around a joint in the sagittal plane.
	Extension: The increasing angle of two (or more) bones around a joint in the sagittal plane.
	Plantar flexion: The decrease in angle between the plantar (bottom) portion of the foot and the posterior shin (understood as ankle extension).
	Dorsiflexion: The decrease in angle between the dorsal (top) portion of the foot and the anterior shin (understood as ankle flexion).
	Scapular anterior tilting (tipping): The movement of the inferior angle of the scapula away from the rib cage.
	Scapular posterior tilting (tipping): The movement of the inferior angle of the scapula toward the rib cage.

SUPERIOR–INFERIOR AXIS →

An imaginary line that passes through a joint from superior to inferior.

JOINT TRANSLATION →

Joint motion where a bone moves along a linear path without any rotation.

CENTRAL NERVOUS SYSTEM (CNS) →

The part of the nervous system consisting of the brain and spinal cord.

PERIPHERAL NERVOUS SYSTEM (PNS) →

The part of the nervous system that connects the rest of the body to the central nervous system.

ACTION POTENTIAL →

Nerve impulse that is relayed from the central nervous system, through the peripheral nervous system, and into the muscle across the neuromuscular junction.

SUPERIOR–INFERIOR AXIS

The **superior–inferior axis**, also known as the axial or vertical axis, is an imaginary line that passes through a joint in a superior to inferior direction, allowing movement in the transverse plane (**Table 6.4**). This axis runs through the length of the spine, which allows for horizontal rotation. The superior–inferior axis also runs through the shoulder joint, which allows for transverse plane horizontal adduction at the glenohumeral joint. Like planes of motion, axes are relative to the body, not the earth. Therefore, the axes will stay the same whether an athlete is lying or standing.

TABLE 6.4 Examples of Superior–Inferior Axis

Axis/Plane	Motion
Superior–inferior axis/ transverse plane	**Horizontal adduction:** The movement of the appendicular skeleton toward the anatomic midline of the body in the transverse plane.
	Horizontal abduction: The movement the appendicular skeleton away from the anatomic midline of the body in the transverse plane.
	Internal (medial) rotation: A rotational movement of the appendicular skeleton toward the anterior midline of the body.
	External (lateral) rotation: A rotational movement of the appendicular skeleton away from the anterior midline of the body.
	Rotation: The rotational movement of the spinal column to either the right or left side.
	Scapular internal rotation: The movement of the medial (vertebral) border of the scapula away from the rib cage.
	Scapular external rotation: The movement of the medial (vertebral) border of the scapula toward the rib cage.

JOINT TRANSLATION

While a large majority of movements in the human body involve rotation about a pivot point, not all do. **Joint translation** is a type of joint motion in which a bone moves along a linear path without any rotation. It involves a displacement of a bone or segment along an axis, typically in a straight line. Joint translation can occur in any direction, including forward and backward, side to side, and up and down. A common example of joint translation occurs at the scapulae (**Table 6.5**).

TABLE 6.5 Joint Motions in Translations

Motion	Description
Scapular elevation	The movement of the scapular superiorly toward the head.
Scapular depression	The movement of the scapular inferiorly toward the pelvis.
Scapular protraction	The movement of the scapula laterally away from the spine.
Scapular retraction	The movement of the scapula medially toward the spine.

LESSON 2: MUSCLE ACTIONS
MUSCLE CONTRACTIONS

For a Sports Performance Coach to understand the roles played by the various muscles in movement, they must have some knowledge of the physiological processes of muscle contractions. The coordination of muscle contractions is controlled by the nervous system, which receives sensory information from both the internal and external environments, processes that information, and replies with a motor response.

The nervous system is divided into two main sections: the **central nervous system (CNS)** and the **peripheral nervous system (PNS)**. The CNS consists of the brain and spinal cord and is considered the body's command center. It receives sensory information from the internal and external environments, processes it, and responds. The PNS is made up of all the peripheral nerves that branch off the CNS. These nerves are considered the transmitters of the nervous systems because they deliver information to and receive information from the CNS.

MUSCLE ACTIVATION

The activation of muscle comprises a complex series of steps beginning with a signal from the brain to engage a muscle. A motor unit sends a nerve impulse called an **action potential** to the muscle, telling it to contract. The electric signal from an action potential turns into a chemical signal, which causes the muscle to release **acetylcholine (ACh)**. The events that take place from the initial electrical signal to the chemical signal to muscle contraction are called **excitation–contraction coupling**.

The functional unit of the muscle is the **sarcomere**, which goes from **Z-disc** to Z-disc (**Figure 6.4**). The Z-discs are what give skeletal muscle their striated appearance. When a

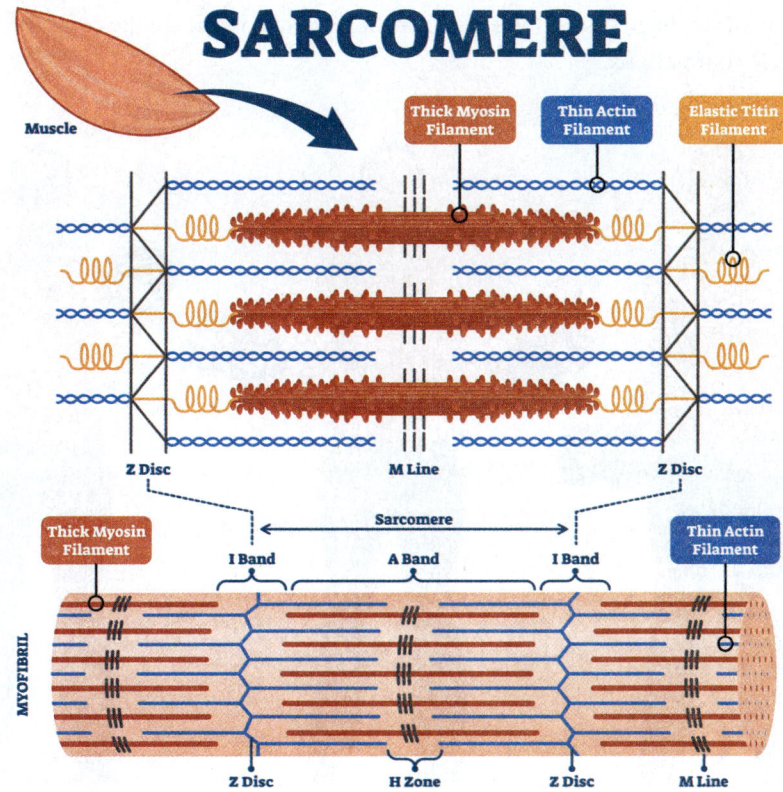

FIGURE 6.4 Sarcomere

© VectorMine/Shutterstock

ACETYL-CHOLINE (ACh) →

A neurotransmitter that helps the action potential cross the synapse into the muscle, which initiates the steps in a muscle contraction.

EXCITATION–CONTRACTION COUPLING →

The physiological process of converting an electrical stimulus into a muscle contraction.

SARCOMERE →

The structural unit of a myofibril, composed of actin and myosin filaments between two Z-lines.

Z-DISC →

A protein structure that serves as a boundary between adjacent sarcomeres in muscle fibers.

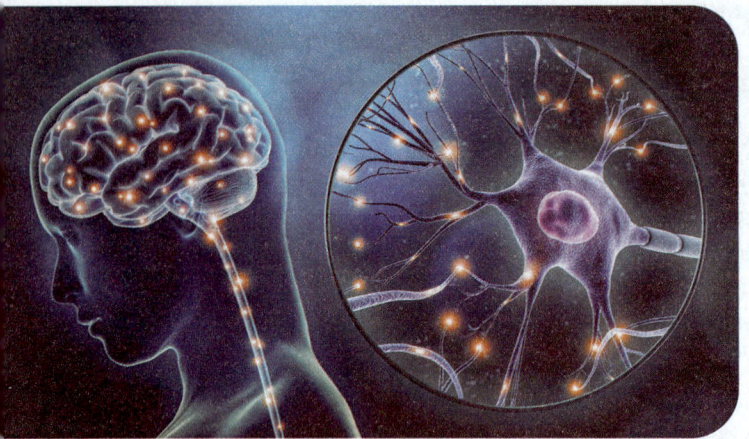

© MattL_Images/Shutterstock

muscle contracts, it brings the Z-discs closer together through a phenomenon known as the sliding filament theory. **Actin** is a thin filament within the sarcomere that attaches to the thicker filament myosin through cross-bridging. **Myosin** heads reach across to connect to the thin actin filament and pull the Z-discs closer together with the help of **adenosine triphosphate (ATP).**

Several proteins—namely, **troponin** and **tropomyosin**—block the actin from making cross-filament connections. When calcium is released, it binds troponin. This binding pulls the other blocking protein, tropomyosin, away from the sites so the myosin heads can connect to the attachment sites on the actin protein.

When the myosin head slides, the actin toward the center of the sarcomere creates the sliding filament. Once the myosin heads attach, they are stuck there unless ATP attaches to the myosin head to release the bond. Then, the myosin head returns to its position, ready to reconnect and pull the actin again. The process in which the myosin cross-bridges continually attach, detach, and reattach is called the ratchet mechanism.

MUSCLE ACTIONS

Three types of muscle contractions occur throughout the HMS to produce, reduce, and stabilize forces: concentric, eccentric, and isometric (**Figure 6.5**). The full range of muscle actions is known as the **muscle action spectrum** (**Table 6.6**). Although skeletal muscle is controlled voluntarily, the athlete rarely thinks about the process. Instead, practice and repetition provide the necessary blueprint for the CNS to coordinate the complex process of all muscle contractions.

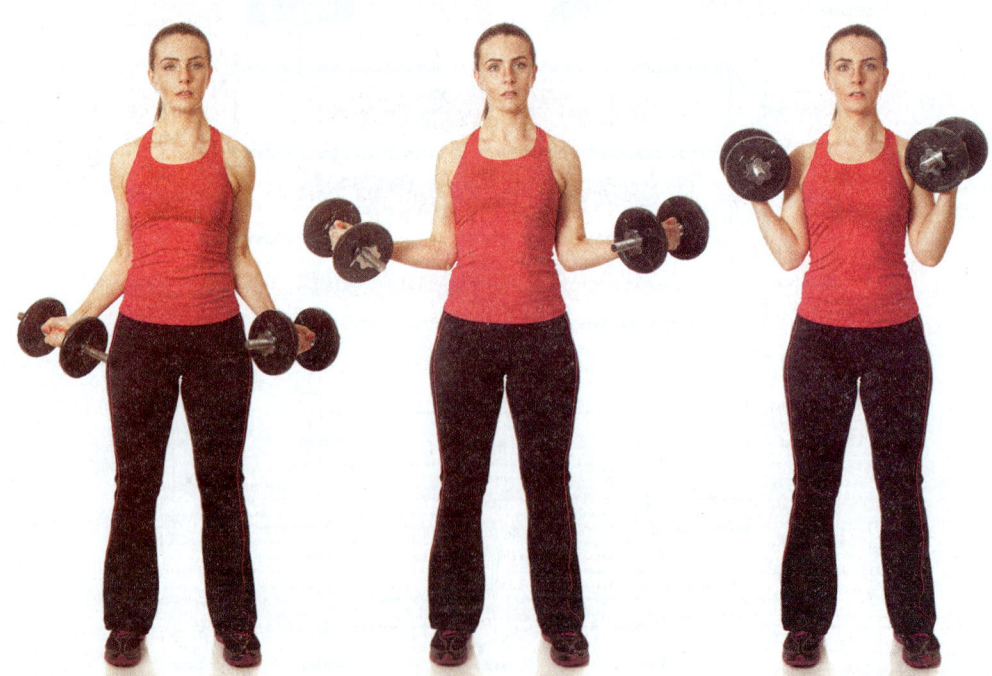

FIGURE 6.5 Muscle Actions
© Nicholas Piccillo/Shutterstock

TABLE 6.6 Muscle Action Spectrum

Concentric	When the proximal and distal ends of the muscle move closer together (i.e., the muscle shortens).
Eccentric	When the proximal and distal ends of the muscle move farther apart (i.e., the muscle lengthens).
Isometric	When a muscle is neither lengthening nor shortening (i.e., the muscle remains the same length).

The muscle actions that contribute to the production of movement in sports and performance are discussed in more detail in the following subsections.

CONCENTRIC

Concentric muscle action occurs when the muscle shortens under tension. For example, in the lifting phase of a squat, the quadriceps concentrically shorten, causing the knee joint to extend as the athlete stands. Concentric contractions increase metabolic demand beyond the demands created by eccentric and isometric contractions—which explains why conditioning activities tend to involve a greater percentage of concentric production. Examples of high concentric to low eccentric and isometric activities include cycling, rope work, and sled pushes and pulls. These activities can increase the athlete's metabolic expenditure while limiting potential soreness and injury from dynamic eccentric muscle movement.

Concentric movements are vital to the way the Sports Performance Coach teaches movement. They include the *lift* while lifting weights and the forward *propulsion* while running along the track. Concentric movements produce vertical jump height and horizontal jump length. However, these concentric muscle actions can often be enhanced through eccentric muscle actions.

ECCENTRIC

Eccentric muscle action involves the lengthening of a muscle while still producing tension. The same muscles that concentrically lift against resistance are usually emphasized during the eccentric portion. For example, in the lowering phase of a squat, the quadriceps eccentrically lengthen as the body lowers. The eccentric phase of the movement is often neglected because most athletes focus on power production rather than the power reduction phase.

Eccentric contractions, however, are vital to conditioning. A meta-analysis showed that eccentric muscle actions, with the appropriate load, can increase muscle strength and size compared to concentric muscle actions, likely due to the higher loads developed during the eccentric phase (Roig et al., 2009). Eccentric muscle actions with a controlled tempo can also increase neuromuscular control and attenuate injury risks (Lepley et al., 2017).

Di Cagno et al. (2020) found eccentric training helped fencers improve technical movements, lunge distance, and advanced lunge distance better than plyometric training. Likewise, Fiorilli et al. (2020) found that overloading multidirectional movements with isoinertial eccentric training improved jump height, linear sprinting, and shooting accuracy to a greater extent than conventional soccer training.

TROPONIN →

A complex of three proteins found in skeletal and cardiac muscle fibers that regulate muscle contraction.

TROPOMYOSIN →

A protein found in muscle fibers that is wound around actin filaments and helps regulate muscle contraction.

MUSCLE ACTION SPECTRUM →

The full range of eccentric, isometric, and concentric muscle contractions required to perform a movement.

CONCENTRIC MUSCLE ACTION →

A muscle action that occurs when a muscle is exerting force greater than the resistive force, resulting in a shortening of the muscle.

ISOMETRIC

An **isometric muscle action** occurs when the muscle remains the same length, but is still producing tension. All muscles have this capacity, but such actions are commonly seen in postural muscles that help maintain erect positions for prolonged periods, such as the erector muscles of the spine that keep the back straight while standing. When engaging in athletic activities such as running, numerous isometric muscle actions work in the frontal and transverse planes to keep the body upright and aligned while moving in a sagittal direction.

Reed et al. (2012) investigated the role of isolated and integrated core stability (isometric) exercises and found these interventions appeared to be beneficial for athletic performance. However, researchers had difficulty precisely ascertaining how beneficial isometric training was because it was part of a comprehensive training program. Doğanay et al. (2020) and Afyon et al. (2018) found that core stability training was beneficial for increasing quickness and agility, but not speed.

ISOTONIC

Isotonic muscle contraction is a type of muscle contraction that involves movement against a constant load or resistance. During isotonic exercises, the tension and resistance on the muscle remain constant throughout the range of motion, and the muscle length changes as it contracts and relaxes. *Isotonic* is a term meaning "the same tension."

Isotonic muscle contraction differs from isometric muscle action in that it refers to the constant tension a muscle maintains while changing positions (**Figure 6.6**). Both concentric and eccentric contractions are isotonic.

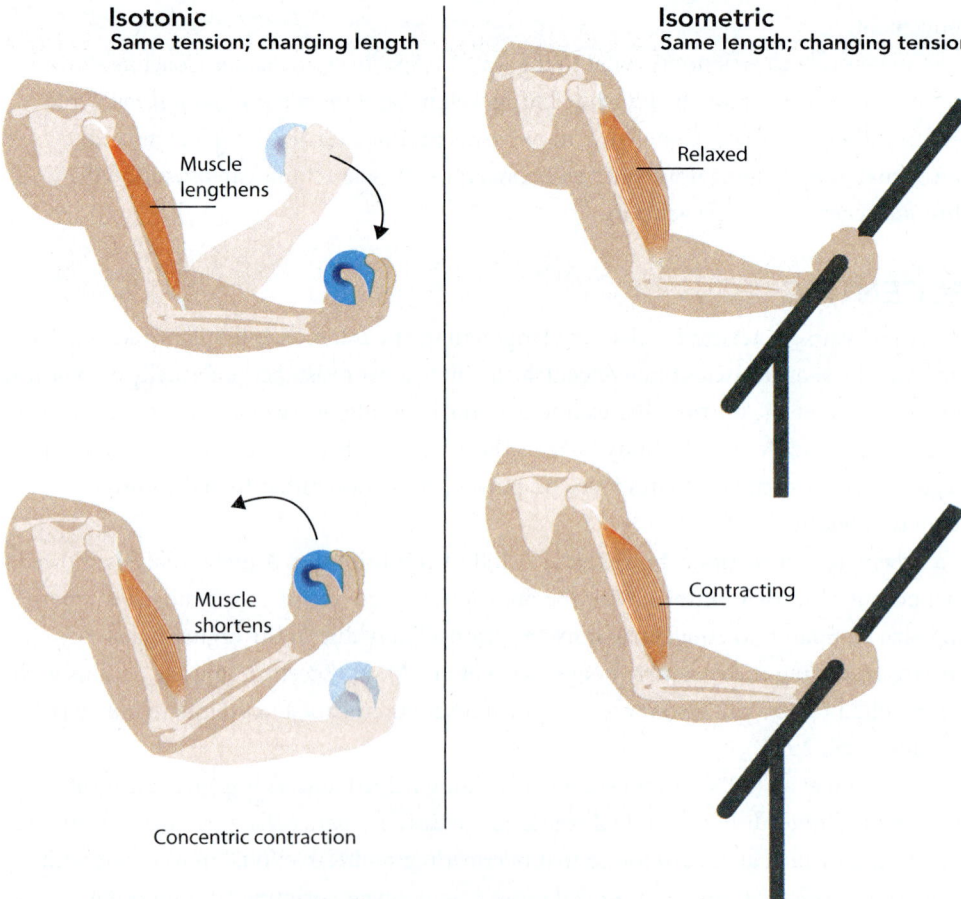

Isotonic
Same tension; changing length

Muscle lengthens

Muscle shortens

Concentric contraction

Isometric
Same length; changing tension

Relaxed

Contracting

FIGURE 6.6 Isotonic Versus Isometric Muscle Action

AMORTIZATION PHASE

The **amortization phase** is the transitional period between the eccentric deceleration of force and the concentric production of force. An example is when an athlete is about to jump and drops eccentrically into a shallow squat. There is a brief moment of dynamic stabilization when the eccentric phase shifts from reducing force during an eccentric load to producing force, which allows the athlete to jump.

Thus, the amortization phase is the period in between the stretch and the shortening of muscles. It is important to minimize the amortization phase to maximize jump height during the stretch–shortening cycle.

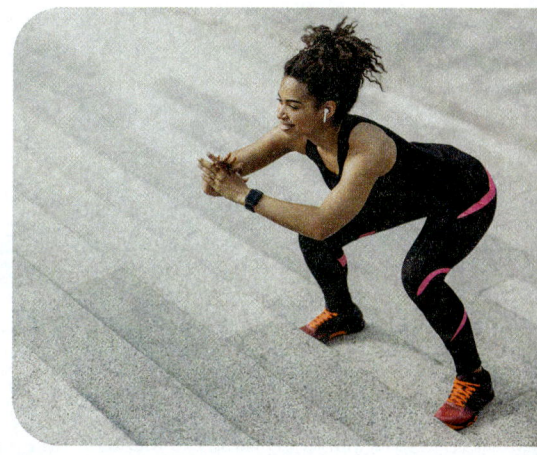

© Prostock-studio/Shutterstock

MUSCLES AS MOVERS

To effectively understand human movement and design effective and safe sports performance programs, the Sports Performance Coach must view the muscular systems' capacity to function as an integrated unit. Muscles work together to provide the human body with various functions that allow for the manipulation of forces placed on the body to produce, reduce, and stabilize movement. During functional movements, a muscle can be categorized as an agonist, synergist, stabilizer, or antagonist, depending on the joint motion performed (**Table 6.7**).

> **AMORTIZATION →**
> **PHASE**
>
> The transition from eccentric loading to concentric unloading during the stretch–shortening cycle.

TABLE 6.7 Muscles as Movers

Muscle	Action	Description
Agonists	Primary movers	The agonist at the hip in the lifting phase of a squat is the gluteus maximus.
Synergists	Muscles that assist the agonist	The synergists at the hip in the lifting phase of the squat are the hamstrings and the posterior fibers of the adductor magnus.
Antagonists	Opposing muscles of a specific joint action	The antagonists at the hip in the lifting phase of a squat are the hip flexors.
Stabilizers	Muscles that contract isometrically to stabilize and limit unwanted motion at the trunk and joints during movement	The stabilizers during a squat are the intrinsic core muscles to maintain spinal alignment and stability.

LEVERS

Leverage in the HMS depends on bones, joints, muscles, and external load. Sometimes leverage is not favorable for lifting weights, but it can be very advantageous for producing speed. Three different classifications are used to describe the **levers** in the human body

> **LEVERS →**
>
> Rigid structures (such as bones) that rotate around a fixed point called a fulcrum in response to the contraction of a muscle.

LOAD →

The external resistance to be moved.

EFFORT →

The internal exertion that muscles produce against an external load.

FULCRUM →

The point of pivot or the axis of rotation.

EFFORT ARM →

The distance from the effort to the fulcrum.

LOAD ARM →

The distance from the load to the fulcrum.

FORCE →

An influence applied by one object to another, resulting in an acceleration or deceleration of the second object.

TORQUE →

A measure of the amount of force on an object that causes the object to rotate.

(**Table 6.8**). Each lever system consists of effort, load, and fulcrum acting on the bone as a lever. The **load** is external resistance. The **effort** is the internal exertion that the muscles produce against the external load. The **fulcrum** is the point of pivot or the axis of rotation.

TABLE 6.8 Lever Classification

Lever Type	Description	Example
First class	The fulcrum (joint) is between the effort (muscle) and the load (external resistance).	Flexion and extension of the head on the neck.
Second class	The load (external resistance) is between the fulcrum and effort (muscle).	Plantar flexion of the foot and ankle.
Third class	The force (muscle) is between the fulcrum and resistance (load).	Flexion of the forearm in a biceps curl.

The distance from the effort to the fulcrum is known as the **effort arm**. In the body, this is the distance between where the muscle inserts onto the bone and the point of pivot (often a joint). The distance from the load to the fulcrum is known as the **load arm**. In the body, this is the distance between the pivot point and the weight or resistance being lifted or moved.

Understanding movement requires a Sports Performance Coach to have some knowledge of force and torque. **Force** is a push or a pull that causes an object with mass to change velocity. Force is applied to the human body externally from an object, such as dumbbells or an opponent. Internally, force is applied back to the object from the contraction of skeletal muscle. The movement of a lever (i.e., bones) around an axis (i.e., joints) produces **torque**, which is the force that causes an object to rotate. Torque generated by a muscle depends on several factors, including the muscle's size, strength, angle of insertion, and the distance between the joint and the muscle's point of attachment. The HMS relies on rotational forces at joints for movement and locomotion.

Because the neuromuscular system is responsible for manipulating force, the amount of leverage the HMS has for any given movement depends on the leverage of the muscles in relation to the resistance. The difference between the distance the weight is from the center of the joint and the muscle's attachment to the joint determines the efficiency with which the muscles manipulate movement. Because attachment sites and lines of pull of muscles through the tendon cannot be altered, the easiest way to alter the amount of torque generated at a joint is to move the load closer to or farther from the point of rotation (the joint).

For example, if an athlete holds a dumbbell straight out to the side at arm's length, the weight is approximately 24 inches from the center of the shoulder joint (fulcrum). The deltoid muscles (agonists for shoulder abduction) attachment is approximately 2 inches from the fulcrum. Therefore, the load arm is roughly 12 times farther from the pivot point than the effort arm. If the weight is moved closer to the joint center, such as to the elbow, the load is now approximately 12 inches from the joint center. With the load arm now only five times greater than the effort arm, the torque required to hold the weight has been essentially reduced by half.

Many people performing side lateral raises with dumbbells inadvertently alter torque in this way by flexing their elbow, bringing the weight closer to the shoulder joint, and effectively reducing the required torque by shortening the load arm. The Sports Performance Coach can use this principle as a regression for exercises that are too demanding, reducing the torque placed on the HMS.

Similarly, an athlete can apply this principle as a progression to increase the torque and place a greater demand on the HMS.

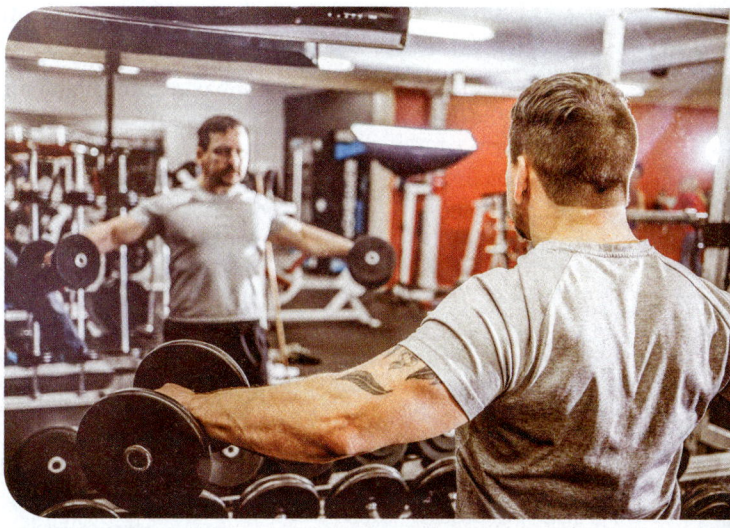

© Benoit Daust/Shutterstock

LENGTH–TENSION RELATIONSHIPS

Length–tension relationships (LTR) refer to the association between a muscle's resting length and the amount of internal tension it can produce (Levangie & Norkin, 2011). Any change in length from the resting position alters the tension that the muscle produces. Maximal force (tension) is produced when the thick myosin filaments develop the most cross-bridges with the thinner actin filament within the sarcomere. The resting length of a muscle is present when the body is standing still; the muscle is neither contracting nor stretching. When muscle activation occurs from either lengthened or shortened positions, fewer cross-bridges and active sites are available, which results in limited force production.

LTR is why deeper squats can be so much more challenging than shallow squats. This concept is also important for understanding the appropriate stabilization muscles, posture, and technique during particular exercises and activities. During a squat, for example, the core stabilizers must optimally perform to protect the spine while loaded. A change in spinal position alters the muscle's ability to develop maximal tension and limits their protective capacities.

Systematized movement assessments allow the Sports Performance Coach to identify movement compensations and implement strategies for the athlete to maximize their performance outcomes while becoming more resilient to dysfunctional movement patterns. During such an assessment, the Sports Performance Coach might identify a muscle as **overactive**. Overactive muscles are also frequently labeled as "shortened." However, it is likely that a neurological hyper-facilitation of the muscle is causing it to shorten due to contraction, rather than a mechanically shortened structure. The antagonist muscle on the other side of the joint may also be affected because it is in a lengthened position. **Reciprocal inhibition** is the phenomenon in which a muscle on one side of a joint contracts and the CNS inhibits the antagonists, limiting the muscle's ability to produce force. In this scenario, the antagonist muscles on the other side of the overactive agonists are considered to be **underactive**. When a muscle on one side of a joint is in a shortened resting length, and the muscles on the other side are in a lengthened resting length, the condition is known as **muscle imbalance**.

It is also important to work a muscle through various ranges of motion to build strength in various positions. A review by Schoenfeld and Grgic (2020) showed that full range-of-motion exercises provide superior hypertrophy in lower-body musculature but might not have the same effects for the upper body. However, shallower squats may increase post-activation potentiation and increase performance in jumps and sprint performance (Seitz & Haff, 2016).

The Sports Performance Coach can use their understanding of LTR to recognize that optimal length can produce optimal strength, and to appreciate that the further the athlete

---

LENGTH–TENSION RELATIONSHIPS (LTR) →

The resting length of a muscle and the tension the muscle can produce at this resting length.

OVERACTIVE →

Increased neural facilitation, causing a muscle to be held in a state of chronic contraction.

RECIPROCAL INHIBITION →

Contraction of an agonist that causes its antagonist to relax, allowing movement at the joint.

UNDERACTIVE →

When neural inhibition of a muscle leads to limited neuromuscular recruitment.

MUSCLE IMBALANCE →

A condition in which the muscles on each side of a joint have altered length–tension relationships.

REGIONAL INTER-DEPENDENCE (RI) MODEL →

A model that proposes problems in one area can lead to compensation patterns and adaptations in other areas, resulting in pain, movement dysfunction, and other symptoms.

deviates from this position, the less force that will be produced. The LTR concept can also be applied to ensure athlete safety. The Sports Performance Coach must understand that imbalances in length and tension can pull joints into suboptimal positions, which can then impact other body regions. More specifically, the **regional interdependence (RI) model** proposes that dysfunction or pain in one area of the body can lead to compensation patterns and adaptation in other areas, resulting in pain and/or movement dysfunction (Sueki et al., 2013).

✓ CHECK IT OUT

Here is one example of how LTR knowledge can be applied: Hold your arm in front of you and make a fist as tightly as you can. Now, flex your wrist and make a fist as tightly as you can. The tension produced is significantly limited. Now try the other three wrist positions: wrist extension, ulnar deviation, and radial deviation. Try to make a fist as tightly as you can. Now go back to your neutral wrist position and compare the strength from the neutral position to the other positions.

FORCE–VELOCITY CURVE

The **force–velocity curve** shows the relationship between force production and speed production depending on the external load. With a relatively light external load, concentric muscle activation moves at relatively high velocities. For example, a baseball player can throw a baseball at incredible speeds with relatively low muscle activation. However, replace the baseball with a 20-pound bowling ball, and the muscle recruitment increases while the velocity of the throw decreases.

Similar examples can be cited when lifting weights (**Figure 6.7**). An athlete can move through squats or bench presses with light external loads quickly with little muscle force. However, as the load increases, the ability to lift the weight concentrically at higher

Strengthening the Force–Velocity Profile of Athletes Using Weightlifting Movements

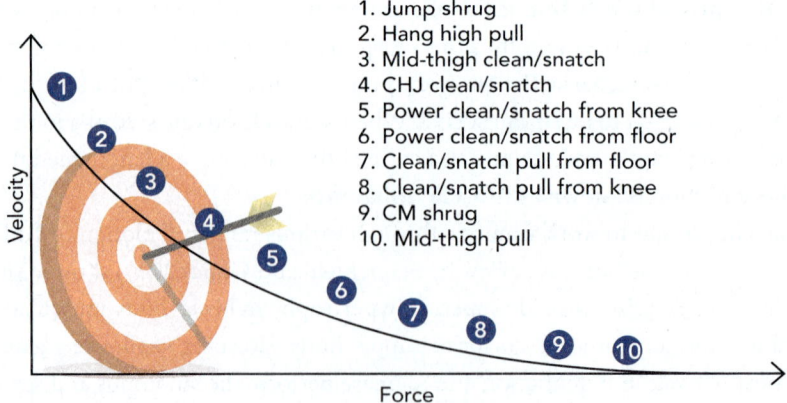

1. Jump shrug
2. Hang high pull
3. Mid-thigh clean/snatch
4. CHJ clean/snatch
5. Power clean/snatch from knee
6. Power clean/snatch from floor
7. Clean/snatch pull from floor
8. Clean/snatch pull from knee
9. CM shrug
10. Mid-thigh pull

FIGURE 6.7 Force–Velocity Profile of Athletes

Based on Suchomel, T. (2017). Enhancing the force velocity profile of athletes using weightlifting derivatives. *Strength and Conditioning Journal, 39*(1), 10-20.

velocities decreases, and the muscle force requirements increase. At certain weights, it does not matter how hard the athlete pushes—the weight cannot be moved quickly, regardless of the amount of force produced.

Plyometric training, using lightweight and high-velocity exercises, help with concentric force production by improving motor unit recruitment and rate coding. During this training, exercises are performed at low repetition ranges (up to 10 repetitions at 30% to 45% 1-repetition maximum [1RM]) to ensure that maximal speeds are always trained. For this reason, it is vital that the Sports Performance Coach limit the number of repetitions when using plyometrics, even if the athlete wishes to do more. The goal is not to practice these movements to exhaustion, but rather to perform them at maximal velocities for each jump or throw, taking advantage of the stretch–shortening cycle.

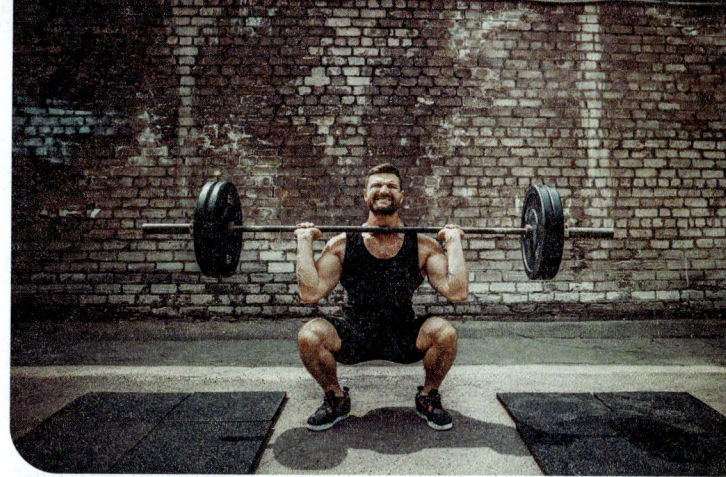

© SOK Studio/Shutterstock

Eccentric muscle activation of the force–velocity curve is the opposite of its concentric counterpart. The lighter the weight, the more slowly the athlete eccentrically decelerates the external load without maximal force production. As the weight gets heavier, the force production increases, and the speed at which the load is decelerated increases. Intuitively, athletes understand that the heavier the weight, the greater the internal force production that is needed to move the load. During the eccentric phase, as the load increases, the muscles must produce greater force. Eventually, as more load is added, the athlete can no longer produce enough internal force to slowly decelerate the load and the weight moves more quickly.

With exercises such as a power clean, often a lighter barbell or dowel is used for technique training. A light load can be added to provide some resistance, but the movement is practiced for speed in this case. As the weight increases, the speed of the lift decreases until the ability to clean the bar is no longer possible.

FORCE–COUPLE RELATIONSHIPS

Different muscles crossing a joint can pull at different vectors, working together to perform a specific joint action. This synergist process of muscles working together to produce movement around a joint is known as a **force–couple relationship**. Depending on the structure of the joints and the angle of pull, these divergent forces work together to produce movement.

Scapular upward rotation is a great example of a force–couple relationship (**Figure 6.8**). The upper trapezius connects along the superior-lateral scapula and pulls superiorly, while the lower trapezius connects to the medial scapula and pulls inferiorly. Lastly, the serratus anterior attaches to the anterior medial border of the scapula and pulls anteriorly. Pulling at different vectors, these three muscles collectively pull the scapula into upward rotation.

By using knowledge of force–couple relationships, the Sports Performance Coach can quickly recognize which muscles are responsible for faulty movement patterns. For example, if a tennis player demonstrates difficulty getting their racquet overhead, the coach will know to perform assessments that test the strength and mobility of the upper and lower trapezius along with the serratus anterior. Or, in this same athlete, the Sports Performance Coach may need to consider the force–couple relationship that produces downward rotation (i.e., levator scapulae, pectoralis minor, rhomboid, and latissimus dorsi), as it could be contributing to the difficulty in upward rotation.

FORCE–VELOCITY CURVE →

A property of skeletal muscle whereby the force in a muscle contraction decreases as the velocity of shortening increases. When this is measured during a complex sport skill, it may be referred to as a force–velocity relationship.

FORCE–COUPLE RELATIONSHIP →

The synergistic action of multiple muscles working together to produce movement around a joint.

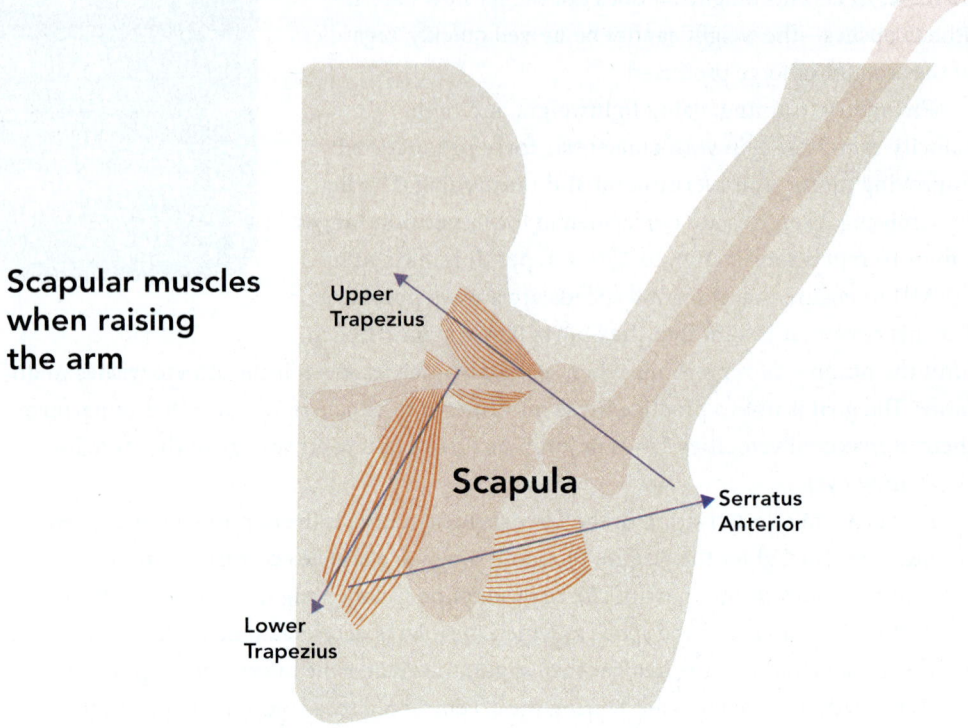

Scapular muscles when raising the arm

Upper Trapezius

Scapula

Serratus Anterior

Lower Trapezius

FIGURE 6.8 Scapular Upward Motion

All human movement uses force–couple relationships to produce and reduce force and to dynamically stabilize the body in multiple planes of motion. The resulting motion depends on factors such as joint type and structure, the direction of pull, attachment sites, and lever type. The Sports Performance Coach needs to understand the integrated nature of human movement and appreciate how to provide stabilization along with dynamic force production and reduction to maximize athletic performance.

LESSON 3: MUSCULAR SYSTEM OF THE BODY

MUSCULAR SYSTEMS

The muscular system comprises more than 600 skeletal muscles that the CNS supports in various ways based on muscle size, fiber type, location, leverage, angle of pull, and task purpose. A landmark paper on spinal stability divided spinal muscular into two distinct yet inter-reliant systems: the global muscular system and the local muscular system (Bergmark, 1989). Each muscle of the lumbo-pelvic-hip complex (LPHC) is designated as global or local based on its mechanical role—that is, whether it transfers load directly between the pelvis and thoracic cage or acts directly on the lumbar spine (Bergmark, 1989). Smaller and deeper muscles that provide intersegmental stability from vertebra to vertebra are considered contributors to the local core muscular system. Larger muscles of the spine that tend to be more superficial and create larger movement patterns are considered part of the global core muscular system. Therefore, any muscle that attaches directly to the LPHC is considered part of the core muscular system, but is subclassified as global or local based on its location and function.

As an athlete moves, these systems work in an interrelated fashion to produce, reduce, and stabilize movement in all three planes of motion to contend with task-related forces of the external environment. With an understanding of the local and global muscular systems, the Sports Performance Coach can better understand how to train local and global muscular systems to provide better stability (Lee et al., 2020), activation (Lee et al., 2019), and performance (Kim et al., 2013; Shin et al., 2013).

LOCAL MUSCULAR SYSTEM

The **local muscular system** is made up of muscles that connect directly to the spine at either the proximal or distal attachment, or both, and work primarily as spinal stabilizers. The psoas muscle connects directly to the spine but is primarily involved in hip flexion, so it is not considered part of the local system in terms of function. The local

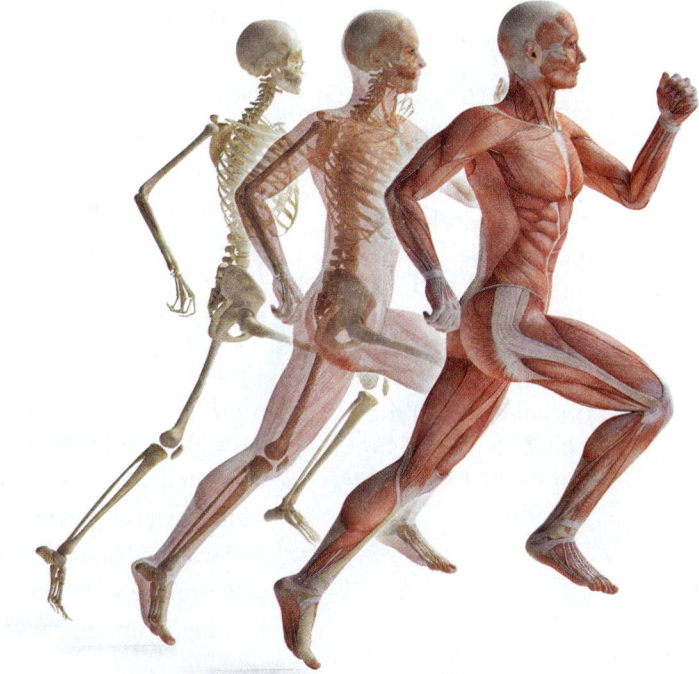

© Adike/Shutterstock

muscular system consists of smaller postural muscles that connect directly to the spine and primarily support spinal stability (Heidari et al., 2015). They predominately consist of type I muscle fibers that work well for endurance, balance, slower motor recruitment, low resistance, and low load (Wilson et al., 2012). The local muscles include the transverse abdominus, multifidi, diaphragm, pelvic floor muscles, and the posterior fibers of the internal obliques.

Core stability is often utilized to supplement and support sports performance. It is frequently described as the ability to control the trunk relative to the pelvis in a manner that allows for energy production, reduction, and transference of distal to proximal segments during the performance of different tasks (Butowicz et al., 2016; Key, 2013; Resende et al., 2020). Traditionally, core stability training is performed in isolation. However, a survey of athletes, coaches, sports scientists, and sports medicine practitioners showed a preference for a more functional approach to core training including loaded, compound, and upright exercises (Clark et al., 2018). For example, a total-body exercise, such as a squat with a cable row, integrates spinal stabilization with lower- and upper-body strength or endurance when performed correctly. Core stability training is associated with increased power production, agility, and dynamic stability during athletic events (Greene et al., 2019).

GLOBAL MUSCULAR SYSTEM

The **global muscular system** is predominately responsible for movement and consists of larger, more superficial muscles that connect the pelvis to the rib cage, the lower extremities, or both. Global muscles have more type II muscle fibers than the local core muscles and are better designed for strength, coordination, agility, and fast-velocity training in which a large variety of movement patterns and parameters of short duration are combined with a spectrum of light to heavy resistance and loads (Wilson et al., 2012). Some of these muscles attach the pelvis to the lower extremities and are essential to locomotion. Others attach the LPHC to the upper extremities to produce, reduce, and transfer forces from the arms to the trunk.

> **LOCAL MUSCULAR SYSTEM** →
>
> Muscles that connect directly to the spine and are predominantly involved in LPHC stabilization.

> **CORE STABILITY** →
>
> The ability of the neuromuscular system to limit unwanted movement of the LPHC.

The local and global systems never work in isolation, so training them in isolation for performance-based outcomes needs to be limited, though not necessarily eliminated. The stabilization system is worked when the global muscular system mobilizes the skeletal system. The global system also helps to stabilize the rib cage, pelvis, and lower and upper extremities. However, the local and global systems' primary roles are not necessarily their exclusive roles. The neuromuscular system works to coordinate the best way for the HMS to produce, reduce, and dynamically stabilize to control for the degrees of freedom needed to accomplish a task.

MOVEMENT SYSTEMS

The global muscular system can be divided into four movement systems or subsystems, which practitioners often refer to as myofascial slings, chains, or meridians (Wilke et al., 2016). Each subsystem connects the LPHC to the lower extremities so that they work together as a functional unit. More than one global subsystem can work at the same time, while the local system works simultaneously to maintain posture and stability. The Sports Performance Coach can use their knowledge of how these subsystems function to help with exercise selection, exercise programming, movement practice, and force–coupling training by linking the dynamics of the lower extremities to and through the LPHC.

DEEP LONGITUDINAL SUBSYSTEM

The deep longitudinal subsystem (DLS) comprises the erector spinae, thoracolumbar fascia, sacrotuberous ligament, biceps femoris, anterior tibialis, and fibularis (peroneus) longus. These muscles work synergistically, primarily during walking and running, to provide a longitudinal means of reciprocal force transmission from the trunk to the ground (**Figure 6.9**). Upon the initial impact in the gait, whether a heel strike or forefoot strike, the anterior tibialis and fibularis longus control the ankle in both the frontal

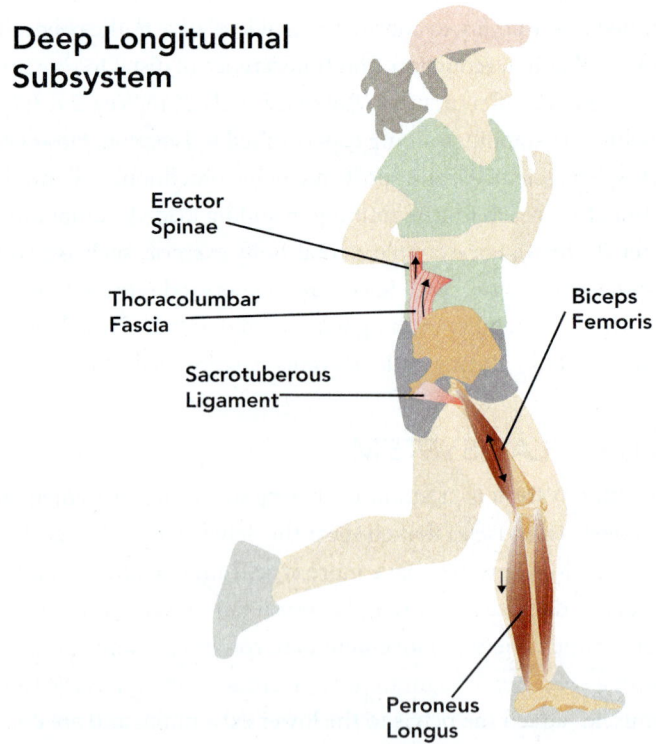

Deep Longitudinal Subsystem

Erector Spinae

Thoracolumbar Fascia

Sacrotuberous Ligament

Biceps Femoris

Peroneus Longus

FIGURE 6.9 The Deep Longitudinal Subsystem: Control of Ground Reaction Forces

(inversion and eversion) and sagittal planes (dorsiflexion and plantar flexion). There is a fascial connection of the fibularis longus with the biceps femoris at the proximal fibular head. The biceps femoris attaches to the ischial tuberosity with a fascial connection with the sacrotuberous ligament. Upon foot strike, the biceps femoris transmits force across the sacrotuberous ligament that crosses from the ischial tuberosity to the sacrum to help stabilize the sacroiliac joint (SIJ). The erector spinae group attaches to the sacrum and runs superiorly through the thoracic region spine and the cervical spine. Upon heel (walking) or forefoot strike (running), the reciprocal force transmission runs through the kinetic chain to stabilize the LPHC, thoracic, and cervical spine.

During walking and running, the biceps femoris eccentrically decelerates knee extension and hip flexion while the anterior tibialis concentrically activates to dorsiflex and invert the foot–ankle complex. Upon heel strike, the anterior tibialis decelerates plantar flexion and eversion. In case of forefoot striking, the fibularis longus decelerates plantar flexion while the anterior tibialis decelerates eversion upon ground contact.

Through forward locomotion, the biceps femoris concentrically flexes the knee and extends the hip while creating tension at the sacrotuberous ligament and the erector spinae. This tensioning creates stabilizing forces at the SIJ and superiorly through the lumbar, thoracic, and cervical vertebrae longitudinally. An athlete can train the DLS in a quadruped position while performing an opposite arm and leg reach. This provides longitudinal stabilization without impacts or reciprocal force transference. A progression to standing could be a single-leg floor bridge while maintaining either plantar flexion or dorsiflexion to engage the muscles from the foot–ankle complex through the hips and spine. A progression to standing can be performed on one leg while the other leg performs repetitive gait swings with or without a resistance band. The stance leg engages the DLS while activating the contralateral swinging leg on the backswing.

POSTERIOR OBLIQUE SUBSYSTEM

The posterior oblique subsystem (POS) is one of the most research-supported global subsystems. The POS comprises the latissimus dorsi and contralateral gluteus maximus (**Figure 6.10**). These two muscles run in similar directions and intersect at the thoracolumbar fascia. A co-contraction of both the latissimus dorsi and gluteus maximus muscles creates a crisscross pattern across the back, pelvis, and hips, creating stabilization forces along the SIJ.

During the individual's gait, the POS works with the DLS to stabilize the SIJ via the backswing of the arm and contralateral hip, facilitated by the latissimus dorsi and contralateral gluteus maximus. Because each new step in the stride creates a backswing, the SIJ is additionally and continually supported. Researchers confirmed this effect in a study in which participants walked on a treadmill at various speeds. The results showed a correlation between the backswing of the arm at the shoulder and the backswing of the contralateral hip (Shin et al., 2013).

Coupling contralateral gluteus maximus and latissimus dorsi activation exercises with the abdominal drawing-in maneuver can produce a significantly greater increase in POS activation (Lee et al., 2020). Drawing-in is not appropriate during many aspects of performance training or game-time activities. Therefore, the Sports Performance Coach might add this exercise into warm-ups and movement preparation. Researchers have also shown that athletes can experience low back pain when the latissimus dorsi is overactive and the gluteus maximus is underactive (Mohamed et al., 2021).

When the gluteus maximus is inhibited, synergists such as the ipsilateral hamstrings, adductor magnus (posterior fibers), and both contralateral and ipsilateral erector spinae

Posterior Oblique Subsystem

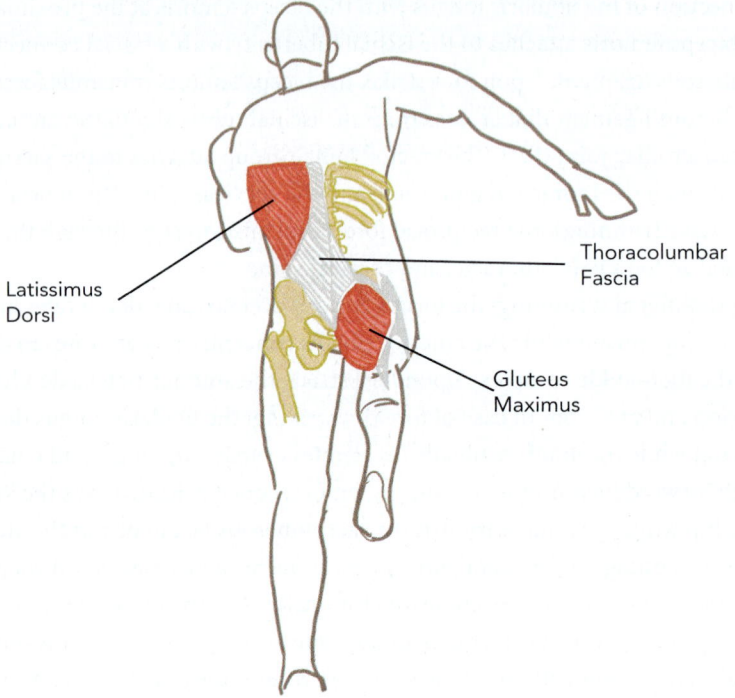

Latissimus Dorsi

Thoracolumbar Fascia

Gluteus Maximus

FIGURE 6.10 The Posterior Oblique Subsystem

muscles are facilitated (Lee et al., 2019), often leading to faulty movement patterns. In such a case, an athlete might need to use self-myofascial rolling (SMR) and static stretching on the facilitated muscles. They can then perform isolated strengthening exercises for the inhibited muscles. However, the athlete should also include an integrated approach to reengage the proper functioning of the POS. An example of a POS-specific exercise is a squat-to-row pattern, which utilizes the latissimus dorsi and gluteus maximus (**Figure 6.11**).

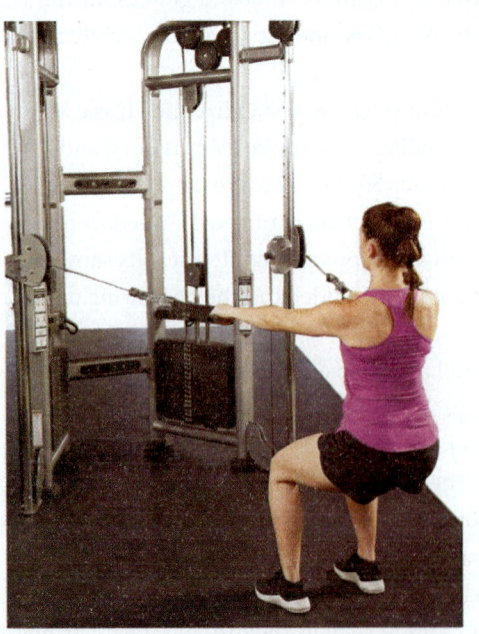
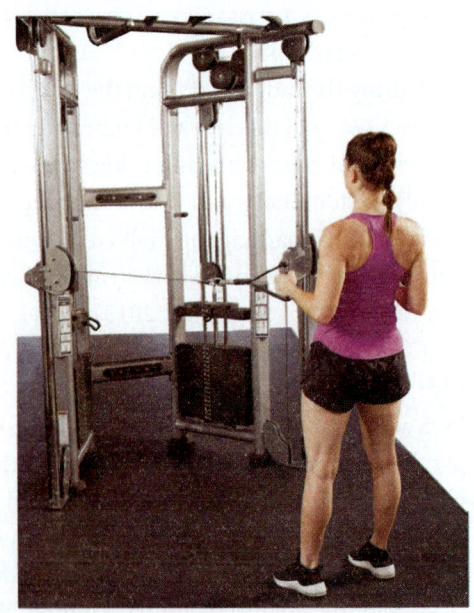

FIGURE 6.11 Squat-to-Row Pattern

Prone hip extension exercises are a great way to work the POS (Lee et al., 2019; Lee et al., 2020). Adding upper-extremity movement will increase the co-contraction of the latissimus dorsi muscles, yielding better results. Research suggests that abduction of the arm to 125 degrees results in activation of the lumbopelvic stabilizing muscles, likely due to the change in lever length and subsequent need for additional stability (Ha & Jeon, 2021). Therefore, a superman exercise using opposing upper- and lower-extremity movement could be beneficial.

📋 COACH'S CORNER

The POS is important in rotationally oriented sports such as baseball, golf, and tennis. For example, a right-handed batter uses the right gluteus maximus and contralateral (left) latissimus dorsi to create rotational power through the swing, while helping stabilize the high-velocity transmission of force through the lumbosacral spine and sacroiliac joint. Running is also heavily reliant on the POS. Therefore, the Sports Performance Coach must consider how muscles work synergistically and select programming and exercise options based on the integrated patterns of core subsystems.

ANTERIOR OBLIQUE SUBSYSTEM

The anterior oblique subsystem (AOS) works concurrently with the POS to produce rotational forces through the transverse plane (**Figure 6.12**). The AOS comprises the external obliques and contralateral adductor complex of the hips. These fibers have similar oblique alignments on opposite sides of the body: The direction of fiber for the external obliques runs from superior-lateral to inferior-medial. The contralateral adductor complex picks up that line of direction as it runs proximal-medial to a relative distal-lateral insertion.

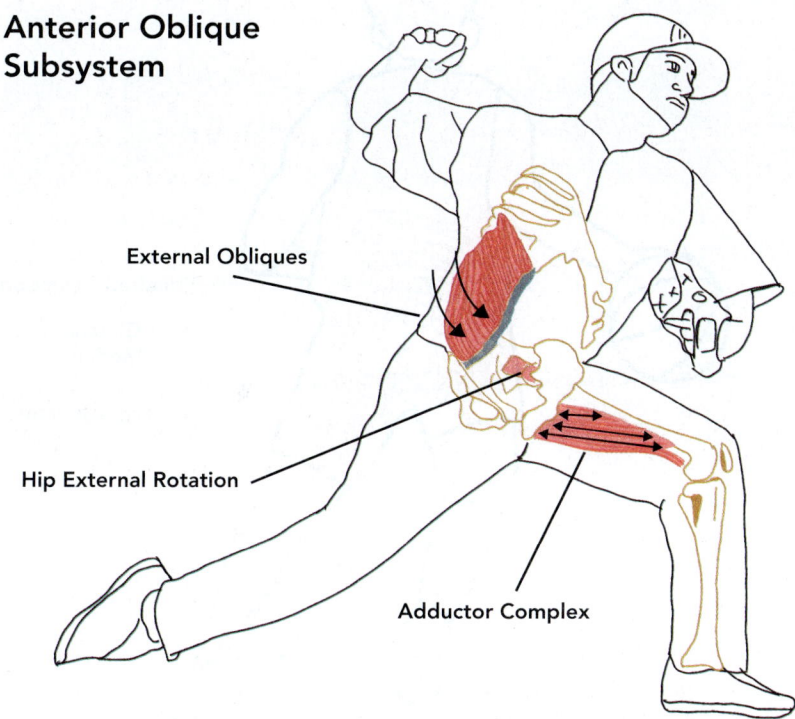

Anterior Oblique Subsystem

External Obliques

Hip External Rotation

Adductor Complex

FIGURE 6.12 The Anterior Oblique Subsystem

This line of pull allows these bodily segments to flex and rotate toward each other. In a right-handed swing, the co-contraction of the right external oblique rotates the spine toward the left side. In a closed chain, the left adductors rotate the pelvis toward the left, creating pelvis-on-femur internal rotation. The AOS works with the POS in different vectors and lines of pull to facilitate similar rotational tasks, such as throwing and swinging.

The AOS can be trained statically prior to progression to movement through a full range of motion and eventually into dynamic movements with speed. Static oblique exercises from either a half-kneeling or a supine position show greater activation patterns of the AOS than either a plank or abdominal crunch (Nakai et al., 2021). Nakai et al. (2021) utilized an isometric half-kneeling oblique exercise in which the participant applied pressure with one arm to the front knee. The AOS is significantly engaged in this exercise as the participant resists hip abduction and trunk rotation. A single-arm standing chest press also isometrically stabilizes the core with the help of the AOS. Dynamically, medicine ball throws, rotational cable chest presses, and swinging patterns rely on the AOS for rotation and core support.

LATERAL SUBSYSTEM

The lateral subsystem (LS) is made up of the gluteus medius, tensor fascia latae (TFL), adductor complex, and contralateral quadratus lumborum (QL) (**Figure 6.13**). These muscles are located either on the medial or the lateral side of the joints and work primarily in the frontal plane to create lateral stability. This LPHC frontal plane stability is essential while standing on a single leg and in other functional activities such as bipedal locomotion (walking or running), climbing stairs, and lunges, or more dynamically in exercises such as ice skating. A single-leg squat is a good assessment to evaluate the LS.

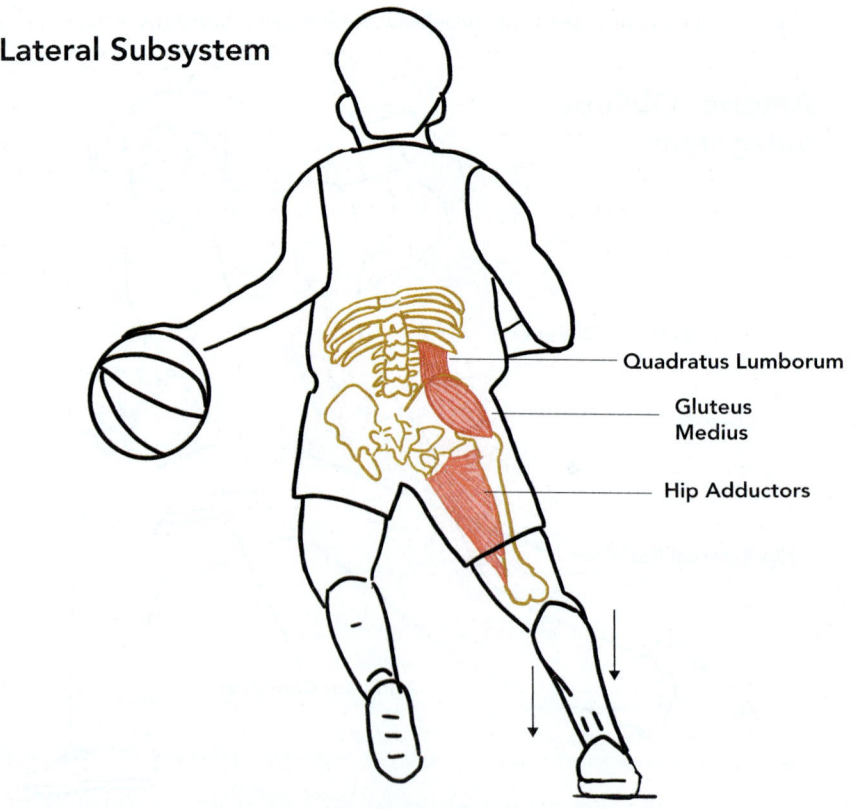

Lateral Subsystem

Quadratus Lumborum

Gluteus Medius

Hip Adductors

FIGURE 6.13 The Lateral Subsystem

Pronation of the foot and valgus of the knee have adverse effects on the production and reduction of force throughout the HMS. Because the deceleration of forces is compounded during sports, especially with activities such as slowing down quickly, it is important that the Sports Performance Coach pays attention to movement patterns and knows how to address deficiencies in the local core systems. Knee valgus moving up the kinetic chain can have adverse effects on both the AOS and POS. These systems work together to stabilize the core while allowing for movement and force production.

One type of engaging exercise for the LS is side planks. This exercise works the QL, gluteus medius, and TFL on the ipsilateral side and the adductors on the contralateral side. Alternatively, an athlete can do an adductor plank by lifting the bottom leg off the floor and using only the forearm and the top leg to lift the LPHC off the ground. Anti-rotational exercises with a lateral pull are also effective facilitators of the LS, as are single-leg balance with excursion exercises.

The four subsystems create movement and provide LPHC stability. These subsystems engage in patterns through chains or slings, but do not work in isolation. Instead, they work concurrently to produce, reduce, and dynamically stabilize forces from the extremities through the LPHC. Although the content presented here in regard to the local core system, the global core system, and the global subsystems has been simplified, the Sports Performance Coach must understand how these systems work and think about ways to program subsystem training into their athletes' programs.

📋 COACH'S CORNER

Designing exercise programs for athletes targeting the four primary subsystems promotes optimal force–couple relationships and joint motion by focusing on specific movement patterns instead of individual muscles. Sports Performance Coaches must design performance programs to improve subsystem functions resulting in properly recruiting muscle synergy. The goal is to improve a client's quality of movement (**Table 6.9**).

TABLE 6.9 Sample Program for Movement Quality

Exercise	Sets	Reps	Tempo	Rest	Subsystem
Frontal plane lunge to balance	2–3	12	Slow–medium	0	LS
Single-leg box jump with stabilization	2–3	12	Slow–medium	0	DLS
Alternating-arm ball cobra	2–3	12	Slow–medium	0	POS
Single-leg cable chop	2–3	12	Slow–medium	60 seconds	AOS

LESSON 4: FUNDAMENTALS OF MOTOR SKILL LEARNING

PRINCIPLES OF MOTOR BEHAVIOR AND SKILL ACQUISITION

Most athletic movement is nothing short of spectacular to spectators. However, human movement, in general, is also quite remarkable. Every mobile joint from the foot and ankle through the knees, hips, and spine has a range of motion that stacks on top of the others. This creates a nearly incalculable number of potential movements that pile atop each other, which must be coordinated and controlled. **Coordination** is the patterning of head, body, and limb movements relative to the patterning of environmental objects and events, regardless of the performer's skill level (McGill, 2011). The CNS receives input from the environment to determine a motor recruitment pattern to move or stabilize joints to reach a desired outcome. In many sports, if the CNS makes even minor miscalculations, the result could be disastrous. For example, if a golfer's club is off by a millimeter in the vertical axis, the ball might end up dozens of yards off target after a 300-yard drive. The studies of motor behavior and motor skill acquisition that have been performed to date help Sports Performance Coaches understand the basic underlying principles of physical performance.

A **motor skill** is an activity or task that requires voluntary movement of the head, body, and limbs to achieve a specific goal (McGill, 2011). Athletes in different sports and in different positions within those sports have different movement requirements to achieve a desired goal. Though similarities exist between swinging a golf club and swinging a baseball bat, these sports require very different skillsets, and there is likely minimal carryover from one to the other. As one example, a golf ball is not moving at a high velocity while the athlete is trying to make contact with it. To better understand skill acquisition, the Sports Performance Coach must understand the components of motor behavior, motor control, motor learning, and motor development.

MOTOR BEHAVIOR IN SPORTS PERFORMANCE TRAINING

Movement is learned, applied, and retained conceptually through motor behavior. **Motor behavior** is the HMS's movement response to internal stimuli and external stimuli. According to Adolph and Franchak (2017), motor behavior includes every kind of movement, from involuntary twitches to goal-directed actions; in every part of the body, from head to toe; in every physical and social context, from solitary play to group interactions.

From another perspective, the study of motor behavior examines how the nervous, muscular, and skeletal systems interact to produce skilled movement using sensory information, the external environmental components of a sport, and the individual athlete's physiology, morphology, and conditioning. Internal stimuli might comprise the CNS's and PNS's interactions with muscles to perform tasks. In contrast, external stimuli might arise from the environment, such as a tennis player responding to a serve or an American football player trying to avoid being tackled while holding onto the ball, ignoring the noise of the crowd, and contending with unfavorable elements of weather (temperature, humidity, or precipitation).

The nervous system must gather all incoming information and interpret it to initiate the appropriate motor response, in a process known as sensory–motor integration

---

COORD-INATION →

The patterning of head, body, and limb movements relative to the patterning of environmental objects and events, regardless of the skill level of the performer.

MOTOR SKILL

An activity or task that requires voluntary movement of the head, body, and limbs to achieve a specific goal.

MOTOR BEHAVIOR

Movement response to internal and external environmental stimuli.

(Coker, 2018; Magill & Anderson, 2021). This integration capitalizes on the ability of the CNS to gather and interpret sensory information and perform the proper motor response. Training with good technique and form is vital to this process because sensorimotor integration is only as effective as the quality of the incoming sensory information (Biedert, 2000; Schmidt & Lee, 2014).

For example, consider a basketball player who jumps for a rebound and lands into a knee valgus position. If this movement pattern is not brought to the athlete's attention through coaching and cueing, the athlete will continue to practice poor movement. The reinforcement of knee valgus movement compensation can limit performance outcomes and lead to issues in the back, knees, and hamstrings (Kay et al., 2017; Sahrmann et al., 2017).

The study of motor behavior combines the disciplines of motor control, motor learning, and motor development (**Figure 6.14**). Each concept plays an important role in how athletes and individuals produce, reduce, and dynamically stabilize forces in multiple planes to achieve goals and acquire—and in some instances, lose—skills.

© Eugene Onischenko/Shutterstock

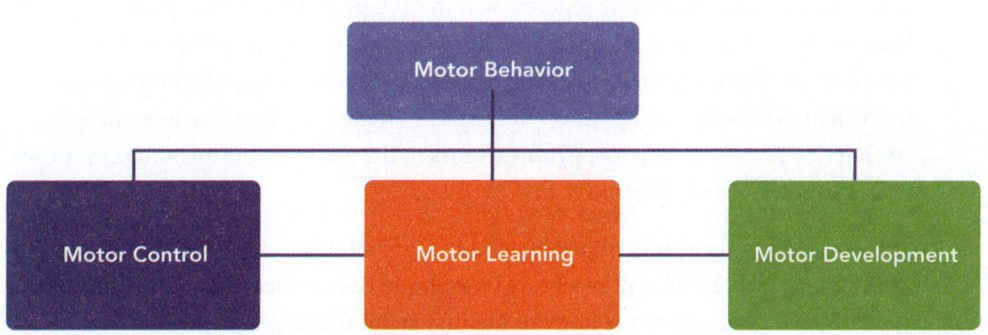

FIGURE 6.14 Motor Behavior Components

MOTOR CONTROL →

How the central nervous system integrates internal and external sensory information with previous experiences to produce a motor response.

THE ROLE OF MOTOR CONTROL IN SKILL ACQUISITION

Motor control is the study of posture and movement and how the CNS assimilates and integrates sensory information with previous experiences to produce a skilled motor response (Fahmy, 2020). For example, a basketball player shooting a free throw must engage the muscles in the correct pattern to produce enough force in the right direction for the ball to go through the hoop. However, if the basketball player adjusts their position, they must then recognize the new distance and recruit the muscles with precise force production in the right direction to make the shot from a new location in space.

This information is received and interpreted, producing a motor response for every shot. The athlete relies on past recruitment patterns and outcomes while also considering the environmental demands to control how the ball leaves their hand and travels through the air at a specific trajectory. Missed shots provide information used to alter the motor recruitment so as to score.

The CNS receives sensory information from the body's position, posture, LTR, touch, and pressure, all while the body moves. These sensory data allow the athlete to understand their head, limb, and trunk orientation and positioning. In addition,

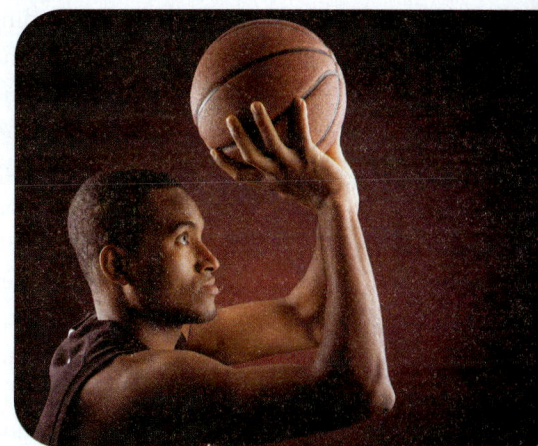

© Cristova/Shutterstock

PERCEPTIONS →

The integration of sensory information with past experiences or memories.

AFFERENT NEURONS →

Sensory neurons that carry signals from sensory stimuli toward the central nervous system.

SENSATIONS →

The ability to detect internal and external physical qualities of the environment. Senses include sight, hearing, touch, taste, and smell.

EFFERENT NEURONS →

Motor neurons that carry signals from the central nervous system toward muscles to create movement.

PROPRIO-CEPTION →

The body's ability to naturally sense its general orientation and relative position of its parts.

sensory input and perceptual inferences allow the athletes to experience the emotional valence (pleasantness or unpleasantness) of what they are touching, such as surface texture (McGlone et al., 2014). **Perceptions** are the integration of sensory information with past experiences or memories (Rose, 1997). The sensory data also allow the player to take in information from the external environment, such as contending with the other team's defenses, crowd noise, speed of play, placement of an object such as a ball, and the surface the athlete is playing on.

An athlete's perception of body positioning and movement, along with their experience of the environment around them, is based on multisensory information (Driver & Spence, 2000). Sensory information is vital in sports for protection, communication, and task execution. The sensory pathways in the body, called **afferent neurons**, allow **sensations** to be received and transferred to the spinal cord for reflexive motor behaviors, to higher cortical areas for processing, or both. **Efferent neurons** are motor neurons that carry the signal from the CNS to the muscles to create movement.

The body uses sensory information in three ways (Rose, 1997):

1. Provide information about the body and its relationship and orientation to the environment before, during, and after movements, such as in a sporting event or training.
2. Assist in planning and executing movement actions, such as how plays will be run and what the individual body segments do in each part of the action plan.
3. Facilitate learning new skills or relearning skills and movement patterns that have become dysfunctional. An example is when Simone Biles pulled out of the individual gymnastics competition in the 2021 Olympic Games due to getting the "twisties," a term referring to a gymnast's loss of the ability to perform flips in the air with twists safely and effectively.

Proprioception is the ability to perceive body segment positions and displacements (Goble & Anguera, 2010). Afferent receptors in multiple tissues such as the skin, muscle, fascia, tendons, and joints allow the body to identify static and dynamic positions, segmental movement and locomotion, and internal tension and force production (Kopeinig et al., 2015). This feedback system is pivotal in maintaining balance and coordination, which enhances injury prevention. Most ACL injuries are noncontact events and can be mitigated by improving balance, lower-extremity biomechanics, muscle activation, functional performance, hip and core strength, power, and decreasing landing impact forces (Padua et al., 2018; Pfeifer et al., 2018). Approximately 70% of noncontact ACL injuries are thought to be preventable with proper biomechanics while moving, landing, decelerating, and changing directions (Myers & Hawkins, 2010).

The nervous system relies on feedback via proprioception, sensations, and perceptions to control various complex ranges of motion throughout the HMS to produce a specific result (Ingram & Wolpert, 2011). For example, swinging a golf club requires the nervous system to simultaneously control multiple joints with various ranges and directions of motion. A novice watching a quality golf swing might think the motion appears simple. However, when a club is put into their hands for the first time, they are likely to hit the turf as often as they connect with the ball. And, when they hit the ball, it likely will not travel in the intended direction. These results occur because the novice has a lack of control over the multiple planes and degrees of motion at the involved joints. This control is developed by refining movement solutions to become more efficient and effective through structuring the environment to reduce the number of potential movement solutions and by engaging in recurrent practice (Ingram & Wolpert, 2011).

An athlete develops efficiency of movement through motor control and learning. The refinement of bodily movement, when presented with a task relative to space and environment, ensures optimal motor behavior and **neuromuscular efficiency**.

THE ROLE OF MOTOR LEARNING IN SKILL ACQUISITION

Skilled motor behavior emerges from interactions between efferent neural pathways that induce muscle contraction and feedback systems that report and refine movement (Azim et al., 2014). The primary purpose of **motor learning** is motor skill acquisition through learning, practice, and experience that leads to relatively permanent change. Motor learning can also include the regaining of skills that are challenging to perform or skills that an athlete could not perform because of injury, aliment, or temporary inability. Proper rehearsal and repetition lead to motor learning; however, an athlete requires feedback to ensure they are optimally learning the skilled movement.

Movement instructions are generated in the CNS and use skeletal muscle to produce an appropriate goal-related change in body position and, if necessary, object manipulation. Feedback is then used to adjust performance as needed to achieve a desired goal. **Feedback** is the utilization of sensory information and sensorimotor integration to aid in the development of permanent neural representations of motor patterns for efficient movement. There are two types of feedback: internal (sensory or task-intrinsic) feedback and external (augmented or task-extrinsic) feedback.

Internal feedback is the sensory feedback that is available while performing a skill. This form of feedback relies on visual, auditory, proprioceptive, and tactile sensory information to monitor action. A **closed-loop control system** allows for task-intrinsic feedback and alterations in movement due to the continuous nature of the movement. Driving a car is a good example of a closed-loop system: The driver uses visual feedback to make minor adjustments to stay in the appropriate lane. In contrast, internal feedback to alter movement is not an option for immediate change in an **open-loop control system**. For example, if a baseball batter swings at a pitch and the ball curves, there is no option for the batter to change the swing to accommodate the curve, even if the batter recognizes that the ball is curving. The same goes for a boxer throwing a punch: If the opponent slips the punch, the direction or trajectory of the jab or cross cannot be changed to follow them. There is no ability to course-correct in an open-loop control system, so the athlete must try again rather than make real-time adjustments.

External feedback is information about the performance of a skill that is external to the person. For example, the Sports Performance Coach can watch the performance of a skill or view external data such as heart rate and biometric monitors and GPS tracking and provide pertinent feedback to the athlete. Additionally, the athlete can watch videos of the performance or even exercise in front of a mirror to get information about movement patterns. This external feedback is added to the internal sensory feedback that the athlete experiences and applied to refine their motor skills.

There are two forms of external feedback: **knowledge of results (KR)** and **knowledge of performance (KP)** (**Table 6.10**). Knowledge of results is external feedback that provides information about an outcome or goal. For example, KR could involve looking at the time after a 100-meter sprint—the clock provides the feedback. Knowledge of performance could be performing an exercise for as many repetitions as possible; in this case the total number of push-ups is the feedback. KP also includes the score of a game, the number of goals made or missed, and all the statistical data showing outcomes that go along with a sport or activity. Such external feedback providing a numerical value related to performance is known as quantitative external feedback.

NEURO-MUSCULAR EFFICIENCY →

The ability of the nervous system to recruit the correct muscles to produce force, reduce force, and dynamically stabilize the body's structure in all three planes of motion.

MOTOR LEARNING →

Integration of motor control processes through learning, practice, and experience, leading to a relatively permanent change in the capacity to produce skilled motor behavior.

FEEDBACK →

The utilization of sensory information and sensorimotor integration to aid in the development of permanent neural representations of motor patterns for efficient movement.

INTERNAL FEEDBACK →

Process whereby sensory information is used by the body to reactively monitor movement and the environment.

CLOSED-LOOP → CONTROL SYSTEM

Task-intrinsic feedback and alterations in movement due to the continuous nature of the movement.

OPEN-LOOP → CONTROL SYSTEM

A control system that does not allow for feedback to alter movement and does not create either immediate change or real-time adjustments.

EXTERNAL → FEEDBACK

Information provided by some external source, such as a coach, video, mirror, or heart rate monitor, to supplement the internal environment.

KNOWLEDGE → OF RESULTS (KR)

Information used after the completion of a movement to inform individuals about the outcome of their performance.

TABLE 6.10 External Feedback

Role	Knowledge of Results (KR)	Knowledge of Performance (KP)
Physical therapist	"You were able to stand up from a seated position without help."	"Grasp the railing overhand rather than underhand to provide greater assistance in your sit-to-stand position."
American football coach	"You couldn't get separation from the defender so the quarterback couldn't get you the ball."	"Come to a quicker stop and fake right before accelerating left to get open."
Youth soccer coach	"Notice how the ball is not going where you want it to go?"	"Strike the ball with the inside of the foot as close to the heel as possible. Be sure to point the toes of your planted foot toward your target."

Knowledge of performance is a form of external feedback that provides information about the movement characteristics and quality that led to the outcome. For example, some athletes review films of performances with coaches so they can get feedback from the coach and watch the video to visually see their performance. As another example, the Sports Performance Coach might have an athlete squat to chair depth while performing the overhead squat assessment. The KR is that the athlete successfully squatted to chair depth; the KP, which looks at the movement quality and characteristics, shows that their feet turned out, knees knocked together, and arms fell forward.

Knowledge of performance can be either descriptive or prescriptive, with each having its own advantages. Descriptive KP is a verbal explanation of an error made during a skill performance. Prescriptive KP is a verbal explanation of an error made during a skill performance and what needs to be done to correct it. For example, a coach might use descriptive KP to inform the athlete of an error and encourage them to determine for themselves what needs to be done for correction. By comparison, prescriptive KP is used to inform an athlete of a situation and how to adjust. For example, between boxing rounds, the ringside coach could bring attention to the boxer's head movement by pointing out that it is difficult to hit a moving target. This kind of information fills the gap created by the lack of internal feedback in open-loop control systems.

Not every repetition will be perfect, and not every sub-par repetition should be addressed. For the skills coach, this is called the performance bandwidth. **Performance bandwidth** occurs when external feedback is not provided because the performance falls within an acceptable range of error for the skill. For example, when a basketball player does not get quite the arc or wrist follow-through in a shot, but it falls within an acceptable range of error, the coach does not always mention it. Further, if external feedback is given too frequently during practice or skill performance, it inhibits learning. Thus, the Sports Performance Coach must always be aware of providing too much criticism and consider verbal feedback as a motivator and not solely a means of pointing out errors and fixes.

Gentile's taxonomy of skill acquisition accounts for the body's position within environmental contexts (Gentile, 2000). It can be used as a framework for developing a systematic progression for skill acquisition. The taxonomy includes two dimensions: the environmental context of the skill and the function of the skill. The environmental context can be further divided into stationary or in-motion conditions, and with or without variability between attempts. Stationary or in-motion conditions refer to changes in the surrounding environment. For example, a basketball player may begin working on drills around cones (stationary condition) before progressing to drills around opponents that move (in-motion condition).

Within stationary and in-motion conditions, the degree of variability between attempts must also be considered. Such variability might include changes in the location of a target, changes in the speed of a moving target, and even fatigue and attentional focus that might fluctuate between attempts. In one example, a bowler will not experience changes in the location or speed of the target. However, they may experience fatigue and distractions as each set progresses.

The function component of skill acquisition suggests that beginner athletes start in a stationary position and then progress to movement. For example, when a basketball player begins learning to dribble, they should do so in a static or stable position first (i.e., standing still), then progress to dribbling while walking and then running. Function can be further divided to address manipulating an object. For example, the basketball player may stand still and imagine or go through the motions of dribbling without a ball; then, the ball can be added as the first progression. This same progression can be used when the athlete adds walking and running—first without a ball and then with a ball.

The Sports Performance Coach can use the template provided in **Table 6.11** to design progressions to optimize skill acquisition.

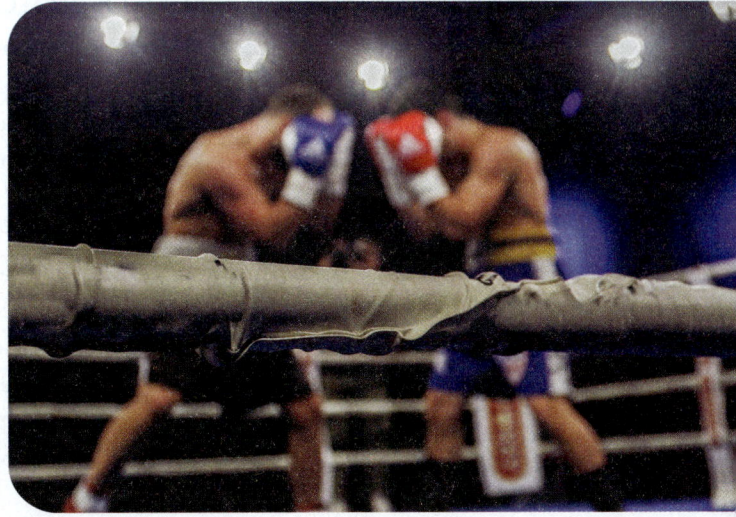
© LorenzoPeg/Shutterstock

KNOWLEDGE OF PERFORMANCE (KP) →

Information about the quality of movement during an action, skill, or performance.

PERFORMANCE BANDWIDTH →

When external feedback like cueing is not provided because the performance falls within an acceptable range of error for the skill.

GENTILE'S TAXONOMY →

A classification of skill progression based on the environment and bodily movement.

TABLE 6.11 Gentile's Taxonomy: Building a Systematic Progression for Skill Acquisition

Environmental Context		Function			
		Body Stability		Body Transport	
		No Object	Object	No Object	Object
Stationary conditions	No variability	1A	1B	1C	1D
	Variability	2A	2B	2C	2D
In-motion conditions	No variability	3A	3B	3C	3D
	Variability	4A	4B	4C	4D

Data from Magill, R. A., Anderson, D. I. (2013). *Motor Learning and Control: Concepts and Applications.* Singapore: McGraw-Hill.

THE ROLE OF MOTOR DEVELOPMENT IN SKILL ACQUISITION

Motor development is the accumulation of motor learning over a lifetime, from infancy through old age. It is often noted in early childhood when pediatricians check children's fine and gross motor development. Fine motor skills include reflexive grasping, a child putting objects in their mouth, and building or stacking. Gross motor development is represented by the child lifting their head, rolling from their back to stomach, standing, and walking. Motor development progresses through life and can include a decline in motor function, mobility, and slowness performing a physical task (Clark et al., 2019). Research shows motor performance increases from childhood (ages 7–9) to young adulthood (ages 19–25) and decreases from young adulthood (ages 19–25) to old age (ages 66–80), with the old age group performing similarly to the childhood group (Leversen et al., 2012). Understanding motor development over the lifespan helps professionals facilitate abilities and performance in people in need of interventions (Leversen et al., 2012).

LESSON 5: UNDERSTANDING CONSTRAINTS IN ATHLETIC PERFORMANCE AND DEVELOPMENT
NEWELL'S MODEL OF CONSTRAINTS

Athletes are limited by multiple constraints when it comes to sports. A constraint is something that eliminates certain possibilities for action. The elimination of options helps determine the behavior and outcome of a situation. The constraints that affect athletes can be classified into three major categories: individual, environmental, and task. Collectively, these categories are known as **Newell's model of constraints** (Newell, 1986, 1991). This model has been used in human movement science and athletic fields throughout the years, including in skill acquisition (Renshaw et al., 2010), motor development (Haywood & Getchell, 2014), motor performance (Glazier & Robins, 2013), medicine (McKeon & Hertel, 2006), physical therapy and rehabilitation (Newell & Valvano, 1998), physical conditioning (Jeffreys, 2011), sports biomechanics (Glazier & Davids, 2009), creative behavior (Stokes, 2008), and sports injuries (Balagué et al., 2019; Pol et al., 2019). The various constraints imposed by the environment, tasks (rules of the game), and the individual limit the options available for an outcome (**Figure 6.15**).

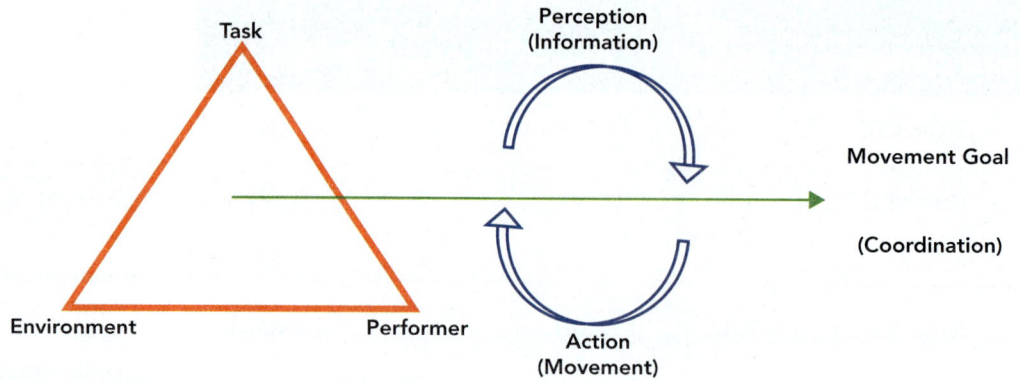

FIGURE 6.15 Newell's Model of Constraints

INDIVIDUAL CONSTRAINTS

Individual constraints limit the athlete based on their physical abilities, such as height, weight (mass), speed, strength, power, and motivation. Constraints related to body structure, such as size and shape, are also known as structural constraints (Haywood & Ge, 2009). Individual constraints are specific to a particular athlete and are generally stable over time. They can affect someone's ability to excel in a specific sport. For example, a shorter basketball player must use a higher arc when releasing the ball to minimize the risk of a taller player blocking the shot. Further, these same players will be constrained to use different angles when passing the ball. Therefore, task constraints are altered based on individual constraints. For example, individual constraints explain why there are weight classes in fight sports.

Some abilities can change over time, such as power, which can compensate for certain structural constraints, such as height, and allow the athlete to better contend with the constraints of a particular sport. Many parasports coaches use a constraint-led approach to work with disability-related nuances and skill development (Dehghansai et al., 2020). Additional individual constraints may include values, fears, motivation, goals, attention, mood, and personality (Balagué et al., 2019). Constraints that deal directly with an athlete's behavior are called functional constraints (Haywood & Getchell, 2009). Coaches and trainers have a significant role to play in reducing the individual constraints of their athletes with both physical and mental directives and support. Having a deeper understanding of individual constraints allows a Sports Performance Coach to provide more descriptive and prescriptive feedback to athletes.

ENVIRONMENTAL CONSTRAINTS

Environmental constraints are the limitations imposed by an individual's surroundings, including natural, sociocultural, and interpersonal factors. These constraints are outside the coach's or athlete's control and can significantly affect performance. In many sports, players are subject to natural constraints such as precipitation, temperature, time of day, elevation, and humidity. While many athletes train in a climate-controlled indoor facility, allowing for increased practice consistency and comfort, they might have difficulty adjusting to temperature and wind changes during outdoor competitions. Therefore, environmental constraints can affect task constraints. Additionally, athletes frequently travel for long distances, which can result in jetlag or travel fatigue. Performing at home is often considered a better environment than playing in an away game because the traveling team must adapt to a new facility and sleep in a hotel room.

The social and psychological aspects of environmental constraints can be referred to as interpersonal constraints. These include relationships with teammates, coaches, family, administrators, opponents, and anyone who has a direct or indirect influence on the athlete. Interpersonal constraints can have either positive or negative effects on performance. For example, a supportive coach or teammate can provide encouragement and motivation, whereas a distracting or hostile opponent can disrupt focus and performance. Similarly, the presence of spectators can create a positive or negative emotional environment that can impact an athlete's performance. For example, a traveling team will likely have to contend with far fewer supporters than the home team.

Regardless of the environment, athletes must be able to demonstrate peak performance. To assist them in achieving this goal, coaches might have athletes review video of an upcoming opponent not only to learn more about their plays and setup, but also to point out potential strengths and weaknesses of the opposing team, and to see the specific environment. This information can then be integrated into training by practicing

---

INDIVIDUAL CONSTRAINTS →

The unique characteristics of an athlete that influence their movement behavior and performance.

ENVIRON-MENTAL CONSTRAINTS →

The external factors in the surrounding environment that can influence an athlete's movement behavior and performance.

in different climates, at different times of day, with or without spectators, or changing playing surfaces if needed (e.g., grass versus turf). However, regardless of the environment, the task is still the same. Therefore, the Sports Performance Coach must enhance factors related to the athlete's individual constraints, such as technical skills, speed, and power, to help offset certain environmental constraints.

TASK CONSTRAINTS

Task constraints are the goals and purpose, rules and regulations, boundaries, space, equipment, and instruction of play that limit participants to specific requirements of the game. They can have a significant impact on movement behavior and performance. For example, the task constraints of basketball (such as the size of the court, the number of players, and the rules) influence the types of movements that are required (such as running, dribbling, and passing) and the strategies that are used to achieve the goal of scoring. Similarly, in weightlifting, the task constraints of the equipment being used (such as the weights and barbell) influence the types of movements that are required (such as lifting, pressing, and pulling) and the strategies that are used to achieve the goal of lifting as much weight as possible.

The task constraints also create the demands that the individual must contend with to be competitive. The individual's skills are honed, and certain physical characteristics may be desired, to meet the task constraints of their sport. For example, being a large, strong male fits the characteristic physical requirements of being an American football lineman. The athlete can learn skills and build greater strength to meet the task of protecting (offense) or pursuing (defense) the quarterback. The task does not change unless the rules change, and the athletes must limit their decisions to align with the task requirement. Different players on the same team will have different constraints based on their position, so each positional role has varying constraints.

CONSTRAINTS-LED APPROACH WITH ATTENTIONAL CUEING

Coaches work directly with players to facilitate progress toward achieving a particular goal in competition or practice environments (Otte et al., 2020). This is done through explicit instruction, with the coach directing the player's attention to focus on a specific attribute of play. However, a **constraints-led approach (CLA)** recognizes that each player has intrinsic abilities to self-regulate and learn to control movement behaviors while performing technical and cognitive skills in a sport.

CLA focuses on creating a learning environment that is tailored to the individual athlete and the specific demands of the task, with the goal of facilitating the emergence of efficient and effective movement patterns (Renshaw et al., 2015). This includes simplifying tasks so that technical skills are easier to acquire and refine through the manipulation of specific and key task constraints such as rules, space, time, and equipment (Renshaw et al., 2015).

Adopting a CLA means the Sports Performance Coach might not need to be as descriptive and prescriptive with their

---

> ### TASK CONSTRAINTS →
>
> The specific requirements, rules, and goals of a sport or task that influence an athlete's movement behavior and performance.

> ### CONSTRAINTS- → LED APPROACH (CLA)
>
> A technique for understanding motor skill acquisition and performance that emphasizes the interaction between the individual, the task, and the environment.

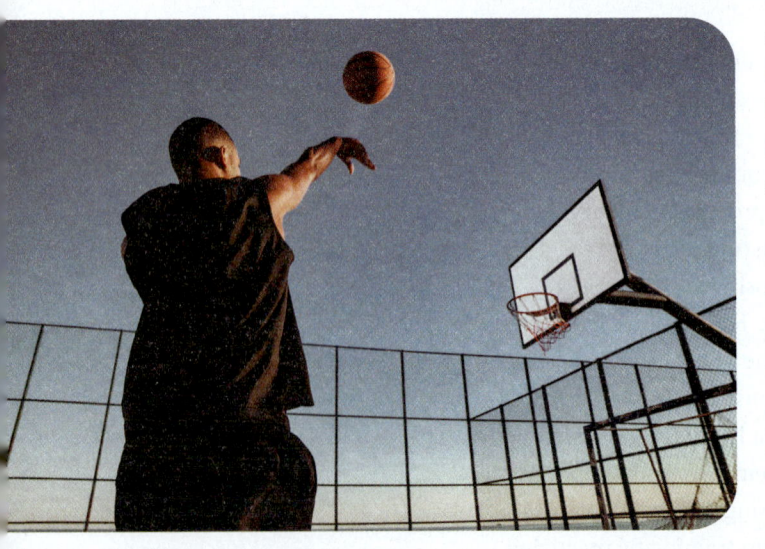

© Dean Drobot/Shutterstock

extrinsic feedback. Instead, they can provide task, environmental, or individual constraints that enable the athlete to explore the task requirements with a nonlinear, individualized, and self-directed approach. For example, rather than providing explicit feedback to a basketball player to catch the ball and shoot more quickly with a higher arc upon release, the coach might use a CLA by stationing a defender near the shooter and instructing them to try to block the shot. The shooter must now catch the ball and release it quickly with a higher shooting arc to avoid the defender's block. Although the shooter might have the first shots blocked, they will likely adapt to the speed and constraints of the task and make intrinsic adjustments to avoid the defender's block. The result is a quicker release of the ball with a higher arc trajectory.

CLA allows task-specific feedback to establish error-correcting capabilities. By manipulating the constraints, coaches and trainers can promote the development of efficient and effective movement patterns and behaviors that are well suited to the demands of the specific sport or activity.

ATTENTIONAL CUEING

Attentional focus is the conscious effort of an individual to focus their attention through explicit thoughts so as to execute a motor skill with superior performance (Benz et al., 2016). **Attentional cueing**, by comparison, is the job of the coach, trainer, and Sports Performance Coach, who directs the attention of the athlete to external or internal foci to produce improved KP or KR. The main goal of verbal feedback and instructions is "to help educate the attention of a learner to perceive and utilize relevant information sources" within skill (acquisition and refinement) training environments (Correia et al., 2019, p. 126).

When providing attentional cueing, the coach will direct the athlete toward either an internal or external focus. With an **internal focus**, the athlete focuses on specific body movements or sensations while performing a skill, such as the movement of the arms during a tennis serve or the contraction of specific muscles during a deadlift. Internal cueing during the deadlift might include "Squeeze the glutes" and "Keep the back straight." Winkelman (2018) has described these as acceptable forms of external augmented feedback for learning techniques in the skill acquisition process. **External focus** refers to directing attention toward external factors in the environment, such as the ball's movement or the position of the goal post. In this case, the athlete focuses on the intention of the movement outcome. External cueing during a deadlift might include statements such as "Drive the floor away" and "Explode upward." Numerous studies have provided converging evidence that an external focus of attention speeds up the learning process so that a higher skill level, characterized by increased effectiveness and efficiency, is achieved sooner (Wulf, 2013; Wulf et al., 2007). An external focus of attention has benefits for the speed of movement execution, and an attentional focus influences movement preparation (Ille et al., 2013).

Table 6.12 summarizes the findings of several studies on attentional cueing, highlighting the differences between internal and external cues and their performance outcomes.

One form of attentional focus, called the quiet eye (QE), addresses the role of visual focus during aiming tasks (Vickers, 1996). Athletes performing aiming tasks are directed to quietly fixate on the target before they initiate action. According to Yoshikawa et al. (2020), QE duration is longer for experts than for novice athletes in various sports and becomes shorter even for experts who choke under pressure during games, resulting in

---

ATTENTIONAL FOCUS →

The conscious effort of an individual to focus their attention through explicit thoughts so as to execute a motor skill with superior performance.

ATTENTIONAL CUEING →

The effort of the coach, trainer, and Sports Performance Coach to direct the attention of the athlete to either an external focus or internal focus to produce improved knowledge of performance or knowledge of results.

INTERNAL FOCUS →

When an athlete focuses on specific body movements or sensations while performing a skill.

EXTERNAL FOCUS →

When an athlete directs attention toward external factors in the environment, focusing on the intention of the movement outcome.

TABLE 6.12 Attentional Cueing

Activity	Internal Cues	External Cues	Outcome	Study
Sprinting	"Push quickly on your legs and keep going as fast as possible while swinging both arms back and forth and raising your knees rapidly."	"Get off the starting blocks as quickly as possible, head toward the finish line rapidly, and cross it as soon as possible."	Reaction and running time were significantly shorter in the external focus condition than in the internal focus condition for both expert and novice participants.	Ille et al., 2013
Sprinting	"Run with maximum effort. Focus on gradually raising your body level and powerfully driving one leg forward and the other leg down and back as quickly as possible."	"Run with maximum effort. Focus on gradually raising up and powerfully driving forward while clawing the floor as quickly as possible."	Trials completed in the external focus condition were significantly faster than trials completed in the internal and control conditions.	Porter et al., 2015
Reducing landing stiffness	"Focus on bending your knees when you land."	"Focus on landing softly."	Instructions promoting an external focus resulted in a reduction in landing stiffness.	Almonroeder et al., 2020

performance deterioration. QE is associated with superior motor control performance in basketball three-point shots (Vickers et al., 2019), basketball free throws (Vickers, 1996), golf driving (Causer et al., 2017), golf putting (Vine et al., 2011), archery (Gonzalez et al., 2017), penalty kicks in soccer (Timmis et al., 2018), and darts (Querfurth et al., 2016). A coach can attentionally cue the athlete, eliciting a QE attentional focus by their athlete when participating in aiming sports.

GETTING TECHNICAL

In a comprehensive review of the published literature on external versus internal feedback, Wulf (2013) identified multiple examples of greater movement effectiveness (e.g., accuracy, consistency, balance), efficiency (e.g., muscular activity, force production, cardiovascular responses), learning advantages, and performance outcomes from external focus. These activities involved multiple skill levels, age groups, and tasks. Tasks comprised balancing on disks, throwing darts, volleyball serve, football and soccer kicks, gymnastics routines, jumping, weightlifting, sprinting, swimming, and more. In 70 of the 78 studies (90%), external feedback led to better outcomes compared to internal feedback. The other eight studies showed no difference between the external and internal feedback groups. None of the studies showed superior benefits from internal feedback for performance tasks.

CONSTRAINTS-LED APPROACH VERSUS CUEING

CLA and cueing are two different approaches to motor learning and performance. CLA has been shown to be more effective than attentional cueing alone for promoting the transfer of learning to new tasks (Gray, 2018). In this study, two groups engaged in a virtual baseball batting task to improve their launch angle over the course of 6 weeks in either a constrained or cued condition. The key difference between the two groups was in the type of feedback they received during training. The CLA group received feedback that was focused on the task constraints (e.g., a barrier was introduced that adjusted based on real-time performance) and encouraged them to adapt their performance to meet these constraints. The attentional cueing group received feedback that was focused on specific technical aspects of batting technique (e.g., position of their feet, how they hold the bat, etc.). Although all groups showed significant improvements in batting performance from pre- to post-training, the CLA group showed the most significant improvement. Further, the researchers concluded that CLA encourages athletes to explore different ways of visualizing the movements, thus resulting in better technique (Gray, 2018).

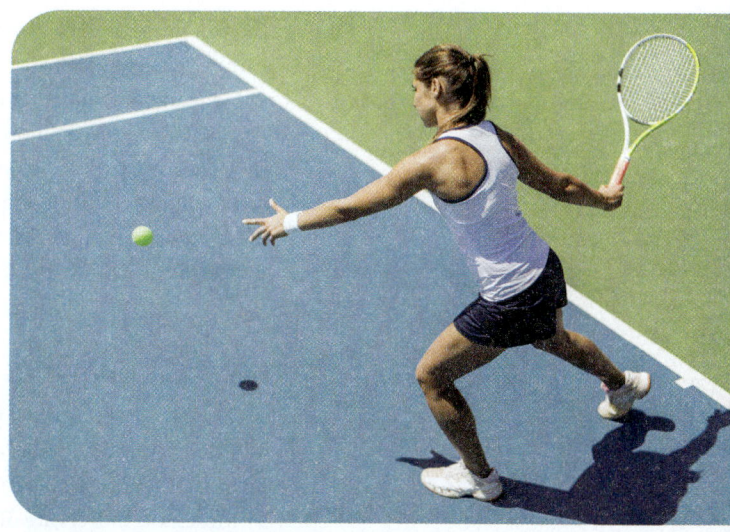

© BGStock72/Shutterstock

COMBINING THE CONSTRAINTS-LED APPROACH AND CUEING

The goal of CLA is to help the athlete to build technical skills by performing the task with constraints that simplify the process by either taking away from or adding to the activity. Cueing can be an effective method for enhancing performance by directing attentional focus toward specific aspects of movement. Verbal cues can be used to direct attention toward the position of the ball or opponents, while visual cues can be used to reinforce correct movement patterns and techniques.

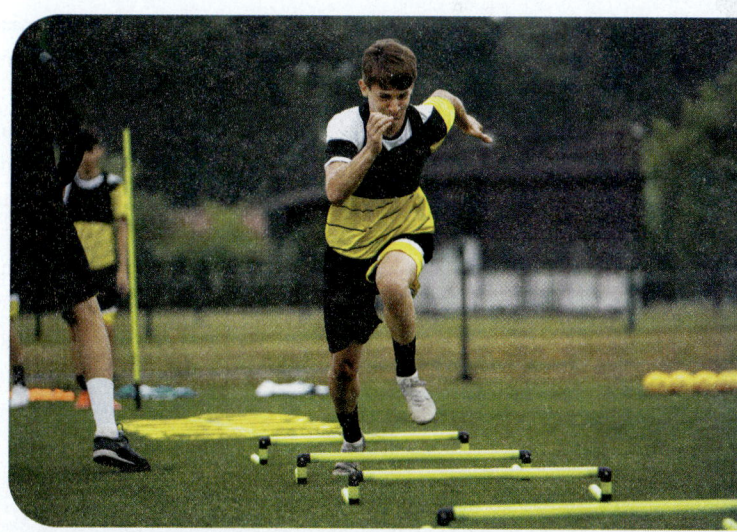

© Matimix/Shutterstock

For example, during the short break between rounds in a boxing or mixed martial arts (MMA) bout, the prescriptive feedback of a coach reminding the athlete to keep their hands up and their chin down offers vital verbal and visual cues (if the coach demonstrates the desired positions). In practice, the combination of attentional focus, feedback, and CLA might be the most valuable to help athletes learn the many complexities of motor behavior.

SUMMARY

Optimal human movement is at the center of the Sports Performance Coach's skillset. When the Sports Performance Coach understands how athletes can maximize performance outcomes and minimize biomechanical dysfunction through skilled movement, the athletes are the true beneficiaries. Using the language of human movement science allows the Sports Performance Coach to be clear and specific about the quality of movement and to identify where issues might exist.

The way the Sports Performance Coach works with athletes is also vital when it comes to motor learning, such as employing Gentile's taxonomy, which provides the Sports Performance Coach with quadrants to add to or take away to progress or regress training. Skill training is also supplemented through movement training by choosing exercises that train the subsystems of the global core to develop and reinforce core support for athletic performance. As the Sports Performance Coach advances in language, motor learning, skill development, exercise selection, and exercise programming, the athletes cultivate their abilities to excel at given roles within sport and performance.

KEY TAKEAWAYS

- There are three cardinal planes of motion: sagittal, frontal, and transverse.
- Each plane of motion is associated with both axes of rotation and joint actions.
- Muscle actions are eccentric, isometric, and concentric.
- Muscles as movers are divided into agonists, antagonists, synergists, and stabilizers to help control and direct human movement.
- Global muscular subsystems help control movement and support the core during dynamic activities. These subsystems include the deep longitudinal subsystem, anterior oblique subsystem, posterior oblique subsystem, and lateral subsystem.
- Leverage systems allow for human movement to occur through three different first-, second-, and third-class levers.
- Motor control, motor learning, and motor development are components of motor behavior. Newell's model of constraints and Gentile's taxonomy allow the Sports Performance Coach to understand motor learning and better coach progress, coordination, and control degrees of freedom.
- A constraints-led approach allows athletes to explore their innate abilities to investigate movement within the realm of the task, environment, and individual constraints.
- Attentional cueing is augmented feedback by the Sports Performance Coach that draws the athlete's attention to components of training or performance to increase knowledge of performance and knowledge of results.

REFERENCES

Adolph, K. E., & Franchak, J. M. (2017). The development of motor behavior. Wiley interdisciplinary reviews. *Cognitive science, 8*(1–2), 10.1002/wcs.1430. https://doi.org/10.1002/wcs.1430

Afyon, Y., Mulazimoglu, O., & Boyacı, A. (2017). The effects of core trainings on speed and agility skills of soccer players. *International Journal of Sports Science, 7*, 239–244. http://article.sapub.org/10.5923.j.sports .20170706.06.html

Almonroeder, T. G., Jayawickrema, J., Richardson, C. T., & Mercker, K. L. (2020). The influence of attentional focus on landing stiffness in female athletes: A cross-sectional study. *International Journal of Sports Physical Therapy, 15*(4), 510–518. https://doi.org/10.26603/ijspt20200510

Azim, E., Fink, A. J., & Jessell, T. M. (2014). Internal and external feedback circuits for skilled forelimb movement. *Cold Spring Harbor Symposia on Quantitative Biology, 79*, 81–92. https://doi.org/10.1101 /sqb.2014.79.024786

Balagué, N., Pol, R., Torrents, C., Ric, A., & Hristovski, R. (2019). On the relatedness and nestedness of constraints. *Sports Medicine, 5*(1), 6. https://doi.org/10.1186/s40798-019-0178-z

Benz, A., Winkelman, N., Porter, J., & Nimphius, S. (2016). Coaching instructions and cues for enhancing sprint performance. *Strength & Conditioning Journal, 38*(1), 1–11. https://doi.org/https://doi.org/10.1519 /ssc.0000000000000185

Bergmark, A. (1989). Stability of the lumbar spine: A study in mechanical engineering. *Acta Orthopaedica Scandinavica Supplementum, 230*, 1–54. https://doi.org/10.3109/17453678909154177

Biedert, R. M. (2000). Contribution of the three levels of nervous system motor control: Spinal cord, lower brain, cerebral cortex. In S. M. Lephart & F. H. Fu (Eds.). *Proprioception and neuromuscular control in joint stability* (pp. 23–29). Human Kinetics.

Butowicz, C. M., Ebaugh, D. D., Noehren, B., & Silfies, S. P. (2016). Validation of two clinical measures of core stability. *International Journal of Sports Physical Therapy, 11*(1), 15–23.

Causer, J., Hayes, S. J., Hooper, J. M., & Bennett, S. J. (2017). Quiet eye facilitates sensorimotor preprograming and online control of precision aiming in golf putting. *Cognitive Processing, 18*(1), 47–54. https://doi .org/10.1007/s10339-016-0783-4

Clark, B. C., Woods, A. J., Clark, L. A., Criss, C. R., Shadmehr, R., & Grooms, D. R. (2019). The aging brain and the dorsal basal ganglia: Implications for age-related limitations of mobility. *Advances in Geriatric Medicine and Research, 1*, e190008. https://doi.org/10.20900/agmr20190008

Clark, D. R., Lambert, M. I., & Hunter, A. M. (2018). Contemporary perspectives of core stability training for dynamic athletic performance: A survey of athletes, coaches, sports science and sports medicine practitioners. *Sports Medicine, 4*(1), 32. https://doi.org/10.1186/s40798-018-0150-3

Coker, C. A. (2018). *Motor learning and control for practitioners* (4th ed.). Routledge.

Correia, V., Carvalho, J., Araújo, D., Pereira, E., & Davids, K. (2019). Principles of nonlinear pedagogy in sport practice. *Physical Education & Sport Pedagogy, 24*, 117–132. https://doi.org/10.1080/17408989.2018.1552673

Dehghansai, N., Lemez, S., Wattie, N., Pinder, R. A., & Baker, J. (2020). Understanding the development of elite parasport athletes using a constraint-led approach: Considerations for coaches and practitioners. *Frontiers in Psychology, 11*, 502981. https://doi.org/10.3389/fpsyg.2020.502981

di Cagno, A., Iuliano, E., Buonsenso, A., Giombini, A., Di Martino, G., Parisi, A., Calcagno, G., & Fiorilli, G. (2020). Effects of accentuated eccentric training versus plyometric training on performance of young elite fencers. *Journal of Sports Science & Medicine, 19*(4), 703–713.

Doğanay, M., Bingül, B. M., & Álvarez-García, C. (2020). Effect of core training on speed, quickness and agility in young male football players. *Journal of Sports Medicine and Physical Fitness, 60*(9). https://doi.org/10.23736 /S0022-4707.20.10999-X

Driver, J., & Spence, C. (2000). Multisensory perception: Beyond modularity and convergence. *Current Biology, 10*, R731–R735.

Fahmy, R. (Ed.). (2020). *NASM essentials of corrective exercise training* (2nd ed.). Jones & Bartlett Learning.

Fiorilli, G., Mariano, I., Iuliano, E., Giombini, A., Ciccarelli, A., Buonsenso, A., Calcagno, G., & di Cagno, A. (2020). Isoinertial eccentric-overload training in young soccer players: Effects on strength, sprint, change of direction, agility and soccer shooting precision. *Journal of Sports Science & Medicine, 19*(1), 213–223.

Gentile, A. M. (2000). Skill acquisition: Action, movement, and neuromotor processes. In J. H. Carr & R. B. Shepard (Eds.). *Movement science: Foundations for physical therapy* (2nd ed., pp. 111–187). Aspen.

Glazier, P. S., & Davids, K. (2009). Constraints on the complete optimization of human motion. *Sports Medicine, 39*(1), 15–28. https://doi.org/10.2165/00007256-200939010-00002

Glazier, P. S., & Robins, M. T. (2013). Self-organisation and constraints in sports performance. In T. McGarry, P. O'Donoghue, & J. Sampaio (Eds.), *Routledge handbook of sports performance analysis* (pp. 42–51). Routledge.

Goble, D. J., & Anguera, J. A. (2010). Plastic changes in hand proprioception following force-field motor learning. *Journal of Neurophysiology, 104*(3), 1213–1215. https://doi.org/10.1152/jn.00543.2010

Gonzalez, C. C., Causer, J., Grey, M. J., Humphreys, G. W., Miall, R. C., & Williams, A. M. (2017). Exploring the quiet eye in archery using field- and laboratory-based tasks. *Experimental Brain Research, 235*(9), 2843–2855. https://doi.org/10.1007/s00221-017-4988-2

Gray, R. (2018). Comparing cueing and constraints interventions for increasing launch angle in baseball batting. *Sport, Exercise, and Performance Psychology, 7*(3), 318–332. https://doi.org/10.1037/spy0000131

Greene, F. S., Perryman, E., Cleary, C. J., & Cook, S. B. (2019). Core stability and athletic performance in male and female lacrosse players. *International Journal of Exercise Science, 12*(4), 1138–1148.

Ha, S. M., & Jeon, I. C. (2021). Comparison of the electromyographic recruitment of the posterior oblique sling muscles during prone hip extension among three different shoulder positions. *Physiotherapy Theory and Practice, 37*(9), 1043–1050. https://doi.org/10.1080/09593985.2019.1675206

Haywood, K., & Getchell, N. (2014). *Life span motor development.* Human Kinetics.

Heidari, P., Farahbakhsh, F., Rostami, M., Noormohammadpour, P., & Kordi, R. (2015). The role of ultrasound in diagnosis of the causes of low back pain: A review of the literature. *Asian Journal of Sports Medicine, 6*(1), e23803. https://doi.org/10.5812/asjsm.23803

Ille, A., Selin, I., Do, M. C., & Thon, B. (2013). Attentional focus effects on sprint start performance as a function of skill level. *Journal of Sports Sciences, 31*(15), 1705–1712. https://doi.org/10.1080/02640414.2013.797097

Ingram, J. N., & Wolpert, D. M. (2011). Naturalistic approaches to sensorimotor control. In *Progress in Brain Research* (Vol. 191, pp. 3–29). Elsevier. https://doi.org/10.1016/B978-0-444-53752-2.00016-3

Jeffreys, I. (2011). A task-based approach to developing context-specific agility. *Strength and Conditioning Journal, 33*, 52–59. https://doi.org/10.1519/SSC.0b013e318222932a

Kay, M. C., Register-Mihalik, J. K., Gray, A. D., Djoko, A., Dompier, T. P., & Kerr, Z. Y. (2017). The epidemiology of severe injuries sustained by National Collegiate Athletic Association student-athletes, 2009–2010 through 2014–2015. *Journal of Athletic Training, 52*(2), 117–128. https://doi.org/10.4085/1062-6050-52.1.01

Key, J. (2013). The core: Understanding it, and retraining its dysfunction. *Journal of Bodywork and Movement Therapies, 17*(4), 541–559. https://doi.org/10.1016/j.jbmt.2013.03.012

Kim, T. Y., Yoo, W. G., An, D. H., Oh, J. S., & Shin, S. J. (2013). The effects of different gait speeds and lower arm weight on the activities of the latissimus dorsi, gluteus medius, and gluteus maximus muscles. *Journal of Physical Therapy Science, 25*(11), 1483–1484. https://doi.org/10.1589/jpts.25.1483

Kopeinig, C., Gödl-Purrer, B., & Salchinger, B. (2015). Fascia as a proprioceptive organ and its role in chronic pain: A review of current literature. *Safety in Health, 1*, A2. https://doi.org/10.1186/2056-5917-1-S1-A2

Lee, J. K., Hwang, J. H., Kim, C. M., Lee, J. K., & Park, J. W. (2019). Influence of muscle activation of posterior oblique sling from changes in activation of gluteus maximus from exercise of prone hip extension of normal adult male and female. *Journal of Physical Therapy Science, 31*(2), 166–169. https://doi.org/10.1589/jpts.31.166

Lee, J. K., Lee, J. H., Kim, K. S., & Lee, J. H. (2020). Effect of abdominal drawing-in maneuver with prone hip extension on muscle activation of posterior oblique sling in normal adults. *Journal of Physical Therapy Science, 32*(6), 401–404. https://doi.org/10.1589/jpts.32.401

Lepley, L. K., Lepley, A. S., Onate, J. A., & Grooms, D. R. (2017). Eccentric exercise to enhance neuromuscular control. *Sports Health, 9*(4), 333–340. https://doi.org/10.1177/1941738117710913

Levangie, P. K., & Norkin, C. C. (2011). *Joint structure and function: A comprehensive analysis* (5th ed.). F. A. Davis.

Leversen, J. S., Haga, M., & Sigmundsson, H. (2012). From children to adults: Motor performance across the life-span. *PLoS One, 7*(6), e38830. https://doi.org/10.1371/journal.pone.0038830

Magill, R. A., & Anderson, D. (2021). *Motor learning and control: Concepts and applications* (12th ed.). McGraw-Hill.

McGill, R. A. (2011). *Motor learning and control: Concepts and applications* (9th ed.). McGraw-Hill.

McGlone, F., Wessberg, J., & Olausson, H. (2014). Discriminative and affective touch: Sensing and feeling. *Neuron, 82*(4), 737–755. https://doi.org/10.1016/j.neuron.2014.05.001

McKeon, P. O., & Hertel, J. (2006). The dynamical-systems approach to studying athletic injury. *Athletic Therapy Today, 11*, 31–33. https://doi.org/10.1123/att.11.1.31

Mohamed, R. R., Abdel-Aziem, A. A., Mohammed, H. Y., & Diab, R. H. (2021). Chronic low back pain changes the latissimus dorsi and gluteus maximus muscles activation pattern and upward scapular rotation: A cross-sectional study. *Journal of Back and Musculoskeletal Rehabilitation*, 10.3233/BMR-200253. https://doi.org/10.3233/BMR-200253

Myers, C. A., & Hawkins, D. (2010). Alterations to movement mechanics can greatly reduce anterior cruciate ligament loading without reducing performance. *Journal of Biomechanics, 43*(14), 2657–2664. https://doi.org/10.1016/j.jbiomech.2010.06.003

Nakai, Y., Kawada, M., Miyazaki, T., Araki, S., Takeshita, Y., & Kiyama, R. (2021). A self-oblique exercise that activates the coordinated activity of abdominal and hip muscles: A pilot study. *PLoS One, 16*(8). https://doi.org/10.1371/journal.pone.0255035

Newell, K. (1986). Constraints on the development of coordination. In M. W. Wade & H. T. A. Whiting (Eds.), *Motor development in children: Aspects of coordination and control* (pp. 341–361). Martinus Nijhoff Publishers.

Newell, K. M. (1991). Motor skill acquisition. *Annual Review of Psychology, 42*, 213–217. https://doi.org/10.1146/annurev.ps.42.020191.001241

Newell, K. M., & Valvano, J. (1998). Movement science: Therapeutic intervention as a constraint in learning and relearning movement skills. *Scandinavian Journal of Occupational Therapy, 5*(2), 51–57. https://doi.org/10.3109/11038129809035730

Otte, F. W., Davids, K., Millar, S. K., & Klatt, S. (2020). When and how to provide feedback and instructions to athletes? How sport psychology and pedagogy insights can improve coaching interventions to enhance self-regulation in training. *Frontiers in Psychology, 11*, 1444. https://doi.org/10.3389/fpsyg.2020.01444

Padua, D. A., DiStefano, L. J., Hewett, T. E., Garrett, W. E., Marshall, S. W., Golden, G. M., Shultz, S. J., & Sigward, S. M. (2018). National Athletic Trainers' Association position statement: Prevention of anterior cruciate ligament injury. *Journal of Athletic Training, 53*(1), 5–19. https://doi.org/10.4085/1062-6050-99-16

Pfeifer, C. E., Beattie, P. F., Sacko, R. S., & Hand, A. (2018). Risk factors associated with non-contact anterior cruciate ligament injury: A systematic review. *International Journal of Sports Physical Therapy, 13*(4), 575–587.

Pol, R., Hristovski, R., Medina, D., & Balague, N. (2019). From microscopic to macroscopic sports injuries: Applying the complex dynamic systems approach to sports medicine: A narrative review. *British Journal of Sports Medicine, 53*(19), 1214–1220. https://doi.org/10.1136/bjsports-2016-097395

Porter, J. M., Wu, W. F., Crossley, R. M., Knopp, S. W., & Campbell, O. C. (2015). Adopting an external focus of attention improves sprinting performance in low-skilled sprinters. *Journal of Strength and Conditioning Research, 29*(4), 947–953. https://doi.org/10.1097/JSC.0000000000000229

Querfurth, S., Schücker, L., de Lussanet, M. H., & Zentgraf, K. (2016). An internal focus leads to longer quiet eye durations in novice dart players. *Frontiers in Psychology, 7*, 633. https://doi.org/10.3389/fpsyg.2016.00633

Reed, C. A., Ford, K. R., Myer, G. D., & Hewett, T. E. (2012). The effects of isolated and integrated 'core stability' training on athletic performance measures: A systematic review. *Sports Medicine, 42*(8), 697–706. https://doi.org/10.2165/11633450-000000000-00000

Renshaw, I., Araújo, D., Button, C., Chow, J. Y., Davids, K., & Moy, B. (2015). Why the constraints-led approach is not teaching games for understanding: A clarification. *Physical Education and Sport Pedagogy, 21*(5), 459–480. https://doi.org/https://doi.org/10.1080/17408989.2015.1095870

Renshaw, I., Davids, K., & Savelsbergh, G. J. P. (2010). *Motor learning in practice: A constraints-led approach.* Routledge.

Resende, R. A., Jardim, S., Filho, R., Mascarenhas, R. O., Ocarino, J. M., & Mendonça, L. M. (2020). Does trunk and hip muscles strength predict performance during a core stability test? *Brazilian Journal of Physical Therapy, 24*(4), 318–324. https://doi.org/10.1016/j.bjpt.2019.03.001

Roig, M., O'Brien, K., Kirk, G., Murray, R., McKinnon, P., Shadgan, B., & Reid, W. D. (2009). The effects of eccentric versus concentric resistance training on muscle strength and mass in healthy adults: A systematic review with meta-analysis. *British Journal of Sports Medicine, 43*(8), 556–568. https://doi.org/10.1136/bjsm.2008.051417

Rose, D. J. (1997). *A multi-level approach to the study of motor control and learning.* Allyn & Bacon.

Sahrmann, S., Azevedo, D. C., & Dillen, L. V. (2017). Diagnosis and treatment of movement system impairment syndromes. *Brazilian Journal of Physical Therapy, 21*(6), 391–399. https://doi.org/10.1016/j.bjpt.2017.08.001

Schmidt, R. A., & Lee, T. D. (2014). *Motor learning and performance: From principles to application* (5th ed.). Human Kinetics.

Schoenfeld, B. J., & Grgic, J. (2020). Effects of range of motion on muscle development during resistance training interventions: A systematic review. *SAGE Open Medicine, 8*, 205031212090155. https://doi.org/10.1177/2050312120901559

Seitz, L. B., & Haff, G. G. (2016). Factors modulating post-activation potentiation of jump, sprint, throw, and upper-body ballistic performances: A systematic review with meta-analysis. *Sports Medicine, 46*(2), 231–240. https://doi.org/10.1007/s40279-015-0415-7

Shin, S. J., Kim, T. Y., & Yoo, W. G. (2013). Effects of various gait speeds on the latissimus dorsi and gluteus maximus muscles associated with the posterior oblique sling system. *Journal of Physical Therapy Science, 25*(11), 1391–1392. https://doi.org/10.1589/jpts.25.1391

Stokes, P. D. (2008). Creativity from constraints: What can we learn from Motherwell? From Modrian? From Klee? *Journal of Creative Behavior, 42*, 223–236. https://doi.org/10.1002/j.2162-6057.2008.tb01297.x

Sueki, D. G., Cleland, J. A., & Wainner, R. S. (2013). A regional interdependence model of musculoskeletal dysfunction: Research, mechanisms, and clinical implications. *Journal of Manual & Manipulative Therapy, 21*(2), 90–102. https://doi.org/10.1179/2042618612Y.0000000027

Timmis, M. A., Piras, A., & van Paridon, K. N. (2018). Keep your eye on the ball; The impact of an anticipatory fixation during successful and unsuccessful soccer penalty kicks. *Frontiers in Psychology, 9*, 2058. https://doi.org/10.3389/fpsyg.2018.02058

Vickers, J. N. (1996). Control of visual attention during the basketball free throw. *American Journal of Sports Medicine, 24*(6 suppl), S93–S97.

Vickers, J. N., Causer, J., & Vanhooren, D. (2019). The role of quiet eye timing and location in the basketball three-point shot: A new research paradigm. *Frontiers in Psychology, 10*, 2424. https://doi.org/10.3389/fpsyg.2019.02424

Vine, S. J., Moore, L. J., & Wilson, M. R. (2011). Quiet eye training facilitates competitive putting performance in elite golfers. *Frontiers in Psychology, 2*, 8. https://doi.org/10.3389/fpsyg.2011.00008

Wilke, J., Krause, F., Vogt, L., & Banzer, W. (2016). What is evidence-based about myofascial chains: A systematic review. *Archives of Physical Medicine and Rehabilitation, 97*(3), 454–461. https://doi.org/10.1016/j.apmr.2015.07.023

Wilson, J. M., Loenneke, J. P., Jo, E., Wilson, G. J., Zourdos, M. C., & Kim, J. S. (2012). The effects of endurance, strength, and power training on muscle fiber type shifting. *Journal of Strength and Conditioning Research, 26*(6), 1724–1729. https://doi.org/10.1519/JSC.0b013e318234eb6f

Winkelman, N. C. (2018). Attentional focus and cueing for speed development. *Strength and Conditioning Journal, 40*(1), 13–25. https://doi.org/10.1519/SSC.0000000000000266

Wulf, G. (2013). Attentional focus and motor learning: A review of 15 years. *International Review of Sport and Exercise Psychology, 6*(1), 77–104. https://doi.org/https://doi.org/10.1080/1750984x.2012.723728

Wulf, G., Töllner, T., & Shea, C. H. (2007). Attentional focus effects as a function of task difficulty. *Research Quarterly for Exercise and Sport, 78*, 257–264.

Yoshikawa, N., Nittono, H., & Masaki, H. (2020). Effects of viewing cute pictures on quiet eye duration and fine motor task performance. *Frontiers in Psychology, 11*, 1565. https://doi.org/10.3389/fpsyg.2020.01565

SECTION 3

ASSESSMENTS, TESTING, AND MONITORING

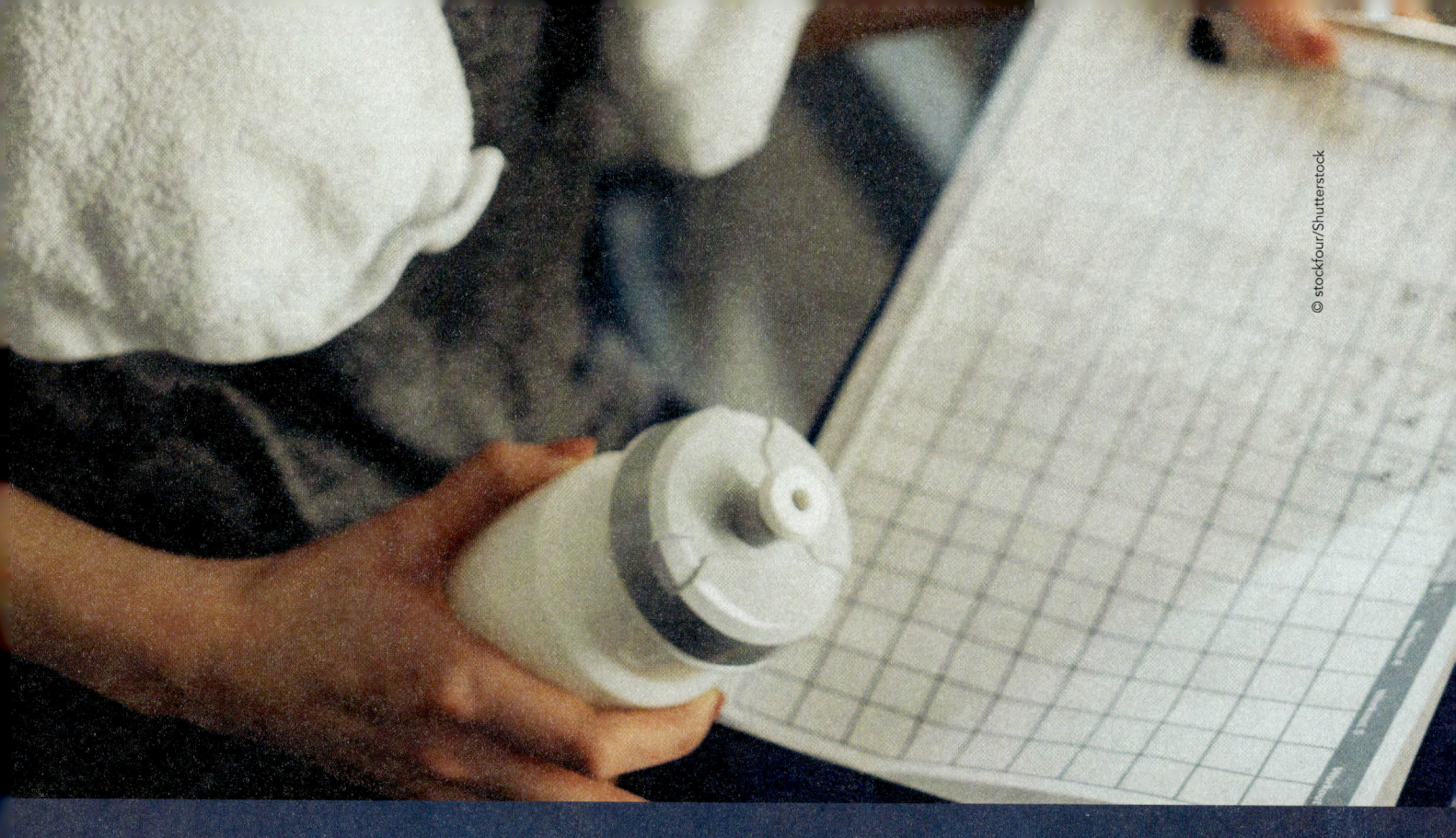

ATHLETE INTAKE AND SPORTS PERFORMANCE ASSESSMENTS

CHAPTER SEVEN

LEARNING OBJECTIVES

Upon completion of this chapter, the Sports Performance Coach will be able to:

- **Explain** the purpose of athlete intake and assessments.
- **Differentiate** between sports performance assessments and sports performance tests.
- **Describe** the athlete intake process.
- **Differentiate** between physiological and anthropometric assessments.
- **Explain** the relationship between transitional, mobility, and dynamic movement assessments.

LESSON 1: SPORTS PERFORMANCE TESTING AND ASSESSMENT OVERVIEW

INTRODUCTION TO ATHLETE INTAKE AND ASSESSMENTS

All athletes need a comprehensive evaluation prior to beginning sports performance training. Much of this entails sports and skill-related performance testing conducted by a coach; other aspects of an evaluation will be conducted by the sports medicine staff. However, a Sports Performance Coach will also conduct a comprehensive evaluation including such elements as intake questionnaires, medical history, physical assessments, and performance testing. These assessments may include gathering information about the athlete's overall health, movement quality, and mobility. The results of the athlete intake and assessments help to inform the selection of additional performance testing and the development of a personalized training plan tailored to the individual needs and goals of the athlete.

SPORTS PERFORMANCE ASSESSMENTS

SPORTS PERFORMANCE ASSESSMENTS →

A comprehensive process that involves gathering information and making decisions (e.g., selecting additional tests, designing programs) about an athlete's physiological, physical, and functional abilities.

Sports performance assessments are a comprehensive process that involves gathering information and making decisions (e.g., selecting additional tests, designing programs) about an athlete's physiological, physical, and functional abilities. Assessments can be conducted using various methods, such as athletes filling out intake forms, performing a needs analysis, and observing general movement patterns, such as a squat. A regular assessment schedule provides an ongoing source of information to modify training as an athlete progresses through an integrated training program. It is important to understand that sports performance assessments are not designed to diagnose any condition, but rather aim to observe each athlete's structural and functional status. Further, these assessments should not replace a medical examination. The Sports Performance Coach must refer the athlete to a qualified medical professional when a medical issue is identified that might put the athlete at risk for injury during training.

PERFORMANCE ASSESSMENTS VERSUS PERFORMANCE TESTS

The terms *assessments* and *tests* are often used interchangeably. Or, sometimes someone may describe a *test* as being designed to *assess* a particulate ability or quality. This usage of the terms is correct. However, in some cases, differences may exist. In this text, the term *sports performance assessments* is generally used to describe a procedure primarily or secondarily concerned with movement quality. For example, the overhead squat assessment (OHSA) primarily evaluates the quality of an athlete's squat. The Sports Performance Coach is asked to select whether an athlete demonstrated deviation from the typical performance during the movement. Another example is the single-leg hop test. The Sports Performance Coach is instructed to quantify the data by measuring the distance the athlete covers, but they also assess the athlete's movement quality. If movement impairments occur, the athlete is instructed to repeat the test. The information obtained from assessments helps the Sports Performance Coach decide on the next assessment or test and helps inform programming strategies. For example, the coach will develop a specific flexibility and strengthening routine that an athlete who demonstrates movement impairments can perform before training.

Conversely, the term **sports performance tests** is generally used to describe procedures primarily focused on quantifiable data with little consideration for movement quality. For example, an athlete's performance on the 300-yard shuttle run is based entirely on the amount of time it takes them to complete the test and does not consider running mechanics. Similarly, a one-repetition maximum bench press quantifies strength via the load the athlete lifts with little concern for how they lift it. Although movement quality should always be a concern for the Sports Performance Coach, performance tests rarely include scoring or evaluation criteria specific to movement quality. Additionally, many sports performance tests have established norms or standards to which an athlete's data can be compared.

SPORTS PERFORMANCE TESTS →

A procedure for measuring performance related to a specific skill or ability (e.g., jump height, strength).

VALIDITY AND RELIABILITY

Sports performance assessments and tests must be valid and reliable to accurately measure the athlete's progress during their training program. Validity is defined as the extent to which the assessment or test accurately measures what it is supposed to measure. Reliability is defined as the ability to consistently reproduce accurate findings over multiple time periods (Currell & Jeukendrup, 2008). For example, the star excursion balance test (SEBT) is a popular choice for assessing dynamic postural control that has documented validity and reliability (Gribble et al., 2012; Powden et al., 2019). The Sports Performance Coach can be confident that the SEBT accurately assesses lower-body dynamic posture, balance, and neuromuscular efficiency and that different fitness professionals can obtain similar results when testing athletes using the same method. The Sports Performance Coach should strive to use valid and reliable performance assessments and tests.

ASSESSMENT SEQUENCING

The Sports Performance Coach needs an organized approach when assessing an athlete. In general, the assessment begins with the athlete intake and needs analysis, which includes a detailed conversation between the parties and specific questionnaires (e.g., the Physical Activity Readiness Questionnaire) for the athlete to fill out. Next, the Sports Performance Coach might conduct other assessments, such as physiological, anthropometric, movement, and mobility assessments. A consistent flow to the assessment approach should be developed to reduce the chances of missing a key assessment (**Figure 7.1**). Further, when conducting movement assessments, the athlete might not perform one or several tests depending on the results of a previous test. For example, if the athlete demonstrates knee valgus during an overhead squat assessment, performing something like the Landing Error Scoring System (LESS) or shark skill test, which further loads the compensation, may not be recommended. However, the choice and sequencing of assessments vary per athlete and are determined during the intake and needs analysis. In some cases, the Sports

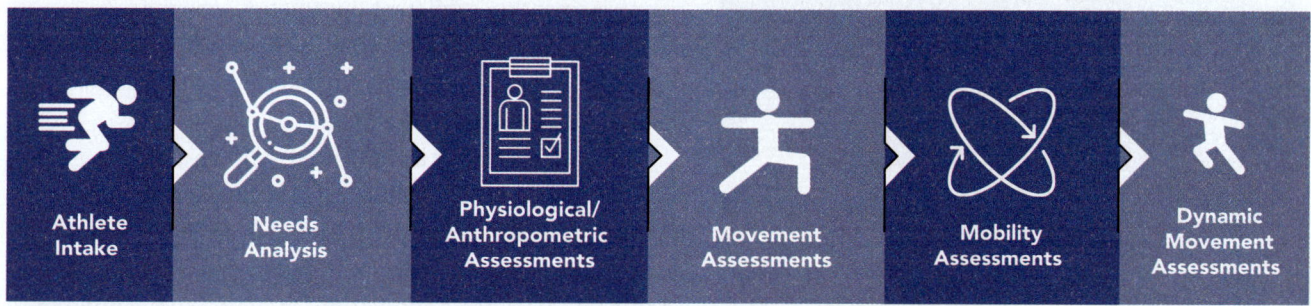

FIGURE 7.1 Consistent Flow for Conducting Movement Assessments

Performance Coach might need to see how the athlete performs under certain conditions, even in the presence of movement impairments.

PERFORMANCE ASSESSMENT COMPONENTS

The sports performance assessment includes a series of tests and measurements to gather information about the athlete. This assessment provides the Sports Performance Coach with a holistic representation of the athlete, offering insights into their past, present, and perhaps future. The assessment includes the following components:

1. Athlete intake
2. Needs analysis
3. Physiological or anthropometric assessments
4. Transitional movement assessments
5. Mobility assessments
6. Dynamic movement assessments

 COACH'S CORNER

It is common for Sports Performance Coaches to work with athletes of different ages. When working with minors, obtaining assent (agreement to participate) and parental or legal guardian consent before beginning any assessment and training is imperative. Written consent forms must outline the performance assessment procedures and training program, and the Sports Performance Coach must have a detailed conversation with all parties outlining the proposed program (Weisleder, 2020). Each state in the United States and different countries have specific laws governing informed consent procedures for minors. The Sports Performance Coach must not use standard consent forms because they might not be legal and valid in every state or country. NASM recommends that the Sports Performance Coach consult a qualified legal professional to understand which forms are needed.

ATHLETE INTAKE

The athlete intake is the initial interview process that the Sports Performance Coach conducts with the athlete. It aims to gather subjective information regarding an athlete's readiness for activity or the health risk assessment. The health risk assessment uses different information, obtained via questionnaire, regarding existing risk factors for participating in athletic activity and exercise to determine the need for medical clearance before training.

The athlete intake is a vital first step in the athlete's preparticipation screening process. The intake needs to be specific to each athlete, with the coach asking relevant questions to gather valuable information that will inform additional assessments and testing, and for accurate program design. Overall, the athlete intake must determine if it is safe

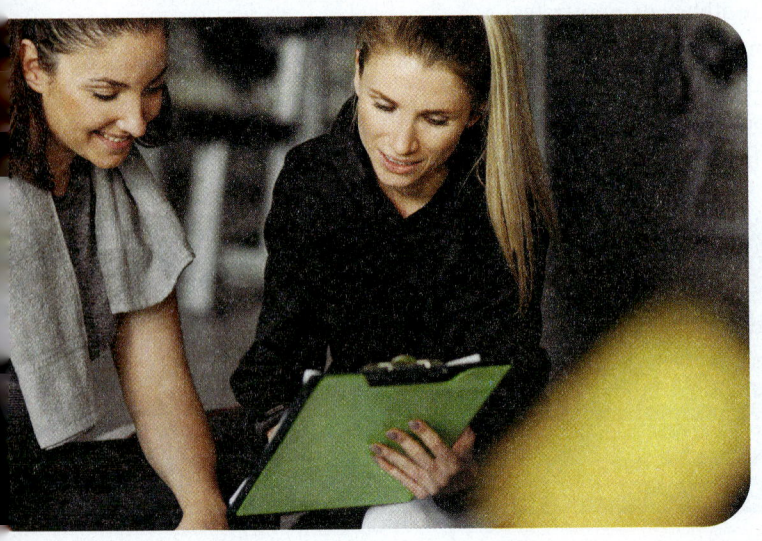

© gpointstudio/Shutterstock

for the athlete to continue with testing and a training program, or if a referral to a medical professional is required. The Sports Performance Coach must also use this time to develop a rapport with the athlete. Each step should be used to engage in conversation with the athlete rather than simply handing over a form for them to complete.

> **⚠ CRITICAL**
>
> Athlete intake might be conducted by a qualified healthcare professional or a member of the sports medicine team in some professional settings. In such settings, the athlete might provide information that falls under the **Health Insurance Portability and Accountability Act (HIPAA)**, which protects the privacy of individuals' health-related information. In this case, the Sports Performance Coach will have limited access to the athlete's health-related information. However, the Sports Performance Coach is responsible for communicating with the sports medicine team to ensure it is safe for the athlete to engage in physical activity. In situations where the Sports Performance Coach is conducting the athlete intake, the athlete's information might be protected under HIPAA and should not be shared without the athlete's consent.

HEALTH INSURANCE PORTABILITY AND ACCOUNTABILITY ACT (HIPAA) →

A federal law that provides privacy and security standards for protected health information.

PHYSICAL ACTIVITY READINESS QUESTIONNAIRE

The **Physical Activity Readiness Questionnaire (PAR-Q+)** is a useful assessment for athletes of all levels as part of the screening process (Maranhao Neto et al., 2013). The Sports Performance Coach must consider the PAR-Q+ as one part of a complex intake process rather than as a final clearance for activity.

Athletes who mark "yes" on any of the questions might need to be referred to a qualified medical professional for clearance (**Figure 7.2**). The full PAR-Q+ can be found in Appendix E.

PHYSICAL ACTIVITY READINESS QUESTIONNAIRE (PAR-Q+) →

A detailed questionnaire designed to assess an individual's physical readiness to engage in structured exercise.

> **📋 COACH'S CORNER**
>
> Most individuals recall as little as one-fifth of the information discussed and immediately forget 40% to 80% of information obtained during a visit to a medical professional (Kessels, 2003; Richard et al., 2017; Sherlock & Brownie, 2014). Given that the athlete might have poor recall, a comprehensive intake process is critical to obtain accurate information about the athlete's health status. Diagnosing an injury is outside the scope of the Sports Performance Coach; thus, the medical history must be used only to shed light on what the athlete and coach might see later.

HEALTH HISTORY QUESTIONNAIRE (HHQ) →

A questionnaire with lists of questions that pertain to health history and habits, such as exercise history, eating behaviors, and general lifestyle.

HEALTH HISTORY QUESTIONNAIRE

A complete pre-exercise **health history questionnaire (HHQ)** collects relevant information on the athlete's past and present health, and serves to complement the PAR-Q+ in expanding the Sports Performance Coach's understanding of the

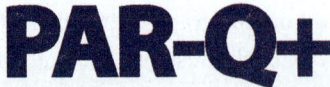

PAR-Q+

The Physical Activity Readiness Questionnaire for Everyone

The health benefits of regular physical activity are clear; more people should engage in physical activity every day of the week. Participating in physical activity is very safe for MOST people. This questionnaire will tell you whether it is necessary for you to seek further advice from your doctor OR a qualified exercise professional before becoming more physically active.

GENERAL HEALTH QUESTIONS

Please read the 7 questions below carefully and answer each one honestly: check YES or NO.	YES	NO
1) Has your doctor ever said that you have a heart condition ☐ **OR** high blood pressure☐?	☐	☐
2) Do you feel pain in your chest at rest, during your daily activities of living, **OR** when you do physical activity?	☐	☐
3) Do you lose balance because of dizziness **OR** have you lost consciousness in the last 12 months? Please answer **NO** if your dizziness was associated with over-breathing (including during vigorous exercise).	☐	☐
4) Have you ever been diagnosed with another chronic medical condition (other than heart disease or high blood pressure)? **PLEASE LIST CONDITION(S) HERE:** _____	☐	☐
5) Are you currently taking prescribed medications for a chronic medical condition? **PLEASE LIST CONDITION(S) AND MEDICATIONS HERE:** _____	☐	☐
6) Do you currently have (or have had within the past 12 months) a bone, joint, or soft tissue (muscle, ligament, or tendon) problem that could be made worse by becoming more physically active? Please answer **NO** if you had a problem in the past, but it **does not limit your current ability** to be physically active. **PLEASE LIST CONDITION(S) HERE:** _____	☐	☐
7) Has your doctor ever said that you should only do medically supervised physical activity?	☐	☐

✅ **If you answered NO to all of the questions above, you are cleared for physical activity.**
Please sign the PARTICIPANT DECLARATION. You do not need to complete Pages 2 and 3.

- ▶ Start becoming much more physically active – start slowly and build up gradually.
- ▶ Follow Global Physical Activity Guidelines for your age (https://www.who.int/publications/i/item/9789240015128).
- ▶ You may take part in a health and fitness appraisal.
- ▶ If you are over the age of 45 yr and NOT accustomed to regular vigorous to maximal effort exercise, consult a qualified exercise professional before engaging in this intensity of exercise.
- ▶ If you have any further questions, contact a qualified exercise professional.

PARTICIPANT DECLARATION
If you are less than the legal age required for consent or require the assent of a care provider, your parent, guardian or care provider must also sign this form.

I, the undersigned, have read, understood to my full satisfaction and completed this questionnaire. I acknowledge that this physical activity clearance is valid for a maximum of 12 months from the date it is completed and becomes invalid if my condition changes. I also acknowledge that the community/fitness center may retain a copy of this form for its records. In these instances, it will maintain the confidentiality of the same, complying with applicable law.

NAME _____ DATE _____

SIGNATURE _____ WITNESS _____

SIGNATURE OF PARENT/GUARDIAN/CARE PROVIDER _____

🛑 **If you answered YES to one or more of the questions above, COMPLETE PAGES 2 AND 3.**

⚠️ **Delay becoming more active if:**

- ✓ You are currently experiencing a temporary illness, such as a cold or fever. It is best to wait until you feel better.
- ✓ You are pregnant. In this case, talk with your health care practitioner, physician, qualified exercise professional, and/or complete the ePARmed-X+ at www.eparmedx.com before becoming more physically active.
- ✓ Your health changes. Answer the questions on Pages 2 and 3 of this document and/or talk to your health care practitioner, physician, or qualified exercise professional before proceeding with any physical activity program.

FIGURE 7.2 PAR-Q+ Questionnaire

Reprinted with permission from the PAR-Q+ Collaboration (www.eparmedx.com) and the authors of the PAR-Q+ (Dr. Darren Warburton, Dr. Norman Gledhill, Dr. Veronica Jamnik, Dr. Roy Shephard, and Dr. Shannon Bredin).

Citations:

Warburton D, Jamnik V, Bredin S, Shephard R, Gledhill N. The 2022 Physical Activity Readiness Questionnaire for Everyone (PAR-Q+) and electronic Physical Activity Readiness Medical Examination (ePARmed-X+). *Health & Fitness Journal of Canada 2022;15*(1):54-57. https://hfjc.library.ubc.ca/index.php/HFJC/article/view/815

Warburton DER, Gledhill N, Jamnik VK, Bredin SSD, McKenzie DC, Stone J, Charlesworth S, Shephard RJ, on behalf of the PAR-Q+ Collaboration. The Physical Activity Readiness Questionnaire for Everyone (PAR-Q+) and electronic Physical Activity Readiness Medical Examination (ePARmed-X+): Summary of consensus panel recommendations. *Health & Fitness Journal of Canada 2011;4*:26-37.

participant's health status. This questionnaire is not usually standardized, but instead is customized to respective sports performance athletes, facilities, or organizations. An HHQ might be accompanied by a verbal discussion with the athlete, with optional additional questionnaires designed to gather more information being administered in some cases.

Athlete Demographic Information

The HHQ typically contains the following athlete information, all of which is considered private and confidential:

- Chronological age
- Gender
- Height
- Weight
- Physician's name and contact information
- Emergency contact information

Medical History

Obtaining the athlete's medical history is a vital part of an HHQ. A medical history provides information about the athlete's past and current health status, as well as any past or recent injuries, surgeries, or chronic health conditions. Gathering this information helps determine if an athlete is ready to participate in a sports performance program or if they need a medical referral first.

Past Injuries and the Kinetic Chain

The athlete's injury history can be discussed as it relates to the sport. This information might help the Sports Performance Coach identify any risk factors for injury. Research shows that prior injury is a risk factor for future injury in some sports (Fulton et al., 2014; Hägglund et al., 2006; Steffen et al., 2008). A prior injury can cause an effect up and down the kinetic chain. For example, an injury at the hip can affect the knee and ankle (Reiman, Bolgla, & Lorenz, 2009; Sueki et al., 2013) and the lumbar spine (Reiman, Weisbach, & Glynn, 2009). In the presence of an injury, the Sports Performance Coach needs to work with the athlete's healthcare team to determine which tasks the athlete can safely perform during their training and competition.

The following are some common injuries and their effects on the human movement system (HMS):

- *Ankle:* **Chronic ankle instability (CAI)** is the tendency of the ankle to give way during routine and sports activity; it can lead to ankle sprains. Research shows that CAI decreases the neural control of the hip abductor (gluteus minimus, medius, and maximus) muscles (Fatima et al., 2020; Friel et al., 2006). This, in turn, can lead to poor control of the lower extremities during functional activities, eventually leading to injury. Researchers have also found that hip abductor muscle weakness is a risk factor for ankle sprains (De Ridder et al., 2017; Kawaguchi et al., 2021; Powers et al., 2017).
- *Knee:* Knee injuries can cause a decrease in the neural control of muscles that stabilize the patellofemoral and tibiofemoral joints and might lead to further injury (Phisitkul et al., 2006; Shanbehzadeh et al., 2017). Knee ligament injuries can also impair adjacent muscle activity above (hip abductors and extensors) and below (ankle plantar flexors) the knee (Thomas et al., 2013). Consequently, impairments

> **CHRONIC ANKLE INSTABILITY (CAI)** →
>
> A condition characterized by recurrent ankle sprains or a feeling of instability in the ankle joint.

at the hip or ankle can also affect knee function, resulting in altered movement and force distribution of the joint, which can eventually result in injury (Chuter & Janse de Jonge, 2012; De Blaiser et al., 2021; Powers, 2010).

- *Low back:* Low back injuries can cause decreased neural control of stabilizing muscles of the core, resulting in poor stabilization of the spine (Chang et al., 2015). This may then lead to dysfunction in the upper and lower extremities because the core muscles are involved with extremity movement and function (De Blaiser et al., 2018; Silfies et al., 2015; Tarnanen et al., 2012).

- *Shoulder:* Shoulder injuries can cause altered neural control of the scapular and rotator cuff muscles, which can lead to instability of the shoulder complex during functional activities (Edouard et al., 2011; Moezy et al., 2014; Paine & Voight, 2013). Shoulder dysfunction associated with previous injuries is linked to reduced thoracic mobility (Haik et al., 2014). For overhead-throwing athletes, past injuries to the shoulder can alter throwing mechanics, leading to further injury (Chu et al., 2016). Poor shoulder motion, such as decreased internal rotation, can affect upper-extremity mechanics and might lead to tennis elbow (Ellenbecker et al., 2012).

- *Other:* Injuries that result from HMS imbalances include repetitive hamstring complex strains, groin strains, patellar tendinitis (jumper's knee), plantar fasciitis (pain in the arch of the foot), posterior tibialis tendinitis (shin splints), biceps tendinitis (shoulder pain), and headaches (Barmherzig & Kingston, 2019; Chalmers et al., 2017; Franklyn-Miller et al., 2017; Mousavi et al., 2019; Opar et al., 2012; Phillips & McClinton, 2017; Van de Velde et al., 2017).

The list of these injuries is not all-inclusive. In all cases, if an athlete presents with an acute injury, they must be referred to a qualified medical professional for evaluation and treatment. In addition, the Sports Performance Coach must consider past injuries when assessing individuals, as the altered neuromuscular control can lead to new muscular imbalances that will manifest over time unless the athlete is giving it proper care.

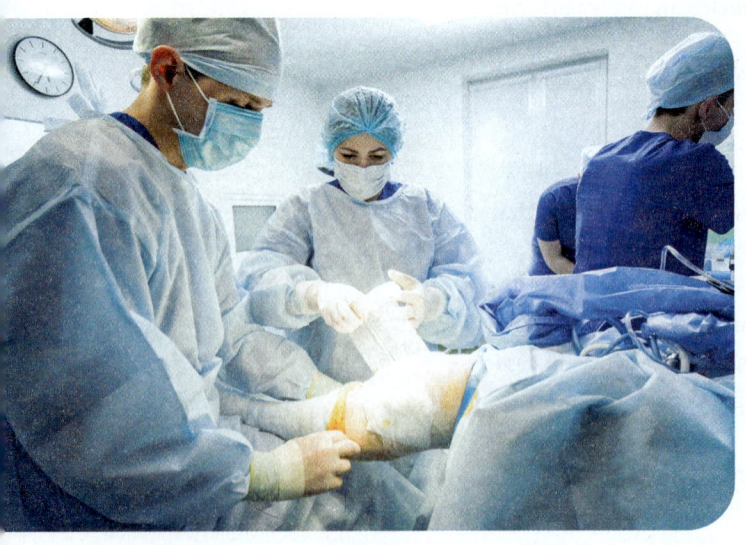

© Roman Zaiets/Shutterstock

KINETIC CHAIN → CHECKPOINT

The five areas of the body that are monitored during movement assessments and exercise: foot/ankle, knees, lumbo-pelvic-hip complex, shoulders, and cervical spine and head.

Past Surgery

Surgical procedures create trauma for the body and have effects similar to those associated with an injury. Previous surgeries can create dysfunction unless they are properly rehabilitated. Some common surgical procedures at each **kinetic chain checkpoint** are described in **Table 7.1**.

In each case, surgery causes pain, inflammation, and psychological and physiological effects, including musculoskeletal denervation, muscle atrophy, depression, stress, and decreased overall mobility. These physiological and psychological effects can directly influence the kinetic chain if not rehabilitated properly. For example, an athlete who undergoes knee anterior cruciate ligament (ACL) repair might experience significant postoperative muscular changes that affect both function and strength (Csapo et al., 2019; Lindström et al., 2013). For this reason, the Sports

TABLE 7.1   Common Surgical Procedures That Affect Kinetic Chain Checkpoints

Checkpoint	Surgical Procedure
Foot and ankle	Achilles' repair
Knee	Knee anterior cruciate ligament repair
Lumbo-pelvic-hip complex (LPHC)	Lumbar disc herniation surgery
Shoulder*	Rotator cuff tear repair
Head and cervical spine	Cervical disc herniation surgery

*Surgery for rotator cuff tears is common among overhead sports (Muto et al., 2017).

Data from Allahabadi et al., 2020; Trofa et a., 2017; Joseph et al., 2013; Mai et al., 2017; Burgmeier & Hsu, 2014; Hsu & Jenkins, 2017; Muto et al., 2017; Leider et al., 2021; Watkins et al., 2018.

Performance Coach must perform movement assessments and integrate the results with the athlete intake to guide exercise programming rather than basing programming solely on athlete intake information.

📋 COACH'S CORNER

The Sports Performance Coach must consider whether an athlete's training program might need to be modified due to prior or current injuries or surgery. The intake results must be carefully considered before the athlete participates in assessments, testing, and training. Prior injuries can be a risk factor for subsequent injury (Fulton et al., 2014; Hägglund et al., 2006). Likewise, prior surgeries are risk factors for later injury (Smith et al., 2017; Teyhen et al., 2015).

Medications

Some athletes might be required to use medications under the guidance of a medical professional. It is not the role of a Sports Performance Coach to administer, prescribe, or educate athletes on the use and effects of any prescribed medications. However, they should have some knowledge of common classifications of medications that affect heart rate and blood pressure (**Table 7.2**). Table 7.2 presents a simplistic overview of medications and should not be considered conclusive evidence regarding the medications or their effects. For complete information regarding medications, contact a qualified healthcare provider.

TABLE 7.2 Common Medications by Classification and Effects on Heart Rate and Blood Pressure

Medication	Basic Function	Heart Rate	Blood Pressure
Beta-blockers (β-blockers)	Generally used as antihypertensive (high blood pressure); might also be prescribed for arrhythmias (irregular heart rate)	↓	↓
Calcium-channel blockers	Generally prescribed for hypertension and angina (chest pain)	↑ ↔ or ↓	↓
Nitrates	Generally prescribed for hypertension and heart failure	↑ ↔	↓ ↔
Diuretics	Generally prescribed for hypertension, heart failure, and peripheral edema	↔	↔ ↓
Bronchodilators	Generally prescribed to correct or prevent bronchial smooth muscle constriction in individuals with asthma and other pulmonary diseases	↔	↔
Vasodilators	Used in the treatment of hypertension and heart failure	↑ ↔ or ↓	↓
Antidepressants	Used in the treatment of various psychiatric and emotional disorders	↑ or ↔	↔ or ↓

Key: ↑ = Increase; ↔ = No effect; ↓ = Decrease

📋 COACH'S CORNER

The Sports Performance Coach needs to become proficient at administering an effective athlete intake interview, which includes engaging in effective communication and active listening. Through a systematically planned conversation, the Sports Performance Coach can acquire important information that reveals potential medical issues and details that can guide the development of the athlete's sports training programming. Effective interviewing is a standard of practice in medicine. A classic medical study in 1975 noted that a good history can determine 83% of diagnoses among medical patients (Hampton et al., 1975). Even today, that statistic is cited by hundreds of studies and is a benchmark for healthcare providers. For Sports Performance Coaches, developing effective communication and active listening skills allows them to connect with athletes, understand their needs, and build professional relationships. While it can take time to develop effective communication and active listening skills, a Sports Performance Coach can begin with these three steps:

1. Focus all attention on the athlete during the interview and reduce any distractions.
2. Be clear and concise.
3. Genuinely care about the athlete's success.

LESSON 2: EVALUATING SPORTS DEMANDS

NEEDS ANALYSIS

The purpose of the **needs analysis** is to gather comprehensive information about the athlete and their sport. This helps the Sports Performance Coach design the most relevant assessment and training program (Scroggs & Simonson, 2021). An efficient needs analysis includes both written and verbal components: Needs analysis questions are presented in writing, such as in the form of a questionnaire, and a verbal discussion also takes place between the Sports Performance Coach and the athlete. The Sports Performance Coach might also gather more information about the athlete's sport through other sources, such as research articles or consultation with other professionals with sport expertise. The Sports Performance Coach should do as much research as possible on the sport and the athlete before the initial meeting to help encourage communication and develop a rapport. The main components of the needs analysis include the sport, position, and athlete profile.

> ### NEEDS ANALYSIS →
>
> Comprehensive written and verbal interview with the athlete to gather more information about their sport, position, and athletic profile.

📋 COACH'S CORNER

The athlete analysis must reflect the individual needs of each athlete, including age. For example, a younger tennis player might need to improve their overall muscular strength, core stability, and motor control, whereas an older athlete might need to refine speed, agility, and quickness for a specific sports position (Zemková & Hamar, 2018). For this reason, the Sports Performance Coach should tailor the athlete assessment to each athlete's needs based on their chronological age, training age, sport, training needs, and goals.

SPORT AND POSITION ANALYSIS

An important component of the athlete analysis is the sport and position analysis. The Sports Performance Coach has to gather information in five key areas related to the athlete's sports and positions (**Figure 7.3**).

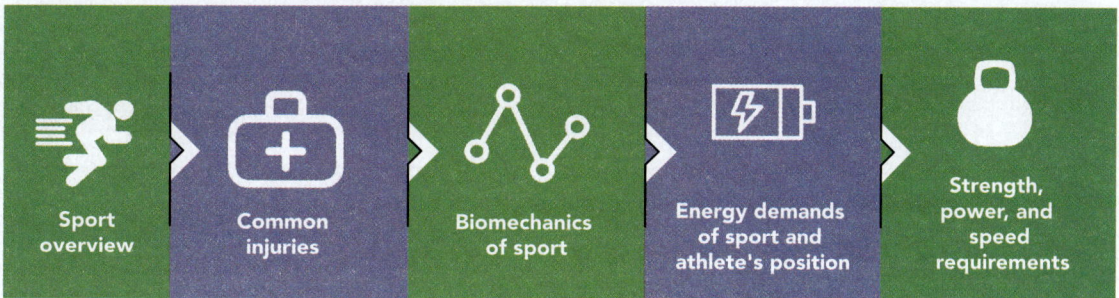

FIGURE 7.3 Components of the Sport and Position Analysis

SPORT OVERVIEW

The first part of the needs analysis includes reviewing the sport, including practice time, competition (game) time, competition schedule or season schedule, relevant rules of play, level of the sport (e.g., collegiate), and an overview of the position(s) played by the athlete and the associated physical demands (e.g., repetitive jumping). This information is essential for the Sports Performance Coach to design the athlete's program. The sport overview also helps the Sports Performance Coach understand how the sport is played in their geographic region. For example, a youth soccer player might be participating in a league with different rules of play compared to leagues in other states or countries. The parameters of the athlete's sport and on-field play influence their training program because the goal of training is to help the athlete perform at the highest level during competition.

COMMON INJURIES

After the sport overview, analysis of common injuries experienced helps the Sports Performance Coach monitor the athlete and design safe and effective exercises. This might include common injuries among different sports, positions, and age groups. Such knowledge helps the coach to effectively monitor the athlete and design safe exercises. Relevant information can be obtained by reading research or consulting with different professionals. For example, the Sports Performance Coach can read the latest injury research for common sports, consult healthcare professionals with sports expertise, or consult sports coaches to understand their perspective on performance training and injury risk.

Table 7.3 lists common sports and injuries related to them (Hootman et al., 2007; Johnson et al., 2017; Kerr et al., 2015; Kerr et al., 2017; Krutsch et al., 2018; Shanley et al., 2011; Weinstein et al., 2019). The Sports Performance Coach needs a comprehensive understanding of these injuries, possible risks, and evidence-based prevention strategies.

TABLE 7.3 Common Sport-Specific Injuries

Sport	Common Injuries
Baseball and softball	Ankle and knee ligament injuries (e.g., ACL), lower-extremity muscle strains (e.g., hamstrings), concussions, contusions, shoulder/elbow ligament sprains or muscle strains, wrist/hand bone fractures
Basketball	Ankle and knee ligament injuries (e.g., ACL), lower-extremity muscle strains (e.g., hamstrings), contusions, concussions, and upper-extremity ligament sprains or muscle strains
Soccer	Ankle and knee ligament injuries (e.g., ACL), lower-extremity muscle strains (e.g., hamstrings), contusions, concussions
Ice hockey and field hockey	Ankle and knee ligament injuries (e.g., ACL), lower-extremity muscle strains (e.g., groin injury), shoulder/elbow ligament sprains or muscle strains, wrist/hand injuries (e.g., bone fracture, muscle strains, ligament sprains, dislocations), concussions, spine injuries
Wrestling	Ankle and knee ligament injuries (e.g., ACL), upper- and lower-extremity muscle strains (e.g., rotator cuff, hamstrings), contusions, concussions, upper-extremity traumatic injuries (e.g., shoulder dislocation, AC joint separation, wrist fracture), spine injuries
Tennis	Ankle and knee ligament injuries (e.g., ACL), upper- and lower-extremity muscle strains (e.g., rotator cuff, hamstrings, calves)
Lacrosse	Ankle and knee ligament injuries (e.g., ACL), upper- and lower-extremity muscle strains (e.g., rotator cuff, hamstrings), concussions, contusions, upper-extremity traumatic injuries (e.g., shoulder dislocation, AC joint separation, wrist fracture)
Gymnastics	Ankle and knee ligament injuries (e.g., ACL), upper- and lower-extremity muscle strains (e.g., rotator cuff, hamstrings), concussions, contusions, upper-extremity traumatic injuries (e.g., shoulder dislocation, AC joint separation, wrist fracture), spine injuries

Sport	Common Injuries
Volleyball	Ankle and knee ligament injury (e.g., ACL), upper- and lower-extremity muscle strains (e.g., rotator cuff, hamstrings), concussions, contusions
Diving and swimming	Spine injuries, upper-extremity injuries (e.g., glenohumeral instability, overuse muscle strains, ligament sprain), postural dysfunctions
Skiing and snowboarding	Ankle and knee ligament injuries (e.g., ACL), lower-extremity muscle strains (e.g., hamstrings), contusions, concussions, upper-extremity traumatic injuries (e.g., shoulder dislocation, AC joint separation, wrist fracture), spine injuries
Cheerleading and dance	Ankle and knee ligament injuries (e.g., ACL), lower-extremity muscle strains (e.g., hamstrings), contusions, concussions, upper-extremity traumatic injuries (e.g., shoulder dislocation, AC joint separation, wrist fracture), spine injuries
Cross-country and running	Lower-extremity overuse injuries (e.g., stress fractures, medial tibial stress syndrome, tendinopathy), lower-extremity muscle strains (e.g., hamstrings), plantar fasciitis

Abbreviations: AC, acromioclavicular; ACL, anterior cruciate ligament.

BIOMECHANICS OF THE SPORT

The next step in the sport and position analysis is analyzing the biomechanics of sport-related movements. This helps to determine which muscles and joint actions and other biomechanical factors contribute to specific movements. The information gained from the sport overview determines which movements are relevant to analyze. Most sports are multidirectional and have unique movement and biomechanical demands (Taylor et al., 2017). For example, a youth soccer athlete might play a midfield position, which requires a high frequency of sprinting, cutting, ball kicking, and passing. The Sports Performance Coach can analyze the biomechanics of these movements to determine the most effective exercises for the athlete's training program.

ENERGY DEMANDS

Understanding the primary energy systems at work during practice and competition can help the Sports Performance Coach determine the most effective training variable (e.g., work-to-rest ratios) for the athlete. The Sports Performance Coach needs a general understanding of the energy demands of common sports for different chronological age groups and levels of play. For example, a collegiate baseball pitcher might play more innings with more intensity and volume (e.g., faster and higher number of pitches) than a high school pitcher. This will require training the energy systems differently due to the sports demands for that age and level of play. **Table 7.4** lists common sports; the full Energy Demand of Sports handout can be found in Appendix E.

STRENGTH, POWER, AND SPEED

The last part of the sport and position analysis includes evaluating the specific strength, power, and speed requirements of an athlete's position. Each sport and position has specific performance demands that require an adequate level of anaerobic and aerobic fitness (**Figure 7.4**). For example, individual sports might have different demands than team sports. These performance demands change in response to such variables as an

TABLE 7.4 Energy Demand of Common Sports

Sport	Phosphagen System	Glycolytic System	Aerobic System
American football	High	Moderate	Low
Baseball	High	Low	—
Basketball	High	Moderate to high	—
Field events (athletics)	High	—	—
Ice hockey	High	Moderate	Moderate
Marathon	Low	Low	High
Powerlifting	High	Low	—
Soccer (football)	High	Moderate	Moderate
Tennis	High	Moderate	Low

Data from from Ostchega, Y., Porter, K. S., Hughes, J., Dillon, C. F., & Nwankwo, T. (2011). Resting pulse rate reference data for children, adolescents, and adults: United States, 1999-2008. *National Health Statistics Report*, (41), 1–16.

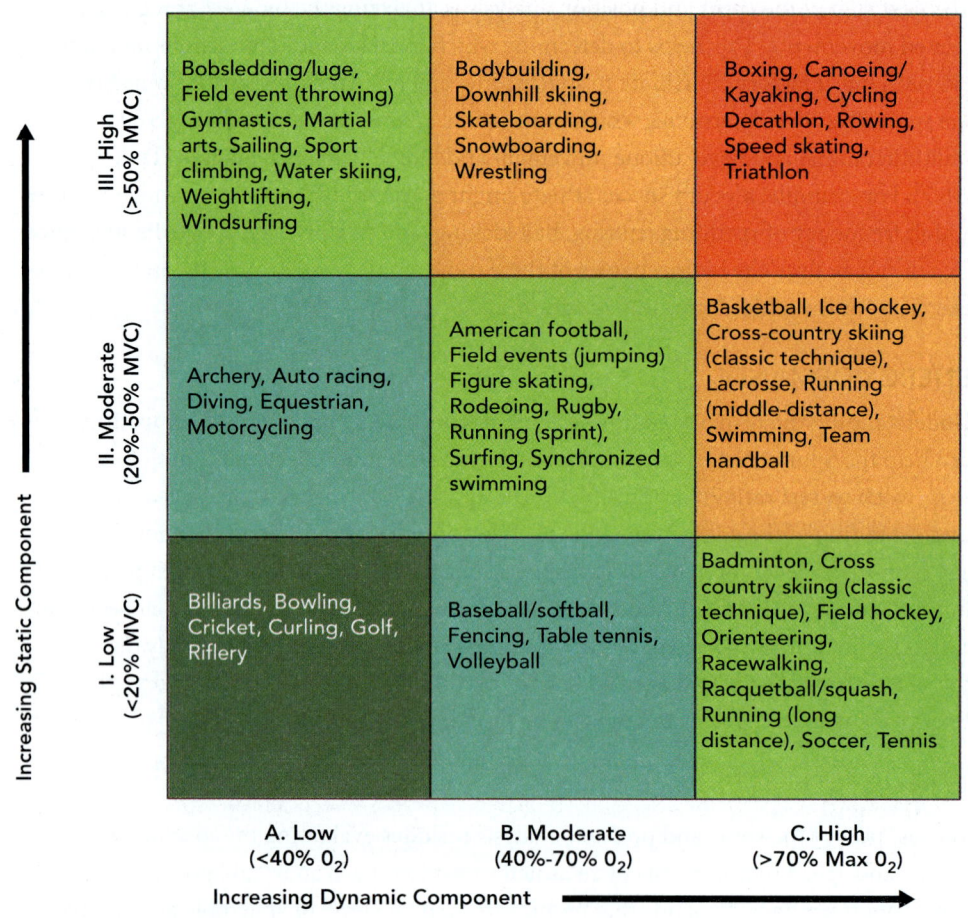

FIGURE 7.4 Classification of Sport Demands

Reproduced from Mitchell, J. H., Haskell, W., Snell, P., & Van Camp, S. P. (2005). Task Force 8: classification of sports. *Journal of the American College of Cardiology, 45*(8), 1364-1367.

increase in chronological age, change in position or game parameters (e.g., competition time, rules of play), or advancing to a higher level of play (e.g., high school to college).

The classification of sport demands is based on the peak static and dynamic components achieved during competition. An athlete might reach higher values during training. The increasing dynamic component is defined in terms of the estimated percentage of maximal oxygen uptake (max O_2) achieved and results in an increased cardiac output. The increasing static component is related to the estimated percentage of maximal voluntary contraction (MVC) reached and results in an increased blood pressure load.

How Sports Performance Coaches record the demands of a sport can vary. **Figure 7.5** shows a simple method of classifying and quantifying the physical demands on professional soccer players by position. Further, Sports Performance Coaches can search for similar information regarding all sports to help support data obtained from athlete interviews and observation.

 COACH'S CORNER

The Sports Performance Coach should consider that an athlete's chronological age has an influence on their athletic profile. Youth athletes might have a different profile due to their training age, level of competition, injury history, and goals. Research shows that sports specialization at a younger age might be necessary for elite-level skills development in some sports (e.g., gymnastics, diving) but can lead to higher rates of injury, psychological stress, and burnout (Jayanthi et al., 2013; Myer et al., 2015). The Sports Performance Coach needs to be aware of such issues with younger athletes to help them and their parents manage any problems that crop up through rest, recovery, cross-training, and participating in other unstructured athletic or sports activities (Myer et al., 2016).

ATHLETE PROFILE

After the sport and position analysis, the Sports Performance Coach gathers more information about the athlete. The athlete profile includes three key components: training age, past and current level of competition, and professional and personal goals (**Figure 7.6**).

TRAINING AGE

The training age represents the number of years the athlete has practiced and played the specific sport and position(s). For example, a 22-year-old volleyball player who has been playing since age 12 has a training age of 10 years. The training age provides important insights into the athlete's physical and mental maturity toward their sport (Myer et al., 2013). The Sports Performance Coach needs to consider training age when working with different athletes because a more mature athlete will respond differently to training than a less mature athlete.

PAST AND CURRENT LEVEL OF COMPETITION

The Sports Performance Coach also needs to discuss the athlete's past and current level of competition. The competition level can be the recreation level or competitive

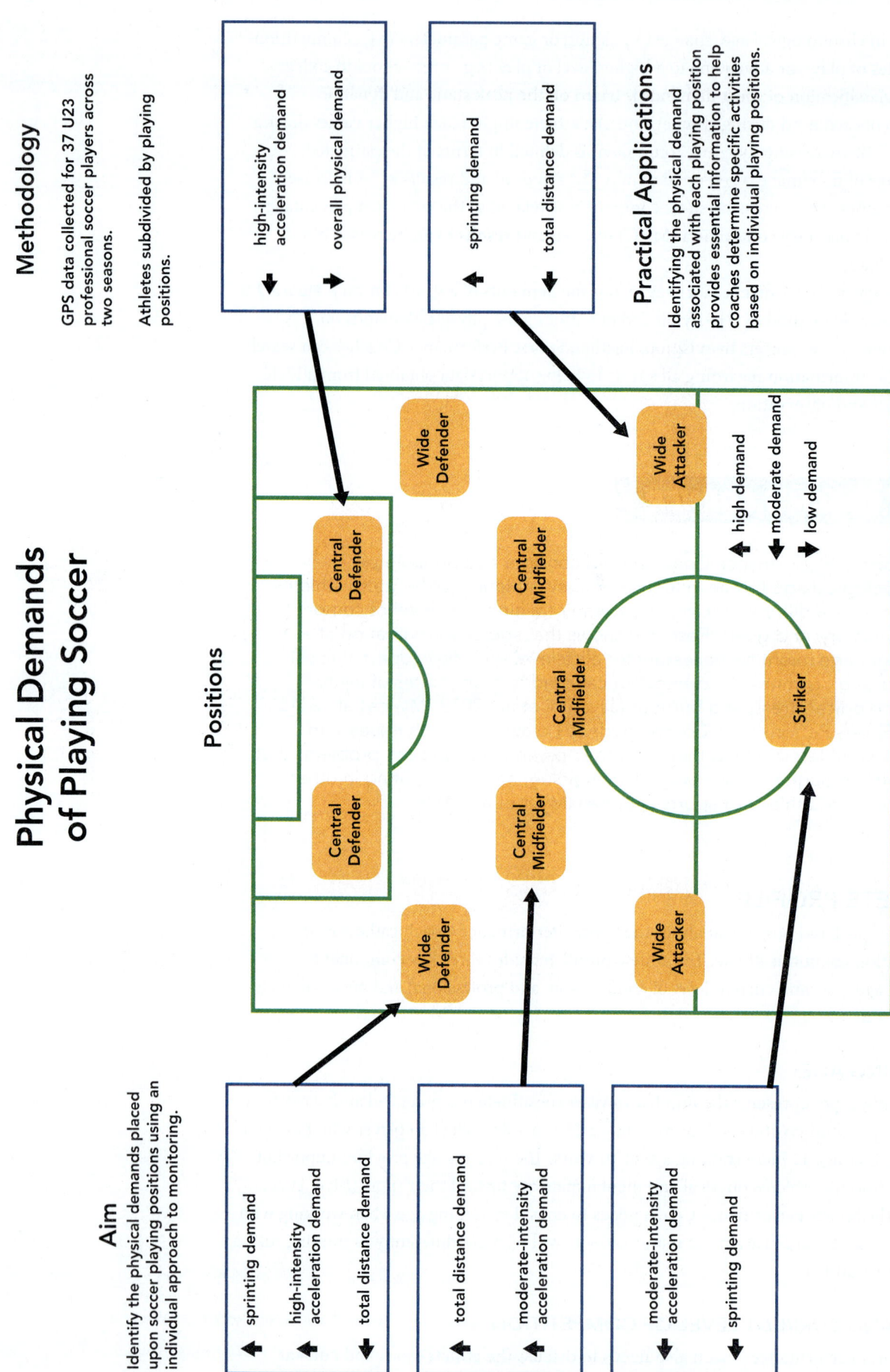

Methodology

GPS data collected for 37 U23 professional soccer players across two seasons.

Athletes subdivided by playing positions.

high-intensity acceleration demand

overall physical demand

sprinting demand

total distance demand

Practical Applications

Identifying the physical demand associated with each playing position provides essential information to help coaches determine specific activities based on individual playing positions.

Physical Demands of Playing Soccer

Aim

Identify the physical demands placed upon soccer playing positions using an individual approach to monitoring.

Positions

Wide Defender

Central Defender

Central Defender

Central Midfielder

Central Midfielder

Wide Defender

Wide Attacker

Striker

Wide Attacker

high demand

moderate demand

low demand

sprinting demand

high-intensity acceleration demand

total distance demand

total distance demand

moderate-intensity acceleration demand

moderate-intensity acceleration demand

sprinting demand

FIGURE 7.5 Physical Demands on Professional Soccer Players

Data from Abbott, W., Brickley, G., & Smeeton, N. J. (2018). Physical demands of playing position within English Premier League academy soccer.

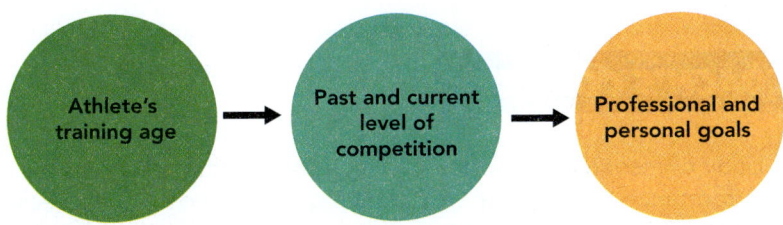

FIGURE 7.6 Components of the Athlete Profile

high school, collegiate, or professional levels. The athlete's competition level influences their training program and adherence. For example, a middle school basketball player might participate in team practice twice per week, whereas a high school player might practice three or more times per week. As a result, the older athlete might be used to a higher frequency of training and games, which can influence their adherence to a multimodal program that includes sports practices, competition, and sports performance training.

Or consider a competitive adult athlete with a full-time job. Their competition level might be high, but their training program might be limited due to their work schedule, which can influence their programming and adherence. In some situations, the athlete's training session time or frequency might need to be modified to accommodate their busy schedule. The Sports Performance Coach might also need to recommend time-efficient training exercises the athlete can do on their own to keep their fitness level and work toward their goals. The Sports Performance Coach must be prepared to work with athletes of all competition levels and be flexible with their weekly schedules and ability to train on multiple days.

PROFESSIONAL AND PERSONAL GOALS

The final component of the athlete profile is professional and personal goals. The Sports Performance Coach needs to help define the athlete's personal and professional goals because they help guide the training program. The Sports Performance Coach is encouraged to use SMART (specific, measurable, attainable, realistic, and timely) goals when establishing training goals collaboratively with the athlete. Professional goals reflect input from the athlete's sports coaches on what needs to be done to improve performance during training and competition. For example, a coach might tell a college volleyball player that they will be playing a new position in the upcoming season that requires a high vertical jump. In turn, the coach and the athlete set a professional goal of increasing the athlete's vertical jump height by a certain distance during the off-season. Personal goals are set by the individual and reflect their needs and desires regarding performance training. For example, the volleyball player might also set a personal goal of stretching weekly to improve their flexibility.

Goal setting is an important component of any athlete's performance training program. Research shows that goal setting helps to improve an athlete's training and competition performance throughout the season (Mellalieu et al., 2006; Simões et al., 2012; Wack et al., 2014).

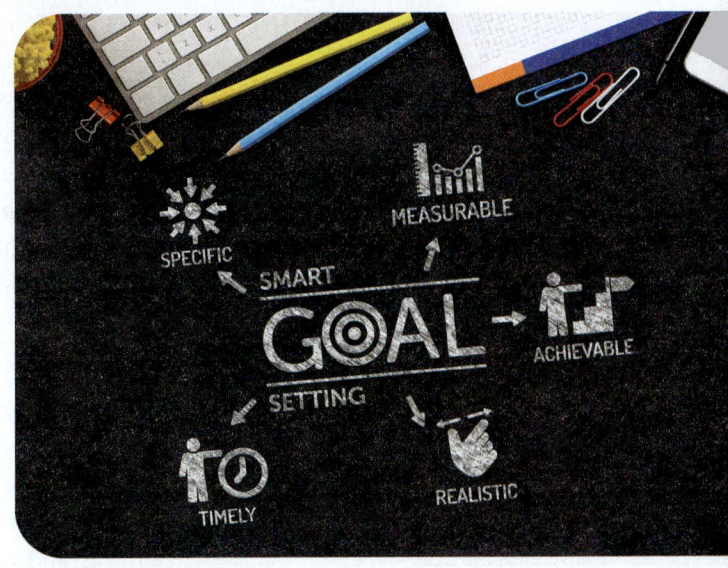

© Garagestock/Shutterstock

LESSON 3: BIOMETRIC ASSESSMENTS

PHYSIOLOGICAL ASSESSMENTS

PHYSIO-LOGICAL ASSESSMENTS →

Measurements of the human body or characteristics, including those obtained from smartwatches and other wearable devices.

Physiological assessments or biometrics provide valuable information about the athlete's overall health. Common methods of assessment include measuring resting heart rate, heart rate variability, oxygen saturation, and blood pressure. The Sports Performance Coach must have a comprehensive understanding of the parameters and normative values for these assessments to accurately monitor the athlete's condition.

RESTING HEART RATE

The resting heart rate (RHR) is taken at the base of the thumb (radial pulse; the preferred location) or on the neck to the side of the windpipe (carotid pulse; use with caution). Typical RHR ranges between 60 and 100 beats per minute (bpm), with an average of 70 bpm for men and 75 bpm for women. A stable assessment of an athlete's RHR is helpful when monitoring training status. If the resting pulse rate continues to decline, it is safe to assume an athlete's fitness is improving (Reimers et al., 2018). Athletes who demonstrate a higher RHR might be overtraining, be stressed, or have an underlying medical issue (Aune et al., 2017; Dressendorfer et al., 1985; Kreher, 2016). If the athlete is not feeling well and demonstrates an atypical RHR, the Sports Performance Coach can further assess and possibly refer the athlete to a qualified healthcare professional. **Table 7.5** provides normative data for adults.

BLOOD PRESSURE

Another common physiological assessment conducted on athletes is blood pressure measurements. Either the Sports Performance Coach or a sports medicine team member can check blood pressure. Current guidelines from the American Heart Association classify the typical blood pressure as a systolic pressure less than 120 millimeters of mercury (mm Hg) and a diastolic pressure less than 80 mm Hg (**Table 7.6**) (Muntner et al., 2019). The Sports Performance Coach must use an accurate digital blood pressure monitor

© Maridav/Shutterstock

TABLE 7.5 Resting Heart Rate Norms for Males and Females (beats per minute)

	Age	Athlete	Very Good	Above Average	Average	Below Average	Poor
Men	12–15	52–59	60–65	65–73	74–82	83–90	91–101
	16–19	46–55	56–60	61–68	69–77	78–86	87–94
	20–39	47–54	55–60	61–68	69–75	76–83	84–94
	40–59	46–54	55–60	61–67	68–76	77–84	85–94
	60–79	45–53	54–59	60–66	67–74	75–83	84–97
Women	12–15	54–62	63–69	70–78	79–86	87–93	94–102
	16–19	50–61	62–68	69–76	77–84	85–93	94–102
	20–39	52–59	60–65	66–73	74–81	82–88	89–98
	40–59	51–58	59–63	64–70	71–78	79–85	86–95
	60–79	52–58	59–63	64–69	70–77	78–85	86–95

Data from from Ostchega, Y., Porter, K. S., Hughes, J., Dillon, C. F., & Nwankwo, T. (2011). Resting pulse rate reference data for children, adolescents, and adults: United States, 1999-2008. *National Health Statistics Report*, (41), 1–16.

TABLE 7.6 Blood Pressure Classification Ranges

Classification	Systolic Blood Pressure (mm Hg)	Diastolic Blood Pressure (mm Hg)	Recommendation
Normal	<120	<80	Maintain
Elevated	120–129	<80	Lifestyle changes
Stage 1 hypertension	130–139	80–89	Lifestyle changes and medical monitoring
Stage 2 hypertension	≥140	≥90	Lifestyle changes, medical monitoring, and medications
Hypertensive crisis	>180	>120	Seek immediate medical attention

Data from: Muntner, P., Shimbo, D., Carey, R. M., Charleston, J. B., Gaillard, T., Misra, S., Myers, M. G., Ogedegbe, G., Schwartz, J. E., Townsend, R. R., Urbina, E. M., Viera, A. J., White, W. B., & Wright, J. T. (2019). Measurement of blood pressure in humans: A scientific statement from the American Heart Association. *Hypertension, 73*(5), e35–e66. https://doi.org/doi:10.1161/HYP.0000000000000087

to obtain the most accurate results (Stergiou et al., 2018). Several commercial brands of monitors meet international standards (Mengden et al., 2000).

For some athletes, monitoring the blood pressure before, during, and after exercise can help coaches gain insight into their cardiac response to exercise. Typically, exercise lowers blood pressure after training in healthy individuals (Carpio-Rivera et al., 2016; Smart et al., 2019). If the athlete presents with elevated blood pressure values, the Sports Performance Coach should suggest they see a qualified healthcare professional.

OXYGEN SATURATION

Oxygen saturation (SpO_2) is reported as a percentage and shows the fraction of oxygenated hemoglobin relative to an athlete's total amount of hemoglobin. Oxygen saturation is often monitored using a pulse oximeter (**Figure 7.7**). In healthy adults, the range for oxygen saturation is 95% to 100% (DeMeulenaere, 2007; Elder et al., 2015). Pulse oximetry is a reliable technology for measuring oxygen saturation (Jubran, 2015). The Sports Performance Coach can use oxygen saturation to monitor the performance of the pulmonary system (e.g., lungs) at rest, during, or after exercise.

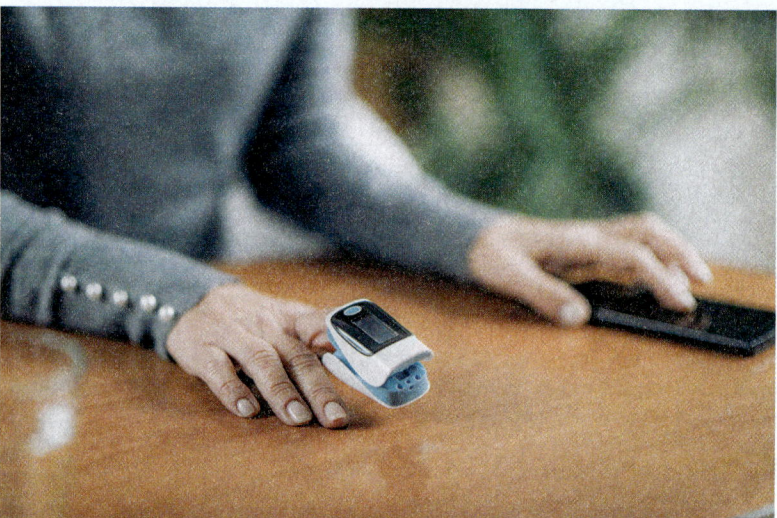

FIGURE 7.7 Pulse Oximetry Measuring SpO_2
© Microgen/Shutterstock

**SYMPATHETIC →
NERVOUS
SYSTEM (SNS)**

Subdivision of the autonomic nervous system that works to increase neural activity and put the body in a heightened state of arousal.

Monitoring an athlete's oxygen saturation is essential because low blood oxygen (hypoxemia) can adversely affect organ systems, including the brain, heart, and kidneys (DeMeulenaere, 2007; Hafen & Sharma, 2021). In general, healthy athletes with normal oxygen saturation values do not recognize significant changes either day to day or over time in response to program progressions.

HEART RATE VARIABILITY

Heart rate variability (HRV) measures the variation in time between each heartbeat; it is commonly reported in milliseconds. HRV provides quantifiable and noninvasive insights into the current state of an athlete's autonomic nervous system (ANS) and its two branches: the **sympathetic nervous system (SNS)** and the **parasympathetic nervous system (PNS)** (Tiwari et al., 2021). The SNS (fight-or-flight) response increases the heart rate, and the PNS (rest-and-digest) response slows the heart rate. HRV is a product of the interaction of these two systems. It is also influenced by variables such as pathology, psychology, environment, lifestyle, and genetics (Tiwari et al., 2021). In general, HRV values fluctuate daily in relation to the current state of the nervous system.

A high HRV is generally a positive sign, indicating that the SNS and PNS are working together to maintain a stable heart rate, which indicates a healthy ANS with good

**PARA-
SYMPATHETIC →
NERVOUS
SYSTEM (PNS)**

Subdivision of the autonomic nervous system that works to decrease neural activity and put the body in a more relaxed state.

adaptability and resilience (Shaffer & Ginsberg, 2017; Tiwari et al., 2021). A high HRV also suggests the cardiac system is able to effectively adjust to different physiological intrinsic (e.g., psychological stress) and extrinsic (e.g., sports training) changes (Fournié et al., 2021).

If an individual has low HRV, then one of the systems is more active—most commonly the SNS. Low HRV during rest indicates that the athlete might be fatigued, stressed, sick, or overtrained (Hourani et al., 2020; Kajaia et al., 2017; Kim et al., 2018; Kreher & Schwartz, 2012). In this case, the Sports Performance Coach might need to adjust the athlete's training program to allow for more rest and recovery. Low HRV is also linked to chronic diseases such as cardiac disease, metabolic syndrome, and chronic respiratory disease (Fournié et al., 2021; Prinsloo et al., 2014).

HRV technology is still emerging, and certain medical conditions can cause low and high HRV responses (Shaffer & Ginsberg, 2017) (**Figure 7.8**). Thus, HRV analysis must not be considered an absolute marker of the athlete's performance and response to training, but instead viewed as one part of the comprehensive sports performance assessment.

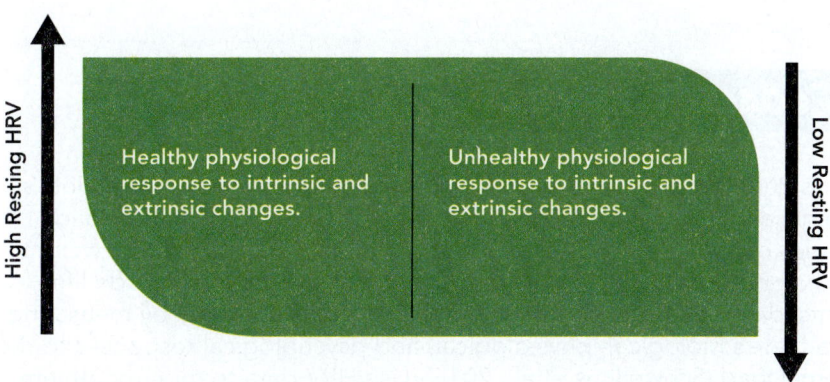

FIGURE 7.8 Resting HRV Responses

📋 COACH'S CORNER

HRV can be a valuable biomarker of an athlete's health and performance (Pagaduan et al., 2020). HRV biofeedback tracks the athlete before, during, and after sports training or competition. The resulting data provide insights into the efficiency of the athlete's body in preparing itself for strenuous activity, maintaining high levels of physiological performance, and adequately recovering. Over the past 5 years, scientists have developed different types of wearable technologies, such as watches, wristbands, and jewelry, that track HRV. The data from these wearable devices might not be as valid and reliable as the gold standard for medical or clinical situations (electrocardiography [EKG]), but they are still accurate enough for general HRV tracking (Dobbs et al., 2019; Stone et al., 2021) and are much more user friendly.

The Sports Performance Coach needs a good understanding of the physiological assessment and normative ranges. This knowledge helps to detect medical issues during the assessment or when the athlete is being monitored. **Table 7.7** summarizes the normative ranges for physiological measurements.

TABLE 7.7 Physiological Assessment Normative Ranges

Biometric	Normative Range	Normal Trend
Resting heart rate (RHR)	60 to 100 beats per minute	Minimal change day to day; steady change over time
Heart rate variability (HRV)	Dependent upon age, gender, physical fitness, and genetics; assessed at individual level	Up to 20% fluctuation day to day; steady change in baseline over time
Oxygen saturation (SpO_2)	95% to 100%	Minimum change day to day or over time
Blood pressure	<120 mm Hg systolic blood pressure <80 mm Hg diastolic blood pressure	Some changes day to day and throughout the day in response to exercise, stress, and diet

📋 COACH'S CORNER

Sports Performance Coaches can also consider monitoring the athlete's external and internal training loads. Measuring external training load includes quantifying the athlete's hours of training, distance run, weight lifted, or number of games played. Other external factors include life events, daily stressors, and travel. Internal load is assessed by measuring the athlete's biological, physiological, and psychological responses to the external load (Schwellnus et al., 2016). Use HRV data to monitor athlete internal loads and adjust the athlete's program accordingly. For example, if an athlete demonstrates a consistent pattern of low HRV during sleep, they might be overtraining and require external load modification.

BODY COMPOSITION ASSESSMENTS

BODY COMPOSITION ASSESSMENTS

Methods used to measure the proportions of different tissues in the body, such as fat, muscle, and bone.

Body composition assessments are methods used to measure the proportions of different tissues in the body, such as fat, muscle, and bone. These measures can be less common among athletes versus a general fitness athlete who needs to lose weight for health reasons, but some sports and positions may have preferred body compositions. Research shows that body composition is related to athletic performance. Low body fat and higher lean muscle mass have positive effects on performance in different sports (Durkalec-Michalski et al., 2019; Turnagöl, 2016). For example, researchers have found that a relatively low body fat percentage and consistent training at a near-race pace are predictors for fast marathon times among competitive runners (Barandun et al., 2012; Thuany et al., 2021). In similar findings, other researchers have reported that reduced body fat and higher lean muscle mass are correlated with improved performance for cross-country skiers, Paralympic swimmers, handball athletes, youth soccer players, military soldiers, and elite track and field athletes (Esco et al., 2018; Hermassi et al., 2020; Högström et al., 2012; Medeiros et al., 2016; Orantes-Gonzalez et al., 2021; Tsukahara et al., 2020). Further, tracking body fat during the offseason is valuable for coaches and the sports medicine team to gain insight into an athlete's overall nutritional and health status.

When an athlete wants to lose body fat, the Sports Performance Coach might need to work with the athlete's healthcare team (e.g., medical doctor, registered dietician) to determine a healthy competitive body composition level. This information can guide the athlete's training program and nutrient intake, with the latter program being led by the registered dietician.

Some common methods for measuring body composition are bioelectrical impedance, air displacement plethysmography, and dual-energy X-ray absorptiometry.

BIOELECTRICAL IMPEDANCE

Bioelectrical impedance analysis (BIA) is an easy body composition assessment that a Sports Performance Coach can administer to athletes. This technology does not require additional hands-on training or tables to reference. In this technique, sensors are applied to the skin, and a weak electrical current runs through the body to estimate the proportion of body fat and lean body mass (Kuriyan, 2018) (**Figure 7.9**). Body weight scales with sensors, as well as handheld devices, are available to conduct this procedure. Given the advances in this technology, it's becoming more commonly used in a variety of athletic settings.

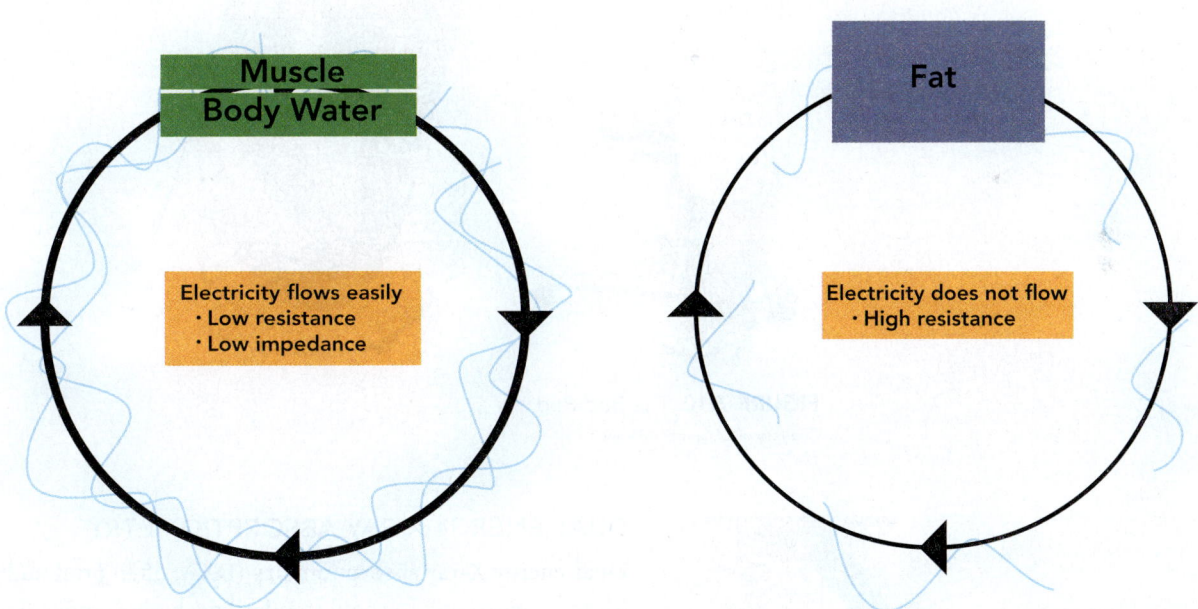

FIGURE 7.9 Bioelectrical Impedance Conduction

However, BIA does have some limitations that can compromise the accuracy of the measurements taken. These limitations include any event where the body retains or loses water (Kyle et al., 2004). Examples include fluctuating hydration levels, dehydration, extreme temperatures, heavy sweat rates, the use of diuretics, and even the volume of urine in the bladder. Further, the quality of the BIA device is an important consideration: Lower-quality devices are more likely to produce inaccurate results versus higher-quality devices that take measurements at both extremities (i.e., hands and feet). However, when the devices are used under consistent conditions, BIA is a reliable method of tracking body fat compared to baseline measures (Kyle et al., 2004).

AIR DISPLACEMENT PLETHYSMOGRAPHY (BOD POD)

Air displacement plethysmography (ADP), or simply "Bod Pod," is another type of body composition measurement that was introduced in 1995 (Ackland et al., 2012; Fields et al., 2004). This technique uses air to measure body composition as a ratio of fat to lean mass. This assessment requires more equipment and setup than BIA. For testing, the athlete sits in a closed chamber that calculates their composition based on the amount of air displaced inside the chamber (Kasper et al., 2021) (**Figure 7.10**). The Bod Pod has good accuracy and is more reliable than BIA, but it lacks portability and time efficiency due to the amount of equipment and setup (Blue et al., 2021; Rumbo-Rodríguez et al., 2021).

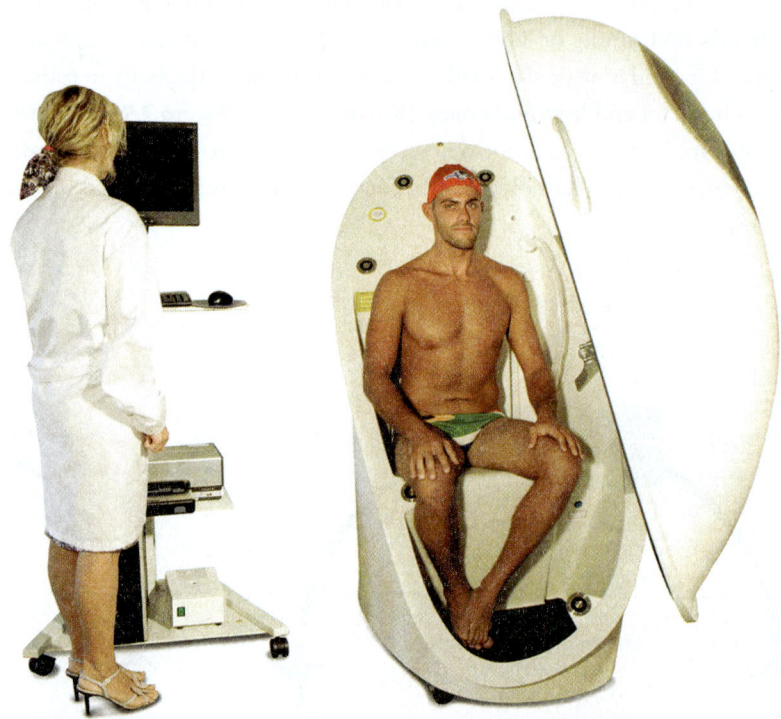

FIGURE 7.10 The Bod Pod

Courtesy of COSMED USA, Inc.

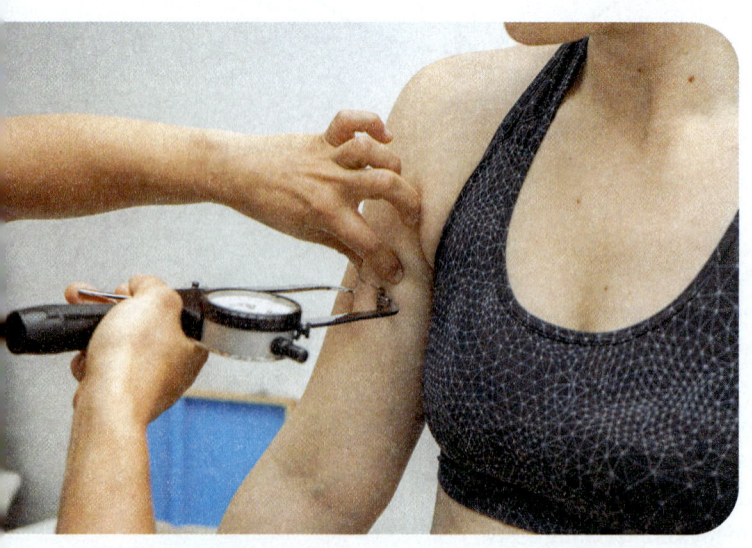

© zkolra/Shutterstock

DUAL-ENERGY X-RAY ABSORPTIOMETRY

Dual-energy X-ray absorptiometry (DXA; often pronounced "dexa") is currently the gold standard for body composition assessment (Shalof et al., 2021). DXA sends a low-energy X-ray beam into the body, which is used to calculate the percentages of tissues making up the body mass, body volume, total body water, and bone mineral density (Smith-Ryan et al., 2017). The DXA measures lean mass indirectly by subtracting the fat tissue mass and bone density from the soft-tissue mass (Li et al., 2021). This technique requires the use of expensive equipment, however, and must be administered by a qualified healthcare professional in a clinical setting (**Figure 7.11**). Despite being a gold standard, DXA is costlier and more challenging to perform versus other forms of body composition testing, such as BIA or the Bod Pod.

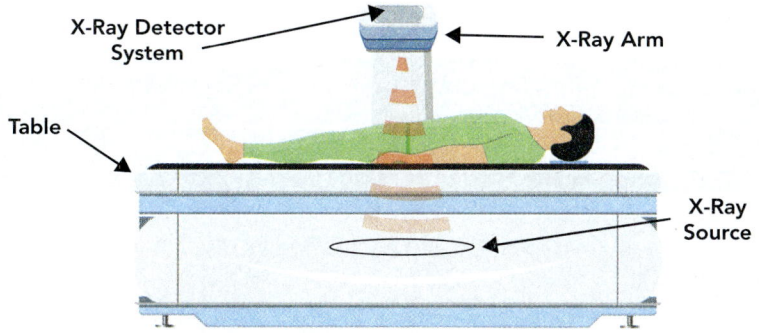

FIGURE 7.11 Dual-Energy X-Ray Absorptiometry

BODY COMPOSITION NORMATIVE DATA

The Sports Performance Coach must consider that common body fat percentage ranges determined over three decades ago are still used as normative values for athletes today (Fleck, 1983; Gibson et al., 2009; Wilmore, 1983). Recent research provides contemporary values for selected sports among biological male and female athletes (Gibson et al., 2009). **Table 7.8** compares the contemporary and traditional body fat percentages for athletes participating in selected sports (Gibson et al., 2009). The normative values presented in the table are for general reference and are not absolutes. Individual variations exist among athletes in different sports and positions. The Sports Performance Coach can work closely with a qualified healthcare professional if a specific body fat percentage range is a performance or training goal for the athlete (Ackland et al., 2012).

TABLE 7.8 Contemporary and Traditional Body Fat Percentages by Sport

Male		
Sport	Contemporary Values* (%)	Traditional Range of Values (%)
Baseball	9	12–15
Basketball	7	7–11
Football	10	9–19
Golf	8	Not reported
Ski	6	7–14
Soccer	5	10
Track	4	6–20
Distance	3	6–13
Sprints	4	8–16
Tennis	6	15–16

(continues)

TABLE 7.8 Contemporary and Traditional Body Fat Percentages by Sport (*continued*)

Female		
Sport	Contemporary Values* (%)	Traditional Range of Values (%)
Softball	24	22
Basketball	18	20–27
Volleyball	21	16–25
Golf	24	Not reported
Ski	19	16–21
Soccer	19	Not reported
Track	17	10–25
Distance	15	10–19
Sprints	16	11–19
Tennis	23	20
Rowing	24	14–18

* Rounded to the closest whole number.

Data from: Gibson, A. L., Mermier, C. M., Wilmerding, M. V., Bentzur, K. M., & McKinnon, M. M. (2009). Body fat estimation in collegiate athletes: An update. *International Journal of Athletic Therapy and Training, 14*(3), 13–16. https://doi.org/10.1123/att.14.3.13

LESSON 4: MOVEMENT ASSESSMENTS

TRANSITIONAL MOVEMENT ASSESSMENTS

**TRANSITIONAL →
MOVEMENT
ASSESSMENT**

An assessment that involves movement without a change in the base of support.

The **transitional movement assessment** is utilized as a part of an athlete's performance assessment to evaluate dynamic posture without changing the athlete's base of support. The Sports Performance Coach assesses the athlete's posture and alignment throughout each movement, viewing it from the front, side, and rear, and noting any movement that deviates from what is considered normal. Transitional movements are completed in a controlled manner, without significant effort by the athlete or feedback or cueing from the Sports Performance Coach, beyond what is needed to set up each assessment. This provides insight into the athlete's ability to perform the movement naturally.

Transitional assessments include movements that do not involve a change in the athlete's base of support. The following assessments are discussed in this section:

- Overhead squat assessment (OHSA)
- OHSA with heels elevated

- OHSA with hands on hips
- Single-leg squat assessment (SLSA)
- Split squat assessment (SSA)
- Star excursion balance test (SEBT)

The Sports Performance Coach is encouraged to have the athlete perform these movements in this order to progressively challenge the athlete. Further, athletes should perform only the assessments deemed necessary based on the assessment of their prior performance (**Figure 7.12**). For example, an athlete who shows no compensations in the OHSA can go directly to the SSA because there is no need to complete the modified OHSA. Conversely, an athlete who demonstrates significant lower-extremity compensation in the OHSA may not be safe completing the SLSA. The Sports Performance Coach must use their discretion during the assessments.

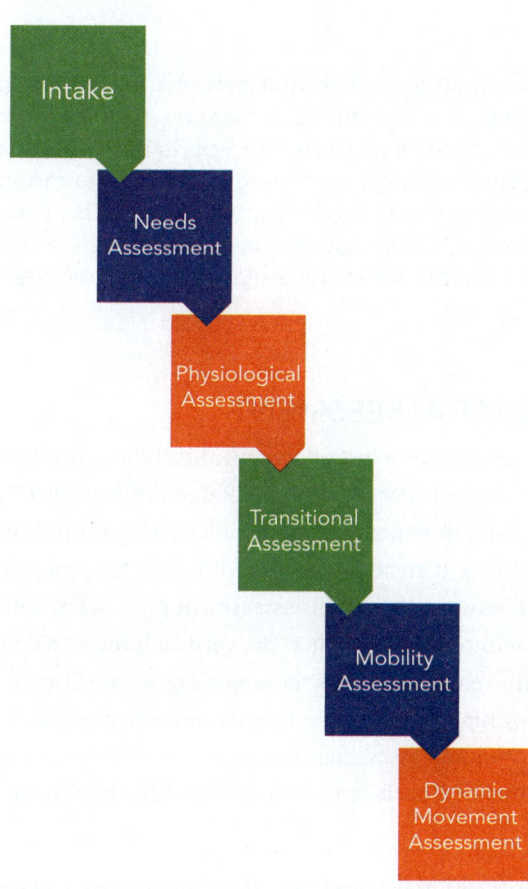

FIGURE 7.12 Transitional Movement Assessments

KINETIC CHAIN CHECKPOINTS

The Sports Performance Coach observes the athlete's movement using five kinetic chain checkpoints (KCCs): foot and ankle, knee, lumbo-pelvic-hip complex (LPHC), shoulder, and head and cervical spine. Observing the KCCs provides observable reference points of specific body regions during movement assessments. This makes it easier to identify movement impairments at a specific body area. **Figure 7.13** details the KCCs from different views.

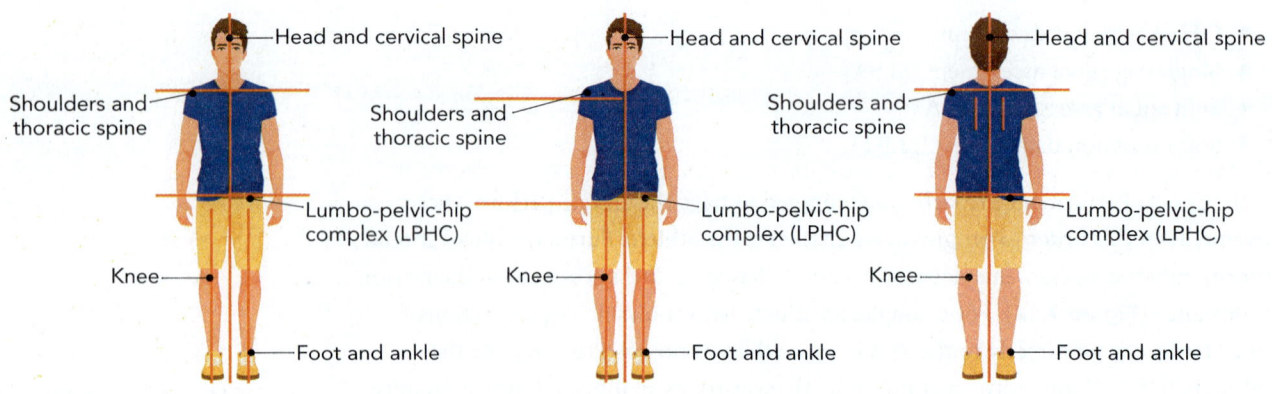

FIGURE 7.13 Kinetic Chain Checkpoint Views

OVERHEAD SQUAT ASSESSMENT

The overhead squat assessment is a test of dynamic flexibility, core strength, balance, and overall neuromuscular control (Post et al., 2017; Rabin & Kozol, 2017), and an accurate and repeatable movement assessment for professionals who administer the test (Post et al., 2017; Rabin & Kozol, 2017). If an athlete works with different professionals, the OHSA can be accurately used between them. This assessment provides an analysis of similar movements used in common sports, such as the vertical jump and defensive stance, or even more advanced movements, such as the single-leg squat (Lisman et al., 2021; Mauntel et al., 2015). The OHSA replicates lower-extremity movement patterns during jump landing tasks (e.g., depth jump assessment) (Goerger et al., 2009). It is a key assessment that the Sports Performance Coach can administer to different athletes (**Figure 7.14**).

STARTING POSITION

1. The athlete stands with their feet hip to shoulder width apart and pointed straight ahead and parallel. The foot and ankle complex are in a neutral position. If possible, the athlete should remove their shoes, so the assessor can view the foot and ankle.
2. The athlete raises their arms overhead, extended and aligned with the torso.

MOVEMENT

1. Instruct the athlete to squat to a depth that brings the femur parallel to the ground, roughly the height of a chair, and then return to the starting position. The athlete can reduce the squat depth if they have discomfort with a deeper squat.
2. Have the athlete repeat the movement for five repetitions for each view, observing from anterior, lateral, and posterior views (**Figure 7.15**).

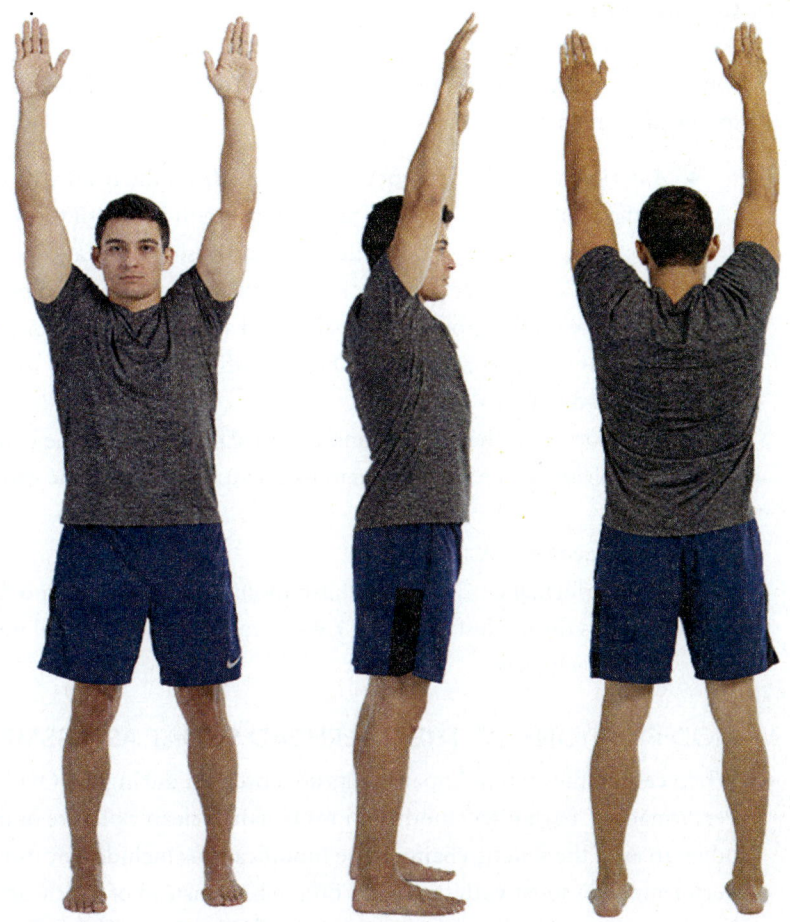

FIGURE 7.14 Overhead Squat Starting Position Views

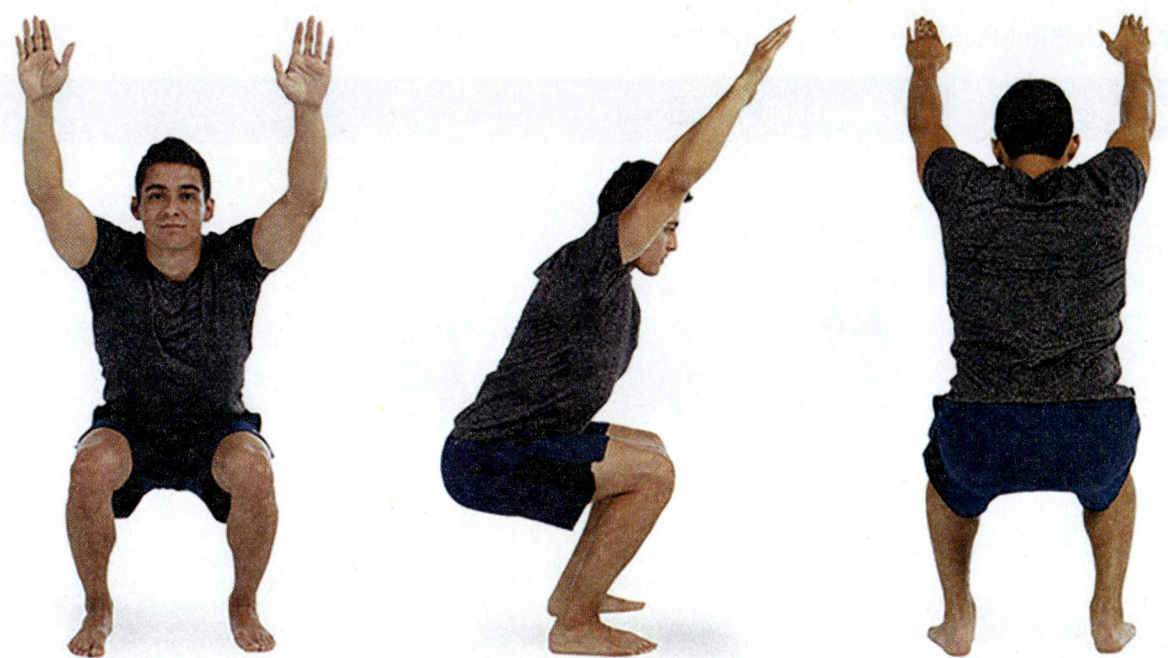

FIGURE 7.15 Overhead Squat Assessment Views

OBSERVATION

Each viewpoint requires the assessor to focus on specific KCCs. The assessor can see some impairments from more than one view. An ideal OHSA performance includes the following elements:

- *Anterior:* View the feet, knees, and LPHC from the front. The feet and hips remain in the sagittal plane with the knees tracking in line with the foot (second and third toes). The LPHC does not shift from side to side or rotate.
- *Lateral:* View the feet, ankles, knees, LPHC, shoulders, and head from the side. The heels stay on the ground. The pelvis and spine remain in a neutral posture. The torso remains in parallel with the tibia while the arms stay in line with the torso. The head remains neutral.
- *Posterior:* View the feet and ankles and shoulders from the back. The arch of the foot and calcaneus (i.e., heel) remain in a neutral position. The shoulders are neutral.

MOVEMENT COMPENSATIONS

The Sports Performance Coach must also monitor for potential movement impairments or compensations during testing. **Table 7.9** summarizes the potential movement impairments observed for each view.

MODIFICATIONS TO THE OVERHEAD SQUAT ASSESSMENT

When certain movement impairments are observed during the OHSA, the Sports Performance Coach offers modifications to gain a clearer picture of the probable causes in other areas of the kinetic chain. These modifications include elevating the athlete's heels or performing the squat with the hands on the hips instead of overhead. These modifications improve an individual's performance of the OHSA (Richards et al., 2016), which is an indication that one or more of the joints impacted by the modification is related to the movement impairment identified in the traditional OHSA.

TABLE 7.9 OHSA: Movement Impairments

Impairment View	Observations
Anterior - Foot and ankle: Feet flatten and turn out - Knee: Valgus or varus	 Feet flatten Feet turn out Knees move inward Knees move outward

Impairment View	Observations

Lateral
 	
• Foot and ankle: Heel rise
 	
• Knee: Knee dominance
 	
• LPHC:
  • Excessive anterior pelvic tilt
  • Excessive posterior pelvic tilt
  • Excessive forward trunk lean
 	
• Shoulder: Arms fall forward
 	
• Head and cervical spine: Forward head
	
	Low back arch Low back round Excessive forward lean Arms fall forward
	
	Forward head

Posterior • Foot and ankle: Excessive foot pronation, heel rise • LPHC: Asymmetrical weight shift	 Feet flatten Heels elevate Asymmetrical weight shift

The modifications systematically remove major joint segments to identify the likely cause of the primary movement impairments. For this reason, NASM recommends performing only one modification at a time to note the influence it has on the rest of the kinetic chain. The modifications should serve as general guidance on the most probable cause of impairments. The Sports Performance Coach can use this information to guide additional testing, such as mobility.

Heels Elevated

If an athlete exhibits movement impairments at the foot and ankle complex, knee, or LPHC, the root cause might be found at the foot and ankle complex or the LPHC. For example, knee valgus might be an impairment caused by a lack of ankle dorsiflexion or muscle imbalances at the hip, such as overactive adductors and underactive gluteals. Elevating the heels during a squat (**Figure 7.16**) places the ankle in plantar flexion, which decreases the extensibility required from the plantar flexor muscles (gastrocnemius, soleus). If the knee valgus is related to ankle dorsiflexion restriction, this modification will improve knee alignment. If the knee valgus is not related to ankle dorsiflexion restriction, this modification will not improve knee alignment.

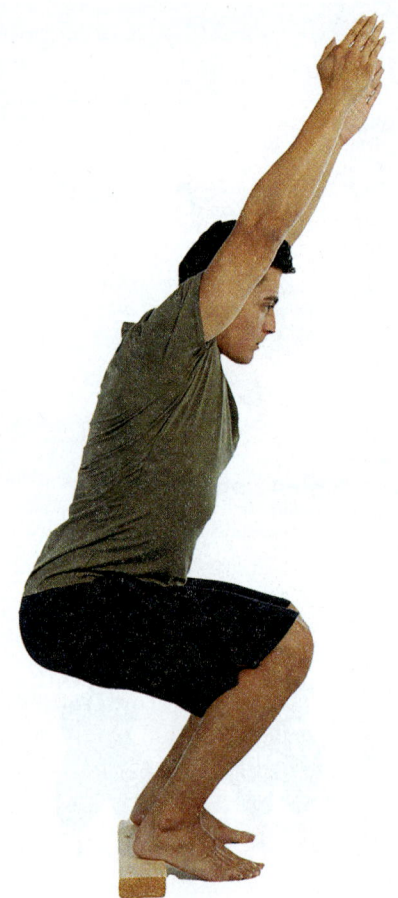

FIGURE 7.16 OHSA with Heels Elevated

Excessive forward trunk lean is another compensation that relates to foot and ankle or LPHC limitations. If the heels-elevated modification improves the squat, then the foot and ankle complex is likely the cause of the excessive forward lean. However, if the modification does not improve the squat, then the cause is likely at the LPHC.

Elevating the heels allows the Sports Performance Coach to see the influence that the ankle has on the individual's deviations (Richards et al., 2016). If an athlete displays a movement impairment during the overhead squat that improves after elevating the heels, then the Sports Performance Coach can include flexibility and activation exercises to improve ankle dorsiflexion prior to more advanced sport movements.

If additional mobility testing is needed, then the Sports Performance Coach should prioritize testing the foot and ankle complex.

Hands on Hips

When the Sports Performance Coach observes an excessive anterior pelvic tilt during the OHSA, the cause may be either above or below the LPHC. The anterior pelvic tilt can be caused by an overactive and short latissimus dorsi pulling upward on the posterior hip when the arms are placed in the overhead position. Conversely, an overactive and short hip flexor complex could pull down on the anterior hip. Placing the hands on the hips directly removes the stretch placed on the latissimus dorsi and other shoulder extensors (**Figure 7.17**), allowing the Sports Performance Coach to see the influence the upper body has on the athlete's impairments (McMillian et al., 2016).

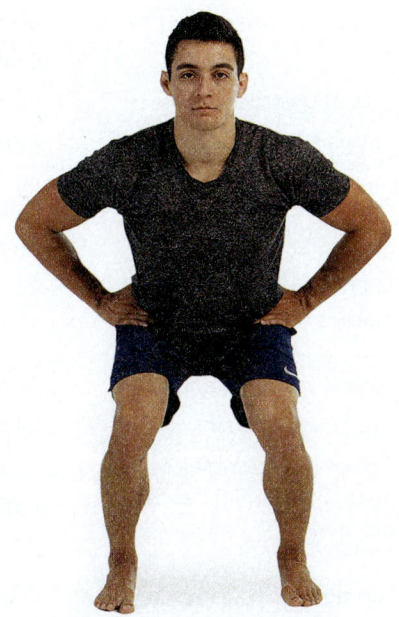

FIGURE 7.17 OHSA with Hands on Hips

If an athlete demonstrates an excessive anterior pelvic tilt during the OHSA, but it is corrected when performing the squat with the hands on the hips, then the primary region that most likely needs to be addressed is the latissimus dorsi. If the impairment still exists with the hands on the hips, then the primary region needing to be addressed is the hip flexor complex.

REPORTING RESULTS

When performing the OHSA or OHSA modifications, the Sports Performance Coach identifies movement impairment at the different KCCs and then records all findings on the Overhead Squat Assessment Observation Findings Template found in Appendix E. Movement assessments reveal the group of overactive and underactive muscles that might potentially relate to a particular movement impairment (**Table 7.10**).

SINGLE-LEG SQUAT ASSESSMENT

The single-leg squat assessment is a progression to the OHSA. This transitional movement assessment also assesses dynamic posture, balance, and neuromuscular control in a more-advanced, single-limb stance. The SLSA is an accurate and repeatable method to identify movement impairments, such as knee valgus, when administered by one or more professionals (Garrick et al., 2018; Räisänen et al., 2016; Ressman et al., 2019;

TABLE 7.10 OHSA: Overactive and Underactive Muscles

View	Checkpoint	Impairment	Probable Overactive Muscles	Probable Underactive Muscles
Anterior	Feet	Turn out	Soleus Lateral gastrocnemius Biceps femoris (short head) Tensor fascia latae (TFL)	Medial gastrocnemius Medial hamstring Gluteus medius/maximus Gracilis, popliteus, sartorius
	Knees	Move inward (valgus)	Adductor complex Biceps femoris (short head) TFL Lateral gastrocnemius Vastus lateralis	Medial hamstring Medial gastrocnemius Gluteus medius/maximus Vastus medialis oblique Anterior/posterior tibialis
		Move outward (varus)	Piriformis Biceps femoris TFL/gluteus minimus and medius	Adductor complex Medial hamstring Gluteus maximus
Lateral	LPHC	Excessive forward lean	Soleus/gastrocnemius Hip flexor complex Abdominal complex (rectus abdominis, external obliques)	Anterior tibialis Gluteus maximus Erector spinae Intrinsic core stabilizers
		Low back arches	Hip flexor Erector spinae Latissimus dorsi	Gluteus maximus Hamstrings Intrinsic core stabilizers
		Low back rounds	Hamstrings Adductor magnus Rectus abdominis External obliques	Gluteus maximus Erector spinae Intrinsic core stabilizers Hip flexor complex Latissimus dorsi
	Shoulders	Arms fall forward	Latissimus dorsi Pectoralis major/minor Coracobrachialis Teres major	Mid/lower trapezius Rhomboids Posterior deltoid Rotator cuff
Posterior	Feet	Flattens	Peroneal complex Lateral gastrocnemius Biceps femoris (short head) TFL	Anterior/posterior tibialis Medial gastrocnemius Gluteus medius
		Heel rises	Soleus	Anterior tibialis

View	Checkpoint	Impairment	Probable Overactive Muscles	Probable Underactive Muscles
	LPHC	Asymmetrical weight shift	Same side of shift • Adductor complex/TFL Opposite side of shift • Gastrocnemius/soleus • Piriformis • Biceps femoris • Gluteus medius	Same side of shift • Gluteus medius Opposite side of shift • Anterior tibialis • Adductor complex

Ugalde et al., 2015). This stance is the most challenging of the lower-extremity transitional assessments due to the single-limb strength and balance required (Agresta et al., 2017; Gianola et al., 2017).

Athletes who perform well during this test also have greater hip abductor strength and activation (Crossley et al., 2011; Garrick et al., 2018). This test is used for athletes who perform the OHSA with optimal form. Additionally, it is used to assess issues of trunk rotation (which typically do not present during the OHSA) or when considering the use of single-leg exercises with athletes, to test their readiness for such single-leg movements.

The SLSA (**Figure 7.18**) is also a good assessment of an individual's ability to balance, which is an important functional consideration for many different sports. Avoid this assessment for athletes who might have an existing lower-extremity injury (e.g., knee injury). Anticipate that athletes who complain of knee pain may display significant compensatory movement impairments at other joints when completing this assessment (Nakagawa et al., 2012).

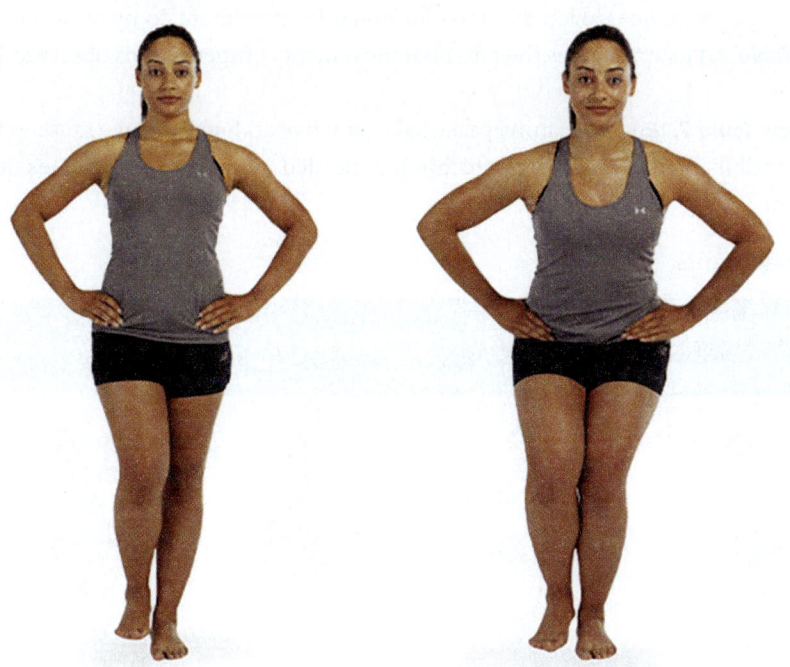

FIGURE 7.18 Single-Leg Squat Assessment

STARTING POSITION

1. Have the athlete stand on one leg with their hands on the hips and eyes focused forward.
2. The stance foot is pointed straight ahead and the foot, ankle, knee, and the LPHC in a neutral position.
3. The non-weight-bearing knee is flexed with the foot next to, but not touching, the stance limb's calf.

MOVEMENT

1. Have the athlete squat as deep as is comfortable and controllable, and return to the starting position.
2. Perform up to five repetitions per view, then repeat on the opposite leg. Perform at a comfortable pace without using momentum to bounce out of the bottom.

OBSERVATION

Each viewpoint requires focus on specific kinetic chain checkpoints. For each, ideal performance of the single-leg squat is represented by the following elements:

- *Anterior:* View the feet, knees, and LPHC from the front. The feet and hips remain in the sagittal plane with the knees tracking in line with the foot (second and third toes). The LPHC remain level and does not rotate or shift from side to side beyond what is needed to first obtain balance.
- *Lateral:* View the feet, ankles, knees, and LPHC from the side. The heel stays on the ground. The pelvis and spine remain in a neutral posture. The torso remains parallel with the tibia.
- *Posterior:* View the feet and ankles from the back. The arch of the foot and calcaneus remain in a neutral position.

MOVEMENT COMPENSATIONS

The Sports Performance Coach monitors for potential movement compensations during testing. **Table 7.11** summarizes the potential movement compensations observed for each view.

Review **Table 7.12** to determine potential overactive and underactive muscles to address flexibility and strengthening techniques needed to improve the athlete's quality of movement.

TABLE 7.11   SLSA: Movement Impairments

Impairment View	Observations
Anterior Knee: Valgus LPHC: Hip hike Hip drop Inward/outward trunk rotation	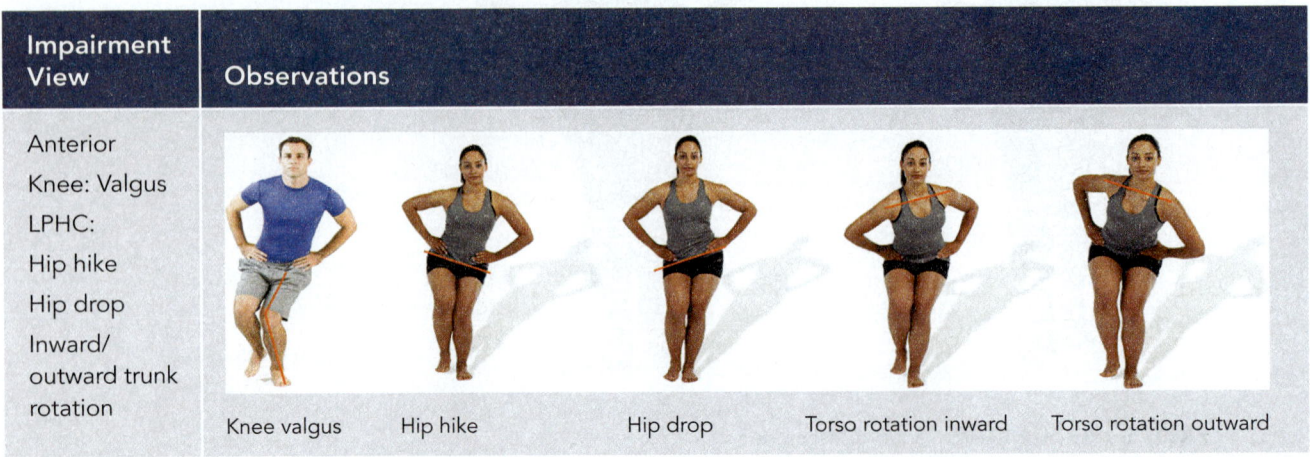 Knee valgus Hip hike Hip drop Torso rotation inward Torso rotation outward

TABLE 7.12 SLSA: Overactive and Underactive Muscles

View	Checkpoint	Impairment	Probable Overactive Muscles	Probable Underactive Muscles
Anterior	Knee	Move inward (valgus)	Adductor complex Biceps femoris (short head) Tensor fascia latae (TFL) Lateral gastrocnemius Vastus lateralis	Medial hamstring Medial gastrocnemius Gluteus medius/maximus Vastus medialis oblique
	LPHC	Hip hike	Quadratus lumborum TFL/gluteus maximus (same side)	Adductor complex (same side) Gluteus medius (same side)
		Hip drop	Adductor complex (same side)	Gluteus medius (same side) Quadratus lumborum (opposite side)
	Upper body	Inward trunk rotation	Internal obliques (same side) External obliques (opposite side) TFL (same side) Adductor complex (same side)	Internal obliques (opposite side) External obliques (same side) Gluteus medius/maximus
		Outward trunk rotation	Internal obliques (opposite side) External obliques (same side) Piriformis (same side)	Internal obliques (same side) External obliques (opposite side) Adductor complex (same side) Gluteus medius/maximus

SPLIT SQUAT ASSESSMENT

The split squat assessment (**Figure 7.19**) is used to assess dynamic posture, balance, and overall neuromuscular control while in a narrow stance. This movement mimics the stance required for a running gait and many other athletic activities (McMillian et al., 2016). The SSA is used in two ways. The first is a regression to the single-leg squat. Some athletes might not have the functional strength to complete a single-leg squat (e.g., when recovering from injury), so the split squat is used to refine observations of unilateral compensations seen during the OHSA. Second, the split squat variation can be used to gain more information for programming decisions related to split-stance movements (e.g., walking lunges, split jumps, Olympic lifting).

Although walking, running, and step lunges are sometimes used as assessments, evidence suggests that a static split squat places less stress on the knee and is safer for athletes, especially those recovering from a knee injury (Escamilla et al., 2010; Jalali et al., 2015). This movement also effectively assesses an individual's balance and hip and knee extensor eccentric strength (Jönhagen et al., 2009).

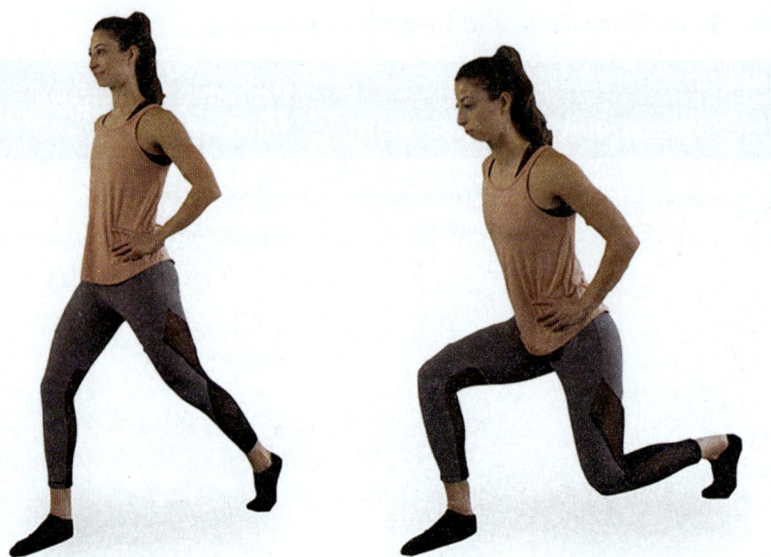

FIGURE 7.19 Split Squat Assessment

The athlete performs the split squat with one foot forward and the other foot back. Then, they switch foot positions and perform the split squat again.

STARTING POSITION

1. Have the athlete stand in a narrow, split stance with the feet parallel (no wider than hip width) and pointed straight ahead. The step length needs to be sufficient for the back knee to contact the ground behind the front foot.
2. Have the athlete place their hands on their hips while standing in an upright position.

MOVEMENT

1. Instruct the athlete to lower to a depth that brings their rear knee just above the ground without touching and return to the starting position. The front foot remains planted on the ground while the rear foot heel is allowed to rise.
2. Repeat the movement for five repetitions, observing from each position (five reps per view). Perform at a comfortable pace without using momentum to bounce out of the bottom.

OBSERVATION

Each viewpoint requires focus on specific KCCs. For each, ideal performance of the SSA is represented by the following elements:

- *Anterior:* View the feet, knees, and LPHC from the front. The feet and hips remain in the sagittal plane with the knees tracking in line with the foot (second and third toes). The LPHC does not shift from side to side or rotate.
- *Lateral:* View the feet, ankles, knees, and LPHC from the side. The front heel stays on the ground. The pelvis and spine remain in a neutral posture.
- *Posterior:* View the feet and ankles from the back. The arch of the foot and calcaneus remain in a neutral position.

MOVEMENT COMPENSATIONS

The Sports Performance Coach monitors the athlete for any movement compensations during testing. **Table 7.13** summarizes the potential movement compensations observed for each view.

TABLE 7.13 Split Squat: Movement Impairments

Impairment View	Observation

Anterior	• Knee: Valgus
	• LPHC:
	  • Asymmetric weight shift
	  • Inward/outward trunk rotation

Lateral	• Foot and ankle: Heel rise • Knee: Knee dominance (front knee) • LPHC: • Excessive forward lean
Posterior	• Foot and ankle: Excessive pronation

REPORTING RESULTS

When performing the SLSA and SSA, the Sports Performance Coach records their findings on the Single-Leg Squat and Split Squat Observational Recording Template found in Appendix E. Mobility assessments in the next stage further distinguish which muscles within a group are the primary contributors to that movement impairment, and if overactivity or underactivity is more responsible for the impairment. These refined observations lead the Sports Performance Coach to select the best exercises to address a given movement pattern or impairment.

✔ CHECK IT OUT

The Sports Performance Coach must also be aware of the foot of the trailing leg. To perform the SSA, the trailing-leg toes demonstrate near-maximal extension. Thus, toe extension restriction can lead to excessive forward trunk lean or the trailing-leg foot turning out. In case of excessive forward lean, the lack of extension prevents the athlete from lowering the rear leg, resulting in their shifting weight forward to descend in the lunge. In case of the toes turning out, an athlete with a lack of extension might allow the heel of the foot to roll inward (turning the toes outward) to move around the limitation.

STAR EXCURSION BALANCE TEST

The star excursion balance test (**Figure 7.20**) is another single-leg assessment that measures dynamic posture and neuromuscular efficiency of the testing leg and establishes objective range of motion measurements during closed-chain functional movements. The SEBT is considered a progression of the SLSA because it challenges the athlete's single-leg dynamic control in multiple positions. It is a valid and reliable movement assessment and a predictor of lower-extremity injury (Dallinga et al., 2012; Grassi et al., 2018; Gribble et al., 2012; Powden et al., 2019).

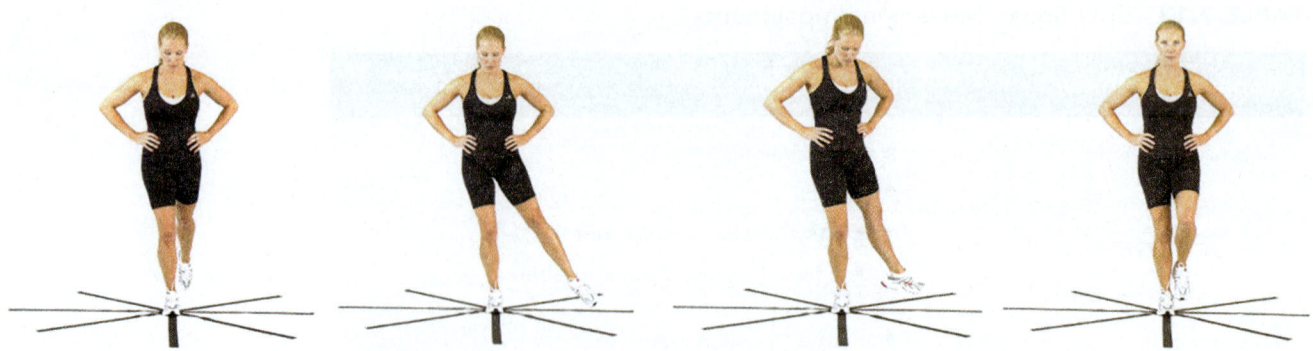

FIGURE 7.20 Star Excursion Balance Test

EQUIPMENT

Tape measure, nonslip surface, roll of tape to mark lines on ground, or star excursion balance test mat.

STARTING POSITION

1. Instruct the athlete to stand barefoot (shoes can be worn if the athlete prefers) on the test leg (stance leg) with the second and third toes on the horizontal line at the center (origin) of the three lines: anterior, posterolateral, and posteromedial. The athlete can also stand in the center of the SEBT mat.
2. Instruct the athlete to squat down as far as they can control with the knee aligned in a neutral position with hands on their hips.

MOVEMENT

1. The athlete performs up to four practice trials prior to final testing on each leg.
2. Conduct up to three recorded trials:
   a. The athlete reaches with their non-stance (opposite) leg along the designated lines.
   b. As the athlete reaches the maximum distance with the non-stance leg, they lightly touch the most distal part of their foot on the designated line while maintaining good dynamic posture.
   c. The Sports Performance Coach marks on the tape or mat where the athlete touched the designated line. The athlete then returns the reaching limb back to the starting position. Instruct the athlete to do this for all three lines.
   d. The athlete should maintain optimal alignment of the stance-leg foot and knee during the recorded trials. The final measurement is how far the athlete reached without any observable movement impairments or loss of balance.
   e. Repeat the movements for each leg.

SCORING

The Sports Performance Coach can score the SEBT using two methods.

- Method 1 (used to objectively measure an increase or decrease in performance over time):
  1. The Sports Performance Coach measures the distance the athlete reached from the horizontal line to where the athlete touched in each direction.
  2. The athlete performs three trials for each direction, and an average score is calculated for each leg.

- Method 2 (a normalized score to compare to existing data): This method requires that the athlete's leg length be measured, from the anterior inferior iliac spine to the medial malleolus.
  1. The Sports Performance Coach measures the distance the athlete reached from the horizontal line to where the athlete touched in each direction.
  2. The athlete performs three trials for each direction, and an average score is calculated for each leg.
  3. A normalized score is calculated for all directions using the following equation:

  $$\text{reach distance} / \text{leg length} \times 100$$

  This measurement is a percentage of the excursion distance in relation to an athlete's height, which allows direct comparison among groups.
  4. The reach distance values are used as an index of dynamic posture control. The farther the athlete reaches, the better their dynamic posture control is.

OBSERVATION

The Sports Performance Coach observes the athlete from the anterior, lateral, and posterior views to identify any movement compensations. During the testing, the coach observes specific KCCs from all viewpoints. For each, ideal performance of the SEBT is represented by the following elements:

- *Anterior:* View the stance foot, knee, and LPHC from the front. The foot and hips remain in the sagittal plane with the knees tracking in line with the foot (second and third toes). The LPHC remains level and does not rotate or shift from side to side beyond what is needed to first obtain balance.
- *Lateral:* View the stance foot, ankle, knee, and LPHC from the side. The heel stays on the ground. The pelvis and spine remain in a neutral posture. The torso remains parallel with the tibia.
- *Posterior:* View the stance foot and ankle from the back. The arch of the foot and calcaneus remain in a neutral position.

RECORDING FINDINGS

MOVEMENT COMPENSATIONS

The Sports Performance Coach measures the athlete's maximum distance for each line and observes the athlete for any movement compensations during testing. **Table 7.14** provides potential movement compensations for the SEBT.

TABLE 7.14   SEBT: Movement Impairments

Impairment View	Observation
Anterior	<ul><li>Knee: Valgus</li><li>LPHC:<ul><li>Asymmetric weight shift</li><li>Inward/outward trunk rotation</li></ul></li></ul>
Lateral	<ul><li>Foot and ankle: Heel rise (stance foot)</li><li>Knee: Knee dominance (stance knee)</li><li>LPHC: Excessive forward lean</li></ul>
Posterior	<ul><li>Foot and ankle: Excessive pronation</li></ul>

The Sports Performance Coach records and calculates the athlete's performance for each leg based on the normalized score, which provides the ability to directly compare legs of other athletes (Gribble & Hertel, 2003). The Sports Performance Coach also records any movement compensations observed during testing on the SEBT Recording Template found in Appendix E.

LESSON 5: RANGE OF MOTION TESTING
MOBILITY ASSESSMENTS

Optimal sports performance and movement require adequate mobility, which depends on a combination of adequate soft tissue extensibility and joint range of motion (ROM). Flexibility is defined as the normal extensibility of all soft tissues (i.e., muscle length) that allows for the full ROM of a joint. However, mobility represents more than just flexibility. It accounts for the entire available joint ROM and the body's neuromuscular control during motion (i.e., muscle length and state of neural activation). For this reason, the Sports Performance Coach can use targeted **mobility assessments** of the specific body segments to focus on and confirm the observations made during the transitional movement assessments. Factors affecting normal mobility include posture, pattern overload movements (e.g., repetitive sports movements), joint structure, age, pain, injury, gender, and psychosocial influences (e.g., stress) (Page et al., 2010). The Sports Performance Coach's ability to identify altered mobility and relate it to a movement dysfunction is vital in developing safe and effective sports performance programs for athletes.

Often, an observed movement impairment results from flexibility limitations due to overactive or shortened muscles or soft tissue, or poor neuromuscular control due to underactive or lengthened muscles. Mobility assessments help direct programming toward flexibility or strengthening strategies to address that impairment.

For example, if the Sports Performance Coach observes a movement impairment during transitional assessments but the mobility assessments do not identify a ROM limitation at the relevant KCC, poor neuromuscular control and underactive or lengthened muscles are more likely to be the culprits. In other words, the muscle underactivity on one side of the joint might be contributing more to the impairment than overactivity on the other side. In this case, the Sports Performance Coach would focus the training program design on activation (isolated strengthening) of those muscles and movement pattern integration. This also assists in avoiding unnecessary stretching techniques for muscles that already have adequate extensibility.

> **MOBILITY ASSESSMENTS** →
>
> A set of assessments designed to observe an individual's ability to move through a range of motion at various joints and segments of the body.

👍 **HELPFUL HINT**

Mobility assessments or tests provide additional valuable insights into the specific movements available at selected joints. However, if time is a constraint or if the Sports Performance Coach is uncomfortable performing mobility assessments, the information gathered from the transitional assessments is adequate for programming. Specifically, the modifications to the OHSA help to identify which major joint segment is the most probable root cause of primary compensations. In addition, the sports medicine team may be responsible for performing these assessments on athletes.

Mobility assessments must be approached within the context of global movement patterns at the five KCCs (Sueki et al., 2013). In other words, an athlete needs more specific mobility testing of a joint only if the transitional movement assessments identify a restriction. If the athlete does not demonstrate any movement impairments at a KCC, specific mobility testing for that checkpoint is not necessary. For example, if an athlete has a movement impairment at the shoulders but has normal lower-extremity dynamic posture, only upper-extremity mobility assessments need to be performed. When observing the mobility of the kinetic chain, just as with transitional movement analysis, the Sports Performance Coach needs to consider that a movement impairment at one KCC can affect adjacent regions or checkpoints (Sueki et al., 2013). Regular mobility assessments serve as feedback regarding the effectiveness of the Sports Performance Coach's programming for the athlete.

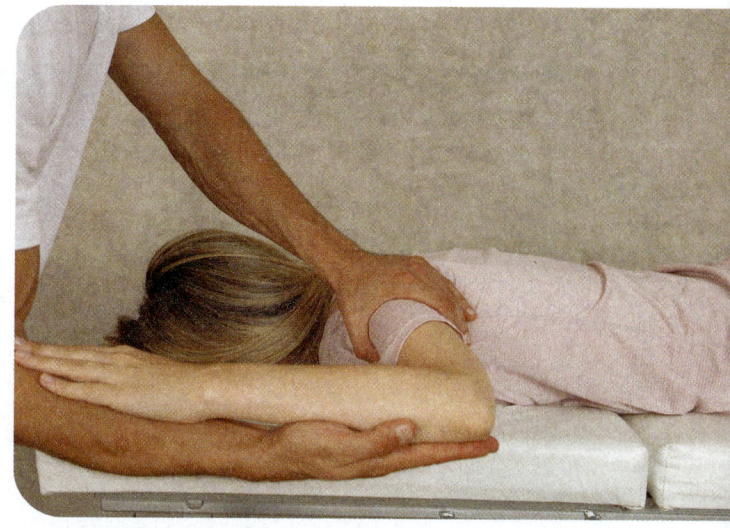

© Albina Gavrilovic/Shutterstock

FOOT AND ANKLE MOBILITY TESTING

Athletes who demonstrate the feet turning out, excessive pronation, knee valgus, or excessive forward trunk lean during the OHSA reveal mobility restrictions at the foot and ankle complex. Additional testing of the ankle can help to identify specific limitations, allowing the Sports Performance Coach to create a more individualized lower-body corrective exercise program for each athlete.

To further investigate the foot and ankle complex, begin by testing ankle dorsiflexion, and then test extension of the first metatarsophalangeal (MTP) joint (Powden et al., 2015; Sánchez-Gómez et al., 2020) (**Table 7.15**). Research shows that ankle dorsiflexion (weight-bearing lunge test) and first MTP extension tests are reliable mobility measures when administered by one or more professionals (Jones & Curran, 2012; Powden et al., 2015).

TABLE 7.15 Foot and Ankle Mobility Tests

Screening Test	Description
Ankle dorsiflexion (weight-bearing lunge test)	**Client position:** • Standing, lunge position, shoes off • Feet straight, heels planted firmly on the ground • Toes positioned approximately 2 inches away from the wall **Type of motion:** • Passive (forward test leg relaxed) **Target motions:** • Client's front (test) leg lunges toward the wall, using the hands for support • Look for the ankle and foot to reach their end range • Back foot is positioned to support overall posture

(continues)

TABLE 7.15 Foot and Ankle Mobility Tests (*continued*)

Screening Test	Description

	Verbal instructions:
	• "Keep your front foot straight and your heel planted firmly on the ground. Then, lunge forward until the first stretch sensation is felt in the back of your front leg. Avoid pushing with your back leg/foot."
	
	Assessment:
	• Normal mobility: Client is able to touch the wall with the forward-bending knee without compression
	• Restricted dorsiflexion: Client is unable to touch the wall, or displays impairments such as:
	  • Heel lift
	  • Foot external rotation
	  • Arch collapse
	  • Knee valgus
	  • Overactive/shortened: Gastrocnemius and soleus

First MTP (big toe) extension
 	
	Client position:
	• Standing or seated
	
	Type of motion:
	• Active target motions:
	  • Client moves the right big toe upward (extension) as far as possible while keeping the other toes and foot stable
	  • Repeat movement with the left big toe
	
	Verbal instructions:
	• "Move your right big toe upward, as far as possible, while keeping everything else still."
	• "Repeat on your left side."
	
	Assessment:
	• Normal mobility: Client is able to extend the big toe above the other toes without compensation
	• Restricted dorsiflexion: Client is unable to extend the big toe above the others, or displays compensation such as:
	  • Movement through the toes
	  • Accessory movement through foot and/or tibia
	  • Overactive/shortened: Flexor hallucis longus

LUMBO-PELVIC-HIP COMPLEX MOBILITY TESTING

If movement impairments are observed at the LPHC or knee, the Sports Performance Coach can test the athlete's trunk mobility. Mobility testing for the lumbar spine and hip helps to identify specific LPHC limitations, allowing the Sports Performance Coach to create a more individualized flexibility and core exercise program for each athlete. The thoracic spine also moves with the lumbar spine and contributes to the overall ROM of the entire spinal column and hip. For that reason, if the Sports Performance Coach identifies lumbar spine mobility impairments, they should perform additional thoracic mobility assessments. To further investigate lumbar spine and hip mobility, the Sports Performance Coach can begin with lumbar spine tests such as active flexion and extension, and then proceed to hip joint tests, such as the modified Thomas test and adductor test. Research shows that the modified Thomas test and the adductor tests are reliable measures of mobility when administered by one or more professionals (Cejudo et al., 2015; Peeler & Anderson, 2008). Other observable tests include passive hip internal rotation and seated hip internal and external rotation (**Table 7.16**).

TABLE 7.16 LPHC Mobility Tests

Screening Test	Description

Lumbar flexion/extension
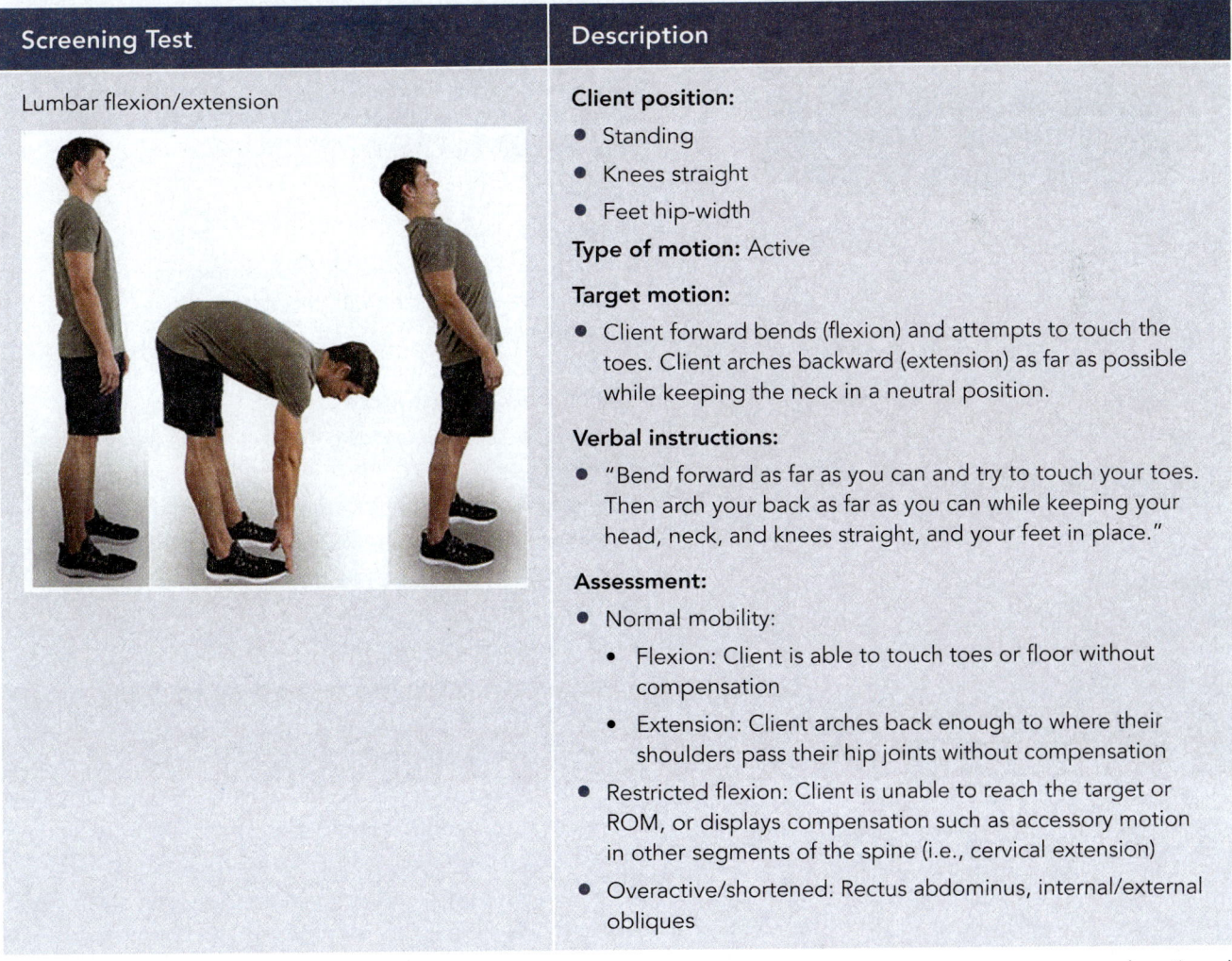
	Client position:
	• Standing
	• Knees straight
	• Feet hip-width
	Type of motion: Active
	
	Target motion:
	• Client forward bends (flexion) and attempts to touch the toes. Client arches backward (extension) as far as possible while keeping the neck in a neutral position.
	
	Verbal instructions:
	• "Bend forward as far as you can and try to touch your toes. Then arch your back as far as you can while keeping your head, neck, and knees straight, and your feet in place."
	
	Assessment:
	• Normal mobility:
	  • Flexion: Client is able to touch toes or floor without compensation
	  • Extension: Client arches back enough to where their shoulders pass their hip joints without compensation
	• Restricted flexion: Client is unable to reach the target or ROM, or displays compensation such as accessory motion in other segments of the spine (i.e., cervical extension)
	• Overactive/shortened: Rectus abdominus, internal/external obliques

(continues)

TABLE 7.16 LPHC Mobility Tests (*continued*)

Screening Test	Description
Hip extension, adduction, and knee flexion (modified Thomas test) 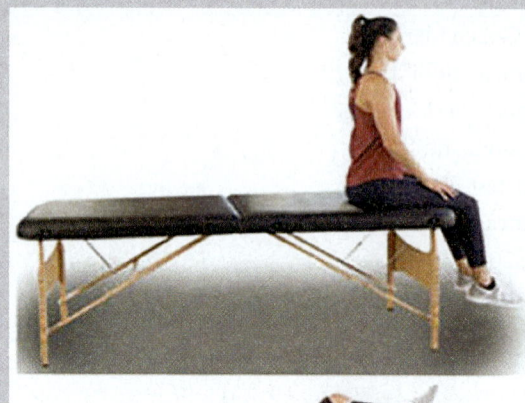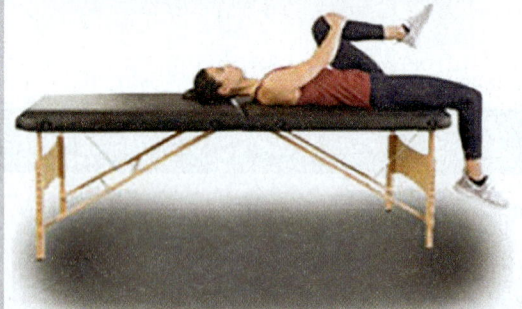	**Client position:** ● Lying supine at the end of a table, both knees bent over the edge of the table **Type of motion:** Passive **Target motion:** ● Client holds the nontesting knee to chest, putting the hip in a maximally flexed position. Lumbar spine and pelvis are flat on the table. Test leg is relaxed on the table. The corrective exercise specialist looks for three movements of the test leg. Repeat on the other side: 　• Hip extension: Assesses psoas length 　• Hip abduction angle: Assesses tensor fascia latae (TFL) length 　• Knee flexion: Assesses rectus femoris length **Verbal instructions:** ● "Sit on the edge of the table and lie back with both knees bent off the table/let your legs hang. Grab your left leg at your knee and pull it toward your chest. Keep your right leg on the table completely relaxed. Repeat that same sequence with the other leg." **Assessment:** ● Normal mobility: 　• Hip extension: The test-side hip and thigh lay flat on the table in line with the torso without compensation 　• Hip adduction: Femur rests in a straight line with torso (not abducted) with no compensation 　• Knee flexion: Knee hangs naturally at 90 degrees off the table edge without compensation ● Restricted hip extension: Test thigh lifts off the table 　• Overactive/shortened: Psoas and rectus femoris ● Restricted hip adduction: Test thigh is abducted and not in line with torso 　• Overactive/shortened: TFL ● Restricted knee flexion: Test knee is slightly extended and not at 90 degrees 　• Overactive/shortened: Rectus femoris

Screening Test	Description
Hip abduction and external rotation (adductor test) 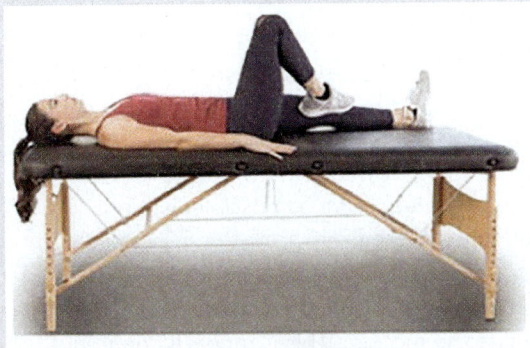 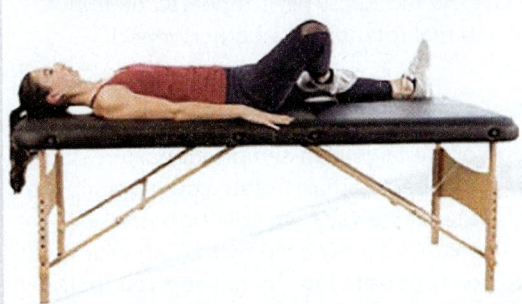	**Client position:** Lying supine on a table **Type of motion:** Passive **Target motion:** • Client lies supine with the test hip and knee bent to 45 degrees, with the foot placed on the medial portion of the opposite leg, between the thigh and shin as needed to achieve the correct angle • The nontesting leg is straight • Client passively relaxes the test leg to let it fall toward the table • Repeat on the opposite side **Verbal instructions:** • "Bend your right leg at the hip and knee to bring your foot against the opposite shin, and then allow your leg to passively relax. Repeat on your other side." **Assessment:** • Normal mobility: Hip and knee on the testing side lay flat on the table without compensation • Restricted abduction: Client is unable to lay the test leg flat on the table, or displays impairments such as accessory motion in the opposite side of the pelvis (i.e., lifts off table) • Overactive/shortened: Hip adductor complex
Passive hip internal rotation 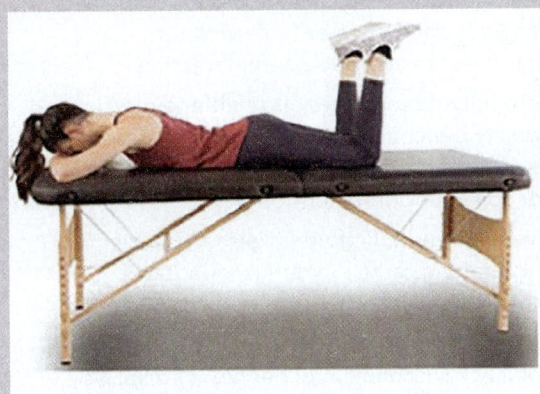 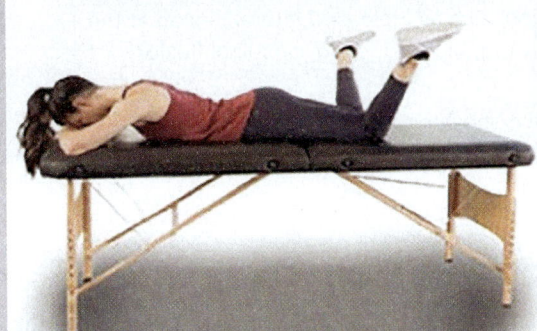	**Client position:** Lying prone on a table with legs together **Type of motion:** Passive **Target motion:** • Client lies prone with both legs together so that knees are in line with the hips, and knees bent to 90 degrees of flexion • The client then passively allows the feet to spread apart (while maintaining bent knees), moving the hips into internal rotation **Verbal instructions:** • "Please bend your knees to 90 degrees. Then, relax and allow your ankles to fall away from each other and lower toward the table." **Assessment:** • Normal mobility: Client can internally rotate the hip until the tibia (shins) are at a 45- degree angle to the table without compensation • Restricted internal rotation: Client is unable to reach the targeted mobility benchmark in either hip, or displays compensation such as knee extension, or lifting or abduction of the hips • Overactive/shortened: Piriformis, quadratus femoris, and gluteus maximus

(continues)

TABLE 7.16 LPHC Mobility Tests (*continued*)

Screening Test	Description

Seated hip internal and external rotation	**Client position:** Seated at the edge of a table with both legs hanging over the side
	
	Type of motion: Active
	
	Target motion:
	
	• Client is seated with an upright posture, hands on hips, and both legs hanging over the side of the table. Client internally rotates one leg, as far as possible, without compensation through the LPHC.
	
	• Then, the client externally rotates the leg as far as possible (the other leg will need to internally rotate to accommodate the motion). This is repeated on the opposite side (internal rotation may be performed bilaterally).
	
	Verbal instructions:
	
	• "Sit at the edge of the table with an upright posture and hands on your hips. Internally rotate your right hip by moving your foot up and away from your opposite leg. Then, externally rotate your right hip by moving your foot up and toward your opposite leg. Try to keep your pelvis level and your back straight. Repeat this on your left side."
	
	Assessment:
	
	• Normal mobility: Client is able to actively rotate the leg at the hip until the tibia (shin) is at an approximately 45-degree angle to the bench or table without compensation for both internal/external rotation
	
	• Restricted internal rotation: Client is unable to reach the targeted mobility benchmark in either hip, or displays impairments such as increased lateral flexion at the spine, hip hiking, or spinal flexion/extension
	
	  • Overactive/shortened: Piriformis, gemellus superior/inferior, obturator internus/externus, quadratus femoris, and gluteus maximus
	
	• Restricted external rotation: Client is unable to reach the targeted mobility benchmark in either hip, or displays compensation such as increased lateral flexion at the spine, hip hiking, hip abduction, or spinal flexion/extension
	
	  • Overactive/shortened: TFL, gluteus minimus and medius (anterior fibers), and hip adductors

SHOULDER AND THORACIC SPINE MOBILITY TESTING

Movement impairment at the shoulders and thoracic spine influences the mobility of the upper extremities. Athletes who demonstrate an upper cross syndrome posture, scapular elevation, or arms falling forward during the OHSA might have flexibility and ROM limitations in the upper body. Decreased mobility at the shoulder and thoracic spine can cause abnormal biomechanical stresses to the upper extremity and can be a potential risk factor for injury in sports involving overhead activity, such as baseball and volleyball (Cools et al., 2015; Heneghan et al., 2019; Ruiz et al., 2020). If the Sports Performance Coach observes such posture and movement impairments, they must also perform a shoulder and thoracic mobility assessment.

To further investigate shoulder and thoracic spine mobility, the Sports Performance Coach can begin with shoulder flexion, retraction, extension, and internal and external rotation. The coach then proceeds to thoracic rotation and extension. These shoulder and thoracic spine tests (**Table 7.17**) are reliable mobility assessments when administered by one or more professionals (Hanney et al., 2011; Johnson et al., 2012; Takatalo et al., 2020).

TABLE 7.17 Shoulder and Thoracic Spine Mobility Tests

Screening Test	Description

Shoulder flexion (lat length test)
 	
	Client position:
	• Standing against a wall or lying supine on the floor, or table, with hips and legs straight
	• If more comfortable, hips flexed, knees bent, feet flat, palms facing each other
	
	Type of motion:
	• Passive (lying)
	• Active (standing)
	
	Target motion:
	• Client brings both arms above the head (flexion), as far as possible, then passively relaxes in that position
	
	Verbal instructions:
	• "Raise both arms above your head, as far as possible, then relax while holding that position."
	
	Assessment:
	• Normal mobility: Upper arms extend directly overhead in line with the lateral midline of the torso without impairment
	• Restricted shoulder flexion: Client is unable to reach their arms in line with their torso, or displays impairments such as:
	  • Elbow flexion
	  • Lumbar extension
	  • Rib cage flaring
	  • Shoulder elevation (shrugging)
	  • Overactive/shortened: Latissimus dorsi, teres major, and pectoralis major (lower fibers)

(continues)

TABLE 7.17   Shoulder and Thoracic Spine Mobility Tests (*continued*)

Screening Test	Description

Shoulder retraction (pectoralis minor test) 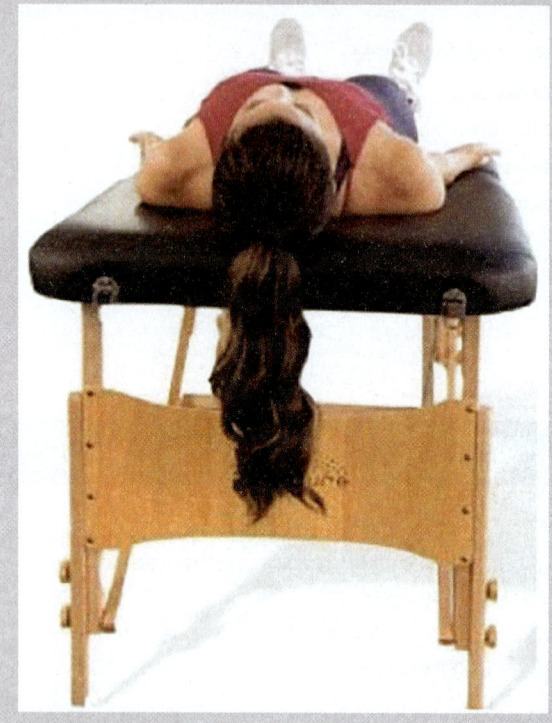	**Client position:** Lying supine on a table with legs extended
	
	Type of motion: Passive
	
	Target motion: Client rests both arms at the side of the body with elbows extended and palms facing upward
	
	Verbal instructions:
	• "Relax both arms at the side of your body with your elbows extended and palms up."
	
	Assessment:
	• Normal mobility: Client can rest their shoulders flat on the table without impairment in other kinetic chain checkpoints
	• Restricted shoulder retraction: Client's shoulders will rest at a level off the table or display an impairment such as:
	   • Lumbar spine extension
	   • Cervical extension
	   • Rib cage flaring
	   • Accessory motion of the arms
	   • Overactive/shortened: Pectoralis minor on the same side as the elevated shoulder or impairment

Shoulder extension 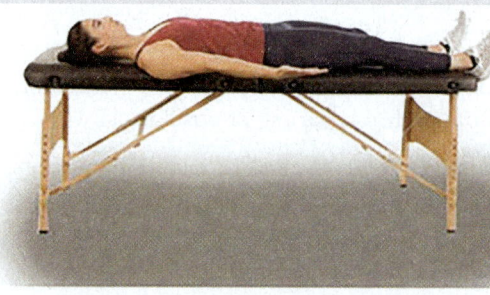 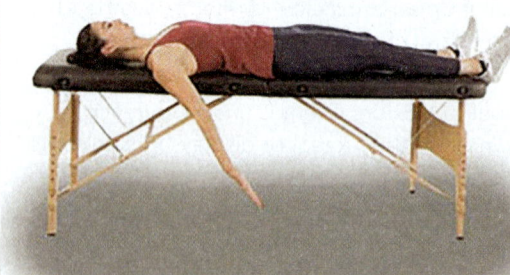	**Client position:** • Standing • Lying supine on a table **Type of motion:** • Passive (lying) • Active (standing) **Target motion:** • Client reaches the arm rearward, as far as is comfortable, while keeping the elbow and wrist straight **Verbal instructions:** • "Reach your arm backward as far as you can, then repeat with the other arm." **Assessment:** • Normal mobility: Client is able to reach just beyond roughly 45 degrees of extension (halfway between the line of the horizon and the wall) without impairment • Restricted flexion: Client is unable to reach the targeted mobility benchmark, or displays impairments such as elbow flexion, shoulder elevation, or the scapula of the test shoulder tilting upward and protracting • Overactive/shortened: Anterior deltoid, pectoralis major (upper fibers), coracobrachialis, biceps brachii

Screening Test	Description

Shoulder internal/external rotation 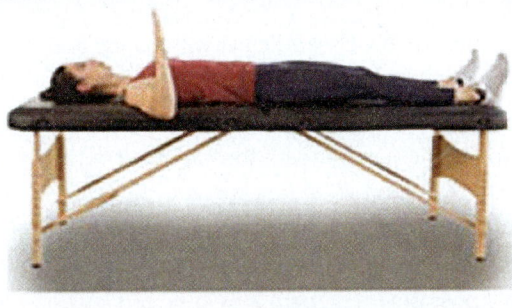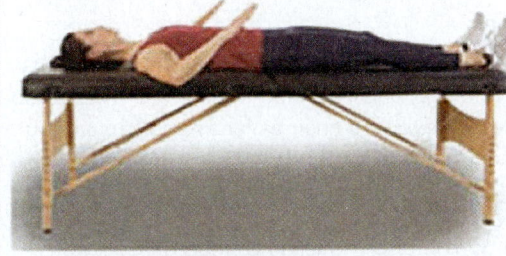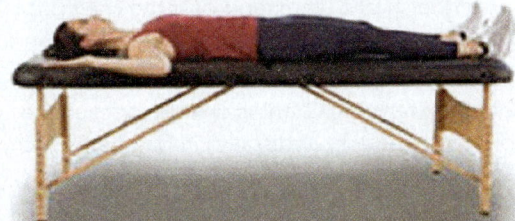	**Client position:**
	• Standing or lying supine on the floor, or a table, with hips and legs straight
	• If they are more comfortable with hips flexed, knees bent and feet flat
	
	Type of motion: Active
	
	Target motion:
	• With shoulders and elbows abducted, and bent to 90 degrees, client rotates arms downward to the table or floor; rotation occurs only at the glenohumeral joint
	• Then, client rotates arms backward, attempting to touch the back of their hand to the plane of the table or to the floor
	
	Verbal instructions:
	• "With your arms out to the side and elbows bent, rotate your arms and hands forward toward the table. Then, rotate your arms and hands backward toward the table."
	
	Assessment:
	• Normal mobility:
	  • Internal rotation: Client can rotate the forearm/hand forward to near the table (roughly halfway between 45 degrees and the table) without impairment
	  • External rotation: Client can rotate the forearm/hand backward to nearly touching or touching the plane of the table without impairment
	• Restricted internal rotation: Client is unable to reach the targeted mobility benchmark, or displays impairments such as the test shoulder elevating and protracting off the table, a change in elbow flexion, or wrist flexion
	  • Overactive/shortened: Teres minor and infraspinatus
	• Restricted external rotation: Client is unable to reach the target mobility benchmark, or displays impairments such as a change in elbow flexion, shoulder elevation, rib cage flaring, or wrist extension
	  • Overactive/shorted: Subscapularis, teres major, latissimus dorsi, and pectoralis major

TABLE 7.17 Shoulder and Thoracic Spine Mobility Tests (*continued*)

Screening Test	Description

Thoracic extension
 	
	Client position:
	
	● Seated on a standard, low-backed chair with hands and arms crossed over chest
	
	● Lumbar and cervical spines neutral throughout
	
	● Chair back should end just beneath the client's shoulder blades
	
	Type of motion: Active
	
	Target motion: Client arches their mid-back over the chair as far as comfortably possible
	
	Verbal instructions:
	
	● "Cross your arms over your chest. While keeping your ribs and low back in place, and your neck in line with your torso, lean your mid-back over the chair as far as you can without tipping the chair."
	
	Assessment:
	
	● Normal mobility: The upper back and head tilt backward, where the tops of the shoulders extend past the chair back (roughly 25 degrees of thoracic extension), and the sternum is nearly parallel to the horizon without impairment
	
	● Restricted thoracic extension: Client is unable to reach the targeted mobility benchmark, or displays impairments such as:
	
	  • Cervical extension
	
	  • Ribs flaring
	
	  • Lumbar extension
	
	    ◦ Overactive/shortened: Rectus abdominis, internal/external obliques

Screening Test	Description

Seated thoracic rotation	**Client position:**
	• Seated with hands crossed in front of body, or crossed with holding a stick or dowel rod
	• Place a medicine ball or foam roller between the knees to stabilize the lower body
	• Ensure the shoulder blades are retracted and depressed
	
	Type of motion: Active
	
	Target motion:
	• Client squeezes the ball or roller between the knees to lock the hips in place
	• Client maintains a neutral cervical spine
	• Client then rotates the upper body to each side, as far as possible
	
	Verbal instructions:
	• "Hold the stick to your chest under your crossed arms. Squeeze the roller between your knees, look forward, and keep your nose in line with your sternum. Rotate your trunk to the right as far as you can. Then, rotate to the left."
	
	Assessment:
	• Normal mobility: The sternum (or stick) rotates roughly 45 degrees from the starting position to each side without impairment
	• Restricted thoracic rotation: Client is unable to reach the targeted mobility benchmark, or displays impairments such as:
	  • Lateral flexion of the spine
	  • Leaning forward or backward
	  • Shoulder protraction
	    • Overactive/shortened: Rectus abdominis, internal/external obliques, and erector spinae on the side opposite of the restriction

RECORDING FINDINGS

The Sports Performance Coach records any mobility impairments and potential overactive muscles on the Mobility Screening Observational Findings Template found in Appendix E. On the template, the coach selects "yes" if the athlete demonstrated adequate ROM or "no" if they did not demonstrate adequate ROM at the selected joints.

> ### ⚠ CRITICAL
>
> As with any movement assessment, the Sports Performance Coach must refer the athlete to a qualified medical provider if a test suggests a possible injury or medical condition. For example, if an athlete reports shoulder pain during the shoulder mobility tests, the test should be stopped immediately and the athlete referred out. Athlete safety is critical during the assessment and training program.

LESSON 6: PERFORMANCE MOVEMENT ASSESSMENTS

DYNAMIC MOVEMENT ASSESSMENTS

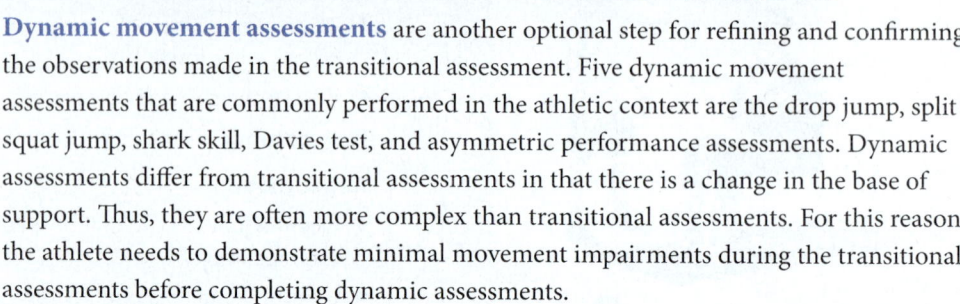

DYNAMIC MOVEMENT ASSESSMENTS →

A set of assessments that involve movement with a change in the base of support.

Dynamic movement assessments are another optional step for refining and confirming the observations made in the transitional assessment. Five dynamic movement assessments that are commonly performed in the athletic context are the drop jump, split squat jump, shark skill, Davies test, and asymmetric performance assessments. Dynamic assessments differ from transitional assessments in that there is a change in the base of support. Thus, they are often more complex than transitional assessments. For this reason, the athlete needs to demonstrate minimal movement impairments during the transitional assessments before completing dynamic assessments.

Athletes should be able to perform the foundational dynamic movement assessments, such as walking or running gait, with minimal concern. However, these dynamic movements emphasize movement speed, dynamic posture, neuromuscular control, and overall performance. For this reason, the Sports Performance Coach needs to take additional care before employing these assessments with athletes. In addition, focus should be directed to movement quality and carefully looking for all movement impairments during the assessments.

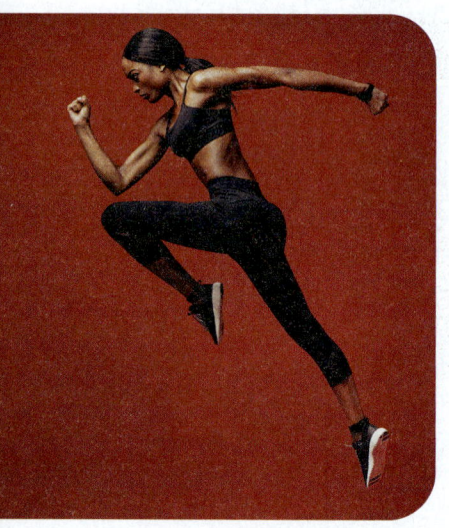

© Jacob Lund/Shutterstock

DROP JUMP ASSESSMENT

The drop jump assessment (also called the depth jump) (**Figure 7.21**) is a dynamic movement assessment used to identify movement impairments during jumping and landing tasks. It is commonly used in clinical, rehabilitation, and sports performance settings. This assessment takes the athlete through the same biomechanical movement pattern as the overhead squat but progresses to a dynamic setting with greater eccentric loading to observe the athlete in a more performance-focused scenario. The drop jump test is a predictor of repeat ACL injuries in athletes who display knee valgus and hip internal rotation (Ekegren et al., 2009; Paterno et al., 2010; Pollard et al., 2017). Research shows that a well-designed sports performance program can effectively reduce movement impairments associated with jumping and landing tasks (DiStefano et al., 2009; Ford et al., 2011).

The Sports Performance Coach should encourage the athlete to perform a maximal vertical jump during the assessment. However, the focus should be on movement quality and control during the assessment to aid in developing a sports performance plan.

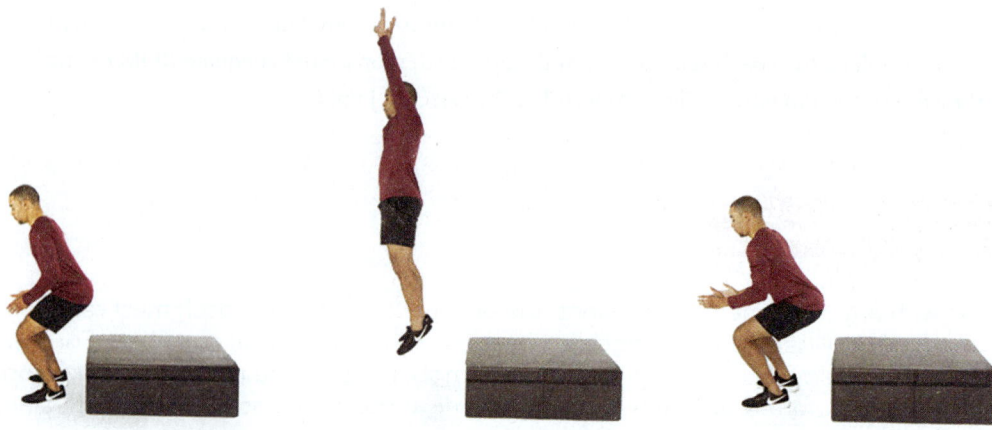

FIGURE 7.21 Drop Jump

EQUIPMENT

Nonslip surface, 12-inch plyometric box, roll of tape to mark lines on ground. The athlete wears athletic clothing and supportive shoes.

STARTING POSITION

1. Have the athlete stand on a 12-inch box.
2. Draw a target line on the floor 12 inches in front of the box.

MOVEMENT

1. Instruct the athlete to jump off the box and land with both feet just after the line.
2. Upon the initial landing, have the athlete quickly jump up for maximum height.
3. The athlete then lands a second time under control.
4. The athlete is allowed up to three practice trials.
5. For testing, the number of repetitions varies for each athlete depending on their ability to perform under fatigue. One to three repetitions per view are recommended as a starting point, following an opportunity to practice the movement after a demonstration.

SCORING

The Sports Performance Coach records any observed movement impairments.

OBSERVATION

The Sports Performance Coach observes the drop jump from anterior and lateral views. Each viewpoint requires a focus on specific KCCs. For each view, ideal performance of the drop jump test is represented by the following elements:

- *Anterior:* View the feet, knees, and LPHC from the front. The feet and hips remain in the sagittal plane, with the knees tracking in line with the foot (second and third toes). The feet are parallel and contact the ground simultaneously. The LPHC does not shift from side to side or rotate.
- *Lateral:* View the feet, ankles, knees, and LPHC from the side. The pelvis and spine remain in a neutral posture. The torso remains parallel with the tibia. The hips, knees, and ankles move through an adequate range of motion for a soft landing.

MOVEMENT COMPENSATIONS

The Sports Performance Coach observes the athlete's drop jump assessment from the anterior and lateral views to identify movement compensations during testing. **Table 7.18** lists potential movement compensations.

TABLE 7.18   Drop Jump: Movement Impairments

Impairment View	Observation
Anterior	<ul><li>Foot and ankle:<ul><li>Excessive pronation</li><li>Asymmetric contact/landing</li></ul></li><li>Knee: Valgus or varus</li><li>LPHC: Asymmetric weight shift</li></ul>
Lateral	<ul><li>Knee:<ul><li>Knee dominance</li><li>Stiff landing</li></ul></li><li>LPHC: Excessive forward lean</li></ul>

RECORDING FINDINGS

The Sports Performance Coach records the athlete's performance on the Drop Jump Observational Findings Template found in Appendix E.

SPLIT SQUAT JUMP ASSESSMENT

The split squat jump assessment (**Figure 7.22**) is a dynamic assessment that progresses from the split squat assessment. The split squat jump challenges the athlete's dynamic posture, balance, and neuromuscular control. This movement is similar to common athletic movements or activities, such as running (McMillian et al., 2016).

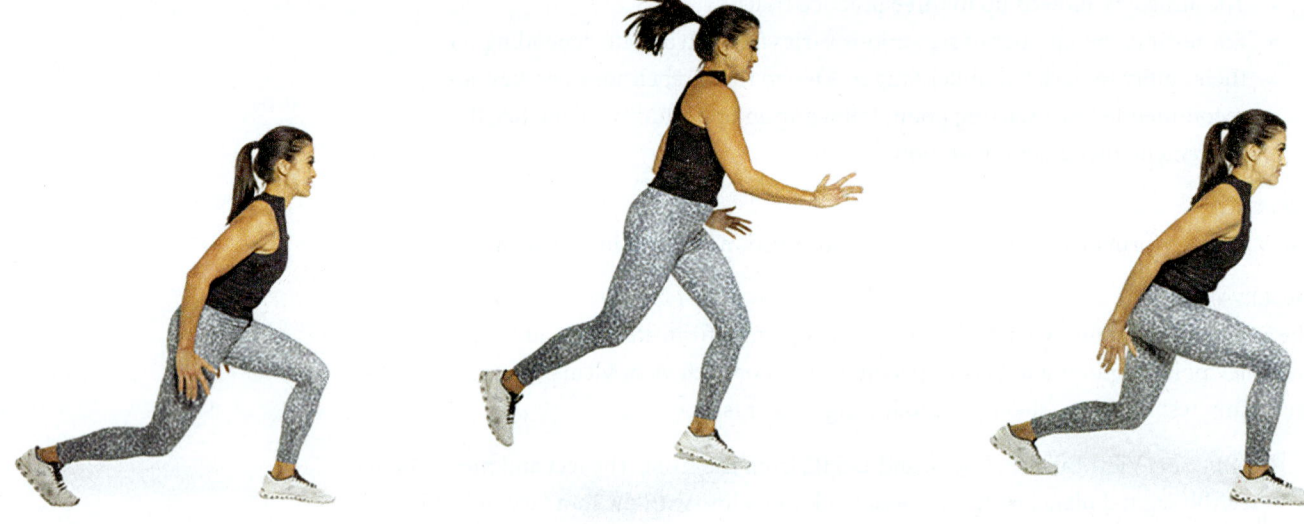

FIGURE 7.22 Split Squat Jump Test

This assessment is considered advanced due to the eccentric load experienced while landing in a staggered stance position. The Sports Performance Coach must monitor the athlete's alignment during the execution of the assessment.

EQUIPMENT
Nonslip surface. The athlete wears athletic clothing and supportive shoes.

STARTING POSITION
Instruct the athlete to stand in a split squat or partial lunge position with one leg in front and one leg in back. The Sports Performance Coach can determine the test leg prior to testing.

MOVEMENT
1. Instruct the athlete to jump up from the split squat position and quickly alternate legs, with the front leg moving to the back and the back leg moving to the front.
2. The athlete is allowed one practice trial prior to testing.
3. Have the athlete perform up to three repetitions per front leg (with the legs alternating, this would be up to six total repetitions).
4. The number of repetitions can vary for each athlete depending on their ability to perform under fatigue.

SCORING
The Sports Performance Coach records any movement impairments.

OBSERVATION

The Sports Performance Coach observes the split squat jump test from the anterior, lateral, and posterior views. For each view, ideal performance of the split squat jump test is represented by the following elements:

- *Anterior:* View the feet, knees, and LPHC from the front. The feet and hips remain in the sagittal plane, with the knees tracking in line with the foot (second and third toes). The LPHC does not shift from side to side or rotate.
- *Lateral:* View the feet, ankles, knees, and LPHC from the side. The front heel stays on the ground and the front knee does not pass the toes. The pelvis and spine remain in a neutral posture.
- *Posterior:* View the feet and ankles from the back. The arch of the foot and the calcaneus remain in a neutral position.

MOVEMENT COMPENSATIONS

The Sports Performance Coach monitors the athlete for movement compensations during testing. **Table 7.19** summarizes the potential movement compensations observed for each view.

TABLE 7.19 Split Squat Jump: Movement Impairments

Impairment View	Observation

Anterior	• Knee: Valgus or varus
	• LPHC:
	  • Asymmetric weight shift
	  • Inward/outward trunk rotation

Lateral	• Foot and ankle: Heel rise (front foot) • Knee: Knee dominance (front knee) • LPHC: Excessive forward lean
Posterior	• Foot and ankle: Excessive pronation

RECORDING FINDINGS

The Sports Performance Coach records any observed movement impairments identified during the split squat jump test on the Split Squat Jump Observational Findings Template found in Appendix E.

SHARK SKILL TEST

The shark skill test is an advanced single-leg assessment that measures dynamic posture, balance, and neuromuscular control. This assessment is considered a progression of the SLSA, providing a unique challenge in different planes of motion, and may not be appropriate for every athlete. The shark skill test has preliminary evidence supporting its use with some athletic populations (Clark, 1998; Tasheva & Mitrev, 2019). Although it is a timed assessment, the Sports Performance Coach should consider and observe the athlete's movement quality. While specific impairments are not noted in scoring the test, the Sports Performance Coach can use this information to determine if this test should be continued and to help design flexibility and strengthening programs.

EQUIPMENT

Nonslip surface, timer, and roll of tape to mark lines on the ground for a grid of nine boxes or a testing mat with boxes. The grid can be numbered to ensure the athlete understands. However, numbering is not required. Place an "X" in the middle box to denote the starting position (**Figure 7.23**).

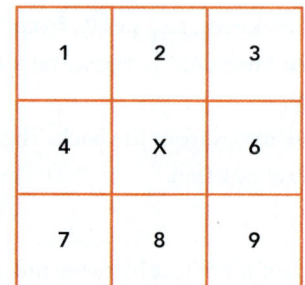

1	2	3
4	X	6
7	8	9

FIGURE 7.23 Shark Skill Test Grid

STARTING POSITION

Position the athlete in the center box of a grid marked "X" with hands on hips and standing on one leg (**Figure 7.24**). Be consistent with the patterns.

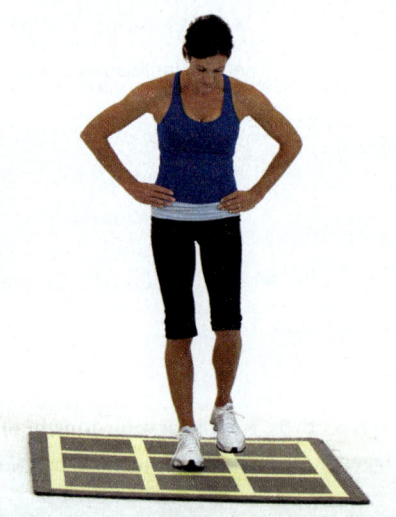

FIGURE 7.24 Shark Skill Test: Starting Position

MOVEMENT

1. Instruct the athlete to hop to each box in succession, beginning with box 1 and then returning to the center box before advancing to the next number (**Figure 7.25**).
2. The athlete can perform one practice trial prior to testing.
3. Conduct two trials per leg for the athlete, totaling four tests. Record the completion time for each trial.

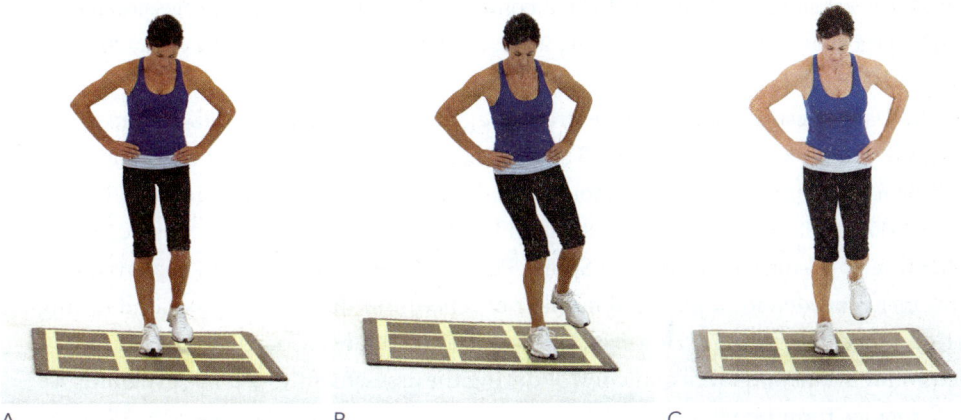

A   B   C

FIGURE 7.25 Shark Skill Test

SCORING

1. Record all times.
2. Add 0.10 second for each of the following faults:
   a. Non-hopping leg touches ground
   b. Hands come off hips
   c. Foot goes into wrong square
   d. Foot does not return to center square

OBSERVATION

The Sports Performance Coach observes the shark skill test from the anterior view and should focus on the relevant KCCs. Note that impairments do not negatively impact the athlete's score, but should be considered for future programming needs. Ideal performance of the shark skills test is represented by the following elements:

- *Anterior:* View the feet, knees, and LPHC from the front. The feet and hips remain in the sagittal plane, with the knees tracking in line with the foot (second and third toes). The LPHC does not shift or drop on the raised leg side.

RECORDING FINDINGS

The Sports Performance Coach records the athlete's performance and time for the shark skill test on the Shark Skill Observational Findings Template found in Appendix E.

DAVIES TEST

The Davies test, also called the closed kinetic chain upper-extremity stability test, is a dynamic movement assessment that identifies impairments during a repetitive, dynamic activity for the upper extremity (**Figure 7.26**) (Heick et al., 2021). Research shows that

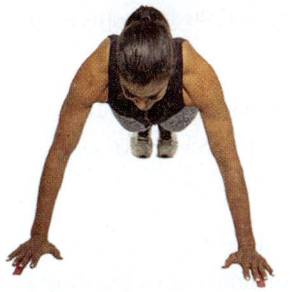 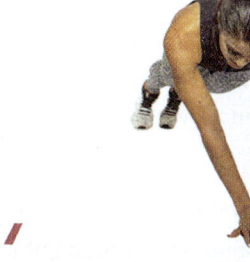 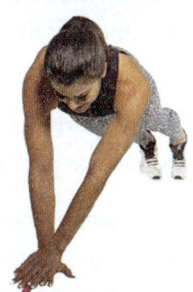

FIGURE 7.26 Davies Test

the Davies test can be reliably used when conducted by more than one professional (de Oliveira et al., 2017; Hollstadt et al., 2020; Sciascia & Uhl, 2015; Tucci et al., 2014; Westrick et al., 2012).

The Davies test requires upper-extremity agility, strength, and stabilization, as well as stability of the trunk and LPHC (Tucci et al., 2014). This assessment might not be suitable for individuals who lack shoulder stability, have current shoulder pain (Tucci et al., 2017), or lack the functional strength to perform a push-up. It is considered a measure of performance, and the Sports Performance Coach needs to explain the movements needed for a maximal number of repetitions during the 15-second testing period (Tucci et al., 2017). However, the Sports Performance Coach also needs to focus on movement quality and control during the assessment to aid in developing a performance training plan.

EQUIPMENT
Two pieces of tape or two cones.

STARTING POSITION
1. Place two pieces of tape on the floor 36 inches (approximately 90 centimeters) apart.
2. Have the athlete assume a push-up position with one hand on each piece of tape and feet together.

MOVEMENT
1. Instruct the athlete to quickly move the right hand to touch the left hand, and then move the left hand to touch the right hand.
2. The individual's body weight shifts over the planted hand so that there is a straight line through the wrist, elbow, and shoulder as they touch it with the floating hand, while maintaining postural control and minimizing unnecessary trunk motion.
3. Perform alternating touching on each side for 15 seconds, and record the number of times a line is touched by both hands and the movement impairments observed.
4. Have the athlete perform three trials. Calculate the average of three trials for the final score.
5. The test ends if the athlete cannot finish or maintain the recommended position during any trial.

SCORING
The Sports Performance Coach records the number of touches and any observed movement impairments.

OBSERVATION
The Sports Performance Coach observes the Davies test primarily from the lateral view. However, they should be located anteriorly enough to accurately count repetitions and watch for alignment of the planted arm. Ideal performance of the Davies test is represented by the following elements:

- *Lateral:* View the LPHC, shoulders, cervical spine, and head from the side. The trunk remains parallel to the ground, with a neutral spine and stable scapulae.

MOVEMENT COMPENSATIONS
The Sports Performance Coach observes the athlete from the lateral view during each trial and counts the repetitions and monitors for movement impairments during testing (**Table 7.20**).

TABLE 7.20 Davies Test: Movement Impairments

Impairment View	Observation
Lateral	LPHC: • Excessive anterior pelvic tilt • Excessive posterior pelvic tilt • Excessive trunk movement
	Shoulder • Scapular elevation • Scapular winging
	Cervical spine: • Excessive cervical extension • Forward head

RECORDING FINDINGS

The Sports Performance Coach records the athlete's performance and identifies movement impairments observed during testing on the Davies Test Observational Findings Template found in Appendix E. **Tables 7.21 and 7.22** provide normative data using Division I athletes for this test.

TABLE 7.21 Normative Data for CKUEST Scores by Number of Touches

Percentile	Men	Women
10	19.0	18.6
20	22.0	20.0
30	23.0	21.0
40	24.0	21.0
50	25.0	23.0
60	26.0	23.0
70	28.0	24.2
80	29.0	26.0
90	30.4	29.0
Mean ± SD	25 ± 4.5	22.9 ± 4.2

Data from Taylor JB, Wright AA, Smoliga JM, DePew JT, Hegedus EJ. Upper-Extremity Physical-Performance Tests in College Athletes. *J Sport Rehabil.* 2016 May;25(2):146-54. doi:10.1123/jsr.2014-0296. Epub 2015 Jan 22.

TABLE 7.22 Normative Data for CKUEST Score by Sport Recorded by Number of Touches

Sport (Number)	Mean (Standard Deviation)
Basketball	
10 male	22.5 (2.7)
15 female	24.7 (6.1)
Baseball	
35 male	22.6 (4.7)
Lacrosse	
26 male	26.5 (3.6)
42 female	22.0 (3.1)
Track and field/cross-country	
34 male	26.6 (4.1)
35 female	21.9 (3.3)
Volleyball	
18 female	24.7 (3.8)
Soccer	
25 female	23.6 (5.3)

Data from Taylor JB, Wright AA, Smoliga JM, DePew JT, Hegedus EJ. Upper-Extremity Physical-Performance Tests in College Athletes. *J Sport Rehabil.* 2016 May;25(2):146-54. doi:10.1123/jsr.2014-0296. Epub 2015 Jan 22.

LESSON 7: BILATERAL ASYMMETRY EVALUATIONS
ASYMMETRICAL PERFORMANCE ASSESSMENTS

ASYMMETRICAL → PERFORMANCE ASSESSMENTS

Dynamic single-leg movements that challenge the dynamic posture, balance, and neuromuscular control of the lower extremity.

Asymmetrical performance assessments are dynamic single-leg movements that challenge an athlete's dynamic posture, balance, and neuromuscular control of the lower extremity. These tests are a progression of the single-leg squat test and might not be appropriate for every athlete due to the advanced movements required. Four commonly performed asymmetrical performance assessments are the single-leg hop, triple hop, triple crossover hop, and 6-meter timed hop test (Janewanitsataporn, 2020; Madsen et al., 2020; Myers et al., 2014). Research shows that single-leg hop tests can be reliably administered by one or more professionals (Dingenen et al., 2019). Although not required, the tests are often done in sequential order, beginning with the single-leg hop (**Figure 7.27**). The Sports Performance Coach will use a tape measure to gather objective (quantitative) data regarding the distance an athlete can jump. In addition, they will obtain subjective (qualitative) data on the athlete's movement quality.

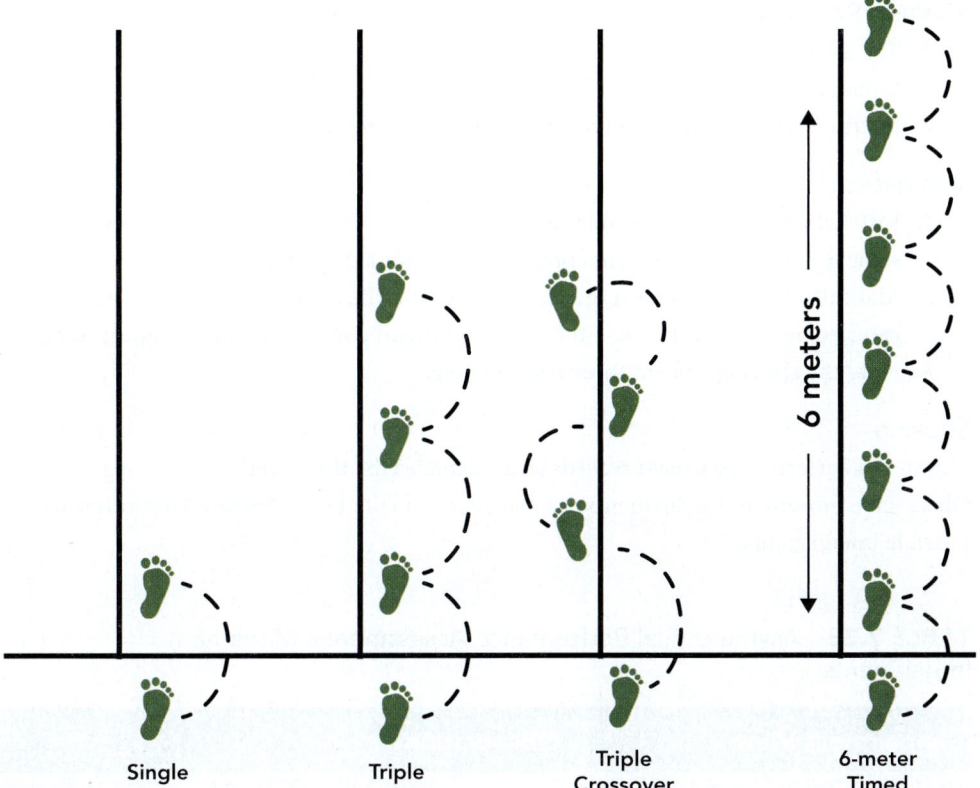

FIGURE 7.27 Four Single-Leg Hop Tests

The labels under the figure read: Single, Triple, Triple Crossover, 6-meter Timed. An arrow marked **6 meters** indicates the distance for the 6-meter Timed test.

EQUIPMENT

Nonslip surface, a roll of tape to mark a 6-meter (approximately 20 feet) line on the ground, tape measure, and timer. The same setup will be used for all of the asymmetrical performance assessments. The timer will be used only on the 6-meter timed hop test.

SINGLE-LEG HOP TEST

The single-leg hop test (**Figure 7.28**) requires the athlete to jump as far as possible and land on the same leg without movement compensations. The athlete can perform three practice trials before testing.

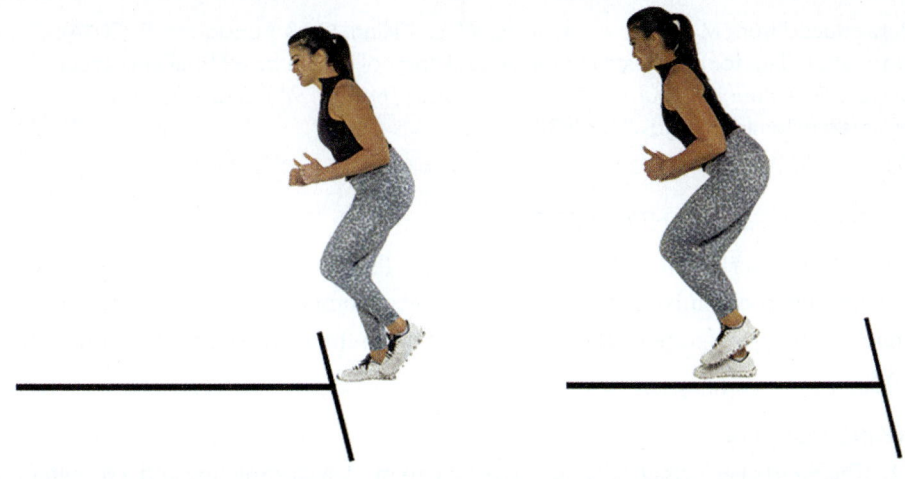

FIGURE 7.28 Single-Leg Hop Test

STARTING POSITION

1. The Sports Performance Coach uses tape to mark a starting line and a 6-meter line.
2. Instruct the athlete to stand on the test leg with toes behind the marked line.

MOVEMENT

1. Instruct the athlete to hop forward one time, as far as possible, and land on the same leg, with no movement compensations, for a 2-second hold.
2. Mark the distance between the starting line and the athlete's heel (measurements can also be taken at the toe—the key is to remain consistent with all repeat tests).
3. Have the athlete perform three trials per leg.

SCORING

The Sports Performance Coach records and calculates the three trials for each leg. Observable movement impairments are considered a failed trial. **Table 7.23** summarizes possible impairments.

TABLE 7.23 Asymmetrical Performance Assessments: Movement Impairments

Impairment View	Observation
Anterior	Foot and ankle: • Feet turn out • Excessive prontation • Asymmetircal contact/landing
Lateral	Knee: • Stiff landing • Knee dominance
	LPHC: • Excessive anterior pelvic tilt • Excessive posterior pelvic tilt • Excessive trunk movement

Reproduced from Myers, B. A., Jenkins, W. L., Killian, C., & Rundquist, P. (2014). Normative data for hop tests in high school and collegiate basketball and soccer players. *International Journal of Sports Physical Therapy, 9*(5), 596–603. https://pubmed.ncbi.nlm.nih.gov/25328822

TRIPLE CROSSOVER HOP TEST

The triple crossover hop test (**Figure 7.29**) assesses the athlete's ability to jump forward and diagonally consecutive times without movement compensations. This test introduces a lateral hopping component. The athlete can perform three practice trials before testing begins.

STARTING POSITION

1. The Sports Performance Coach uses tape to mark a starting line and a 6-meter line.
2. Instruct the athlete to stand on the test leg with toes behind the marked line.

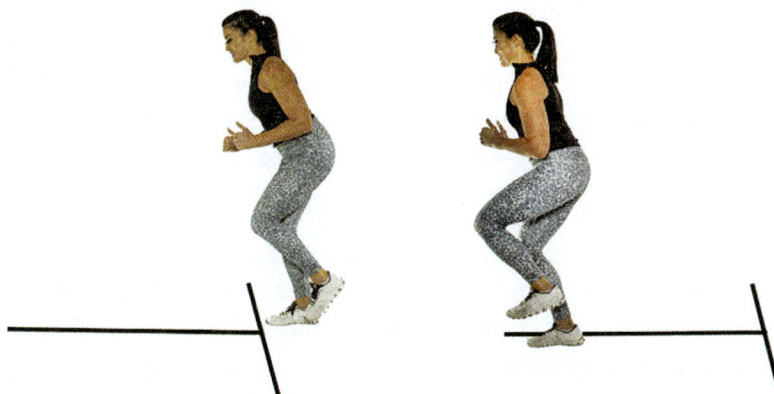

FIGURE 7.29 Triple Crossover Hop Test

MOVEMENT

1. Instruct the athlete to jump forward and diagonally over the 6-meter line for three consecutive times, as far as possible, and then land on the same leg without any movement compensations.
2. Mark the distance between the starting line and the athlete's heel (measurements can also be taken at the toe—the key is to remain consistent with all repeat tests).
3. Have the athlete perform three trials for each leg.

SCORING

The Sports Performance Coach records and calculates the data for the three trials for each leg. Observable movement compensations are considered a failed trial. Table 7.23 summarizes possible impairments.

TRIPLE HOP TEST

The triple hop test (**Figure 7.30**) requires the athlete to jump as far as possible consecutive times and land on the same leg without movement compensations. The athlete can perform three practice trials before testing begins.

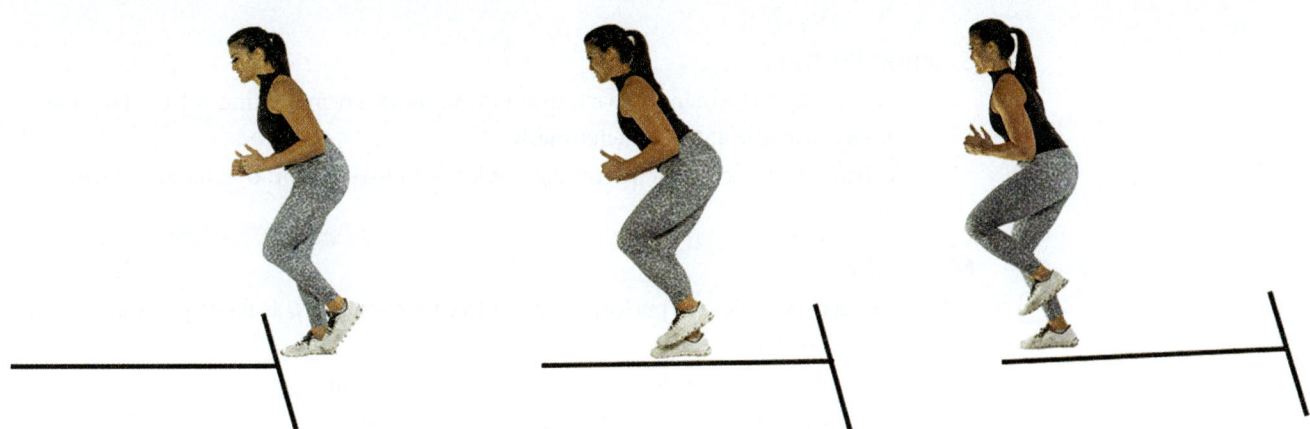

FIGURE 7.30 Triple Hop Test

STARTING POSITION

1. The Sports Performance Coach uses tape to mark a starting line and a 6-meter line.
2. Instruct the athlete to stand on the test leg with toes behind the marked line.

MOVEMENT

1. Instruct the athlete to jump forward three consecutive times, as far as possible, and then land on the same leg without any movement compensations.
2. Mark the distance between the starting line and the athlete's heel (measurements can also be taken at the toe—the key is to remain consistent with all repeat tests).
3. Have the athlete perform three trials per leg.

SCORING

The Sports Performance Coach records and calculates the data for the three trials for each leg. Any observable movement compensations are considered a failed trial. Table 7.23 summarizes possible impairments.

SIX-METER TIMED HOP TEST

The 6-meter timed hop test (**Figure 7.31**) requires the athlete to jump forward consecutively, as far as possible, over a distance of 6 meters without any movement compensations. The athlete can perform one practice trial before testing begins.

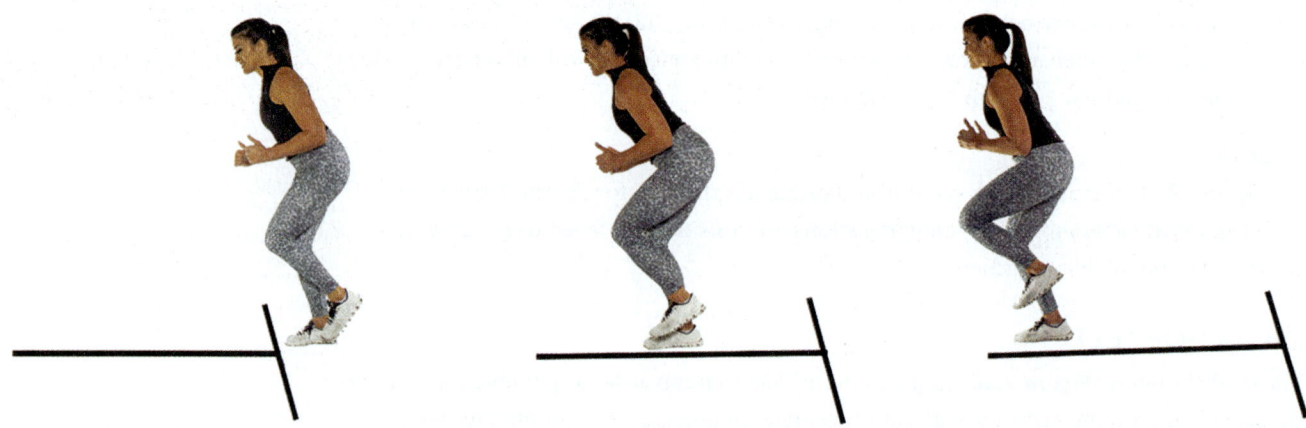

FIGURE 7.31 Six-Meter Timed Hop Test

STARTING POSITION

1. The Sports Performance Coach uses tape to mark a 6-meter line with a start line and a finish line at the 6-meter mark.
2. Instruct the athlete to stand on the test leg with toes behind the marked starting line.

MOVEMENT

1. Instruct the athlete to perform consecutive forward hops, as far as possible, over a 6-meter distance.
2. Start the timer when the athlete begins the movement.
3. Stop the timer when the athlete passes the finish line.
4. Have the athlete performs three trials per leg.

SCORING

The Sports Performance Coach records and calculates the data for the three trials for each leg. Any observable movement compensations are considered a failed trial. Table 7.23 summarizes possible impairments.

OBSERVATION

The Sports Performance Coach observes all four single-leg hop tests from anterior and lateral views. The Sports Performance Coach should stand diagonally to the athlete so as to observe both viewpoints simultaneously. Each one requires a focus on specific KCCs. For each view, ideal performance of the single-leg hop is represented by the following elements:

- *Anterior:* View the test foot, knee, and LPHC from the front. The foot and hip remain in the sagittal plane, with the knee tracking in line with the foot (second and third toes). The foot is parallel and contacts the ground. The LPHC does not shift from side to side or rotate.
- *Lateral:* View the test foot, ankle, knee, and LPHC from the side. The pelvis and spine remain in a neutral posture. The torso remains parallel with the tibia. The hip, knee, and ankle move through an adequate range of motion for a soft landing.

MOVEMENT COMPENSATIONS

The Sports Performance Coach observes for movement impairments that occurred during testing. Table 7.23 summarizes possible impairments.

RECORDING FINDINGS

The Sports Performance Coach records the athlete's distance and time, and identifies any movement impairments observed during testing, on the Asymmetrical Performance Tests Observational Findings Template found in Appendix E. **Table 7.24** provides normative data for all asymmetrical performance assessment tests.

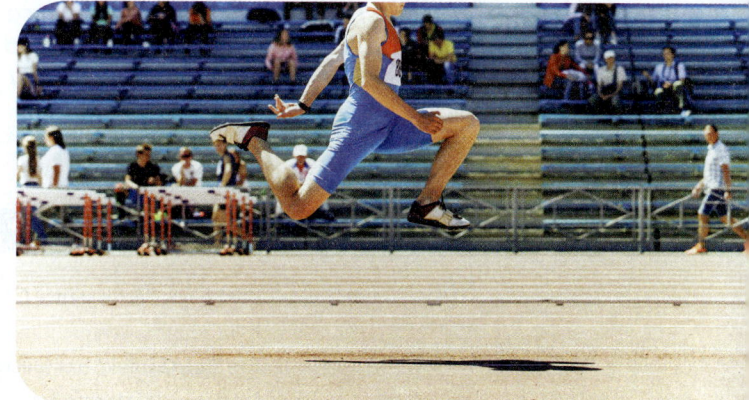

© Real Sports Photos/Shutterstock

TABLE 7.24 Normative Values for Asymmetrical Performance Assessments

Test	Male College Athlete	Female College Athlete
Single-leg hop (cm)	192 ± 20	149 ± 17
Triple hop (cm)	632 ± 72	470 ± 53
Triple crossover hop (cm)	570 ± 75	406 ± 54
Six-meter timed hop (sec)	1.74 ± 0.21	21.3 ± 0.20
Test	**Male High School Athlete**	**Female High School Athlete**
Single-leg hop (cm)	181 ± 20	129 ± 18
Triple hop (cm)	583 ± 77	428 ± 54
Triple crossover hop (cm)	522 ± 77	375 ± 60
Six-meter timed hop (sec)	1.91 ± 0.23	2.25 ± 0.24

Hop test norms for college and high school basketball and soccer players from Myers et al., 2014.

The single-leg hop tests are considered a set of valid and reliable functional tests for the lower extremities in healthy individuals and in athletes post-injury (e.g., post–ACL reconstruction) (Janewanitsataporn, 2020; Madsen et al., 2020). For athletes recovering from an injury, healthcare professionals often calculate the limb symmetry index (LSI), which is a measure of performance for the injured and noninjured limbs (Myers et al., 2014). For example, the LSI for the distance single-leg hop tests (single and triple) is calculated using the following equation: LSI = shortest-performing limb mean/farthest-performing limb mean. The LSI ranges from 0 to 100%. Researchers have used 80% to 90% as a common benchmark for athletes recovering from lower-extremity injury. Thus, for an athlete to be cleared to return to practice or competition, the injured extremity must perform at 80% or higher of the value for the noninjured extremity (Madsen et al., 2020). The Sports Performance Coach needs a good understanding of the LSI because it is commonly used to measure an athlete's function and ability to return to activity after an injury.

SUMMARY

The Sports Performance Coach must perform a comprehensive assessment of athletes at all levels. A thorough assessment may include athlete intake, needs analysis, and movement assessments. The athlete intake has several important components, such as the PAR-Q+ and HHQ, that help determine if it is safe for the athlete to participate in testing and training. The needs analysis provides more in-depth information about the athlete's sport, position, and athletic profile. Physiological and body composition assessments provide information about the athlete's resting cardiorespiratory function and ratios of body tissues, such as fat mass to lean mass. Additionally, movement assessments provide vital information about an athlete's neuromuscular control, flexibility, and strength. If needed, mobility assessments can help further confirm observations from the transitional assessment and determine whether a mobility intervention is warranted. Lastly, dynamic postural assessments are considered a progression from the transitional assessment and provide information about more complex movement patterns when the base of support is changing. These assessments can help determine if more sport-specific testing is required.

The intake and assessment process described in this chapter is not all-inclusive—many other methods of assessment exist. The choice of assessments should match the athlete's individual needs. Further, different professional settings might determine which assessments the Sports Performance Coach will perform. The Sports Performance Coach is encouraged to have a comprehensive understanding of the information in this chapter but to also study other methods to have a broad understanding of this topic.

KEY TAKEAWAYS

- A comprehensive sports performance assessment is needed to help the Sports Performance Coach design an individualized program that aligns with the athlete's goals and abilities and the needs of the athlete's sport.
- Sports performance testing is a systematic approach to problem solving that provides the Sports Performance Coach with foundational information for making educated decisions about exercise and acute training variable selection.

- Sports performance tests should be valid and reliable. Validity is defined as the extent to which the testing method accurately measures what is intended; reliability is defined as the ability to reproduce the test results consistently over time.
- NASM recommends developing a consistent flow to the assessment approach to reduce the chances of missing a key assessment. In addition, when conducting movement assessments, the athlete might not perform one or several tests depending on the results of a prior test.
- The sports performance assessment generally includes a series of tests and measurements that provide insights about the athlete's health status and abilities. Performing these tests accurately and thoroughly is vital to the overall success of a sports performance improvement program. The assessment components should include:
  - Athlete intake
  - Needs analysis
  - Physiological and anthropometric assessments
  - Transitional movement assessments
  - Mobility assessments
  - Dynamic movement assessments
  - Asymmetrical performance assessments

REFERENCES

Abbott, W., Brickley, G., & Smeeton, N. J. (2018). Physical demands of playing position within English Premier League academy soccer. *Journal of Human Sport and Exercise, 13*(2), https://doi.org/10.14198/jhse.2018.132.04

Ackland, T. R., Lohman, T. G., Sundgot-Borgen, J., Maughan, R. J., Meyer, N. L., Stewart, A. D., & Müller, W. (2012). Current status of body composition assessment in sport: Review and position statement on behalf of the ad hoc research working group on body composition health and performance, under the auspices of the I.O.C. Medical Commission. *Sports Medicine, 42*(3), 227–249. https://doi.org/10.2165/11597140-000000000-00000

Agresta, C., Church, C., Henley, J., Duer, T., & O'Brien, K. (2017). Single-leg squat performance in active adolescents aged 8–17 years. *Journal of Strength and Conditioning Research, 31*(5), 1187–1191. https://doi.org/10.1519/jsc.0000000000001617

Alizadeh, S., & Mattes, K. (2019). How anterior pelvic tilt affects the lower extremity kinematics during the late swing phase in soccer players while running: A time series analysis. *Human Movement Science, 66*, 459–466. https://doi.org/10.1016/j.humov.2019.06.001

Allahabadi, S., Amendola, A., & Lau, B. C. (2020). Optimizing return to play for common and controversial foot and ankle sports injuries. *JBJS Review, 8*(12), e20.00067. https://doi.org/10.2106/jbjs.Rvw.20.00067

Aune, D., Sen, A., Ó'Hartaigh, B., Janszky, I., Romundstad, P. R., Tonstad, S., & Vatten, L. J. (2017). Resting heart rate and the risk of cardiovascular disease, total cancer, and all-cause mortality: A systematic review and dose-response meta-analysis of prospective studies. *Nutrition Metabolism & Cardiovascular Diseases, 27*(6), 504–517. https://doi.org/10.1016/j.numecd.2017.04.004

Barandun, U., Knechtle, B., Knechtle, P., Klipstein, A., Rüst, C. A., Rosemann, T., & Lepers, R. (2012). Running speed during training and percent body fat predict race time in recreational male marathoners. *Open Access Journal of Sports Medicine, 3*, 51–58. https://doi.org/10.2147/OAJSM.S33284

Barmherzig, R., & Kingston, W. (2019). Occipital neuralgia and cervicogenic headache: Diagnosis and management. *Current Neurology Neuroscience Report, 19*(5), 20. https://doi.org/10.1007/s11910-019-0937-8

Blue, M. N. M., Tinsley, G. M., Ryan, E. D., & Smith-Ryan, A. E. (2021). Validity of body-composition methods across racial and ethnic populations. *Advances in Nutrition, 12*(5), 1854–1862. https://doi.org/10.1093/advances/nmab016

Burgmeier, R. J., & Hsu, W. K. (2014). Spine surgery in athletes with low back pain: Considerations for management and treatment. *Asian Journal of Sports Medicine, 5*(4), e24284. https://doi.org/10.5812/asjsm.24284

Carpio-Rivera, E., Moncada-Jiménez, J., Salazar-Rojas, W., & Solera-Herrera, A. (2016). Acute effects of exercise on blood pressure: A meta-analytic investigation. *Arquivos Brasileiros de Cardiologia, 106*(5), 422–433. https://doi.org/10.5935/abc.20160064

Cejudo, A., Ayala, F., De Baranda, P. S., & Santonja, F. (2015). Reliability of two methods of clinical examination of the flexibility of the hip adductor muscles. *International Journal of Sports Physical Therapy, 10*(7), 976–983.

Chalmers, P. N., Wimmer, M. A., Verma, N. N., Cole, B. J., Romeo, A. A., Cvetanovich, G. L., & Pearl, M. L. (2017). The relationship between pitching mechanics and injury: A review of current concepts. *Sports Health, 9*(3), 216–221. https://doi.org/10.1177/1941738116686545

Chang, W.-D., Lin, H.-Y., & Lai, P.-T. (2015). Core strength training for patients with chronic low back pain. *Journal of Physical Therapy Science, 27*(3), 619–622. https://doi.org/10.1589/jpts.27.619

Chu, S. K., Jayabalan, P., Kibler, W. B., & Press, J. (2016). The kinetic chain revisited: New concepts on throwing mechanics and injury. *PM&R, 8*(3 suppl), S69–77. https://doi.org/10.1016/j.pmrj.2015.11.015

Chuter, V. H., & Janse de Jonge, X. A. (2012). Proximal and distal contributions to lower extremity injury: A review of the literature. *Gait Posture, 36*(1), 7–15. https://doi.org/10.1016/j.gaitpost.2012.02.001

Clark, M. A. (1998). *Test–retest reliability of the shark skill test: A clinical neuromuscular control test.* https://books.google.com/books?id=ErDztgAACAAJ

Cools, A. M., Johansson, F. R., Borms, D., & Maenhout, A. (2015). Prevention of shoulder injuries in overhead athletes: A science-based approach. *Brazilian Journal of Physical Therapy, 19*(5), 331–339. https://doi.org/10.1590/bjpt-rbf.2014.0109

Crossley, K. M., Zhang, W. J., Schache, A. G., Bryant, A., & Cowan, S. M. (2011). Performance on the single-leg squat task indicates hip abductor muscle function. *American Journal of Sports Medicine, 39*(4), 866–873. https://doi.org/10.1177/0363546510395456

Csapo, R., Hoser, C., Gföller, P., Raschner, C., & Fink, C. (2019). Fitness, knee function and competition performance in professional alpine skiers after ACL injury. *Journal of Science and Medicine in Sport, 22*(suppl 1), S39–S43. https://doi.org/10.1016/j.jsams.2018.06.014

Currell, K., & Jeukendrup, A. E. (2008). Validity, reliability and sensitivity of measures of sporting performance. *Sports Medicine, 38*(4), 297–316. https://doi.org/10.2165/00007256-200838040-00003

Dallinga, J. M., Benjaminse, A., & Lemmink, K. A. (2012). Which screening tools can predict injury to the lower extremities in team sports? A systematic review. *Sports Medicine, 42*(9), 791–815. https://doi.org/10.1007/bf03262295

Daneshmandi, H., Harati, J., Fahim, S., & Be, P. (2017). Bodybuilding links to upper crossed syndrome. *Physical Activity Review, 5.* https://doi.org/10.16926/par.2017.05.17

De Blaiser, C., Roosen, P., Willems, T., Danneels, L., Bossche, L. V., & De Ridder, R. (2018). Is core stability a risk factor for lower extremity injuries in an athletic population? A systematic review. *Physical Therapy in Sport, 30*, 48–56. https://doi.org/10.1016/j.ptsp.2017.08.076

De Blaiser, C., Roosen, P., Willems, T., De Bleecker, C., Vermeulen, S., Danneels, L., & De Ridder, R. (2021). The role of core stability in the development of non-contact acute lower extremity injuries in an athletic population: A prospective study. *Physical Therapy in Sport, 47*, 165–172. https://doi.org/10.1016/j.ptsp.2020.11.035

DeMeulenaere, S. (2007). Pulse oximetry: Uses and limitations. *Journal for Nurse Practitioners, 3*(5), 312–317. https://doi.org/https://doi.org/10.1016/j.nurpra.2007.02.021

de Oliveira, V. M., Pitangui, A. C., Nascimento, V. Y., da Silva, H. A., Dos Passos, M. H., & de Araújo, R. C. (2017). Test–retest reliability of the Closed Kinetic Chain Upper Extremity Stability Test (CKCUEST) in adolescents: Reliability of CKCUEST in adolescents. *International Journal of Sports Physical Therapy, 12*(1), 125–132.

De Ridder, R., Witvrouw, E., Dolphens, M., Roosen, P., & Van Ginckel, A. (2017). Hip strength as an intrinsic risk factor for lateral ankle sprains in youth soccer players: A 3-season prospective study. *American Journal of Sports Medicine, 45*(2), 410–416. https://doi.org/10.1177/0363546516672650

Dingenen, B., Truijen, J., Bellemans, J., & Gokeler, A. (2019). Test–retest reliability and discriminative ability of forward, medial and rotational single-leg hop tests. *Knee, 26*(5), 978–987. https://doi.org/10.1016/j.knee.2019.06.010

DiStefano, L. J., Padua, D. A., DiStefano, M. J., & Marshall, S. W. (2009). Influence of age, sex, technique, and exercise program on movement patterns after an anterior cruciate ligament injury prevention program in youth soccer players. *American Journal of Sports Medicine 37*(3), 495–505. https://doi.org/10.1177/0363546508327542

Dobbs, W. C., Fedewa, M. V., MacDonald, H. V., Holmes, C. J., Cicone, Z. S., Plews, D. J., & Esco, M. R. (2019). The accuracy of acquiring heart rate variability from portable devices: A systematic review and meta-analysis. *Sports Medicine, 49*(3), 417–435. https://doi.org/10.1007/s40279-019-01061-5

Dressendorfer, R. H., Wade, C. E., & Scaff, J. H., Jr. (1985). Increased morning heart rate in runners: A valid sign of overtraining? *Physician and Sportsmedicine, 13*(8), 77–86. https://doi.org/10.1080/00913847.1985.11708858

Durkalec-Michalski, K., Nowaczyk, P. M., Podgórski, T., Kusy, K., Osiński, W., & Jeszka, J. (2019). Relationship between body composition and the level of aerobic and anaerobic capacity in highly trained male rowers. *Journal of Sports Medicine and Physical Fitness, 59*(9), 1526–1535. https://doi.org/10.23736/s0022-4707 .19.08951-5

Edouard, P., Degache, F., Beguin, L., Samozino, P., Gresta, G., Fayolle-Minon, I., Farizon, F., & Calmels, P. (2011). Rotator cuff strength in recurrent anterior shoulder instability. *Journal of Bone and Joint Surgery, 93*(8), 759–765. https://doi.org/10.2106/jbjs.I.01791

Ekegren, C. L., Miller, W. C., Celebrini, R. G., Eng, J. J., & Macintyre, D. L. (2009). Reliability and validity of observational risk screening in evaluating dynamic knee valgus. *Journal of Orthopaedic & Sports Physical Therapy, 39*(9), 665–674. https://doi.org/10.2519/jospt.2009.3004

Elder, J. W., Baraff, S. B., Gaschler, W. N., & Baraff, L. J. (2015). Pulse oxygen saturation values in a healthy school-aged population. *Pediatric Emergency Care, 31*(9), 645–647. https://doi.org/10.1097/pec.0000000000000331

Ellenbecker, T. S., Nirschl, R., & Renstrom, P. (2012). Current concepts in examination and treatment of elbow tendon injury. *Sports Health, 5*(2), 186–194. https://doi.org/10.1177/1941738112464761

Escamilla, R. F., Zheng, N., Macleod, T. D., Imamura, R., Edwards, W. B., Hreljac, A., Fleisig, G. S., Wilk, K. E., Moorman, C. T., 3rd, Paulos, L., & Andrews, J. R. (2010). Cruciate ligament forces between short-step and long-step forward lunge. *Medicine & Science in Sports & Exercise, 42*(10), 1932–1942. https://doi.org/10.1249 /MSS.0b013e3181d966d4

Esco, M. R., Fedewa, M. V., Cicone, Z. S., Sinelnikov, O. A., Sekulic, D., & Holmes, C. J. (2018). Field-based performance tests are related to body fat percentage and fat-free mass, but not body mass index, in youth soccer players. *Sports (Basel), 6*(4), 105. https://doi.org/10.3390/sports6040105

Fatima, S., Bhati, P., Singla, D., Choudhary, S., & Hussain, M. E. (2020). Electromyographic activity of hip musculature during functional exercises in participants with and without chronic ankle instability. *Journal of Chiropractic Medicine, 19*(1), 82–90. https://doi.org/10.1016/j.jcm.2019.07.002

Fields, D. A., Higgins, P. B., & Hunter, G. R. (2004). Assessment of body composition by air-displacement plethysmography: Influence of body temperature and moisture. *Dynamic Medicine, 3*(1), 3–3. https://doi.org /10.1186/1476-5918-3-3

Fleck, S. J. (1983). Body composition of elite American athletes. *American Journal of Sports Medicine, 11*(6), 398–403. https://doi.org/10.1177/036354658301100604

Ford, K. R., Myer, G. D., Schmitt, L. C., Uhl, T. L., & Hewett, T. E. (2011). Preferential quadriceps activation in female athletes with incremental increases in landing intensity. *Journal of Applied Biomechanics, 27*(3), 215–222. https://doi.org/10.1123/jab.27.3.215

Fournié, C., Chouchou, F., Dalleau, G., Caderby, T., Cabrera, Q., & Verkindt, C. (2021). Heart rate variability biofeedback in chronic disease management: A systematic review. *Complementary Therapies in Medicine, 60*, 102750. https://doi.org/https://doi.org/10.1016/j.ctim.2021.102750

Franklyn-Miller, A., Richter, C., King, E., Gore, S., Moran, K., Strike, S., & Falvey, E. C. (2017). Athletic groin pain (part 2): A prospective cohort study on the biomechanical evaluation of change of direction identifies three clusters of movement patterns. *British Journal of Sports Medicine, 51*(5), 460–468. https://doi.org/10.1136 /bjsports-2016-096050

Friel, K., McLean, N., Myers, C., & Caceres, M. (2006). Ipsilateral hip abductor weakness after inversion ankle sprain. *Journal of Athletic Training, 41*(1), 74–78. https://pubmed.ncbi.nlm.nih.gov/16619098

Fulton, J., Wright, K., Kelly, M., Zebrosky, B., Zanis, M., Drvol, C., & Butler, R. (2014). Injury risk is altered by previous injury: A systematic review of the literature and presentation of causative neuromuscular factors. *International Journal of Sports Physical Therapy, 9*(5), 583–595. https://pubmed.ncbi.nlm.nih.gov/25328821

Garrick, L. E., Alexander, B. C., Schache, A. G., Pandy, M. G., Crossley, K. M., & Collins, N. J. (2018). Athletes rated as poor single-leg squat performers display measurable differences in single-leg squat biomechanics compared with good performers. *Journal of Sport Rehabilitation, 27*(6), 546–553. https://doi.org/10.1123 /jsr.2016-0208

Gianola, S., Castellini, G., Stucovitz, E., Nardo, A., & Banfi, G. (2017). Single leg squat performance in physically and non-physically active individuals: A cross-sectional study. *BMC Musculoskeletal Disorders, 18*(1), 299. https://doi.org/10.1186/s12891-017-1660-8

Gibson, A. L., Mermier, C. M., Wilmerding, M. V., Bentzur, K. M., & McKinnon, M. M. (2009). Body fat estimation in collegiate athletes: An update. *International Journal of Athletic Therapy and Training, 14*(3), 13–16. https://doi.org/10.1123/att.14.3.13

Goerger, B., Norcross, M., Blackburn, T., & Padua, D. (2009). Lower extremity kinematics of a double leg jump landing task and overhead squat are correlated. *Medicine & Science in Sports & Exercise, 41*. https://doi.org /10.1249/01.MSS.0000354724.83015.61

Grassi, A., Alexiou, K., Amendola, A., Moorman, C. T., Samuelsson, K., Ayeni, O. R., Zaffagnini, S., & Sell, T. (2018). Postural stability deficit could predict ankle sprains: A systematic review. *Knee Surgery, Sports Traumatology, Arthroscopy, 26*(10), 3140–3155. https://doi.org/10.1007/s00167-017-4818-x

Gribble, P. A., & Hertel, J. (2003). Considerations for normalizing measures of the star excursion balance test. *Measurement in Physical Education and Exercise Science, 7*(2), 89–100. https://doi.org/10.1207/S15327841MPEE0702_3

Gribble, P. A., Hertel, J., & Plisky, P. (2012). Using the star excursion balance test to assess dynamic postural-control deficits and outcomes in lower extremity injury: A literature and systematic review. *Journal of Athletic Training, 47*(3), 339–357. https://doi.org/10.4085/1062-6050-47.3.08

Hafen, B. B., & Sharma, S. (2021). Oxygen saturation. In *StatPearls*. StatPearls Publishing. http://www.ncbi.nlm.nih.gov/books/NBK525974/

Hägglund, M., Waldén, M., & Ekstrand, J. (2006). Previous injury as a risk factor for injury in elite football: A prospective study over two consecutive seasons. *British Journal of Sports Medicine, 40*(9), 767–772. https://doi.org/10.1136/bjsm.2006.026609

Haik, M. N., Alburquerque-Sendín, F., Silva, C. Z., Siqueira-Junior, A. L., Ribeiro, I. L., & Camargo, P. R. (2014). Scapular kinematics pre- and post-thoracic thrust manipulation in individuals with and without shoulder impingement symptoms: A randomized controlled study. *Journal of Orthopaedic & Sports Physical Therapy, 44*(7), 475–487. https://doi.org/10.2519/jospt.2014.4760

Hampton, J. R., Harrison, M. J., Mitchell, J. R., Prichard, J. S., & Seymour, C. (1975). Relative contributions of history-taking, physical examination, and laboratory investigation to diagnosis and management of medical outpatients. *British Medical Journal 2*(5969), 486–489. https://doi.org/10.1136/bmj.2.5969.486

Hanney, W., Kolber, M., & Marshall, J. (2011). The reliability of clinical measurements designed to quantify shoulder mobility. *Physical Therapy Reviews, 16*, 413–422. https://doi.org/10.1179/1743288X11Y.0000000023

Heick, J. D., Haggerty, J., & Manske, R. C. (2021). A comparison of resting scapular posture and the Davies closed kinetic chain upper extremity stability test. *International Journal of Sports Physical Therapy, 16*(3), 835–843. https://doi.org/10.26603/001c.23425

Heneghan, N., Webb, K., Mahoney, T., & Rushton, A. (2019). Thoracic spine mobility, an essential link in upper limb kinetic chains in athletes: A systematic review. *Translational Sports Medicine, 2*(6), 305–315. https://doi.org/10.1002/tsm2.109

Hermassi, S., Bragazzi, N. L., & Majed, L. (2020). Body fat is a predictor of physical fitness in obese adolescent handball athletes. *International Journal of Environmental Research and Public Health, 17*(22). https://doi.org/10.3390/ijerph17228428

Högström, G. M., Pietilä, T., Nordström, P., & Nordström, A. (2012). Body composition and performance: Influence of sport and gender among adolescents. *Journal of Strength and Conditioning Research, 26*(7), 1799–1804. https://doi.org/10.1519/JSC.0b013e318237e8da

Hollstadt, K., Boland, M., & Mulligan, I. (2020). Test–retest reliability of the Closed Kinetic Chain Upper Extremity Stability Test (CKCUEST) in a modified test position in Division I collegiate basketball players. *International Journal of Sports Physical Therapy, 15*(2), 203–209.

Hootman, J. M., Dick, R., & Agel, J. (2007). Epidemiology of collegiate injuries for 15 sports: summary and recommendations for injury prevention initiatives. *Journal of Athletic Training, 42*(2), 311–319. https://pubmed.ncbi.nlm.nih.gov/17710181

Hourani, L. L., Davila, M. I., Morgan, J., Meleth, S., Ramirez, D., Lewis, G., Kizakevich, P. N., Eckhoff, R., Morgan, T., Strange, L., Lane, M., Weimer, B., & Lewis, A. (2020). Mental health, stress, and resilience correlates of heart rate variability among military reservists, guardsmen, and first responders. *Physiology & Behavior, 214*, 112734. https://doi.org/10.1016/j.physbeh.2019.112734

Hsu, W. K., & Jenkins, T. J. (2017). Management of lumbar conditions in the elite athlete. *Journal of the American Academy of Orthopaedic Surgeons, 25*(7), 489–498. https://doi.org/10.5435/jaaos-d-16-00135

Jalali, M., Farahmand, F., Mousavi, S. M., Golestanha, S. A., Rezaian, T., Shirvani Broujeni, S., Rahgozar, M., & Esfandiarpour, F. (2015). Fluoroscopic analysis of tibial translation in anterior cruciate ligament injured knees with and without bracing during forward lunge. *Iranian Journal of Radiology, 12*(3), e17832. https://doi.org/10.5812/iranjradiol.17832v2

Janewanitsataporn, S. (2020). The functional tests after ACL reconstruction with and without meniscal repair. *Journal of Health Science and Medical Research, 38*. https://doi.org/10.31584/jhsmr.2020726

Jayanthi, N., Pinkham, C., Dugas, L., Patrick, B., & Labella, C. (2013). Sports specialization in young athletes: Evidence-based recommendations. *Sports Health, 5*(3), 251–257. https://doi.org/10.1177/1941738112464626

Johnson, B. K., Brou, L., Fields, S. K., Erkenbeck, A. N., & Comstock, R. D. (2017). Hand and wrist injuries among US high school athletes: 2005/06–2015/16. *Pediatrics, 140*(6). https://doi.org/10.1542/peds.2017-1255

Johnson, K. D., Kim, K. M., Yu, B. K., Saliba, S. A., & Grindstaff, T. L. (2012). Reliability of thoracic spine rotation range-of-motion measurements in healthy adults. *Journal of Athletic Training, 47*(1), 52–60. https://doi.org/10.4085/1062-6050-47.1.52

Jones, A. M., & Curran, S. A. (2012). Intrarater and interrater reliability of first metatarsophalangeal joint dorsiflexion: Goniometry versus visual estimation. *Journal of the American Podiatric Medical Association, 102*(4), 290–298. https://pubmed.ncbi.nlm.nih.gov/22826327/

Jönhagen, S., Ackermann, P., & Saartok, T. (2009). Forward lunge: A training study of eccentric exercises of the lower limbs. *Journal of Strength & Conditioning Research, 23*(3), 972–978. https://doi.org/10.1519/JSC.0b013e3181a00d98

Joseph, A. M., Collins, C. L., Henke, N. M., Yard, E. E., Fields, S. K., & Comstock, R. D. (2013). A multisport epidemiologic comparison of anterior cruciate ligament injuries in high school athletics. *Journal of Athletic Training, 48*(6), 810–817. https://doi.org/10.4085/1062-6050-48.6.03

Jubran, A. (2015). Pulse oximetry. *Critical Care, 19*(1), 272–272. https://doi.org/10.1186/s13054-015-0984-8

Kajaia, T., Maskhulia, L., Chelidze, K., Akhalkatsi, V., & Kakhabrishvili, Z. (2017). The effects of non-functional overreaching and overtraining and overtraining on autonomic nervous system function in highly trained athletes. *Georgian Medical News, 264*, 97–103.

Kamali, F., Sinaei, E., & Morovati, M. (2019). Comparison of upper trapezius and infraspinatus myofascial trigger point therapy by dry needling in overhead athletes with unilateral shoulder impingement syndrome. *Journal of Sport Rehabilitation, 28*(3), 243–249. https://doi.org/10.1123/jsr.2017-0207

Kasper, A. M., Langan-Evans, C., Hudson, J. F., Brownlee, T. E., Harper, L. D., Naughton, R. J., Morton, J. P., & Close, G. L. (2021). Come back skinfolds, all is forgiven: A narrative review of the efficacy of common body composition methods in applied sports practice. *Nutrients, 13*(4), 1075. https://doi.org/10.3390/nu13041075

Kawaguchi, K., Taketomi, S., Mizutani, Y., Inui, H., Yamagami, R., Kono, K., Takagi, K., Kage, T., Sameshima, S., Tanaka, S., & Haga, N. (2021). Hip abductor muscle strength deficit as a risk factor for inversion ankle sprain in male college soccer players: A prospective cohort study. *Orthopaedic Journal of Sports Medicine, 9*(7). https://doi.org/10.1177/23259671211020287

Kerr, Z. Y., Baugh, C. M., Hibberd, E. E., Snook, E. M., Hayden, R., & Dompier, T. P. (2015). Epidemiology of National Collegiate Athletic Association men's and women's swimming and diving injuries from 2009/2010 to 2013/2014. *British Journal of Sports Medicine, 49*(7), 465–471. https://doi.org/10.1136/bjsports-2014-094423

Kerr, Z. Y., Roos, K. G., Djoko, A., Dalton, S. L., Broglio, S. P., Marshall, S. W., & Dompier, T. P. (2017). Epidemiologic measures for quantifying the incidence of concussion in National Collegiate Athletic Association sports. *Journal of Athletic Training, 52*(3), 167–174. https://doi.org/10.4085/1062-6050-51.6.05

Kessels, R. P. (2003). Patients' memory for medical information. *Journal of the Royal Society of Medicine, 96*(5), 219–222. https://www.ncbi.nlm.nih.gov/pmc/articles/PMC539473/

Kim, H. G., Cheon, E. J., Bai, D. S., Lee, Y. H., & Koo, B. H. (2018). Stress and heart rate variability: A meta-analysis and review of the literature. *Psychiatry Investigation, 15*(3), 235–245. https://doi.org/10.30773/pi.2017.08.17

Kreher, J. B. (2016). Diagnosis and prevention of overtraining syndrome: An opinion on education strategies. *Open Access Journal of Sports Medicine, 7*, 115–122. https://doi.org/10.2147/OAJSM.S91657

Kreher, J. B., & Schwartz, J. B. (2012). Overtraining syndrome: A practical guide. *Sports Health, 4*(2), 128–138. https://doi.org/10.1177/1941738111434406

Krutsch, W., Krutsch, V., Hilber, F., Pfeifer, C., Baumann, F., Weber, J., Schmitz, P., Kerschbaum, M., Nerlich, M., & Angele, P. (2018). 11.361 sports injuries in a 15-year survey of a Level I emergency trauma department reveal different severe injury types in the 6 most common team sports. *Sportverletz Sportschaden, 32*(2), 111–119. https://doi.org/10.1055/s-0583-3792

Kuriyan, R. (2018). Body composition techniques. *Indian Journal of Medical Research, 148*(5), 648–658. https://doi.org/10.4103/ijmr.IJMR_1777_18

Kyle, U. G., Bosaeus, I., De Lorenzo, A. D., Deurenberg, P., Elia, M., Gómez, J. M., Heitmann, B. L., Kent-Smith, L., Melchior, J. C., Pirlich, M., Scharfetter, H., Schols, A. M., & Pichard, C. (2004). Bioelectrical impedance analysis: Part I: Review of principles and methods. *Clinical Nutrition, 23*(5), 1226–1243. https://doi.org/10.1016/j.clnu.2004.06.004

Laudner, K. G., Wenig, M., Selkow, N. M., Williams, J., & Post, E. (2015). Forward shoulder posture in collegiate swimmers: A comparative analysis of muscle-energy techniques. *Journal of Athletic Training, 50*(11), 1133–1139. https://doi.org/10.4085/1062-6050-50.11.07

Leider, J., Piche, J. D., Khan, M., & Aleem, I. (2021). Return-to-play outcomes in elite athletes after cervical spine surgery: A systematic review. *Sports Health, 13*(5), 437–445. https://doi.org/10.1177/19417381211007813

Li, G. H.-Y., Lee, G. K.-Y., Au, P. C.-M., Chan, M., Li, H.-L., Cheung, B. M.-Y., Wong, I. C.-K., Lee, V. H.-F., Mok, J., Yip, B. H.-K., Cheng, K. K.-Y., Wu, C.-H., & Cheung, C.-L. (2021). The effect of different measurement modalities in the association of lean mass with mortality: A systematic review and meta-analysis. *Osteoporos Sarcopenia, 7*(suppl 1), S13–S18. https://doi.org/10.1016/j.afos.2021.02.004

Lindström, M., Strandberg, S., Wredmark, T., Felländer-Tsai, L., & Henriksson, M. (2013). Functional and muscle morphometric effects of ACL reconstruction: A prospective CT study with 1 year follow-up. *Scandinavian Journal of Medicine & Science, 23*(4), 431–442. https://doi.org/10.1111/j.1600-0838.2011.01417.x

Lisman, P., Wilder, J. N., Berenbach, J., Foster, J. J., & Hansberger, B. L. (2021). Sex differences in lower extremity kinematics during overhead and single leg squat tests. *Sports Biomechanics*, 1–14. https://doi.org/10.1080/14763141.2020.1839124

Madsen, L. P., Booth, R. L., Volz, J. D., & Docherty, C. L. (2020). Using normative data and unilateral hopping tests to reduce ambiguity in return-to-play decisions. *Journal of Athletic Training, 55*(7), 699–706. https://doi.org/10.4085/1062-6050-0050.19

Mai, H. T., Chun, D. S., Schneider, A. D., Erickson, B. J., Freshman, R. D., Kester, B., Verma, N. N., & Hsu, W. K. (2017). Performance-based outcomes after anterior cruciate ligament reconstruction in professional athletes differ between sports. *American Journal of Sports Medicine, 45*(10), 2226–2232. https://doi.org/10.1177/0363546517704834

Maranhao Neto, G. A., Luz, L. G., & Farinatti, P. T. (2013). Diagnostic accuracy of pre-exercise screening questionnaire: Emphasis on educational level and cognitive status. *Archives of Gerontology and Geriatrics, 57*(2), 211–214. https://doi.org/10.1016/j.archger.2013.03.008

Mauntel, T. C., Post, E. G., Padua, D. A., & Bell, D. R. (2015). Sex differences during an overhead squat assessment. *Journal of Applied Biomechanics, 31*(4), 244–249. https://doi.org/10.1123/jab.2014-0272

McMillian, D. J., Rynders, Z. G., & Trudeau, T. R. (2016). Modifying the functional movement screen deep squat test: The effect of foot and arm positional variations. *Journal of Strength and Conditioning Research, 30*(4), 973–979. https://doi.org/10.1519/jsc.0000000000001190

Medeiros, R. M., Alves, E. S., Lemos, V. A., Schwingel, P. A., da Silva, A., Vital, R., Vieira, A. S., Barreto, M. M., Rocha, E. A., Tufik, S., & de Mello, M. T. (2016). Assessment of body composition and sport performance of Brazilian paraolympic swim team athletes. *Journal of Sports Rehabilitation, 25*(4), 364–370. https://doi.org/10.1123/jsr.2015-0036

Mellalieu, S. D., Hanton, S., & O'Brien, M. (2006). The effects of goal setting on rugby performance. *Journal of Applied Behavior Analysis, 39*(2), 257–261. https://doi.org/10.1901/jaba.2006.36-05

Mengden, T., Chamontin, B., Phong Chau, N., Luis Palma Gamiz, J., & Chanudet, X. (2000). User procedure for self-measurement of blood pressure: First International Consensus Conference on Self Blood Pressure Measurement. *Blood Pressure Monitoring, 5*(2), 111–129.

Mitchell, J. H., Haskell, W., Snell, P., & Van Camp, S. P. (2005). Task force 8: Classification of sports. *Journal of the American College of Cardiology, 45*(8), 1364–1367. https://doi.org/10.1016/j.jacc.2005.02.015

Moezy, A., Sepehrifar, S., & Solaymani Dodaran, M. (2014). The effects of scapular stabilization based exercise therapy on pain, posture, flexibility and shoulder mobility in patients with shoulder impingement syndrome: A controlled randomized clinical trial. *Medical Journal of the Islamic Republic of Iran, 28*, 8. https://pubmed.ncbi.nlm.nih.gov/25664288

Mousavi, S. H., Hijmans, J. M., Rajabi, R., Diercks, R., Zwerver, J., & van der Worp, H. (2019). Kinematic risk factors for lower limb tendinopathy in distance runners: A systematic review and meta-analysis. *Gait and Posture, 69*, 13–24. https://doi.org/10.1016/j.gaitpost.2019.01.011

Muntner, P., Shimbo, D., Carey, R. M., Charleston, J. B., Gaillard, T., Misra, S., Myers, M. G., Ogedegbe, G., Schwartz, J. E., Townsend, R. R., Urbina, E. M., Viera, A. J., White, W. B., & Wright, J. T. (2019). Measurement of blood pressure in humans: A scientific statement from the American Heart Association. *Hypertension, 73*(5), e35–e66. https://doi.org/doi:10.1161/HYP.0000000000000087

Muto, T., Inui, H., Ninomiya, H., Tanaka, H., & Nobuhara, K. (2017). Characteristics and clinical outcomes in overhead sports athletes after rotator cuff repair. *Journal of Sports Medicine (Hindawi Publishing Corp.)*, 5476293. https://doi.org/10.1155/2017/5476293

Myer, G. D., Jayanthi, N., Difiori, J. P., Faigenbaum, A. D., Kiefer, A. W., Logerstedt, D., & Micheli, L. J. (2015). Sport specialization: Part I: Does early sports specialization increase negative outcomes and reduce the opportunity for success in young athletes? *Sports Health, 7*(5), 437–442. https://doi.org/10.1177/1941738115598747

Myer, G. D., Jayanthi, N., DiFiori, J. P., Faigenbaum, A. D., Kiefer, A. W., Logerstedt, D., & Micheli, L. J. (2016). Sports specialization: Part II: Alternative solutions to early sport specialization in youth athletes. *Sports Health, 8*(1), 65–73. https://doi.org/10.1177/1941738115614811

Myer, G. D., Lloyd, R. S., Brent, J. L., & Faigenbaum, A. D. (2013). How young is "too young" to start training? *ACSMs Health and Fitness Journal, 17*(5), 14–23. https://doi.org/10.1249/FIT.0b013e3182a06c59

Myers, B. A., Jenkins, W. L., Killian, C., & Rundquist, P. (2014). Normative data for hop tests in high school and collegiate basketball and soccer players. *International Journal of Sports Physical Therapy, 9*(5), 596–603. https://pubmed.ncbi.nlm.nih.gov/25328822

Nakagawa, T. H., Moriya É, T., Maciel, C. D., & Serrão, A. F. (2012). Frontal plane biomechanics in males and females with and without patellofemoral pain. *Medicine & Science in Sports & Exercise, 44*(9), 1747–1755. https://doi.org/10.1249/MSS.0b013e318256903a

Opar, D. A., Williams, M. D., & Shield, A. J. (2012). Hamstring strain injuries: Factors that lead to injury and re-injury. *Sports Medicine, 42*(3), 209–226. https://doi.org/10.2165/11594800-000000000-00000

Orantes-Gonzalez, E., Heredia-Jimenez, J., & Escabias, M. (2021). Body mass index and aerobic capacity: The key variables for good performance in soldiers. *European Journal of Sports Science*, 1–8. https://doi.org/10.1080/17461391.2021.1956599

Ostchega, Y., Porter, K. S., Hughes, J., Dillon, C. F., & Nwankwo, T. (2011). Resting pulse rate reference data for children, adolescents, and adults: United States, 1999–2008. *National Health Statistics Report, 41*, 1–16.

Pagaduan, J. C., Chen, Y.-S., Fell, J. W., & Wu, S. S. X. (2020). Can heart rate variability biofeedback improve athletic performance? A systematic review. *Journal of Human Kinetics, 73*, 103–114. https://www.ncbi.nlm.nih.gov/pmc/articles/PMC7386140/

Page, P., Frank, C. C., & Lardner, R. (2010). *Assessment and treatment of muscle imbalance: The Janda approach*. Human Kinetics.

Paine, R., & Voight, M. L. (2013). The role of the scapula. *International Journal of Sports Physical Therapy, 8*(5), 617–629. https://pubmed.ncbi.nlm.nih.gov/24175141

Paterno, M. V., Schmitt, L. C., Ford, K. R., Rauh, M. J., Myer, G. D., Huang, B., & Hewett, T. E. (2010). Biomechanical measures during landing and postural stability predict second anterior cruciate ligament injury after anterior cruciate ligament reconstruction and return to sport. *American Journal of Sports Medicine, 38*(10), 1968–1978. https://doi.org/10.1177/0363546510376053

Peeler, J. D., & Anderson, J. E. (2008). Reliability limits of the modified Thomas test for assessing rectus femoris muscle flexibility about the knee joint. *Journal of Athletic Training, 43*(5), 470–476. https://doi.org/10.4085/1062-6050-43.5.470

Phillips, A., & McClinton, S. (2017). Gait deviations associated with plantar heel pain: A systematic review. *Clinical Biomechanics, 42*, 55–64. https://doi.org/10.1016/j.clinbiomech.2016.12.012

Phisitkul, P., James, S. L., Wolf, B. R., & Amendola, A. (2006). MCL injuries of the knee: Current concepts review. *Iowa Orthopedic Journal, 26*, 77–90.

Pollard, C. D., Sigward, S. M., & Powers, C. M. (2017). ACL injury prevention training results in modification of hip and knee mechanics during a drop-landing task. *Orthopaedic Journal of Sports Medicine, 5*(9), 2325967117726267. https://doi.org/10.1177/2325967117726267

Post, E. G., Olson, M., Trigsted, S., Hetzel, S., & Bell, D. R. (2017). The reliability and discriminative ability of the overhead squat test for observational screening of medial knee displacement. *Journal of Sport Rehabilitation, 26*(1). https://doi.org/10.1123/jsr.2015-0178

Powden, C. J., Dodds, T. K., & Gabriel, E. H. (2019). The reliability of the star excursion balance test and lower quarter Y-balance test and lower quarter Y-balance test in healthy adults: A systematic review. *International Journal of Sports Physical Therapy, 14*(5), 683–694. https://pubmed.ncbi.nlm.nih.gov/31598406

Powden, C. J., Hoch, J. M., & Hoch, M. C. (2015). Reliability and minimal detectable change of the weight-bearing lunge test: A systematic review. *Manual Therapy, 20*(4), 524–532. https://doi.org/10.1016/j.math.2015.01.004

Powers, C. M. (2010). The influence of abnormal hip mechanics on knee injury: A biomechanical perspective. *Journal of Orthopaedic & Sports Physical Therapy, 40*(2), 42–51. https://doi.org/10.2519/jospt.2010.3337

Powers, C. M., Ghoddosi, N., Straub, R. K., & Khayambashi, K. (2017). Hip strength as a predictor of ankle sprains in male soccer players: A prospective study. *Journal of Athletic Training, 52*(11), 1048–1055. https://doi.org/10.4085/1062-6050-52.11.18

Prinsloo, G. E., Rauch, H. G., & Derman, W. E. (2014). A brief review and clinical application of heart rate variability biofeedback in sports, exercise, and rehabilitation medicine. *The Physician and Sportsmedicine, 42*(2), 88–99. https://doi.org/10.3810/psm.2014.05.2061

Rabin, A., & Kozol, Z. (2017). Utility of the overhead squat and forward arm squat in screening for limited ankle dorsiflexion. *Journal of Strength and Conditioning Research, 31*(5), 1251–1258. https://doi.org/10.1519/jsc.0000000000001580

Räisänen, A., Pasanen, K., Krosshaug, T., Avela, J., Perttunen, J., & Parkkari, J. (2016). Single-leg squat as a tool to evaluate young athletes' frontal plane knee control. *Clinical Journal of Sport Medicine, 26*(6), 478–482. https://doi.org/10.1097/jsm.0000000000000288

Reiman, M. P., Bolgla, L. A., & Lorenz, D. (2009). Hip function's influence on knee dysfunction: A proximal link to a distal problem. *Journal of Sport Rehabilitation, 18*(1), 33–46. https://doi.org/10.1123/jsr.18.1.33

Reiman, M. P., Weisbach, P. C., & Glynn, P. E. (2009). The hip's influence on low back pain: A distal link to a proximal problem. *Journal of Sport Rehabilitation, 18*(1), 24–32. https://doi.org/10.1123/jsr.18.1.24

Reimers, A. K., Knapp, G., & Reimers, C.-D. (2018). Effects of exercise on the resting heart rate: A systematic review and meta-analysis of interventional studies. *Journal of Clinical Medicine, 7*(12), 503. https://doi.org/10.3390/jcm7120503

Ressman, J., Grooten, W. J. A., & Rasmussen Barr, E. (2019). Visual assessment of movement quality in the single leg squat test: A review and meta-analysis of inter-rater and intrarater reliability. *BMJ Open Sport & Exercise Medicine, 5*(1), e000541. https://doi.org/10.1136/bmjsem-2019-000541

Richard, C., Glaser, E., & Lussier, M.-T. (2017). Communication and patient participation influencing patient recall of treatment discussions. *Health Expectations, 20*(4), 760–770. https://doi.org/https://doi.org/10.1111/hex.12515

Richards, J., Selfe, J., Sinclair, J., May, K., & Thomas, G. (2016). The effect of different decline angles on the biomechanics of double limb squats and the implications to clinical and training practice. *Journal of Human Kinetics, 52*, 125–138. https://www.ncbi.nlm.nih.gov/pmc/articles/PMC5260524/

Ruiz, J., Feigenbaum, L., & Best, T. M. (2020). The thoracic spine in the overhead athlete. *Current Sports Medicine Reports, 19*(1), 11–16. https://doi.org/10.1249/jsr.0000000000000671

Rumbo-Rodríguez, L., Sánchez-SanSegundo, M., Ferrer-Cascales, R., García-D'Urso, N., Hurtado-Sánchez, J. A., & Zaragoza-Martí, A. (2021). Comparison of body scanner and manual anthropometric measurements of body shape: A systematic review. *International Journal of Environmental Research and Public Health, 18*(12). https://doi.org/10.3390/ijerph18126213

Sánchez-Gómez, R., Becerro-de-Bengoa-Vallejo, R., Losa-Iglesias, M. E., Calvo-Lobo, C., Navarro-Flores, E., Palomo-López, P., Romero-Morales, C., & López-López, D. (2020). Reliability study of diagnostic tests for functional hallux limitus. *Foot & Ankle International, 41*(4), 457–462. https://doi.org/10.1177/1071100719901116

Schwellnus, M., Soligard, T., Alonso, J.-M., Bahr, R., Clarsen, B., Dijkstra, H. P., Gabbett, T. J., Gleeson, M., Hägglund, M., Hutchinson, M. R., Janse Van Rensburg, C., Meeusen, R., Orchard, J. W., Pluim, B. M., Raftery, M., Budgett, R., & Engebretsen, L. (2016). How much is too much? (Part 2) International Olympic Committee consensus statement on load in sport and risk of illness. *British Journal of Sports Medicine, 50*(17), 1043–1052. https://doi.org/10.1136/bjsports-2016-096572

Sciascia, A., & Uhl, T. (2015). Reliability of strength and performance testing measures and their ability to differentiate persons with and without shoulder symptoms. *International Journal of Sports Physical Therapy, 10*(5), 655–666. https://pubmed.ncbi.nlm.nih.gov/26491616

Scroggs, K., & Simonson, S. R. (2021). Writing a needs analysis: Exploring the details. *Journal of Strength and Conditioning Research.* https://journals.lww.com/nsca-scj/Fulltext/9000/Writing_a_Needs_Analysis__Exploring_the_Details.99182.aspx

Shaffer, F., & Ginsberg, J. P. (2017). An overview of heart rate variability metrics and norms [Review]. *Frontiers in Public Health, 5*(258). https://doi.org/10.3389/fpubh.2017.00258

Shalof, H., Dimitri, P., Shuweihdi, F., & Offiah, A. C. (2021). Which skeletal imaging modality is best for assessing bone health in children and young adults compared to DXA? A systematic review and meta-analysis. *Bone, 150*, 116013. https://doi.org/10.1016/j.bone.2021.116013

Shanbehzadeh, S., Mohseni Bandpei, M. A., & Ehsani, F. (2017). Knee muscle activity during gait in patients with anterior cruciate ligament injury: A systematic review of electromyographic studies. *Knee Surgery, Sports Traumatology, Arthroscopy, 25*(5), 1432–1442. https://doi.org/10.1007/s00167-015-3925-9

Shanley, E., Rauh, M. J., Michener, L. A., & Ellenbecker, T. S. (2011). Incidence of injuries in high school softball and baseball players. *Journal of Athletic Training, 46*(6), 648–654. https://doi.org/10.4085/1062-6050-46.6.648

Sherlock, A., & Brownie, S. (2014). Patients' recollection and understanding of informed consent: A literature review. *ANZ Journal of Surgery, 84*(4), 207–210. https://doi.org/10.1111/ans.12555

Silfies, S. P., Ebaugh, D., Pontillo, M., & Butowicz, C. M. (2015). Critical review of the impact of core stability on upper extremity athletic injury and performance. *Brazilian Journal of Physical Therapy, 19*(5), 360–368. https://doi.org/10.1590/bjpt-rbf.2014.0108

Simões, P., Vasconcelos-Raposo, J., Silva, A., & Fernandes, H. M. (2012). Effects of a process-oriented goal setting model on swimmer's performance. *Journal of Human Kinetics, 32*, 65–76. https://www.ncbi.nlm.nih.gov/pmc/articles/PMC3590857/

Smart, N. A., Way, D., Carlson, D., Millar, P., McGowan, C., Swaine, I., Baross, A., Howden, R., Ritti-Dias, R., Wiles, J., Cornelissen, V., Gordon, B., Taylor, R., & Bleile, B. (2019). Effects of isometric resistance training on resting blood pressure: Individual participant data meta-analysis. *Journal of Hypertension, 37*(10), 1927–1938. https://doi.org/10.1097/hjh.0000000000002105

Smith, M. V., Nepple, J. J., Wright, R. W., Matava, M. J., & Brophy, R. H. (2017). Knee osteoarthritis is associated with previous meniscus and anterior cruciate ligament surgery among elite college American football athletes. *Sports Health, 9*(3), 247–251. https://doi.org/10.1177/1941738116683146

Smith-Ryan, A. E., Mock, M. G., Ryan, E. D., Gerstner, G. R., Trexler, E. T., & Hirsch, K. R. (2017). Validity and reliability of a 4-compartment body composition model using dual energy x-ray absorptiometry-derived body volume. *Clinical Nutrition, 36*(3), 825–830. https://doi.org/10.1016/j.clnu.2016.05.006

Steffen, K., Myklebust, G., Andersen, T. E., Holme, I., & Bahr, R. (2008). Self-reported injury history and lower limb function as risk factors for injuries in female youth soccer. *American Journal of Sports Medicine, 36*(4), 700–708. https://doi.org/10.1177/0363546507311598

Stergiou, G. S., Alpert, B., Mieke, S., Asmar, R., Atkins, N., Eckert, S., Frick, G., Friedman, B., Graßl, T., Ichikawa, T., Ioannidis, J. P., Lacy, P., McManus, R., Murray, A., Myers, M., Palatini, P., Parati, G., Quinn, D., Sarkis, J., . . . O'Brien, E. (2018). A universal standard for the validation of blood pressure measuring devices: Association for the Advancement of Medical Instrumentation/European Society of Hypertension/International Organization for Standardization (AAMI/ESH/ISO) collaboration statement. *Hypertension, 71*(3), 368–374. https://doi.org/10.1161/hypertensionaha.117.10237

Stone, J. D., Ulman, H. K., Tran, K., Thompson, A. G., Halter, M. D., Ramadan, J. H., Stephenson, M., Finomore, V. S., Jr., Galster, S. M., Rezai, A. R., & Hagen, J. A. (2021). Assessing the accuracy of popular commercial technologies that measure resting heart rate and heart rate variability. *Frontiers in Sports and Active Living, 3*, 585870. https://doi.org/10.3389/fspor.2021.585870

Sueki, D. G., Cleland, J. A., & Wainner, R. S. (2013). A regional interdependence model of musculoskeletal dysfunction: Research, mechanisms, and clinical implications. *Journal of Manual & Manipulative Therapy, 21*(2), 90–102. https://doi.org/10.1179/2042618612Y.0000000027

Takatalo, J., Ylinen, J., Pienimäki, T., & Häkkinen, A. (2020). Intra- and inter-rater reliability of thoracic spine mobility and posture assessments in subjects with thoracic spine pain. *BMC Musculoskeletal Disorders, 21*(1), 529. https://doi.org/10.1186/s12891-020-03551-4

Tarnanen, S. P., Siekkinen, K. M., Häkkinen, A. H., Mälkiä, E. A., Kautiainen, H. J., & Ylinen, J. J. (2012). Core muscle activation during dynamic upper limb exercises in women. *Journal of Strength and Conditioning Research, 26*(12), 3217–3224. https://doi.org/10.1519/JSC.0b013e318248ad54

Tasheva, R., & Mitrev, G. (2019). Effect of hip adductors on basketball players balance. *Journal of Applied Sports Sciences, 1*, 85–90. https://doi.org/10.37393/jass.2019.01.8

Taylor, J. B., Wright, A. A., Smoliga, J. M., DePew, J. T., & Hegedus, E. J. (2016). Upper-extremity physical-performance tests in college athletes. *Journal of Sport Rehabilitation, 25*(2), 146–154. https://doi.org/10.1123/jsr.2014-0296

Taylor, J. B., Wright, A. A., Dischiavi, S. L., Townsend, M. A., & Marmon, A. R. (2017). Activity demands during multi-directional team sports: A systematic review. *Sports Medicine, 47*(12), 2533–2551. https://doi.org/10.1007/s40279-017-0772-5

Teyhen, D. S., Shaffer, S. W., Butler, R. J., Goffar, S. L., Kiesel, K. B., Rhon, D. I., Williamson, J. N., & Plisky, P. J. (2015). What risk factors are associated with musculoskeletal injury in US Army Rangers? A prospective prognostic study. *Clinical Orthopaedics and Related Research, 473*(9), 2948–2958. https://doi.org/10.1007/s11999-015-4342-6

Thomas, A. C., Villwock, M., Wojtys, E. M., & Palmieri-Smith, R. M. (2013). Lower extremity muscle strength after anterior cruciate ligament injury and reconstruction. *Journal of Athletic Training, 48*(5), 610–620. https://doi.org/10.4085/1062-6050-48.3.23

Thuany, M., de Souza, R. F., Hill, L., Mesquita, J. L., Rosemann, T., Knechtle, B., Pereira, S., & Gomes, T. N. (2021). Discriminant analysis of anthropometric and training variables among runners of different competitive levels. *International Journal of Environmental Research and Public Health, 18*(8), 42–48. https://doi.org/10.3390/ijerph18084248

Tiwari, R., Kumar, R., Malik, S., Raj, T., & Kumar, P. (2021). Analysis of heart rate variability and implication of different factors on heart rate variability. *Current Cardiology Reviews, 17*(5). https://doi.org/10.2174/1573403x16999201231203854

Trofa, D. P., Miller, J. C., Jang, E. S., Woode, D. R., Greisberg, J. K., & Vosseller, J. T. (2017). Professional athletes' return to play and performance after operative repair of an Achilles tendon rupture. *American Journal of Sports Medicine, 45*(12), 2864–2871. https://doi.org/10.1177/0363546517713001

Tsukahara, Y., Torii, S., Yamasawa, F., Iwamoto, J., Otsuka, T., Goto, H., Kusakabe, T., Matsumoto, H., & Akama, T. (2020). Changes in body composition and its relationship to performance in elite female track and field athletes transitioning to the senior division. *Sports (Basel), 8*(9). https://doi.org/10.3390/sports8090115

Tucci, H. T., Felicio, L. R., McQuade, K. J., Bevilaqua-Grossi, D., Camarini, P. M., & Oliveira, A. S. (2017). Biomechanical analysis of the Closed Kinetic Chain Upper-Extremity Stability Test. *Journal of Sport Rehabilitation, 26*(1), 42–50. https://doi.org/10.1123/jsr.2015-0071

Tucci, H. T., Martins, J., Sposito, G. d. C., Camarini, P. M. F., & de Oliveira, A. S. (2014). Closed Kinetic Chain Upper Extremity Stability test (CKCUES test): A reliability study in persons with and without shoulder impingement syndrome. *BMC Musculoskeletal Disorders, 15*(1), 1. https://doi.org/10.1186/1471-2474-15-1

Turnagöl, H. H. (2016). Body composition and bone mineral density of collegiate American football players. *Journal of Human Kinetics, 51*, 103–112. https://www.ncbi.nlm.nih.gov/pmc/articles/PMC5260544/

Ugalde, V., Brockman, C., Bailowitz, Z., & Pollard, C. D. (2015). Single leg squat test and its relationship to dynamic knee valgus and injury risk screening. *PM&R Journal, 7*(3), 229–235. https://doi.org/10.1016/j.pmrj.2014.08.361

Van de Velde, M., Matricali, G. A., Wuite, S., Roels, C., Staes, F., & Deschamps, K. (2017). Foot segmental motion and coupling in stage II and III tibialis posterior tendon dysfunction. *Clinical Biomechanics, 45*, 38–42. https://doi.org/10.1016/j.clinbiomech.2017.04.007

Wack, S. R., Crosland, K. A., & Miltenberger, R. G. (2014). Using goal setting and feedback to increase weekly running distance. *Journal of Applied Behavior Analysis, 47*(1), 181–185. https://doi.org/10.1002/jaba.108

Watkins, R. G. T., Chang, D., & Watkins, R. G., 3rd. (2018). Return to play after anterior cervical discectomy and fusion in professional athletes. *Orthopaedic Journal of Sports Medicine, 6*(6), 2325967118779672. https://doi.org/10.1177/2325967118779672

Weinstein, S., Khodaee, M., & VanBaak, K. (2019). Common skiing and snowboarding injuries. *Current Sports Medicine Reports, 18*(11), 394–400. https://doi.org/10.1249/jsr.0000000000000651

Weisleder, P. (2020). Helping them decide: A scoping review of interventions used to help minors understand the concept and process of assent. *Frontiers in Pediatrics, 8*, 25. https://doi.org/10.3389/fped.2020.00025

Westrick, R. B., Miller, J. M., Carow, S. D., & Gerber, J. P. (2012). Exploration of the Y-balance test for assessment of upper quarter closed kinetic chain performance. *International Journal of Sports Physical Therapy, 7*(2), 139–147.

Wilmore, J. H. (1983). Body composition in sport and exercise: Directions for future research. *Medicine & Science in Sports & Exercise, 15*(1), 21–31.

Zemková, E., & Hamar, D. (2018). Sport-specific assessment of the effectiveness of neuromuscular training in young athletes. *Frontiers in Physiology, 9*, 264. https://doi.org/10.3389/fphys.2018.00264

Żuk, B., Sutkowski, M., Paśko, S., & Grudniewski, T. (2019). Posture correctness of young female soccer players. *Scientific Reports, 9*(1), 11179. https://doi.org/10.1038/s41598-019-47619-1

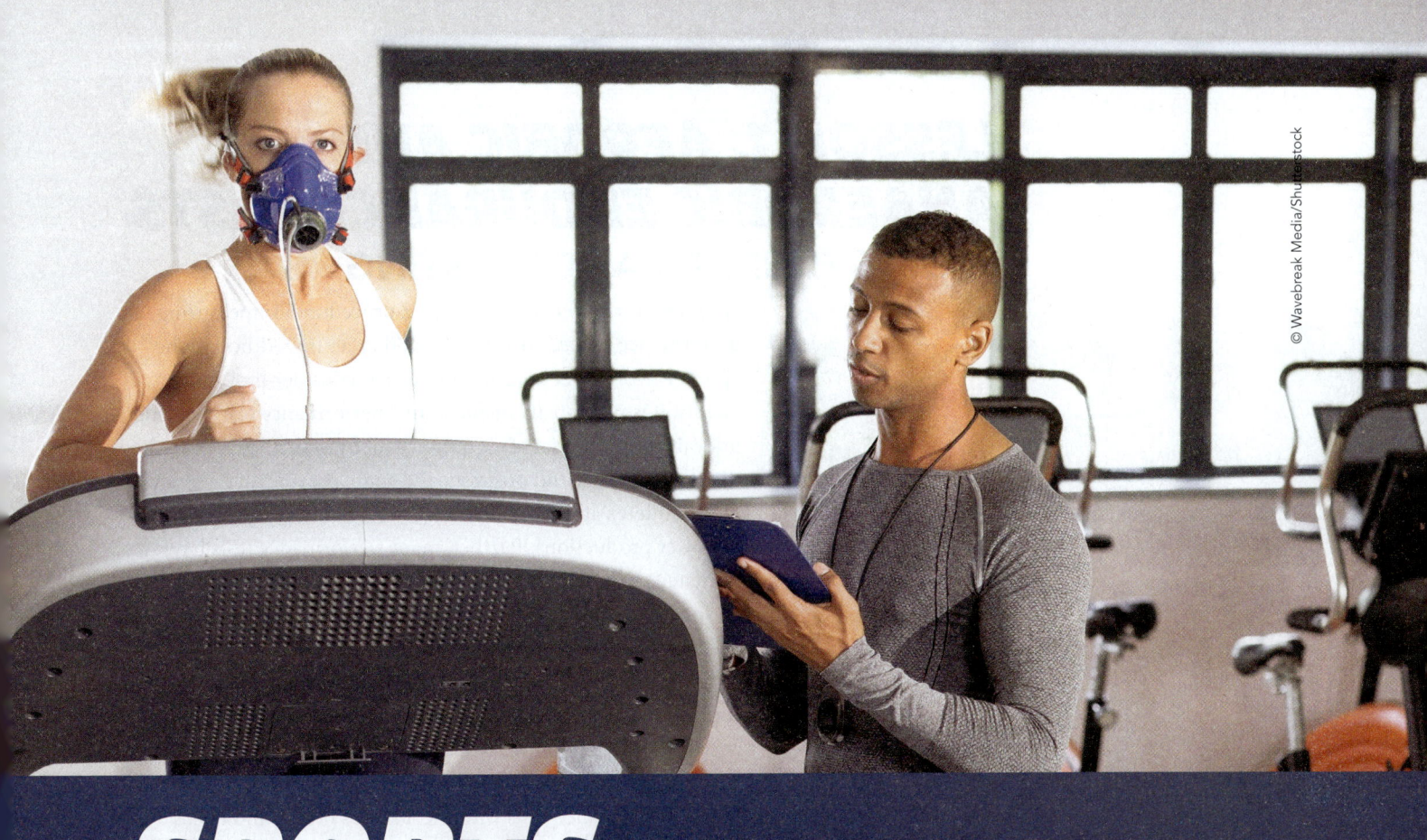

SPORTS PERFORMANCE TESTING AND EVALUATION

LEARNING OBJECTIVES

Upon completion of this chapter, the Sports Performance Coach will be able to:

- **Describe** the purpose of sports performance testing.
- **Explain** the importance of using appropriate sports performance tests.
- **Differentiate** between cardiovascular, strength, power, and speed, agility, and quickness (SAQ) performance tests.
- **Prioritize** performance testing results based on individual needs and sport-specific demands.
- **Evaluate** the findings of assessments and tests.

LESSON 1: AEROBIC AND ANAEROBIC ENDURANCE TESTS

SPORTS PERFORMANCE TESTING

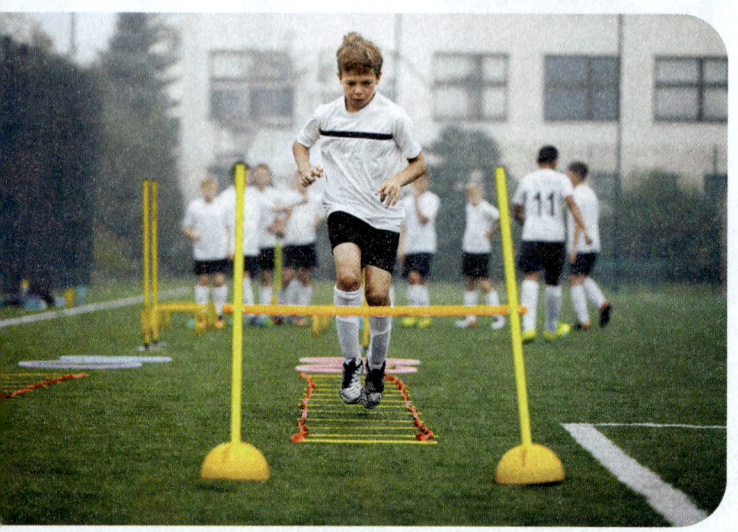

© Matimix/Shutterstock

Sports performance tests describe a procedure for measuring performance related to a specific skill or ability. Although the Sports Performance Coach must always consider movement quality, it is not usually included in a performance test's scoring or evaluation criteria. Most performance tests are specific to the athlete's sport and position, and some provide an overview of the athlete's athletic ability (e.g., vertical jump as a measure of power production). Further, many performance tests have validated evaluation criteria with which to compare an athlete's performance. Such data allow a coach or trainer to see where an athlete ranks compared to similar-age athletes if needed.

The Sports Performance Coach should also carefully consider the information obtained from the athlete intake, needs analysis, and movement assessments when deciding which sports tests are best for the athlete. Matching the correct sports performance tests with the athlete's profile and needs will yield the most accurate information (Currell & Jeukendrup, 2008).

The information necessary to create the right program for a specific individual or team comes through proper sports performance testing. A regular schedule of assessments and tests provides the Sports Performance Coach with an ongoing source of information to modify training and move an athlete through an integrated training program. Additionally, it enables the coach to continuously monitor the athlete's needs, functional capabilities, and physiological effects of exercise, enabling the athlete to reach peak performance.

It is important to understand that sports performance testing is not designed to diagnose any condition, but rather is conducted to observe each athlete's ability to perform a specific skill or task. Further, sports performance testing is not intended to replace a medical examination. The Sports Performance Coach must refer the athlete to a qualified medical professional when a medical issue is identified that might put the athlete at risk for injury during training.

PRETEST PROCEDURES

Sports performance testing requires the athlete to demonstrate maximal ability on each specific test. For example, a 40-yard dash requires maximal running speed. Given the all-out effort required during such tests, the Sports Performance Coach should develop consistent preparation procedures for athletes before testing. Establishing pretest procedures helps to decrease certain injury risks and standardizes the athlete's testing preparation. For example, if the athlete always performs 5 minutes of myofascial rolling followed by 5 minutes of dynamic stretching, then performance tests over time can be reliably compared. Conversely, if an athlete decides to warm up one time with myofascial rolling and dynamic stretching, but the next time with a stationary bike and plyometrics, it will be challenging to determine if and to what extent the warm-up affected the testing results.

WARM-UP AND COOL-DOWN

The Sports Performance Coach instructs the athlete to sufficiently warm up before any upper-body or lower-body testing to avoid the risk of injury (Davis et al., 2021; Herman et al., 2012). This differs from other types of movement assessments, such as the overhead squat assessment, in which the athlete does not warm up prior to testing. The warm-up also helps the athlete to mentally focus on the upcoming test, which can be beneficial for them (Van Raalte et al., 2019). The warm-up should include predetermined practice trials of the specific test to familiarize the athlete with the testing procedures and movements.

The athlete should also cool down after completing the testing to allow for a safe and adequate recovery. The type of warm-up and cool-down, including training variables (e.g., time), varies for each athlete and the tests that were administered. A general recommendation is 5 to 10 minutes for the warm-up and 5 to 10 minutes for the cool-down.

AEROBIC AND ANAEROBIC ENDURANCE TESTS

Sports Performance Coaches conduct aerobic assessments to measure an athlete's VO_2 max or aerobic fitness level. Additionally, anaerobic assessments are conducted to assess an athlete's anaerobic endurance.

AEROBIC TESTS

Aerobic tests evaluate an athlete's aerobic fitness level and capacity for performing work (Kenney et al., 2019). Common aerobic tests include the treadmill, bike, and different field tests. Anaerobic tests are used to evaluate an athlete's anaerobic capacity (Moore & Murphy, 2003). The Sports Performance Coach should include aerobic and anaerobic tests within the athlete's performance testing to identify the starting exercise intensity and appropriate modes of exercise.

VO₂ MAX

Maximal oxygen consumption (VO_2 max) testing is the most valid measure of aerobic fitness (**Figure 8.1**). A higher score reflects greater oxygen utilization and a greater

> **AEROBIC TESTS** →
>
> Tests used to evaluate an athlete's aerobic fitness level and capacity to perform work.

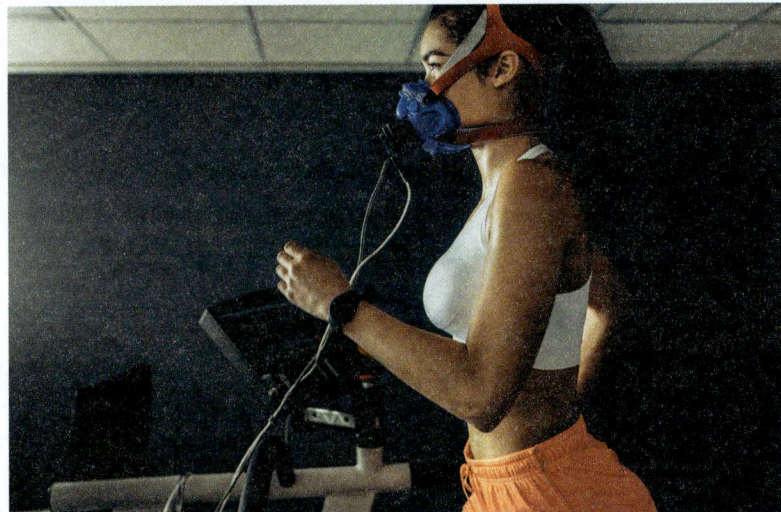

FIGURE 8.1 VO₂ Max Testing
© Jacob Lund/Shutterstock

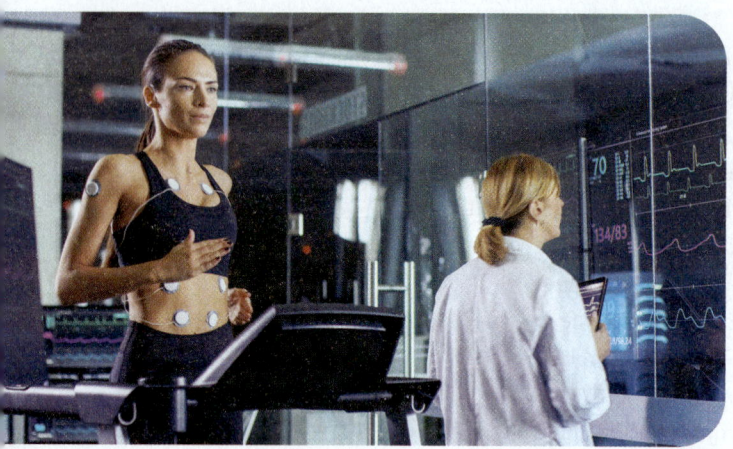
© Gorodenkoff/Shutterstock

capacity for physical work. VO_2 max peaks around age 25 into the early 30s, but it is highly trainable, implying that athletic individuals in their 40s could have higher scores than during their sedentary 20s. VO_2 max scores decrease by approximately 5% per decade in fit individuals (an average of 0.5% per year) and approximately 10% per decade in unfit individuals (an average of 1.0% per year) (Kenney et al., 2019).

VO_2 max testing can be either direct or indirect. Direct testing is not always practical because it requires specific equipment requirements, such as a treadmill, computer equipment, an oxygen/carbon dioxide analyzer, and an electrocardiograph machine or heart rate monitor. Conversely, indirect tests estimate VO_2 max based on submaximal exercise performance and other physiological measures such as heart rate, blood lactate, and respiratory exchange ratio. This type of VO_2 max testing is often preferred for determining aerobic fitness because it is easier to administer, less expensive, and provides valid predictions of VO_2 max (Al-horani, 2019; Bennett et al., 2016). Indirect testing can be performed using field-based tests such as the 1.5-mile run.

📋 COACH'S CORNER

Sports performance tests are valid and reliable procedures commonly used by sports performance professionals. Many of the tests have reference scores that list the most recent values for these tests and are specific to age groups, biological sex, and sports. The Sports Performance Coach must consider using the data as a comparison for their athlete's performance on the specific test and to help guide their performance exercise programming.

Åstrand Treadmill Test

The Åstrand treadmill test is an aerobic treadmill test to estimate VO_2 max (Kang et al., 2001).

EQUIPMENT

Treadmill, stopwatch, recording sheet, heart rate monitor.

INSTRUCTIONS

1. The athlete warms up and performs practice trials as needed.
2. The athlete runs at a constant 5 mph (8 kph) pace throughout the test while going through different stages of treadmill elevation.
3. The athlete begins with a 3-minute run at 0% elevation.
4. The athlete keeps the same speed while running at 2.5% elevation for 2 minutes.
5. Every 2 minutes, increase the treadmill elevation by 2.5% until the athlete cannot continue (**Table 8.1**).
6. The test is complete when the athlete reaches exhaustion.
7. The athlete cools down as needed.
8. Record the stage time (minutes) and elevation (percentage).
9. Calculate the VO_2 max prediction with the following equation:
   VO_2 max = (time $\times$ 1.444) + 14.99.

TABLE 8.1 Åstrand Treadmill Test Stages

Stage	Treadmill Speed	Stage Time (minutes)	Elevation (%)
1	5 mph (8 kph)	3	0
2	5 mph (8 kph)	2	2.5
3	5 mph (8 kph)	2	5.0
4	5 mph (8 kph)	2	7.5
5	5 mph (8 kph)	2	10.0
6	5 mph (8 kph)	2	12.5
7	5 mph (8 kph)	2	15.0
8	5 mph (8 kph)	2	17.5
9	5 mph (8 kph)	2	20.0
10	5 mph (8 kph)	2	22.5

✔ **CHECK IT OUT**

The Åstrand treadmill test and cycle ergometer test are both valid and reliable assessments for measuring predicted VO_2 max (Hoehn et al., 2015; Kang et al., 2001). However, these tests require more equipment and monitoring of the athlete (e.g., heart rate, blood pressure) than other aerobic field tests. Therefore, they might not be ideal to conduct in some performance training situations due to availability of equipment, setup time, and efficiency of testing multiple athletes. The Sports Performance Coach must consider such factors prior to testing based on the setting.

Cycle Ergometer Test (Åstrand-Rhyming)

The cycle ergometer test is an aerobic cycle test to measure estimated VO_2 max (Acevedo & Starks, 2011; Cink & Thomas, 1981; Hoehn et al., 2015).

EQUIPMENT

Cycle ergometer, recording sheet, stopwatch, heart rate monitor, optional blood pressure monitor.

INSTRUCTIONS

1. Adjust the cycle ergometer so the athlete sits upright with the knee slightly bent when the foot is at the bottom of the pedaling stroke.
2. The athlete warms up for 2 to 3 minutes by pedaling 50 revolutions per minute (rpm) to achieve a heart rate (HR) greater than 120 beats per minute (bpm) to determine test intensity.
3. The athlete performs a 6-minute test.

4. Set the initial resistance based on the athlete's biological sex and conditioning:
   - Males (unconditioned): 300 to 600 kilogram-meters per minute (kg-m/min) (50 to 100 watts)
   - Males (conditioned): 600 to 900 kg-m/min (100 to 150 watts)
   - Females (unconditioned): 300 to 450 kg-m/min (50 to 75 watts)
   - Females (conditioned): 450 to 600 kg-m/min (75 to 100 watts)
5. During the 6-minute testing period:
   - After the first and second minute, measure the athlete's heart rate and adjust the resistance accordingly:
     - Increase the resistance if the HR is less than 120 bpm.
     - Decrease the intensity if the HR is greater than 170 bpm.
   - Record HR and rate of perceived exertion (RPE) each minute to ensure the athlete is in a safe target HR range. Covert the HR to minutes.
   - Optionally assess blood pressure at the 2- or 4-minute mark.
   - The average HR at 5 and 6 minutes determines VO_2 max.
6. The athlete does one of the following steps:
   - After the 6-minute testing period, if the athlete has reached an average target HR of between 125 and 170 bpm, begin a 4-minute cool-down with 0 resistance. The Sports Performance Coach records HR, blood pressure, and RPE after each minute.
   - If the athlete has not reached an average target HR of between 125 and 170 bpm, continue the test for an additional 1 minute, increasing the resistance until the athlete reaches an HR of at least 125 bpm. At the end of each minute, the Sports Performance Coach records HR and blood pressure. After the athlete reaches an average target HR of between 125 and 170 bpm, begin a 4-minute cool-down with 0 resistance. Record HR, blood pressure, and RPE after each minute.
7. Refer to the Maximal Oxygen Uptake Score in Appendix E to obtain the maximal oxygen uptake (L/min) for the athlete based on the 5- and 6-minute averages. If step 6, part 2, was taken, take the average from the last 2 minutes.
8. Correct the value obtained from the Maximal Oxygen Uptake Score for age using the factor given in **Table 8.2**.

TABLE 8.2 Correction Factors for Predicted Maximal Oxygen Uptake

Age (years)	Factor	Maximum Heart Rate (bpm)	Factor
15	1.10	210	1.12
25	1.00	200	1.00
35	0.87	190	0.93
40	0.83	180	0.83
45	0.78	170	0.75
50	0.75	160	0.69
55	0.71	150	0.64
60	0.68		
65	0.65		

Factor to use to correct predicted maximal oxygen uptake when (a) the participant is older than 30–35 years of age or (b) the participant's maximum heart rate is known. Multiply the factor by value obtained from Maximal Oxygen Uptake Score.

Adapted from Acevedo & Starks, 2011.

9. After obtaining the athlete's results, determine the relative maximal oxygen uptake. Refer to **Table 8.3** to determine the subject's aerobic fitness level.

TABLE 8.3 Classification of Maximal Oxygen Uptake (Maximal Aerobic Power) by Age Group

Age (years)	Low	Somewhat Low	Average	High	Very High
Men					
20–29	≤2.79	2.80–3.09	3.10–3.69	3.70–3.99	≥4.00
	≤38	39–43	48–51	52–56	≥57
30–39	≤2.49	2.50–2.79	2.80–3.39	3.40–3.69	≥3.70
	≤34	35–39	40–47	48–51	≥52
40–49	≤2.19	2.20–2.49	2.50–3.09	3.10–3.39	≥3.40
	≤30	31–35	36–43	44–47	≥48
50–59	≤1.89	1.90–2.19	2.20–2.79	2.80–3.09	≥3.10
	≤25	26–31	32–39	40–43	≥44
60–69	≤1.59	1.60–1.89	1.90–2.49	2.50–2.79	≥2.80
	≤21	22–26	27–35	36–39	≥40
Women					
20–29	≤1.69	1.70–1.99	2.00–2.49	2.50–2.79	≥2.80
	≤28	29–34	35–43	44–48	≥49
30–39	≤1.59	1.60–1.89	1.90–2.39	2.40–2.69	≥2.70
	≤27	28–33	34–41	42–47	≥48
40–49	≤1.49	1.50–1.79	1.80–2.29	2.30–2.59	≥2.60
	≤25	26–31	32–40	41–45	≥46
50–65	≤1.29	1.30–1.59	1.60–2.09	2.10–2.39	≥2.40
	≤21	22–28	29–36	37–41	≥42

The upper number refers to maximal oxygen uptake in L/min; the lower number refers to maximal oxygen uptake in kg-m/min. In these tests, 58-kg weights were used for women; 72-kg weights were used for males.

Adapted from Acevedo & Starks, 2011.

12-Minute Run Test

The 12-minute run test is an aerobic test to measure predicted VO_2 max (Alvero-Cruz et al., 2017; Bandyopadhyay, 2015).

EQUIPMENT

Timer; recording sheet; running track (400 meter or ¼ mile), flat-looped course with markers every 100 meter, or treadmill.

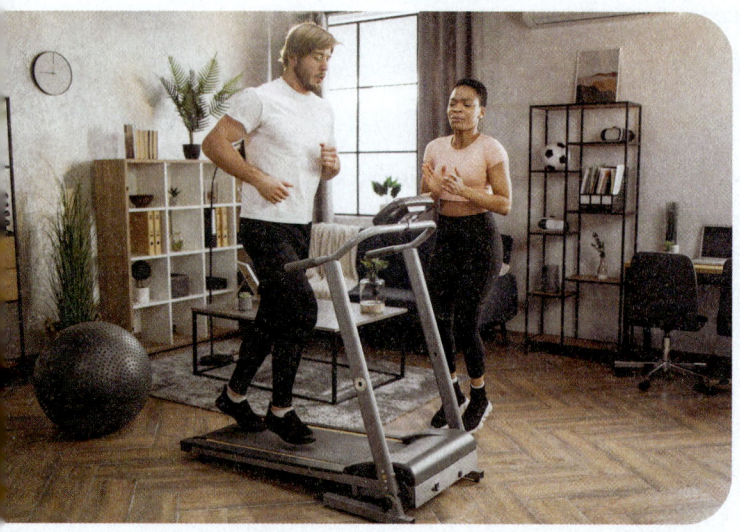

© SofikoS/Shutterstock

1. The athlete warms up as needed.
2. The athlete stands at the starting line ready to run.
3. Upon the signal (e.g., "Go!"), the athlete begins the run, and the Sports Performance Coach starts the timer at the same time.
4. The athlete runs for 12 minutes, and the total distance is recorded from that time. The score is converted to miles or kilometers.
5. The athlete cools down as needed.
6. The athlete's predicted VO_2 max is calculated using miles or kilometers:
   - VO_2 max = (35.971 × distance in miles) – 11.288
   - VO_2 max = (22.351 × distance in kilometers) – 11.288 (distance in meters is converted to kilometers)
7. The Sports Performance Coach can also calculate the distance from laps (laps × 400 m or total meters). The distance is converted to kilometers or miles. The Percentile Ranks for the 12-Minute Run (Appendix E) provide reference scores for this test based on the distance covered.

1.5-Mile Run Test

The 1.5-mile run test is an aerobic test to measure estimated VO_2 max (Alvero-Cruz et al., 2017; Bandyopadhyay, 2015).

EQUIPMENT

Timer; recording sheet; running track (400 meter or ¼ mile), 1.5-mile flat-looped course, or treadmill.

INSTRUCTIONS

1. The athlete warms up as needed.
2. The athlete stands at the starting line, ready to run.
3. Upon the signal (e.g., "Go!"), the athlete begins the run, and the Sports Performance Coach starts the timer at the same time.
4. The athlete runs 1.5 miles in the shortest amount of time possible.
5. Record the time after the athlete completes the distance.
6. Calculate the athlete's predicted VO_2 max using the following equation:
   - VO_2 max = (483 / time) + 3.5.
7. The athlete cools down as needed.
8. The Sports Performance Coach can also compare the athlete's completion time to the 1.5-Mile Run Test Reference Scores in Appendix E.

Ventilatory Threshold Test

The ventilatory threshold (VT1) test is a low- to moderate-workload aerobic test that gradually progresses in intensity level and relies on the interpretation of the way an athlete talks to determine a specific event at which the body's metabolism undergoes a significant change. Because it is an aerobic test, the athlete must attain a steady-state (SS) heart rate before the Sports Performance Coach performs any assessment of talking.

The following factors should be considered when conducting the ventilatory threshold (VT1) test:

- Determine the preference for increasing workloads (e.g., speed, grade, wattage). A range of 0.5 to 1 mph increases or 1% to 2% inclines are used for treadmills, 15- to 25-watt increases are used for cycling, and 10- to 15-watt increases are used for arm ergometers.
- Determine the duration of each stage. Stages usually last between 1 and 3 minutes to ensure that the athlete attains an SS heart rate. Larger increases in intensity require longer durations to attain a SS heart rate and are not recommended. SS heart rate implies a visible leveling of the athlete's heart rate at each stage, rather than continuing to climb upward.
- Conduct the continuous talk test once a SS heart rate is attained. The continuous talk test involves speaking continuously for about 20 seconds, although the Sports Performance Coach can observe the talking challenge within 10 seconds. The continuous talk test must be continuous and recited from memory—for example, the phonetic alphabet: "A is for apple, B is for boy, C is for cat." Another option is to have the athlete share information regarding their typical morning routine, detailing the steps involved in getting ready for work or school. The dialogue they provide needs to be continuous.

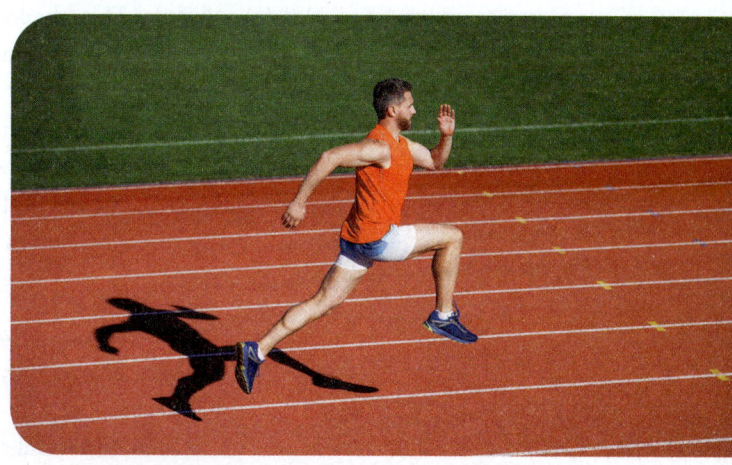

© Just dance/Shutterstock

EQUIPMENT

Treadmill or bicycle or arm ergometer, heart rate monitor, recording sheet.

INSTRUCTIONS

1. Have the athlete begin the test at an intensity considered light to easy, and gradually progress through incremental stages.
2. Perform the continuous talk test toward the end of each stage after the athlete attains a SS heart rate, as determined by using a heart rate monitor or another tracking device.
3. Repeat the continuous talk test until the talk test becomes challenging, but not difficult, for the athlete. This is a sign that the athlete has reached VT1. At this moment, record the athlete's heart rate and speed, grade, or wattage, depending on which type of equipment is being used.
4. Evaluate the challenge of continuous talking:
   - Observe the athlete's ability to speak continuously at a conversational pace (e.g., smooth, streamlined, and continuous versus choppy, interrupted, and disjointed).
   - Ask the individual to rate the challenge (e.g., an easy, small challenge; an uncomfortable, challenging task; or a difficult, nearly impossible task); VT1 is marked as uncomfortable or challenging.
   - Listen to the athlete's breathing sounds; VT1 occurs when their breathing becomes clearly audible with visible signs of rib cage elevation.
5. Consider continuing one stage beyond the suspected VT1 stage to validate the assessment.
6. Repeat this test within 2 to 3 days for purposes of reliability. Use the average physiological response to notate the athlete's VT1.

Ventilatory Threshold (VT2) Test

The ventilatory threshold (VT2) test is a higher workload aerobic test that relies on the interpretation of the way an athlete talks. The VT2 talk test measures the level at which the body can work at its highest sustainable SS intensity for more than a few minutes. At this level, the body relies heavily on the anaerobic energy systems, which begin to overwhelm the blood's lactic acid buffering capacity.

The following factors should be considered when conducting the ventilatory threshold (VT2) test:

1. VT2 testing is recommended only for individuals with suitable performance goals, given the purpose, nature, and intensity required for measuring this physiological marker.
2. Although several standardized field tests exist (e.g., 60-minute rides, 30- or 60-minute runs), they demand a lot of time and are tedious to administer.
3. A modified test, such as a 20-minute run or ride test protocol, provides a viable alternative, and is easier to conduct than the standardized 30- or 60-minute protocols.
4. The test requires the subject to maintain their highest-sustainable pace for 20 minutes and the fitness professional to record the athlete's heart rate and marker of performance (e.g., RPE, speed, wattage) over the last 5 minutes.

EQUIPMENT
Treadmill or bicycle, recording sheet.

INSTRUCTIONS
1. To start, increase the intensity to a predetermined pace. Some careful programming is required to determine this pace, but the test allows for some minor adjustments during the first few minutes of the trial. Remember that the athlete needs to hold this pace for 20 minutes; it needs to be the most intense pace they can safely handle.
2. Record the athlete's heart rate and marker of performance (e.g., speed, wattage, RPE) during the last 5 minutes of the trial.
3. Use the average heart rates collected over the last 5 minutes, and then correct that number by 95% to estimate the athlete's VT2. This 5% correction is needed because a 20-minute pace is usually more intense than when an athlete is performing a 30- to 60-minute test.

Beep Test (20-Meter Shuttle Run)

The beep test (20-meter shuttle run) is an aerobic field test to measure repeated intense exercise and predicted VO_2 max (Mayorga-Vega et al., 2015; Tomkinson et al., 2017).

EQUIPMENT
Timer, recording sheet, cones, beep test audio app, speaker to play audio, flat nonslip surface.

INSTRUCTIONS
1. The athlete warms up and performs practice trials as needed.
2. The Sports Performance Coach sets up two lines of cones 20 meters apart (**Figure 8.2**).
3. The athlete stands behind one of the lines facing the other line, ready to run.
4. When signaled, the athlete runs at the start of the first beep.
5. The first level of beeps are in 1-minute increments, and the beeps become shorter as the stages increase.
6. The athlete continues running between the two lines, beginning each run when signaled by the recorded beeps.

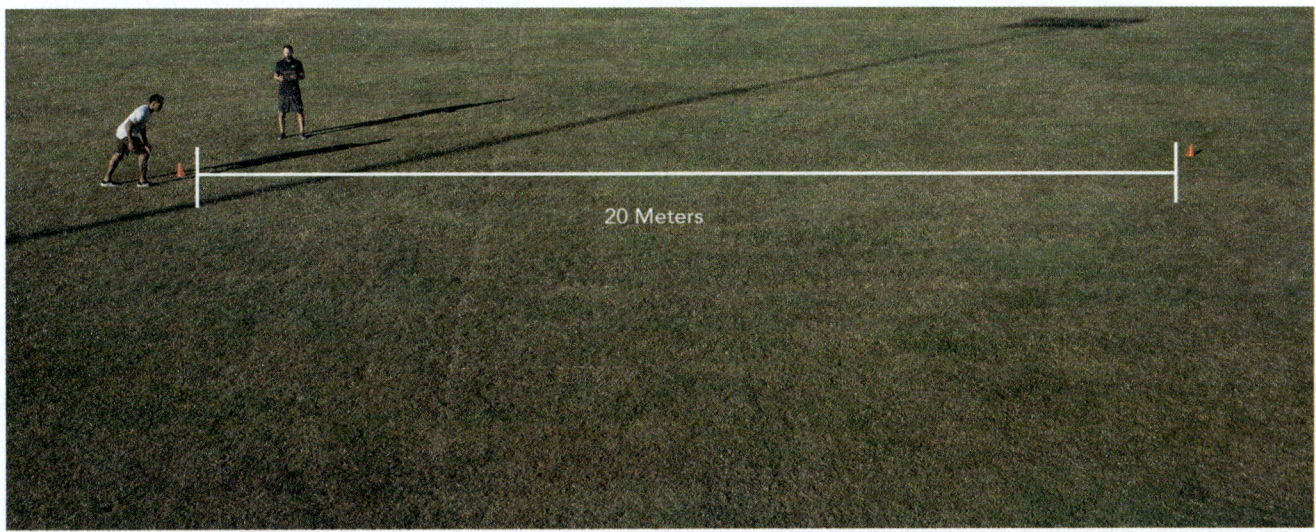

FIGURE 8.2 Beep Test Setup

7. If the athlete does not make it to the other side before the beep, they must try to catch up before the next beep.
8. Testing is completed when the athlete cannot complete two consecutive shuttles in time.
9. The athlete cools down as needed.
10. The athlete's final score is the stage and number of laps they reached before they were unable to keep up with the beeping.
11. Record the results. Beep Test Shuttle Reference Scores can be found in Appendix E.
12. The Sports Performance Coach can also calculate the athlete's predicted VO_2 max from the results. Several available apps and tables can convert the values.

Yo-Yo Intermittent Recovery Test

The yo-yo intermittent recovery test is an aerobic field test to measure repeated intense exercise and predicted VO_2 max.

EQUIPMENT

Timer, measuring tape at least 30 meters in length, eight marker cones, recording sheet, audio software for test, speaker, nonslip flat surface of sufficient distance.

INSTRUCTIONS

1. The athlete warms up and performs practice trials as needed.
2. Marker cones are placed over a 20-meter test area, two apart, to mark the start line and the turning line of the course. Cones are also placed 5 meters behind the start line (**Figure 8.3**).

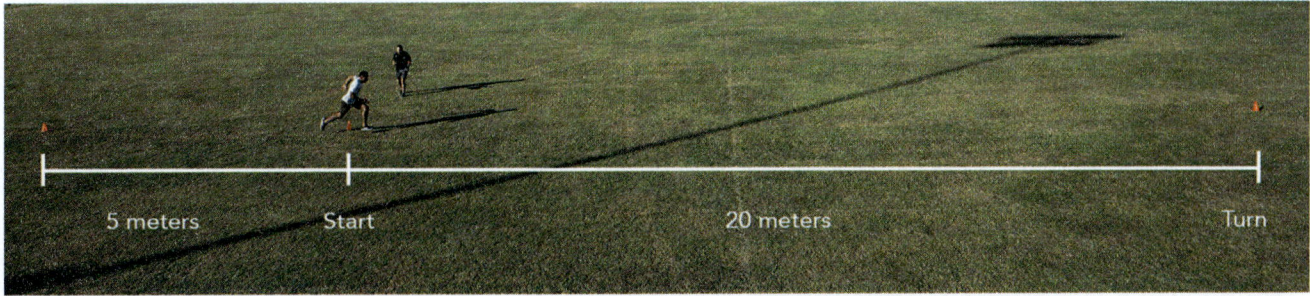

FIGURE 8.3 Yo-Yo Intermittent Recovery Test

3. The athlete begins at the starting line, ready to run.
4. When signaled (e.g., "Go!"), the athlete runs until they reach the turning line. At the next auditory signal, the athlete turns and runs back to the starting line before the next auditory signal.
5. The athlete can jog past the starting line for recovery but must return to the starting line and wait for the next auditory signal.
6. The athlete must place one foot on or over the starting or turning line at the auditory signal.
7. The time between auditory signals decreases as the stages increase and the athlete runs for as long as they can.
8. The test is complete when the athlete cannot maintain the running pace for two trials. The athlete is warned the first time they cannot reach the start or turn line in time.
9. The last level and number of laps (2 × 20 meters) is recorded as their final test score. Descriptive Data Results or Yo-Yo Within Various Sports can be found in Appendix E.
10. The athlete cools down as needed.
11. Calculate the athlete's predicted VO_2 max using the following equation (Bangsbo et al., 2008): VO_2 max (mL/min/kg) = IR1 distance (m) × 0.0084 + 36.4.

ANAEROBIC ENDURANCE

Anaerobic tests maximally stress the body's energy systems. It is common for sports to require an athlete to perform at a maximal level for short periods and with short periods of recovery. Numerous tests for anaerobic endurance are available, but the 300-yard shuttle run is a popular test used for different sports due to the repeated use of short distances with little rest between bouts. The Sports Performance Coach should consider other available anaerobic tests if this test is not applicable to a specific athlete.

300-YARD SHUTTLE RUN

The 300-yard shuttle run is an anaerobic field test that estimates lower-body anaerobic capacity (Sporis et al., 2008).

EQUIPMENT
Timer, measuring tape, two marker cones, recording sheet, a flat grass surface or nonslip indoor surface of sufficient distance.

INSTRUCTIONS
1. The athlete warms up and performs practice trials as needed.
2. Marker cones and lines are placed 25 yards apart to indicate the sprint.
3. The athlete starts with a foot on one line, ready to run. When signaled (e.g., "Go!"), the athlete runs to the opposite 25-yard line, touches it with their foot, turns, and runs back to the start (**Figure 8.4**).
4. The athlete repeats this action six times without stopping, covering 300 yards total.
5. The athlete performs two trials.
6. The athlete takes a 5-minute rest and performs the second trial.
7. The athlete cools down as needed.
8. The average of two trials is recorded as the final test score. **Table 8.4** provides reference scores for this test. The Percentile Ranks for 300-Yard Shuttle Run for NCAA Athletes can be found in Appendix E.

ANAEROBIC TESTS →

Tests that evaluate an athlete's anaerobic fitness and maximally stress the energy systems of the body.

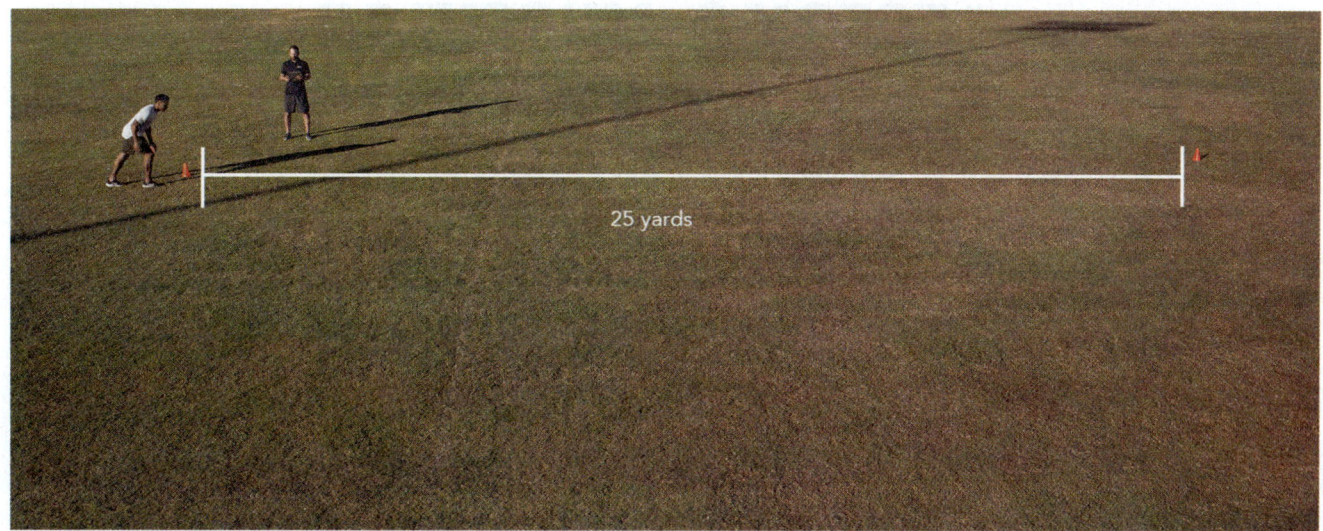

FIGURE 8.4 300-Yard Shuttle Run

TABLE 8.4 Descriptive Data for 300-Yard Shuttle Test

Group, Sport, or Position	Number of Athletes	Time (seconds)
High school volleyball (women) (98)	27	68.0 ± 6.3
NCAA Division 1 volleyball (women) (98)	26	67.7 ± 3.8
National soccer (men) (107)	18	56.7 ± 1.7
Recreational men and women (121)	81	72.8 ± 9.1
National badminton (men) (120)	12	73.3 ± 3.4

The values listed are means ± standard deviation. The data are based on research studies and are descriptive, not normative. Use these numbers for reference only.

Reproduced from Haff, G. & Triplett, T. (2015). *Essentials of strength training and conditioning* (4th Ed.). Human Kinetics.

📋 **COACH'S CORNER**

When administering sports performance tests to large groups of athletes, the Sports Performance Coach must make sure there are an adequate setup, pretest procedures, and test administration. One or more coaches might be required to organize the groups and record each athlete's results. This teamwork helps the group assessment to run efficiently, especially if multiple tests are administered.

LESSON 2: MUSCULAR ENDURANCE AND STRENGTH TESTS

MUSCULAR ENDURANCE TESTS

Muscular endurance tests are bodyweight performance tests that evaluate specific muscle groups. Muscular endurance is an important aspect of athletic performance that must be considered in any performance training program.

PUSH-UP TEST

The push-up test is a muscular endurance field test of the upper extremities (Hashim et al., 2018). The goal is to complete as many repetitions as possible, with good form, usually for a predetermined length of time (Saint Romain & Mahar, 2001). A variety of methods may be used to conduct this test, depending on the type of athlete (e.g., older adults, youths, military) (Haff & Dumke, 2021).

EQUIPMENT

Exercise mat or comfortable surface, recording sheet, timer.

INSTRUCTIONS

1. The athlete warms up and performs practice trials as needed.
2. The athlete begins by assuming a push-up position with their hands slightly outside of shoulder-width apart, elbows and knees fully extended, and spine in a neutral position (**Figure 8.5**). If the athlete is not able to perform a standard push-up or demonstrates poor form, they can complete testing from a kneeling position.
3. When signaled (e.g., "Go!"), the athlete lowers their body to achieve 90 degrees of elbow flexion before returning to the start position. They repeat this pattern for 60 seconds or until exhaustion.
4. Count all repetitions completed to the full depth during the 60-second testing period (Acevedo & Starks, 2011).
5. The athlete is allowed to rest, but only in the "up" position.
6. The athlete cools down as needed.
7. The Sports Performance Coach reassesses the athlete at regular intervals (e.g., 4 to 6 weeks) to evaluate progress. **Table 8.5** presents reference scores for this test.

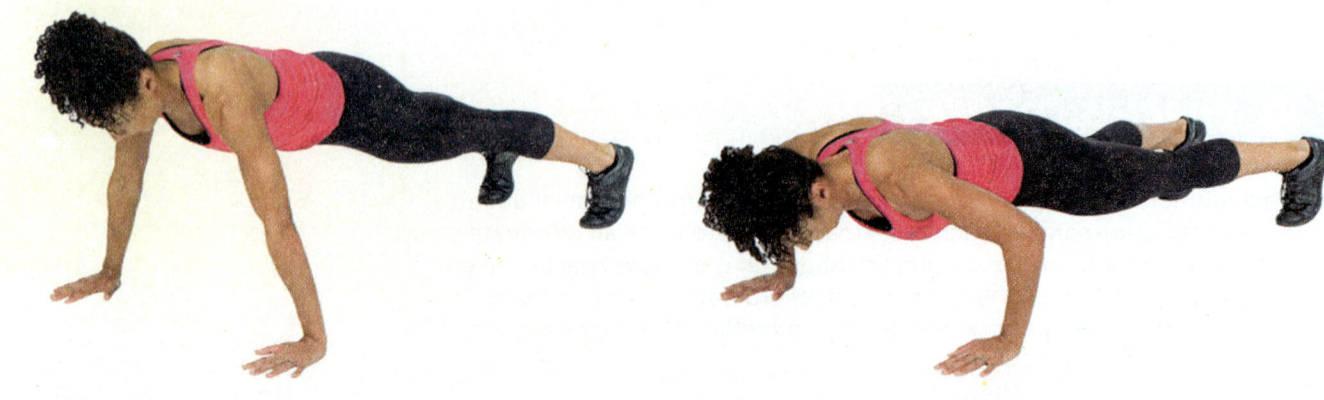

FIGURE 8.5 Push-Up Test

TABLE 8.5 Push-Up Test Reference Scores

Age (years)	15–19	20–29	30–39	40–49	50–59	60–69
Men						
Excellent	≥39	≥36	≥30	≥25	≥21	≥18
Very good	29–38	29–35	22–29	17–24	13–20	11–17
Good	23–28	22–28	17–21	13–16	10–12	8–10
Fair	18–22	17–21	12–16	10–12	7–9	5–7
Needs improvement	≤17	≤16	≤11	≤9	≤6	≤4
Women						
Excellent	≥33	≥30	≥27	≥24	≥21	≥17
Very good	25–32	21–29	20–26	15–23	11–20	12–16
Good	18–24	15–20	13–19	11–14	7–10	5–11
Fair	12–17	10–14	8–12	5–10	2–6	2–4
Needs improvement	≤11	≤9	≤7	≤4	≤1	≤1

The Canadian Physical Activity, Fitness and Lifestyle Approach: CSEP-Health and Fitness Program's Health-Related Appraisal and Counselling Strategy, 3rd Edition © 2003. Adapted with permission of the Canadian Society for Exercise Physiology.

PULL-UP TEST

The pull-up test is a muscular endurance field test of the upper extremities (Hewit et al., 2018). A variety of methods can be used to conduct this test (Burnstein et al., 2011; Rutherford & Corbin, 1994).

EQUIPMENT
Pull-up bar, recording sheet, timer.

INSTRUCTIONS

1. The athlete warms up and performs practice trials as needed.
2. The athlete hangs from a horizontal bar at a height where their arms are fully extended and their feet free from the floor. The athlete uses an overhead grip (palms facing away) to perform a standard pull-up (**Figure 8.6**).
3. When signaled (e.g., "Go!"), the athlete pulls themselves up until their chin clears the horizontal bar and then lowers themselves back to the starting position.
4. The athlete keeps their legs and trunk straight and avoids kicking their legs or swinging their body.
5. The athlete repeats this pattern for 60 seconds or until exhaustion. The athlete is allowed to rest in the up or down position, but cannot rest with their chin supported on the bar.

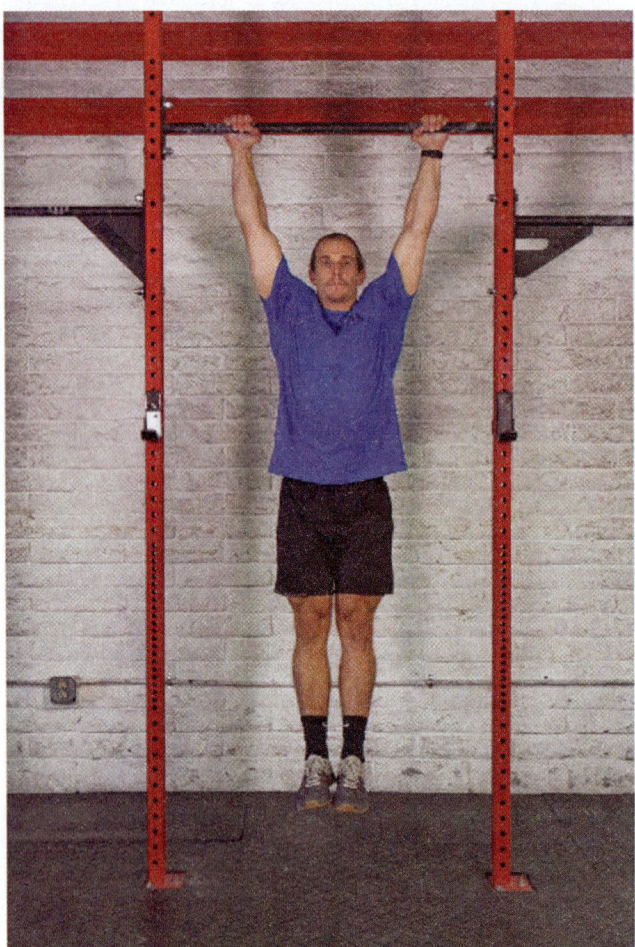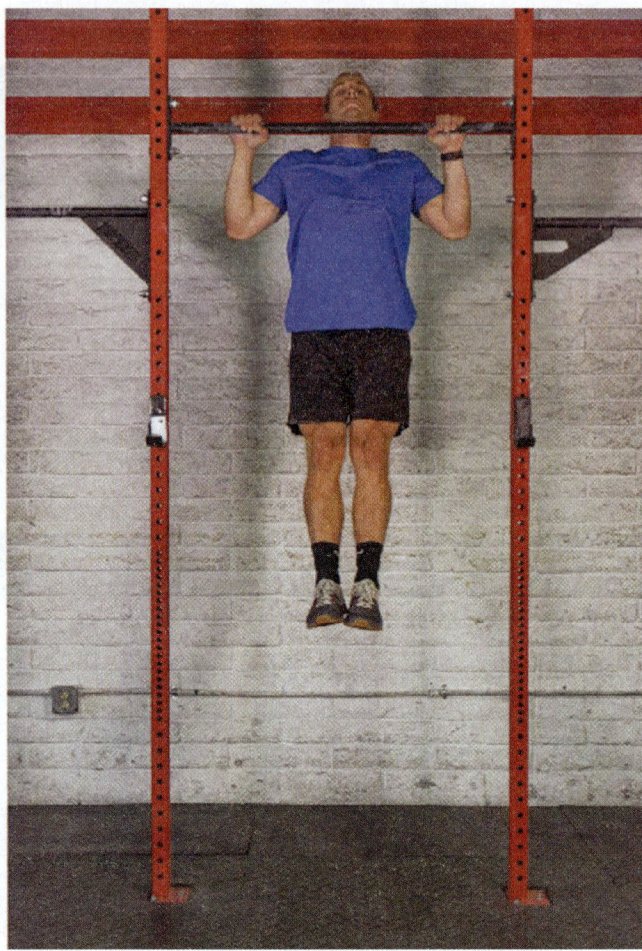

FIGURE 8.6 Palm Forward Grip

6. Count all completed repetitions during the 60-second testing period.
7. The athlete cools down as needed.
8. The Sports Performance Coach reassesses the athlete at regular intervals (e.g., 4 to 6 weeks) to evaluate progress. **Table 8.6** provides reference scores for this test.

TABLE 8.6 Pull-Up Test Reference Scores

	Males				Females			
Age (years)	20–29	30–39	40–49	50–59	20–29	30–39	40–49	50–59
Excellent	>10	>9	>7	>4	>3	>3	>3	>3
Good	9–10	8–9	6–7	3–4	3	3	3	3
Fair	7–8	6–7	4–5	2	2	2	2	2
Poor	5–6	3–5	2–3	1	1	1	1	1
Needs improvement	<5	<3	<2	<1	<1	<1	<1	<1

CURL-UP TEST

The curl-up test is a muscular endurance field test of the anterior abdominals. This test is considered both valid and reliable (Davoli et al., 2018; Knudson, 2001). As with other endurance tests, a variety of methods may be used to conduct this test (Haff & Dumke, 2021).

Equipment

Exercise mat or comfortable surface, recording sheet, tape measure, timer.

Instructions

1. The athlete warms up and performs practice trials as needed.
2. Place a strip of masking tape on the floor at the fingertips, and then place a second strip of tape approximately 5 inches (12 cm) (age < 45 years) or 3 inches (8 cm) (age ≥ 45 years) beyond the first strip, toward the athlete's heels (**Figure 8.7**).
3. The athlete lies supine on the floor with knees bent and feet flat. The athlete places the arms at the sides.
4. When signaled (e.g., "Go!"), the athlete performs controlled curl-ups, lifting the shoulder blades off the mat and returning to the start position after each repetition.
5. The athlete touches their fingertips to the second strip of tape to successfully complete a repetition. The athlete's trunk must return to flat on the mat before each new curl-up.
6. The athlete repeats this pattern for 60 seconds or until exhaustion.
7. Count all successful curl-ups during the 60-second testing period.
8. The athlete cools down as needed. **Table 8.7** provides reference scores for this test.

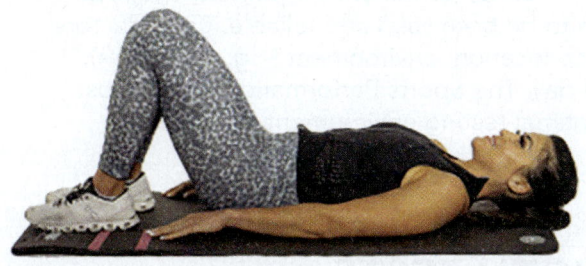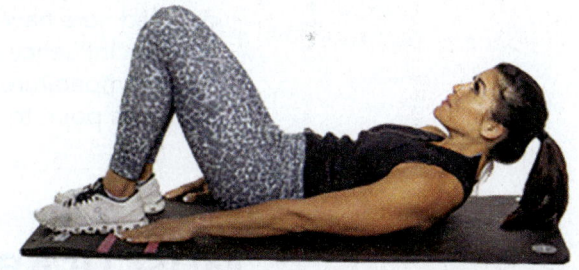

FIGURE 8.7 Curl-Up Position

TABLE 8.7   Curl-Up Test Reference Scores

Age (years)	15–19	20–29	30–39	40–49	50–59	60–69
Men						
Excellent	25	25	25	25	25	25
Very good	23–24	21–24	18–24	18–24	17–24	16–24
Good	21–22	16–20	15–17	13–17	11–16	11–15
Fair	16–20	11–15	11–14	6–12	8–10	6–10
Needs improvement	≤15	≤10	≤10	≤5	≤7	≤5

(continues)

TABLE 8.7 Curl-Up Test Reference Scores (*continued*)

Age (years)	15–19	20–29	30–39	40–49	50–59	60–69
Women						
Excellent	25	25	25	25	25	25
Very good	22–24	18–24	19–24	19–24	19–24	17–24
Good	17–21	14–17	10–18	11–18	10–18	8–16
Fair	12–16	5–13	6–9	4–10	6–9	3–7
Needs improvement	≤11	≤4	≤5	≤3	≤5	≤2

The Canadian Physical Activity, Fitness and Lifestyle Approach: CSEP-Health and Fitness Program's Health-Related Appraisal and Counselling Strategy, 3rd Edition © 2003. Adapted with permission of the Canadian Society for Exercise Physiology.

📋 COACH'S CORNER

The accuracy of a performance test is dependent on two main factors: validity and reliability. Test validity is the level of accuracy for the test. Test reliability is how well the test can be consistently repeated. The tests detailed here have been shown to be both valid and reliable. Other factors that can influence testing include location, environment (e.g., loud gym), room temperature, and time of day. The Sports Performance Coach must make it a point to create the optimal testing environment for athletes.

MUSCULAR STRENGTH TESTS

Muscular strength tests are foundational measures of athletic ability. These tests provide information on how strong the athlete is in regard to specific movements and related muscle groups. Several standard tests have been developed based on the repetition maximum. Maximal strength is best obtained by using a one-repetition maximum test. However, performing a true one-repetition maximum test might not be practical for all populations. For this reason, the Sports Performance Coach can have an athlete perform anywhere from one to five repetitions during maximal testing, and refer to the proper conversion chart. However, some error is introduced when calculating maximal strength using several repetitions.

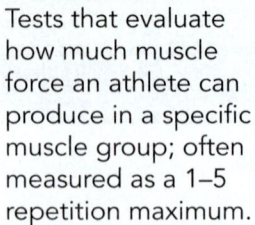

MUSCULAR STRENGTH TESTS →

Tests that evaluate how much muscle force an athlete can produce in a specific muscle group; often measured as a 1–5 repetition maximum.

GRIP STRENGTH TEST

The grip strength test is a measurement of the maximum strength of the hand and forearm muscles. Hand grip strength is a valid and reliable test (Cronin et al., 2017; Nikodelis et al., 2021). Several different testing methods may be used for determining grip strength. The following information utilizes a common testing protocol and related reference values for the United States (Perna et al., 2016; Wang et al., 2018; Wong, 2016). Hand grip strength is important in most sports that require use of the upper extremities and is related to optimal shoulder function. Specific testing is valuable for athletes in sports that require repetitive gripping, such as golf and racquet sports (Mohamed et al., 2014; Torres-Ronda et al., 2011).

EQUIPMENT
Hand dynamometer.

INSTRUCTIONS
1. The athlete warms up and performs practice trials as needed.
2. The athlete stands with their arms at their sides with their elbows straight and forearms neutral.
3. The dynamometer is gripped between the palm at the base of the thumb and the second joint of the fingers (**Figure 8.8**).
4. When signaled (e.g., "Go!"), the athlete squeezes the dynamometer with maximum effort.
5. The athlete repeats the test three times on each hand, alternating hands, with a 60-second rest between testing bouts.
6. The maximum contraction of each hand over three trials is summed for the right and left hands. Then, the Sports Performance Coach calculates and records a combined grip strength score from both hands and can compare it to United States Max Grip Strength Scores found in Appendix E (Perna et al., 2016).
7. The athlete cools down as needed.

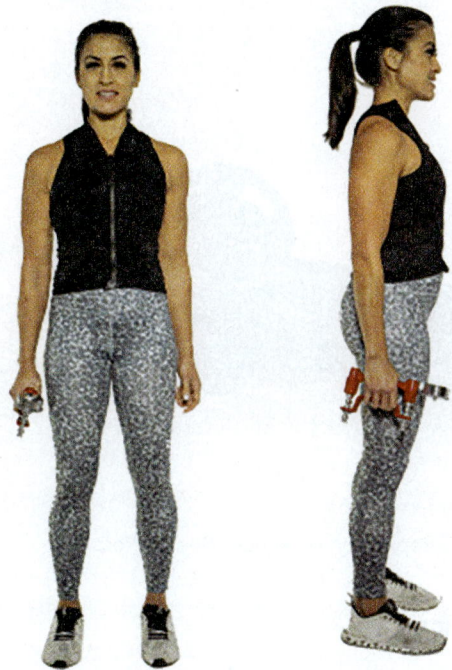

FIGURE 8.8 Hand Grip Position

1–5 RM BENCH PRESS TEST

The 1–5 RM bench press test is a maximum strength test of the upper body (McMaster et al., 2014). Maximum strength is often measured by a 1–5 repetition maximum (RM). This test is considered an advanced assessment for strength-specific goals and, as such, might not be suitable for all athletes, especially those who have limited experience with resistance training.

EQUIPMENT
Chest press bench, Olympic barbell, recording sheet, weighted plates.

1. The athlete warms up and performs practice trials as needed. A comfortable weight is used for the warm-up and initial repetitions of the testing.
2. The athlete lies on their back on a weight-lifting bench. The lower back is in a neutral position, avoiding excessive arching. Both feet are planted on the ground.
3. The athlete grasps the barbell with hands slightly greater than shoulder-width apart (**Figure 8.9**).
4. The athlete, with assistance, unracks the weighted barbell, lowers it to their chest, and presses it back into full elbow extension. After completing five repetitions, they re-rack the weight. The Sports Performance Coach must properly spot the athlete during the testing.
5. The athlete takes a 2-minute rest.
6. The Sports Performance Coach increases the load by 5% to 10% of the initial weight for the next bout of testing.
7. The athlete continues with testing until they are no longer comfortable adding weight or cannot complete a minimum of five repetitions.
8. The athlete cools down as needed.
9. Use the One Repetition Maximum Conversion Chart (Appendix E) to calculate the athlete's final 1 RM.
10. The Sports Performance Coach reassesses the athlete at regularly scheduled intervals to measure progress.

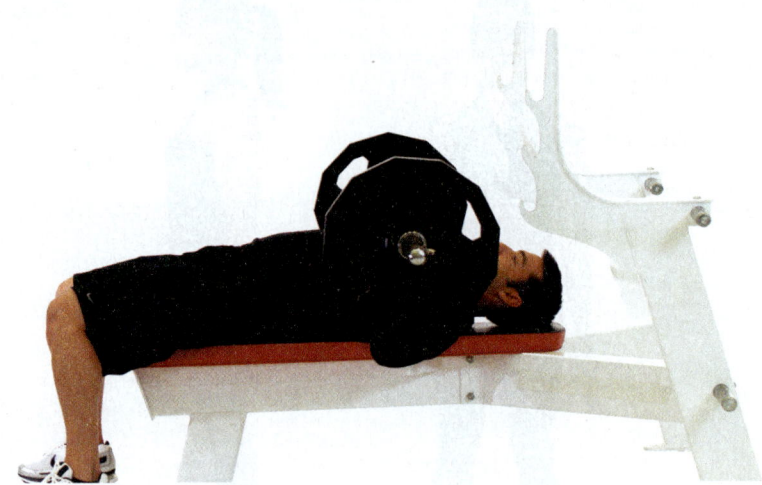

FIGURE 8.9 1–5 Repetition Maximum Bench Press Test

1–5 RM SQUAT TEST

The 1–5 RM squat test is a maximum strength test of the lower body (McMaster et al., 2014). Maximum strength is often measured by a 1–5 RM. This test is considered an advanced assessment for strength-specific goals and, as such, might not be suitable for all athletes, especially those with limited experience with resistance training.

EQUIPMENT
Squat rack, Olympic bar, weighted plates.

INSTRUCTIONS

1. The athlete warms up and performs practice trials as needed. A comfortable weight is used for the warm-up and initial repetitions of the testing.

2. The athlete stands in a standardized starting position. The exact position may vary with each athlete. However, the Sports Performance Coach should ensure there is little to no variability between tests of the same athlete.

3. The athlete lowers themselves under the racked barbell, placing it on their shoulders and grasping the barbell with their hands. The Sports Performance Coach must properly spot the athlete during the testing.

4. The athlete unracks the weighted barbell and steps away from the squat rack. The athlete lowers into a squatting position. Movement proficiency must be maintained for the test to be valid. The depth of squat can be adjusted as needed (e.g., one-fourth squat, full squat). The athlete returns to the starting position (**Figure 8.10**).

5. After completing five repetitions, the athlete re-racks the weight.

6. The athlete takes a 2-minute rest.

7. The Sports Performance Coach increases the load by 5% to 10% of the initial weight for the next bout of testing.

8. The athlete repeats the motion until they are no longer comfortable adding weight or cannot complete a minimum of five repetitions.

9. The athlete cools down as needed.

10. Use the One Repetition Maximum Conversion Chart (Appendix E) to calculate the athlete's final 1 RM.

11. The Sports Performance Coach reassesses the athlete at regularly scheduled intervals to measure progress.

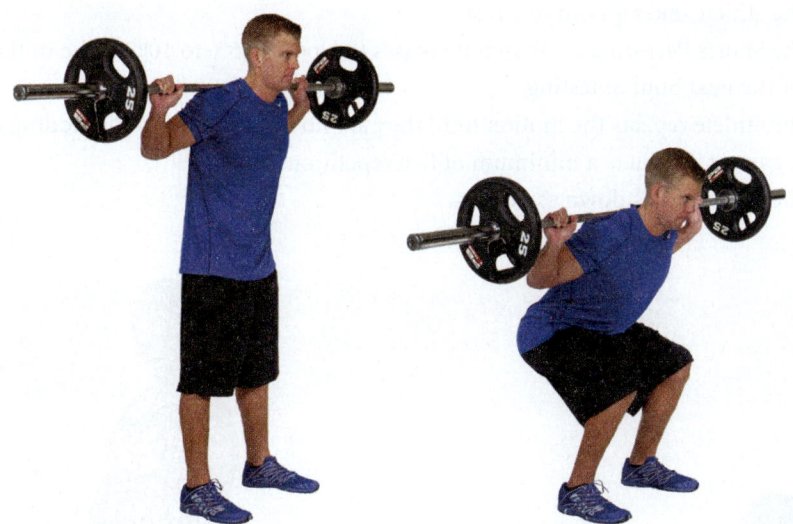

FIGURE 8.10 1–5 Repetition Maximum Squat Test

📋 COACH'S CORNER

The depth of the squat descent varies among athletes and must be based on their training goals, health status, and functional abilities. A common recommendation is for individuals to perform either partial squats with a 40-degree knee angle, or parallel or half squats with a 70- to 100-degree knee angle (Schoenfeld, 2010). The Sports Performance Coach is referred to the NASM Squat Movement: Evidence Based Review manuscript for a more in-depth discussion on this topic.

1–5 RM DEADLIFT TEST

The 1–5 RM deadlift test is a maximum strength test of the lower body (Bishop et al., 2014). Maximum strength is often measured by a 1–5 RM. This test is considered an advanced assessment for strength-specific goals and, as such, might not be suitable for all athletes.

EQUIPMENT
Squat rack (optional), Olympic bar, recording sheet, weighted plates.

INSTRUCTIONS
1. The athlete warms up and performs practice trials as needed. A comfortable weight is used for the warm-up and initial repetitions of the testing.
2. The weighted bar is placed on the ground. The athlete stands in a standardized starting position. The exact position may vary with each athlete. However, the Sports Performance Coach should ensure there is little to no variability between tests of the same athlete.
3. The athlete reaches forward and grabs the weighted barbell with arms straight at a shoulder-width grip.
4. The athlete bends knees until their shins touch the bar.
5. The athlete then stands up with the weight by straightening their hips and knees to full extension, avoiding locking out. The Sports Performance Coach must properly spot the athlete during the testing (**Figure 8.11**).
6. After completing five repetitions, the athlete lowers the weight to the ground.
7. The athlete takes a 2-minute rest.
8. The Sports Performance Coach increases the load by 5% to 10% of the initial weight for the next bout of testing.
9. The athlete repeats the motion until they are no longer comfortable adding weight or cannot complete a minimum of five repetitions.
10. The athlete cools down as needed.

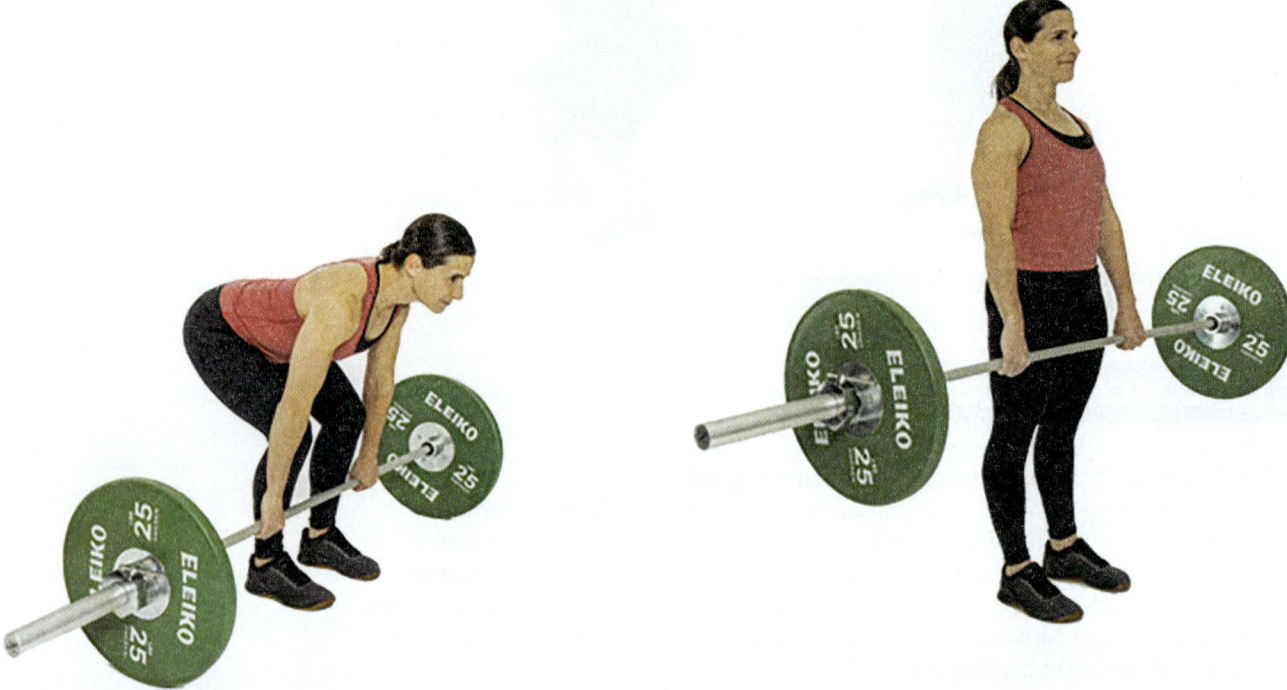

FIGURE 8.11 1–5 Repetition Maximum Deadlift Test

11. Use the One Repetition Maximum Conversion Chart (Appendix E) to calculate the athlete's final 1 RM.
12. The Sports Performance Coach reassesses the athlete at regularly scheduled intervals to measure progress (Martín-Fuentes et al., 2020).

📋 COACH'S CORNER

The Sports Performance Coach must always remember to provide proper spotting techniques during maximum strength testing to ensure the athlete's safety. Using one or more professionals to spot the athlete during the movement or using safety equipment (e.g., squat rack spotter arms or safety straps) helps create a safe testing environment.

NORDIC HAMSTRING LOWERING TEST

The Nordic hamstring lowering test is a maximal eccentric strength test of the hamstring (Sconce et al., 2015). This test is considered an advanced assessment for strength-specific goals and, as such, might not be suitable for all athletes.

EQUIPMENT
Comfortable surface or exercise mat, recording sheet, optional camera.

INSTRUCTIONS
1. The athlete warms up and performs practice trials as needed.
2. The athlete begins by kneeling in an upright position on a comfortable surface or exercise mat. The athlete keeps their hips fixed in line with the knee and shoulder joints throughout the movement.
3. One Sports Performance Coach sits behind the athlete and stabilizes their legs above the ankles (**Figure 8.12**).

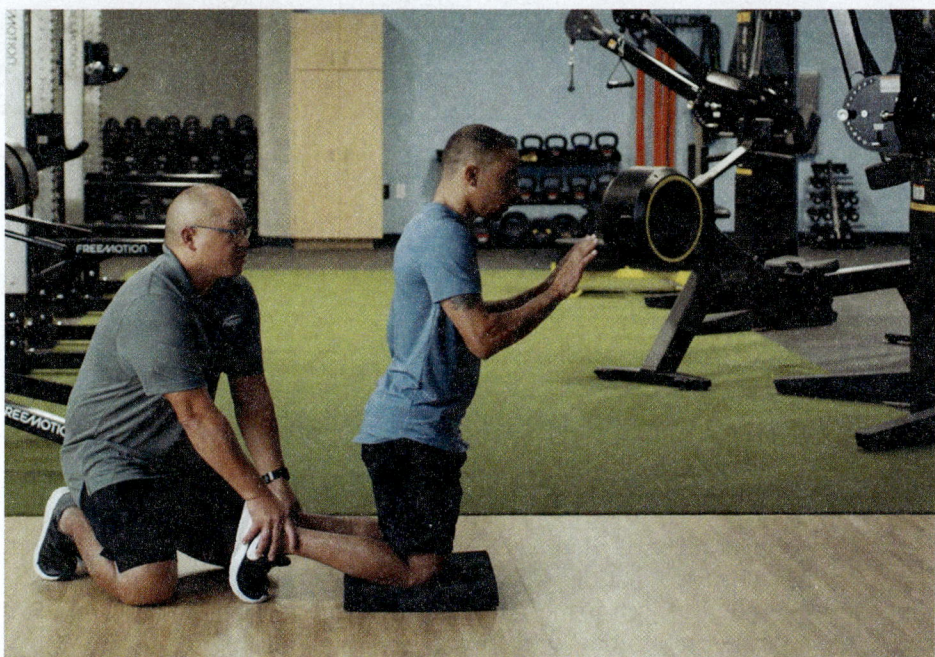

FIGURE 8.12 Nordic Hamstring Lowering Start

4. When signaled (e.g., "Go!"), the athlete attempts to slowly lower themselves to the ground.

5. A camera can be used (optimal) to record the movement for more precise measuring of the breakpoint. The breakpoint is the angle where the athlete can no longer control the movement, causing them to fall forward to the ground and catch themselves (**Figure 8.13**).

6. The athlete gets three attempts, and the best breakpoint angle is documented (lowest, closest to the floor) as the reference score.

7. The athlete cools down as needed.

8. To date, there are no reference scores available for this test. The Sports Performance Coach uses the initial test to establish a baseline for each athlete and track performance over time.

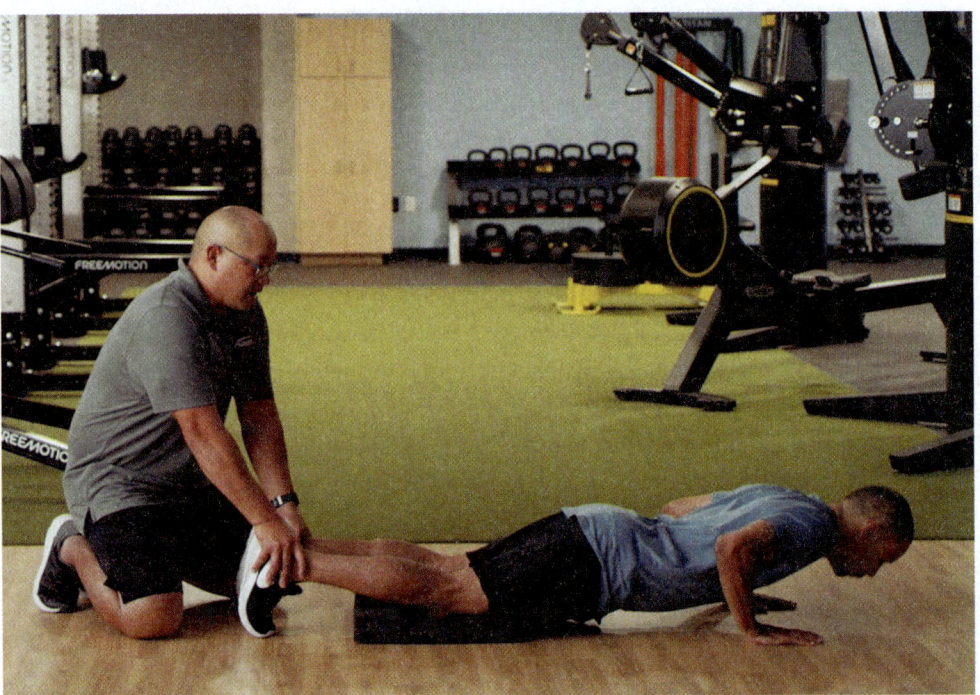

FIGURE 8.13 Nordic Hamstring Lowering After Breakpoint

🤖 GETTING TECHNICAL

The Nordic hamstring exercise is a popular exercise that effectively prevents hamstring injuries in such sports as soccer and track and field (Al Attar et al., 2017; Tsaklis et al., 2015; van der Horst et al., 2015). The Nordic hamstring lowering test is an emerging field test that measures the eccentric strength of the hamstrings (Sconce et al., 2015). The Sports Performance Coach must consider that this field test does not replace more scientific strength testing, such as isokinetic strength testing. More studies are needed to validate this field test for different athletes and sports.

LESSON 3: TESTING POWER
POWER TESTS

The Sports Performance Coach must consider that specific **power tests** might provide valuable information about the athlete's ability to explosively exert force in the shortest time. Power tests include the vertical jump test, horizontal broad jump, and power clean, and the medicine ball rotational, soccer, and overhead throws.

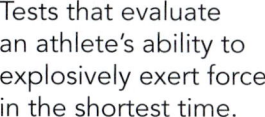

POWER TESTS →

Tests that evaluate an athlete's ability to explosively exert force in the shortest time.

VERTICAL JUMP TEST (DOUBLE-LEG)

The vertical jump test (double-leg) is a lower-body power test for both legs (Rodríguez-Rosell et al., 2017).

EQUIPMENT
Vertec or similar measurement device, scoring form, nonslip surface.

INSTRUCTIONS
1. The athlete warms up and performs practice trials as needed.
2. Measure the standing reach of the athlete with one arm fully extended upward. The testing equipment is adjusted so that when the athlete jumps, they do not jump higher or lower than the testing device.
3. When signaled (e.g., "Go!"), the athlete jumps and touches the highest possible vane without any preliminary steps (**Figure 8.14**). No shuffle step, sidestep, drop step, or gather steps are allowed. The jump is straight up and straight down.
4. Measure the height difference between the athlete's standing reach and their jumping height.
5. The athlete gets two attempts. If on the second attempt, the athlete reaches a new height, they are awarded a third attempt.
6. The athlete cools down as needed.
7. Record the athlete's final score. A Percentile Breakdown of Vertical Jump Height by Five-Year Groups can be found in Appendix E.

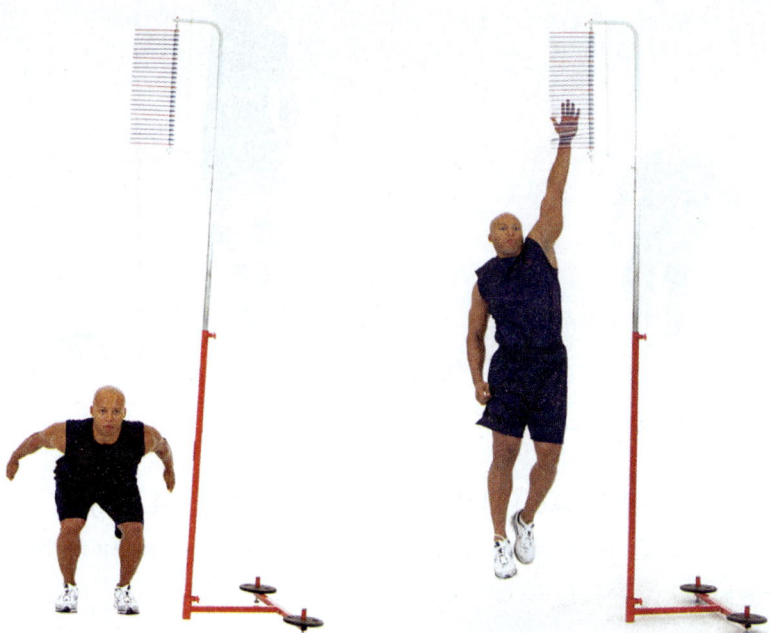

FIGURE 8.14 Vertical Jump Test (Double-Leg)

VERTICAL JUMP TEST (SINGLE-LEG)

The vertical jump test (single-leg) is a lower-body power test for one leg (Rodríguez-Rosell et al., 2017).

EQUIPMENT

Vertec or similar measurement device, scoring form, nonslip surface.

INSTRUCTIONS

1. The athlete warms up and performs practice trials as needed.
2. Measure the standing reach of the athlete with one arm fully extended upward. The testing equipment is adjusted so that when the athlete jumps, they do not jump higher or lower than the testing device.
3. The athlete balances on one leg.
4. When signaled (e.g., "Go!"), the athlete jumps on the balance leg and touches the highest possible vane, then lands on the same leg (**Figure 8.15**). No shuffle step, sidestep, drop step, or gather steps are allowed. The jump is straight up and straight down.
5. Measure the height difference between the standing reach and jumping height.
6. The athlete gets two attempts per leg. If on the second attempt, the athlete reaches a new height, they are awarded a third attempt.
7. The athlete cools down as needed.
8. Record the athlete's final score. To date, no reference scores are available for this test. The Sports Performance Coach uses the initial test to establish a baseline for each athlete.

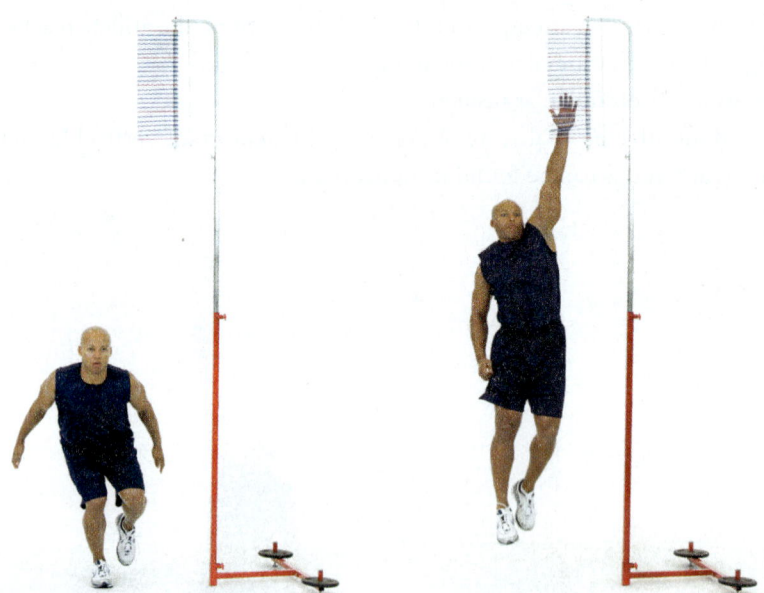

FIGURE 8.15 Vertical Jump Test (Single-Leg)

HORIZONTAL (BROAD) JUMP TEST (DOUBLE-LEG)

The horizontal (broad) jump test (double-leg) is a lower-body power test for both legs (Zhou et al., 2020).

EQUIPMENT

Nonslip surface, tape measure, recording form, marking tape.

1. Tape is used to mark off a starting line.
2. The athlete warms up and performs practice trials as needed.
3. The athlete stands on the line and jumps forward as far as possible (**Figure 8.16**).
4. The athlete gets three attempts.
5. Record the relative distance (in inches or centimeters) from the edge of the starting line (the edge closest to the landing point) to the athlete's heel or closest body part. If the athlete falls forward or backward, record the distance from the heel or body part nearest the starting line. Horizontal Jump Reference Scores and Percentile Rankings can be found in Appendix E.
6. The athlete cools down as needed.

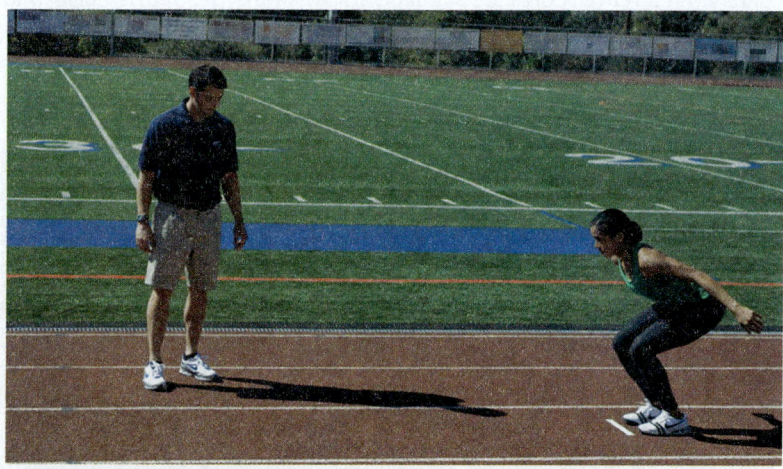

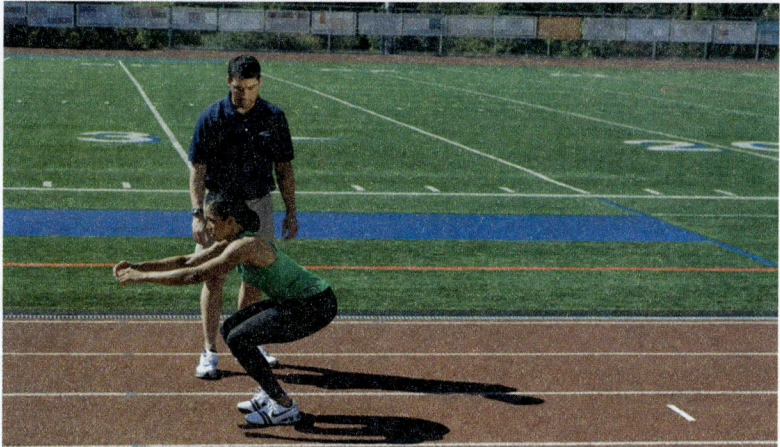

FIGURE 8.16 Horizontal Jump Assessment (Double-Leg)

HORIZONTAL (BROAD) JUMP TEST (SINGLE-LEG)

The horizontal (broad) jump test (single-leg) is a lower-body power test for one leg (Zhou et al., 2020).

EQUIPMENT

Nonslip surface, tape measure, recording form, marking tape.

INSTRUCTIONS

1. Tape is used to mark off starting line.
2. The athlete warms up and performs practice trials as needed.
3. The athlete stands on the line and jumps forward as far as possible with one leg, landing on the same leg (**Figure 8.17**).
4. Record the relative distance from the edge of the starting line (the edge closest to the landing point) to the athlete's heel or closest body part. This test differs from the single-leg hop test in that the focus is solely on the distance jumped rather than lower-body alignment.
5. The athlete gets three attempts.
6. If the athlete falls backward, record the distance from the body part nearest the starting line.
7. The athlete cools down as needed.
8. To date, no reference scores are available for this test. The Sports Performance Coach uses the initial test to establish a baseline for each athlete. This test can be performed in all planes of motion.

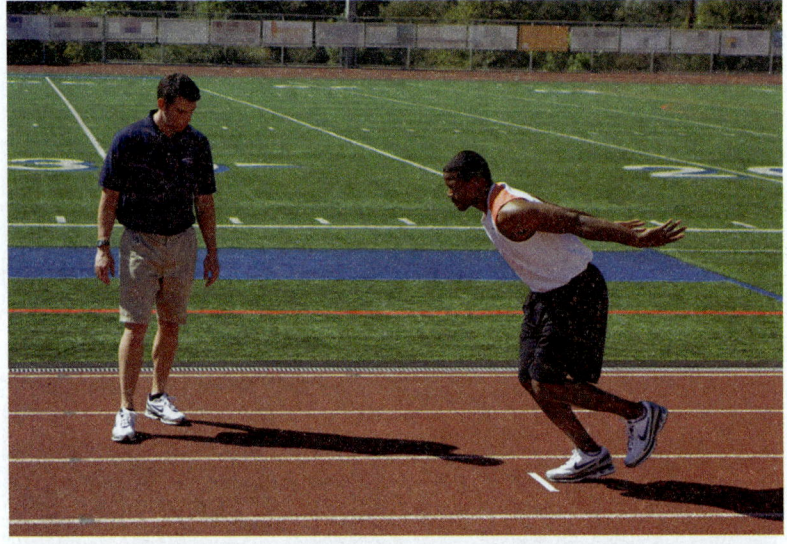

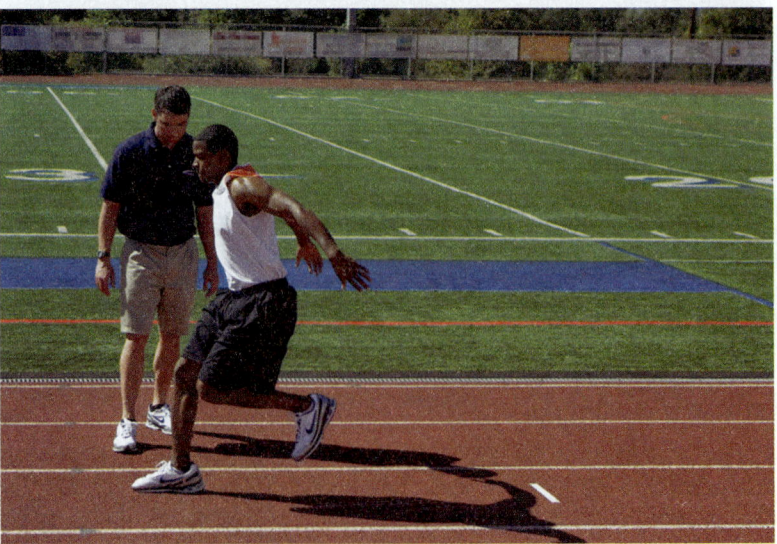

FIGURE 8.17 Horizontal Jump Assessment (Single-Leg)

POWER CLEAN TEST

The power clean test is an upper- and lower-body power test. This test is used to determine the training intensities of Olympic lifts. Prior to testing, athletes need proper training and must demonstrate technical proficiency with the movement.

EQUIPMENT

Optional squat rack, Olympic bar, recording form, weighted plates.

INSTRUCTIONS

1. The athlete warms up and performs practice trials as needed.
2. The athlete is positioned in the starting position for a power clean exercise. The Sports Performance Coach provides close supervision and spots the athlete during the test.
3. The athlete performs the power clean movement. After completing five repetitions, they lower the weight to the ground (**Figure 8.18**).
4. The athlete takes a 2-minute rest.
5. Increase the load by 5% to 20% of the initial weight for the next bout of testing.
6. The athlete repeats the power cleans until they are no longer comfortable adding weight or cannot complete a minimum of five repetitions. Power Clean Percentile Rankings can be found in Appendix E.
7. The athlete cools down as needed.

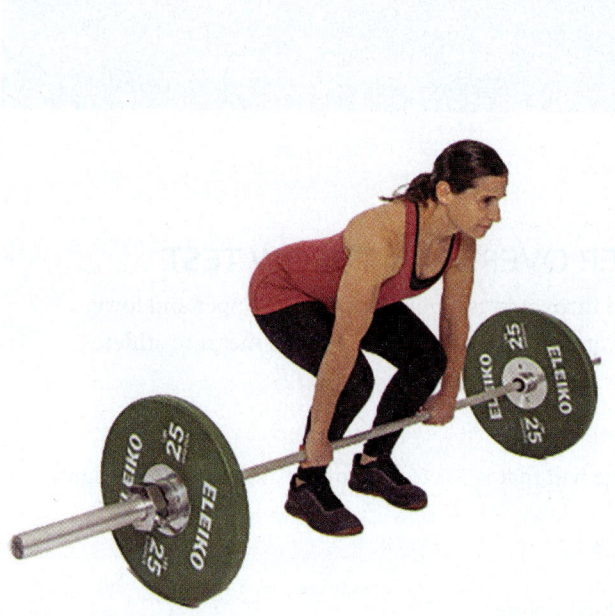
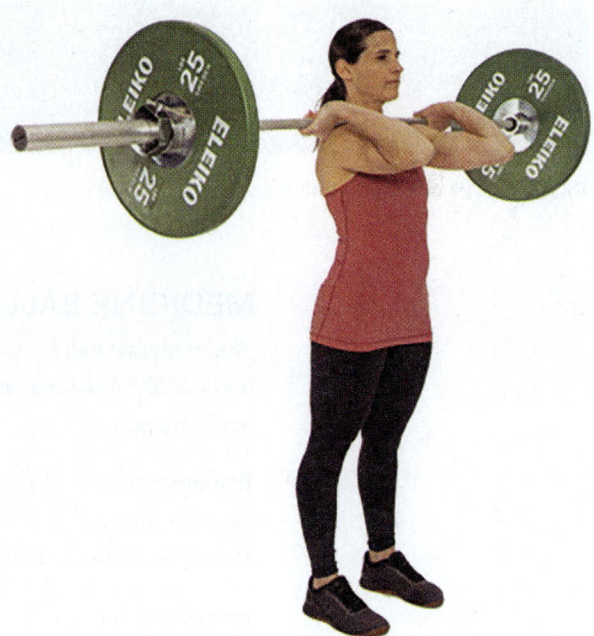

FIGURE 8.18 Power Clean Assessment

ROTATIONAL MEDICINE BALL THROW TEST

The rotational medicine ball throw test is a power test of the upper and lower body.

EQUIPMENT

Nonslip surface, weighted medicine ball that is 5% to 10% of the athlete's body weight, recording form, tape measure.

1. Tape is used to mark off a starting line.
2. The athlete warms up and performs practice trials as needed.
3. The athlete stands at the line and begins perpendicular to the throwing zone, with feet pointing straight ahead.
4. The athlete holds a medicine ball with both hands.
5. When signaled (e.g., "Go!"), the athlete rotates through the hips as in a golf swing, loading the back leg, with the ball at approximately hip level. The athlete quickly rotates the other way, throwing the medicine ball like a shot put as far as possible (**Figure 8.19**).
6. The athlete gets two attempts for the right and left sides. Measure the distance thrown to the nearest foot or centimeter, and record the farthest distance for each side. To date, no reference scores are available for this test. The Sports Performance Coach uses the initial test to establish a baseline for each athlete.
7. The athlete cools down as needed.

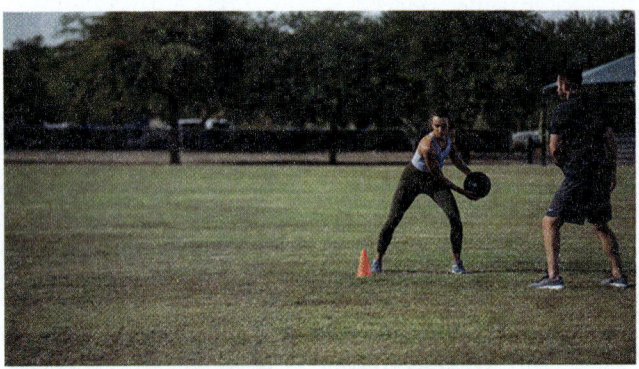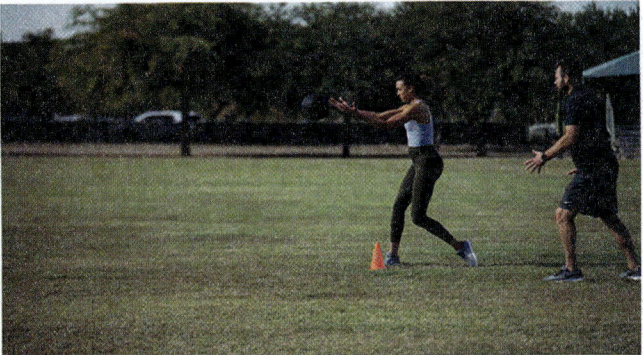

FIGURE 8.19 Medicine Ball Rotational Throw

MEDICINE BALL SOCCER OVERHEAD THROW TEST

The medicine ball soccer overhead throw test is a power test of the upper and lower body. Multiple sports, such as soccer and tennis, utilize this test to measure athlete performance.

EQUIPMENT

Nonslip surface, weighted medicine ball that is 5% to 10% of the athlete's body weight, recording form, tape measure.

INSTRUCTIONS

1. Tape is used to mark off a starting line.
2. The athlete warms up and performs practice trials as needed.
3. The athlete stands at the line with their feet staggered and facing the direction in which they will throw the ball. The front of the forward foot touches the line.
4. The athlete holds the medicine ball, centered above their head.
5. When signaled (e.g., "Go!"), the athlete throws the medicine ball forward using a proper soccer throw-in technique as far as possible without taking any steps (**Figure 8.20**). The athlete is allowed to shift their weight onto the forward foot, but they cannot take any steps.
6. The athlete has two attempts.

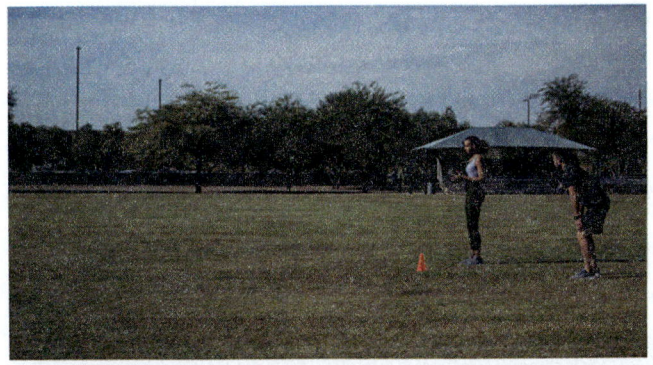
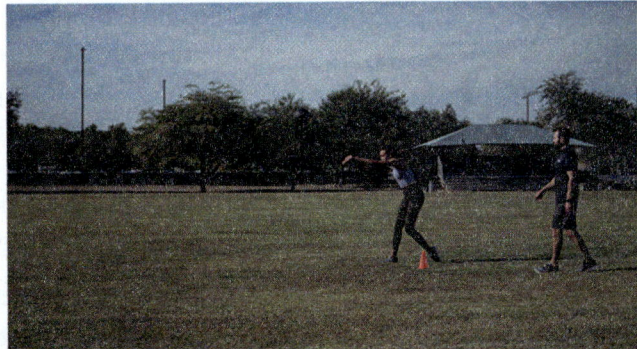

FIGURE 8.20 Medicine Ball Soccer Throw Test

7. Measure the distance thrown; the farthest distance is recorded to the nearest 0.5 foot or 10 cm. Only Male and Female Youth Tennis Player Reference Values (Appendix E) are currently available for this test (Fernandez-Fernandez et al., 2014).
8. The athlete cools down as needed.

REVERSE OVERHEAD MEDICINE BALL THROW TEST

The reverse overhead medicine ball throw test is a power test of the upper and lower body (Manske & Reiman, 2013).

EQUIPMENT
Nonslip surface, weighted medicine ball that is 5% to 10% of the athlete's body weight, recording form, tape measure.

INSTRUCTIONS

1. Tape is used to mark off a starting line.
2. The athlete warms up and performs practice trials as needed.
3. The athlete stands facing away from the start line with their heels at the line. The athlete holds a medicine ball, arms extended, at chest level.
4. When signaled (e.g., "Go!"), the athlete squats down, brings the ball between their legs, then explosively throws the medicine ball up and back overhead for a maximal distance (**Figure 8.21**). The athlete is allowed to step or fall back over the line, but is not allowed to jump.

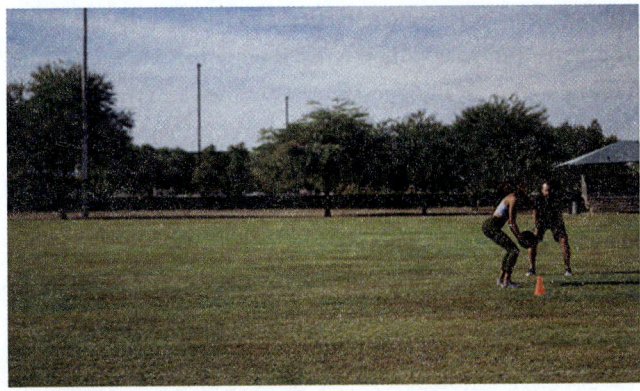
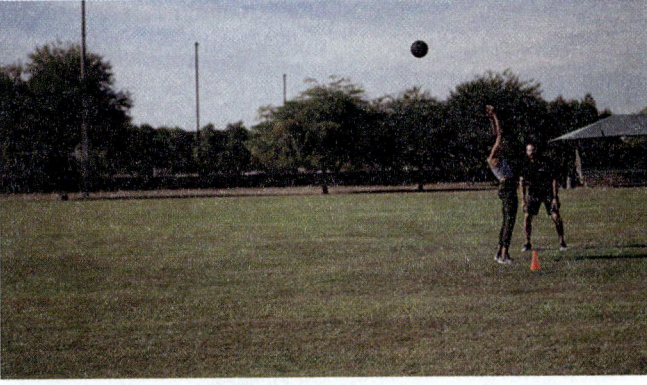

FIGURE 8.21 Overhead Medicine Ball Throw

5. The athlete has two attempts.
6. Measure the distance thrown to the nearest foot or centimeter; the farthest distance is recorded. **Table 8.8** provides scores for different sports for this test (Cornell et al., 2015; Duncan & Hankey, 2010; Mayhew et al., 2005; Stockbrugger & Haennel, 2001).
7. The athlete cools down as needed.

TABLE 8.8 Reverse Overhead Medicine Ball Throw Test Scores

Sport or Occupation	Average Distance
Average Population	
Collegiate football players (male)	10.41 ± 1.45 m
Volleyball (male)	15.4 ± 1.1 m
Wrestlers (male)	14.2 ± 1.8 m
Firefighters (male)	12.62 ± 1.76 m
Adolescents (mean age 12.7 ± 1.5 years)	5.6 ± 1.3m

Reproduced from from Hoffman, J. (2006). *Norms for fitness, performance, and health.* Human Kinetics.

LESSON 4: TESTING SPEED, AGILITY, AND QUICKNESS
SPEED, AGILITY, AND QUICKNESS TESTS

SPEED, AGILITY, AND QUICKNESS (SAQ) TESTS →

Speed, agility, and quickness (SAQ) tests are fundamental qualities of sports performance (Trecroci et al., 2016). SAQ tests can help Sports Performance Coaches identify an athlete's strengths and weaknesses in terms of ability to move the body as fast as possible in one direction (speed); ability to accelerate, decelerate, stabilize, and quickly change directions with proper posture (agility); and react and change body position with a maximum rate of force production (quickness). By understanding an athlete's current abilities, more effective programs can be designed that target specific areas for improvement. By improving SAQ, athletes can perform better in their sport and reduce the risk of injury. The Sports Performance Coach can use specific tests to measure the athlete's SAQ performance, including the 10- to 40-yard sprint test, lower-extremity functional test, 5–10–5 test, T-test, and 5–0–5 test.

Tests that evaluate an athlete's ability to move the body as fast as possible in one direction (speed); ability to accelerate, decelerate, stabilize, and quickly change directions with proper posture (agility); and react and change body position with a maximum rate of force production (quickness).

10- TO 40-YARD SPRINT TEST

The 10- to 40-yard sprint test, also frequently called the "dash," measures reaction capabilities and acceleration and speed for 10, 20, 30, or 40 yards.

EQUIPMENT

Nonslip surface, timer, measurement tape, recording form, two cones.

1. Determine which distance to test, and set up cones at 10, 20, 30, or 40 yards as appropriate.
2. The athlete warms up and performs practice trials as needed.
3. The athlete stands at the starting mark, the first cone.
4. The Sports Performance Coach stands at the finishing mark, the second cone, either 10, 20, 30, or 40 yards from the starting mark.
5. The athlete sprints to the finishing mark.
6. The timer is started on the first movement and stopped after the athlete hits the finishing mark (**Figure 8.22**).
7. Record the score for each distance tested. The athlete can perform one or more trials. Percentile Ranks for the 40-Yard Sprint in Male Youth and Speed Test Norms for Various Sports can be found in Appendix E.
8. The athlete cools down as needed.

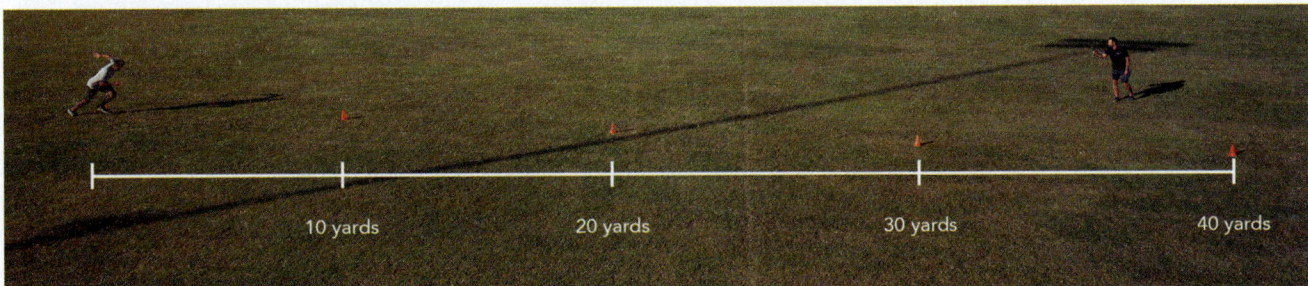

FIGURE 8.22 10- to 40-Yard Sprint

📋 COACH'S CORNER

The Sports Performance Coach chooses the sprint distance based on the athlete's sport and position. For example, the 40-yard sprint is commonly used to test football players as part of the National Football League (NFL) combined preseason athlete assessment (Clark et al., 2019), and the 30-yard sprint is baseball-specific because the distance between bases is 30 yards (Brasch et al., 2019; Kohmura et al., 2008).

LOWER-EXTREMITY FUNCTIONAL TEST

The lower-extremity functional test (LEFT) measures multi-plane speed and agility.

EQUIPMENT
Timer, measurement tape, recording form, two cones.

INSTRUCTIONS
1. Place two cones 10 yards apart.
2. The athlete warms up and performs practice trials as needed.
3. The athlete stands at the starting mark, the first cone (**Figure 8.23**).
4. The Sports Performance Coach stands at the second cone. When signaled (e.g., "Go!"), the athlete begins. The timer begins at the first movement and ends when the athlete crosses the imaginary line between the coach and the second cone.

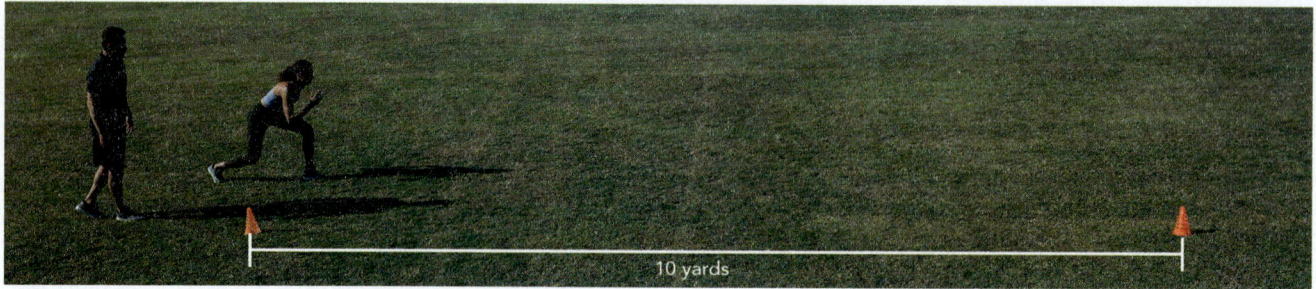

FIGURE 8.23 Lower-Extremity Functional Test Starting Position

5. The athlete runs the following sequence (**Figure 8.24**):
   - Forward sprint to second cone; touch cone.
   - Backpedal to first cone; touch cone.
   - Side shuffle to second cone; touch cone.
   - Side shuffle to first cone; touch cone.
   - Carioca to second cone; touch cone.
   - Carioca to first cone; touch cone.
   - Forward sprint to second cone.
6. Record the athlete's time. The athlete can perform one or more trials. **Table 8.9** provides reference scores for this test (Brumitt et al., 2016).
7. The athlete cools down as needed.

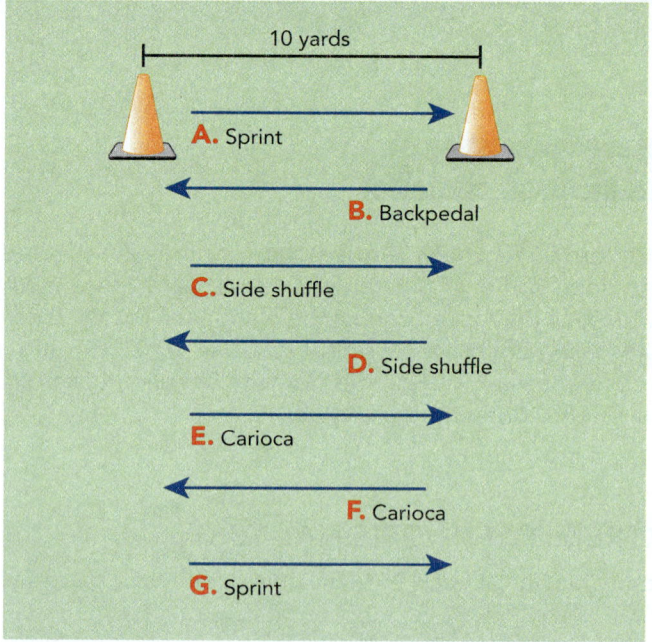

FIGURE 8.24 Lower-Extremity Functional Test

5–10–5 TEST (PRO AGILITY TEST)

The 5–0–5 test (pro agility test) measures an athlete's ability to quickly accelerate, decelerate, and change direction.

EQUIPMENT

Nonslip surface, timer, measurement tape, recording form, three cones, adhesive tape.

TABLE 8.9 LEFT Reference Average Scores

Sex	Average Times
Average Population	
Men	100 seconds (range, 90–125 seconds)
Women	135 seconds (range, 120–150 seconds)
NCAA College Athletes	
Men	105 ± 9 seconds
Women	117 ± 10 seconds

INSTRUCTIONS

1. Two cones are placed 10 yards apart, with a third cone in the middle of the two. Have pre-marked lines at each cone or use adhesive tape to mark a line on the ground.
2. The athlete warms up and performs practice trials as needed.
3. The athlete stands at the middle line and the starting mark (the first cone) in an athletic stance, touching the line on the ground. Their hand on the ground at the starting mark represents the direction in which they will go (e.g., if they are going to run to the left, they place their left hand on the ground). The Sports Performance Coach faces the middle cone to time the run at the first cone. The athlete faces the coach (**Figure 8.25**).
4. When signaled (e.g., "Go!"), the athlete sprints to the second cone and touches the line with their left hand. The timer starts on the first movement.
5. The athlete changes direction and sprints to the third cone and touches the line with their right hand, then changes direction and sprints past the first cone (**Figure 8.26**).
6. The athlete can go to the right or left but must use coordinated hand placement with each direction.
7. The timer stops after the athlete passes the first cone. The Sports Performance Coach records the final time. The athlete can perform one or more trials in each direction. Percentile Rankings for Pro Agility Test in NCAA Athletes and College Football Players Participating in the NFL are found in Appendix E.
8. The athlete cools down as needed.

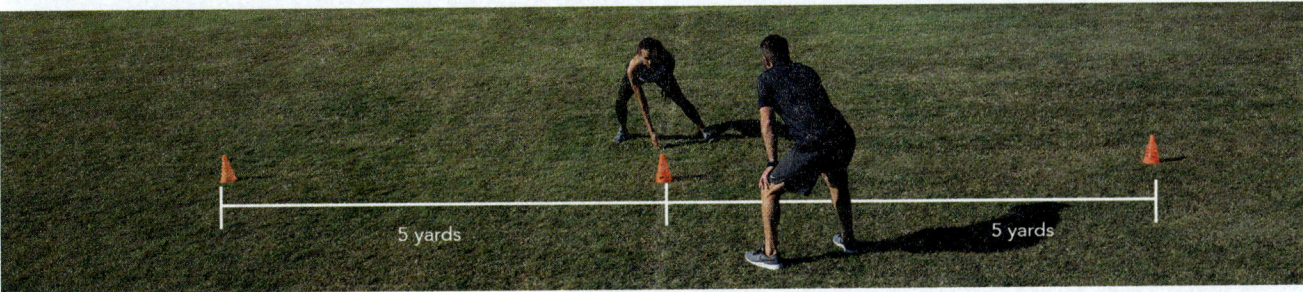

FIGURE 8.25 5–10–5 Test Starting Position

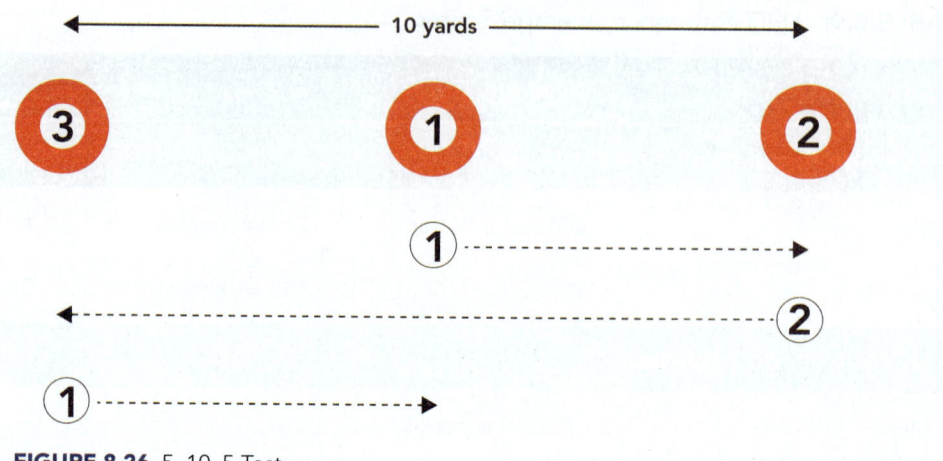

FIGURE 8.26 5–10–5 Test

T-TEST

The T-test measures an athlete's ability to sprint forward, side shuffle, and run backward (Pauole et al., 2000).

EQUIPMENT

Nonslip surface, timer, measurement tape, recording form, four cones.

INSTRUCTIONS

1. Four cones are positioned in the shape of a T. The leg of the T is 10 yards in length, and the cross piece of the T is 10 yards. **Figure 8.27** labels the cone placements.
2. The athlete warms up and performs practice trials as needed.
3. The athlete stands ready to run at the first cone (Figure 8.27).

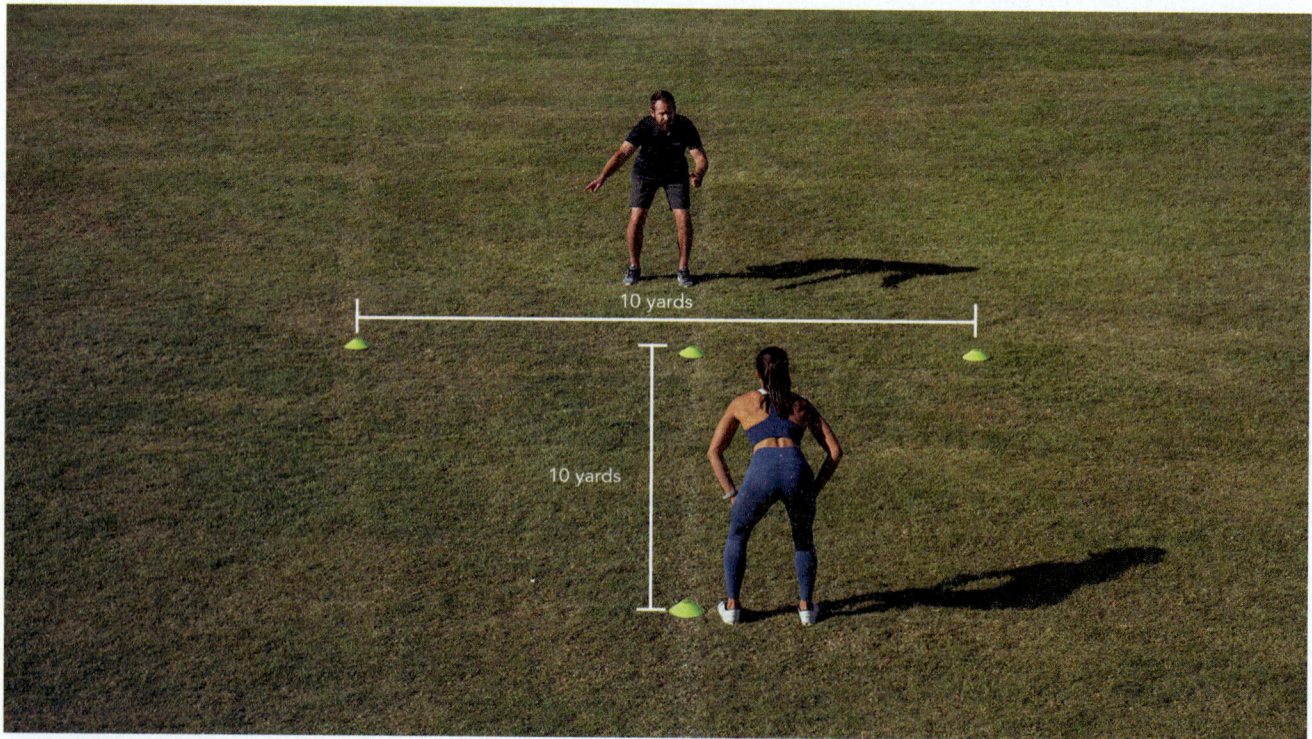

FIGURE 8.27 T-Test Starting Position

4. When signaled (e.g., "Go!"), the athlete runs 10 yards to the second cone (center cone) and touches the base of the cone with their right hand. Timing starts at the first movement.
5. The athlete side shuffles left 5 yards to the third cone, and touches the cone base with the left hand.
6. The athlete cariocas right 10 yards to the fourth cone, and touches the cone base with the right hand.
7. The athlete side shuffles 5 yards back to the second cone (center cone), and touches the base with the left hand.
8. The athlete backpedals to the starting cone (**Figure 8.28**).
9. The athlete has three attempts. The final score is the average of all three or of the closest two times. **Table 8.10** provides performance normative scores for this test. T-Test Reference Scores Among Different Sports are found in Appendix E.
10. The athlete cools down as needed.

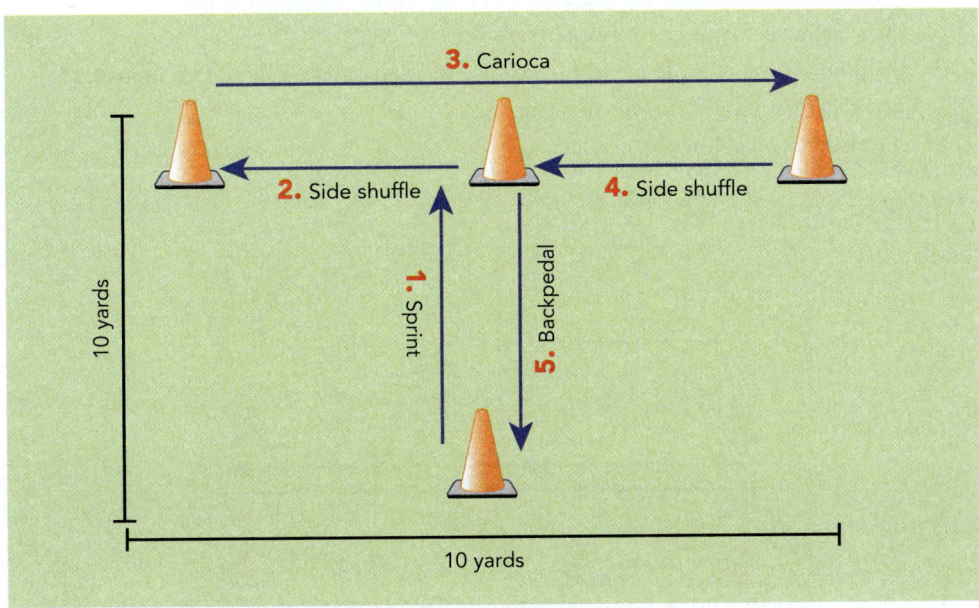

FIGURE 8.28 T-Test Pattern

TABLE 8.10 T-Test Performance Scores

Ranking	Male (seconds)	Female (seconds)
Excellent	<9.50	<10.50
Good	9.51–10.50	10.51–11.50
Average	10.51–11.50	11.51–12.50
Poor	>11.50	>12.50

Data from Hoffman, J. (2006). *Norms for fitness, performance, and health*. Human Kinetics.

5–0–5 DRILL

The 5–0–5 drill measures an athlete's ability to change direction at high velocities, and the ability to maintain high velocity after a change of direction.

EQUIPMENT

Nonslip surface, timer, measurement tape, recording form. Three cones or six cones may be used to mark both sides if desired (**Figure 8.29**).

INSTRUCTIONS

1. A start–stop line and four cones—two at 5 meters and two at 10 meters—are marked off.
2. The athlete warms up and performs practice trials as needed.
3. The athlete begins on the start line, ready to run. When signaled (e.g., "Go!"), the athlete sprints forward, passing through the start–stop line (10 meters) to the turning point. The timer starts as the athlete passes the start–stop line (**Figure 8.30**).
4. At the turning point (5 meters), the athlete performs a cutting maneuver off the right or left leg, and one foot must be on or over the line.
5. The athlete sprints back through the start–stop line. The timer stops.
6. The athlete performs one or more trials for each leg.
7. The final time is recorded, and the average of trials can be calculated. **Table 8.11** provides reference scores for this test.
8. The athlete cools down as needed.

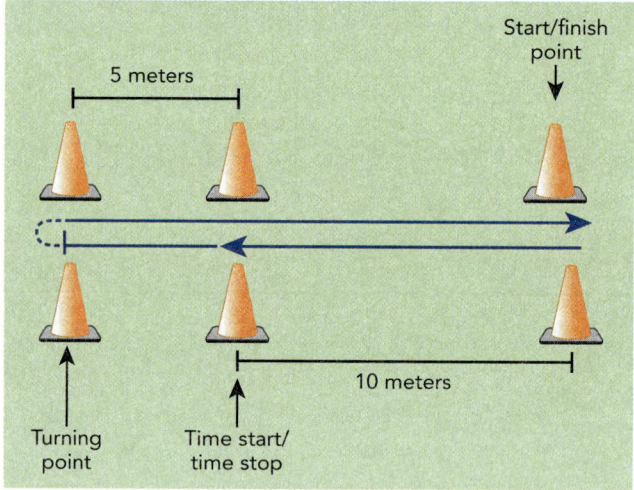

FIGURE 8.29 5–0–5 Test

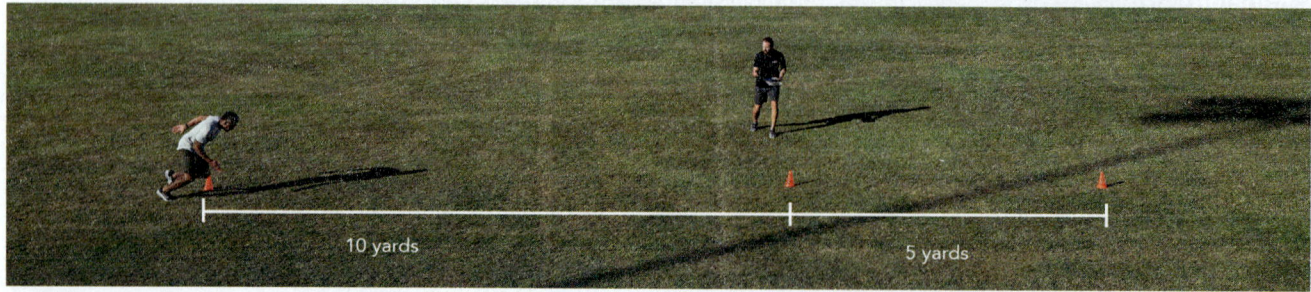

FIGURE 8.30 5–0–5 Test Starting Position

TABLE 8.11 5–0–5 Drill Performance Scores Among Different Sports

Group, Sport, or Position	Number of Athletes	Time (seconds)
National softball (women)	10	2.66 ± 0.14
National basketball (women)	12	2.69 ± 0.28
High school rugby league (men)	870	2.51 ± 0.15

The values listed are means ± standard deviation. The data are based on research studies and are descriptive, not normative. Use these numbers for reference only.

Data from Haff, G. & Triplett, T. (2015). *Essentials of strength training and conditioning* (4th Ed.). Human Kinetics.

📋 **COACH'S CORNER**

For some of these assessments, both descriptive and normative data may be collected. Descriptive data describe the performance of an individual or a specific group of athletes. Normative data rank or measure the athlete's performance on a test, which can be used as a basis of comparison for individuals or teams. A great example is the T-test. This test has descriptive data, which describe how different athletes performed, as well as normative data, which are used to create specific rankings (e.g., poor, average, good, excellent). The Sports Performance Coach can use normative data when measuring the athlete's performance over time as needed and when comparing the athlete's performance against that of other athletes. The Sports Performance Coach can use descriptive data to understand the average performance among different sports.

LESSON 5: EVALUATION AND REASSESSMENT

RESULTS EVALUATION AND REASSESSMENT

It is important for the Sports Performance Coach to understand that the primary purpose of all assessments and testing is to guide programming. As the saying goes, "If you're not assessing, then you're guessing." In some sports, the required testing might not appear to line up with on-field or on-court performance and programming, such as the bench press test used in the NFL. Critics of this test claim that lying supine on a bench and pressing a specific weight upward for a specific number of repetitions does not relate to on-field performance. However, studies support that the bench press test correlates with strength and endurance in the sport (Mann et al., 2014). Therefore, the Sports Performance Coach needs to investigate not only the demands of the sport but also the testing requirements of the sport before beginning assessments and performance-based tests.

Performance tests often serve more than one goal. First, they uncover areas of opportunity for program design. For example, a basketball player who scores high on the

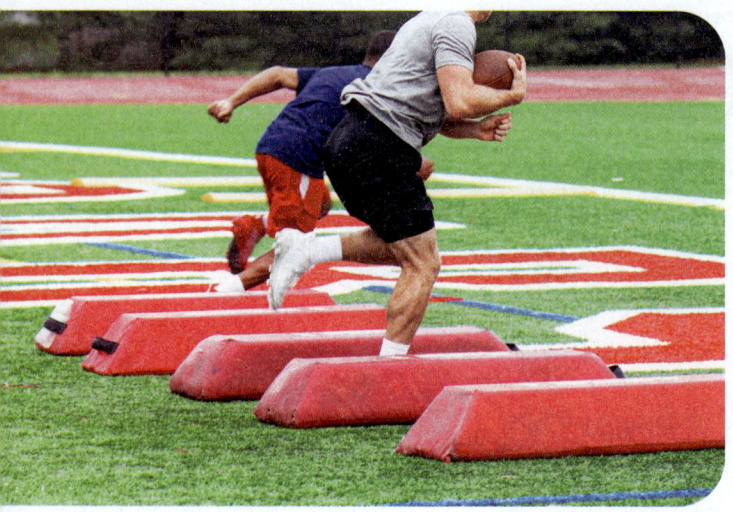

© WoodysPhotos/Shutterstock

T-test but low on the 5–10–5 pro agility test might need to focus on developing lateral speed and decelerative ability rather than forward acceleration. If an athlete performs well on the bench press test but poorly on the push-up test, they might need to focus on upper-extremity muscular endurance. All test results must be examined in the context of the chosen sport, because linear speed and muscular endurance might not be vital biomotor abilities for an athlete's success.

Performance tests also serve as objective measures of improvement. Many performance tests have reference scores that can be used to compare athletes to other athletes in the same sport, which helps the athlete understand where they fall in terms of performance. For example, the 40-yard dash is a measure of linear acceleration and is timed, with reference data available for males and females of various ages. Thus, if an 18-year-old male athlete runs 40 yards in 5.46 seconds and desires to be in the 90th percentile by age, he must improve by 0.7 second. Similarly, the vertical jump test is a measure of lower-body power. If a 30-year-old female basketball player has a vertical jump of 12.5 inches and desires to be in the 90th percentile, she needs to improve her jump by 5 inches. Armed with this information, the Sports Performance Coach can develop a program that focuses on components of power production.

Further, even if reference data are not available for a particular test, improvement in that test can measure an improvement in performance. For example, no reference data are available for the bench press tests, so an athlete cannot compare their results with those of other athletes in the same sport. However, an athlete knows that by improving the one repetition maximum in 4 weeks of training, they have improved their upper-body maximal strength. These objective measures can help the Sports Performance Coach and athlete to set clear goals with distinct timelines and direction for improvement, such as improving strength, agility, or power production.

In most cases, performance tests are used in combination with performance assessments. All data and results must, therefore, be analyzed collectively rather than isolating specific tests. For example, if an athlete demonstrates multiple movement impairments during the overhead squat and the single-leg squat assessments, and then performs poorly on the vertical jump test, the Sports Performance Coach should first focus on improving movement quality before improving power production. In many cases, improving the overhead squat immediately impacts the athlete's performance.

From one perspective, impairments in foundational movements, such as the squat, may be seen as energy leaks. For example, an athlete who demonstrates knee valgus during the squat will likely demonstrate knee valgus during the loading phase of the vertical jump, and force will not be directed entirely in a vertical direction. Designing a program to improve strength and power production in this athlete will produce positive results, but the athlete will likely be limited in this area and such a program might increase the risk of certain injuries. As another example, an athlete who demonstrates lower back extension with shoulder flexion during the overhead squat assessment might have impaired performance on the medicine ball soccer throw test. Taking these results together, the Sports Performance Coach must design a program that focuses on improving shoulder flexion and core stability before beginning upper-body strengthening and power training.

Certain performance movements should not necessarily be left out of an athlete's program; rather, the goal is to ensure the program aligns with NASM methodologies.

The athlete with knee valgus in the overhead squat and vertical jump, for example, could still include squat jumps in the training program, but the initial focus should be on technique, deceleration, and stabilization rather than obtaining a maximal height. As the athlete develops neuromuscular control, the Sports Performance Coach can introduce additional lower-body strength and power exercises.

The Sports Performance Coach can develop programs to improve strength, power, and multidirectional agility if an athlete does not demonstrate impairments during movement assessments. It is important to understand the goals of each performance test so the coach can apply the results to specific aspects of training. For example, if an athlete's most essential issue is lack of speed (e.g., low 40-yard dash score), which is vital to success in their sport, the programming needs to focus on components of speed development before addressing other markers of low performance.

The Sports Performance Coach must also establish designated reassessment periods to retest the athlete with the same movement assessments and performance tests administered at baseline (**Figure 8.31**). This is a vital aspect of all training programs because it allows the Sports Performance Coach to document and track an athlete's

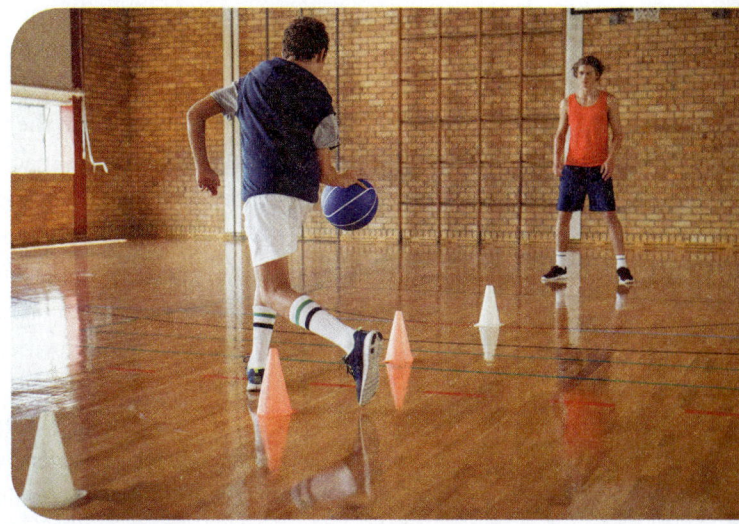

© WBMUL/Shutterstock

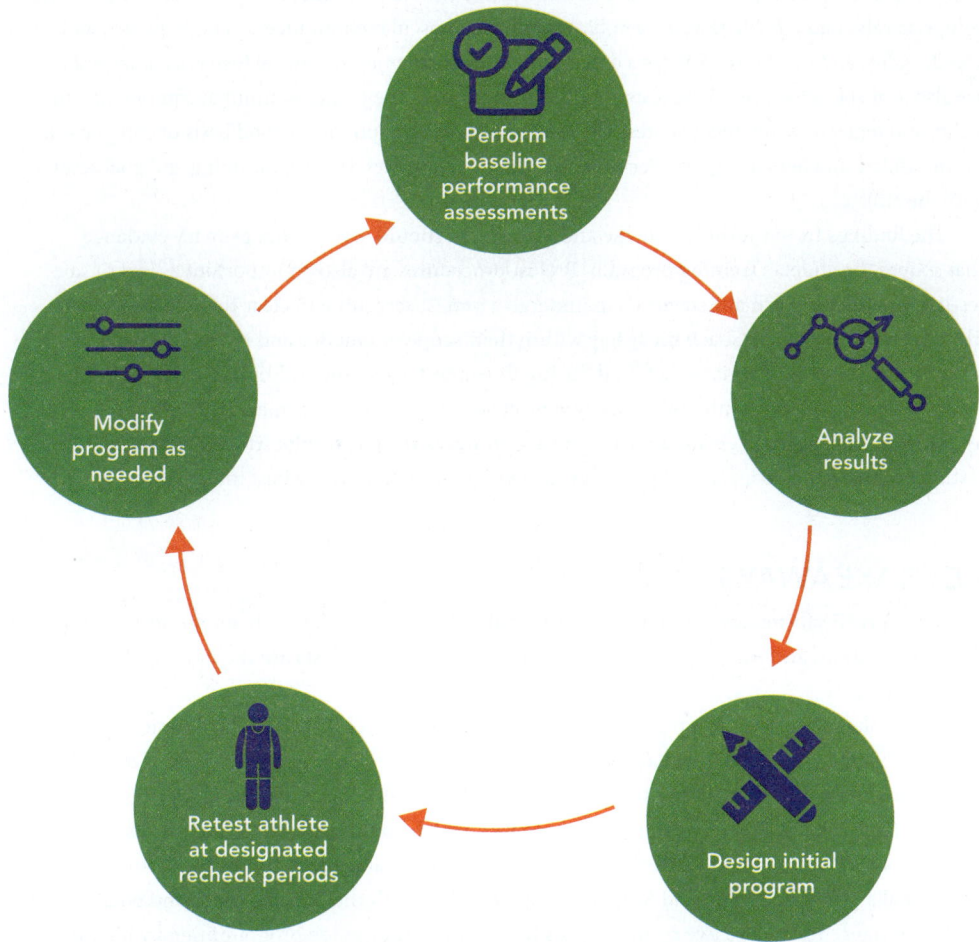

FIGURE 8.31 Assessment and Reassessment Process

progress and modify programs as needed. Reassessments generally follow mesocycles using traditional methods of periodization, which are often set up in 4-week blocks.

Additionally, 4 weeks between tests is enough time for the athlete to experience some adaptations to the training stimulus, allowing for noticeable improvements when retesting. However, spacing retesting out to every 4 weeks is not a requirement. The Sports Performance Coach must base any testing on the specific needs of the athlete. When reassessing for movement quality, for example, the Sports Performance Coach may want the athlete to perform the overhead and single-leg squats more regularly to assist in making minor adjustments to training programs. It is essential that all assessments and testing are performed consistently by following the recommended and standardized procedures for each test.

The Sports Performance Coach needs a comprehensive understanding of common sports performance tests related to the population of athletes with whom the coach is working. Having a solid understanding of these tests, including the athlete's retest ability, enhances the reliability of the assessment and supports a more effective sports performance program. Lastly, it should be recognized that the selected tests discussed in this chapter are not all-inclusive, and that other sports performance tests are available.

SUMMARY

Performance tests are, in part, a continuation of performance assessments, which a Sports Performance Coach introduces during the comprehensive athlete intake and assessment process. Performance tests comprise valid and reliable tests for aerobic endurance, muscular endurance, strength, power, and speed, agility, and quickness. The tests described in this chapter are not all-inclusive, as other tests are also available. However, these tests are easy to administer, they require minimal equipment and setup, and many have reference scores. The reference scores can provide a good basis of comparison for the athlete and help the Sports Performance Coach create exercise programming and goal setting with the athlete.

The findings from the athlete intake and assessment should serve as the primary evidence that shapes the athlete's training program. Pretest procedures are also an important aspect of safe testing for athletes. Each athlete needs to undergo a pretest screening to clear them to participate. The Sports Performance Coach must stay within their scope of practice and refer the athlete to a healthcare provider if an issue is found during the pretest screening. Additionally, the Sports Performance Coach must attempt to become proficient at specific performance pretest and assessment procedures to ensure that any testing produces reliable results. This improves overall testing accuracy and ensures the Sports Performance Coach obtains the best information.

KEY TAKEAWAYS

- The Sports Performance Coach must consider all information obtained from the athlete intake, needs analysis, and movement assessments to determine which tests are the most applicable for the athlete.
- Each athlete should warm up prior to performing performance tests. This preparation differs from that for other movement assessments, such as the overhead squat assessment, where the athlete does not warm up prior to testing. The warm-up can reduce the risk of injuries and help the athlete mentally focus on the upcoming tasks, which could improve testing results.
- The Sports Performance Coach should choose the aerobic, anaerobic, muscular endurance, muscular strength, power, and SAQ tests that best align with the athlete's needs and goals.
- Performance tests serve two primary goals for training: They guide programming by identifying areas of opportunity, and they serve as objective measures of performance improvement.

- The Sports Performance Coach should analyze and collect performance tests and movement assessment data as a whole rather than isolating certain tests. When able to do so, an athlete should demonstrate control and coordination in the movement assessments prior to attempting to demonstrate maximal performance during performance testing.

REFERENCES

Acevedo, E. O., & Starks, M. A. (2011). *Exercise testing and prescription lab manual*. Human Kinetics.

Al Attar, W. S. A., Soomro, N., Sinclair, P. J., Pappas, E., & Sanders, R. H. (2017). Effect of injury prevention programs that include the Nordic hamstring exercise on hamstring injury rates in soccer players: A systematic review and meta-analysis. *Sports Medicine, 47*(5), 907–916. https://doi.org/10.1007/s40279-016-0638-2

Al-horani, R. (2019). The validity of submaximal cycle ergometer test to predict maximal oxygen consumption. *International Journal of Coaching Science, 13*, 36–46.

Alvero-Cruz, J. R., Giráldez García, M. A., & Carnero, E. A. (2017). Reliability and accuracy of Cooper's test in male long distance runners. *Revista Andaluza de Medicina del Deporte, 10*(2), 60–63. https://doi.org /https://doi.org/10.1016/j.ramd.2016.03.001

Bandyopadhyay, A. (2015). Validity of Cooper's 12-minute run test for estimation of maximum oxygen uptake in male university students. *Biology of Sport, 32*(1), 59–63. https://www.ncbi.nlm.nih.gov/pmc/articles /PMC4314605/

Bangsbo, J., Iaia, F., & Krustrup, P. (2008). The yo-yo intermittent recovery test: A useful tool for evaluation of physical performance in intermittent sports. *Sports Medicine, 38*, 37–51.

Bennett, H., Parfitt, G., Davison, K., & Eston, R. (2016). Validity of submaximal step tests to estimate maximal oxygen uptake in healthy adults. *Sports Medicine, 46*(5), 737–750. https://doi.org/10.1007/s40279-015-0445-1

Bishop, A., DeBeliso, M., Sevene, T. G., & Adams, K. J. (2014). Comparing one repetition maximum and three repetition maximum between conventional and eccentrically loaded deadlifts. *Journal of Strength and Conditioning Research, 28*(7), 1820–1825. https://doi.org/10.1519/jsc.0000000000000315

Brasch, M. T., Neeld, K. L., Konkol, K. F., & Pettitt, R. W. (2019). Value of wellness ratings and countermovement jumping velocity to monitor performance. *International Journal of Exercise Science, 12*(4), 88–99. https:// pubmed.ncbi.nlm.nih.gov/30761203

Brumitt, J., Heiderscheit, B. C., Manske, R. C., Niemuth, P., Mattocks, A., & Rauh, M. J. (2016). The lower-extremity functional test and lower-quadrant injury in NCAA Division III athletes: A descriptive and epidemiologic report. *Journal of Sport Rehabilitation, 25*(3), 219–226. https://doi.org/10.1123/jsr.2014-0316

Burnstein, B. D., Steele, R. J., & Shrier, I. (2011). Reliability of fitness tests using methods and time periods common in sport and occupational management. *Journal of Athletic Training, 46*(5), 505–513. https:// doi.org/10.4085/1062-6050-46.5.505

Cink, R. E., & Thomas, T. R. (1981). Validity of the Åstrand-rhyming nomogram for predicting maximal oxygen intake. *British Journal of Sports Medicine, 15*, 182–185.

Clark, K. P., Rieger, R. H., Bruno, R. F., & Stearne, D. J. (2019). The National Football League combine 40-yd dash: How important is maximum velocity? *Journal of Strength and Conditioning Research, 33*(6), 1542–1550. https://doi.org/10.1519/jsc.0000000000002081

Cornell, D., Gnacinski, S., Langford, M., Mims, J., & Ebersole, K. (2015). Backwards overhead medicine ball throw and countermovement jump performance among firefighter candidates. *Journal of Trainology, 4*, 11–14. https://doi.org/10.17338/trainology.4.1_11

Cronin, J., Lawton, T., Harris, N., Kilding, A., & McMaster, D. T. (2017). A brief review of handgrip strength and sport performance. *Journal of Strength and Conditioning Research, 31*(11), 3187–3217. https://doi.org /10.1519/jsc.0000000000002149

Currell, K., & Jeukendrup, A. E. (2008). Validity, reliability and sensitivity of measures of sporting performance. *Sports Medicine, 38*(4), 297–316. https://doi.org/10.2165/00007256-200838040-00003

Davis, A. C., Emptage, N. P., Pounds, D., Woo, D., Sallis, R., Romero, M. G., & Sharp, A. L. (2021). The effectiveness of neuromuscular warmups for lower extremity injury prevention in basketball: A systematic review. *Sports Medicine Open, 7*(1), 67. https://doi.org/10.1186/s40798-021-00355-1

Davoli, G., Augustemak de Lima, L., & Silva, D. (2018). Abdominal muscular endurance in Brazilian children and adolescents: A systematic review of cross-sectional studies. *Revista Brasileira de Cineantropometria e Desempenho Humano, 20*, 483–496.

Duncan, M., & Hankey, J. (2010). Concurrent validity of the backwards overhead medicine ball throw as a test of explosive power in adolescents. *Medicina Sportiva, 14*, 103–107. https://doi.org/10.2478/v10036-010-0019-0

Fernandez-Fernandez, J., Ulbricht, A., & Ferrauti, A. (2014). Fitness testing of tennis players: How valuable is it? *British Journal of Sports Medicine, 48*(suppl 1), i22–i31. https://doi.org/10.1136/bjsports-2013-093152

Haff, G. G., & Dumke, C. (2021). *Laboratory manual for exercise physiology*. Human Kinetics.

Haff, G., & Triplett, T. (2015). *Essentials of strength training and conditioning* (4th ed.). Human Kinetics.

Hashim, A., Ariffin, A., Hashim, A. T., & Yusof, A. B. (2018). Reliability and validity of the 90° push-ups test protocol. *International Journal of Scientific Research and Management, 6*(06). https://doi.org/10.18535/ijsrm/v6i6.pe01

Herman, K., Barton, C., Malliaras, P., & Morrissey, D. (2012). The effectiveness of neuromuscular warm-up strategies, that require no additional equipment, for preventing lower limb injuries during sports participation: A systematic review. *BMC Medicine, 10*, 75. https://doi.org/10.1186/1741-7015-10-75

Hewit, J. K., Jaffe, J. A., & Crowder, T. (2018). A comparison of muscle activation during the pull-up and three alternative pulling exercises. *Journal of Physical Fitness, Medicine & Treatment in Sports, 5*(4). https://doi.org/10.19080/JPFMTS.2018.05.555669

Hoehn, A. M., Mullenbach, M. J., & Fountaine, C. J. (2015). Actual versus predicted cardiovascular demands in submaximal cycle ergometer testing. *International Journal of Exercise Science, 8*(1), 4–10. https://pubmed.ncbi.nlm.nih.gov/27182410

Hoffman, J. (2006). *Norms for fitness, performance, and health*. Human Kinetics.

Kang, J., Chaloupka, E. C., Mastrangelo, M. A., Biren, G. B., & Robertson, R. J. (2001). Physiological comparisons among three maximal treadmill exercise protocols in trained and untrained individuals. *European Journal of Applied Physiology, 84*(4), 291–295. https://doi.org/10.1007/s004210000366

Kenney, W. L., Wilmore, J. H., & Costill, D. L. (2019). *Physiology of sport and exercise*. Human Kinetics.

Knudson, D. (2001). The validity of recent curl-up tests in young adults. *Journal of Strength and Conditioning Research, 15*(1), 81–85.

Kohmura, Y., Aoki, K., Yoshigi, H., Sakuraba, K., & Yanagiya, T. (2008). Development of a baseball-specific battery of tests and a testing protocol for college baseball players. *Journal of Strength and Conditioning Research, 22*(4), 1051–1058. https://doi.org/10.1519/JSC.0b013e31816eb4ef

Mann, J. B., Ivey, P. J., Brechue, W. F., & Mayhew, J. (2014). Reliability and smallest worthwhile difference of the NFL-225 test in NCAA Division I football players. *Journal of Strength and Conditioning Research, 28*, 1427–1432.

Manske, R., & Reiman, M. (2013). Functional performance testing for power and return to sports. *Sports Health, 5*(3), 244–250. https://doi.org/10.1177/1941738113479925

Martín-Fuentes, I., Oliva-Lozano, J. M., & Muyor, J. M. (2020). Electromyographic activity in deadlift exercise and its variants: A systematic review. *PLoS One, 15*(2), e0229507–e0229507. https://doi.org/10.1371/journal.pone.0229507

Mayhew, J. L., Bird, M., Cole, M. L., Koch, A. J., Jacques, J. A., Ware, J. S., Buford, B. N., & Fletcher, K. M. (2005). Comparison of the backward overhead medicine ball throw to power production in college football players. *Journal of Strength and Conditioning Research, 19*(3), 514–518. https://pubmed.ncbi.nlm.nih.gov/16095399/

Mayorga-Vega, D., Aguilar-Soto, P., & Viciana, J. (2015). Criterion-related validity of the 20-M shuttle run test for estimating cardiorespiratory fitness: A meta-analysis. *Journal of Sports Science and Medicine, 14*(3), 536–547. https://pubmed.ncbi.nlm.nih.gov/26336340

McMaster, D. T., Gill, N., Cronin, J., & McGuigan, M. (2014). A brief review of strength and ballistic assessment methodologies in sport. *Sports Medicine, 44*(5), 603–623. https://doi.org/10.1007/s40279-014-0145-2

Mohamed, M., Kadir, Z., Md Yusof, S., Mazaulan, M., & Adnan, M. (2014). Relationship between handgrip strength on muscular strength among racquet sport athletes. *Proceedings of the International Colloquium on Sports Science, Exercise, Engineering and Technology*, 259–266. https://doi.org/10.1007/978-981-287-107-7_27

Moore, A., & Murphy, A. (2003). Development of an anaerobic capacity test for field sport athletes. *Journal of Science and Medicine in Sport, 6*(3), 275–284. https://doi.org/10.1016/s1440-2440(03)80021-x

Nikodelis, T., Savvoulidis, S., Athanasakis, P., Chalitsios, C., & Loizidis, T. (2021). Comparative study of validity and reliability of two handgrip dynamometers: K-Force Grip and Jamar. *Biomechanics, 1*(1), 73–82. https://www.mdpi.com/2673-7078/1/1/6

Pauole, K., Madole, K. D., Garhammer, J. J., Lacourse, M. G., & Rozenek, R. (2000). Reliability and validity of the T test as a measure of agility, leg power, and leg speed in college-aged men and women. *Journal of Strength and Conditioning Research, 14*, 443–450.

Perna, F. M., Coa, K., Troiano, R. P., Lawman, H. G., Wang, C.-Y., Li, Y., Moser, R. P., Ciccolo, J. T., Comstock, B. A., & Kraemer, W. J. (2016). Muscular grip strength estimates of the U.S. population from the National Health and Nutrition Examination Survey 2011–2012. *Journal of Strength and Conditioning Research, 30*(3), 867–874. https://doi.org/10.1519/JSC.0000000000001104

Rodríguez-Rosell, D., Mora-Custodio, R., Franco-Márquez, F., Yáñez-García, J. M., & González-Badillo, J. J. (2017). Traditional vs. sport-specific vertical jump tests: Reliability, validity, and relationship with the legs strength and sprint performance in adult and teen soccer and basketball players. *Journal of Strength and Conditioning Research, 31*(1), 196–206. https://doi.org/10.1519/jsc.0000000000001476

Rutherford, W. J., & Corbin, C. B. (1994). Validation of criterion-referenced standards for tests of arm and shoulder girdle strength and endurance. *Research Quarterly for Exercise and Sport, 65*(2), 110–119. https://doi.org/10.1080/02701367.1994.10607605

Saint Romain, B., & Mahar, M. T. (2001). Norm-referenced and criterion-referenced reliability of the push-up and modified pull-up. *Measurement in Physical Education and Exercise Science, 5*(2), 67–80. https://doi.org/10.1207/S15327841MPEE0502_1

Schoenfeld, B. J. (2010). Squatting kinematics and kinetics and their application to exercise performance. *Journal of Strength and Conditioning Research, 24*(12), 3497–3506. https://doi.org/10.1519/JSC.0b013e3181bac2d7

Sconce, E., Jones, P., Turner, E., Comfort, P., & Graham-Smith, P. (2015). The validity of the Nordic hamstring lower for a field-based assessment of eccentric hamstring strength. *Journal of Sports Rehabilitation, 24*(1), 13–20. https://doi.org/10.1123/jsr.2013-0097

Sporis, G., Ruzic, L., & Leko, G. (2008). The anaerobic endurance of elite soccer players improved after a high-intensity training intervention in the 8-week conditioning program. *Journal of Strength and Conditioning Research, 22*, 559–566. https://doi.org/10.1519/JSC.0b013e3181660401

Stockbrugger, B. A., & Haennel, R. G. (2001). Validity and reliability of a medicine ball explosive power test. *Journal of Strength and Conditioning Research, 15*(4), 431–438. https://journals.lww.com/nsca-jscr/Fulltext/2001/11000/Validity_and_Reliability_of_a_Medicine_Ball.6.aspx

Tomkinson, G. R., Lang, J. J., Tremblay, M. S., Dale, M., LeBlanc, A. G., Belanger, K., Ortega, F. B., & Léger, L. (2017). International normative 20 m shuttle run values from 1,142,026 children and youth representing 50 countries. *British Journal of Sports Medicine, 51*(21), 1545–1554. https://doi.org/10.1136/bjsports-2016-095987

Torres-Ronda, L., Sánchez-Medina, L., & González-Badillo, J. J. (2011). Muscle strength and golf performance: A critical review. *Journal of Sports Science and Medicine, 10*(1), 9–18. https://pubmed.ncbi.nlm.nih.gov/24149290

Trecroci, A., Milanović, Z., Rossi, A., Broggi, M., Formenti, D., & Alberti, G. (2016). Agility profile in sub-elite under-11 soccer players: Is SAQ training adequate to improve sprint, change of direction speed and reactive agility performance? *Research in Sports Medicine, 24*(4), 331–340. https://doi.org/10.1080/15438627.2016.1228063

Tsaklis, P., Malliaropoulos, N., Mendiguchia, J., Korakakis, V., Tsapralis, K., Pyne, D., & Malliaras, P. (2015). Muscle and intensity based hamstring exercise classification in elite female track and field athletes: Implications for exercise selection during rehabilitation. *Open Access Journal of Sports Medicine, 6*, 209–217. https://doi.org/10.2147/oajsm.S79189

van der Horst, N., Smits, D. W., Petersen, J., Goedhart, E. A., & Backx, F. J. (2015). The preventive effect of the Nordic hamstring exercise on hamstring injuries in amateur soccer players: A randomized controlled trial. *American Journal of Sports Medicine, 43*(6), 1316–1323. https://doi.org/10.1177/0363546515574057

Van Raalte, J. L., Brewer, B. W., Cornelius, A. E., Keeler, M., & Gudjenov, C. (2019). Effects of a mental warmup on the workout readiness and stress of college student exercisers. *Journal of Functional Morphology and Kinesiology, 4*(3). https://doi.org/10.3390/jfmk4030042

Wang, Y.-C., Bohannon, R. W., Li, X., Sindhu, B., & Kapellusch, J. (2018). Hand-grip strength: Normative reference values and equations for individuals 18 to 85 years of age residing in the United States. *Journal of Orthopaedic & Sports Physical Therapy, 48*(9), 685–693. https://doi.org/10.2519/jospt.2018.7851

Wong, S. L. (2016). Grip strength reference values for Canadians aged 6 to 79: Canadian Health Measures Survey, 2007 to 2013. *Health Report, 27*(10), 3–10.

Zhou, H., Yu, P., Thirupathi, A., & Liang, M. (2020). How to improve the standing long jump performance? A mininarrative review. *Applied Bionics and Biomechanics, 2020*, 8829036–8829036. https://doi.org/10.1155/2020/8829036

SECTION 4

COMPONENTS OF THE INTEGRATED TRAINING MODEL

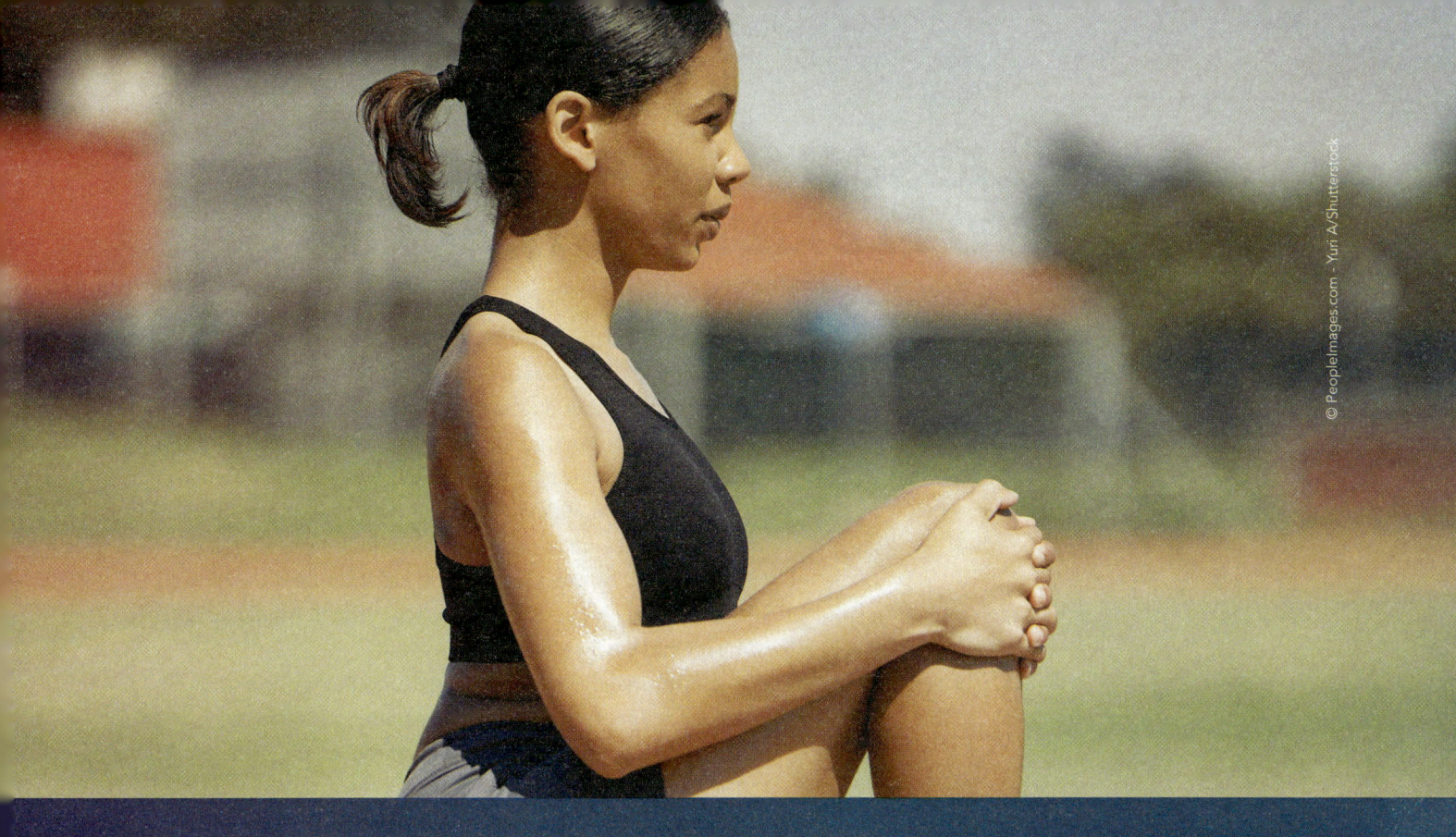
© PeopleImages.com - Yuri A/Shutterstock

FLEXIBILITY TRAINING FOR SPORTS PERFORMANCE

CHAPTER NINE

LEARNING OBJECTIVES

Upon completion of this chapter, the Sports Performance Coach will be able to:

- **Summarize** the importance of flexibility training for athletes with differing performance-related goals.

- **Explain** the scientific rationale for flexibility training.

- **Describe** the different flexibility and mobility techniques used within performance training.

- **Identify** appropriate acute training variables for flexibility training.

- **Select** flexibility programs or techniques based on a needs analysis.

LESSON 1: INTRODUCTION TO FLEXIBILITY TRAINING

INTRODUCTION

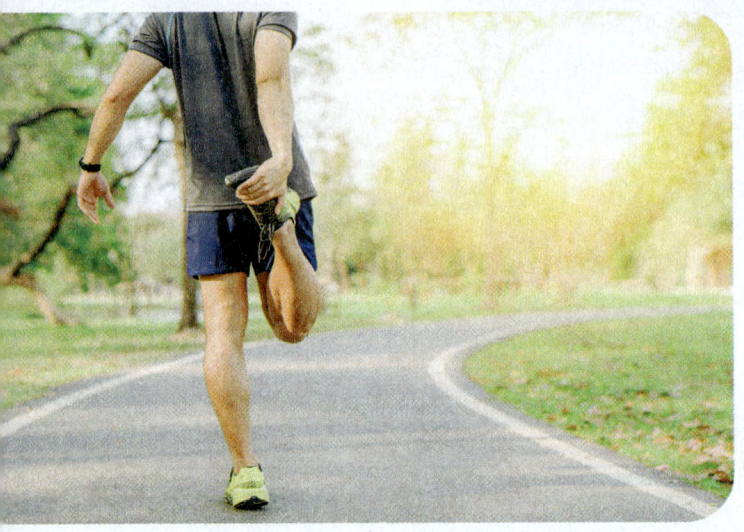

© Interstid/Shutterstock

Sports Performance Coaches have long viewed improving flexibility as a vital part of the training process because increased flexibility may help reduce musculotendinous injuries and improve athletic performance. Most sports are strenuous, dynamic activities by their very nature, so having the optimal level of flexibility required for the sport will ensure that soft tissues are compliant enough to reduce the risk of injury caused by excessive mechanical strain. Also, ideal flexibility may reduce unnecessary movement impairments that impact movement efficiency.

Unfortunately, the correct application of the scientific principles underpinning flexibility training is often misunderstood by professionals and athletes alike. Therefore, informed guidance from the Sports Performance Coach is necessary to achieve the desired results.

FLEXIBILITY VERSUS RANGE OF MOTION

The scientific literature provides different definitions of flexibility. Some resources focus on the **range of motion (ROM)** of a joint, and describe flexibility as the ROM allowed in each plane of motion at a specific joint (Hall, 2019). Other definitions focus on the extent to which soft tissues can lengthen; in such cases, flexibility refers to the intrinsic properties of the tissue that determine maximal joint ROM without causing injury (Holt et al., 1996; Knudson et al., 2000). Knudson (2021) provides a definition that considers both ROM and tissue properties as inseparable components of flexibility, describing it as the ability of a joint or groups of joints to allow motion without injury. Integrating these understandings, this chapter will define **flexibility** as the normal extensibility of soft tissues that allow for the full range of motion of a joint.

The terms *flexibility* and *ROM* are frequently used interchangeably and are generally considered synonymous. However, it is important to note that the definition of flexibility refers to tissue extensibility, whereas ROM refers to joint motion. Of course, one does impact the other. For example, a lack of tissue extensibility will reduce joint ROM. Similarly, a lack of joint ROM (e.g., from arthritis, surgical hardware) can impede tissue extensibility. Therefore, it is vital to clarify terms when speaking with other performance professionals.

ROM can be subdivided into active ROM and passive ROM (Hoppenbrouwers et al., 2006; López-Bedoya et al., 2013; Sands et al., 2008). **Active ROM** is the amount of movement a person can produce voluntarily using muscular contractions. Active ROM measures the motion that an athlete can achieve on their own, without any external assistance. It may be a more accurate reflection of functional ability and the ability to perform specific movements in a sport than passive ROM. Further, active ROM may have a greater carryover to sports performance.

Passive ROM is the amount of movement a joint can display when an external force is applied to relaxed muscles. This force is usually applied by an individual with

RANGE OF MOTION (ROM) →

The degree to which specific joints or body segments can move; often measured in degrees.

FLEXIBILITY →

The normal extensibility of soft tissues that allows for the full range of motion of a joint.

ACTIVE ROM →

The range of motion achieved with voluntary muscular contractions.

the necessary skills and education. For example, a physical therapist or athletic trainer can use passive ROM during testing to identify joint limitations such as stiffness or adhesions. A trained practitioner can categorize limitations based on how the joints and tissues feel as they move through a specific ROM.

Active ROM is associated with active flexibility, which is usually of greater interest to the performance client because it correlates more strongly with athletic ability than does passive flexibility (Verkhoshansky & Siff, 2009). Passive ROM is associated with passive flexibility, which is usually greater than active flexibility due to the additional force applied. Therefore, it is often necessary to use passive flexibility under the guidance of a trained professional to improve passive ROM, which in turn may increase active ROM.

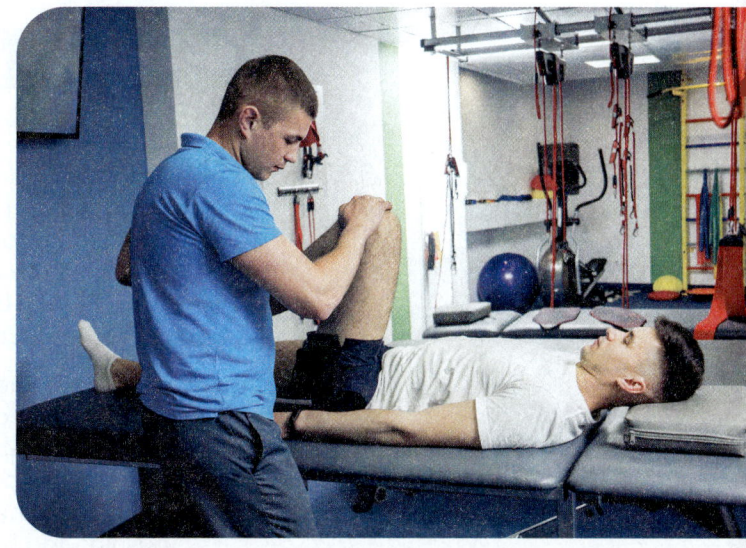

© Roman Zaiets/Shutterstock

THE ROLE OF FLEXIBILITY IN PERFORMANCE

Flexibility plays a crucial role in athletic performance because it allows the athlete to perform the necessary movements for the specific sport more safely. For example, a Taekwondo athlete will not score highly in a match if they do not have the flexibility to kick their opponent in the head. The extent to which flexibility affects performance depends on the nature of the sport, the type of flexibility, the training method, and individual factors related to the client, such as age, sex, occupation, injury history, and training experience.

Nuzzo (2020) recently challenged the assumption that flexibility is important to performance. However, this author utilized the sit-and-reach test, which is simply a way to measure flexibility, as a demonstration of flexibility itself. Nuzzo found that the sit-and-reach test had little specificity to many functional activities and, therefore, suggested that flexibility training (especially passive flexibility) should be de-emphasized in training programs.

In other words, Nuzzo argued that flexibility is not important simply because some researchers used one particular flexibility test that had little relevance to activities in which improving flexibility would still be helpful. This conclusion is a broad generalization that neglects the value of focused flexibility training tailored toward the client's specific sports performance goals.

It may be tempting to focus solely on active ROM because of its greater carryover to performance, but passive ROM remains important. A joint will typically exhibit a greater passive ROM than active ROM because a small amount of motion cannot be voluntarily controlled (Günal et al., 1996; James & Parker, 1989), due in part to the muscles' ability to lengthen more than they can shorten (Vander et al., 2001). In addition, a reserve of passive flexibility may provide the tissues with a buffer against excessive strain when external forces push a person's limbs beyond their normal ROM, such as when slipping on wet grass during a soccer match or being caught in an awkward tackle during a rugby game.

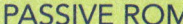

PASSIVE ROM →

The range of motion achieved in the absence of muscular contractions, with assistance from a coach or trainer.

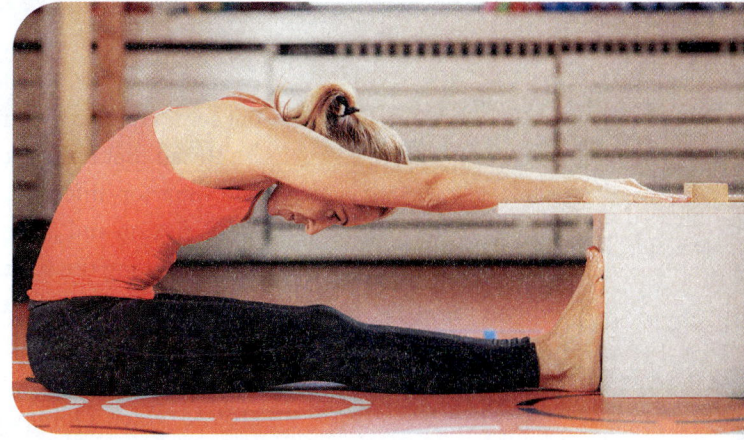

© Microgen/Shutterstock

Sometimes, people are unwilling to move into a particular ROM because of psychological barriers such as fear and anxiety. This fear is often driven primarily by concerns about a previous injury.

The Sports Performance Coach should provide clear verbal guidance and reassurance, so the athlete understands any potential risk when accessing their active ROM. Here are a few tips coaches can use when working with an athlete who is reluctant to participate in a flexibility program:

- Emphasize the benefits of stretching, such as increased flexibility and ROM, reduced risk of injury, and improved performance.
- Remind the athlete that stretching can be a form of stress relief and a way to relax both the mind and the body.
- Encourage the athlete to stretch within their comfort zone and avoid pushing too hard.
- Highlight the fact that stretching helps to reduce the risk of injuries by improving flexibility and mobility.

MOBILITY VERSUS FLEXIBILITY

The terms *mobility* and *flexibility* are generally used interchangeably by many sports performance professionals. However, the Sports Performance Coach should be aware of the distinct differences in how these terms may be used in various healthcare and performance settings. *Mobility* is used in a majority of the scientific literature and by the World Health Organization to describe and assess a person's ability to complete many types of tasks, such as standing up from sitting, walking, and performing normal activities of daily living (Boonen & Maksymowych, 2010).

In contrast, in many performance and fitness settings, **mobility** refers to the ability of a joint to move through its full ROM with control and stability. It is a measure of the joint's overall function and is influenced by factors such as joint structure, muscle strength, and neural control. Mobility exercises focus on improving the quality and range of movement at a joint and often involve active movements and exercises that challenge joint stability and control at different degrees.

Mobility has also been used in the biomechanics literature for more than a century to refer to the **degrees of freedom (DOF)** available at a given joint (Bernstein, 2020). DOF refers to the number of independent directions in which a joint can move (Scheck, 2018). In many cases, DOF is described as the number of axes around which a joint can rotate; but some complexities may exist.

Recall that there are three axes of rotation (anterior–posterior, mediolateral, and superior–inferior). The knee, as an example, may be described as having three DOF: flexion and extension along the mediolateral axis, internal and external rotation along the superior–inferior axis when the knee is flexed, and a slight degree of abduction and adduction along the anterior–posterior axis. However, if joint translation is included, the knee will demonstrate six DOF (Komdeur et al., 2002) (**Figure 9.1**). Be aware that DOF is not the same as ROM; DOF is the number of axes around which a joint can rotate, and ROM is how far the joint can rotate around each of those axes.

MOBILITY

The ability of a joint to move through its full range of motion with control and stability; the ability to move freely.

DEGREES OF FREEDOM (DOF) →

The number of independent directions in which a joint can move.

Degrees of Freedom (DOF) at the Knee Joint

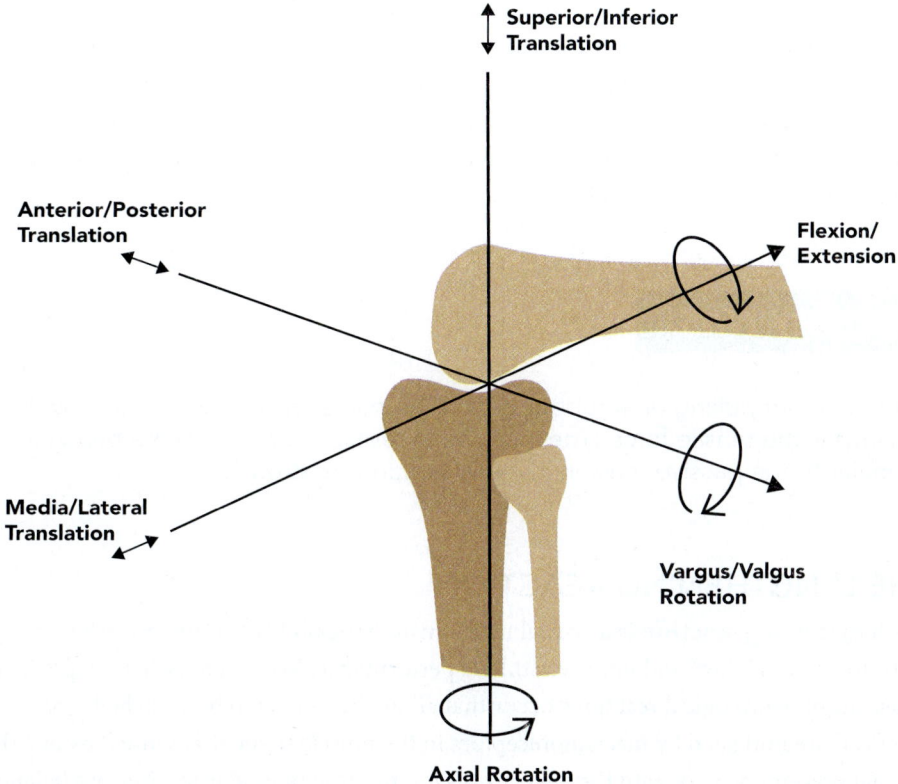

FIGURE 9.1 Degrees of Freedom (DOF) at the Knee Joint

HYPER-MOBILITY →

Increased movement and functionality of a joint beyond normal range of motion.

ELASTICITY →

The ability of soft tissues to return to resting length after being stretched.

PLASTICITY →

The ability of soft tissues to permanently change shape or deform.

Mobility has also often been described in the context of **hypermobility** studies (Al-Rawi et al., 1985; Jaffe et al., 1988; Seow et al., 1999). In the clinical sense, hypermobility is a rheumatological multisystemic, hereditary, connective tissue disorder characterized by joint instability and chronic pain (Atwell et al., 2021; Simmonds & Keer, 2007).

While both mobility and flexibility are essential for optimal function and performance, they target different aspects of movement and may be addressed by different exercises. For example, mobility exercises aim to improve joint function and stability, whereas flexibility exercises aim to improve tissue extensibility and ROM. Therefore, a comprehensive performance program should include exercises that target both of these aspects to improve overall movement quality and reduce the risk of injury.

SCIENTIFIC PRINCIPLES OF FLEXIBILITY

The scientific principles of flexibility involve understanding the physiological and biomechanical factors that contribute to flexibility, as well as the principles of training and adaptation that can be used to improve flexibility. Flexibility is influenced by a combination of factors, including the **elasticity** and **plasticity** of muscles, tendons, and other connective tissues, as well as the ROM of joints.

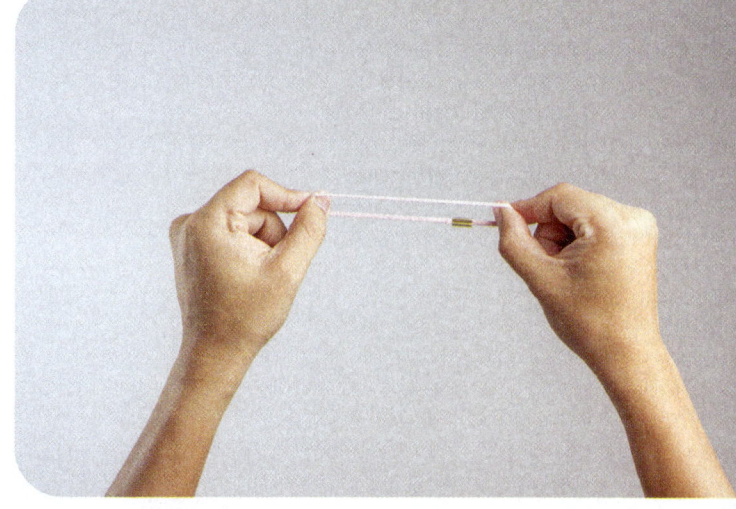

© BonNontawat/Shutterstock

Another important consideration is that the limits of motion are established by the reaction of the neuromuscular system when the body is exposed to forces. Tensile forces are of primary interest when discussing flexibility because these forces are applied in opposite directions to stretch or elongate a tissue. Understanding the subsequent responses of the body to these forces helps the Sports Performance Coach better tailor flexibility training to the specific needs of each athlete. The various physiological responses and principles, such as the lengthening reaction, autogenic and reciprocal inhibition, and stretch tolerance, are discussed in this section.

> **⚙ TRY THIS**
>
> Think about pulling on a rubber band: The pull exerted on the band by the hands is the tensile force. The increase in resistance felt from the band is similar to the passive tension in muscles during a stretch.

THE LENGTHENING REACTION

The **lengthening reaction** is a crucial mechanism in flexibility training for athletes, as it helps to prevent injury and improve athletic performance. When a muscle is lengthened, a cascade of neurological reactions occur that allow the muscle to be stretched. These reactions are mitigated by mechanoreceptors in the muscle tissue that sense tension. These mechanoreceptors work with the nervous system to sense muscular tension and balance the tasks of preventing injury (from excessive contraction or lengthening) and allowing for a fully functional ROM.

The relaxation and lengthening of muscles after prolonged tension occurs primarily due to specialized mechanoreceptors called **Golgi tendon organs (GTOs)** located in muscle tissue, near the muscle–tendon junction, and within the joint capsule (**Figure 9.2**). When high levels of muscular tension are detected, GTOs produce reflexive relaxation via inhibitory interneurons to save the muscle from potential injury. This reflex is also called the inverse stretch reflex (Fehr, 2012).

LENGTHENING → REACTION

When a muscle is lengthened, the cascade of neurological reactions that occur to allow the muscle to be stretched.

GOLGI → TENDON ORGANS (GTOS)

Specialized sensory receptors located in the musculotendinous junction that are sensitive to changes in tension and the rate of tension change.

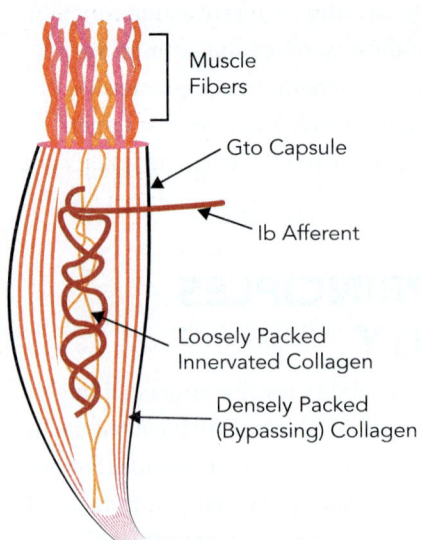

Muscle Fibers

Gto Capsule

Ib Afferent

Loosely Packed Innervated Collagen

Densely Packed (Bypassing) Collagen

FIGURE 9.2 Golgi Tendon Organ (GTO) Anatomy

Furthermore, the lengthening reaction helps to prevent injury by reducing the likelihood of muscle strains and tears. When a muscle is stretched beyond its normal limits without the lengthening reaction, it can become strained or torn. However, by promoting the lengthening reaction through stretching exercises, athletes can minimize the risk of injury and recover more quickly from any injuries that do occur.

AUTOGENIC INHIBITION

Autogenic inhibition plays a part in the lengthening reaction and flexibility training. This process generally involves an isometric contraction of the stretched muscle. Methods that utilize autogenic inhibition may have different names in the literature, including "hold–relax" and "contract–relax," but are collectively categorized as neuromuscular stretching methods. Regardless of the name used, the basic premise is the same: A muscle is placed into a passive stretch, then undergoes an isometric contraction to cause subsequent muscle relaxation, before being held at the same ROM or moved into a greater passive stretch (Cayco et al., 2019; Nakamura et al., 2020).

Autogenic inhibition plays a role in the inhibitory function of GTOs within the muscle that is stretching and contracting. However, evidence is lacking as to whether this reflex activity is important in neuromuscular stretching (Chalmers, 2004; Hindle et al., 2012; Sharman et al., 2006). GTOs are primarily active *during* a contraction, so the inhibitory effect will subside almost immediately after cessation of the stimulus (Behm, 2019).

However, while holding the muscle in a stretched position, there is a substantial temporary decrease in motor neuron excitability, which may act in the same manner as static stretching. Additionally, increases in ROM during neuromuscular techniques may be partly explained by changes in stretch tolerance and thixotropic characteristics of tissues (e.g., the viscosity of tissues decreasing).

Athletes who engage in regular stretching exercises promoting autogenic inhibition can benefit from increased ROM, which can lead to improved athletic performance. For example, a gymnast who can stretch their hamstrings to a greater degree may be able to perform more advanced tumbling and acrobatic skills.

RECIPROCAL INHIBITION

Reciprocal inhibition is a neurological process that plays a significant role in flexibility training. It refers to the phenomenon in which the activation of one muscle (agonist) leads to the relaxation of its opposing muscle (antagonist). This process is governed by the nervous system, specifically through the actions of agonist and antagonist muscles and their corresponding motor neurons. Put simply, reciprocal inhibition is the process that enables normal functional movements to occur.

During flexibility training, reciprocal inhibition is employed to facilitate deeper stretches and to improve overall flexibility. When a muscle is stretched, its antagonist muscle is activated, causing the stretched muscle to relax, which allows for a greater ROM. This process can be utilized in various stretching techniques, such as static stretching, dynamic stretching, and proprioceptive neuromuscular facilitation stretching.

For example, when stretching the hamstrings, the quadriceps (the antagonist muscles) are activated, which leads to the relaxation of the hamstrings, allowing for a deeper stretch (**Figure 9.3**). This process helps to reduce the risk of injury, enhance muscle coordination, and improve overall flexibility.

Reciprocal inhibition happens because the commands from the central nervous system (CNS) that activate the motor neurons of the agonist's muscle also excite Ia-inhibitory

AUTOGENIC INHIBITION →

The process by which neural impulses that sense tension are greater than the impulses that cause muscles to contract, providing an inhibitory effect to the muscle spindles.

RECIPROCAL INHIBITION →

When an agonist contracts causing its antagonist to relax to allow movement at the joint.

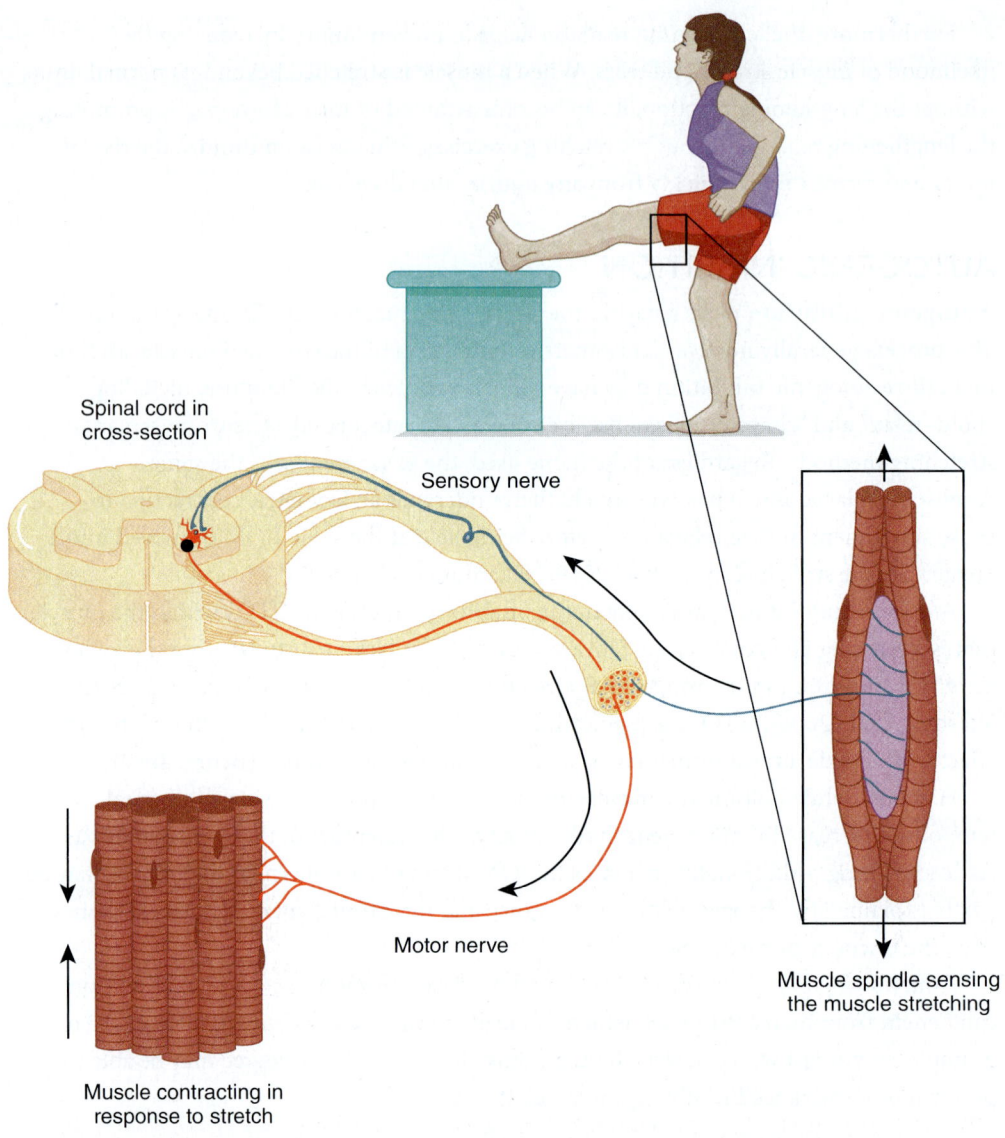

FIGURE 9.3 Anatomy Involved During Reciprocal Inhibition

Spinal cord in cross-section

Sensory nerve

Motor nerve

Muscle contracting in response to stretch

Muscle spindle sensing the muscle stretching

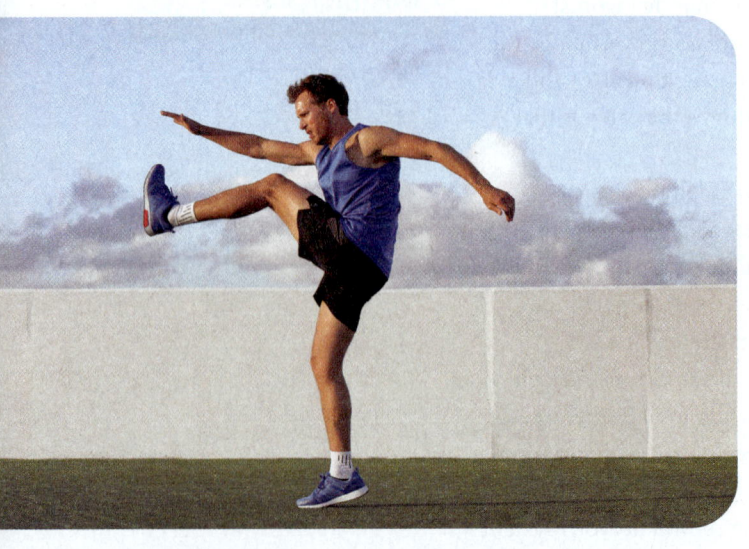

interneurons that synapse (connect with) the motor neurons of the antagonist muscle (Sharman et al., 2006). This phenomenon prevents a reflexive contraction of the antagonist muscle fibers, ensuring that the agonist–antagonist pair do not fight against themselves during movement. Reciprocal inhibition is often cited as the underlying mechanism for the more significant gains in ROM that are achieved in stretches featuring a shortening contraction of the opposing muscle group (Entyre & Abraham, 1986; Ferber et al., 2002).

Sharman et al. (2006) acknowledged that evidence exists to support the notion that greater activation of the opposing muscle group will result in greater relaxation of the target muscle via Ia-afferent presynaptic inhibition. However, they asserted that clinical research data are lacking to support the idea that such a mechanism plays a substantial role in neuromuscular-style stretching that involves activation of the antagonist muscle. Some questions regarding technique may arise in research involving reciprocal inhibition, such as how long the stretches were held and how often the stretches were repeated. Regardless, it has been well documented during dynamic activities, so its effect will likely be most significant during dynamic-type stretches.

INHIBITION VERSUS DISFACILITATION

The terms *inhibition* and *disfacilitation* are often used interchangeably. Although both result in a form of inhibition, one is active and the other passive. **Inhibition** is an active process that results from stimulation of inhibitory neurons. When excited, these inhibitory interneurons can prevent motoneurons from firing. For example, when performing an active stretch, contraction of an antagonist muscle sends a barrage of signals that actively inhibit the target muscle to be stretched.

In contrast, with **disfacilitation**, motor neuron inhibition results from a lack of, or decrease in, input into the sensory neurons. This happens when someone performs a passive stretch and holds it for a prolonged period of time.

For an analogous example, consider that if a cyclist slowed their pedaling rate or stopped rotating the crank altogether to coast, they would decrease the input activity and the bicycle's speed would be effectively *disfacilitated*. However, if the cyclist applied their brakes, they would actively be slowing the bike, effectively *inhibiting* the bike's speed.

MUSCLE SPINDLE DISFACILITATION

ROM is highly related to the extent of muscle resistance caused by **tonic reflexes** (Guissard & Duchateau, 2006). Whereas dynamic stretching can excite the neuromuscular system, static stretching can decrease or disfacilitate (downregulate) the stretch reflex (Behm & Chaouachi, 2011; Behm et al., 2001; Behm et al., 2004; Behm et al., 2016).

With passive static stretching, which is often used during assisted stretching, the muscle is typically extended at a slow to moderate rate and then held for an extended period, typically 15 to 60 seconds (Alter, 2004; Behm et al., 2016). Naturally, once the stretch reaches the maximum ROM, the stretch rate will no longer change. Within seconds, structures within the muscle spindles, called nuclear bag fibers, will begin to decrease their discharge rate, diminishing the stretch reflex (disfacilitation). As a stretch is held in this position for a prolonged period (typically 15 to 60 seconds), the nuclear bag fibers accommodate this new position and decrease their discharge frequency (disfacilitation). For example, 1 hour of repeated passive stretching of the plantar flexors (calves) has been shown to reduce stretch reflexes by 44% to 85% (Avela et al., 1999).

This decreased discharge frequency can be partially attributed to the actions of the nervous system, which attempts to return the muscle spindles to their normal resting length (Matthews, 1982). By decreasing the spindle length, the nuclear chain fibers decrease their discharge rate, and the stretch reflex contractions decrease further, leading to more relaxation of the muscle.

STRETCH TOLERANCE

Stretch tolerance refers to a theoretical model of learned dissociation between the discomfort of stretching and injury. In simple terms, the nervous system learns over repeated applications of stretching that the high levels of passive tension do not cause injury, and thus it lowers its perception of the stimulus as being potentially harmful. In other words, the tolerance to stretching forces gradually increases over time. This theory arose out of several studies that showed the mechanical properties of soft tissues remained

INHIBITION →

The suppression or reduction of activity in motor neurons via activation of inhibitory neurons.

DIS-FACILITATION →

The reduction of excitatory input to specific motor neurons.

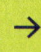

TONIC REFLEXES →

Involuntary, automatic muscle responses to specific sensory stimuli, such as changes in body position or muscle length.

STRETCH TOLERANCE →

The ability to experience the physical sensations of stretching to reduce the discomfort felt at the end range of motion.

unchanged following several weeks of stretching, even though ROM changed (Ben & Harvey, 2010; LaRoche & Connolly, 2006; Mitchell et al., 2007).

Improving stretch tolerance allows athletes to stretch their muscles further, for longer durations, and more effectively, leading to increased flexibility, greater performance, and decreased chances of some injuries. However, the Sports Performance Coach must ensure that each flexibility program is individualized for each athlete. Stretching further and for longer may not be necessary for all athletes in all sports.

> ### 🤖 GETTING TECHNICAL
>
> Recent research has suggested that stretch tolerance may be linked with the endogenous modulation of pain, and it may be a useful indicator of pain sensitivity during rehabilitation for musculoskeletal injuries (Støve et al., 2021). In practical terms, a client or athlete who is struggling to regain lost ROM following an injury can engage their body's endogenous pain inhibitory mechanisms, either by performing exercise or by introducing a painful competing stimulus (such as pressing a massage tool into sensitive areas of the affected muscle group), thereby taking advantage of the increased stretch tolerance to move into a deeper ROM.

LESSON 2: STRUCTURE AND FUNCTION OF THE NEUROMUSCULAR SYSTEM
NEUROMUSCULAR ANATOMY STRUCTURE AND FUNCTION

In the past several decades, research has placed increasingly greater emphasis on the importance of the neuromuscular system in governing ROM. Nearly every study that has demonstrated effective flexibility training methods has suggested that the neuromuscular system must be involved for joint ROM to improve. This phenomenon reflects that the nervous and muscular systems are vastly different in form and function. As such, each is considered an individual system given the unique physiological responses that occur in response to flexibility training. Developing an understanding of the neuromuscular system and its subsystems will only improve programming quality for the performance client.

THE NERVOUS SYSTEM

The nervous system plays a critical role in an athlete's level of flexibility because it is the body's command, control, and communication system. One function of the nervous system pertinent to flexibility training is **proprioception**.

Sensory information is collected from specialized receptors called **mechanoreceptors**, which relay information to the CNS. Mechanoreceptors are located throughout the

---

PROPRIO-CEPTION →

The body's ability to naturally sense its general orientation and relative position of its parts.

MECHANO-RECEPTORS →

Specialized structures that respond to mechanical forces (touch and pressure) within tissues and then transmit signals through sensory nerves.

musculoskeletal system and convert mechanical signals into information useful to the CNS. When a joint moves, its surrounding tissues and receptors are affected by stretching and relaxation in relation to the range and direction of the joint's motion.

For example, during knee flexion, the quadriceps muscles and associated tendons, the anterior aspect of the knee joint capsule, and the skin covering these structures are stretched. In contrast, tissues located on the posterior of the thigh, such as the hamstrings muscle group, are shortened. The CNS uses these kinds of changes in the shape and length of the surrounding tissues to develop a sense of how far the joint has moved through its ROM and to determine whether increased muscle tone is required to provide stability or prevent the joint from moving further.

Flexibility training is primarily affected by mechanoreceptors found in the muscle (muscle spindles), tendonous connections (Golgi tendon organs), the joint capsule (joint receptors), and the skin (cutaneous receptors). Mechanical information is transduced via these receptors and sent to the CNS, where an internal picture of joint movement is created (**Figure 9.4**) (Tuthill & Azim, 2018). The CNS combines these proprioceptive signals with information from other senses, such as sight and hearing, to create an internal motor landscape that tells an individual which physical actions they are likely capable of performing within the current environment.

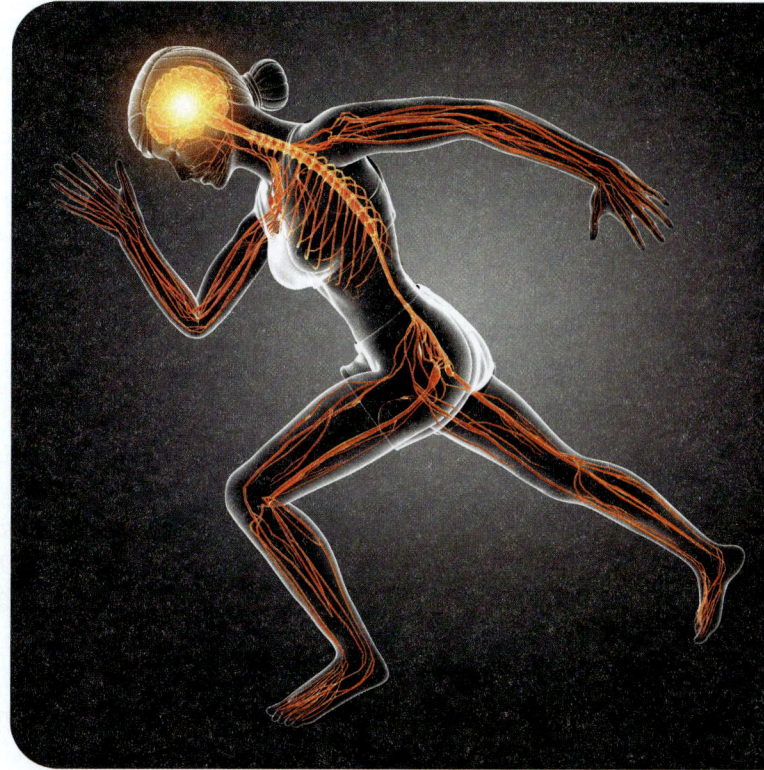
© S K Chavan/Shutterstock

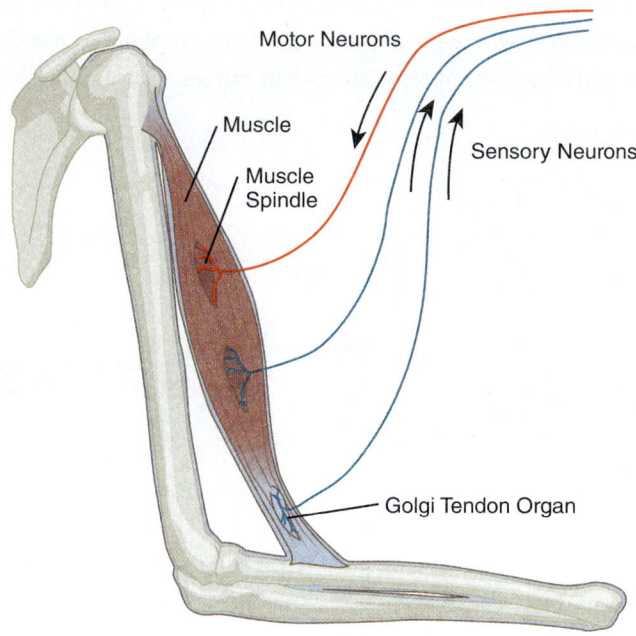

FIGURE 9.4 Neuromuscular Interaction

Based on Tuthill, J. C. & Azim, E. (2018). Proprioception. Current Biology, 28(5), R194-R203.

🤖 *GETTING TECHNICAL*

The process by which cells in the body convert mechanical signals into electrochemical information is called **mechanotransduction**. When muscles compress and lengthen during movement, the affected cells detect these mechanical changes via the deformation of their membranes and the extracellular environment. Those changes stimulate essential biochemical processes such as protein synthesis and hormone production.

MUSCLE SPINDLES

Muscle spindles can be regarded as both a protective and a proprioceptive system. As a protective system, if the muscle is rapidly elongated to the end or near the end of the ROM, then a reflexive signal will be sent to the spinal cord to contract the stretched muscle (Myers et al., 2003). This reflex contraction of the elongated muscle, known as the **stretch reflex**, helps prevent the joint skeletal structures (bones and cartilage) and ligaments from exceeding the joint's normal ROM, which in turn helps prevent damage or injury.

Muscle spindles are located within, and lie parallel to, the power-generating muscle fibers. They are called intrafusal fibers because they are located within the muscle fibers themselves, as opposed to the regular muscle fibers, which are called extrafusal fibers (**Figure 9.5**).

Intrafusal fibers are entwined with sensory nerve endings and are responsible for sending information about muscle length to the CNS. In contrast, extrafusal fibers are the standard muscle fibers that generate force and cause muscle contractions. They are the primary components of skeletal muscles and are responsible for our ability to move and maintain posture.

Flexibility's velocity-dependent nature might help explain a common phenomenon in sports such as martial arts, where people can reach large amplitudes of motion in static positions such as splits, but cannot replicate similar ranges of motion in dynamic actions

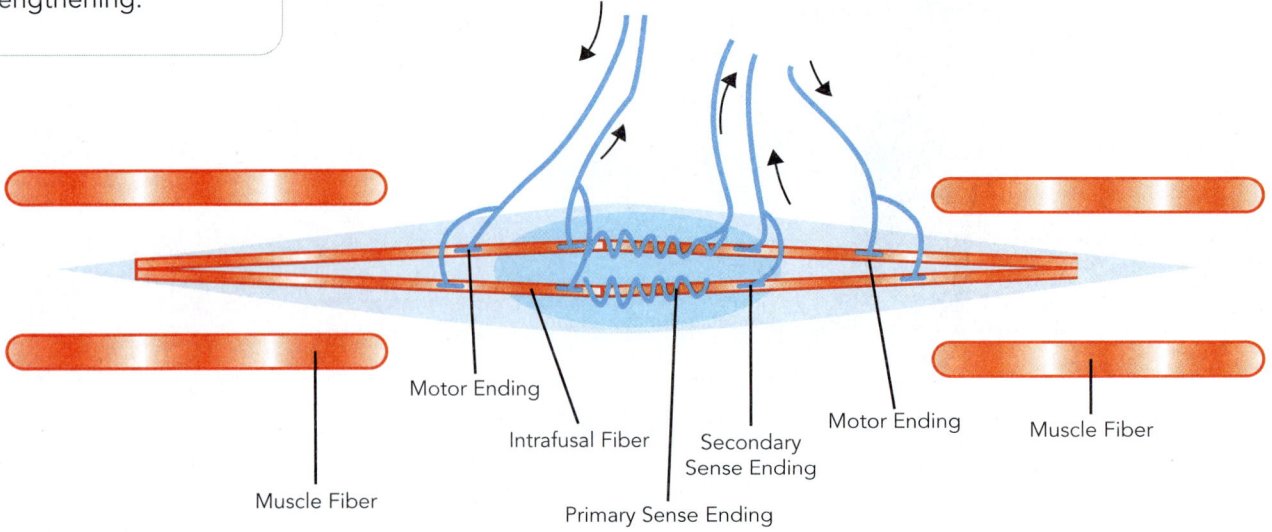

Motor Ending

Intrafusal Fiber

Secondary
Sense Ending

Motor Ending

Muscle Fiber

Muscle Fiber

Primary Sense Ending

FIGURE 9.5 Anatomy of a Typical Muscle Spindle

such as high kicks. The large gap between static and dynamic flexibility is often reduced with dedicated, dynamic stretching practice, but more research is needed to confirm the underlying mechanisms.

The muscle spindle contains primary and secondary nerve endings that respond to different stimuli. Primary nerve endings, called dynamic fibers, are sensitive to changes in the magnitude (amount) and rate (velocity) of the muscle length. Secondary endings, called static fibers, are much less sensitive to the rate of change, but provide information about static muscle length in the absence of movement. Therefore, the greatest contribution from secondary endings is to position sense instead of movement (Proske & Gandevia, 2009).

This division of sensory fibers into dynamic and static types means that the stretch reflex can also be categorized as either dynamic or static (Levin & Feldman, 1994). The SAID principle (principle of specificity) dictates that the body's neuromuscular system will adapt based on the stresses placed on it. Therefore, specific adaptations following flexibility training are likely to be velocity-dependent, as is the case for resistance training (Behm & Sale, 1993).

GOLGI TENDON ORGANS

Golgi tendon organs are located at the junctions between skeletal muscle fibers and the tendons. Approximately 5 to 25 muscle fibers enter each GTO's capsule and attach to collagen bundles; the collagen bundles exit the other side of the capsule to converge with the tendon (Jami, 1988). Within the capsule, large sensory neurons are interweaved with collagen bundles in a configuration resembling a braided spiral (**Figure 9.6**).

When the muscle stretches, the distance between these neurons and collagen fibers decreases, causing the collagen fibers to compress the GTOs (Swett & Schoultz, 1975). The signals that travel from the GTOs to the CNS provide information about the amount of force exerted by the muscle. In contrast, when a muscle contracts, it generates tension and pulls on the tendon, increasing the distance between the neurons and collagen fibers. If the GTOs sense too much tension, the CNS will engage an inhibitory reflex telling the contracting muscle to relax. This action is known as autogenic inhibition or the inverse myotatic reflex.

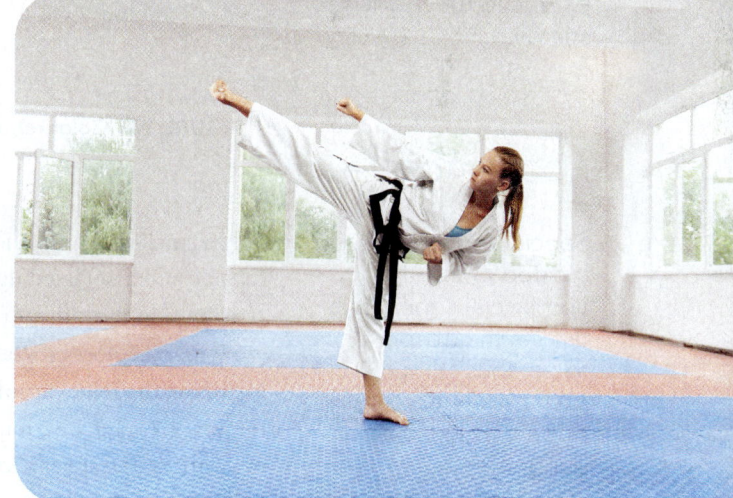

© Serhii Bobyk/Shutterstock

JOINT RECEPTORS

Mechanoreceptors exist in both the joint capsule and its corresponding ligaments, but their role in regular movement is minimal and often exaggerated. **Joint receptors** are all but inactive during movements in the mid-ROM, and they are most strongly stimulated when a joint moves close to its physiological limits (Latash, 2008). Therefore, the role of joint receptors is primarily to detect the limits of motion. Although joint receptors have

> **JOINT RECEPTORS** →
>
> Receptors located in and around the joint capsule that respond to pressure, acceleration, and deceleration of the joint.

RUFFINI ENDINGS →

Slow-adapting, encapsulated receptors found in the dermis, subcutaneous tissues, and some connective tissues, which respond to skin stretch.

FREE NERVE ENDINGS →

Unencapsulated sensory nerve endings found in the skin, ligaments, tendons, and joint capsule, which detect temperature and pressure changes, pain, and mechanical stimuli.

NOCICEPTORS →

Specialized structures located in the skin and fascial connective tissues that respond to noxious stimuli, such as damage, pain, or perceptions of danger.

CUTANEOUS RECEPTORS →

Specialized sensory nerve endings found in the skin that detect and respond to various types of external stimuli.

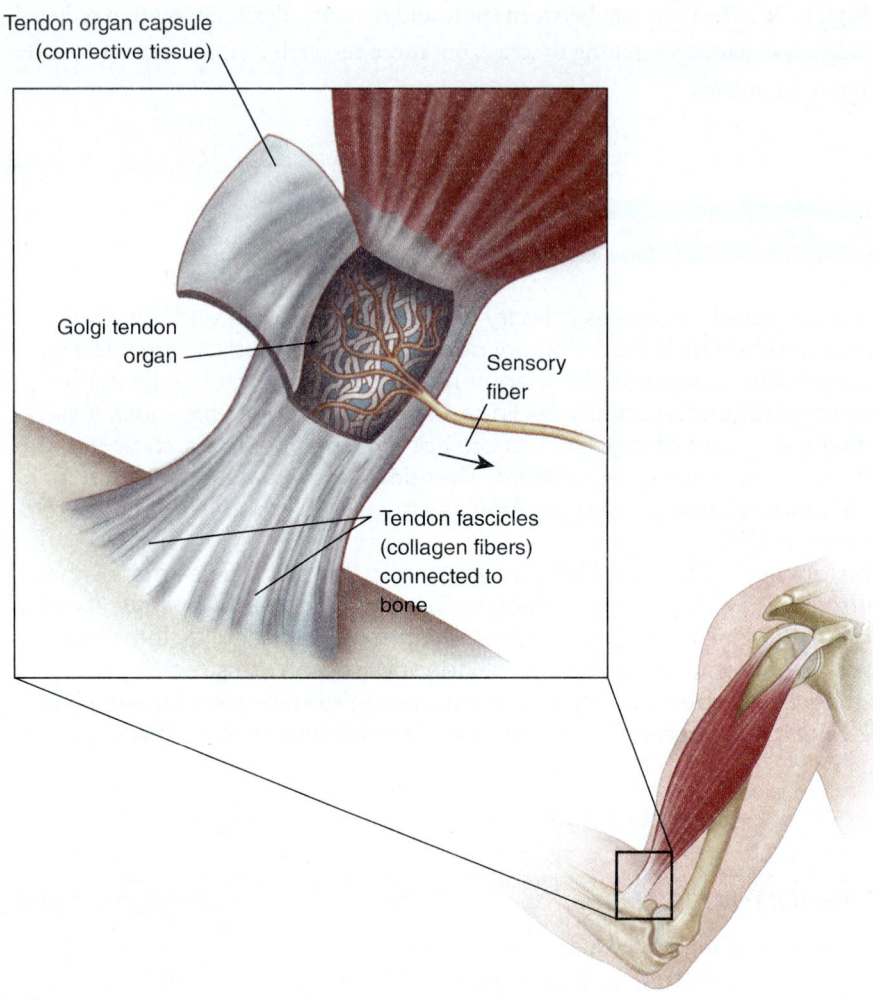

FIGURE 9.6 Golgi Tendon Organ

only a small role until a joint approaches its end ROM, it is worth noting that the joint capsule and associated ligaments have been found to contribute as much as 47% of the resistance to movement (Alter, 2004).

Joint receptors are found in various parts of the joint capsule and associated structures, including the joint capsule, ligaments, tendons, and surrounding connective tissues (**Figure 9.7**). The distribution of these receptors varies depending on the specific type of joint and the specific receptor involved. The joint capsule is a fibrous structure that surrounds and encloses the joint, providing stability and protection. Free nerve endings and **Ruffini endings** are primarily found in the joint capsule; they detect changes in joint position, movement, and pressure.

FREE NERVE ENDINGS

Free nerve endings (bare nerve endings with no fibrous capsule) are found in the joint capsule but are also spread throughout the muscle and its associated connective tissue elements. These nerve endings are mainly composed of type III and type IV (small-diameter myelinated and unmyelinated, respectively) afferent fibers. They are considered **nociceptors** that send signals to the CNS only when a stimulus is strong enough to potentially cause harm to the tissues. The extent to which free nerve endings influence flexibility is primarily determined by an athlete's experience relating to the

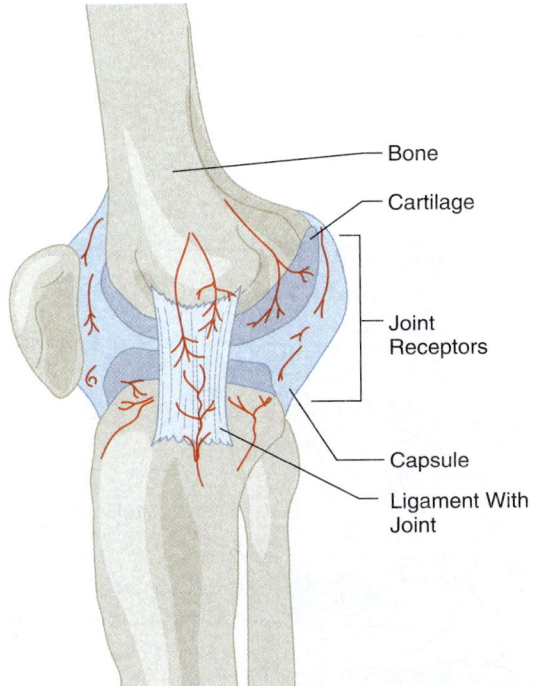

FIGURE 9.7 Joint Receptors

safety of a particular movement and their level of stretch tolerance. If a stretch exceeds an athlete's tolerance, free nerve endings may be stimulated, which then inhibits the full stretch capacity or triggers a withdrawal reflex.

CUTANEOUS RECEPTORS

Cutaneous receptors (also known as skin receptors) provide the CNS with information about the body's internal and external environments (**Figure 9.8**). Cutaneous receptors are predominantly type II (slowly adapting) sensory receptors that contribute to the body's ability to detect the magnitude and direction of joint movement by sensing changes in skin tension patterns (Grigg, 1994; Johansson & Flanagan, 2009). Because the skin contributes only approximately 2% of joint resistance to movement, the extent to which cutaneous receptors limit flexibility is likely small (Alter, 2004).

THE MUSCULAR SYSTEM

Skeletal muscle structure is of significant functional importance in flexibility training. Its properties can generally be divided into active and passive components (Knudson, 2021). A typical skeletal muscle is composed of numerous distinctive bundles of fibers called **fascicles**, and each bundle is surrounded by a sheath of connective tissue called **perimysium**. The whole muscle is also surrounded by a connective tissue sheath called **epimysium**, which packages all the fascicles into a collective functional unit (**Figure 9.9**).

Hundreds of muscle fibers are present within each fascicle, and each individual muscle fiber is considered a muscle cell. Each muscle fiber has its own connective tissue sheath called **endomysium**. These coverings of connective tissue at each organizational layer of the muscle, which are collectively known as the **parallel elastic component (PEC)**, contribute to the passive tension that arises in stretched muscles. The PEC gradually blends to form a discrete tendon that blends in with the connective tissue covering bone.

FASCICLE

A bundle of muscle fibers surrounded by perimysium.

PERIMYSIUM →

Connective tissue surrounding a muscle fascicle.

EPIMYSIUM →

Connective tissue surrounding and enclosing an entire skeletal muscle.

ENDOMYSIUM

Connective tissue that wraps around individual muscle fibers within a fascicle.

PARALLEL **ELASTIC COMPONENT (PEC)**

The passive elastic properties of a muscle that are attributed to the connective tissue elements running parallel to the muscle fibers.

Skin Sensory Receptors

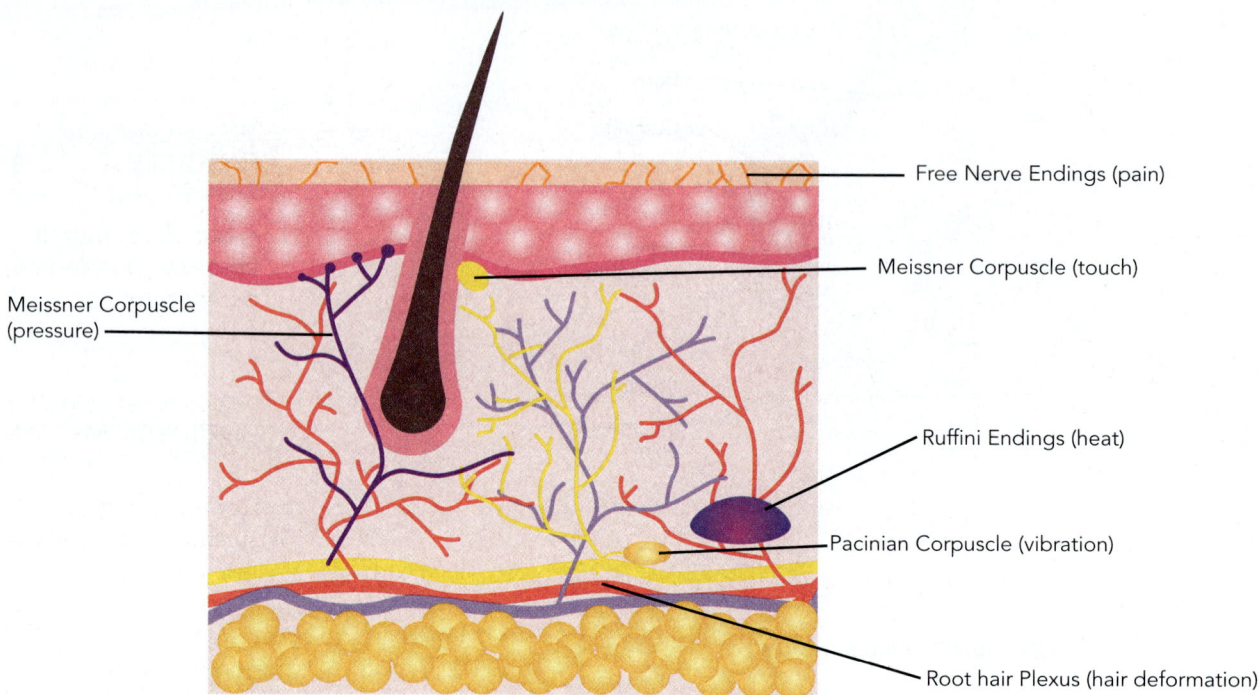

FIGURE 9.8 Receptors in the Skin

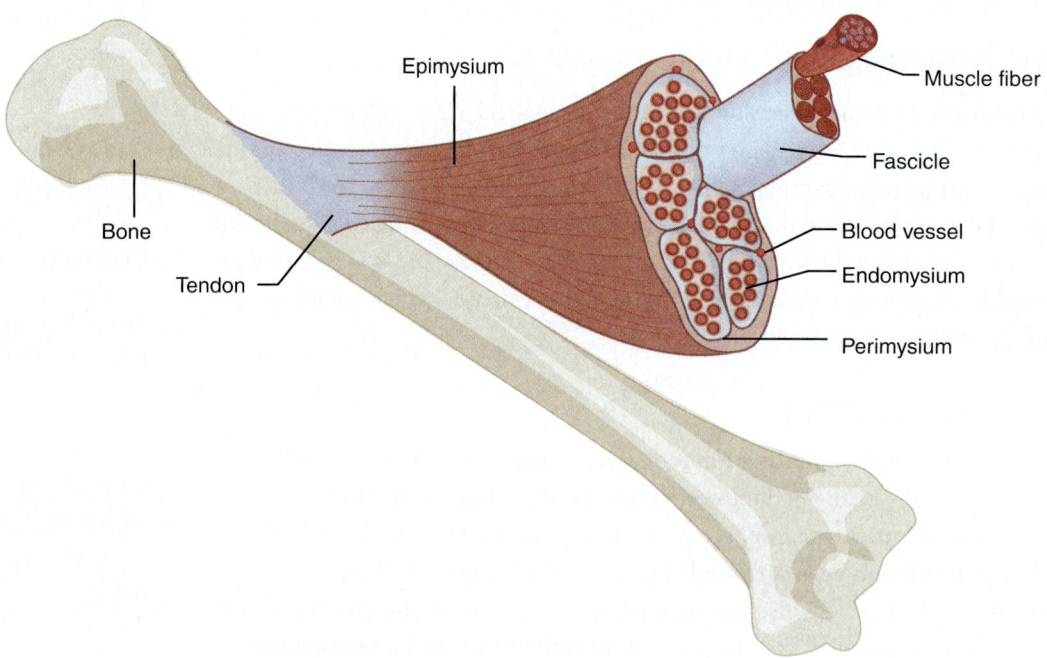

FIGURE 9.9 Structure of Skeletal Muscle

MUSCLE FIBER ARRANGEMENT

The arrangement of a muscle's fascicles has a considerable influence on its potential ROM and force production (Lieber & Friden, 2000). Muscle fibers can be categorized as parallel or pennate arrangements (**Figure 9.10**). In parallel muscles, the fascicles run parallel to the

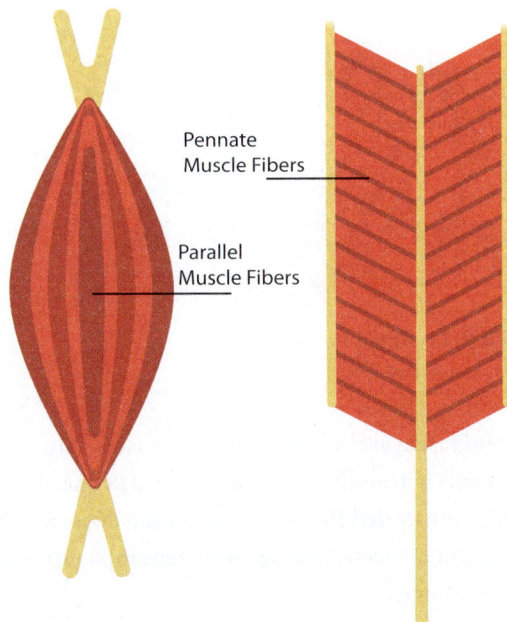

FIGURE 9.10 Parallel Versus Pennate Muscle

muscle's long axis. The biceps brachii of the upper arm is perhaps the best-known example of a muscle with a parallel arrangement.

In contrast, fibers in pennate muscles are aligned at an oblique angle to the line of pull. A simple way to visualize pennate muscles is to think of the vanes on feathers (*pennate* originates from the Latin *pennatus*, meaning "winged"). Pennate muscles can be further organized into unipennate, bipennate, and multipennate muscles.

ROM is greater in parallel muscles compared to those with a pennate fiber arrangement but at the cost of force development; conversely, pennate muscles favor force development over ROM (Hamill et al., 2021). On the one hand, due to their lower passive resistance, parallel muscles may respond more favorably to passive stretching. On the other hand, pennate muscles may respond better to active stretching methods that utilize isometric contractions because of their ability to produce greater tension levels. Due to their greater physiological cross-sectional area, stronger contractions result in a greater depression in stretch sensitivity, enabling the joint to move further into the ROM (Kurz, 2003).

THE FASCIAL SYSTEM

The previously mentioned sheaths of connective tissue that surround the components of muscle at its different layers (endomysium, perimysium, and epimysium) belong to a category of soft tissue known as **fascia** (Stecco et al., 2006). Fascia is essentially a collective name for all the connective tissues that envelop and surround the contractile components of the muscle fibers, and it is made up of a relatively simple mixture of cells, fibers, and amorphous (shapeless) gel-like material called ground substance (**Figure 9.11**).

Fascial cells consist primarily of fibroblasts (produce connective tissue fibers), fasciacytes (produce hyaluronan, which facilitates sliding between fascial surfaces), and adipocytes (stores of fat within connective tissue). Fibers produced by fibroblasts are mainly **elastin** and **collagen**. Elastin facilitates connective tissue lengthening, whereas collagen provides structure and stability. The quality of fascial surface sliding and the quantity of elastin content influence fascial mobility, which is integral for normal, healthy musculoskeletal functioning (Langevin, 2021).

FASCIA →

Connective tissue that surrounds muscles and bones.

ELASTIN →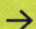

A protein that provides elasticity to skin, tendons, ligaments, and other structures.

COLLAGEN →

A protein found in connective tissue, muscles, and skin that provides strength and structure; the most abundant protein in the human body.

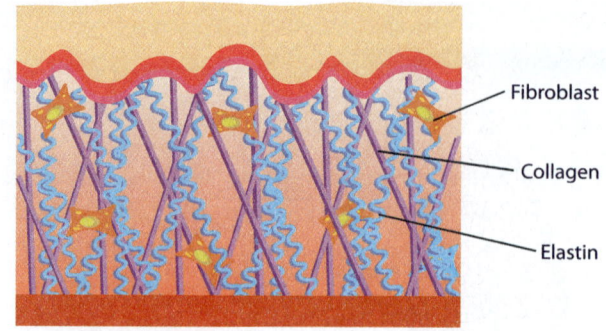

FIGURE 9.11 Structure of Fascia

© Sofia Bessarab/Shutterstock

Collectively, muscle and fascia are referred to as myofascia. Notably, most of the stiffness (resistance to stretch) within the myofascia comes primarily from the fascia. Konrad and Tilp (2014) demonstrated that static stretching does not affect tendon stiffness; such findings suggest a necessity to separate tendinous structures from the PEC in discussions of "muscle" stiffness.

MYOFASCIAL LINES

Myofascial lines are whole-body linkages of fascia that some anatomists have documented during cadaveric dissection (**Figure 9.12**). The continuity of these myofascial lines has been suggested as a mechanism that can explain how flexibility exercises can improve ROM in distal areas not directly exposed to stretching forces (Wilke et al., 2016).

However, it is important to remember that popular fascial models based on the concept of myofascial continuity remain theoretical, and further evidence is required to support their applicability in living humans (Bordoni & Myers, 2020). The fascial elements within the muscle–tendon unit contribute a large proportion of the passive resistance to stretch, which can be plotted on a passive length–tension curve. With training, connective tissues can become less resistant to stretching at a certain point in the ROM.

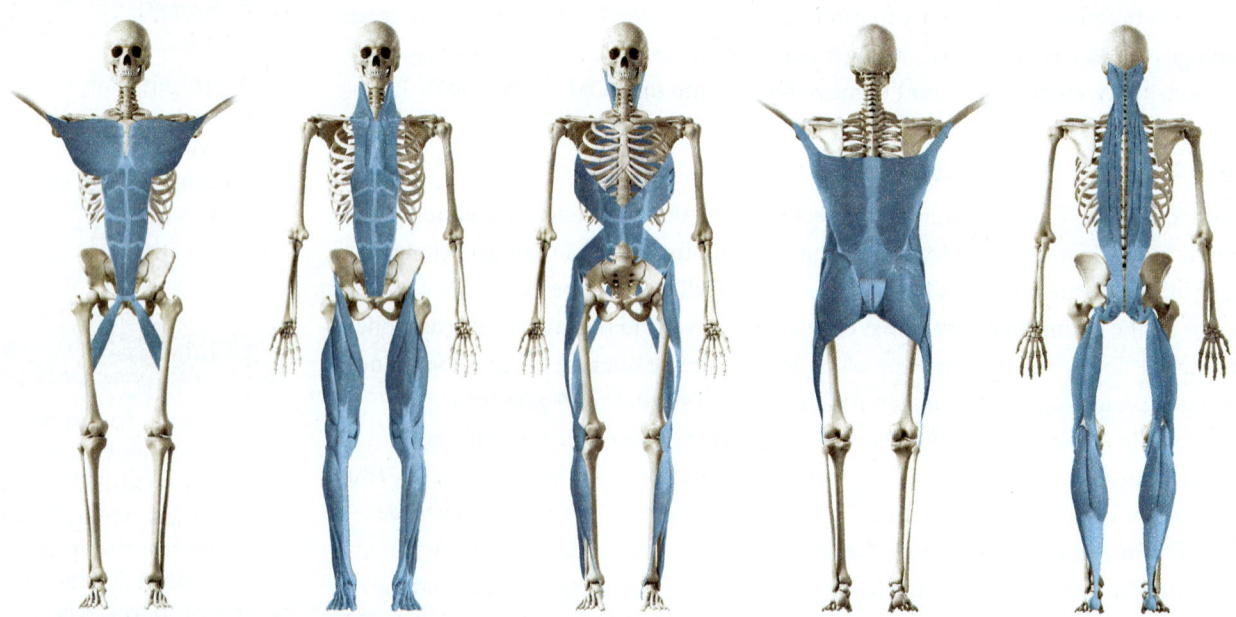

FIGURE 9.12 Common Myofascial Lines

The effect of passive tension is particularly apparent in multi-joint muscles when a muscle is stretched across multiple joints. For example, when lying in the supine position, flexing the knee will produce much greater hip flexion ROM compared to when the knee is extended. The reduction in ROM when the knee is extended during hip flexion is caused by the hamstrings muscle group extending simultaneously across both joints, resulting in an inability to lengthen and thus limiting ROM fully. This phenomenon is known as **passive insufficiency**, and it can generally be improved by making the tissues more extensible with regular stretching training.

LESSON 3: THE SCIENCE OF FLEXIBILITY TRAINING
SCIENTIFIC RATIONALE FOR FLEXIBILITY TRAINING

It is not uncommon for an athlete to hire a sports and performance professional with the singular goal of improving fitness for athletic purposes. There are several reasons why integrated flexibility training is beneficial for athletic performance. Most important are pattern overload that the athlete can experience and the cumulative injury cycle.

PATTERN OVERLOAD

Pattern overload describes how muscle groups may become imbalanced by constant repetition of similar sequences of joint actions and muscular contractions, which may occur in specific sporting activities, such as endurance running, or in occupations that involve repetitive tasks (McDonald et al., 2019; Sugimoto et al., 2019). Other sport-specific examples include elbow valgus extension overload in baseball pitchers (Paulino et al., 2016) and intersection syndrome in golf (Balakatounis et al., 2017).

Such overload occurs frequently in sports because many athletes perform the same routines that stress the same lines of tension with minimal movement variation. However, pattern overload is not necessarily restricted to movement patterns; maintaining a constant static posture, such as prolonged sitting, may also be considered a repetitive *pattern* and contribute to musculoskeletal symptoms in the shoulders, low back, thighs, and knees (Daneshmandi et al., 2017).

For example, freestyle wrestlers demonstrate a higher degree of kyphosis than Greco-Roman wrestlers owing to spending more time in a hunched-shoulders position (Rajabi et al., 2008). Continuous exposure to loads by way of repetitive muscular contractions during dynamic motions or prolonged static loads during sustained postures with minimal rest may also result in localized ischemic effects and elevated fatigue levels.

CUMULATIVE INJURY CYCLE

Poor posture and repetitive, overuse movements can create dysfunction within the connective tissue of the human body (Iqbal & Alghadir, 2017). These dysfunctions can eventually lead to an injury and a repair response by the body termed

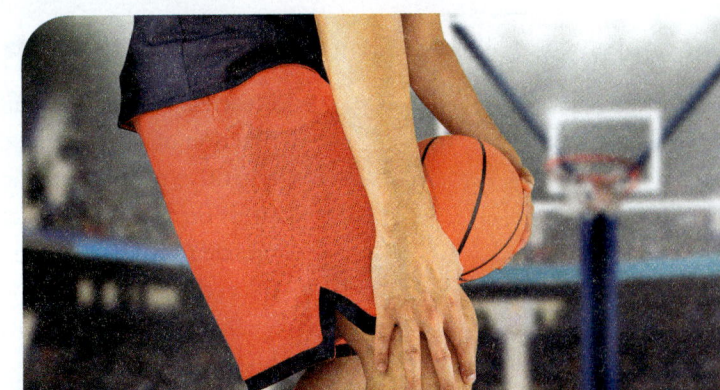

PASSIVE INSUFFICIENCY →

The inability of a biarticular muscle to stretch or lengthen sufficiently across both joints simultaneously. This phenomenon occurs when a muscle reaches its maximum length and can no longer generate effective passive tension.

PATTERN OVERLOAD →

Consistently repeating the same pattern of motion over long periods of time, leading to dysfunction or injury.

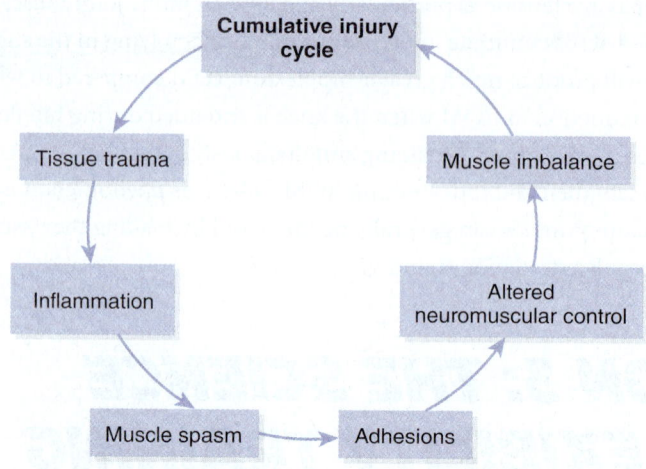

FIGURE 9.13 Cumulative Injury Cycle

the **cumulative injury cycle** (**Figure 9.13**). This pattern of disrepair can occur after physical damage to the body. It is a vicious cycle in which myofascial adhesions and muscle imbalances form due to tissue trauma, increasing the risk of future injury or dysfunction.

Additionally, pain receptors in the affected areas may become oversensitive to chemicals released from damaged or overloaded cells. This process may contribute to the onset of pain in response to stimuli that otherwise would not be perceived as painful (Visser & van Dieën, 2006) and may contribute to an exaggerated response to pain. Subsequently, fear avoidance may worsen physical symptoms (Vlaeyen & Linton, 2000). This fear avoidance can cause athletes to stop training or reduce their training load, leading to stiff fibrotic tissue development between connective tissues that should otherwise demonstrate extensibility.

Repeated injuries or trauma to an area will affect the quality of soft tissues, leading to the deposition of stiff and inelastic fibrotic tissue that interferes with athletic performance. For example, immobilization of a limb following an injury often results in a loss of ROM and an increase in sensations of tightness. This phenomenon may be caused by a loss of sarcomeres (the functional units in a muscle contraction) in series or by persistent neurological guarding as the CNS continues to believe that it needs to protect the area.

MUSCLE IMBALANCES

Muscle imbalances occur when there is a discrepancy in the strength, flexibility, or function of antagonistic or synergistic muscle groups. These imbalances can result from repetitive patterns or lead to abnormal movement patterns, altered biomechanics, and stress on the musculoskeletal system. Similarly, the cumulative injury cycle could cause muscle imbalances to develop over time, or chronic muscle imbalances could initiate the cycle.

Two hypotheses have been proposed to explain the source of muscle imbalances. The first hypothesis is that muscle imbalance has a biomechanical origin caused by repetitive movements and prolonged static postures. The biomechanical origin hypothesis states that consistently performing the same movement patterns or maintaining the same postures for long periods can cause adaptations in muscle length and strength, which may lead to dysfunction throughout the kinetic chain (Sahrmann et al., 2017).

Consequently, joints may be exposed to higher risks of injury due to being subjected to abnormal stress patterns. This problem could lead to sport-specific pattern overload injuries discussed previously.

The second hypothesis is that a person may have a neurological predisposition to muscle imbalance (Page et al., 2010). The neurological origin hypothesis began with Czech physician Vladimir Janda. Although he recognized that biomechanical factors may cause muscle imbalances, Janda (1978) postulated that an impaired relationship between tight or short muscles and excessively inhibited muscles might also be a contributing factor. Muscle imbalances may also occur between muscle groups on opposite sides of the body, such as substantial differences in dominant-side versus nondominant-side hip abductor strength in young adults (Jacobs et al., 2005). Such a difference in muscle function on opposite sides of the body may adversely affect gait in a way that presents an increased risk of injury.

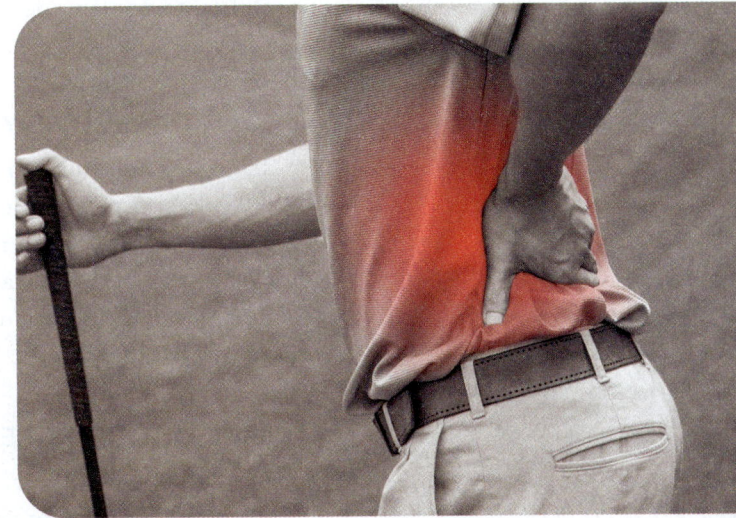

© Sattahipbeach/Shutterstock

COMMON CAUSES OF MUSCLE IMBALANCES

Given the two hypotheses, it is likely that muscle imbalances are caused by a combination of biomechanical and neurological factors, including pattern overload, poor technical skill, aging, lack of recovery, and lack of core strength (Sueki et al., 2013). If left unattended, such imbalances may result in altered reciprocal inhibition, synergistic dominance, and joint dysfunction. These imbalances can produce poor neuromuscular efficiency, negatively affecting the function of the human movement system and resulting in decreased performance.

POOR TECHNICAL SKILL

An inability to execute skilled movements results in inefficient use of energy and excessive overloading of specific muscles, leading to regional tightness. Underused muscles that become weak may compound the problem. This dysfunction is seen in athletes who develop "bad habits" in their fundamentals. Initially, the suboptimal movement pattern might get the job done, but optimizing form will inevitably allow higher performance levels in the long run. Flexibility training to correct muscle imbalances will allow full ROM and a more biomechanically efficient form. Movements such as a golf swing and throwing mechanics are particularly susceptible to this problem.

AGING

Among the various age-related physiological changes that impact flexibility are loss of muscle elasticity and mass, joint degeneration, and a loss of motor neurons. These factors contribute to the inevitable decline in physical capacities that occurs with senescence. Flexibility training can play a significant role in helping to restore or maintain the optimal tissue extensibility needed to continue competing in selected sports and improve activities of daily living.

Additionally, older athletes seeking performance improvements may have many years of "bad form habits" stacked up along with the potential for many injuries over the years. For this reason, a full range of postural assessments should be used with older-adult athletes to develop a flexibility training program that meets both their performance and everyday needs.

LACK OF RECOVERY

Taking too little time to rest between training sessions impedes recovery, making it difficult for tissues stressed during physical activity to adequately regenerate in time for the next session. Tissues may become overactive and shortened as a consequence. Such overactivity inevitably leads to the underactivity of the antagonist's muscles (altered reciprocal inhibition) and muscle imbalances, and the risk of entering the cumulative injury cycle increases.

LACK OF CORE STRENGTH

A sufficiently strong core enables the athlete to properly distribute their weight and absorb and transfer forces appropriately. This development improves critical athletic qualities such as strength, speed, and power. Conversely, a lack of adequate core strength may interfere with these processes in a way that causes muscle imbalances. Specifically, a lack of core strength, particularly in the lumbar multifidus and transverse abdominis, is a primary contributor to muscle imbalances that cause an anterior pelvic tilt and excessive lumbar extension (Takaki et al., 2016). Maintaining proper ROM and core strength throughout the lumbo-pelvic-hip complex is essential for getting the most out of performance training.

ALTERED RECIPROCAL INHIBITION

Reciprocal inhibition is an essential part of the human sensorimotor system that contributes to postural and movement control by means of task-dependent muscle activation, enabling the body to maintain a relative balance between agonist and antagonist muscle groups (Yavuz et al., 2018). However, the functioning of this mechanism can become abnormal in case of altered reciprocal inhibition, which occurs when overactive muscles cause their antagonists to become underactive. The mechanism of reciprocal inhibition was discussed earlier in the chapter.

SYNERGISTIC DOMINANCE

In addition to their agonist and antagonist roles, muscles can act as synergists. Synergist muscles create forces to assist prime movers, but are not intended to be the primary force producers for a given joint motion (Hamill et al., 2021). For example, the hamstring complex and the erector spinae are synergistic with the gluteus maximus during hip extension.

Synergistic dominance occurs when the synergist takes over (dominants) as the primary mover for a specific motion. In simple terms, synergists "pick up the slack" because other muscles (agonists) are not doing their job. For example, if the prime hip extensors (gluteus maximus and hamstrings group) cannot adequately fulfill their role during the initial swing phases of the running gait cycle, the lumbar extensors may be recruited to complete the movement by increasing an anterior pelvic tilt. Synergistic dominance may cause a number of issues, such as abnormal kinematics that stress the joint and its associated soft-tissue structures (i.e., capsule, ligaments, tendons, and muscles), potentially leading to strains, sprains, and overuse symptoms.

Altered reciprocal inhibition and synergistic dominance are the result of muscle imbalances. For example, a common muscle imbalance in the hips is overactive hip flexors causing underactive hip extensors. This may result from or cause the common postural impairment of an anterior pelvic tilt. The chronic contraction of the hip flexor group causes chronic inhibition (altered reciprocal inhibition) of the hip extensor group (Mills et al., 2015). Thus, during a movement that requires hip extension, such as running or jumping, the primary hip extensor (gluteus maximus) may be unable to maintain optimal force production. In this case, contraction of the synergist (hamstrings) will increase in an attempt to meet the force production demands (synergistic dominance).

The Sports Performance Coach must be able to connect the dots when faced with these issues. For example, if an athlete has decreased gluteus maximus function and complains of "tight" hamstrings, then it is likely that optimal gluteal strength will need to be restored to help reduce the sensations of tightness in the synergists.

JOINT DYSFUNCTION

Joint movement can be described as either osteokinematic or arthrokinematic motion. **Osteokinematic** motion, also known as "real motion," consists of the observable movements of bony segments—for example, flexion, extension, abduction, adduction, and rotation of the limbs (**Figure 9.14**). **Arthrokinematic** motion involves the movement of one articulating surface relative to the other surface within the joint (**Figure 9.15**). These movements, which consist mainly of rolls, slides, and spins, cannot be actively controlled or observed.

Joint movement is affected by both the joint structure and the muscle forces acting on it. If the muscles are not functioning optimally, the nature of the forces they produce will cause alterations in the movements produced. In the case of synergistic dominance, joint dysfunction is produced by the synergist contributing more force than the prime mover, which alters the ideal movement. For example, an excessive anterior pelvic tilt that reduces gluteus maximus function and increases the demand for the hamstrings is likely to alter motion at the iliofemoral and tibiofemoral joints.

OSTEO-KINEMATIC

Movement of a limb that is visible.

ARTHRO-KINEMATIC

The description of joint surface movement; consists of three major types—roll, slide, and spin.

Joint dysfunction is the next step in the movement dysfunction cycle and can be the direct result of synergistic dominance. Think of it this way: Muscle imbalances cause altered postural alignment and altered reciprocal inhibition; then altered reciprocal inhibition causes synergistic dominance; and finally, synergistic dominance means that a synergist is applying more force to the bone than the prime mover is, causing joint dysfunction.

The Sports Performance Coach must be able to continue connecting the dots. For example, if an athlete has "tight" hamstrings and underactive gluteal muscles, they may also demonstrate altered motion at the iliofemoral joint. Consider this fact: The arrangement of fibers and the insertion of the gluteus maximus help it to stabilize the iliofemoral joint while also producing hip extension. Unfortunately, the hamstrings do not serve this same stabilization role for the joint. Therefore, if the hamstrings are dominant over the gluteals for hip extension, then aberrant motion at the iliofemoral joint is likely to occur.

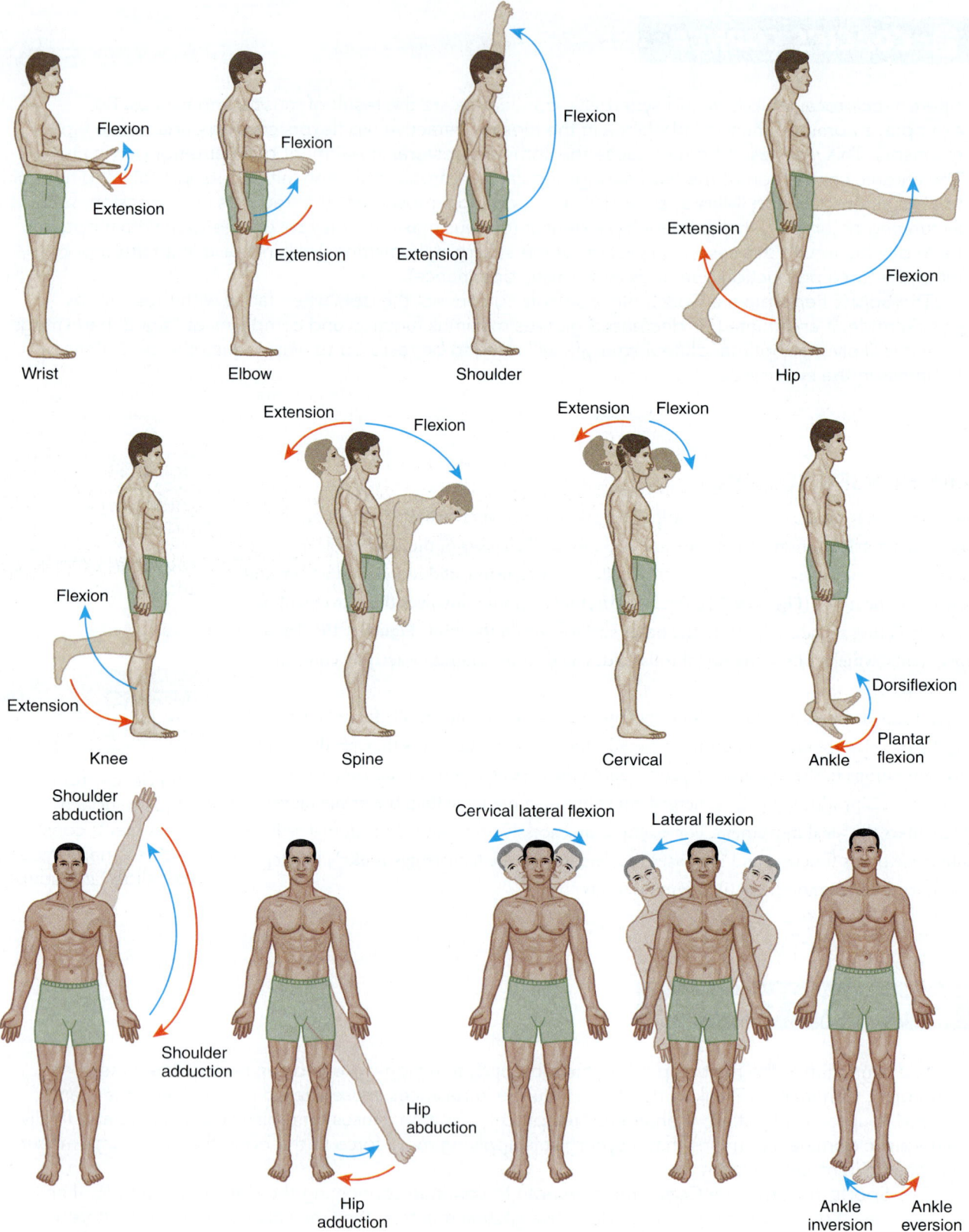

FIGURE 9.14 Osteokinematic Motions

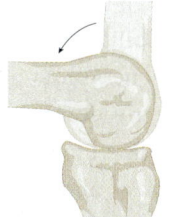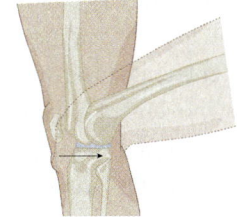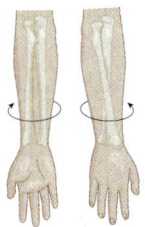

FIGURE 9.15 Arthrokinematic Motions

POOR NEUROMUSCULAR EFFICIENCY

Neuromuscular efficiency is characterized by the ability of the nervous system to activate the correct muscles with appropriate levels of force to meet the unique demands of the task and environment (Shumway-Cook & Woollacott, 2017). Poor neuromuscular efficiency can promote compensatory movement strategies that increase the risk of musculoskeletal injuries (Gutierrez et al., 2009; Hewett et al., 2005; Padua et al., 2015; Paterno et al., 2010). Such compensatory movement strategies may present as inappropriate landing mechanics, insufficient postural control, and abnormal muscle activation patterns caused by changes in the CNS that adversely affect the athlete's ability to control their musculoskeletal system (Riemann et al., 2002).

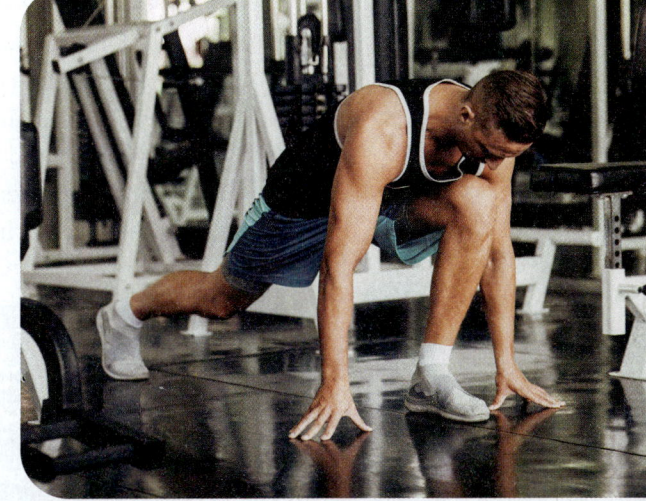

© I AM NIKOM/Shutterstock

Muscle imbalances can negatively impact neuromuscular efficiency by altering muscle recruitment patterns, leading to inefficient and uncoordinated movements. The presence of imbalances can cause the body to develop compensatory movement patterns, which can place undue stress on other muscles, joints, and connective tissues, potentially leading to further imbalances and increasing the risk of injury.

Additionally, muscle imbalances can affect joint stability and reduce proprioception, decreasing the body's awareness of its position and movements in space. Imbalances can also impair the ability of muscles to generate force effectively, reducing overall performance and increasing the risk of injury.

Flexibility training can play a vital role in correcting muscle imbalances, and thereby reducing altered reciprocal inhibition, synergistic dominance, joint dysfunction, and poor neuromuscular efficiency. By incorporating targeted stretching exercises and dynamic mobility drills, flexibility training helps to lengthen short, overactive muscles and improve overall muscle balance. This restoration of balance can alleviate altered reciprocal inhibition, allowing underactive muscles to function properly and preventing synergistic muscles from taking over the role of the inhibited muscles. As a result, joint stability and function improve, reducing the risk of joint dysfunction and injury.

LESSON 4: PRINCIPLES OF FLEXIBILITY TRAINING
FLEXIBILITY TRAINING GUIDELINES

Flexibility training is an essential aspect of any comprehensive training program, as it not only bolsters performance but also mitigates the risk of injury. This lesson explores evidence-based guidelines for flexibility training tailored to athletes across a spectrum of skill levels and disciplines. The importance of conducting a thorough needs analysis and utilizing assessment information to create an individualized flexibility program is addressed as part of the discussion. Integrated self-myofascial techniques; static, active, and dynamic stretching techniques; movement preparation; and effective warm-ups are other integral components of a well-rounded training approach. By adhering to these guidelines, athletes can maximize their ROM, unlock their full potential, and lay the foundation for a sustainable athletic career.

NEEDS ANALYSIS AND ASSESSMENT INFORMATION

Flexibility training programs must be intentional and specific to the athlete to realize their optimal benefits. Flexibility is joint-, position-, and speed-specific (Kurz, 2003). In turn, flexibility training should be guided by the demands of these factors as they relate to the athlete's chosen sport or activities. For example, a Taekwondo athlete needs to perform rapid high kicks during a contest. A flexibility training program for such a client would most certainly involve dynamic stretches of the hips in the planes of flexion, extension, and abduction, as these actions are all present in the sport (front kicks, back kicks, and sidekicks, respectively). However, many athletes need to start with foundational levels of flexibility before progressing to sport-specific flexibility.

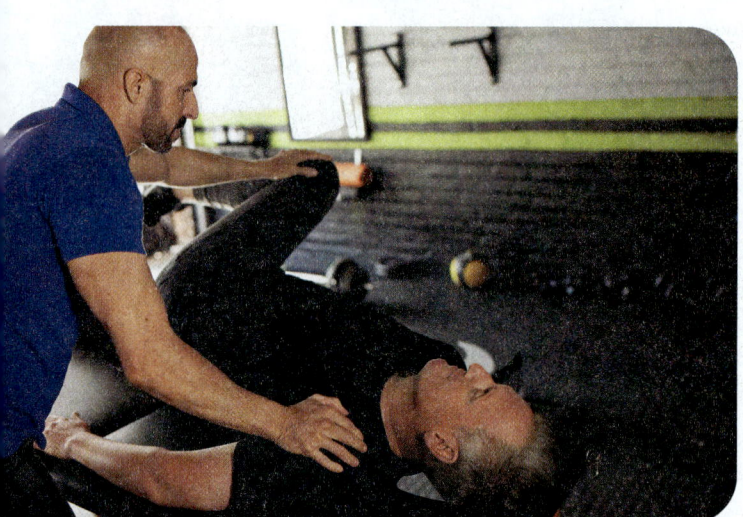

© Jono Erasmus/Shutterstock

A needs analysis is a crucial step in designing an effective flexibility program. It helps identify specific areas of focus and allows for the creation of personalized plans that cater to an athlete's unique requirements. The needs analysis is essential to understand the demands of the athlete's sport and specific position, as different sports require varying levels of flexibility and ROM. Conducting a comprehensive assessment of the athlete's current flexibility, such as via the overhead squat with and without modifications, and mobility testing, if necessary, will provide a baseline for designing the program and tracking progress. The assessment data should be reviewed to identify any flexibility limitations, asymmetries, or muscle imbalances that may predispose the athlete to injury or hinder performance.

Additionally, the athlete's injury history must be considered, as it may necessitate modifications or additional focus on particular areas to prevent reinjury and promote overall musculoskeletal health. Athletes should be assessed at the beginning of the program to establish their relevant baseline capacities, and progress can be monitored with frequent assessments.

Although standard assessments can be utilized, assessments can also be tailored to match the performance demands of each athlete. For example, an athlete who utilizes Olympic weightlifting movements could perform a regular overhead squat and also a modification to a deep overhead squat while holding a PVC pipe or an empty barbell. The purpose of such a modification is to give the Sports Performance Coach additional insight into how the athlete performs sport-specific movements.

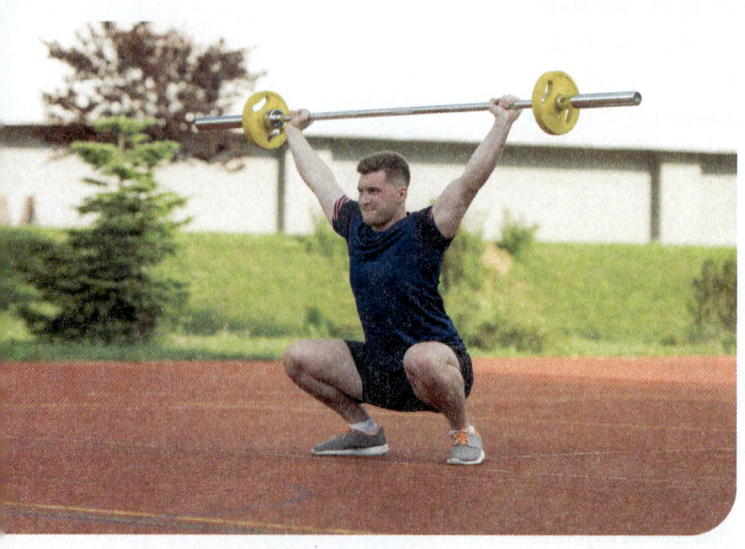

© Jasminko Ibrakovic/Shutterstock

FLEXIBILITY TRAINING TECHNIQUES

Flexibility training is a critical element in all training programs. It offers numerous benefits—for example, correcting muscle imbalances, augmenting joint ROM, enhancing muscle extensibility, and boosting neuromuscular efficiency (Floyd, 2018; Kenney et al., 2019). A diverse array of flexibility training techniques exist, encompassing self-myofascial techniques, and static, active, dynamic, and neuromuscular stretching, which can be seamlessly integrated into any performance training routine. The primary objective of flexibility training is to improve tissue extensibility and joint ROM, particularly in overactive tissues identified during the assessment process, ultimately optimizing an individual's athletic performance and overall physical well-being.

FLEXIBILITY TRAINING AND ATHLETIC PERFORMANCE

It is often mistakenly believed that stretching—specifically, static stretching—before athletic activities can hinder performance, prompting some athletes to avoid it altogether. However, this is not a universal truth. Research on the impact of stretching on athletic performance is less clear than the evidence supporting the ROM benefits from flexibility protocols.

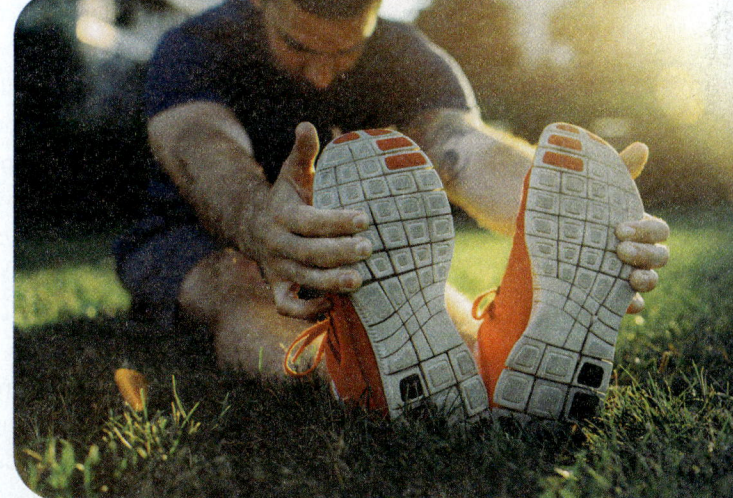

© AnastasiaDudka/Shutterstock

Numerous studies have found that pre-exercise stretching does not acutely impair strength or power. It is generally recommended that static stretching should be performed for less than 60 seconds per muscle before athletic activities to prevent performance decrements, though dynamic and ballistic stretching do not have the same impacts. Dynamic stretching as part of a warm-up improves performance in countermovement jumping (Carvalho et al., 2012; Holt & Lambourne, 2008; Perrier et al., 2011), and performing dynamic stretches at game-like speeds appears to have a greater carryover effect to on-field performance (Neeham et al., 2009).

Further, recent research indicates that the risk of performance impairments is minimal when static or neuromuscular stretching is integrated into a proper warm-up. To mitigate potential adverse effects on performance, a warm-up protocol that includes dynamic activity immediately after stretching is advised to reduce muscle injuries, increase joint ROM, and maintain athletic performance capabilities.

INTEGRATION OF TECHNIQUES FOR MAXIMAL PERFORMANCE

Each flexibility technique can be beneficial to athletes, depending on their needs. For example, an athlete who demonstrates significant movement impairments and muscle imbalances would benefit greatly from self-myofascial techniques (SMT) and static stretches in the initial phases of training. A primary goal for this athlete would be to improve movement patterns prior to engaging in more demanding and higher-intensity training. The standard recommendation of holding static stretches for no more than 60 seconds during a warm-up (Behm et al., 2016) will likely improve ROM. Further, evidence has documented that static stretching can reduce the incidence of lower-body muscle and tendon injuries, especially with high-velocity contractions and rapid change of direction activities (Behm et al., 2016; McHugh & Cosgrave, 2009).

Studies involving a full warm-up that integrates various flexibility techniques generally do not report performance decrements, and sometimes even indicate performance

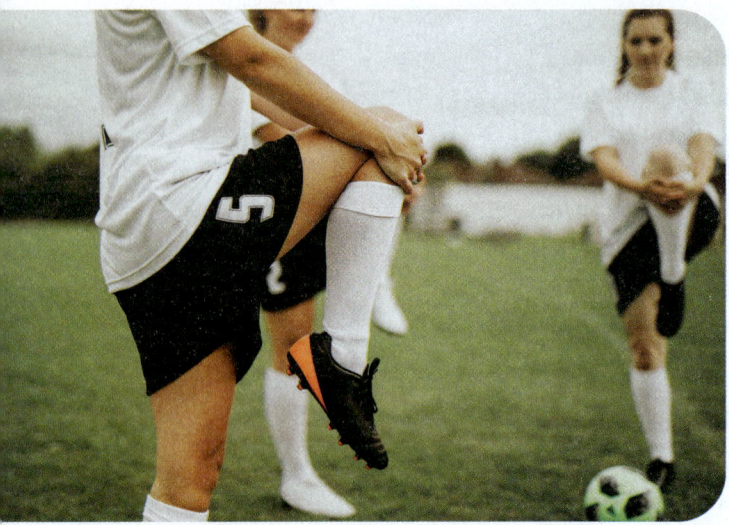
© Rawpixel.com/Shutterstock

improvements. The absence of static stretching deficits when a full warm-up is included could be attributed to the **post-activation potentiation** effects of dynamic activities. Furthermore, incorporating static or dynamic stretching into a warm-up can boost athletes' confidence in their subsequent sports performance, which is crucial for optimal performance. As such, integrating short-to-moderate durations of static stretching (less than 60 seconds) into a comprehensive warm-up prior to competition can be beneficial.

MOVEMENT PREPARATION

Movement preparation, also known as movement prep or dynamic warm-up, is a series of exercises designed to prepare the body for physical activity. It helps to increase blood flow, improve joint mobility, enhance muscle flexibility, and activate the nervous system, ultimately optimizing athletic performance and reducing the risk of injury. Movement preparation is an essential component of any workout, sport, or physical activity, as it sets the stage for the body to perform optimally during the main activity.

Movement prep should be tailored to the individual athlete and follow a sequence of flexibility techniques—for example, SMT; static stretching if needed; and then progressive, dynamic stretching before activity. SMT is well known to improve blood flow and joint ROM without negatively impacting performance. Then, if an athlete demonstrates movement impairments caused by muscle imbalances, static stretching can be used specifically on the muscles identified as overactive. Finally, general dynamic exercises, such as air squats and lunges, can be performed.

Table 9.1 provides an example movement prep program for a general athlete. Dynamic stretching could be progressed to serve as a rehearsal of the skill(s) performed during the central part of the training session for certain athletes (Young & Behm, 2002). The types of exercises that should be selected for the athletes' movement prep should be based on the demands of the sport(s) and individual assessment results. For example, a Taekwondo

---

POST-ACTIVATION POTENTIATION →

The phenomenon in which acute muscle force generation is increased as a result of the inner contraction of the muscle.

TABLE 9.1   Example Movement Prep Program

Technique	Exercise	Variables
Self-myofascial techniques (SMT)	Calves Hip flexors Upper back	1 set Hold tender spots for 30–60 seconds
Static stretching	Wall calf stretch Kneeling hip flexor stretch Seated thoracic rotation	2 sets Hold at the first point of tension for 45 seconds
Dynamic stretching	Air squat Lunge with medicine ball rotation Multiplanar hip swings	2 sets 10 reps each

athlete could perform static hamstring stretches, followed by hip swings in all directions before practicing their specific kicking skills.

WARM-UP CONSIDERATIONS

The potential effects of warming up before exercise are summarized in **Table 9.2** (Bishop, 2003).

TABLE 9.2 Benefits of a Warm-up

Temperature Related	Non-Temperature Related
Decreased muscle and joint resistance	Increased blood flow to muscles
Greater release of oxygen from hemoglobin and myoglobin	Elevation of baseline oxygen consumption
Speeding of metabolic reactions	Post-activation potentiation
Increased nerve conduction rate	Psychological effects and increased preparedness
Increased thermoregulatory strain	

An effective warm-up will often include aerobic exercise, stretching, and sport-specific movements (Haff & Triplett, 2016). As presented in Table 9.1, NASM recommends a movement prep program that consists of SMT, various forms of stretching as needed, and dynamic movements. In many cases, a series of six to eight dynamic movements can fulfill the role of aerobic exercise. However, the Sports Performance Coach and the athlete are encouraged to include appropriate aerobic exercise if necessary. The period of aerobic exercise should typically last at least 5 minutes to elevate the heart rate, increase body temperature, and reduce joint and soft-tissue viscosity (deVries & Housh, 1995).

ACUTE TRAINING VARIABLES FOR FLEXIBILITY TRAINING

Most Sports Performance Coaches are familiar with the acute training variables, such as sets, repetitions, intensity, volume, and frequency. Flexibility is no different, in the sense that it requires attention to be given to the finer details of each exercise: how long it is performed, how many times, the amount of rest between exercises, the sequence of efforts within the workout, and so on. These details are covered in the following section.

SETS AND REPETITIONS

Just as the number of repetitions and the amount of time a muscle is under tension are important in strength training, they are also critical considerations in flexibility training (**Table 9.3**).

- SMT can vary based on the equipment used and experience. However, general recommendations are one set per body part and rolling an area for 30 to 60 seconds. Total rolling time per muscle group should not exceed 120 seconds.

TABLE 9.3 Sets and Repetitions for Flexibility Training

Type of Stretch	Sets	Repetitions/Duration
Self-myofascial techniques (SMT)	1 set	30–60 seconds; not to exceed 120 seconds
Static	1–3 sets	Hold each stretch for 30 seconds
Active	1–3 sets	Hold each stretch for 1–2 seconds and repeat for 5–10 repetitions
Dynamic	1–2 sets	10–15 repetitions 3–10 exercises

- Static stretching is the process of passively taking a muscle to the point of tension and holding the stretch for a minimum of 30 seconds (Behm & Chaouachi, 2011). Typical static stretch routines reflected in the research literature are usually held for 10 to 30 seconds per muscle group, for two to three sets (Sim et al., 2009). However, guidelines suggest 30- to 60-second static stretches are most optimal prior to exercise or athletic activity (Behm & Chaouachi, 2011; Kay & Blazevich, 2012).
- Active stretches are suggested for pre-activity warm-ups, such as before sports competitions or high-intensity exercises. If an individual possesses muscle imbalances, active stretching should be performed after SMT and static stretching for muscles determined to be overactive during the assessment process. Typically, 5 to 10 repetitions of each stretch are performed and held for 1 to 2 seconds each.
- Dynamic stretching uses the concept of reciprocal inhibition to improve soft-tissue extensibility (Kenney et al., 2019). Athletes are recommended to perform one set of 10 repetitions using 3 to 10 dynamic stretches.

INTENSITY

Stretch intensity appears to play an even larger role than duration in determining the effectiveness of stretching. For example, Fukaya et al. (2020) showed that high-intensity, short-duration stretching was more effective than low-intensity, long-duration stretching in bringing about greater changes in ROM. Subjective levels of discomfort are used to measure stretch intensity. However, duration and intensity seem to confer different benefits: Longer stretch durations result in lower passive torque, whereas higher stretch intensities seem to create greater increases in joint angle (Freitas et al., 2015).

However, applying higher stretch intensities may not be effective for everyone. Behm (2019) suggested it is unnecessary to stretch to the point of discomfort (100% intensity, or the most discomfort the person can tolerate in that particular exercise). Some studies have shown improvements even when stretching at 30% to 40% of maximal intensity, but stretching at 60% to 85% intensity provides substantial benefits (Behm, 2018). The Sports Performance Coach is advised to use a level of intensity that is tolerable for the athlete (mild discomfort), which also confers steady improvements in ROM. In other words, the athlete should be able to relax throughout the duration of the stretch.

The difference in benefits conferred by variables such as intensity may depend on the individual's training experience. In untrained individuals, it has been shown that performing stretching exercises at high or low intensity promotes similar gains in flexibility (Santos et al., 2020). Clients should probably perform only as many sets as it takes to stop seeing increases in ROM—in other words, when their current stretching set

TABLE 9.4 General Intensities for Flexibility Training

Type of Stretch	Intensity
Self-myofascial techniques (SMT)	Some discomfort. Athlete should be able to breathe normally and appear relaxed.
Static	Hold stretch at the first point of resistance (tension). Mild discomfort may be appropriate for some athletes.
Active	Hold stretch at the first point of resistance (tension). Mild discomfort may be appropriate for some athletes.
Dynamic	Bodyweight.

does not elicit any further flexibility gains than the previous set. **Table 9.4** provides general recommendations for stretch intensity.

TRAINING FREQUENCY

The optimal number of times to stretch per week has not been thoroughly investigated, but it likely depends on the intensity of the stretching technique. Even static stretching can cause delayed-onset muscle soreness (Smith et al., 1993), which is a sign of muscle damage and a need to permit sufficient time off between stretching applications for the body to recover. However, substantial evidence supports the notion that stretching more than one time per week is more effective than a single training session.

For example, Nakamura et al. (2021) reported that ankle dorsiflexion ROM was increased, and muscle stiffness was decreased significantly, in people who stretched three times per week compared to once per week. Cipriani et al. (2012) showed that daily stretching produced greater ROM increases than stretching three times per week. These findings suggest that higher frequencies of stretching may be more effective. Combining this evidence with the previously cited studies, a stretching routine performed once per day, five to six days per week, is likely in the optimal training zone for many athletes.

Regarding SMT, at present there are no known reasons why myofascial rolling cannot be performed daily or most days of the week. This is the current practice of NASM with apparently healthy athletes. However, this will ultimately be determined by the athlete, any possible precautions that exist, and the advice of a licensed medical professional.

TRAINING VOLUME

Some practitioners have demonstrated that it is not necessarily the time per stretch that matters, but rather the weekly volume. For example, Thomas et al. (2018) showed that a minimum of 5 minutes of stretching per week is more effective than a lower weekly volume, but stretching more than 10 minutes per week seems to result in minimal additional benefits. Ryan et al. (2014) reported that performing a dynamic stretching routine lasting 6 to 12 minutes improved flexibility more than in a control group, but cautioned that longer durations of dynamic stretching might impair performance in repetitive high-intensity activities. Regarding SMT, the total duration should be between 5 and 10 minutes, with 90 to 120 seconds per muscle group. **Table 9.5** provides an overview of the common frequency and volume recommendations.

TABLE 9.5 Frequency and Volume Recommendations for Flexibility Training

Type of Stretch	Frequency	Volume
Self-myofascial techniques (SMT)	Daily or most days of the week	Total duration between 5 and 10 minutes per session
Static	2–6 days per week	5–10 minutes per week per muscle group
Active	2–6 days per week	5–10 minutes per week per muscle group
Dynamic	2–6 days per week	6–10 minutes per session

EXERCISE SELECTION

The choice of stretching exercises will depend on when the athlete wishes to conduct their flexibility training program and how well they can perform the exercises without supervision. It is good coaching practice to supervise the athlete's flexibility training to ensure proper form and execution.

The decision of which muscles to target during the static stretching portion of the routine should be based on the results of a comprehensive assessment. Muscles identified as overactive during movement assessments (i.e., overhead squat assessment) take priority in a stretching routine to correct muscle imbalances and altered length–tension relationships.

👍 HELPFUL HINT

If the athlete is stretching primarily at home, at away games, at an airport, or on the bus ride to and from games, exercise programming will need to take into account such factors as the amount of space they have available, the type of surface on which they will be stretching (e.g., carpet and vinyl flooring have vastly different frictional characteristics that will affect the ability to slide the feet when increasing a stretch), and potential hazards and distractions such as pets and family members.

It is illogical and possibly counterproductive to stretch underactive/lengthened muscles in which no ROM deficits are apparent. **Table 9.6** provides a summary of muscles to target based on common movement impairments.

Additionally, sport-specific stretches should target the muscle groups that are most relevant to the athlete's performance, ideally in positions that mimic the actions of their sport. For example, poor hamstrings extensibility may limit a hurdler's ability to flex the hip. Therefore, hamstrings stretches performed in a position that mimics the primary actions of their sport will likely have a greater transfer of training effect to their athletic

TABLE 9.6 Flexibility Exercises for Common Movement Impairments

Movement Impairment	Potential Overactive Muscle	Recommended Stretch
Feet turn out	Gastrocnemius Soleus Biceps femoris	Wall calf stretch Supine lateral hamstring stretch
Knee valgus	Gastrocnemius Adductors Tensor fascia latae	Wall calf stretch Standing adductor stretch Half-kneeling hip flexor stretch
Anterior pelvic tilt	Hip flexor complex Erector spinae Latissimus dorsi	Half-kneeling hip flexor stretch Seated spinal rotation Ball latissimus stretch
Arms fall forward	Latissimus dorsi Pectorals major/minor Thoracic spine	Ball latissimus stretch Ball pectoral stretch T-spine extension

performance. A suitable stretching sequence may begin with SMT, then static hamstring stretches, followed by anterior–posterior leg swings and practicing the actual hurdle gait used during competition.

EXERCISE ORDER

The sequence of body parts to stretch does not appear to matter. However, athletes should be encouraged to develop a routine that progresses from the feet upward or the neck downward. Doing so may preserve time and help athletes ensure they do not skip vital areas. Consistency is the key to reliable progress, so the athlete can use any approach they wish as long as it is one they can stick with.

However, one pertinent consideration is whether performing a specific stretch will allow the following stretch to be more effective. For example, if an athlete demonstrates the feet turning out and an anterior pelvic tilt, performing a wall calf stretch might be advantageous before performing a standing hip flexor stretch. Doing so may allow the athlete to more effectively target the hip flexors during the standing stretch.

As mentioned earlier, NASM recommends an integrated flexibility program. Therefore, the Sports Performance Coach is encouraged to develop programs that begin with SMT, then static stretching in the presence of muscle imbalances, and finally dynamic and then sport-specific stretches as necessary (**Table 9.7**).

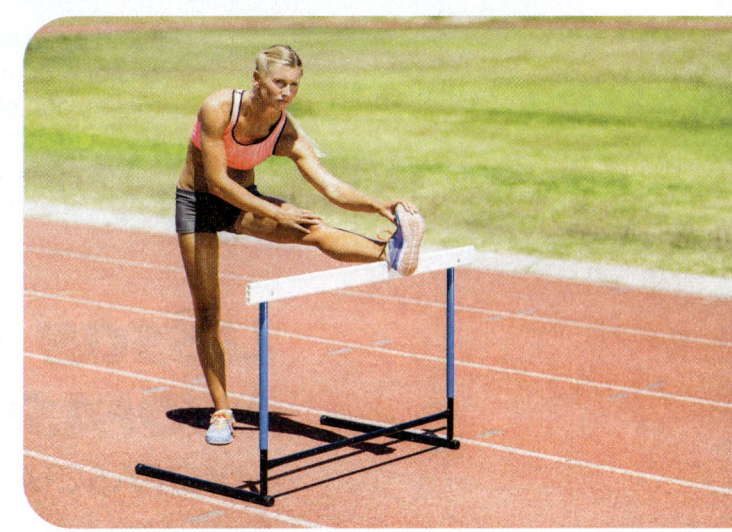
© Wavebreakmedia/Shutterstock

TABLE 9.7 Flexibility Exercise Order

Movement Impairment	Recommended Sequence	Example Routine for Taekwondo Athlete
Feet turn out and anterior pelvic tilt	SMT > static > dynamic > sport/skill-specific	1. SMT: Calves, quadriceps, and hip flexor group 2. Static: Wall calf stretch and standing hip flexor stretch 3. Dynamic: Multiplanar lunge with rotation and leg swings 4. Skill-specific: Rapid high kicks

✔ **CHECK IT OUT**

Static Stretching's Influence on Strength and Power

There has been much debate in the research and sport science communities regarding the effects of static stretching on strength and athletic performance. Some studies have found that static stretching impairs strength and power, and recommend avoiding this technique prior to exercise or sport competition (Haddad et al., 2014).

Looking at the research more closely, static stretching, when performed acutely and in isolation, can temporarily impair muscular power due to its relaxation response. This is especially true when stretches are held for extended periods (2 minutes or longer), are performed in an acute fashion (every now and again), and are the only form of exercise performed prior to maximal effort (sprinting or jumping). However, static stretches, when performed for 30 to 60 seconds in a chronic fashion (included prior to every workout) and followed by dynamic activities, do not impair athletic performance (Behm et al., 2016; Kay & Blazevich, 2012; Reid et al., 2018).

As such, NASM recommends performing static stretching, especially when individuals exhibit limited joint ROM or muscle imbalances. The following are some recommendations for static stretches:

- Should be held for 30 to 60 seconds
- Used only on muscles identified as overactive during the assessment process, or if certain joints require additional ROM due to sport-specific needs
- Followed by additional warm-up protocols, such as dynamic stretching, to regain motor neuron excitability

LESSON 5: MODALITIES FOR MYOFASCIAL TECHNIQUES
MYOFASCIAL TECHNIQUES

Myofascial techniques are a set of manual therapy methods that focus on addressing the myofascial system. These techniques aim to increase flexibility and mobility and enhance overall function by addressing issues in the fascial system, such as restrictions or imbalances. Several different myofascial techniques exist—for example, self-myofascial rolling (SMR) using a traditional myofascial roller, balls, or handheld devices, as well as percussion massage guns and instrument-assisted soft-tissue mobilization. These may be used in combination or individually, depending on the needs of the client.

Certain techniques require that the practitioner receive specialized education or maintain specific state licensure. Further, many athletes are best suited to learn how to apply practical techniques by themselves to use when the coach, trainer, or practitioner is not available. Therefore, NASM recommends that the Sports Performance Coach teach athletes various **self-myofascial techniques (SMT)**.

SMT refers to a method of training that is reported to mobilize restrictions within myofascial tissues that arise from adhesions, to reduce pain and muscle spasms, and to increase ROM (Škarabot et al., 2015). NASM has moved away from using the term "myofascial release"; it can be misleading given the lack of evidence to support the proposed mechanisms of releasing fascia that often accompany this type of training. Instead, neurological effects such as changes in parasympathetic-induced muscle tone, reflexes, and pain tolerance are more plausible explanations for the observed changes in ROM and pain (Behm & Wilke, 2019).

SELF-MYOFASCIAL TECHNIQUES (SMT) →

Techniques for addressing and breaking up adhesions of the fascia and the surrounding muscle tissues that can be applied and directed by the user; examples include foam rolling and self-massage.

MYOFASCIAL ROLLING

Many SMT methods are available for sports performance professionals and athletes. However, the foam roller seems to be the most popular among fitness and medical professionals (Cheatham, 2019; Cheatham et al., 2018). Foam rollers come in many shapes, sizes, and densities.

Myofascial rolling focuses on the nervous and fascial systems. It may produce both a mechanical response and a neurophysiological response that influences tissue relaxation and pain in the local and surrounding tissues by activating sensory pathways of the CNS (Grabow et al., 2018; Young et al., 2018). In the mechanical effect, the direct roller compression may relax the local myofascia by increasing local blood flow and reducing myofascial restriction and adhesions (Jay et al., 2014; Kelly & Beardsley, 2016). In the neurophysiological effect, the direct roller compression may influence tissue relaxation

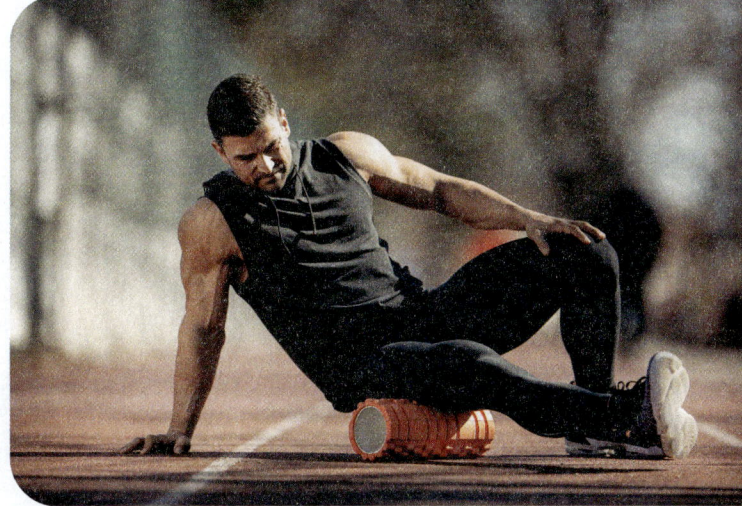

© Just Life/Shutterstock

and pain in the local and surrounding tissues by stimulating local mechanoreceptors and pain receptors. These receptors send inhibitory signals to the CNS, triggering a cascade of tissue-relaxation and pain-blocking responses that affect the tissues being compressed by the roller (Aboodarda et al., 2015; Young et al., 2018).

Myofascial rolling can be done during a warm-up and has been reported to provide similar increases in ROM as stretching (Wilke et al., 2020) with minimal to no negative impact on subsequent performance (Halperin et al., 2014). It may also be performed at the end of a workout to potentially reduce the effect of delayed-onset muscle soreness after exercise (Jay et al., 2014). It is crucial to note that when a person is using a foam roller, they should find a tender spot and sustain pressure on that spot for a minimum of 30 seconds, which will increase the relaxation response. The effect may sometimes take longer to occur, depending on the client's ability to consciously relax. Self-myofascial rolling is suggested before stretching because it may improve the effectiveness of static stretching techniques (Škarabot et al., 2015).

SMR TECHNIQUES

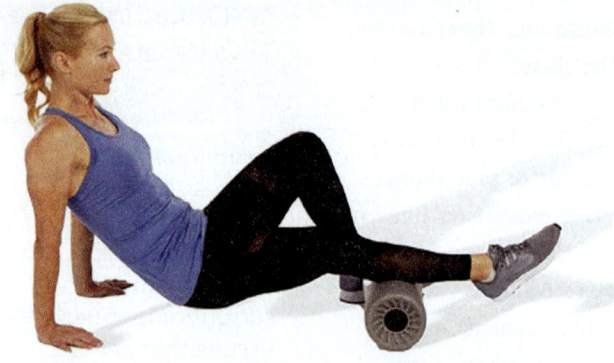

Calves

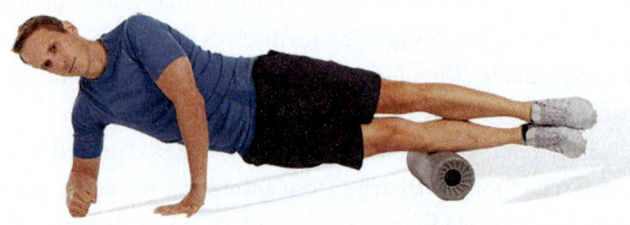

Peroneals

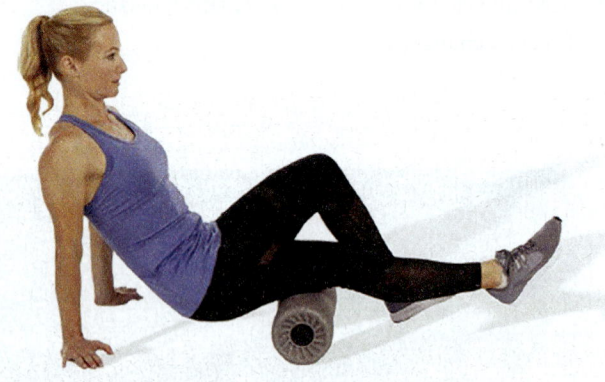

Hamstrings

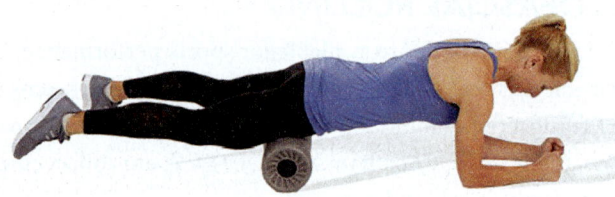

Quadriceps

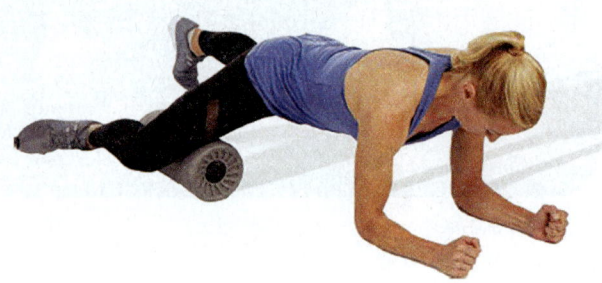

Adductors

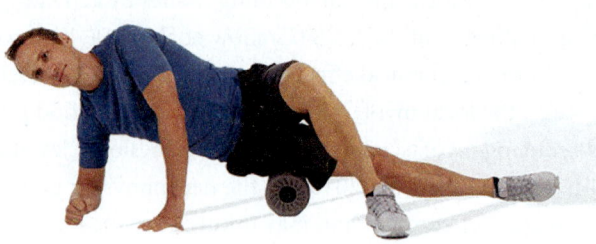

Lateral Thigh

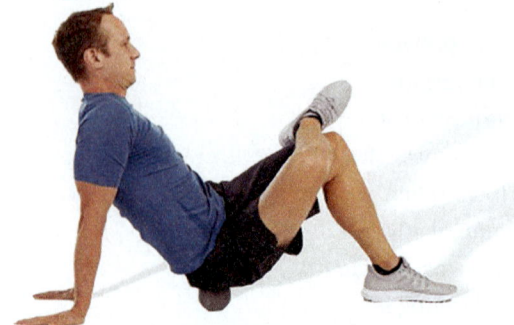

Gluteal Complex

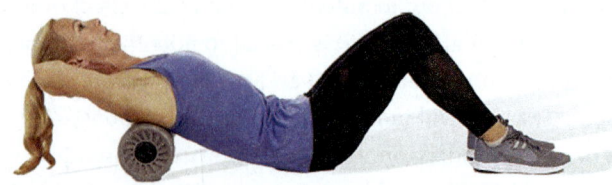

Thoracic Spine

MYOFASCIAL BALLS

The use of objects such as tennis balls to perform myofascial self-massage provides a portable and inexpensive way to elicit many of the same benefits as myofascial rolling that can be done anywhere. Sets and repetition duration are the same as for myofascial rolling.

HANDHELD MYOFASCIAL ROLLERS

Handheld rollers are constructed of various materials. They come in varying sizes, but are generally smaller than cylindrical foam rollers. Because handheld rollers are guided by the user, size and density are less of a concern because the pressure may be easily changed by increasing or decreasing the force. Handheld rollers are a suitable option for users who cannot get on the ground to use a traditional roller.

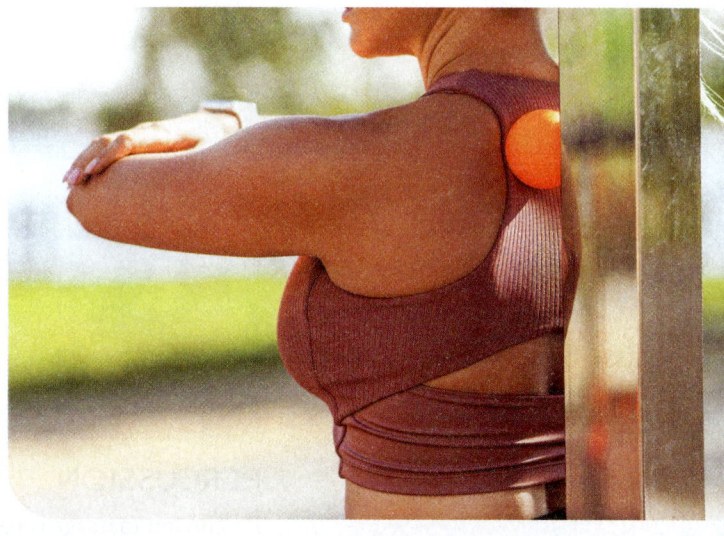
© Khosro/Shutterstock

However, handheld rollers do have a few limitations. First, use of those that require both hands may be limited to the lower extremities. Second, their use is limited by body positioning. Many users may struggle to reach certain muscle groups while maintaining a safe posture. Third, the amount of pressure applied is limited by upper-body strength. Athletes may need to apply more pressure than they can, whether due to an upper-extremity injury or just a simple lack of strength, to achieve the desired effect. Therefore, if the user can get on the ground, use of a cylindrical myofascial roller is preferred over a handheld one. If the user cannot get on the ground, then the handheld device is a suitable alternative.

Some handheld rollers can be compressed into a shorter length and, therefore, may be more convenient for travel than a typical foam roller. Also, it is recommended that Sports Performance Coaches not use a handheld roller to apply pressure on their athletes. Instead, the athlete should always be in control of the pressure; this enhances the safety of the technique and teaches the athlete to be self-reliant.

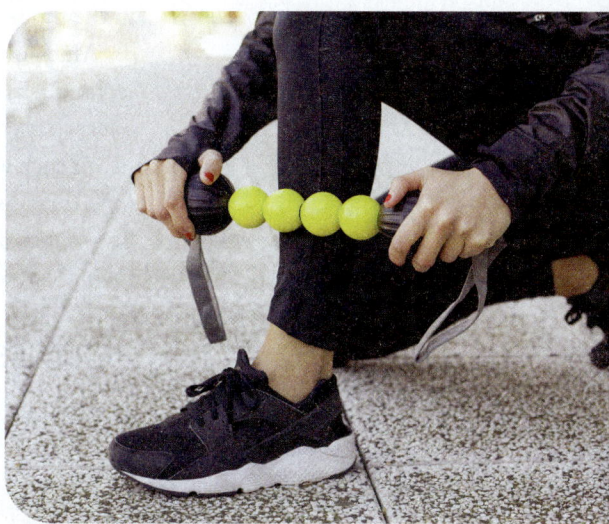
© Luna Vandoorne/Shutterstock

VIBRATION

The therapeutic effects of vibration are well known (Dong et al., 2019; Games et al., 2015; Park et al., 2018). However, much of the research into this technique has used vibration plates or whole-body vibration. The use of vibration delivered via a more targeted device, such as a myofascial roller, also appears to be effective, but the specific ramifications are less well known. In a study comparing a myofascial roller with vibration to the same roller without vibration, those in the vibration group experienced greater improvements in flexibility and mobility (Cheatham, Stull, & Kolber, 2017; Han et al., 2017; Lim & Park, 2019; Romero-Moraleda et al., 2019) and reduction in the perception of pain (Cheatham, Stull, & Kolber, 2017; Han et al., 2017; Romero-Moraleda et al., 2019). Further, such improvements appeared to occur without negative effects on performance (Lim & Park, 2019; Romero-Moraleda et al., 2019; Sağiroğlui, 2017).

Notably, these studies utilized different vibrating myofascial rollers that vibrate at different frequencies and with different amplitudes. Thus, the research is currently unable to prescribe a specific roller or frequency for a specific outcome. For example, using a

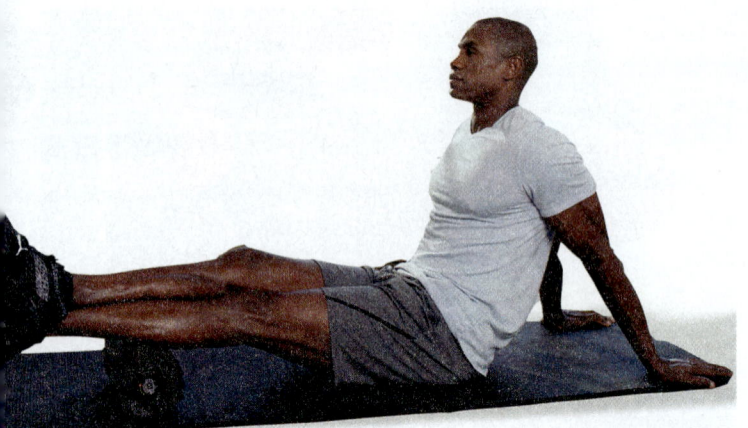

lower setting on a multispeed vibration roller does not appear to produce a different result than using a higher frequency. More research is needed on vibration rollers before program standards can be recommended.

A key takeaway from the current vibration roller research is the influence on the perception of pain. The vibration likely mitigates pain through an effect called vibratory analgesia (Hollins et al., 2014). Put simply, vibratory analgesia occurs when the vibration stimulates certain mechanoreceptors that temporarily interfere with the sensation of pain.

PERCUSSION

Percussion massage is gaining much popularity with the recent introduction of percussion massage guns. Such devices resemble a hardware tool, and they deliver a percussive impact via a pneumatic arm with a PVC attachment, which contacts the soft tissues at rates often in the thousands of revolutions per minute (rpm).

Much of the initial literature regarding percussive massage guns suggests that this technique is quite promising. For example, Konrad et al. (2020) noted that, while the effects of percussive devices are similar to those produced by a massage therapist, the use of such a handheld tool can provide similar increases in ROM without the need for a therapist and with no negative effect on muscle strength. Percussive devices may be a viable alternative for athletes who cannot tolerate the discomfort and exertion of myofascial rolling.

PERCUSSION TECHNIQUES

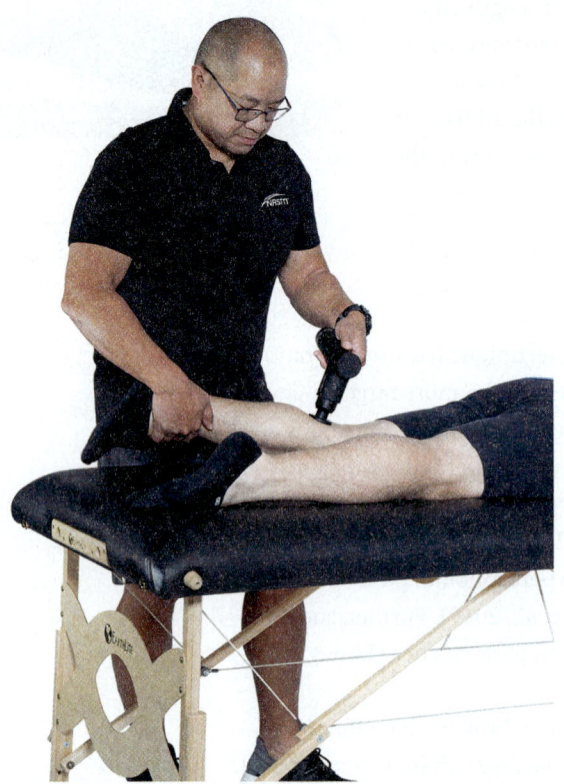

Calf Complex

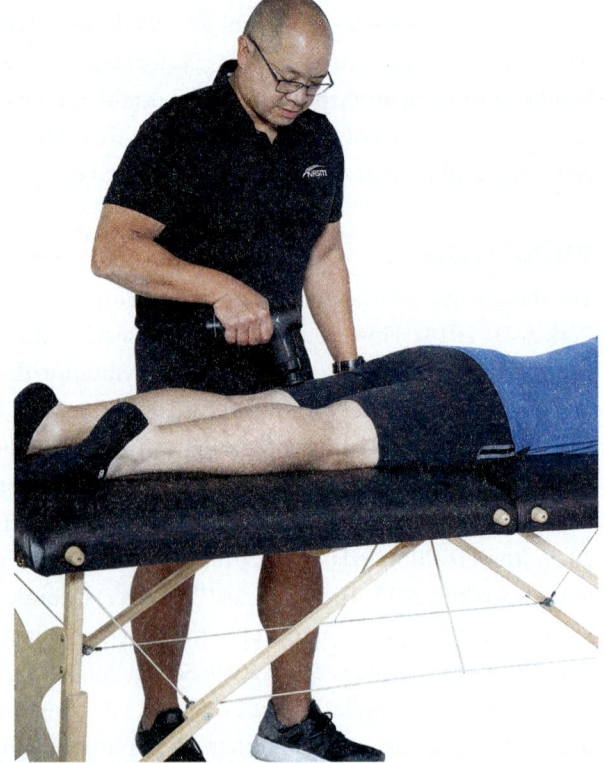

Hamstrings

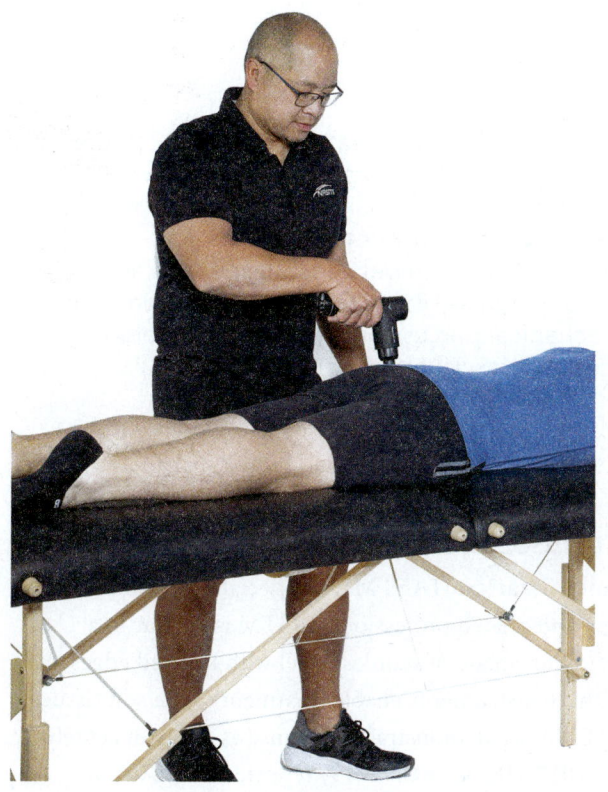

Gluteals

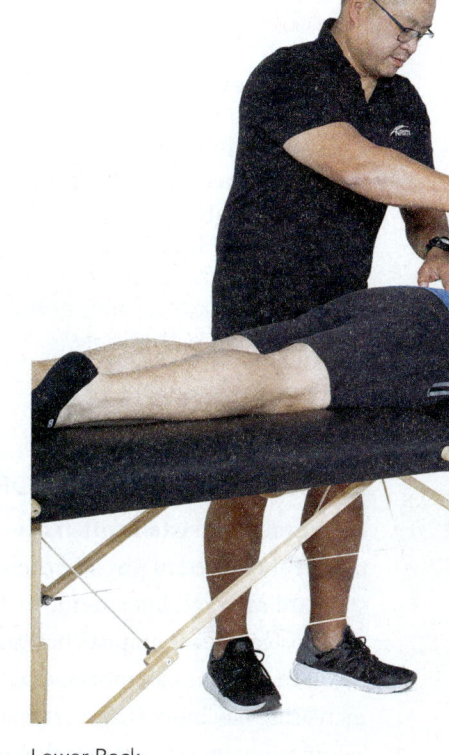

Lower Back

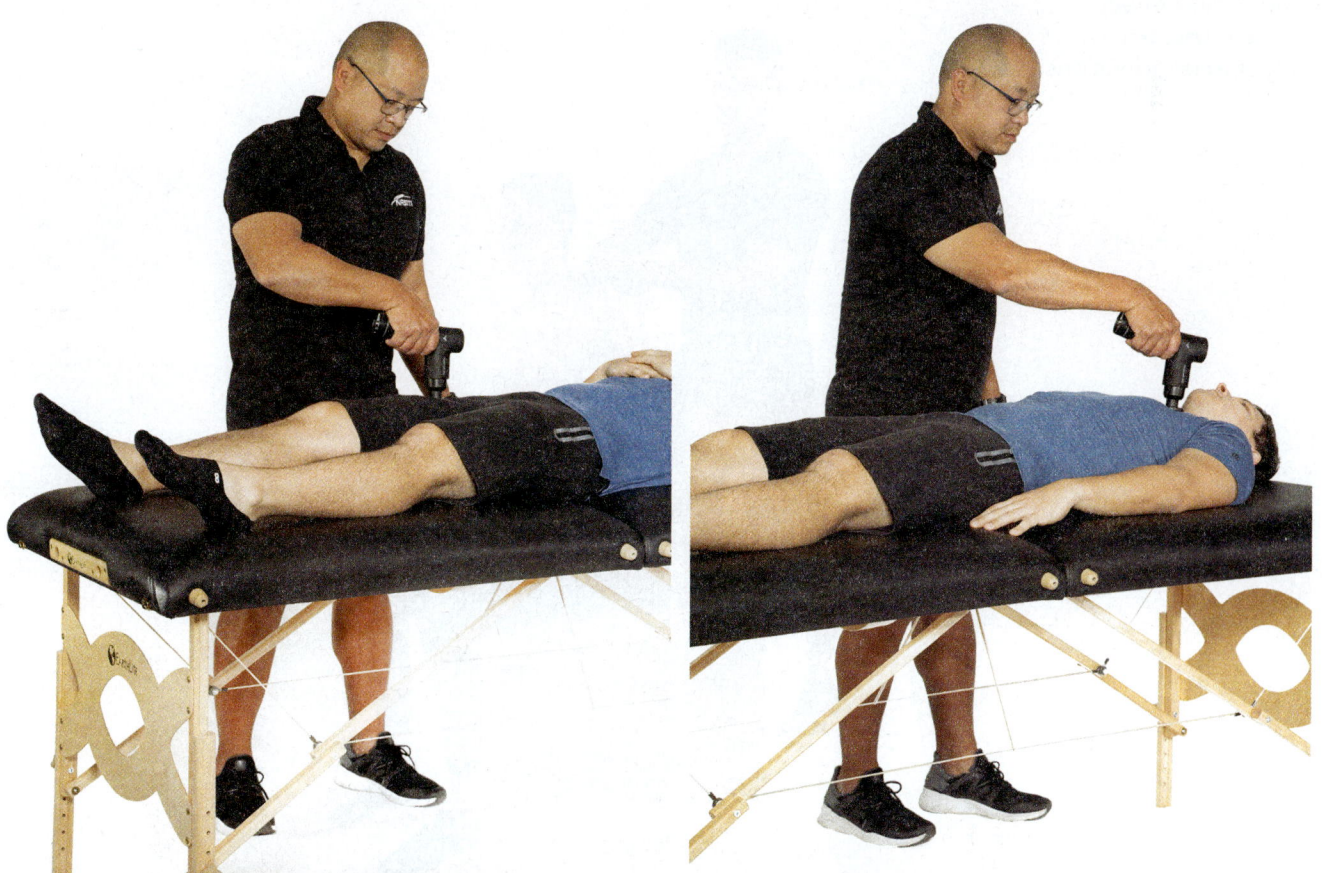

Quadriceps

Pectorals

In a survey of 425 professionals conducted by Cheatham et al. (2021), the researchers reported that most respondents used a medium and low device speed setting for pre- and post-exercise (62%), pain modulation (59%), and myofascial mobility (52%). Approximately one-third to one-half of the respondents employed a total treatment time between 30 seconds and 3 minutes (36% to 48%) or 3 to 5 minutes (18% to 22%). Most respondents (54% to 69%) believed that mechanical percussion increased local blood flow, modulated pain, enhanced myofascial mobility, and reduced myofascial restrictions.

INSTRUMENT-ASSISTED SOFT-TISSUE MOBILIZATION

INSTRUMENT-ASSISTED SOFT-TISSUE MOBILIZATION (IASTM) →

Use of specially designed instruments to provide a mobilizing effect to scar tissue and myofascial adhesions.

Instrument-assisted soft-tissue mobilization (IASTM) is a specialized myofascial intervention used in physical therapy and related professions. IASTM is similar to a standard massage, but specific instruments made of stainless steel with beveled edges are used instead of a therapist's hands. These instruments enable treatment of the soft tissues involved with human movement. IASTM has demonstrated promise as a way of acutely increasing flexibility (Lambert et al., 2017). Ikeda et al. (2019) reported that IASTM significantly increased ankle dorsiflexion with a 5-minute application of the technique to the posterior aspect of the lower leg.

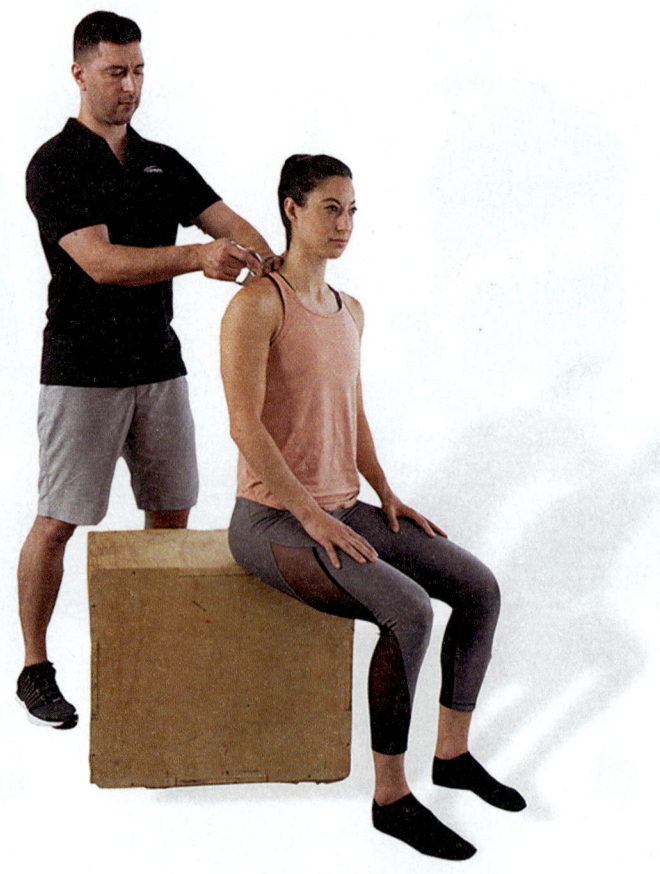

Instrument-Assisted Soft-Tissue Mobilization (IASTM)

Table 9.8 provides an overview of general training variables that can be applied to the various myofascial techniques. The Sports Performance Coach is encouraged to choose the best method for each athlete based on the assessment results and needs analysis. It is common for performance professionals and athletes to have a wide variety of myofascial tools available for different circumstances.

TABLE 9.8 Summary of Myofascial Techniques Variables

Technique	Repetitions	Repetition Duration	Total Duration
Roller/ball	1–3	2–4 seconds	30–120 seconds
Vibration	3–6	30–120 seconds	6–12 minutes
Percussion	1–2	30–60 seconds	3–5 minutes
Instrument-assisted soft-tissue mobilization (IASTM)	1	5 minutes	Variable

LESSON 6: STATIC, ACTIVE, AND DYNAMIC STRETCHING TECHNIQUES

STATIC STRETCHING

Static stretching involves passively extending a muscle to the point of tension and maintaining the stretch for at least 30 seconds (Behm & Chaouachi, 2011). This traditional stretching technique, which is perhaps the most popular form of stretching, combines low force with longer durations (Thomas et al., 2018). Holding the muscle in an elongated position for an extended time inhibits the muscle spindle, triggering a relaxation response and enabling better muscle lengthening (**Table 9.9**) (Thomas et al., 2018).

Static stretching may affect numerous sensory mechanisms within the nervous system, promoting increased stretch tolerance. Additionally, contracting the opposing muscles while holding the stretch can lead to reciprocal inhibition of the stretched muscle, enhancing stretch effectiveness. For instance, during a kneeling hip flexor stretch, an individual can engage

> **STATIC STRETCHING** →
>
> A type of stretch in which the muscle is passively lengthened to the point of tension and held for a sustained amount of time.

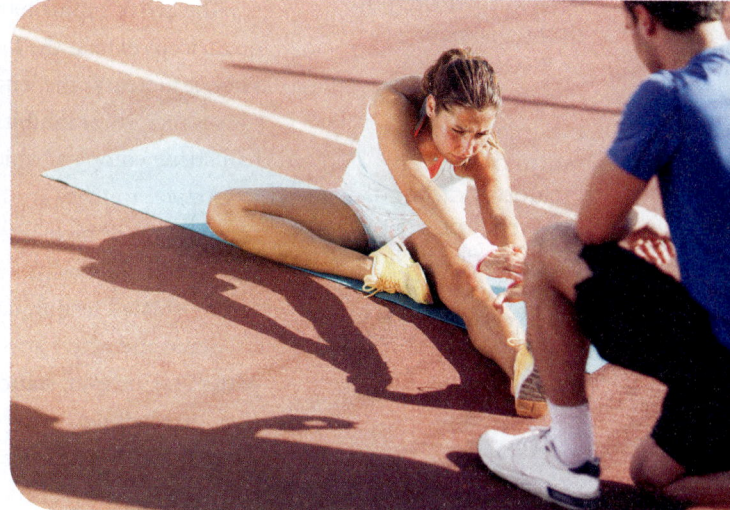
© BGStock72/Shutterstock

TABLE 9.9 Acute Training Variables for Static Stretching

Repetition Duration	Repetitions	Sets
30–60 seconds	1–3	1–3

the hip extensors (gluteus maximus) to reciprocally inhibit the hip flexors (psoas, rectus femoris), resulting in greater muscle lengthening (Lempke et al., 2018). Another example is activating the quadriceps during a hamstring stretch. Static stretching is recommended for reducing muscle spindle activity in overactive muscles both before and after activity.

Several mechanisms have been proposed to explain the increases in ROM following bouts of static stretching, including a reduction in the excitation of motor neurons innervating the stretched muscles (neural inhibition and disfacilitation; Guissard et al., 2001), increased muscle fascicle length (Freitas & Mil-Homens, 2015; Simpson et al., 2017), and altered stretch tolerance (Larouche et al., 2020). As discussed earlier in the chapter, static stretching is often avoided before physical activity due to potential adverse effects on performance. However, when used as part of an integrated warm-up or movement prep session, these adverse effects are eliminated before the athlete engages in more intense physical activity.

> ✔ **CHECK IT OUT**
>
> The effects of a static stretch may be enhanced by actively contracting its antagonist while holding the stretch, such as tensing the quadriceps during a hamstring stretch, which purportedly activates reciprocal inhibition pathways (Blazevich et al., 2012).

ACTIVE STRETCHING

<aside>
ACTIVE STRETCHING →

A type of stretching that uses agonists and synergists to dynamically move the joint into a range of motion; includes holding the stretched position for 1 to 2 seconds and repeating for 5 to 10 repetitions.
</aside>

Active stretching is the process of using agonists and synergists to dynamically move the joint into the ROM (Vernetta-Santana et al., 2015). This form of stretching increases motor neuron excitability, creating reciprocal inhibition of the muscle being stretched (Kenney et al., 2019).

The active supine hamstring stretch is a good example of active stretching. The quadriceps extend the knee, which enhances the stretch of the hamstrings in two ways. First, it increases the length of the hamstrings. Second, the contraction of the quadriceps causes reciprocal inhibition (decreased neural drive and muscle spindle excitation) of the hamstring complex, which allows it to elongate (Vernetta-Santana et al., 2015).

Active stretches are suggested for pre-activity warm-up, such as before sports competition or high-intensity exercise. Typically, 5 to 10 repetitions of each stretch are performed and held for 1 to 2 seconds each (**Table 9.10**). Detailed explanations of various active-isolated techniques are provided in the next section.

Static and active stretches typically require the same body position and movement patterns. However, static stretches involve holding each stretch for a specific time period (e.g., 30 seconds), whereas active stretches require holding the stretch for only 1 to 2 seconds and repeating the motion for 5 to 10 repetitions. Active stretching can be considered a progression from static stretching.

TABLE 9.10 Acute Training Variables for Active Stretching

Type of Stretch	Mechanism of Action	Training Variables
Active stretch	Reciprocal inhibition	1–3 sets Hold each stretch for 1–2 seconds and repeat for 5–10 repetitions

STATIC AND ACTIVE STRETCHING EXERCISES

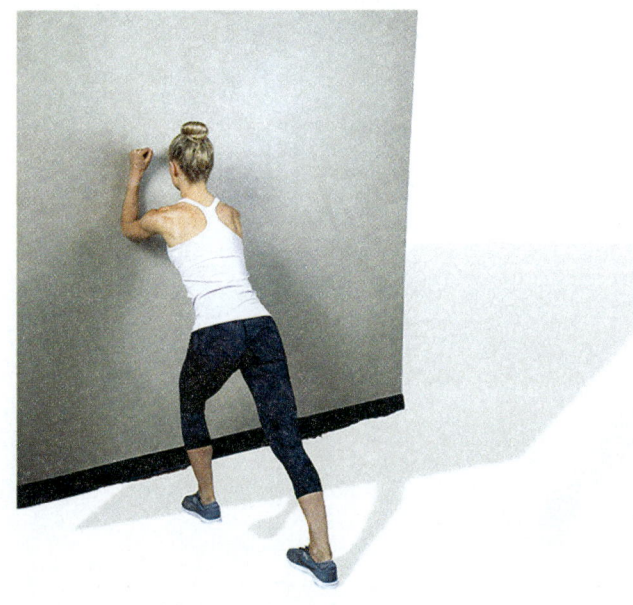

Gastrocnemius

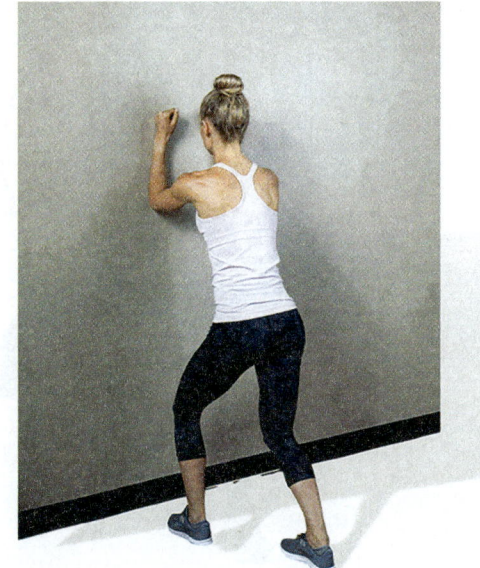

Soleus

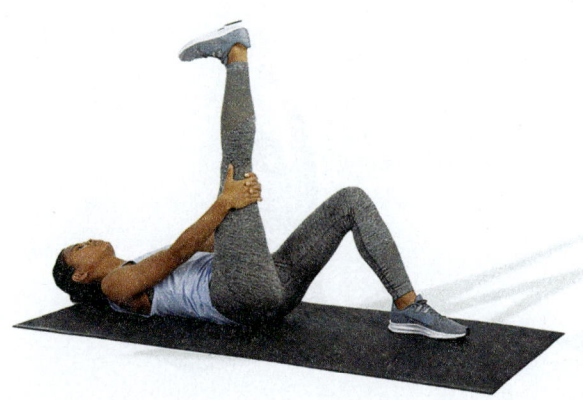

Hamstring

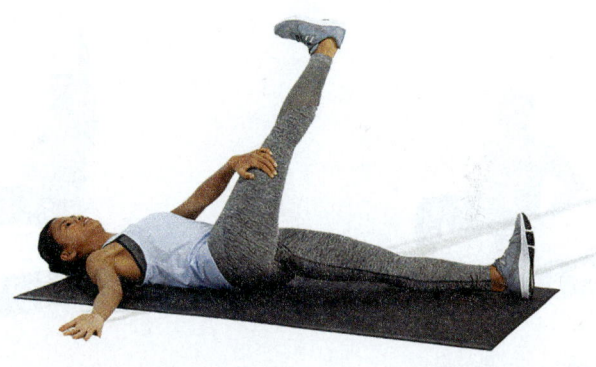

Supine Lateral Hamstring

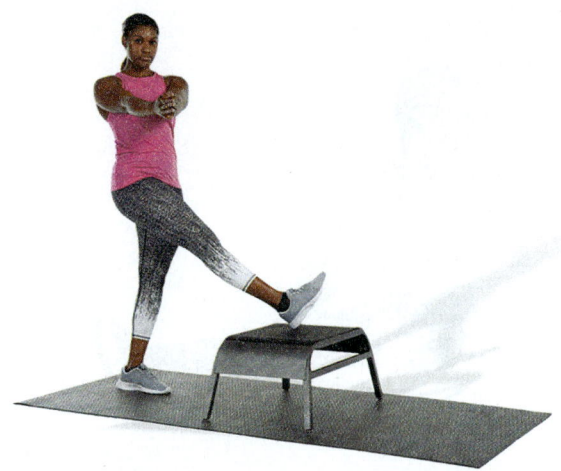

Standing Lateral Hamstring

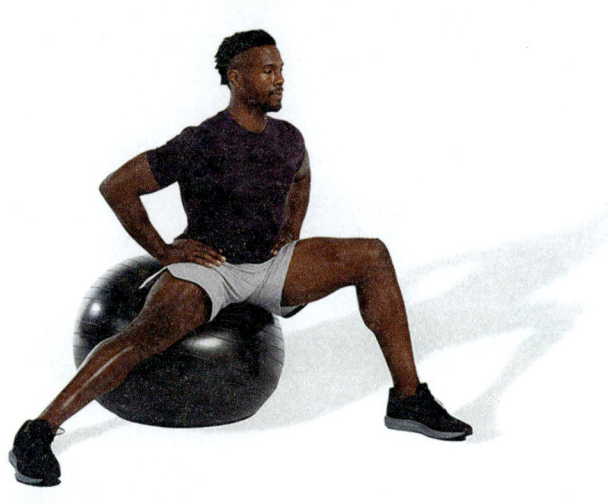

Seated Adductor

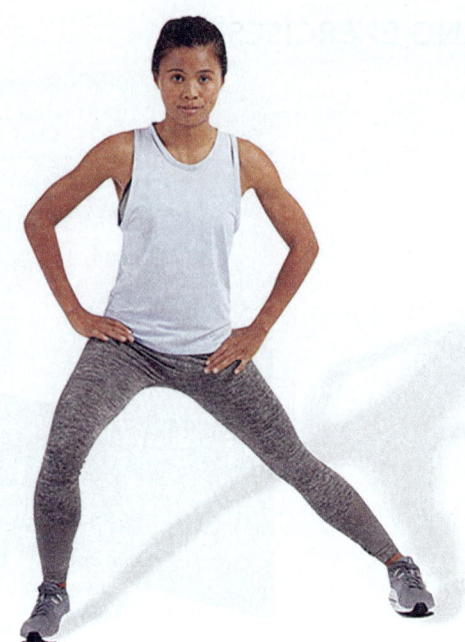

Standing Adductor

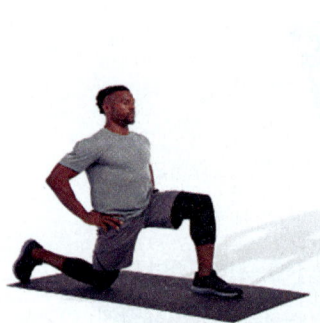
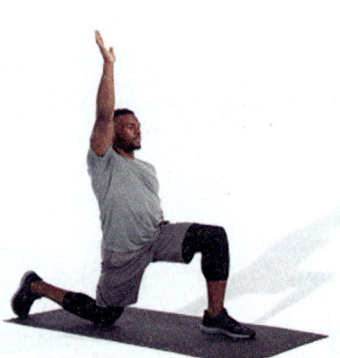
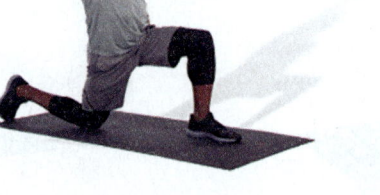
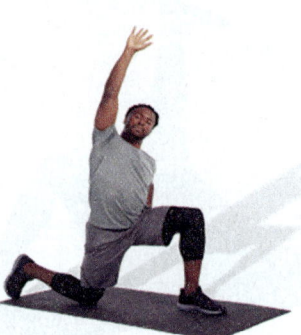

Kneeling Hip Flexor

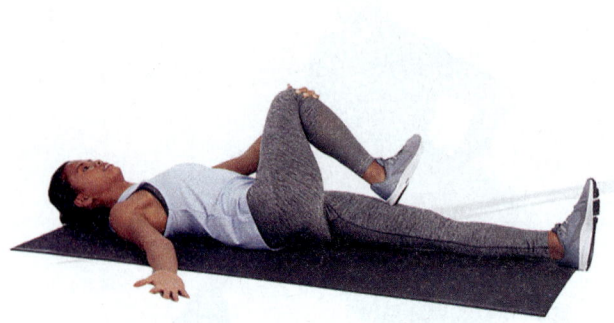

Supine Piriformis

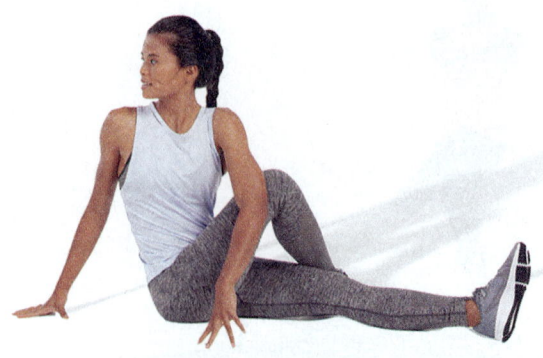

Seated Erector Spinae

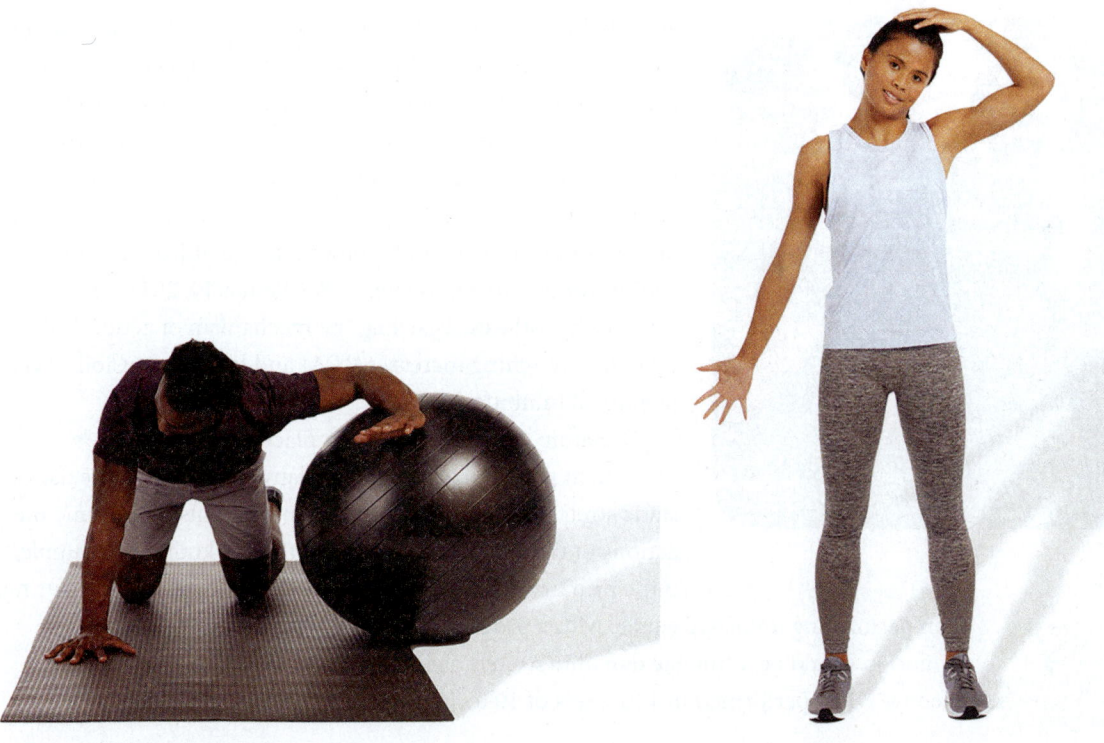

Chest

Upper Trap/Scalene

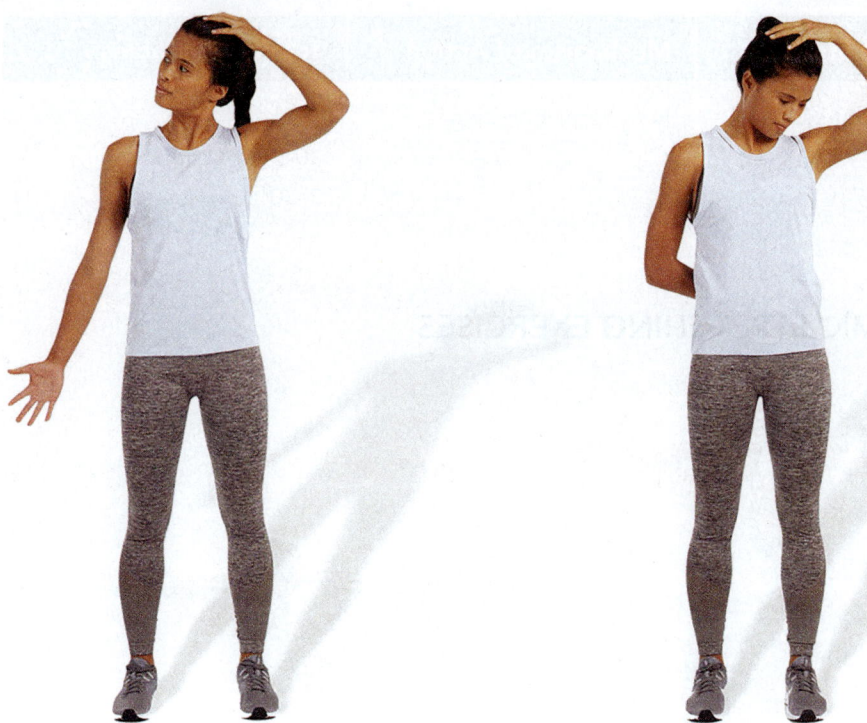

Sternocleidomastoid

Levator Scapulae

DYNAMIC STRETCHING

Dynamic stretching is most often performed as an active movement, with the intention of stretching the muscle–tendon unit at speed. This type of stretching has been shown to improve strength and power when performed immediately before activity and is recommended as part of a comprehensive warm-up to reduce muscle injuries (Behm et al.,

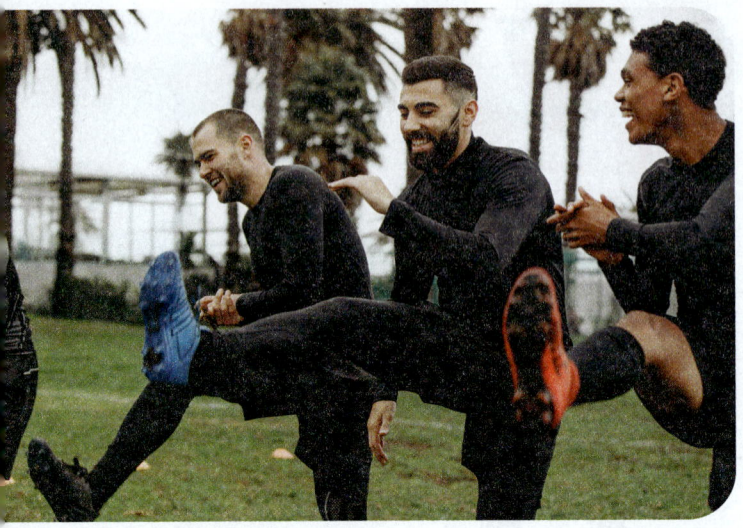
© Jacob Lund/Shutterstock

2016; Behm et al., 2021; Behm & Chaouachi, 2011). For example, club head speeds and ball speeds in golf are improved when golf play is preceded by dynamic stretching (Moran et al., 2009).

Dynamic stretching may be divided into static and active types. Nevertheless, the method referred to in the literature is almost always the active type, whereby concentric contractions of the agonist muscles and momentum are utilized to move a joint through its ROM (Behm & Chaouachi, 2011). The primary hypothesis regarding the mechanism of action is that dynamic stretching increases ROM and tissue extensibility via reciprocal inhibition.

Dynamic stretches are ideally placed into an athlete's movement prep program and, in many cases, follow the use of static stretches. They generally use movements that mimic the actions of the sport or main task of the workout. For example, if the primary goal of a training session is to work on squatting, then performing unloaded squats with a progressively larger amplitude and higher rate of motion would be a suitable dynamic stretching intervention. Dynamic stretches are effective when performed in 1 to 2 sets of 10 to 15 repetitions (**Table 9.11**).

DYNAMIC STRETCHING →

A type of stretching that uses the force production of a muscle and the body's momentum to take a joint through the full available range of motion.

TABLE 9.11   Acute Training Variables for Dynamic Active Stretching

Type of Stretch	Mechanism of Action	Training Variables
Dynamic stretching	Reciprocal inhibition	1 set 10–15 repetitions 3–10 exercises

DYNAMIC STRETCHING EXERCISES

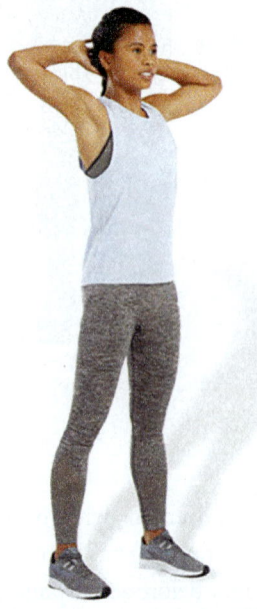
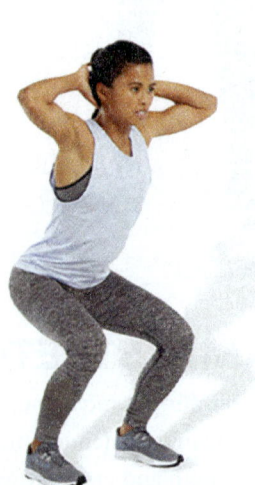

Bodyweight Squat

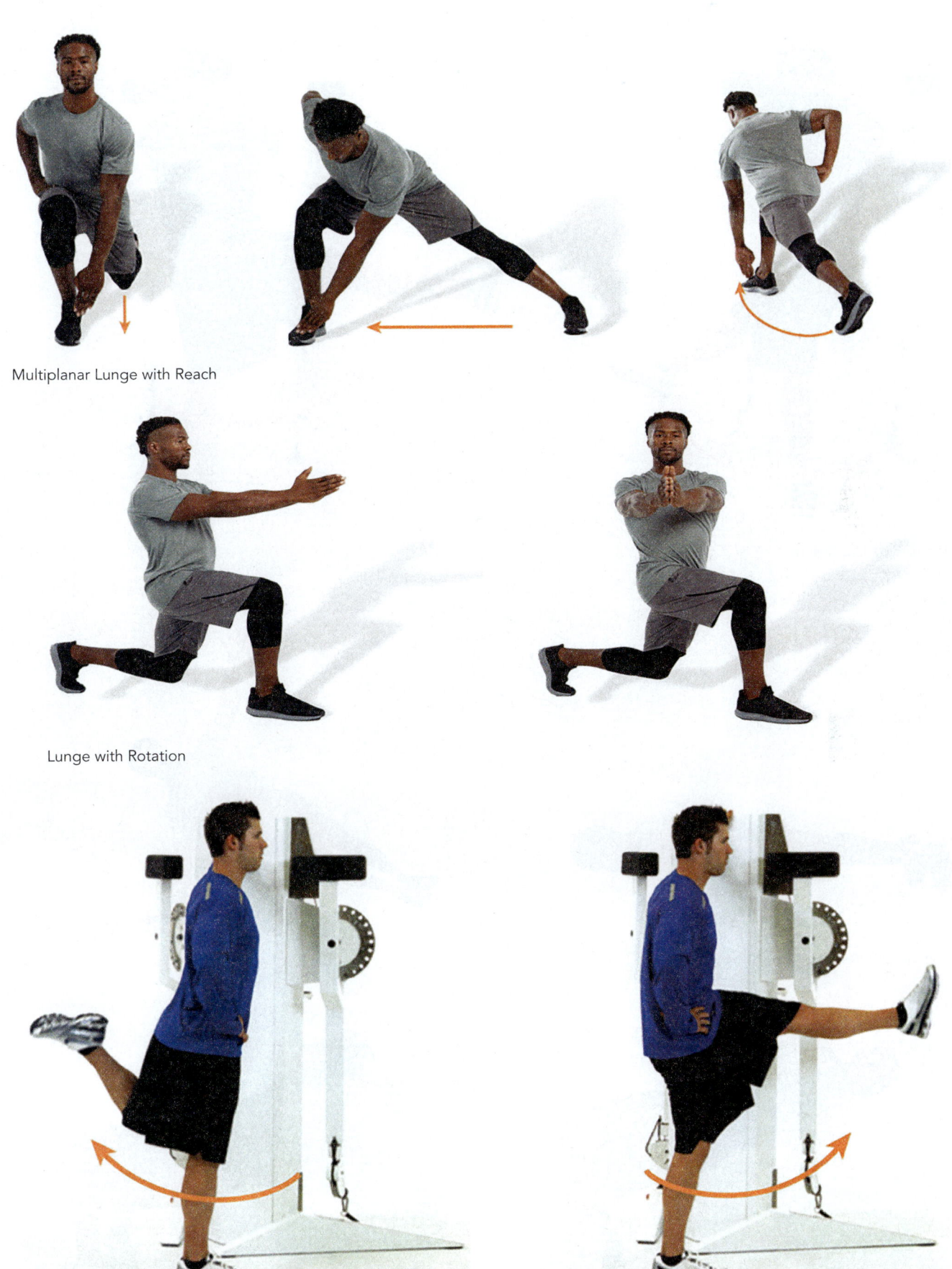

Multiplanar Lunge with Reach

Lunge with Rotation

Front-to-Back Leg Swings

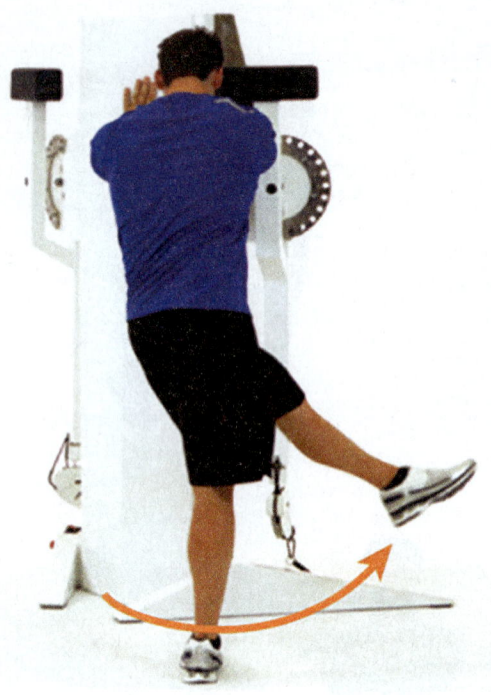
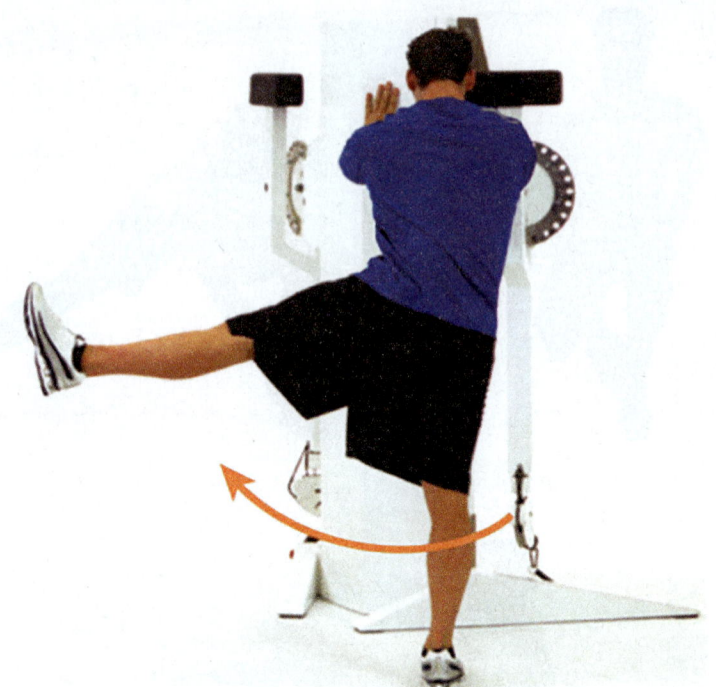

Side-to-Side Leg Swings

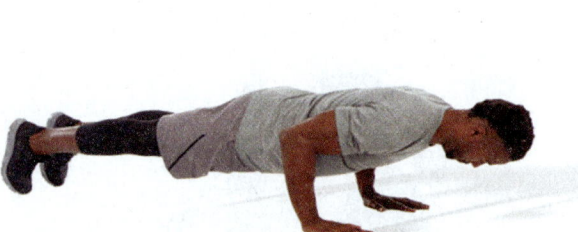
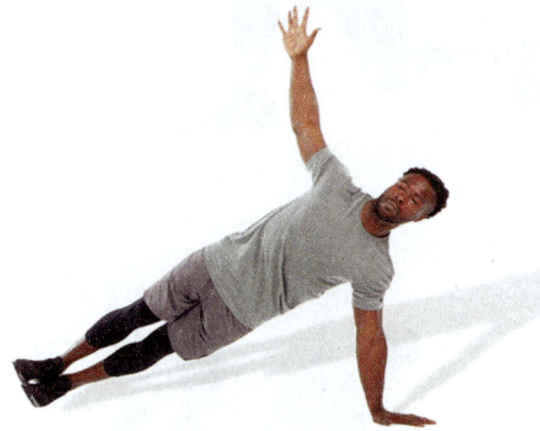

Push-up with Rotation

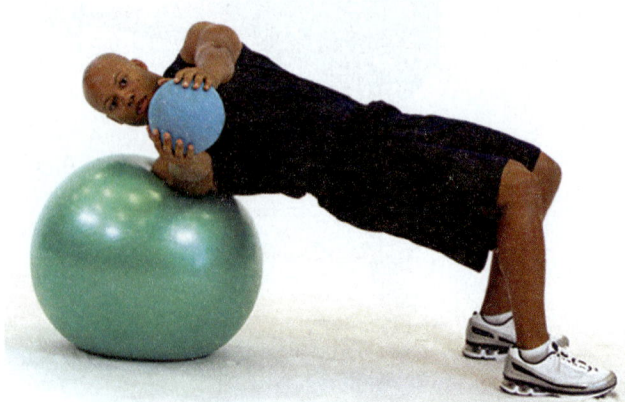
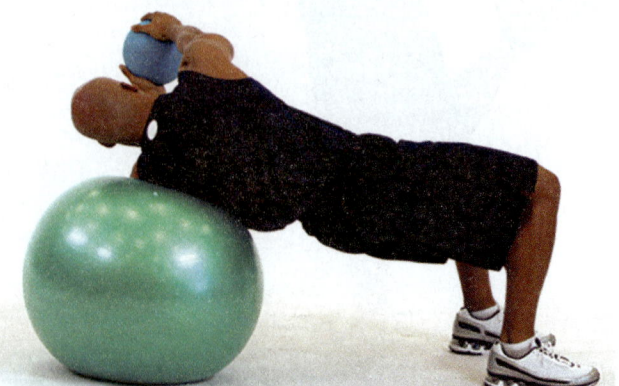

Russian Twist

LESSON 7: ADDITIONAL FLEXIBILITY PRACTICES
ADVANCED FLEXIBILITY TECHNIQUES

This lesson on advanced flexibility techniques builds upon the foundational methods taught in previous lessons. While several techniques exist, this lesson introduces Stick Mobility and assisted stretching techniques.

STICK MOBILITY

Stick Mobility is a system of flexibility, strength, and coordination training that takes advantage of the increased neuromuscular drive to attain greater mobility and stability benefits compared to traditional stretching alone (Stick Mobility, 2021b). Stick Mobility techniques adhere to dynamic stretching guidelines, but they can be performed as static and active techniques as well. This type of training utilizes the body as a form of resistance along with a flexible rod, and does not appear too dissimilar from the traditional flexibility training used in martial arts, dance, and gymnastics. In addition, by coordinating the muscles and joints as a unified system, the entire kinetic chain becomes better balanced, thereby improving performance and decreasing the risk of injury.

Although some exercises may vary, general acute training variables are found in **Table 9.12**. The system is built on several core principles:

- Mechanical leverage
- Stable training positions
- Visual and kinesthetic feedback
- Irradiation (tensing one muscle recruits neighboring muscles into the task)
- Varying types of isometric contractions
- Neural coordination

TABLE 9.12 Acute Training Variables for Stick Mobility

Type of Stretch	Mechanism of Action	Training Variables
Stick Mobility	Reciprocal inhibition	1 set 8–10 repetitions 1- to 2-second hold at end range 3–10 exercises

ASSISTED STRETCHING

Assisted stretching is a type of flexibility training in which an individual receives help from a Sports Performance Coach, athletic training staff member, or team physical therapist to perform a stretch more effectively. The assistance provided can enhance the stretch, allowing the individual to reach a greater ROM, improve flexibility, and achieve better results than they might achieve through unassisted or self-administered stretches.

A primary advantage of partner-assisted stretching is that contractions of the agonist or antagonist muscles can be included while a stretch is held. This approach is traditionally known as proprioceptive neuromuscular facilitation (PNF) stretching (Sharman et al., 2006;

> **ASSISTED STRETCHING** →
>
> A type of flexibility training in which an individual receives help from a partner, coach, trainer, or physical therapist to perform a stretch more effectively.

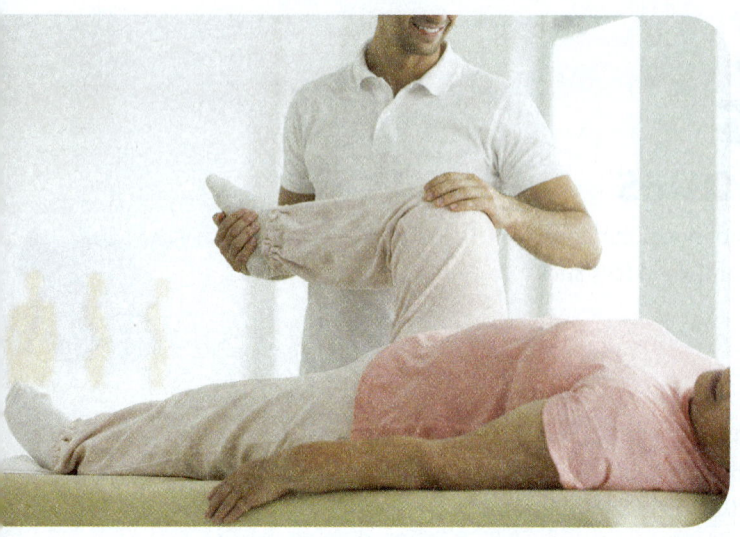

© Ground Picture/Shutterstock

Victoria et al., 2013). The proposed mechanisms for the increase in ROM include autogenic inhibition, thixotropic characteristics of tissues, and altered stretch tolerance (Sharman et al., 2006).

PNF stretches are generally divided into three named categories: hold–relax (HR), contract–relax (CR), and contract–relax–activate–contract (CRAC). HR has been described as the application of an isotonic contraction of the stretched muscle(s) resisted by a third party (strength coach or therapist); CR involves a self-applied isometric contraction of the stretched muscle(s) (Cayco et al., 2019).

CRAC, a very popular method of PNF stretching, is the primary focus of this section. It utilizes a subsequent contraction of the opposing (shortened) muscle group after the contraction of the lengthened muscle group is released. In theory, this technique is able to utilize reciprocal inhibition as the joint is moved into a greater ROM while the shortened muscle group contracts.

Lim (2018) suggests that a moderate level of contraction intensity (20% to 40% of the maximum voluntary isometric contraction) can create a tangible training effect while minimizing the burden on the myofascial tissues. However, the intensity used can vary per practitioner and per athlete. Kurz (2003) recommends that PNF-style stretching be done in 2 to 5 sets of 3 to 5 contractions per muscle group, performed 2 to 4 days per week (**Table 9.13**). Based on the research, the following protocols are recommended:

1. Taking the muscle to its end ROM (point of joint compensation)
2. Active contraction of the muscle to be stretched (20% to 40% of the maximum voluntary isometric contraction)
3. Passively (or actively) moving to a new end ROM
4. Statically holding the new position for 20 to 30 seconds and repeating 3 to 5 times

TABLE 9.13   Acute Training Variables for Assisted Stretching

Type of Stretch	Mechanism of Action	Training Variables
Assisted stretching using CRAC	Autogenic and reciprocal inhibition	2–5 sets 3–5 contractions per muscle group 20%–40% intensity Hold new position for 20–30 seconds 3–10 muscle groups

SUMMARY

Flexibility is an important motor quality that is fundamental for the development and expression of other motor qualities, including strength, speed, and endurance. It improves performance and reduces risk of injury by resolving muscle imbalances, reducing joint dysfunctions, enabling the development of strength at ranges of motion specific to the athlete's sport, and improving compliance in soft tissues such as muscles, fascia, and tendons.

Despite its fundamental importance to healthy posture, functional movement, and athletic performance, flexibility is an oft-neglected aspect of training. Athletes often present with inadequate soft-tissue extensibility and joint ROM, and improving flexibility should be a priority for such individuals. Those athletes who require relatively normal levels of ROM will often obtain much of their flexibility training in the course of practicing their regular physical activities, but may still need guidance on how to warm up appropriately and resolve tender zones with self-myofascial techniques.

Contrary to popular opinion, performing static stretches during a warm-up is not harmful when limited to 60 seconds' duration per muscle group and followed up with dynamic stretches, and it may even afford some protection against muscle injuries caused by lack of soft-tissue compliance. Stretching is the most common way to improve ROM, with methods to achieve this goal including self-myofascial techniques, static stretching, active stretching, dynamic stretching, and partner-assisted stretching.

KEY TAKEAWAYS

- Flexibility is defined as the range of motion available at a joint or group of joints. It is influenced by several factors, including the ability of peripheral soft tissues to lengthen (extensibility), the compliance of joint structures such as ligaments and capsules, and the shape and geometry of bones that make up the joint.
- Several mechanisms have been proposed to explain how and why flexibility improves with training. However, the scientific literature is full of conflicting data, and more research is needed to verify the competing hypotheses.
- A lack of flexibility may lead to compensatory movement strategies that contribute to aberrant neuromuscular issues such as pattern overload, muscle imbalances, synergistic dominance, and joint dysfunction.
- Flexibility can increase even with a single short-duration stretch, but consistent training inputs over a long period of time are required to make lasting change.
- There are many ways to develop flexibility, including static passive, static active, and dynamic active stretching, as well as self-myofascial techniques (i.e., soft-tissue mobilization exercises).
- The literature offers guidelines on the optimal number of sets, repetitions, intensity, volume, and frequency of flexibility training exercises, but the dose–response relationship will be highly individual to each person and must be determined by trial and error.

REFERENCES

Aboodarda, S. J., Spence, A. J., & Button, D. C. (2015). Pain pressure threshold of a muscle tender spot increases following local and non-local rolling massage. *BMC Musculoskeletal Disorders, 16*, 265. https://doi.org/10.1186/s12891-015-0729-5

Al-Rawi, Z. S., Al-Aszawi, A. J., & Al-Chalabi, T. (1985). Joint mobility among university students in Iraq. *Rheumatology, 24*(4), 326–331.

Alter, M. (2004). *Science of flexibility* (3rd ed.). Human Kinetics.

Atwell, K., Michael, W., Dubey, J., James, S., Martonffy, A., Anderson, S., Rudin, N., & Schrager, S. (2021). Diagnosis and management of hypermobility spectrum disorders in primary care. *Journal of the American Board of Family Medicine, 34*(4), 838–848. https://doi.org/10.3122/jabfm.2021.04.200374

Avela, J., Kyröläinen, H., Komi, P. V., & Rama, D. (1999). Reduced reflex sensitivity persists several days after long-lasting stretch-shortening cycle exercise. *Journal of Applied Physiology, 86*(4), 1292–1300. https://doi.org/10.1152/jappl.1999.86.4.1292

Balakatounis, K., Angoules, A. G., Angoules, N. A., & Panagiotopoulou, K. (2017). Synthesis of evidence for the treatment of intersection syndrome. *World Journal of Orthopedics, 8*(8), 619–623. https://doi.org/10.5312/wjo.v8.i8.619

Behm, D. G. (2019). *The science and physiology of flexibility and stretching: Implications and applications in sport performance and health*. Routledge.

Behm, D. G., Bambury, A., Cahill, F., & Power, K. (2004). Effect of acute static stretching on force, balance, reaction time, and movement time. *Medicine & Science in Sports & Exercise, 36*(8), 1397–1402. https://doi.org/10.1249/01.MSS.0000135788.23012.5F

Behm, D. G., Blazevich, A. J., Kay, A. D., & McHugh, M. (2016). Acute effects of muscle stretching on physical performance, range of motion, and injury incidence in healthy active individuals: A systematic review. *Applied Physiology, Nutrition, and Metabolism, 41*(1), 1–11.

Behm, D. G., Button, D. C., & Butt, J. C. (2001). Factors affecting force loss with prolonged stretching. *Canadian Journal of Applied Physiology, 26*(3), 262–272. https://doi.org/10.1139/h01-017

Behm, D. G., & Chaouachi, A. (2011). A review of the acute effects of static and dynamic stretching on performance. *European Journal of Applied Physiology, 111*(11), 2633–2651. https://doi.org/10.1007/s00421-011-1879-2

Behm, D. G., Kay, A. D., Trajano, G. S., & Blazevich, A. J. (2021). Mechanisms underlying performance impairments following prolonged static stretching without a comprehensive warm-up. *European Journal of Applied Physiology, 121*(1), 67–94. https://doi.org/10.1007/s00421-020-04538-8

Behm, D. G., & Sale, D. G. (1993). Velocity specificity of resistance training. *Sports Medicine, 15,* 374–388.

Behm, D. G., & Wilke, J. (2019). Do self-myofascial release devices release myofascia? Rolling mechanisms: A narrative review. *Sports Medicine, 49*(8), 1173–1181. https://doi.org/10.1007/s40279-019-01149-y

Ben, M., & Harvey, L. A. (2010). Regular stretch does not increase muscle extensibility: A randomized controlled trial. *Scandinavian Journal of Medicine & Science in Sports, 20*(1), 136–144. https://doi.org/10.1111/j.1600-0838.2009.00926.x

Bernstein, N. (2020). *Biomechanics for Instructors.* Springer Nature.

Bishop, D. (2003). Warm up I: Potential mechanisms and the effects of passive warm up on exercise performance. *Sports Medicine, 33*(6), 439–454. https://doi.org/10.2165/00007256-200333060-00005

Blazevich, A. J., Kay, A. D., Waugh, C., Fath, F., Miller, S., & Cannavan, D. (2012). Plantarflexor stretch training increases reciprocal inhibition measured during voluntary dorsiflexion. *Journal of Neurophysiology, 107*(1), 250–256. https://doi.org/10.1152/jn.00407.2011

Boonen, A., & Maksymowych, W. P. (2010). Measurement: Function and mobility (Focusing on the ICF framework). *Best Practice & Research Clinical Rheumatology, 24*(5), 605–624. https://doi.org/10.1016/j.berh.2010.05.008

Bordoni, B., & Myers, T. (2020). A review of the theoretical fascial models: Biotensegrity, fascintegrity, and myofascial chains. *Cureus.* https://doi.org/10.7759/cureus.7092

Carvalho, F. L. P., Carvalho, M. C. G. A., Simão, R., Gomes, T. M., Costa, P. B., Neto, L. B., Carvalho, R. L. P., & Dantas, E. H. M. (2012). Acute effects of a warm-up including active, passive, and dynamic stretching on vertical jump performance. *Journal of Strength and Conditioning Research, 26*(9), 2447–2452. https://doi.org/10.1519/JSC.0b013e31823f2b36

Cayco, C. S., Labro, A. V., & Gorgon, E. J. R. (2019). Hold–relax and contract–relax stretching for hamstrings flexibility: A systematic review with meta-analysis. *Physical Therapy in Sport, 35,* 42–55. https://doi.org/10.1016/j.ptsp.2018.11.001

Chalmers, G. (2004). Re-examination of the possible role of Golgi tendon organ and muscle spindle reflexes in proprioceptive neuromuscular facilitation muscle stretching. *Sports Biomechanics, 3*(1), 159–183. https://doi.org/10.1080/14763140408522836

Cheatham, S. W. (2019). Roller massage: A descriptive survey of allied health professionals. *Journal of Sports Rehabilitation, 28*(6), 640–649. https://doi.org/10.1123/jsr.2017-0366

Cheatham, S. W., Baker, R. T., Behm, D. G., Stull, K., & Kolber, M. J. (2021). Mechanical percussion devices: A survey of practice patterns among healthcare professionals. *International Journal of Sports Physical Therapy, 16*(3). https://doi.org/10.26603/001c.23530

Cheatham, S. W., Stull, K. R., & Ambler-Wright, T. (2018). Roller massage: Survey of physical therapy professionals and a commentary on clinical standards: Part II. *International Journal of Sports Physical Therapy, 13*(5), 920–930. https://doi.org/10.26603/ijspt20180920

Cheatham, S. W., Stull, K. R., & Kolber, M. J. (2017). Comparison of a vibrating foam roller and a non-vibrating foam roller intervention on knee range of motion and pressure pain threshold: A randomized controlled trial. *Journal of Sport Rehabilitation, 28*(1), 1–23. https://doi.org/10.1123/jsr.2017-0164

Cipriani, D. J., Terry, M. E., Haines, M. A., Tabibnia, A. P., & Lyssanova, O. (2012). Effect of stretch frequency and sex on the rate of gain and rate of loss in muscle flexibility during a hamstring-stretching program: A randomized single-blind longitudinal study. *Journal of Strength and Conditioning Research, 26*(8), 2119–2129. https://doi.org/10.1519/JSC.0b013e31823b862a

Daneshmandi, H., Choobineh, A., Ghaem, H., & Karimi, M. (2017). Adverse effects of prolonged sitting behavior on the general health of office workers. *Journal of Lifestyle Medicine, 7*(2), 69–75. https://doi.org/10.15280/jlm.2017.7.2.69

deVries, H. A., & Housh, T. J. (1995). *Physiology of exercise for physical education, athletics and exercise science* (5th ed.). Brown.

Dong, Y., Wang, W., Zheng, J., Chen, S., Qiao, J., & Wang, X. (2019). Whole body vibration exercise for chronic musculoskeletal pain: A systematic review and meta-analysis of randomized controlled trials. *Archives of Physical Medicine and Rehabilitation, 100*(11), 2167–2178. https://doi.org/10.1016/j.apmr.2019.03.011

Entyre, B. R., & Abraham, L. D. (1986). Gains in range of ankle dorsiflexion using three popular stretching techniques. *American Journal of Physical Medicine and Rehabilitation, 65*(4), 189–196.

Fehr, J. (2012). Spinal reflexes. In *Quantitative human physiology* (2nd ed.). Academic Press.

Ferber, R., Osternig, L. R., & Gravelle, D. C. (2002). Effect of PNF stretch techniques on knee flexor muscle EMG activity in older adults. *Journal of Electromyography and Kinesiology, 12*(5), 391–397. https://doi.org/10.1016/S1050-6411(02)00047-0

Floyd, R. T. (2018). *Manual of structural kinesiology* (20th ed.). New York, NY: McGraw-Hill.

Freitas, S. R., & Mil-Homens, P. (2015). Effect of 8-week high-intensity stretching training on biceps femoris architecture. *Journal of Strength and Conditioning Research, 29*(6), 1737–1740. https://doi.org/10.1519/JSC.0000000000000800

Freitas, S. R., Vilarinho, D., Vaz, J. R., Bruno, P. M., Costa, P. B., & Mil-homens, P. (2015). Responses to static stretching are dependent on stretch intensity and duration. *Clinical Physiology and Functional Imaging, 35*(6), 478–484. https://doi.org/10.1111/cpf.12186

Fukaya, T., Kiyono, R., Sato, S., Yahata, K., Yasaka, K., Onuma, R., & Nakamura, M. (2020). Effects of static stretching with high-intensity and short-duration or low-intensity and long-duration on range of motion and muscle stiffness. *Frontiers in Physiology, 11*, 601912. https://doi.org/10.3389/fphys.2020.601912

Games, K. E., Sefton, J. M., & Wilson, A. E. (2015). Whole-body vibration and blood flow and muscle oxygenation: A meta-analysis. *Journal of Athletic Training, 50*(5), 542–549. https://doi.org/10.4085/1062-6050-50.2.09

Grabow, L., Young, J. D., Alcock, L. R., Quigley, P. J., Byrne, J. M., Granacher, U., Škarabot, J., & Behm, D. G. (2018). Higher quadriceps roller massage forces do not amplify range-of-motion increases nor impair strength and jump performance. *Journal of Strength and Conditioning Research, 32*(11), 3059–3069. https://doi.org/10.1519/JSC.0000000000001906.

Grigg, P. (1994). Peripheral neural mechanisms in proprioception. *Journal of Sports Rehabilitation, 3*(1), 2–17.

Guissard, N., & Duchateau, J. (2006). Neural aspects of muscle stretching. *Exercise and Sport Sciences Reviews, 34*(4), 154–158. https://doi.org/10.1249/01.jes.0000240023.30373.eb

Guissard, N., Duchateau, J., & Hainaut, K. (2001). Mechanisms of decreased motoneuron excitation during passive muscle stretching. *Experimental Brain Research, 137*(2), 163–169. https://doi.org/10.1007/s002210000648

Günal, I., Köse, N., Erdogan, O., Göktürk, E., & Seber, S. (1996). Normal range of motion of the joints of the upper extremity in male subjects, with special reference to side. *Journal of Bone & Joint Surgery, 78*(9), 1401–1404. https://doi.org/10.2106/00004623-199609000-00017

Gutierrez, G. M., Kaminski, T. W., & Douex, A. T. (2009). Neuromuscular control and ankle instability. *PM&R, 1*(4), 359–365. https://doi.org/10.1016/j.pmrj.2009.01.013

Haddad, M., Dridi, A., Chtara, M., Chaouachi, A., Wong, D. P., Behm, D., & Chamari, K. (2014). Static stretching can impair explosive performance for at least 24 hours. *Journal of Strength and Conditioning Research, 28*, 140–146. https://doi.org/10.1519/JSC.0b013e3182964836.

Haff, G. G., & Triplett, N. T. (Eds.). (2016). *NSCA's essentials of strength training and conditioning*. Human Kinetics.

Hall, S. (2019). *Basic biomechanics* (8th ed.). McGraw-Hill Education.

Halperin, I., Aboodarda, S. J., Button, D. C., Andersen, L. L., & Behm, D. G. (2014). Roller massager improves range of motion of plantar flexor muscles without subsequent decreases in force parameters. *International Journal of Sports Physical Therapy, 9*(1), 92–102. https://www.ncbi.nlm.nih.gov/pmc/articles/PMC3924613/

Hamill, J., Knutzen, K., & Derrick, T. (2021). *Biomechanical basis of human movement* (5th ed.). Wolters Kluwer Health.

Han, S.-W., Lee, Y.-S., & Lee, D. J. (2017). The influence of the vibration form roller exercise on the pains in the muscles around the hip joint and the joint performance. *Journal of Physical Therapy Science, 29*(10), 1844–1847. https://doi.org/10.1589/jpts.29.1844

Hewett, T. E., Myer, G. D., Ford, K. R., Heidt, R. S., Colosimo, A. J., McLean, S. G., Van Den Bogert, A. J., Paterno, M. V., & Succop, P. (2005). Biomechanical measures of neuromuscular control and valgus loading of the knee predict anterior cruciate ligament injury risk in female athletes: A prospective study. *American Journal of Sports Medicine, 33*(4), 492–501. https://doi.org/10.1177/0363546504269591

Hindle, K., Whitcomb, T., Briggs, W., & Hong, J. (2012). Proprioceptive neuromuscular facilitation (PNF): Its mechanisms and effects on range of motion and muscular function. *Journal of Human Kinetics, 31*(2012), 105–113.

Hollins, M., McDermott, K., & Harper, D. (2014). How does vibration reduce pain? *Perception, 43*(1), 70–84. https://doi.org/10.1068/p7637

Holt, J., Holt, L. E., & Pelham, T. W. In T. Bauer (Ed.), *Biomechanics in sports XIII* (pp. 170–174). Lakehead University; 1996.

Holt, B. W., & Lambourne, K. (2008). The impact of different warm-up protocols on vertical jump performance in male collegiate athletes. *Journal of Strength and Conditioning Research, 22*(1), 226–229. https://doi.org/10.1519/JSC.0b013e31815f9d6a

Hoppenbrouwers, M., Eckhardt, M. M. E. M., Verkerk, K., & Verhagen, A. (2006). Reproducibility of the measurement of active and passive cervical range of motion. *Journal of Manipulative and Physiological Therapeutics, 29*(5), 363–367. https://doi.org/10.1016/j.jmpt.2006.04.007

Ikeda, N., Otsuka, S., Kawanishi, Y., & Kawakami, Y. (2019). Effects of instrument-assisted soft tissue mobilization on musculoskeletal properties. *Medicine and Science in Sports and Exercise, 51*(10), 2166–2172. https://doi.org/10.1249/MSS.0000000000002035

Iqbal, Z. A., & Alghadir, A. H. (2017). Cumulative trauma disorders: A review. *Journal of Back and Musculoskeletal Rehabilitation, 30*(4), 663–666. https://doi.org/10.3233/bmr-150266

Jacobs, C., Uhl, T. L., Seeley, M., Sterling, W., & Goodrich, L. (2005). Strength and fatigability of the dominant and nondominant hip abductors. *Journal of Athletic Training, 40*(3), 203–206. https://www.ncbi.nlm.nih.gov/pmc/articles/PMC1250264/

Jaffe, M., Tirosh, E., Cohen, A., & Taub, Y. (1988). Joint mobility and motor development. *Archives of Disease in Childhood, 63*(2), 159–161. https://doi.org/10.1136/adc.63.2.159

James, B., & Parker, A. W. (1989). Active and passive mobility of lower limb joints in elderly men and women. *American Journal of Physical Medicine & Rehabilitation, 68*(4), 162–167.

Jami, L. (1988). Functional properties of the Golgi tendon organs. *International Archives of Physiology & Biochemistry, 96*(4), A363–A378.

Janda, V. (1978). Muscles, central nervous motor regulation and back problems (pp. 27–41). In L. M. Korr (Ed.), *The neurobiologic mechanisms in manipulative therapy*. Springer.

Jay, K., Sundstrup, E., Søndergaard, S. D., Behm, D., Brandt, M., Sųrvoll, C. A., Jakobsen, M. D., & Andersen, L. L. (2014). Specific and cross over effects of massage for muscle soreness: Randomized controlled trial. *International Journal of Sports Physical Therapy, 9*(1), 82–91. https://www.ncbi.nlm.nih.gov/pmc/articles/PMC3924612/

Johansson, R. S., & Flanagan, J. R. (2009). Coding and use of tactile signals from the fingertips in object manipulation tasks. *Nature Reviews Neuroscience, 10*(5), 345–359. https://doi.org/10.1038/nrn2621

Kay, A. D., & Blazevich, A. J. (2012). Effect of acute static stretch on maximal muscle performance: A systematic review. *Medicine & Science in Sports & Exercise, 44*(1), 154–164. https://doi.org/10.1249/MSS.0b013e318225cb27

Kelly, S., & Beardsley, C. (2016). Specific and cross-over effects of foam rolling on ankle dorsiflexion range of motion. *International Journal of Sports Physical Therapy, 11*(4), 544–551.

Kenney, W. L., Wilmore, J. H., & Costill, D. L. (2019). *Physiology of sport and exercise* (7th ed.). Human Kinetics.

Komdeur, P., Pollo, F. E., & Jackson, R. W. (2002). Dynamic knee motion in anterior cruciate impairment: A report and case study. *Baylor University Medical Center Proceedings, 15*(3), 257–259. https://doi.org/10.1080/08998280.2002.11927850

Knudson, D. (2021). *Fundamentals of biomechanics* (3rd ed.). Springer Nature.

Knudson, D., Magnusson, P., & McHugh, M. (2000). Current issues in flexibility fitness. *President's Council on Physical Fitness and Sports Research Digest, 3*(10), 1–8.

Konrad, A., Glashüttner, C., Reiner, M. M., Bernsteiner, D., & Tilp, M. (2020). The acute effects of a percussive massage treatment with a hypervolt device on plantar flexor muscles' range of motion and performance. *Journal of Sports Science & Medicine, 19*(4), 690–694. https://www.ncbi.nlm.nih.gov/pmc/articles/PMC7675623/

Konrad, A., & Tilp, M. (2014). Increased range of motion after static stretching is not due to changes in muscle and tendon structures. *Clinical Biomechanics, 29*(6), 636–642. https://doi.org/10.1016/j.clinbiomech.2014.04.013

Kurz, T. (2003). *Stretching scientifically: A guide to flexibility training* (4th ed.). Stadion Publishing.

Lambert, M., Hitchcock, R., Lavallee, K., Hayford, E., Morazzini, R., Wallace, A., Conroy, D., & Cleland, J. (2017). The effects of instrument-assisted soft tissue mobilization compared to other interventions on pain and function: a systematic review. *Physical Therapy Reviews, 22*, 76–85. https://doi.org/10.1080/10833196.2017.1304184

Langevin, H. M. (2021). Fascia mobility, proprioception, and myofascial pain. *Life, 11*(7), 668.

LaRoche, D. P., & Connolly, D. A. J. (2006). Effects of stretching on passive muscle tension and response to eccentric exercise. *American Journal of Sports Medicine, 34*(6), 1000–1007. https://doi.org/10.1177/0363546505284238

Larouche, M.-C., Camiré Bernier, S., Racine, R., Collin, O., Desmons, M., Mailloux, C., & Massé-Alarie, H. (2020). Stretch-induced hypoalgesia: A pilot study. *Scandinavian Journal of Pain, 20*(4), 837–845. https://doi.org/10.1515/sjpain-2020-0018

Latash, M. (2008). *Neurophysiological basis of movement* (2nd ed.). Human Kinetics.

Lempke, L., Wilkinson, R., Murray, C., & Stanek, J. (2018). The effectiveness of PNF versus static stretching on increasing hipflexion range of motion. *Journal of Sport Rehabilitation, 27*(3), 289–294. https://doi.org/10.1123/jsr.2016-0098

Levin, M. F., & Feldman, A. G. (1994). The role of stretch reflex threshold regulation in normal and impaired motor control. *Brain Research, 657*(1–2), 23–30. https://doi.org/10.1016/0006-8993(94)90949-0

Lieber, R. L., & Frieden, J. (2000). Functional and clinical significance of skeletal muscle architecture. *Muscle and Nerve, 23*(11), 1647–1666.

Lim, J.-H., & Park, C.-B. (2019). The immediate effects of foam roller with vibration on hamstring flexibility and jump performance in healthy adults. *Journal of Exercise Rehabilitation, 15*(1), 50–54. https://doi.org/10.12965/jer.1836560.280

Lim, W. (2018). Optimal intensity of PNF stretching: Maintaining the efficacy of stretching while ensuring its safety. *Journal of Physical Therapy Science, 30*(8), 1108–1111. https://doi.org/10.1589/jpts.30.1108

López-Bedoya, J., Vernetta-Santana, M., Robles-Fuentes, A., & Ariza-Vargas, L. (2013). Effect of three types of flexibility training on active and passive hip range of motion. *Journal of Sports Medicine and Physical Fitness, 53*(3), 304–311.

Matthews, P. B. C. (1982). Where does Sherrington's "muscular sense" originate? Muscles, joints, corollary discharges? *Annual Review of Neuroscience, 5*(1), 189–218. https://doi.org/10.1146/annurev.ne.05.030182.001201

McDonald, A. C., Mulla, D. M., & Keir, P. J. (2019). Muscular and kinematic adaptations to fatiguing repetitive upper extremity work. *Applied Ergonomics, 75*, 250–256. https://doi.org/10.1016/j.apergo.2018.11.001

McHugh, M. P., & Cosgrave, C. H. (2009). To stretch or not to stretch: The role of stretching in injury prevention and performance. *Scandinavian Journal of Medicine & Science in Sports.* https://doi.org/10.1111/j.1600-0838.2009.01058.x

Mills, M., Frank, B., Goto, S., Blackburn, T., Cates, S., Clark, M., Aguilar, A., Fava, N., & Padua, D. (2015). Effect of restricted hip flexor muscle length on hip extensor muscle activity and lower extremity biomechanics in college-aged female soccer players. *International Journal of Sports Physical Therapy, 10*(7), 946–954.

Mitchell, U. H., Myrer, J. W., Hopkins, J. T., Hunter, I., Feland, J. B., & Hilton, S. C. (2007). Acute stretch perception alteration contributes to the success of the PNF "contract–relax" stretch. *Journal of Sport Rehabilitation, 16*(2), 85–92. https://doi.org/10.1123/jsr.16.2.85

Moran, K., McGrath, T., Marshall, B., & Wallace, E. (2009). Dynamic stretching and golf swing performance. *International Journal of Sports Medicine, 30*(02), 113–118. https://doi.org/10.1055/s-0028-1103303

Myers, J. B., Riemann, B. L., Ju, Y.-Y., Hwang, J.-H., McMahon, P. J., & Lephart, S. M. (2003). Shoulder muscle reflex latencies under various levels of muscle contraction: *Clinical Orthopaedics and Related Research, 407*, 92–101. https://doi.org/10.1097/00003086-200302000-00017

Nakamura, M., Sato, S., Hiraizumi, K., Kiyono, R., Fukaya, T., & Nishishita, S. (2020). Effects of static stretching programs performed at different volume-equated weekly frequencies on passive properties of muscle–tendon unit. *Journal of Biomechanics, 103*, 109670. https://doi.org/10.1016/j.jbiomech.2020.109670

Nakamura, M., Sato, S., Kiyono, R., Yahata, K., Yoshida, R., Fukaya, T., & Konrad, A. (2021). Comparison of the acute effects of hold–relax and static stretching among older adults. *Biology, 10*(2), 126. https://doi.org/10.3390/biology10020126

Needham, R. A., Morse, C. I., & Degens, H. (2009). The acute effect of different warm-up protocols on anaerobic performance in elite youth soccer players. *Journal of Strength and Conditioning Research, 23*(9), 2614–2620. https://doi.org/10.1519/JSC.0b013e3181b1f3ef

Nuzzo, J. L. (2020). The case for retiring flexibility as a major component of physical fitness. *Sports Medicine (Auckland, N.Z.), 50*(5), 853–870. https://doi.org/10.1007/s40279-019-01248-w

Padua, D. A., DiStefano, L. J., Beutler, A. I., de la Motte, S. J., DiStefano, M. J., & Marshall, S. W. (2015). The landing error scoring system as a screening tool for an anterior cruciate ligament injury-prevention program in elite-youth soccer athletes. *Journal of Athletic Training, 50*(6), 589–595. https://doi.org/10.4085/1062-6050-50.1.10

Page, P., Frank, C. C., & Lardner, R. (2010). *Assessment and treatment of muscle imbalance: The Janda approach.* Human Kinetics.

Park, Y. J., Park, S. W., & Lee, H. S. (2018). Comparison of the effectiveness of whole body vibration in stroke patients: A meta-analysis. *BioMed Research International, 2018*, 5083634. https://doi.org/10.1155/2018/5083634

Paterno, M. V., Schmitt, L. C., Ford, K. R., Rauh, M. J., Myer, G. D., Huang, B., & Hewett, T. E. (2010). Biomechanical measures during landing and postural stability predict second anterior cruciate ligament injury after anterior cruciate ligament reconstruction and return to sport. *American Journal of Sports Medicine, 38*(10), 1968–1978. https://doi.org/10.1177/0363546510376053

Paulino, F. E., Villacis, D. C., & Ahmad, C. S. (2016). Valgus extension overload in baseball players. *American Journal of Orthopedics (Belle Mead, N.J.), 45*(3), 144–151.

Perrier, E. T., Pavol, M. J., & Hoffman, M. A. (2011). The acute effects of a warm-up including static or dynamic stretching on countermovement jump height, reaction time, and flexibility. *Journal of Strength and Conditioning Research, 25*(7), 1925–1931. https://doi.org/10.1519/JSC.0b013e3181e73959

Proske, U., & Gandevia, S. C. (2009). The kinesthetic senses. *Journal of Physiology, 587*(17), 4139–4146.

Rajabi, R., Doherty, P., Goodarzi, M., & Hemayattalab, R. (2008). Comparison of thoracic kyphosis in two groups of elite Greco-Roman and freestyle wrestlers and a group of non-athletic participants. *British Journal of Sports Medicine, 42*(3), 229–232; discussion 232. https://doi.org/10.1136/bjsm.2006.033639

Reid, J. C., Greene, R., Young, J. D., Hodgson, D. D., Blazevich, A. J., & Behm, D. G. (2018). The effects of different durations of static stretching within a comprehensive warm-up on voluntary and evoked contractile properties. *European Journal of Applied Physiology, 118*(7), 1427–1445. https://doi.org/10.1007/s00421-018-3874-3

Riemann, B. L., Myers, J. B., & Lephart, S. M. (2002). Sensorimotor system measurement techniques. *Journal of Athletic Training, 37*(1), 85–98. https://www.ncbi.nlm.nih.gov/pmc/articles/PMC164313/

Romero-Moraleda, B., González-García, J., Cuéllar-Rayo, Á., Balsalobre-Fernández, C., Muñoz-García, D., & Morencos, E. (2019). Effects of vibration and non-vibration foam rolling on recovery after exercise with induced muscle damage. *Journal of Sports Science and Medicine, 18*(1), 172–180. https://www.ncbi.nlm.nih.gov/pmc/articles/PMC6370959/

Ryan, E. D., Everett, K. L., Smith, D. B., Pollner, C., Thompson, B. J., Sobolewski, E. J., & Fiddler, R. E. (2014). Acute effects of different volumes of dynamic stretching on vertical jump performance, flexibility and muscular endurance. *Clinical Physiology and Functional Imaging, 34*(6), 485–492. https://doi.org/10.1111/cpf.12122

Sağiroğlui, İ. (2017). Acute effects of applied local vibration during foam roller exercises on lower extremity explosive strength and flexibility performance. *European Journal of Physical Education and Sport Science, 3*(1), 20–31. https://oapub.org/edu/index.php/ejep/article/view/1041

Sahrmann, S., Azevado, D. C., & Van Dillen, L. (2017). Diagnosis and treatment of movement impairment syndromes. *Brazilian Journal of Physical Therapy, 21*(6), 391–399.

Sands, W. A., McNeal, J. R., Stone, M. H., Kimmel, W. L., Gregory Haff, G., & Jemni, M. (2008). The effect of vibration on active and passive range of motion in elite female synchronized swimmers. *European Journal of Sport Science, 8*(4), 217–223. https://doi.org/10.1080/17461390802116682

Santos, C. X., Beltrão, N. B., Pirauá, A. L. T., Durigan, J. L. Q., Behm, D., & de Araújo, R. C. (2020). Static stretching intensity does not influence acute range of motion, passive torque, and muscle architecture. *Journal of Sport Rehabilitation, 29*(1), 1–6. https://doi.org/10.1123/jsr.2018-0178

Scheck, F. (2018). *Mechanics: From Newton's laws to deterministic chaos* (6th ed.). Springer Nature.

Seow, C. C., Chow, P. K., & Khong, K. S. (1999). A study of joint mobility in a normal population. *Annals of the Academy of Medicine, Singapore, 28*(2), 231–236.

Sharman, M. J., Cresswell, A. G., & Riek, S. (2006). Proprioceptive neuromuscular facilitation stretching: Mechanisms and clinical implications. *Sports Medicine, 36*(11), 929–939. https://doi.org/10.2165/00007256-200636110-00002

Shumway-Cook, A., & Woollacott, M. (2017). *Motor control* (5th ed.). Wolters Kluwer.

Sim, A. Y., Dawson, B. T., Guelfi, K. J., Wallman, K. E., & Young, W. B. (2009). Effects of static stretching in warm-up on repeated sprint performance. *Journal of Strength and Conditioning Research, 23*(7), 2155–2162.

Simmonds, J. V., & Keer, R. J. (2007). Hypermobility and the hypermobility syndrome. *Manual Therapy, 12*(4), 298–309.

Simpson, C. L., Kim, B. D. H., Bourcet, M. R., Jones, G. R., & Jakobi, J. M. (2017). Stretch training induces unequal adaptation in muscle fascicles and thickness in medial and lateral gastrocnemii. *Scandinavian Journal of Medicine & Science in Sports, 27*(12), 1597–1604. https://doi.org/10.1111/sms.12822

Škarabot, J., Beardsley, C., & Štirn, I. (2015). Comparing the effects of self-myofascial release with static stretching on ankle range-of-motion in adolescent athletes. *International Journal of Sports Physical Therapy, 10*(2), 203–212.

Smith, L. L., Brunetz, M. H., Chenier, T. C., McCammon, M. R., Houmard, J. A., Franklin, M. E., & Israel, R. G. (1993). The effects of static and ballistic stretching on delayed onset muscle soreness and creatine kinase. *Research Quarterly for Exercise and Sport, 64*(1), 103–107. https://doi.org/10.1080/02701367.1993.10608784

Stecco, C., Porzionato, A., Macchi, V., Tiengo, C., Parenti, A., Aldegheri, R., Delmas, V., & De Caro, R. (2006). Histological characteristics of the deep fascia of the upper limb. *Italian Journal of Anatomy and Embryology/Archivio Italiano Di Anatomia Ed Embriologia, 111*(2), 105–110.

Stick Mobility. (2021a). *Free workout videos.* https://www.stickmobility.co.uk/pages/free-workout-videos

Stick Mobility. (2021b). *FAQ.* https://stickmobility.com/pages/faq

Støve, M. P., Hirata, R. P., & Palsson, T. S. (2021). The tolerance to stretch is linked with endogenous modulation of pain. *Scandinavian Journal of Pain, 21*(2), 355–363. https://doi.org/10.1515/sjpain-2020-0010

Sueki, D. G., Cleland, J. A., & Wainner, R. S. (2013). A regional interdependence model of musculoskeletal dysfunction: Research, mechanisms, and clinical implications. *Journal of Manual & Manipulative Therapy, 21*(2), 90–102. https://doi.org/10.1179/2042618612Y.0000000027

Sugimoto, D., Jackson, S. S., Howell, D. R., Meehan, W. P., & Stracciolini, A. (2019). Association between training volume and lower extremity overuse injuries in young female athletes: Implications for early sports specialization. *Physician and Sports Medicine, 47*(2), 199–204. https://doi.org/10.1080/00913847.2018.1546107

Swett, J. E., & Schoultz, T. W. (1975). Mechanical transduction in the Golgi tendon organ: A hypothesis. *Archives Italiennes De Biologie, 113*(4), 374–382.

Takaki, S., Kaneoka, K., Okubo, Y., Otsuka, S., Tatsumura, M., Shiina, I., & Miyakawa, S. (2016). Analysis of muscle activity during active pelvic tilting in sagittal plane. *Physical Therapy Research, 19*(1), 50–57. https://doi.org/10.1298/ptr.E9900

Thomas, E., Bianco, A., Paoli, A., & Palma, A. (2018). The relation between stretching typology and stretching duration: The effects on range of motion. *International Journal of Sports Medicine, 39*(4), 243–254. https://doi.org/10.1055/s-0044-101146

Tuthill, J. C., & Azim, E. (2018). Proprioception. *Current Biology, 28*(5), R194–R203.

Vander, A. J., Sherman, J. H., & Luciano, D. S. (2001). *Human physiology: The mechanisms of body function.* McGraw-Hill.

Verkhoshansky, Y., & Siff, M. (2009). *Supertraining* (6th ed.). Verkhoshansky SSTM.

Vernetta-Santana, M., Ariza-Vargas, L., Robles-Fuentes, A., & López-Bedoya, J. (2015). Acute effect of active isolated stretching technique on range of motion and peak isometric force. *Journal of Sports Medicine and Physical Fitness, 55*(11), 1299–1309.

Victoria, G. D., Carmen, E., Alexandru, S., Florin, C., & Daniel, D. (2013). The PNF (proprioceptive neuromuscular facilitation) stretching technique: A brief review. *Science, Movement and Health, 13*(2), 623–628.

Visser, B., & van Dieën, J. H. (2006). Pathophysiology of upper extremity muscle disorders. *Journal of Electromyography & Kinesiology, 16*(1), 1–16.

Vlaeyen, J. W. S., & Linton, S. J. (2000). Fear-avoidance and its consequences in chronic musculoskeletal pain: A state of the art. *Pain, 85*(3), 317–332. https://doi.org/10.1016/S0304-3959(99)00242-0

Wilke, J., Müller, A.-L., Giesche, F., Power, G., Ahmedi, H., & Behm, D. G. (2020). Acute effects of foam rolling on range of motion in healthy adults: A systematic review with multilevel meta-analysis. *Sports Medicine, 50*(2), 387–402. https://doi.org/10.1007/s40279-019-01205-7

Wilke, J., Niederer, D., Vogt, L., & Banzer, W. (2016). Remote effects of lower limb stretching: Preliminary evidence for myofascial connectivity? *Journal of Sports Sciences, 34*(22), 2145–2148. https://doi.org/10.1080/02640414.2016.1179776

Yavuz, U. Ş., Negro, F., Diedrichs, R., & Farina, D. (2018). Reciprocal inhibition between motor neurons of the tibialis anterior and triceps surae in humans. *Journal of Neurophysiology, 119*(5), 1699–1706. https://doi.org/10.1152/jn.00424.2017

Young, J. D., Spence, A. J., & Behm, D. G. (2018). Roller massage decreases spinal excitability to the soleus. *Journal of Applied Physiology, 124*(4), 950–959. https://doi.org/10.1152/japplphysiol.00732.2017

Young, W. B., & Behm, D. G. (2002). Should static stretching be used during a warm-up for strength and power activities? *Strength and Conditioning Journal, 24*(6), 33–37. https://doi.org/10.1519/00126548-200212000-00006

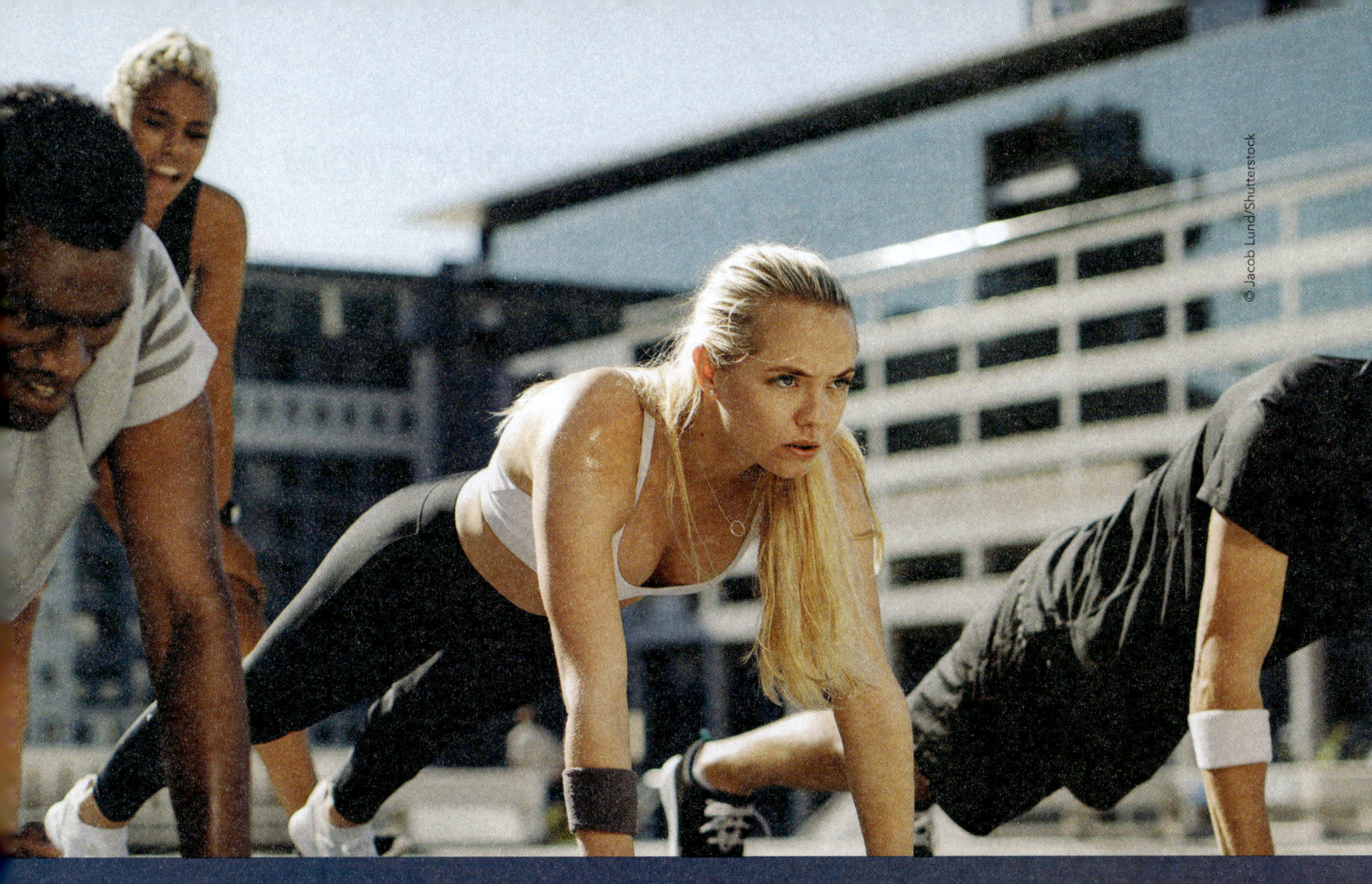

CORE TRAINING FOR SPORTS PERFORMANCE

CHAPTER TEN

LEARNING OBJECTIVES

Upon completion of this chapter, the Sports Performance Coach will be able to:

- **Summarize** the importance of core training for athletes with differing performance-related goals.

- **Explain** the scientific rationale for core training.

- **Describe** different core training techniques used within performance training.

- **Identify** appropriate acute training variables for core training.

- **Select** core training programs or techniques based on athlete needs.

LESSON 1: INTRODUCTION TO CORE TRAINING

INTRODUCTION

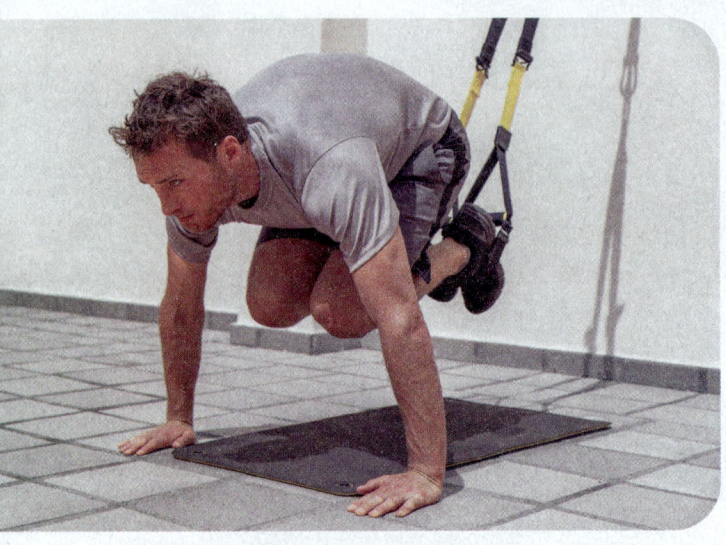

© Maridav/Shutterstock

Core training is essential for athletes across all sports and disciplines, as it plays a crucial role in overall performance, injury prevention, and maintaining good posture. The core, which consists of muscles in the abdomen, lower back, hips, and pelvis, serves as the body's central region; these muscles work together to stabilize and support the spine. One of the main benefits of core training is improved stability and balance. A strong core provides a stable foundation for athletic movements, enabling better control and coordination during sports activities. This can lead to enhanced performance and reduced risk of falls or other accidents. Thus, training the core is an established strength and conditioning pillar, and well-developed core musculature has been shown to reduce injury risk and maximize athletic performance (Alentorn-Geli et al., 2009).

An optimally functioning core provides a stable but versatile platform for the limbs to operate from to generate, resist, and absorb motion forces so the body can efficiently produce, coordinate, and control the movements required for daily living or sport performance (Kamal, 2015). Core training exercises are used for many purposes. For example, fitness enthusiasts may perform core training to acquire a flat midsection. In contrast, a physical therapist may prescribe specific core exercises for patients with lower back issues (Chang et al., 2015). The Sports Performance Coach, however, must understand all core training concepts and apply them within a sporting context to prepare athletes for their sport. In addition, understanding the functional characteristics of the core ensures the Sports Performance Coach is equipped to design and deliver a core training program specific to the athlete's performance needs and reduce the athlete's injury risk.

OVERVIEW OF CORE FUNCTIONALITY

The **core**, also known as the lumbo-pelvic-hip complex (LPHC), includes a space within the body that lies inferior to the diaphragm, and is surrounded by the abdominal muscles anteriorly and laterally, the lumbar spine and gluteal muscles posteriorly, and the pelvic floor and hip musculature inferiorly (Huxel Bliven & Anderson, 2013). Recall that optimal neuromuscular control is the coordinated action of the muscles firing at the right time and with the appropriate force for a specific task. This core musculature coordination is vital for an athlete to demonstrate **core stability**, **core endurance**, **core strength**, and **core power**. All of these attributes are foundational to athletic performance.

For example, in everyday activities such as walking, the core isometrically stabilizes the LPHC with low levels of muscular contractions to maintain the desired posture. The lower stiffness levels allow for the necessary torsion (twisting) of the LPHC required for efficient, fluid locomotion. Conversely, when the athlete is attempting a heavy lift, such as a deadlift, or experiences the impact of striking an opponent during a contact sport, the core should

---

CORE →

The structures that make up the lumbo-pelvic-hip complex (LPHC), including the lumbar spine, pelvic girdle, abdomen, and hip joint.

CORE STABILITY →

The ability of the neuromuscular system to limit unwanted movement of the lumbo-pelvic-hip complex.

engage with much higher levels of contraction for increased spinal stiffness.

The optimal level of spinal stiffness is modulated by the central nervous system (CNS) and is based on previous experience and expected demand. For example, experienced athletes rarely have to consciously engage core muscles during an event. However, inappropriate core stiffness modulation (high-level stiffness for low-level tasks) can cause excessive rigidity and lead to movement inefficiency with low-force-related tasks (Comerford & Mottram, 2012). At the other end of the spectrum, low-level stiffness for high-level tasks can result in poor performance and increased injury risks.

THE IMPORTANCE OF CORE STABILITY

Core stability is vital for all athletes. During athletic activities, the core stabilizes the LPHC to assist with balance and alignment of limbs during weight transfer, and propulsion to ensure forward (sagittal plane) motion occurs with limited (unwanted) frontal and transverse plane motion at the LPHC. In addition, with vertical pressing, pushing, or pulling actions, the core isometrically controls (prevents) unwanted flexion, extension, rotation, and lateral movements of the LPHC. This isometric contraction helps protect the joints, ligaments, and discs from shear, overstrain, stretch, or overcompression forces. Moreover, an optimal functioning core provides a stable base so the limbs can absorb impact and generate the required force without movement leaking through the LPHC (Hewett et al., 2002; Hodges & Richardson, 1996; Leetun et al., 2004; Nadler, Malanga, Bartoli, et al., 2002; Nadler, Moley, et al., 2002; O'Sullivan et al., 1997).

Many athletes train for hours every day. However, they still lead modern lives that may be largely sedentary or encourage poor posture when not training. Therefore, athletes' resting or standing habits can influence their core stabilization capabilities.

For example, sustained postures, such as swayback posture (**Figure 10.1**) when standing or slouching when sitting, can negatively impact core-stabilizing muscle function. Holding these postures puts the deep core muscles in stretched positions for extended periods (Sahrmann, 2002). The deep core stabilizing muscles adapt to the stretched positions—such as by increasing muscle sarcomere length, thereby altering the amount of tension that can be produced while at this resting length (Williams & Goldspink, 1978). Consequently, stabilizing muscles can lack optimal force production in specific positions, reducing their ability to provide necessary core control and alignment during postural situations.

Even with these changes, many athletes can still demonstrate high performance because the superficial core muscles (frequently called the "mirror muscles") can compensate for poor core stability. However, this effect is temporary and comes with a cost. Over time, the superficial core muscles become shortened and overactive. This phenomenon reduces the core movement system's ability to be explosive, as it develops the rigidity necessary to perform the postural stabilizer role (Comerford & Mottram, 2012; Lewis et al., 2009; Sahrmann, 2002). Educating athletes about the adverse effects of poor postural habits in everyday living can help them avoid these detrimental changes in core function and maximize their core training programs (Comerford & Mottram, 2001).

CORE ENDURANCE →

The ability to control the motion of the spine over a given longer duration.

CORE STRENGTH →

The ability to control the motion of the spine.

CORE POWER →

The ability to control rapid force acceleration and deceleration of the spine.

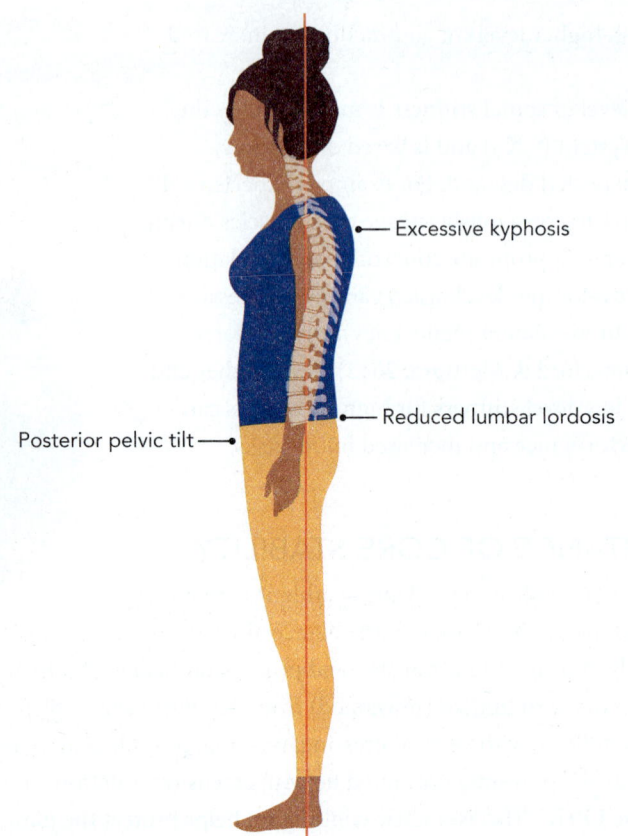

Excessive kyphosis

Reduced lumbar lordosis

Posterior pelvic tilt

FIGURE 10.1 Swayback Posture

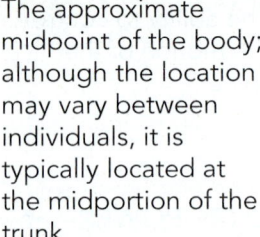

CENTER OF GRAVITY →

The approximate midpoint of the body; although the location may vary between individuals, it is typically located at the midportion of the trunk.

BASE OF SUPPORT →

The area beneath a person that consists of every point of contact made between the body and the support surface.

CORE FUNCTION DURING SPORT

Every sport has specific actions that are rarely performed in the same way as in other sports, whether those actions involve running, jumping, landing, kicking, striking, or throwing. An optimally functioning core allows the athlete to control, adjust, and disassociate the various columns of the body (upper body, torso, lower body) to cope with the varying situations they may face when playing their sport and execute that action with the highest quality (Putnam, 1993). This capability is especially significant in sports that involve a lot of unpredictability, such as basketball or soccer, where the athlete needs to make the appropriate decisions (receive and process information, select an appropriate action, and adjust as needed) and then respond quickly to that situation with good execution.

For example, a defender in soccer requires quick reflexes and bodily control. They rely heavily on their core's capabilities to control their **center of gravity** and the trunk's momentum over a changing **base of support** in the direction of their opponent to guard a shot on goal. In this example, it is also essential for the athlete to be isometrically strong enough to control their center of mass and limit momentum to stay centered and balanced to reduce their risk of injury.

If athletes become "off-balance" from poor momentum control, they leave themselves open to injury, particularly noncontact injury. Noncontact injury can occur in various body regions through predictable patterns of motion that create overstretching or compression of muscles or joints. For example, overstretching the hip can lead to an adductor muscle strain or overcompression of the lower back, leading to a facet joint sprain (Hewett et al., 2002; Hodges & Richardson, 1996; Leetun et al., 2004; Nadler, Moley, et al., 2002).

In addition, there are significant differences in how the core functions for various performance tasks. For example, some performance tasks require maximal muscle activation and force from the core (e.g., a dunk or posting up in basketball). In contrast, other tasks require less force but high precision of movement for accuracy (e.g., putting in golf). Furthermore, sometimes the athlete needs both power and precision concurrently (e.g., kicking a ball for a long-range pass in soccer). All of these actions require modulation of the core activation and recruitment strategies of the various muscle groups (Comerford & Mottram, 2012).

An optimally functioning core provides the athlete with the tools to efficiently and effectively execute all actions in all situations, whether a skill-based sport or not. It assists the athlete in holding the ideal biomechanical position so that sport-specific actions can be performed with the highest quality for better generation of force and speed from the extremities, while simultaneously protecting the athlete's joints and ligaments from overstrain or overcompression. Appropriate core muscle activation provides neuromuscular control, stability (local and global), and movement (strength and power) for efficient skills such as kicking (Putnam, 1993), throwing (Hirashima et al., 2007), and serving in tennis (Kibler et al., 1996; Marshall & Elliott, 2000). For example, when sprinting, stopping, jumping, or landing, the core is responsible for stabilizing the LPHC, contributes to the alignment of the upper and lower limbs, and plays a fundamental role in the quality of movement (Hodges & Richardson, 1996; Leetun et al., 2004; Nadler, Malanga, Bartoli, et al., 2002; Nadler, Moley, et al., 2002).

Athletes with enough core strength to stabilize their LPHC when running maintain ideal pelvic alignment and trunk positioning. At the same time, their nervous system adjusts the core musculature activation to modulate spinal stiffness, so that torso rotation occurs. However, unwanted motion, such as excessive low-back extension, lateral spinal flexion, or hip adduction (Bosch & Klomp, 2005), is prevented. Poor core stabilization and an unstable pelvis can lead to overstriding, decreased running efficiency, and increased risk of injury (Bosch & Klomp, 2005).

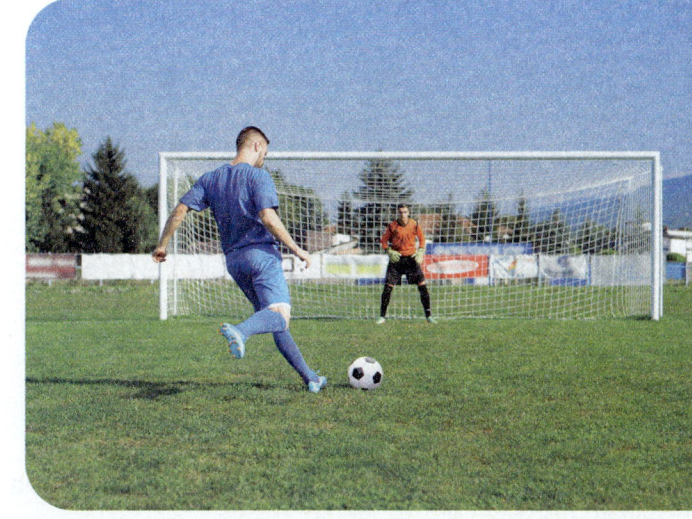

© BRG.photography/Shutterstock

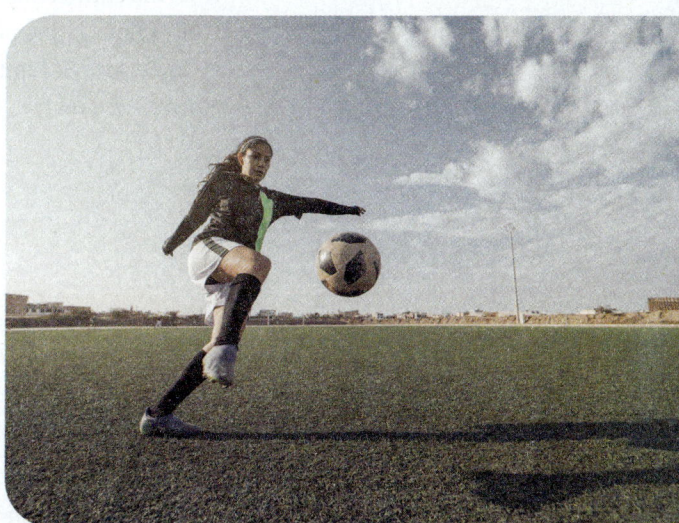

© Cavan Images - Offset/Shutterstock

LESSON 2: STRUCTURE AND FUNCTION OF THE CORE
ANATOMY OF THE CORE

The core is the central region of the body and comprises the structures of the LPHC. It is utilized in all daily living and sporting activities by controlling the motion of the trunk through layers of musculature and connecting the upper and lower extremities through various fascial connections (**Figure 10.2**). The layers of core musculature are divided into the local stabilization system, global stabilization system, and movement system.

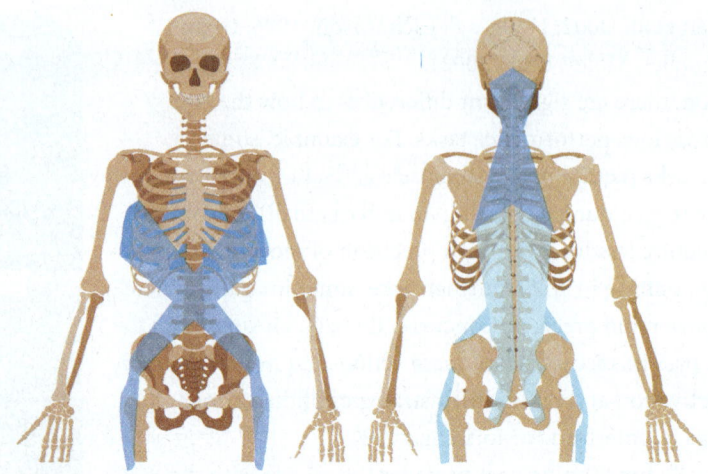

FIGURE 10.2 Fascial Connections

The entire body can also be viewed as a series of columns to help visualize how the various layers play a unique but integrated role in providing dynamic stabilization (Comerford & Mottram, 2012). From the ground up, the columns are described as the lower legs and feet, thighs, trunk and pelvis, and head and neck (**Figure 10.3**).

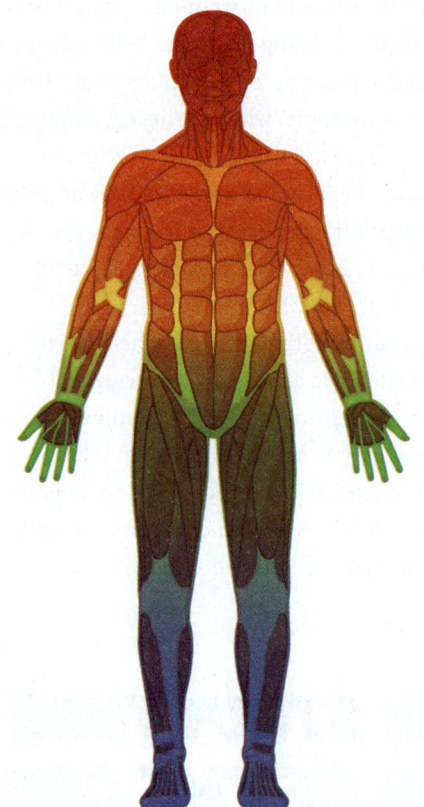

FIGURE 10.3 Kinetic Chain Columns

The deeper muscles of the stabilization system are positioned closer to the spine and offer better alignment and stability of the columns, whereas the more superficial muscles of the movement system span multiple columns and create motion. An optimally functioning core allows the athlete to fully control, produce, reduce, and transfer motion through the LPHC. It enables the athlete to adjust and respond to situations efficiently and produce motion most appropriately, maximizing their ability to perform their sporting actions.

FUNCTIONAL ANATOMY OF THE CORE

To fully understand how to program and train an athlete's core, the Sports Performance Coach can use the athlete's sport-specific actions as the starting point. Understanding a sport's specific movement characteristics and the role of the core during these movements is essential. Moreover, the coach must fully understand the importance of the functional anatomy and the difference between exercises designed to train the neurological and musculoskeletal systems. Both systems are equally necessary, yet it is impossible to perform an exercise that isolates training for only one of them.

Even so, some exercises can be designed to improve the cognitive control and coordination of the core stability muscles, which can be considered a "software upgrade" within the neurological system. Other exercises can focus more on increasing hypertrophy, strength, and power, which can be considered a "hardware upgrade" to the musculoskeletal system. Reviewing the key core musculature and its role in sport-specific functions enables the Sports Performance Coach to develop an integrated core training program.

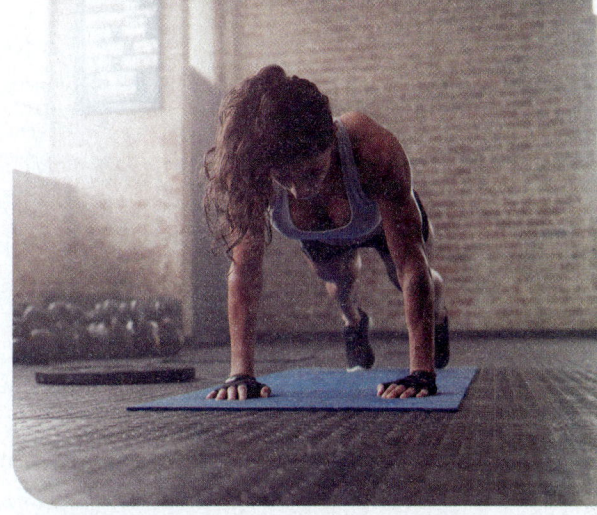

© Jacob Lund/Shutterstock

LOCAL CORE STABILIZERS

The **local core stabilizers** (**Figure 10.4**) are the deepest layer of muscles, which are located closest to the joints of the LPHC. These muscles are primarily slow-twitch type I fibers with a high density of muscle spindles and broad muscle attachments. They usually span only a single joint and are disadvantaged biomechanically in movement production

> **LOCAL CORE STABILIZERS** →
>
> The deepest layer of muscles, which are located closest to the joints of the lumbo-pelvic-hip complex.

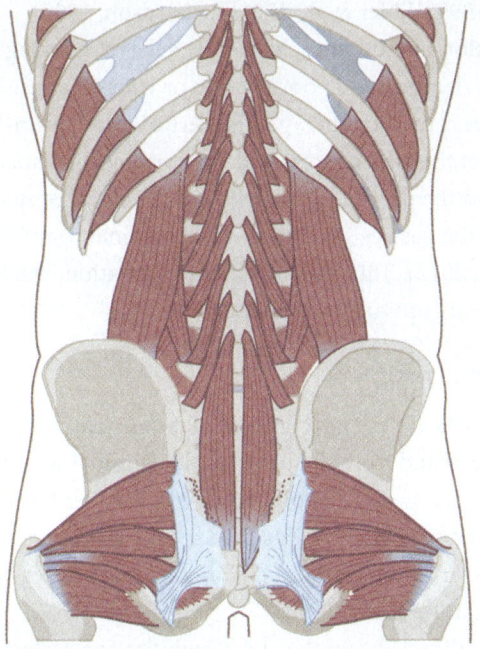

FIGURE 10.4 Local Core Musculature

due to their short lever length (Comerford & Mottram, 2012). However, their proximity to the joints and attachments makes them effective at providing compressive stability to prevent excessive translatory shear of the joint surfaces. The high density of muscle spindles aids in proprioceptive feedback (McGill, 2001). The primary muscles that make up the local stabilization system of the lumbopelvic region are listed in **Table 10.1**.

TABLE 10.1   Local Core Stabilizers

- Transversus abdominis
- Quadratus lumborum
- Deep multifidus
- Pelvic floor musculature
- Diaphragm
- Deep segmental muscle fibers of the psoas
- Deep hip rotators

FEED-FORWARD ACTIVATION →

When a muscle is automatically activated in anticipation of a movement.

These muscles have also been shown to provide a **feed-forward activation** mechanism. This mechanism creates spinal stiffness in preparation for movement by increasing intra-abdominal pressure (IAP) and generating tension in the thoracolumbar fascia (TLF), facilitating a proximal to distal sequencing of core muscle activation (Crisco & Panjabi, 1991; Hodges, 1999; Kibler et al., 2006; Richardson, 1999).

The core uses this "proximal to distal" feed-forward activation sequence to efficiently respond during reactive situations that consistently occur in sports. This consideration is especially important for athletes who play sports that present frequent unpredictable situations. The core can quickly respond and provide stiffness to the LPHC to rapidly facilitate control of the athlete's center of mass momentum. For example, proximal to distal muscle sequencing is a critical core function for throwing and kicking actions in sports. It creates stiffness in the connective tissues and fascia through the LPHC just before the movement, allowing for the efficient transfer of force through the extremities (Crisco & Panjabi, 1991; Hodges, 1999; Kibler et al., 2006; Richardson, 1999).

The timing of activation in these muscles can be delayed, altering ideal muscle sequences when athletes demonstrate poor posture or when they are in pain. Therefore, exercises for these muscles are often therapeutic. Perturbation or unstable-based training is a method used to target the anticipatory feed-forward mechanism and increase the sensitivity of activation of the deeper core stabilizers in neutral or midrange positions to avoid any reliance on the passive structures, such as spinal ligaments, for stabilization (Comerford & Mottram, 2012). This leads to quicker activation, resulting in more initial spinal stiffness and allowing optimal movement.

GLOBAL CORE STABILIZERS →

Muscles spanning over the lumbo-pelvic-hip complex, attaching from the pelvis to the spine and from the pelvis to the femur.

GLOBAL CORE STABILIZERS

The **global core stabilizers** are the next layer of muscles spanning the LPHC, attaching from the pelvis to the spine and from the pelvis to the femur. These muscles are also predominantly slow-twitch type I fiber dominant, with broader attachments. However, these muscles span farther over LPHC joints than the local deeper core stabilizers, providing them with longer lever lengths and giving them a greater biomechanical advantage in controlling movement.

The primary muscles that make up the global stabilization system are listed in **Table 10.2**. The muscle fibers of this group are obliquely oriented, giving them the

TABLE 10.2   Global Core Stabilizers

- Superficial multifidus
- Psoas major
- Iliacus
- External obliques
- Internal obliques
- Gluteus medius
- Medial gluteus medius
- Proximal adductor complex

greatest ability to decelerate and eccentrically control motion in the transverse and frontal planes. The eccentric deceleration in all planes is significant for most athletes, given the rotational nature of human movement. The oblique fiber alignment also equips this group of core muscles to coordinate the alignment of columns of the body (Comerford & Mottram, 2012).

The global core stabilizers influence the alignment of the pelvis and hips, which has a continued effect on the alignment of the lower legs and feet. Similarly, they coordinate the alignment of the upper back, which has a continued effect on the arms and head position. One athletic performance function closely aligned with the global core stabilizing muscles is **dissociation**, when one part of the body can perform a separate task from what the rest is doing, such as looking back to catch a football while running accurately in the opposite direction.

Optimal functioning of the global stabilizer muscles allows the athlete to dissociate the various columns of the body in the transverse plane without losing control of the center of mass in the frontal or sagittal planes. Dissociating the columns above or below the LPHC is a movement skill that aids in distributing load through each column and is extremely important for athletic movement efficiency. However, the inability to dissociate motion in the transverse plane can lead to unwanted motion in the frontal plane, increasing the risk of injury (Comerford & Mottram, 2012; Crisco & Panjabi, 1991; Hodges, 1999; Kibler et al., 2006; Richardson, 1999).

For instance, a defender in soccer may need to guard a player by moving in one direction while watching the ball roll across the field in the opposite direction. If the player cannot dissociate the upper- and lower-body movements, compensatory action often follows, negatively impacting the player's ability to control their center of mass. Consequently, the player's ability to adjust their body in this situation is impeded, and their risk of injury increases with increased trunk lateral momentum (Paillard, 2019).

The global stabilizer muscles can be targeted using exercises focusing on dissociation and asymmetrical challenge exercises with slow, controlled speeds coupled with low force. An oblique twist as well as anti-rotation exercises like the Pallof press with upper-body rotation (keeping the LPHC still) and the prone plank with hip extension (preventing motion at the lower back) are examples of exercises that focus on dissociation and asymmetrical challenges.

DISSOCIATION →

The ability for one region of the body to perform a task separate from what the rest of the body is doing.

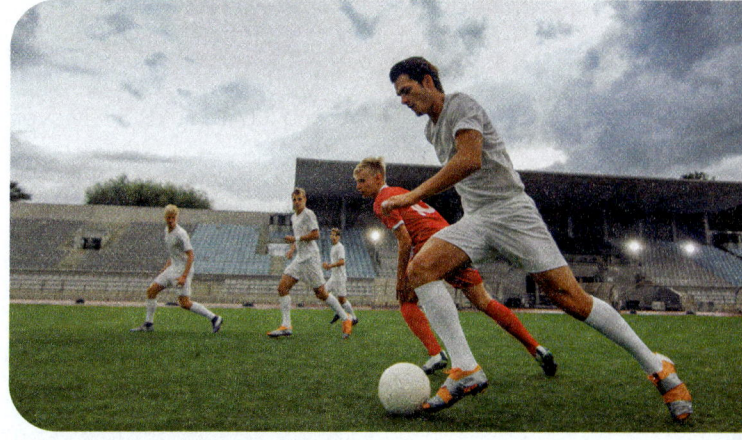

© Gorodenkoff/Shutterstock

MOVEMENT → SYSTEM

Superficial core muscles that attach the spine and pelvis to the extremities.

MOVEMENT SYSTEM

The **movement system** includes the layer of superficial core muscles that attach the spine and pelvis to the extremities. These muscles are predominantly fast-twitch type II fibers and have narrower attachments in many cases (**Figure 10.5**). They span farther over LPHC joints than the global core stabilizers, providing them with significantly longer lever lengths and making them more biomechanically advantaged in accelerating and decelerating joints and producing high-force motion. In addition, their structure helps stabilize the LPHC and move the extremities during high-force, sagittally oriented actions such as sprinting. As a result, the movement system can create the most force output.

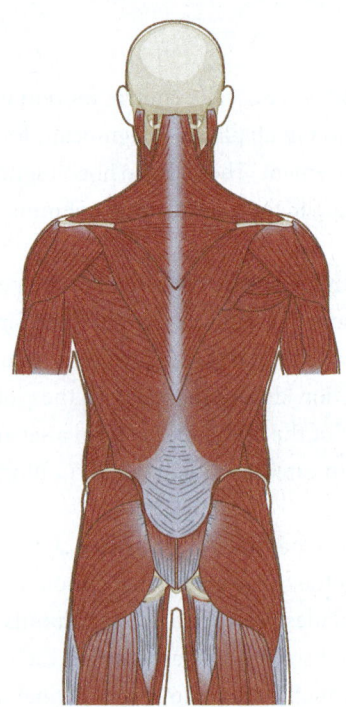

FIGURE 10.5 Movement System

The primary muscles that make up the movement system are provided in **Table 10.3**. These muscles are dominant in maximal explosive sporting actions in the sagittal plane, such as those performed by a sprinter or an offensive tackle in American football blocking the opponent. As previously mentioned, shortening the movement system muscles through poor postural habits can reduce their explosive power and outer range strength

TABLE 10.3 Movement System

- Erector spinae
- Rectus abdominis
- Latissimus dorsi
- Hip flexors
- Superficial gluteus maximus
- Hamstrings
- Quadriceps

and create joint mobility issues as they develop reduced flexibility. This can hinder an athlete's ability to dissociate the columns of the body in the transverse plane through inappropriate levels of stiffness created by the movement system muscle loss of flexibility (Comerford & Mottram, 2012; Crisco & Panjabi, 1991; Hodges, 1999; Kibler et al., 2006; Richardson, 1999).

Dissociation exercises (in the transverse plane, specifically) that bias the global core stabilizer muscles can help break up these rigidity patterns formed over time by the core movement system from poor sustained postural habits (Comerford & Mottram, 2012). The movement system muscles can be targeted by using symmetrical exercises in the sagittal plane with high force or fast speed, such as slow bilateral triple-extension exercises such as a squat thrust or an overhead medicine ball soccer throw.

FASCIAL SLINGS

All of the aforementioned core muscle groups work synergistically to provide dynamic stabilization and neuromuscular control of the entire LPHC (Sung et al., 2016). The core muscle system integrates with the kinetic chain via a network of noncontractile connective tissue (fascia) that spans LPHC. These **fascial slings** cross-link the upper and lower extremities. From this, various functional systems are created, such as the anterior, posterior, and lateral sling systems that facilitate LPHC stability and coordinate the cross-patterning function that is so vital to athlete performance (**Figure 10.6**). In addition, the fascial slings help transfer loads between the upper and lower extremities, relying on proximal to distal sequencing of core muscle activation to provide stability between the pelvis and spine and to utilize the core's elastic potential during sporting actions (Neumann, 2017).

The anterior oblique sling links the adductors with the ipsilateral internal obliques crossing over to the contralateral external oblique, shoulder, and arm. Increased proximal stiffness through the core stabilizers facilitates increased fascial tension to maximize elastic potential energy transfer between contralateral extremities through the core.

**DISSOCIATION →
EXERCISES**

Exercises that require the athlete to process separate tasks for different regions of the body, such as running while catching a pass from the side.

**FASCIAL →
SLINGS**

The interconnected chains of muscles, fascia, and other soft tissues that link the upper and lower extremities together.

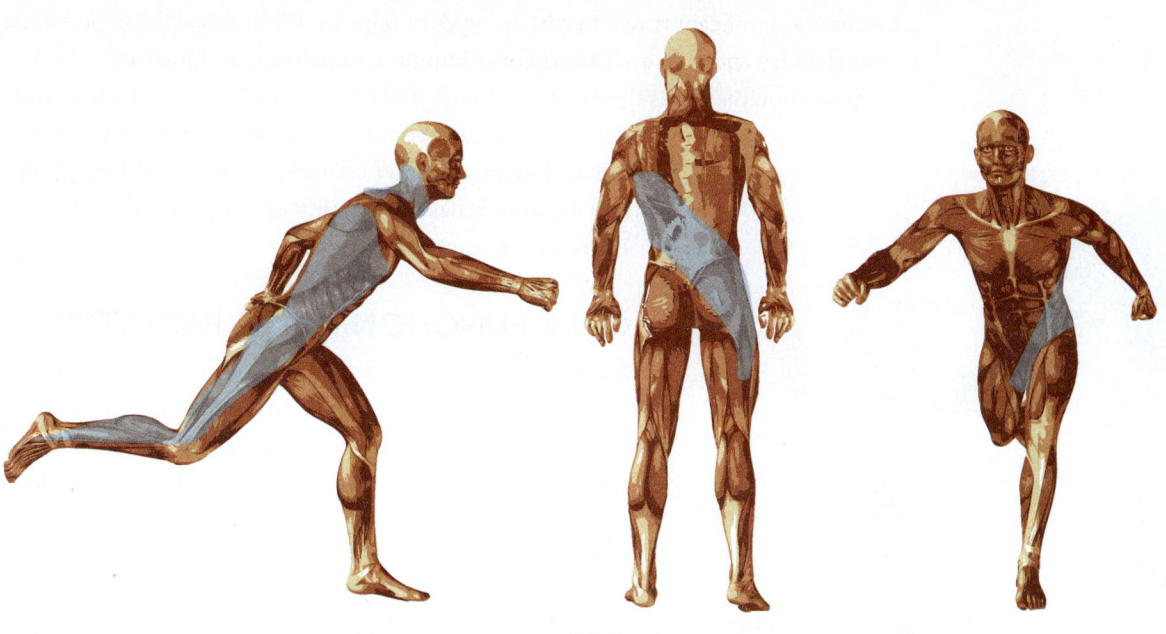

Lateral Sling   Posterior Oblique Sling   Anterior Oblique Sling

FIGURE 10.6 Functional Systems

The posterior oblique sling links the latissimus dorsi, thoracolumbar fascia, and contralateral gluteus maximus. This sling helps coordinate upper- and lower-body movements, transfers force, and provides stability during various activities, such as walking, running, and throwing.

The lateral sling comprises the gluteus medius, gluteus minimus, tensor fascia latae, and iliotibial band (ITB). These structures work together to stabilize the pelvis during weight-bearing activities, particularly when the body is on one leg—for example, when walking, running, or standing on one foot.

The fascial sling system can be integrated into core training exercises by adding bands around the extremities that link to the core to facilitate the fascial tension and enhance dynamic core stabilization and single-leg exercises (Neumann, 2017). For instance, medicine ball lifts and chops (with bands that attach to the core and diagonally to the extremities) can facilitate fascial sling function and enhance elastic energy transfer through the core.

LESSON 3: THE SCIENCE OF CORE TRAINING
SCIENTIFIC RATIONALE FOR CORE TRAINING

Core training is widely recognized as essential to athletic performance and injury prevention. The scientific rationale behind core training for athletes lies in the understanding that the core is the central link connecting the upper and lower extremities. A strong and stable core enables efficient force transfer between these regions, contributing to optimal performance in sports and activities. Incorporating core training into an athlete's regimen promotes better biomechanics, balance, and stability during dynamic movements during sport-specific skills and while training. However, a poor-performing core poses a significant threat to certain types of injuries. Within the athlete population, previous injury and pain are factors contributing to impaired core function.

This section discusses the impact of injury and pain on core muscle function and examines how a suboptimal functioning core can lead to reduced neuromuscular control and increased risk of injury. It also explores how core training can improve the function of the LPHC and minimize injury risk.

CORE FUNCTION IN THE PAIN STATE

Many athletes train their core muscles inadequately by targeting specific muscle functions. Additionally, some athletes do not address dysfunction caused by previous injuries or the particular needs of their sport (Hamza, 2013). As previously mentioned, understanding how the core muscles function during an athlete's sporting movements is critical for the Sports Performance Coach when preparing a training program, especially when determining how to reduce the risk of injury.

The prevalence of lower back pain (LBP) among athletes varies depending on the specific sport, the level of competition,

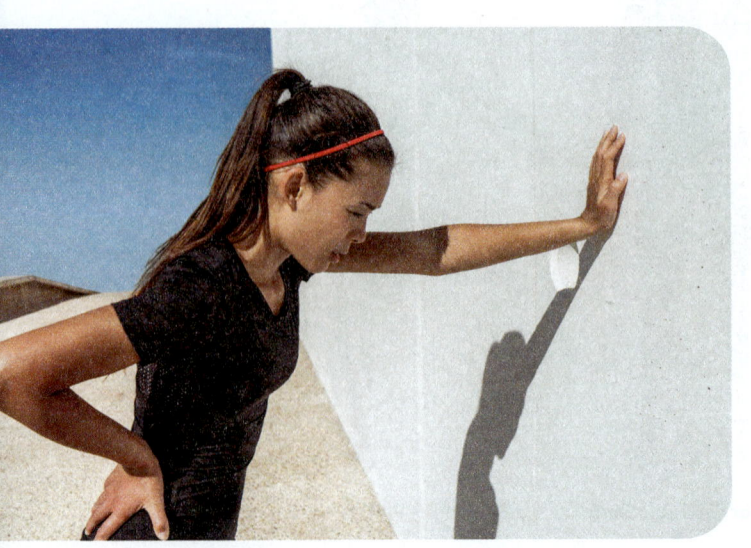

© Maridav/Shutterstock

and the population being studied. However, LBP is a common issue among athletes, especially those involved in sports that require repetitive movements, heavy lifting, or twisting motions. Chronic LBP has been shown to delay the timing and impair the activation of the core stabilizer muscles such as the transversus abdominis, internal oblique, and multifidus during low-threshold tasks (Hodges et al., 1996; O'Sullivan et al., 1998; Richardson et al., 2002).

In addition, in individuals with LBP, core movement system muscles such as erector spinae or the hamstring muscles can go into a protective spasm to brace and prevent additional movement that may irritate the injured area. Concurrently, the activation of deep local core stabilizers can be impaired due to their proximity to the inflamed joints. Unfortunately, these protective mechanisms and altered muscle recruitment strategies sometimes persist even when LBP has ceased and the individual has recovered from the injury (Hodges et al., 1996; O'Sullivan et al., 1998; Richardson et al., 2002).

Hungerford et al. (2003) found a delay in firing of the internal oblique, multifidus, and gluteus maximus in the stance leg of patients with sacroiliac joint pain. Laasonen (1984) found 10% to 30% more paraspinal atrophy in patients with LBP on the affected side compared to the unaffected side. In addition, it has been demonstrated that the multifidus atrophies on the affected side in patients with LBP (Hides et al., 1996; Rantanen et al., 1993).

The loss of muscle size in the core region has been associated with more severe injuries. In one study, a motor control exercise that increased the size and function of the multifidus resulted in fewer games missed due to injury in Australian rules football (Hrysomallis, 2013). Several studies have also demonstrated that individuals with LBP have weaker back extensor muscles (Iwai et al., 2004) and decreased muscle endurance (Jørgensen & Nicolaisen, 1987; McGill, 2002).

Moreover, core muscle weakness is a known risk factor for developing LBP (Lee et al., 1999). However, the Sports Performance Coach must be aware that focusing on core strengthening in isolation may not be adequate for reducing the risk of LBP. Including exercises that improve the reaction speed and proprioception of the core muscles may also be necessary when developing a core program for an athlete, especially one who has recently recovered from a lower back injury.

There is also a close link between core stabilization and posture, balance, and proprioception of the LPHC. Individuals with LBP have altered postural control when compared to healthy controls. Notably, the single-leg balance in individuals with LBP is less efficient and effective than in healthy controls (Ebenbichler et al., 2001). In fact, individuals with LBP have failure rates more than four times that of controls in tasks involving bilateral standing with closed eyes (Mok et al., 2004).

Individuals with LBP also perform more poorly on unexpected balance challenges. With unexpected perturbations (balance challenges), the lumbar paraspinal muscles in individuals with LBP react significantly more slowly than those in healthy controls owing to their altered feed-forward mechanisms (Wilder et al., 1996). It has also been demonstrated that individuals with LBP have altered spinal proprioception (Leinon et al., 2003; O'Sullivan et al., 1998; O'Sullivan et al., 2002).

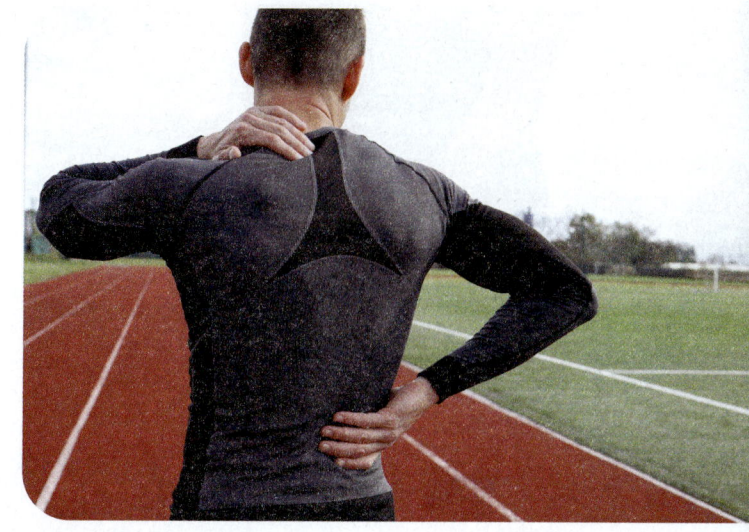

© Albina Gavrilovic/Shutterstock

Accordingly, the Sports Performance Coach must recognize the impact of pain from a previous injury on core muscle function and its influence on exercise selection when programming. As just discussed, altered core muscle recruitment strategies from protective mechanisms may persist in an athlete when pain is no longer present and the athlete has fully recovered from the injury. If not addressed, these altered strategies can reduce the athlete's available movement options due to the inappropriate bracing, reducing their ability to adjust their actions to the varying situations they face.

The Sports Performance Coach can restore movement capabilities after injury by including exercises focusing on movement skills and coordination, such as dissociation exercises. In addition, they should collaborate with the sports medicine staff when training an athlete who has recently recovered from an LPHC injury. Exercises that are integrated with the medical team's approach and avoidance of too advanced or inappropriate exercises should be part of the program. Creating a core training program with targeted exercises that address the negative impact of a previous injury will help restore core function and avoid future injury.

CORE TRAINING FOR INJURY RESISTANCE

Poor control of the LPHC through suboptimal core muscle performance has been shown to influence the risk of injury (Hewett et al., 2009; Hughes, 2014; Jamison et al., 2012; Jamison et al., 2013; Noehren et al., 2014; Paterno et al., 2010; Read et al., 2016; Taylor et al., 2017). Reduced ability of the core to control movements of the LPHC while landing or changing direction in cutting scenarios increases spine and knee loading, increasing the risk of anterior cruciate ligament (ACL) injuries. The hip musculature is a critical component of the LPHC, and poor hip flexion control deficits (hip extensor weakness) are a risk factor for developing LBP (Nadler, Malanga, Feinberg, et al., 2002).

Deficits of as much as 26% of hip abductor strength and 36% of hip external rotator strength, causing reduced control of hip internal rotation, have been identified as a factor in females with knee pain (Ireland et al., 2003). Decreased hip abduction strength and poor hip adduction control usually follow a simple ankle sprain (Friel et al., 2006).

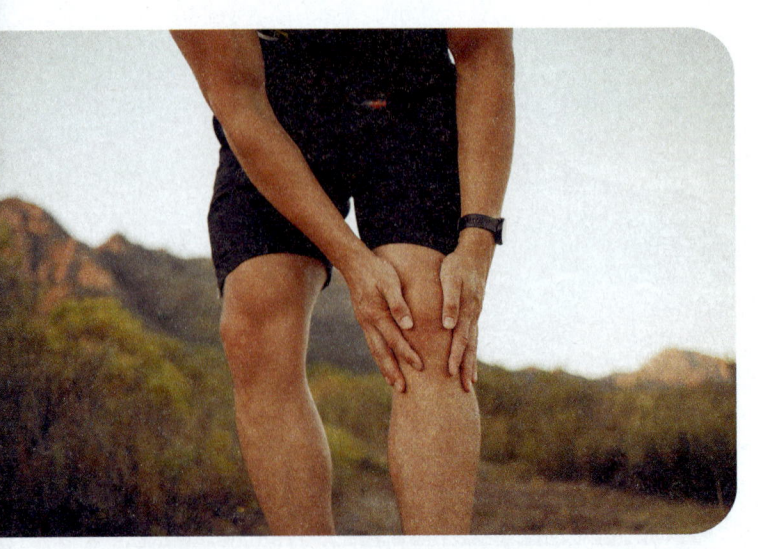

Concurrently, suboptimal neural control of the LPHC through a weakness in hip external rotators can cause reduced relative tibial external rotation control, leading to increased subtalar joint pronation and potential ankle and foot issues (Khamis & Yizhar, 2007; Youdas et al., 2006). Fredericson et al. (2000) also reported that runners with ITB syndrome had weaker hip abduction strength than healthy controls.

Poor performance in LPHC movement control tests is associated with an increased risk of dancers' lower-extremity and lumbar spine injuries (Roussel et al., 2009). In this highly interdependent system, an inability to control motion in one region of the LPHC in a specific direction can lead to a predictable injury pattern in another region. Given this relationship, an athlete with optimal core control of the LPHC can reduce the risk of injury in other areas of their body. This factor has important implications when designing a sports performance training program. The program should address direction-specific movement control deficits and target the appropriate core muscles.

DRAWING IN AND ABDOMINAL BRACING

Drawing-in (abdominal hollowing), also known as the **drawing-in maneuver**, is used to recruit the local core stabilizers by pulling the navel in toward the spine. This technique increases the activation of the local spinal stabilizers (Kim & Oh, 2015; Lee et al., 2013; Lee et al., 2016; Suehiro et al., 2014) and enhances lumbopelvic stability by creating tension in the thoracolumbar fascia (**Figure 10.7**), while simultaneously minimizing the activation of global muscle activity during exercise (Kahlaee et al., 2017; Suehiro et al., 2014).

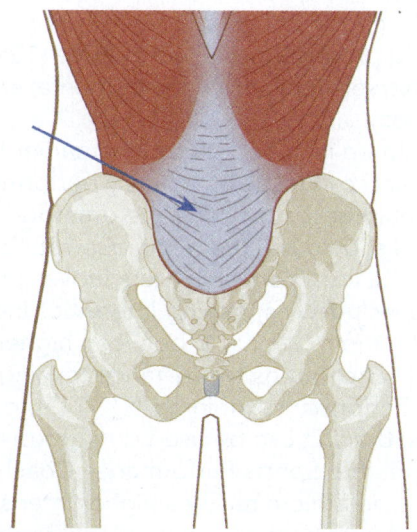

FIGURE 10.7 Thoracolumbar Fascia

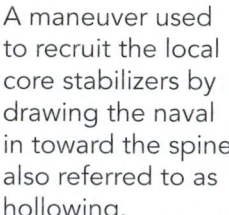

DRAWING-IN →
MANEUVER

A maneuver used to recruit the local core stabilizers by drawing the naval in toward the spine; also referred to as hollowing.

Bracing is a core stabilization technique that contracts the local and global muscles at the same time. Bracing is performed by stiffening the abdominal wall and pushing the abdomen out externally (Barnett & Gilleard, 2005). When it is performed correctly, the athlete uses the breath to increase intra-abdominal pressure, resulting in increased spinal stabilization.

Some researchers have claimed that bracing results in greater spinal stabilization than the drawing-in maneuver (Grenier & McGill, 2007). For example, Urquhart et al. (2005) found that bracing resulted in greater activation of the external obliques and rectus abdominis and caused a co-contraction of multiple core muscles during specific exercises. However, bracing alone may not simultaneously activate critical local core muscles. Indeed, Allison et al. (1998) found greater transverse abdominis and internal oblique activation in subjects performing the drawing-in maneuver compared to bracing.

Bracing is a core stabilization technique that inherently goes together with increased training loads. For example, athletes performing very heavy lifts for minimal repetitions frequently hold their breath at specific points in the movement—a process known as the **Valsalva maneuver**. Hackett and Chow (2013) suggested that loads more than 80% of maximal intensity generally require a brief moment of holding breath to generate a spike in intra-abdominal pressure that allows the athlete to exert more force and increase spinal stability and trunk rigidity.

BRACING →

A core stabilization technique that contracts the local and global muscles at the same time by stiffening the abdominal wall and pushing the abdomen out externally.

VALSALVA →
MANEUVER

A process that involves expiring against a closed windpipe, creating additional intra-abdominal pressure and spinal stability.

The drawing-in maneuver and abdominal bracing are frequently used during core training and can positively impact spinal stability and pain management. In addition, both are widely used by therapists, physicians, and Sports Performance Coaches to benefit individuals with lumbar instability (Vaičienė et al., 2018). These techniques provide spinal stability via different mechanisms, and both should be included in the overall integrated training program.

The drawing-in maneuver should be used initially to increase the awareness and function of local core stabilizers. Ideally, local core stabilizers, such as the transverse abdominis, should function subconsciously, providing the stability needed for any given task. However, due to the sedentary nature of modern society (even some of the most active athletes may still be considered "sedentary" when considering the abundance of movement that humans are capable of), the local core stabilizers may begin to lose the ability to respond quickly. The local core stabilizers are not a muscle group that needs to be inherently strong. Instead, they should produce low levels of force (10% to 25% of maximal voluntary contraction [MVC]) quickly, providing intervertebral and intersegmental stability before any other movement (i.e., proximal to distal stabilization).

For this reason, the drawing-in maneuver should be included during the earlier training phases, when the athlete is exposed to lighter intensities and can focus on actively performing the technique. In many cases, the Sports Performance Coach should begin teaching the drawing-in maneuver with the athlete in a supine and calm position, and should link the technique with breathing. When performed appropriately, over time, activation of the local core stabilizers moves from a conscious to a subconscious level, making way for bracing to be included as training intensities increase.

The Sports Performance Coach should consider the relationship between higher-intensity lifting and bracing when designing core training programs. Higher-intensity resistance training is generally not experienced in the early phases of the Optimum Performance Training™ (OPT) Model. Thus, bracing is not required or suggested during these phases. Bracing can be used during resistance training exercises that exceed approximately 75%. However, the Sports Performance Coach can begin teaching the bracing technique during core training before the athlete reaches higher intensities. Generally, after an athlete progresses through many ground-based core exercises (e.g., plank, bridge) and reaches loaded core training in functional positions (e.g., farmer's carry, landmines), bracing should be the recommended core stabilization technique.

LESSON 4: PRINCIPLES OF CORE TRAINING

CORE TRAINING GUIDELINES

Research has demonstrated that specific core training programs can decrease pain and improve both function and performance (Smart et al., 2011). Numerous studies support the role of core training in injury prevention and rehabilitation. Core stabilizer–specific exercises restore the size, activation, and endurance of the multifidus in individuals with LBP (Hides et al., 2001). Using exercises that bias the core global stabilizer muscles to address direction-specific motion control deficits of the LPHC (such as a low back extension or lateral flexion) has been shown to significantly improve LPHC motion after a six-week program (Mendiguchia et al., 2021).

NEEDS ANALYSIS AND ASSESSMENT INFORMATION

Core training should be based on a needs analysis to ensure that the exercises and interventions are tailored to an athlete's specific requirements, goals, and limitations.

An individualized approach helps optimize the training process, improving core strength, stability, and overall performance.

A needs analysis is also a vital step in designing an effective core training program because it helps the Sports Performance Coach understand the unique demands of the athlete's sport and position. Further, conducting movement assessments and sport-specific testing can help identify which core capabilities (stabilization, endurance, strength, or power) an athlete may need to focus on.

Lastly, an athlete's injury history must be considered. As mentioned earlier, either previous or current LBP may adversely affect core muscle activation and timing.

© Matimix/Shutterstock

PROGRESSING CORE TRAINING

An effective core training program should incorporate a diverse range of techniques in a structured and progressive manner. This comprehensive approach progresses through a **neural continuum** (**Table 10.4**), encompassing various stages through the manipulation of training variables. In simple terms, the neural continuum suggests that exercises should begin easy and progress to continually challenge the athlete by increasing their difficulty and complexity through manipulating planes and range of motion (ROM), types of resistance, body position, speed, duration, frequency, and intensity. Collectively, the continuum allows for a wide array of exercises that can be adjusted to progress any level of athlete. (Note that this is not an exhaustive list of all potential training variables.)

> **NEURAL CONTINUUM** →
>
> A spectrum of neural involvement in muscular activation, ranging from low to high levels of neural drive.

TABLE 10.4 Example of Core Training Variables

Exercise Selection	Variables
• Safe	• Plane of motion
• Progressive	• Range of motion
• Simple to complex	• Type of resistance
• Stable to unstable	• Stability ball
• Static to dynamic	• Cable
• Known to unknown	• Tubing
• Single task to dual task	• Medicine ball
• Activity/goal-specific	• Dumbbells
• Proprioceptively challenging	• Body position
• Floor	• Supine
• Foam pad	• Prone
• Half foam roll	• Kneeling
• Stability ball	• Half kneeling
• Wobble board	• Standing
• Rotation discs	• Feedback
	• External feedback
	• Internal feedback

Four distinct stages can be implemented to fully harness the advantages of the neural continuum. Stage 1 focuses on foundational motor control core training, stage 2 provides advanced motor control core training, stage 3 emphasizes strength-biased core training, and stage 4 comprises integrated core training.

STAGE 1: FOUNDATIONAL MOTOR CONTROL CORE TRAINING

This stage aims to help the athlete "find" and increase their awareness of the local and global stabilizer muscles through cognitive activation, dissociation, and unstable surface exercises. Such training increases the dominance of stabilizer muscles with stabilizing tasks and improves proximal to distal activation sequencing, reaction speed, and proprioceptive awareness to maintain a core neutral position.

Attaining reasonable motor control ensures that the athlete can maintain intervertebral stability. In addition, the athlete must activate the core stabilizer muscles and be able to dissociate the columns without losing the core's neutral position before loading in a stable position. Progressions within this stage include increasing complexity with decreased stability, movement of limbs, and dissociation exercises.

STAGE 2: ADVANCED MOTOR CONTROL CORE TRAINING

Once an athlete can effectively activate the core stabilizer muscles to control the neutral position, the global stabilizer and movement system muscles can be trained using load to increase core strength without compromising stability. This stage can be described as consisting of two phases, which ensure ideal sequencing to optimize function. Advanced motor control builds upon motor control core training by enhancing the athlete's ability to isometrically resist forces in all planes of motion without losing intervertebral stability and keeping a neutral position. This helps to improve the athlete's core stiffness and momentum control. Progressions in this stage include increasing external load and decreasing external stabilization.

STAGE 3: STRENGTH-BIASED CORE TRAINING

Once the athlete develops isometric strength in the neutral position, strengthening out of the neutral position can be introduced. This develops the athlete's ability to control forces, thereby enhancing lumbopelvic stability and improving movement competency through a full range of spinal motion. Developing core strength through a full range of motion is also crucial to adequately prepare the athlete for power-based core exercises that utilize explosive movements that can transfer to the athlete's sport-specific actions. Progressions in this stage include increasing complexity of the movement and external load.

STAGE 4: INTEGRATION-BIASED CORE TRAINING

This stage aims to transfer core activation and strength adaptations to functional activities. The athlete must be able to load the core in stable positions and effectively control forces through the appropriate ranges of motion before transferring them into functional patterns. Exercises that train proximal to distal firing patterns and maximize facial sling tension should be integrated with this stage to optimize the core's elastic power, which should transfer specifically to the athlete's sport-specific actions to increase their explosivity. Progressions in this stage include adjusting the specificity of the movements to translate to the athlete's sport.

ACUTE TRAINING VARIABLES FOR CORE TRAINING

The Sports Performance Coach must ensure that all programs follow recommended acute training variables for core training.

SETS AND REPETITIONS

Sets and repetitions are vital components of core training for athletes, as they determine the volume and structure of the workout, directly impacting the development of strength, endurance, and overall performance. By incorporating a well-designed combination of sets and repetitions into their training, athletes can effectively target specific muscle groups and tailor their training program to meet the unique demands of their respective sport(s). Adhering to appropriate sets and repetitions ensures that core training remains challenging yet manageable, allowing for consistent progress while minimizing the risk of overtraining or injury. Carefully planned sets and repetitions during core training contribute to an athlete's ability to build a strong, stable, and efficient core, which is essential for optimal performance across a wide range of sports. **Table 10.5** provides an overview of set and repetition guidelines for core training.

TABLE 10.5 Sets and Repetitions for Core Training

Stage of Core Training	Sets	Repetitions/Duration
Stage 1: Foundational motor control core training	1–3	12–20 repetitions; <10-second holds for isometrics
Stage 2: Advanced motor control training	2–3	12–20 repetitions; 30- to 90-second holds for isometrics
Stage 3: Strength-biased core training	2–4	8–12 repetitions
Stage 4: Integration-biased core training	1–4	8–12 repetitions Sport-specific training: 4–6 explosive repetitions

INTENSITY

The intensity of core training plays a crucial role in achieving the desired performance outcomes, as it directly influences development of muscle stabilization, endurance, and strength. By progressively challenging the core muscles with an appropriate level of intensity, athletes can stimulate muscle adaptation and growth, leading to improved stability, posture, and overall performance. Moreover, working at an optimal intensity helps to prevent plateaus in progress, ensuring continuous improvements in performance. However, it is essential to balance intensity with proper form and technique to minimize the risk of injury and maximize the effectiveness of each exercise. Recommended intensities vary based on athlete experience, injury history, and assessment results. In most cases, the intensity of core exercises should be increased by adjusting the complexity of the exercise, neural demand, spinal ROM, and tempo rather than increasing load. **Table 10.6** provides general recommendations.

TABLE 10.6 General Intensities for Core Training

Stage of Core Training	Intensity
Stage 1: Foundational motor control core training	Bodyweight activation; <25% maximal contraction.
Stage 2: Advanced motor control core training	Bodyweight activation; <25% maximal contraction. Intensity is increased by altering body position or adding external equipment.
Stage 3: Strength-biased core training	Bodyweight. Increased spinal ROM. External load can be increased when using equipment (e.g., cables).
Stage 4: Integration-biased core training	Medicine ball <10% bodyweight. Intensity is increased through increased tempo, rate of force production, and complexity of exercises.

TRAINING FREQUENCY

A well-planned training schedule ensures that core muscles are consistently and progressively challenged, allowing for the necessary adaptations to occur, while also providing ample time for recovery and repair. By striking the right balance between training and recovery, athletes can prevent overtraining, reduce the risk of injuries, and maximize the benefits of core training. In essence, the frequency of core training is a critical factor in enabling athletes to achieve peak performance, enhance their competitive edge, and maintain a high level of functional fitness.

TRAINING VOLUME

The volume of core training is a key factor for athletes, as it determines the overall workload. A well-calibrated training volume ensures that core muscles are sufficiently stimulated to trigger necessary adaptations, while allowing for adequate recovery and repair. By finding the optimal balance between training intensity and volume, athletes can experience continuous progress in their core development, leading to improved performance across a wide range of sports. Moreover, appropriate training volume helps to prevent overtraining, reduces the risk of injuries, and contributes to a more sustainable and effective core training program.

The Sports Performance Coach must recognize that the core muscles are subject to load and stress during the duration of training sessions. For example, a traditional strength development exercise, such as a deadlift, requires significant core muscle activation. Therefore, the general frequency and volume guidelines recommended in **Table 10.7** must be adjusted for each athlete to reflect their total training demand. For this reason, many Sports Performance Coaches may choose to alternate core training and other resistance training days.

TABLE 10.7   Frequency and Volume for Core Training

Stage of Core Training	Frequency	Volume
Stage 1: Foundational motor control core training	2–3 times per day 4–6 variable sessions per week	36–75 repetitions per exercise
Stage 2: Advanced motor control core training	5–7 variable sessions per week	36–75 repetitions per exercise
Stage 3: Strength-biased core training	2–5 variable sessions per week	18–24 repetitions per exercise
Stage 4: Integration-biased core training	2–5 variable sessions per week	15–30 repetitions per exercise

LESSON 5: MOTOR CONTROL AND STRENGTH-BIASED CORE TRAINING

FOUNDATIONAL MOTOR CONTROL CORE TRAINING

The starting point of all core training is to teach the athlete how to "find" the neutral core position and activate the core stabilizers using the drawing-in maneuver. The drawing-in maneuver increases self-awareness of the local and global stabilizers and improves their function to enhance intervertebral stability. This maneuver should be performed in various positions. In this stage, it is best to begin in a supine or crook-lying position. The crook-lying position is supine with knees bent and feet flat on the floor, which takes the tension off the hip flexors, potentially making it easier for the athlete to maintain a neutral pelvis.

Once the athlete can activate the local core muscles, they should progress by extending the legs while maintaining a neutral pelvis and spine position. One way to find the neutral core position is to have the athlete fully anterior tilt the pelvis (create a gap between the floor and the lower back) and then posteriorly tilt the pelvis (flatten the lower back, so there is no gap), and then find the midpoint between the two positions. Once the core neutral position has been found, the athlete can perform a slight drawing-in of the abdominals (approximately 25% MVC) to increase the activation of transversus abdominis, internal oblique, and tensioning of the thoracolumbar fascia (TLF), which connects into the deep multifidus.

The athlete can begin by working on drawing in and then holding while they breathe normally. This will aid in improving the sensitivity of proximal to distal activation sequencing of the core stabilizers and targets slow-twitch fibers and muscular endurance adaptations of these deep core muscles (like a software upgrade). Once 10-second holds with relaxed breathing can be achieved, progressions can include performing in different positions, such as bridging, side-lying, prone, quadruped, quadruped rocking, sitting, and standing in the universal athletic position.

The next progression within motor control core training is to challenge the athlete in the core neutral position by introducing activation of the global stabilizers through asymmetrical limb loading and dissociation exercises. Asymmetrical limb loading exercises can be performed in supine or crook-lying (hook-lying) positions and include bent knee fallouts, leg slides, dead bugs, and bridge variations or from a quadruped position with bird dog variations. Dissociation exercises include several variations and can be performed from any position, such as thoracic spine rotation over a stationary pelvis, flexion and extension of the thoracic spine over a stationary pelvis, and lateral flexion of the thoracic spine over a stationary pelvis.

Another variation of dissociation exercise involves rotating the hips and pelvis under a stationary thoracic spine. However, the athlete must continue to focus on core activation during asymmetrical limb loading or dissociation exercises rather than shifting focus to the movement. Again, the goal is to introduce variations, allowing the athlete to maintain optimal activation and positioning.

The last progression for motor control core training is designed to improve proprioception, especially the deep core stabilizers' feed-forward activation mechanism (reaction speed). This is accomplished by adding an unstable base, such as foam rollers, wobble boards, or rotation discs, under the athlete's base of support. These exercises all have a low threshold and are designed to progress by challenging motor control and muscular endurance.

Progressions in motor control core training should not be fatiguing. Ideally, exercises should be recommended more frequently throughout the day rather than a high volume performed all at once. Having an athlete perform these exercises two to three times per day on four to six days per week, with up to ten 10-second repetitions, is generally sufficient. Further, these exercises must be performed slowly with ideal posture while breathing diaphragmatically.

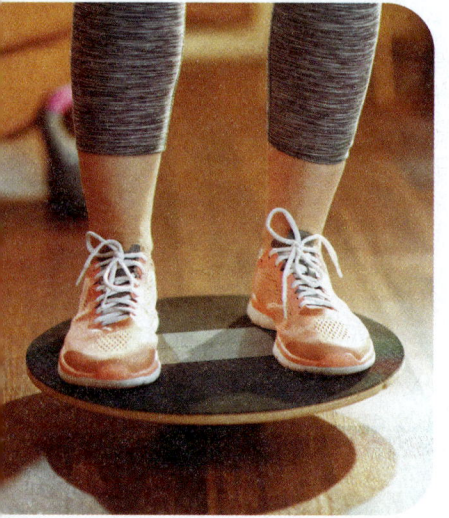

© Alliance Images/Shutterstock

FOUNDATIONAL MOTOR CONTROL CORE TRAINING EXERCISES

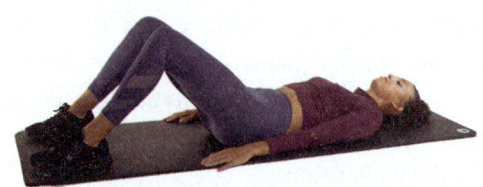

Crook-Lying Core Activation

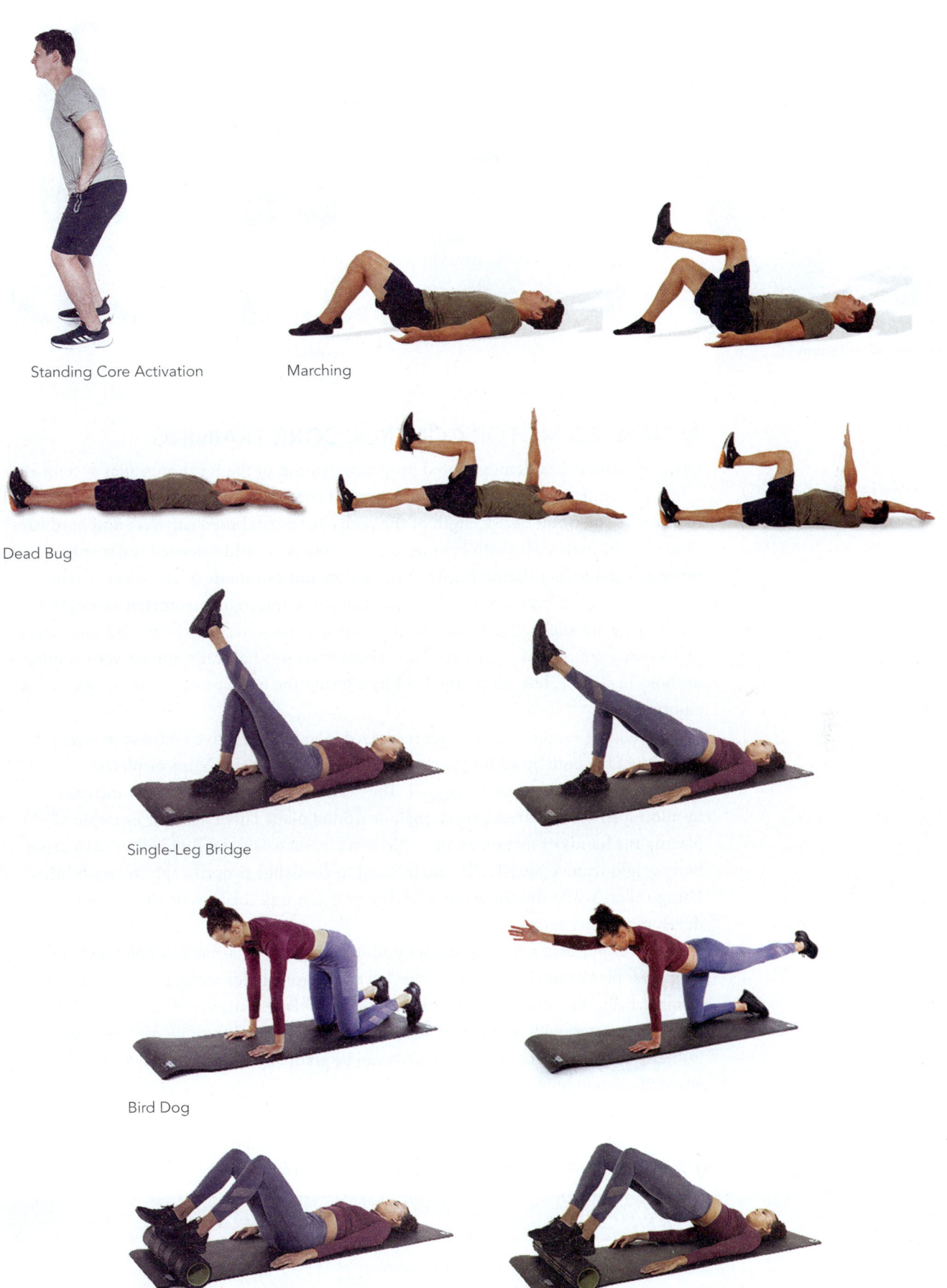

Standing Core Activation

Marching

Dead Bug

Single-Leg Bridge

Bird Dog

Bridge Feet on Roller with Hip Abduction

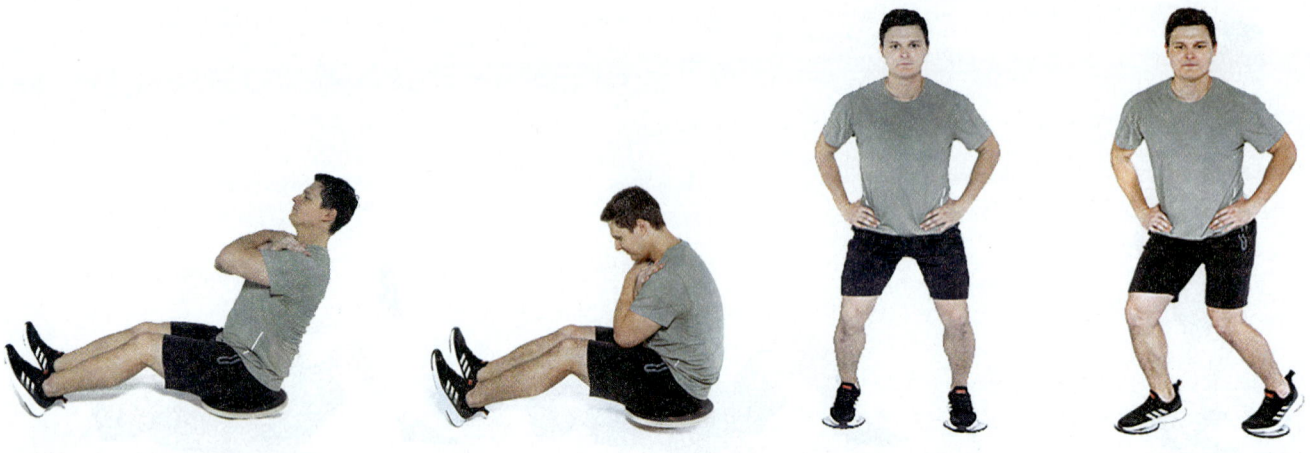

Wobble Board Seated Crunch

Standing Bilateral Hip Rotation

ADVANCED MOTOR CONTROL CORE TRAINING

Once the athlete has demonstrated proper activation of the local muscular system and achieved competency in maintaining a neutral core position, exercises can be designed to improve the isometric strength of the core (like a combined software and hardware upgrade). Isometric strength is imperative in sports, as athletes need the trunk to serve as a stable foundation for force reduction and production. Therefore, these exercises focus on keeping the LPHC neutral while improving isometric strength; side-lying clam shells, fire hydrants, quadruped variations, and short- and long-lever planks are examples of these exercises. These exercises naturally appear very similar to those in stage 1, but add to the load by altering the body position or using external equipment.

These same exercises can target increased isometric reactive stiffness or strength capacity of the core by adding perturbation or load, such as chains or plates, depending on the programming goal. They can bias the global stabilizer muscles by adding an asymmetrical, rotational, or frontal plane challenge. For example, placing the hands or feet on an unstable surface, such as a stability ball or suspension bodyweight trainer (i.e., TRX), can be used to challenge proprioception capabilities. Using rollers while simultaneously flexing or extending the hips or shoulders helps develop core strength.

These exercises can be progressed by adding longer lever arms. Examples include long-lever plank exercises and fixed-feet lateral or prone holds using a BOSU ball or a Roman chair. These exercises target isometric muscular endurance of the core and, for this purpose, can start with 30 seconds of isometric holds or until the core neutral position is lost. Two to three sets of 30-second holds can be gradually built up to two to three sets of 60- to 90-second holds (**Table 10.8**).

TABLE 10.8 Acute Training Variables for Advanced Motor Control Core Training

Focus of Exercise	Primary Action	Training Variables
Isometric strength and endurance	Core stabilization: drawing-in maneuver	1–4 exercises 2–3 sets of 30- to 90-second holds, or 12–20 reps

The last progression of advanced motor control core training is to further challenge isometric strength in functional positions. It is beneficial for athletes to perform core exercises in a standing position because these motor patterns are commonly used in sporting activities. These exercises develop the athlete's ability to isometrically resist, reduce, or produce forces in all three planes in an upright position. The single-arm farmer's carry is an excellent example of an exercise to develop core neutral control against lateral forces. The Pallof press with resistance bands or cables also develops core neutral strength to control lateral and rotational forces, which is essential for most athletes. Resistance can also be increased with this exercise to elicit further strength adaptations. Again, two to three sets of 12 to 20 repetitions are appropriate. This exercise can also be modified into an LPHC rotation dissociation exercise by holding the press position while keeping the LPHC completely still and moving the upper back into rotation or lateral flexion. Exercises that target isometric reactive stiffness against momentum during functional movement patterns include side steps, drop steps, and lunges using slosh pipes or aqua bags across the shoulders. These tools create perturbation that challenges the core to control momentum forces; the ability to control momentum is an essential quality for an athlete to develop.

ADVANCED MOTOR CONTROL CORE TRAINING EXERCISES

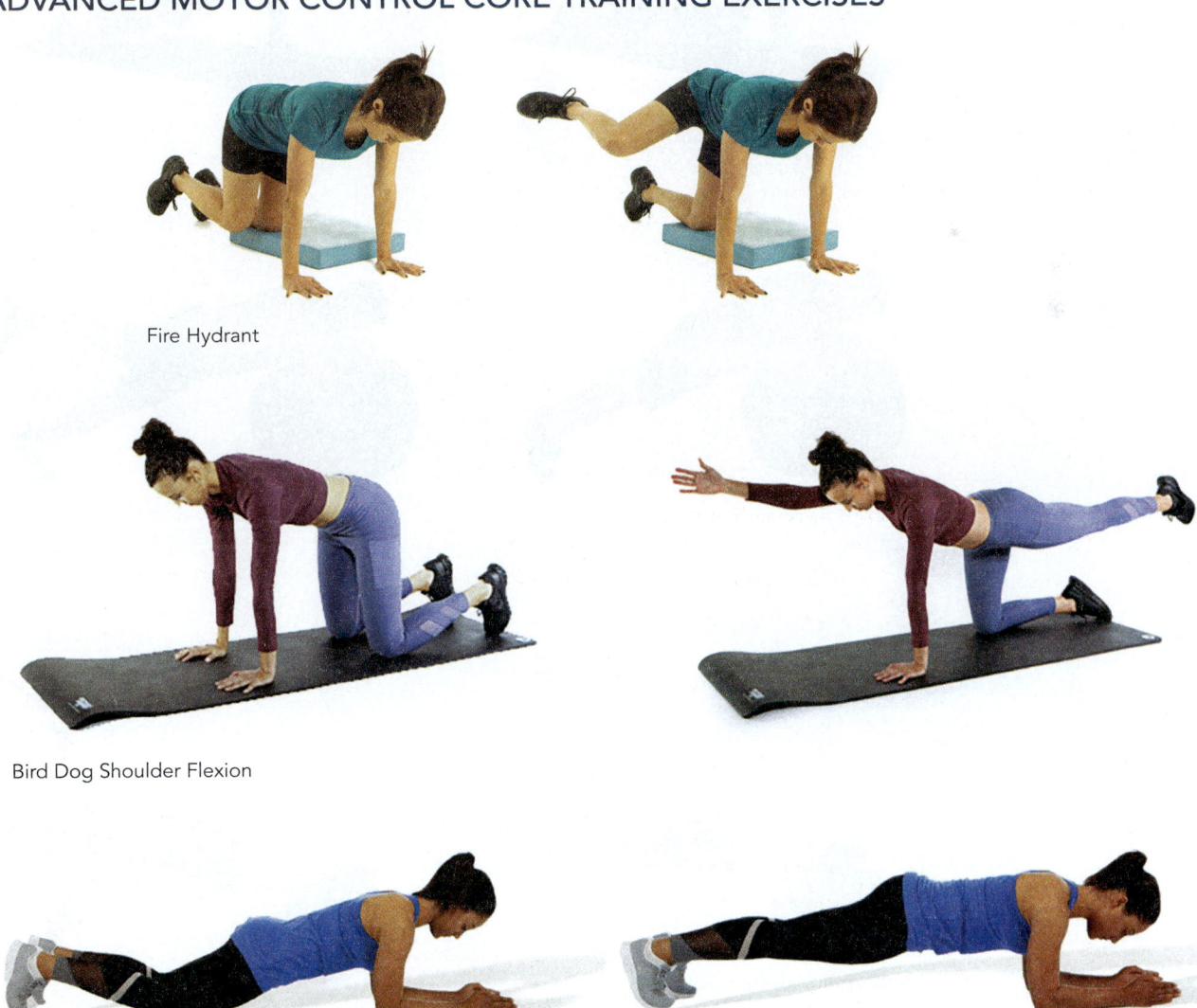

Fire Hydrant

Bird Dog Shoulder Flexion

Plank

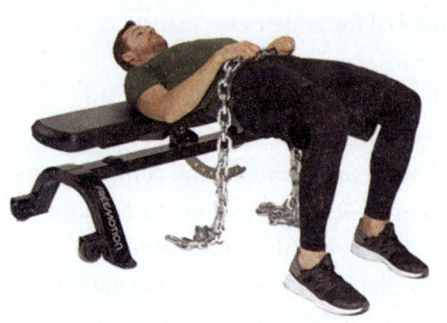
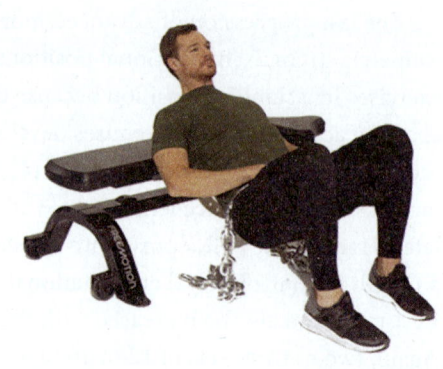

Bench Bridge Chains over Waist

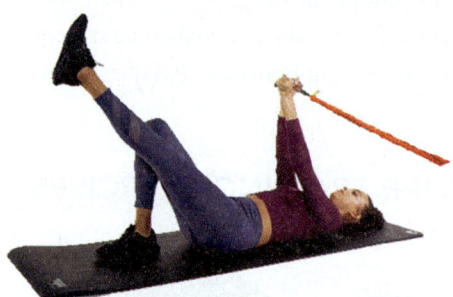
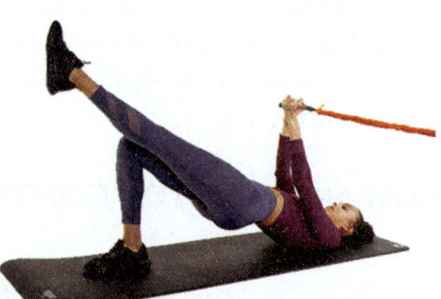

Single-Leg Bridge Perturbation

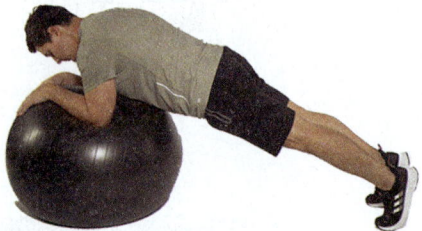
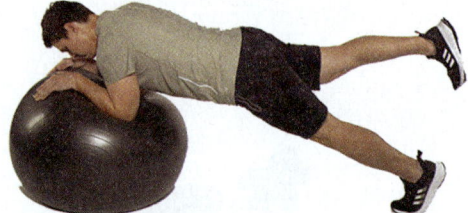

Stability Ball Plank Progression

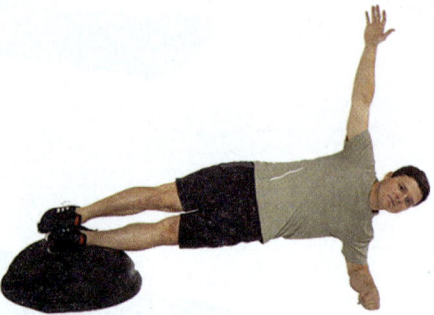
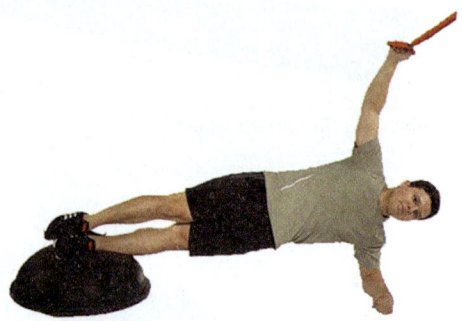

Side Plank with Perturbation

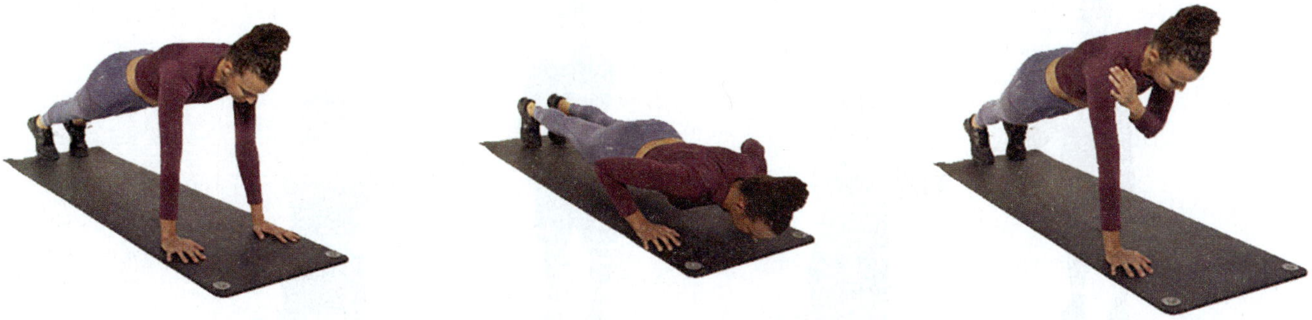

Shoulder Tap Push-ups

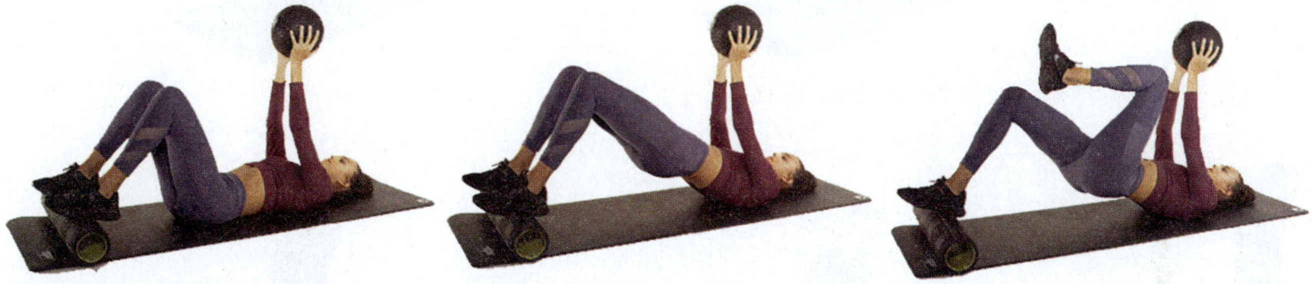

Feet Roller Medicine Ball Stabilization

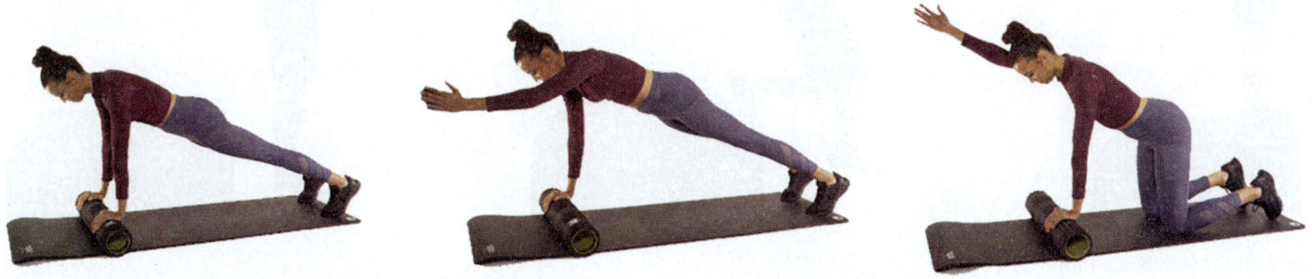

Hands on Roller with Shoulder Flexion

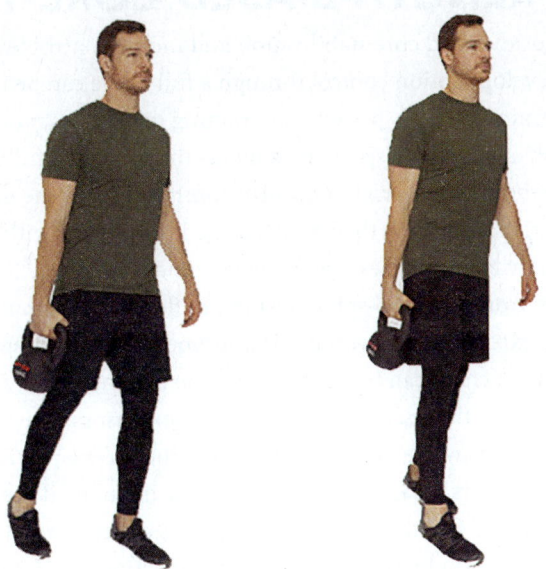

Single-Arm Farmer's Carry

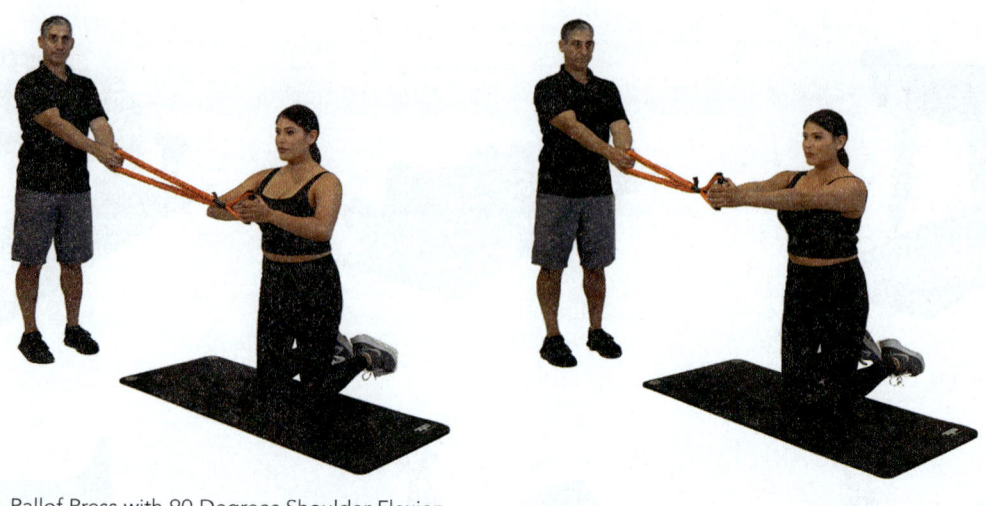

Pallof Press with 90 Degrees Shoulder Flexion

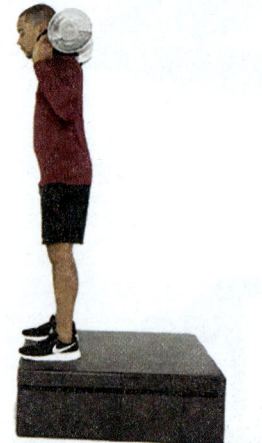
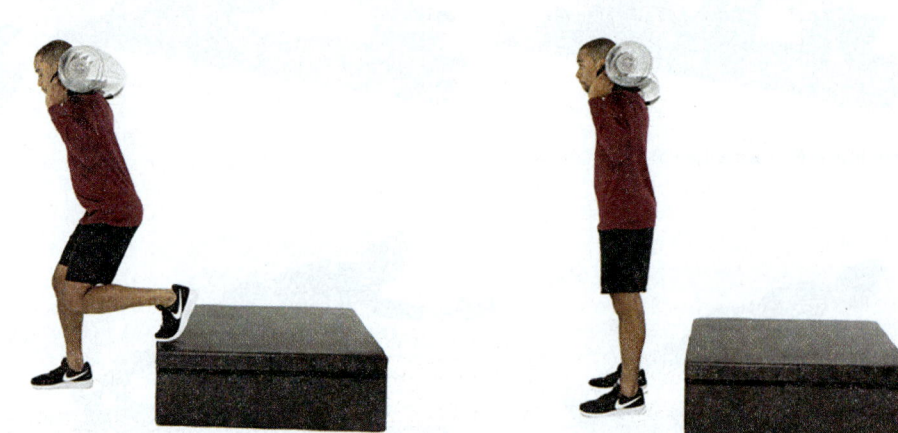

Drop Steps with Aqua Bag

STRENGTH-BIASED CORE TRAINING

Once advanced core stabilization and motor control levels have been achieved, exercises to develop motion control through a full range can be integrated into the athlete's training program. Strength-biased core training introduces more traditional core strengthening involving dynamic spine movements throughout a full ROM. These exercises can also help the athlete learn to optimize control of the spine in various positions that may be experienced during their sport. Seated roll-downs with or without holding a medicine ball, stability ball crunches, and reverse crunches are excellent ways to train the abdominals to move from a neutral spine position to flexed, or from flexed to a neutral spine position. Back extensions and variations of prone positions integrating a sturdy object, such as a Roman chair, can be used to train the core in prone, supine, or lateral positions to strengthen the abdominals or the back extensors. The athlete must learn to perform these movements while maintaining the stability of the pelvis.

Transverse plane exercises should be included if the athlete demonstrates adequate sagittal and frontal plane control. Diagonal band or cable chops from low to high, or from high to low, in bilateral or split stance positions train the oblique abdominal core muscle to control rotational forces. Landmines are also a great way to train lateral flexion strength. These core exercises should be performed at a slow to moderate tempo with control to increase the time under tension and develop strength and peak force output (**Table 10.9**).

TABLE 10.9   Acute Training Variables for Strength-Biased Core Training

Focus of Exercise	Primary Action	Training Variables
Core strength	Dynamic eccentric and concentric movements	1–4 exercises 2–4 sets of 8–12 reps

✔ CHECK IT OUT

Diagonal bands, cable chops, and landmines can fit into strength-biased or advanced motor control core training. When these exercises are used in the strength-biased stage, the Sports Performance Coach should teach the athlete to include movement in the spine through an adequate ROM. Thus, for a cable chop, the rotation will be generated through the spine while the shoulders and arms remain relatively still. Similarly, the landmine should include lateral spinal flexion during the exercise. Conversely, when used in the advanced motor control stage, the athlete will demonstrate little to no movement in the spine during these exercises. Instead, the movement will be generated at the shoulder and arms, thereby increasing the stabilization demand of the local core musculature.

STRENGTH-BIASED CORE EXERCISES TRAINING

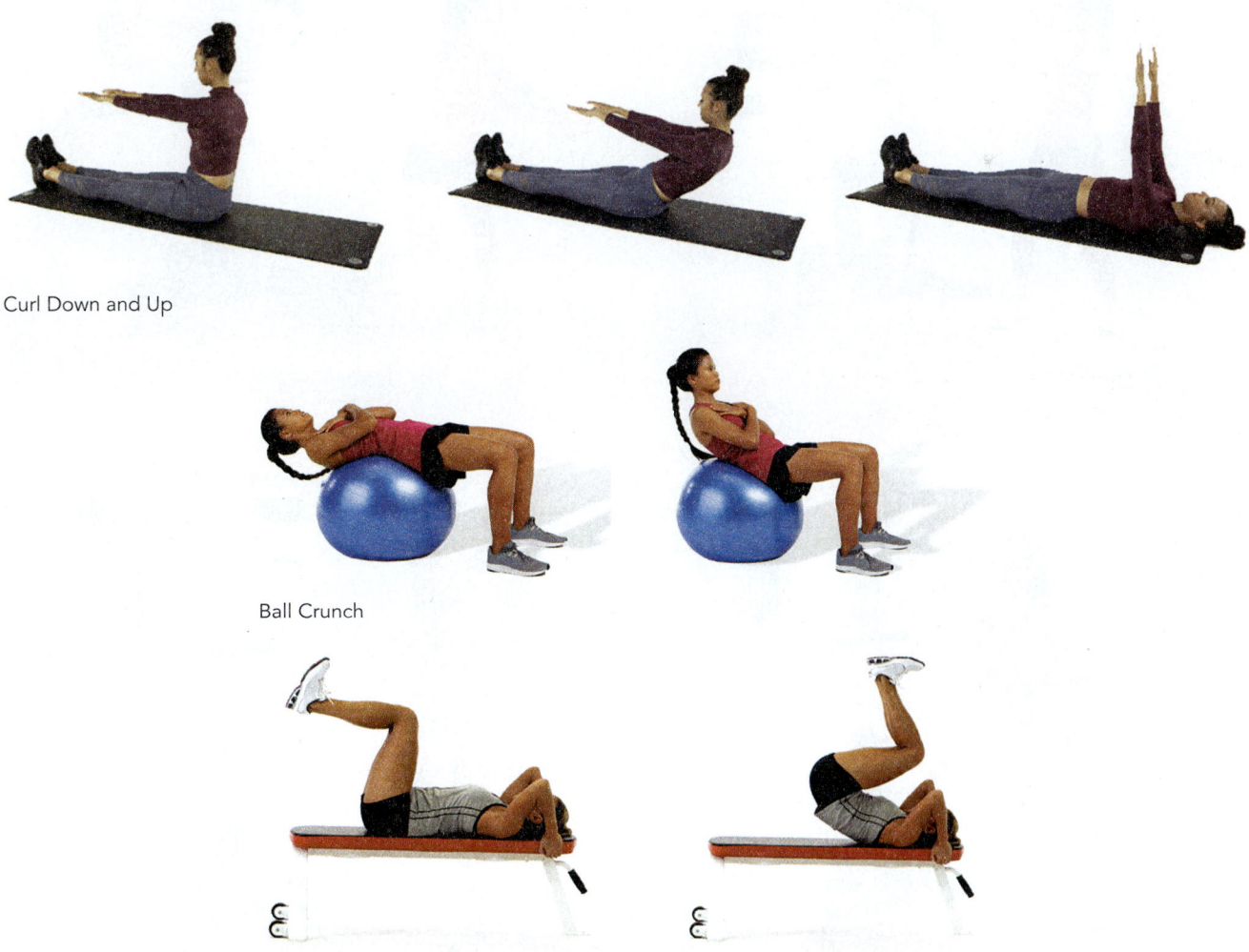

Curl Down and Up

Ball Crunch

Reverse Crunch

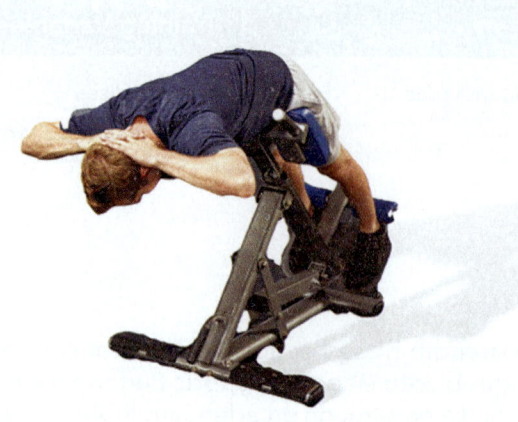
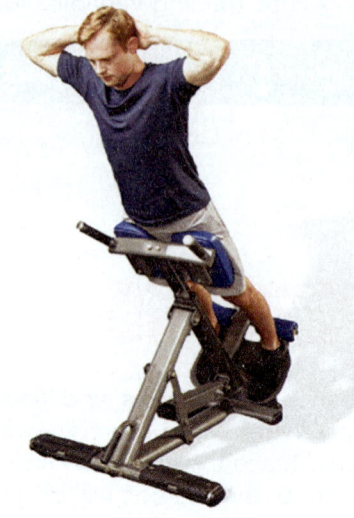

Back Extension

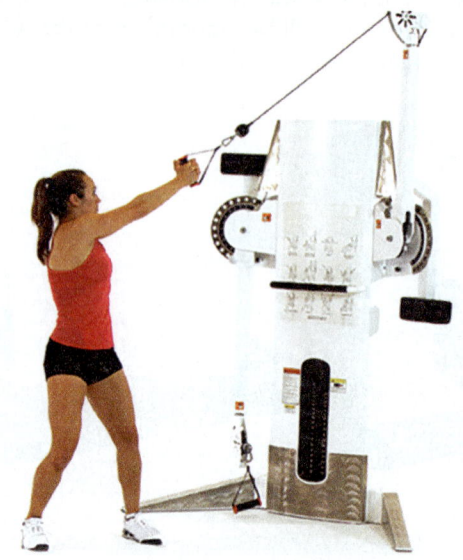
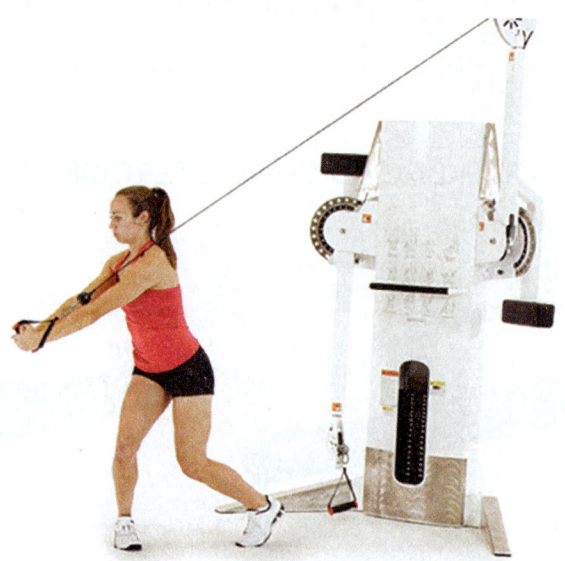

Cable Chop

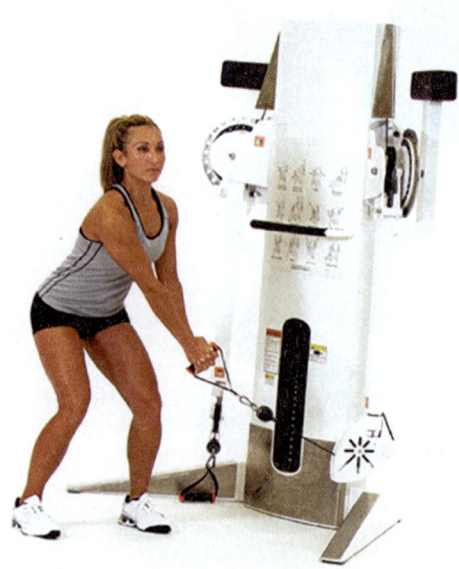
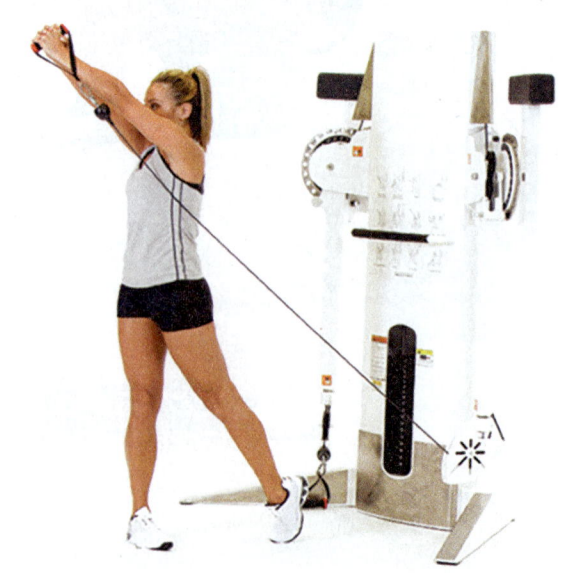

Cable Lift

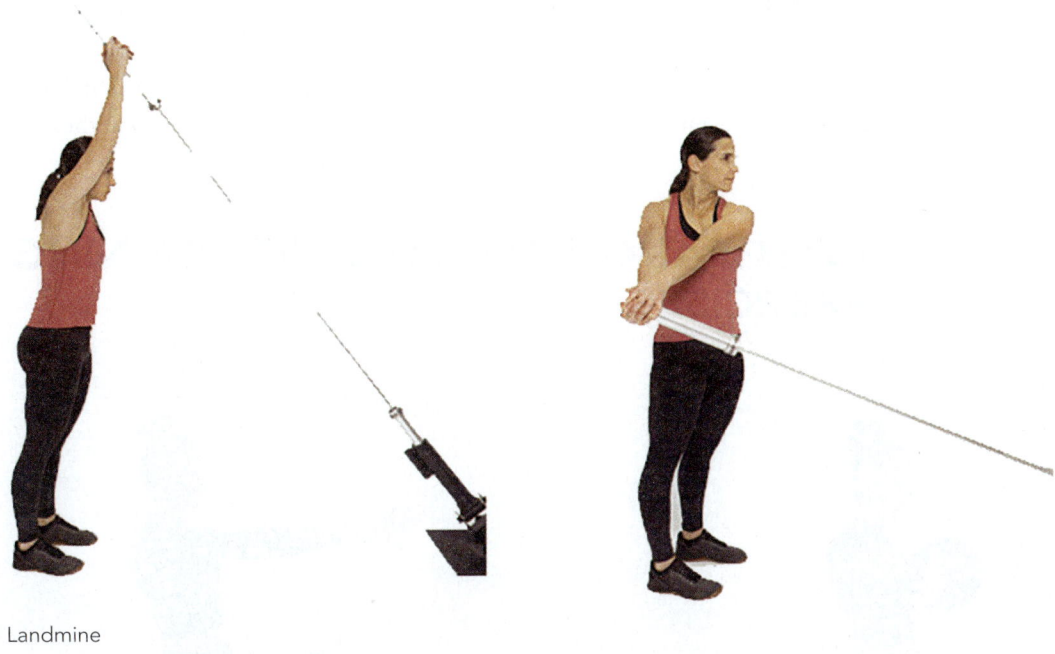

Landmine

LESSON 6: CORE TRAINING FOR SPORTS

INTEGRATION-BIASED CORE TRAINING

Integration-biased training focuses on applying the concepts of motor control and strength-biased core training to sport-specific actions. The progressions used in this stage focus on improving the rate of force production and the movement efficiency of the core musculature and extremities. This form of core training prepares athletes to dynamically stabilize and generate forces at speeds that more closely mimic those experienced in sports (Butcher et al., 2007). Exercises that develop power with the integration of proximal to distal firing transfer better to explosive sporting actions. Power can be developed in the core musculature with medicine ball exercises, such as rotation chest passes, soccer throws, woodchop throws, and back extension throws. These exercises aim to begin from a stationary position and then generate power to move the medicine ball toward a reinforced wall or another sturdy object. The focus must be on rapid power production by moving as explosively as the athlete can control (**Table 10.10**).

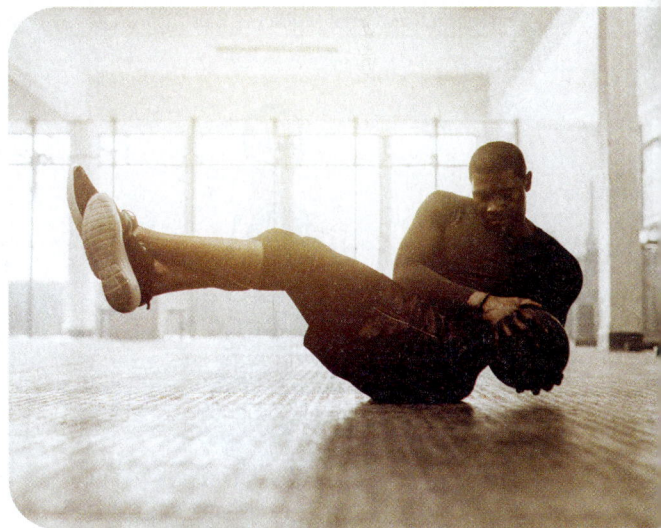

© Jacob Lund/Shutterstock

TABLE 10.10 Acute Training Variables for Integration-Biased Core Training

Focus of Exercise	Primary Action	Training Variables
Core power	Dynamic stabilization and rate of force production	1–4 exercises 1–3 sets of 8–12 reps

JUMPING–LANDING

Integration-biased core training can progress to assist in developing basic sports actions (e.g., jumping–landing, acceleration, deceleration) in all planes of motion. For example, these exercises might include a sagittal plane jump with a medicine ball chest pass upon landing.

INTEGRATION-BIASED CORE TRAINING EXERCISES

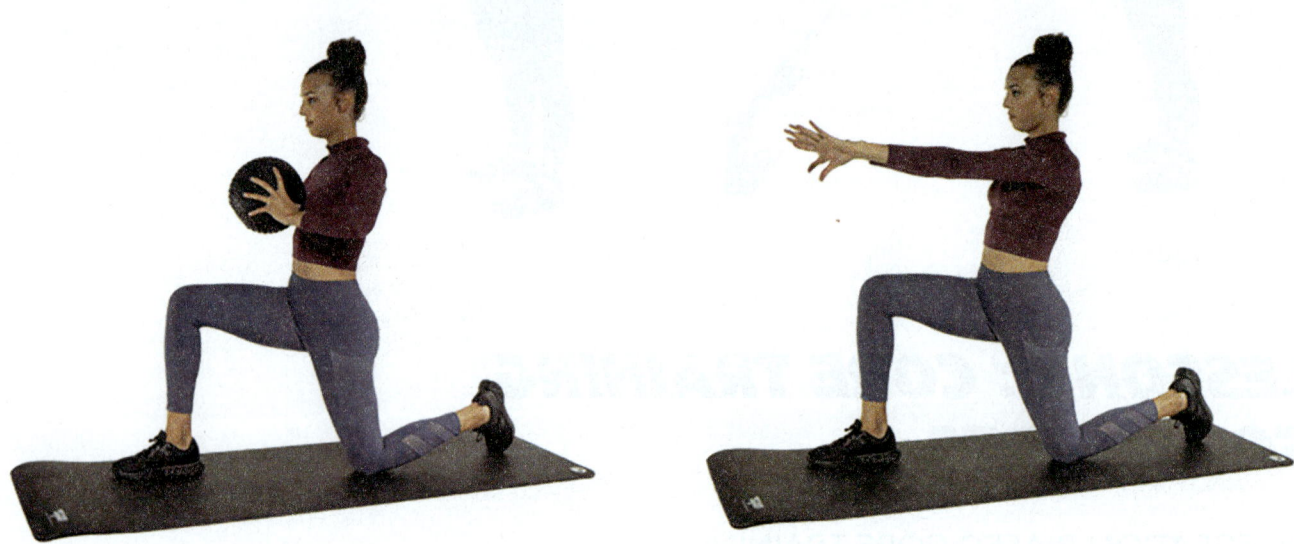

Kneeling Rotational Medicine Ball Toss

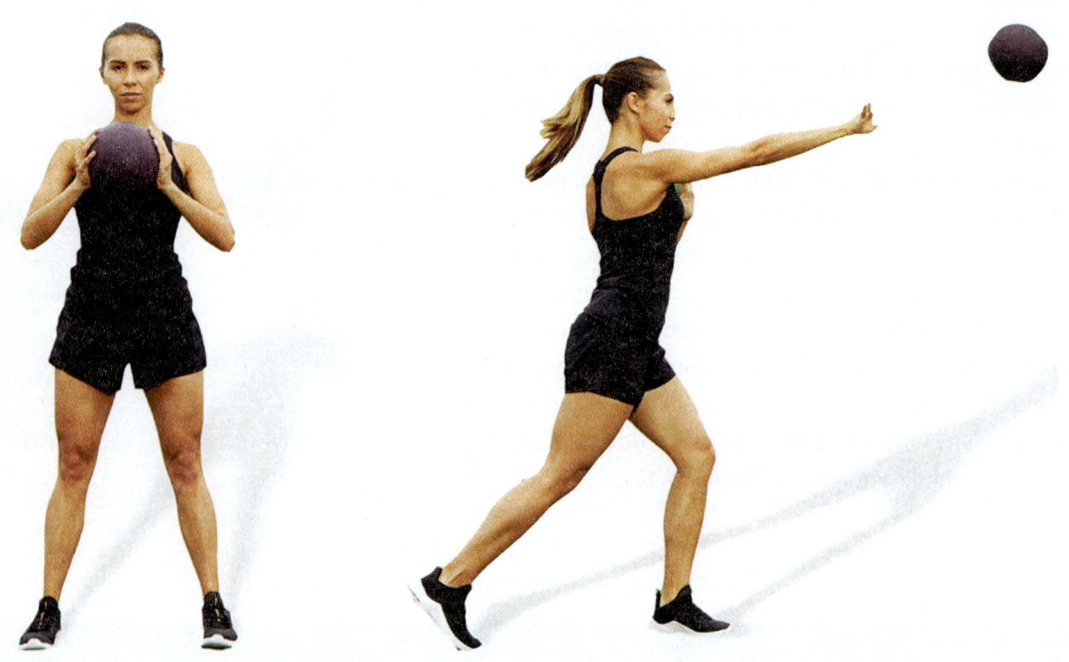

Medicine Ball Rotational Chest Pass

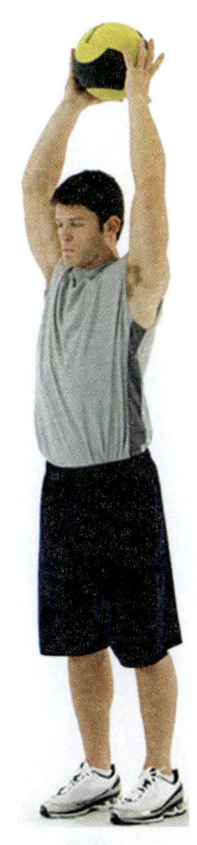
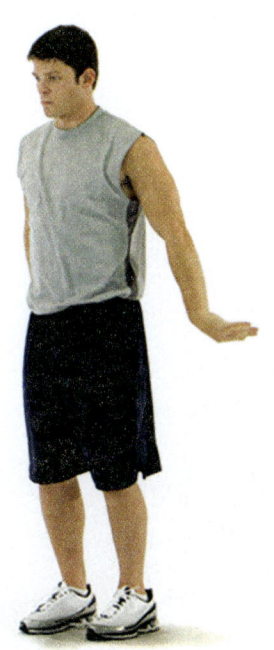

Medicine Ball Soccer Throw

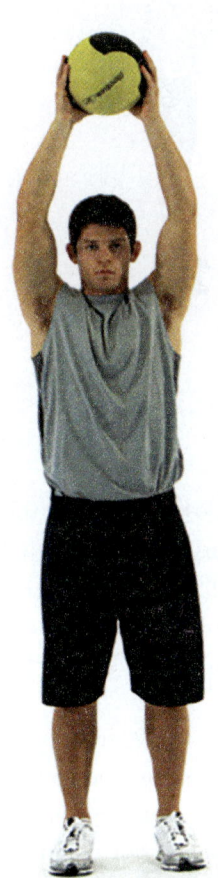
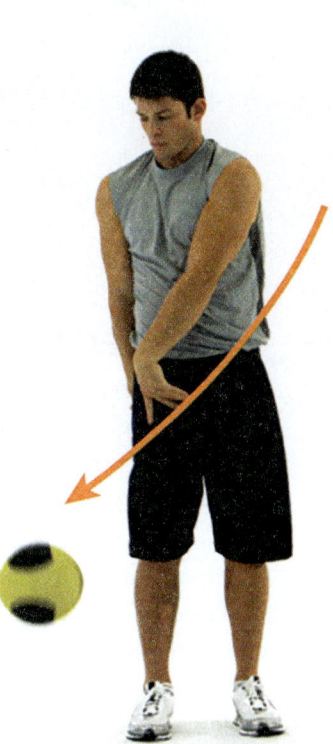

Medicine Ball Woodchop Throw

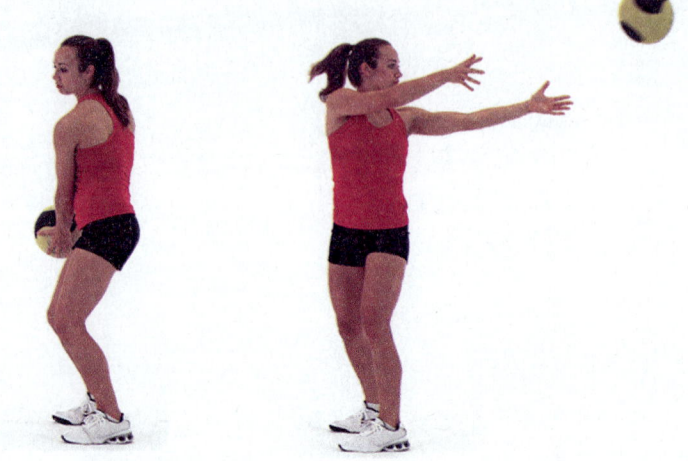

Medicine Ball Back Extension Throw

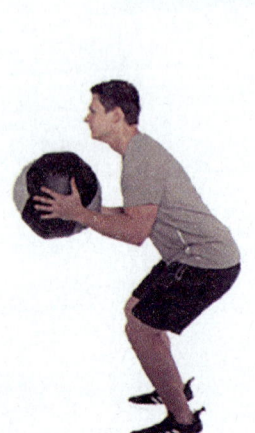
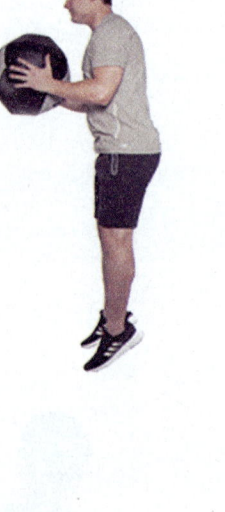
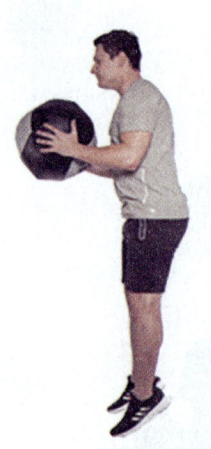
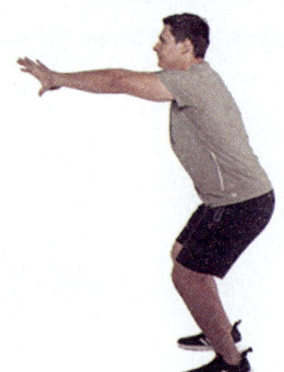

Medicine Ball with Landing Chest Pass

SPORT-SPECIFIC MOVEMENT

Lastly, athletes must be able to transfer power development into actions specific to their sports. In most cases, power generation occurs beginning with the lower extremities, through the core, and is outwardly expressed in the upper extremity in the transverse plane. This process is seen in hitting and throwing, or in the lower extremity in kicking or pivoting. The athlete can use resistance bands or medicine balls to perform explosive actions that mimic the sport (**Table 10.11**).

Power exercises with bands attached to the LPHC from behind create resistance around the core, increase core muscle activation, and facilitate proximal to distal movement generation with exercises related to sport-specific actions. For example, an explosive upper-body rotational exercise such as a side oblique medicine ball throw is a similar movement pattern to a tennis forehand shot.

TABLE 10.11 Explosive Sports Actions

Upper-Body Rotation	
Sport	**Action**
Tennis	Serve: Cross-body high–low Forehand: Cross-body low–high
Baseball	Hitting Pitching
Golf	Driving
Basketball	Rip through
Football	Throwing
Hockey	Passing and shooting
Lower-Body Rotation	
Sport	**Action**
Soccer	Striking ball Defending opponent
Basketball	Pivot Step back
Martial arts	Roundhouse kick
Football	Field goal and kickoff kicking

These exercises should be performed at maximal speed while maintaining ideal form and technique. Therefore, there needs to be a good amount (minimum 10 seconds) of recovery between reps. For example, the athlete should perform no more than four to six reps and two to four sets, with at least 2 minutes of recovery between sets (**Table 10.12**).

TABLE 10.12 Acute Training Variables for Integration-Biased Sport-Specific Core Training

Focus of Exercise	Primary Action	Training Variables	Rest
Core power	Dynamic stabilization and rate of force production with additional resistance	1–4 exercises 2–4 sets of 4–6 reps	Minimum of 2 minutes between sets

SPORT-SPECIFIC EXERCISES

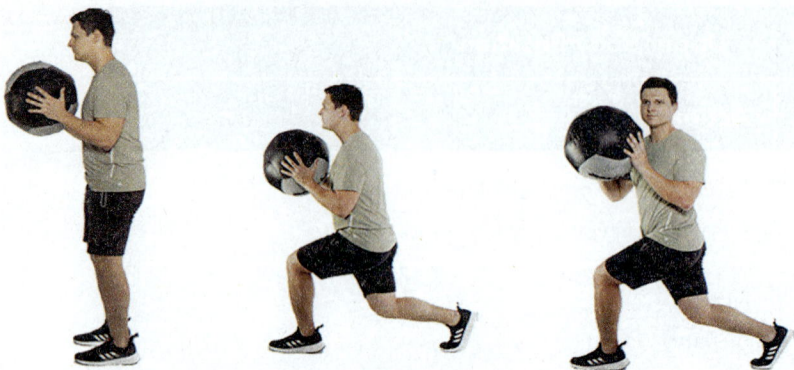

Medicine Ball Lunge with Rotation Chest Pass

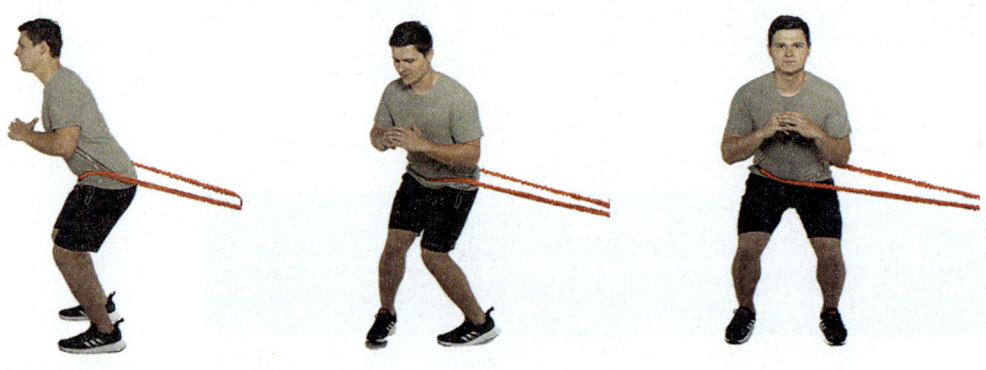

Resisted Pivots

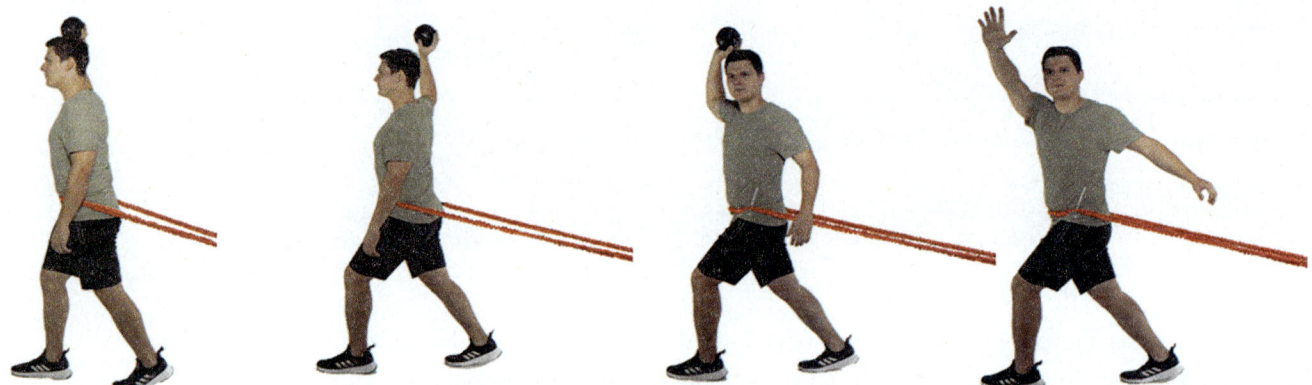

Resisted Lunge Overhead Throw

SUMMARY

Core training is a fundamental component of all integrated sports performance training programs. A comprehensive core training program enables an athlete to achieve optimal neuromuscular control of the LPHC and achieve optimal performance, and is a factor in injury prevention. The core musculature helps protect the spine from harmful forces during functional activities. Effective core training optimizes core stability, endurance, strength, and power. Focusing on each of these components is essential for ensuring that athletes can effectively stabilize their core and forcefully move their trunks.

The core's local, global, and movement muscles must be trained to effectively acquire core stability, endurance, strength, and power adaptations. In addition, local muscles generally provide dynamic control of spinal segments important for core stability.

The primary muscles that make up the movement system include the erector spinae, rectus abdominis, latissimus dorsi, hip flexors, superficial gluteus maximus, hamstrings, and quadriceps. Sports Performance Coaches should ensure that local muscles effectively stabilize the spine when introducing more advanced core exercises that use global and movement muscles to move the trunk. Additionally, it is critical to ensure local, global, and movement core muscles demonstrate adequate endurance due to the continuous need for optimal spinal stability and precise trunk movements during many sporting activities.

KEY TAKEAWAYS

- In sports and activities of daily living, locomotion requires force transfer through a stable and relatively stiff torso. Inappropriate stiffness can lead to a loss of energy transfer if there is too little stiffness or if there is movement inefficiency with too much stiffness.
- An athlete's resting daily habits can influence core stabilization capabilities. Despite training volume, poor posture can result in a loss of optimal core function.
- Many sports involve a high degree of unpredictability, requiring the athlete to quickly change direction based on incoming information. Therefore, optimal core function is vital in the athlete's dissociating columns of the body to allow for efficient movement.
- The Sports Performance Coach must understand the demands of each sport to understand the core's role.
- Many athletes suffer from lower back pain (LBP) at some stage in their career due to the varying levels and types of forces to which their LPHC tissues are exposed in their sport. Chronic LBP has been shown to delay the timing (a feed-forward mechanism) and impairs the activation of the core stabilizer muscles, such as the transversus abdominis, internal oblique, and multifidus, during low-threshold tasks. Therefore, core training is vital for all athletes.
- A comprehensive core training program for an athlete should account for all exercise training variables and include four progressive stages:
  - Stage 1: Foundational motor control core training
  - Stage 2: Advanced motor control core training
  - Stage 3: Strength-biased core training
  - Stage 4: Integration-biased core training

REFERENCES

Alentorn-Geli, E., Myer, G. D., Silvers, H. J., Samitier, G., Romero, D., Lázaro-Haro, C., & Cugat, R. (2009). Prevention of non-contact anterior cruciate ligament injuries in soccer players. Part 1: Mechanisms of injury and underlying risk factors. *Knee Surgery, Sports Traumatology, Arthroscopy, 17*(7), 705–729. https://doi.org/10.1007/s00167-009-0813-1

Allison, G. T., Godfrey, P., & Robinson, G. (1998). EMG signal amplitude assessment during abdominal bracing and hollowing. *Journal of Electromyography and Kinesiology: Official Journal of the International Society of Electrophysiological Kinesiology, 8*(1), 51–57. https://doi.org/10.1016/s1050-6411(97)00004-7

Barnett, F., & Gilleard, W. (2005). The use of lumbar spinal stabilization techniques during the performance of abdominal strengthening exercise variations. *Journal of Sports Medicine and Physical Fitness, 45*(1), 38–43.

Bosch, F., & Klomp, R. (2005). *Running: Biomechanics and exercise physiology applied in practice.* Elsevier Churchill Livingstone.

Butcher, S. J., Craven, B. R., Chilibeck, P. D., Spink, K. S., Grona, S. L., & Sprigings, E. J. (2007). The effect of trunk stability training on vertical takeoff velocity. *Journal of Orthopaedic and Sports Physical Therapy, 37*(5), 223–231. https://doi.org/10.2519/jospt.2007.2331

Chang, W.-D., Lin, H.-Y., & Lai, P.-T. (2015). Core strength training for patients with chronic low back pain. *Journal of Physical Therapy Science, 27*(3), 619–622. https://doi.org/10.1589/jpts.27.619

Comerford, M. J., & Mottram, S. L. (2001). Movement and stability dysfunction: Contemporary developments. *Manual Therapy, 6*(1), 15–26. https://doi.org/10.1054/math.2000.0388

Comerford, M., & Mottram, S. (2012). *Kinetic control: The management of uncontrolled movement* (1st ed.). Churchill Livingstone/Elsevier Australia.

Crisco, J. J., & Panjabi, M. M. (1991). The intersegmental and multisegmental muscles of the lumbar spine. A biomechanical model comparing lateral stabilizing potential. *Spine, 16*(7), 793–799. https://doi.org/10.1097/00007632-199107000-00018

Ebenbichler, G. R., Oddsson, L. I., Kollmitzer, J., & Erim, Z. (2001). Sensory-motor control of the lower back: Implications for rehabilitation. *Medicine & Science in Sports & Exercise, 33*(11), 1889–1898. https://doi.org/10.1097/00005768-200111000-00014

Fredericson, M., Cookingham, C. L., Chaudhari, A. M., Dowdell, B. C., Oestreicher, N., & Sahrmann, S. A. (2000). Hip abductor weakness in distance runners with iliotibial band syndrome. *Clinical Journal of Sport Medicine, 10*(3), 169–175. https://doi.org/10.1097/00042752-200007000-00004

Friel, K., McLean, N., Myers, C., & Caceres, M. (2006). Ipsilateral hip abductor weakness after inversion ankle sprain. *Journal of Athletic Training, 41*(1), 74–78. https://www.ncbi.nlm.nih.gov/pmc/articles/PMC1421486/

Grenier, S. G., & McGill, S. M. (2007). Quantification of lumbar stability by using 2 different abdominal activation strategies. *Archives of Physical Medicine and Rehabilitation, 88*(1), 54–62. https://doi.org/10.1016/j.apmr.2006.10.014

Hackett, D. A., & Chow, C. M. (2013). The Valsalva maneuver: Its effect on intra-abdominal pressure and safety issues during resistance exercise. *Journal of Strength and Conditioning Research, 27*(8), 2338–2345. https://doi.org/10.1519/JSC.0b013e31827de07d

Hamza, A. (2013). The effects of core strength training (with and without suspension) on lipid peroxidation and lunge speed for young fencers. *Ovidius University Annals, Series Physical Education and Sport/Science, Movement and Health, 13*(S2), 129–136.

Hewett, T. E., Paterno, M. V., & Myer, G. D. (2002). Strategies for enhancing proprioception and neuromuscular control of the knee. *Clinical Orthopaedics and Related Research, 402*, 76–94. https://doi.org/10.1097/00003086-200209000-00008

Hewett, T. E., Torg, J. S., & Boden, B. P. (2009). Video analysis of trunk and knee motion during non-contact anterior cruciate ligament injury in female athletes: Lateral trunk and knee abduction motion are combined components of the injury mechanism. *British Journal of Sports Medicine, 43*(6), 417–422. https://doi.org/10.1136/bjsm.2009.059162.

Hides, J. A., Jull, G. A., & Richardson, C. A. (2001). Long-term effects of specific stabilizing exercises for first-episode low back pain. *Spine, 26*(11), E243–E248. https://doi.org/10.1097/00007632-200106010-00004

Hides, J. A., Richardson, C. A., & Jull, G. A. (1996). Multifidus muscle recovery is not automatic after resolution of acute, first-episode low back pain. *Spine, 21*(23), 2763–2769. https://doi.org/10.1097/00007632-199612010-00011

Hirashima, M., Kudo, K., Watarai, K., & Ohtsuki, T. (2007). Control of 3D limb dynamics in unconstrained overarm throws of different speeds performed by skilled baseball players. *Journal of Neurophysiology, 97*(1), 680–691. https://doi.org/10.1152/jn.00348.2006

Hodges, P. W. (1999). Is there a role for transversus abdominis in lumbo-pelvic stability? *Manual Therapy, 4*(2), 74–86. https://doi.org/10.1054/math.1999.0169

Hodges, P. W., & Richardson, C. A. (1996). Inefficient muscular stabilization of the lumbar spine associated with low back pain: A motor control evaluation of transversus abdominis. *Spine, 21*(22), 2640–2650. https://doi.org/10.1097/00007632-199611150-00014

Hodges, P., Richardson, C., & Jull, G. (1996). Evaluation of the relationship between laboratory and clinical tests of transversus abdominis function. *Physiotherapy Research International: The Journal for Researchers and Clinicians in Physical Therapy, 1*(1), 30–40. https://doi.org/10.1002/pri.45

Hrysomallis, C. (2013). Injury incidence, risk factors and prevention in Australian rules football. *Sports Medicine (Auckland, NZ), 43*(5), 339–354. https://doi.org/10.1007/s40279-013-0034-0

Hughes, G. (2014). A review of recent perspectives on biomechanical risk factors associated with anterior cruciate ligament injury. *Research in Sports Medicine, 22*(2), 193–212. https://doi.org/10.1080/15438627.2014.881821.

Hungerford, B., Gilleard, W., & Hodges, P. (2003). Evidence of altered lumbopelvic muscle recruitment in the presence of sacroiliac joint pain. *Spine, 28*(14), 1593–1600.

Huxel Bliven, K. C., & Anderson, B. E. (2013). Core stability training for injury prevention. *Sports Health, 5*(6), 514–522. https://doi.org/10.1177/1941738113481200

Ireland, M. L., Willson, J. D., Ballantyne, B. T., & Davis, I. M. (2003). Hip strength in females with and without patellofemoral pain. *Journal of Orthopaedic and Sports Physical Therapy, 33*(11), 671–676. https://doi.org/10.2519/jospt.2003.33.11.671

Iwai, K., Nakazato, K., Irie, K., Fujimoto, H., & Nakajima, H. (2004). Trunk muscle strength and disability level of low back pain in collegiate wrestlers. *Medicine & Science in Sports & Exercise, 36*(8), 1296–1300. https://doi.org/10.1249/01.mss.0000135791.27929.c1

Jamison, S. T., McNally, M. P., Schmitt, L. C., & Chaudhari, A. M. (2013). The effects of core muscle activation on dynamic trunk position and knee abduction moments: Implications for ACL injury. *Journal of Biomechanics, 46*(13), 2236–2241. https://doi.org/10.1016/j.jbiomech.2013.06.021

Jamison, S. T., Pan, X., & Chaudhari, A. M. (2012). Knee moments during run-to-cut maneuvers are associated with lateral trunk positioning. *Journal of Biomechanics, 45*(11), 1881–1885. https://doi.org/10.1016/j.jbiomech.2012.05.031

Jørgensen, K., & Nicolaisen, T. (1987). Trunk extensor endurance: Determination and relation to low-back trouble. *Ergonomics, 30*(2), 259–267. https://doi.org/10.1080/00140138708969704

Kahlaee, A. H., Ghamkhar, L., & Arab, A. M. (2017). Effect of the abdominal hollowing and bracing maneuvers on activity pattern of the lumbopelvic muscles during prone hip extension in subjects with or without chronic low back pain: A preliminary study. *Journal of Manipulative and Physiological Therapeutics, 40*(2), 106–117. https://doi.org/10.1016/j.jmpt.2016.10.009

Kamal, O. (2015). Effects of core strength training on karate spinning wheel kick and certain physical variables for young female. *Ovidius University Annals, Series Physical Education and Sport/Science, Movement and Health, 15*(2), 504–509.

Khamis, S., & Yizhar, Z. (2007). Effect of feet hyperpronation on pelvic alignment in a standing position. *Gait & Posture, 25*(1), 127–134. https://doi.org/10.1016/j.gaitpost.2006.02.005

Kibler, W. B., Chandler, T. J., Livingston, B. P., & Roetert, E. P. (1996). Shoulder range of motion in elite tennis players. Effect of age and years of tournament play. *American Journal of Sports Medicine, 24*(3), 279–285. https://doi.org/10.1177/036354659602400306

Kibler, W. B., Press, J., & Sciascia, A. (2006). The role of core stability in athletic function. *Sports Medicine (Auckland, NZ), 36*(3), 189–198. https://doi.org/10.2165/00007256-200636030-00001

Kim, M.-H., & Oh, J.-S. (2015). Effects of performing an abdominal hollowing exercise on trunk muscle activity during curl-up exercise on an unstable surface. *Journal of Physical Therapy Science, 27*(2), 501–503. https://doi.org/10.1589/jpts.27.501

Laasonen, E. M. (1984). Atrophy of sacrospinal muscle groups in patients with chronic, diffusely radiating lumbar back pain. *Neuroradiology, 26*(1), 9–13. https://doi.org/10.1007/BF00328195

Lee, A. Y., Kim, E. H., Cho, Y. W., Kwon, S. O., Son, S. M., & Ahn, S. H. (2013). Effects of abdominal hollowing during stair climbing on the activations of local trunk stabilizing muscles: A cross-sectional study. *Annals of Rehabilitation Medicine, 37*(6), 804–813. https://doi.org/10.5535/arm.2013.37.6.804

Lee, J. H., Hoshino, Y., Nakamura, K., Kariya, Y., Saita, K., & Ito, K. (1999). Trunk muscle weakness as a risk factor for low back pain: A 5-year prospective study. *Spine, 24*(1), 54–57. https://doi.org/10.1097/00007632-199901010-00013

Leetun, D. T., Ireland, M. L., Willson, J. D., Ballantyne, B. T., & Davis, I. M. (2004). Core stability measures as risk factors for lower extremity injury in athletes. *Medicine & Science in Sports & Exercise, 36*(6), 926–934. https://doi.org/10.1249/01.mss.0000128145.75199.c3

Leinonen, V., Kankaanpää, M., Luukkonen, M., Kansanen, M., Hänninen, O., Airaksinen, O., & Taimela, S. (2003). Lumbar paraspinal muscle function, perception of lumbar position, and postural control in disc herniation–related back pain. *Spine, 28*(8), 842–848.

Lewis, C. L., Sahrmann, S. A., & Moran, D. W. (2009). Effect of position and alteration in synergist muscle force contribution on hip forces when performing hip strengthening exercises. *Clinical Biomechanics, 24*(1), 35–42.

Marshall, R. N., & Elliott, B. C. (2000). Long-axis rotation: The missing link in proximal-to-distal segmental sequencing. *Journal of Sports Sciences, 18*(4), 247–254. https://doi.org/10.1080/026404100364983

McGill, S. M. (2001). Low back stability: From formal description to issues for performance and rehabilitation. *Exercise and Sport Sciences Reviews, 29*(1), 26–31. https://doi.org/10.1097/00003677-200101000-00006

McGill, S. M. (2002). *Low back stability: Myths and realities in low back disorders: Evidence-based prevention and rehabilitation.* Human Kinetics.

Mendiguchia, J., Gonzalez De la Flor, A., Mendez-Villanueva, A., Morin, J. B., Edouard, P., & Garrues, M. A. (2021). Training-induced changes in anterior pelvic tilt: Potential implications for hamstring strain injuries management. *Journal of Sports Sciences, 39*(7), 760–767. https://doi.org/10.1080/02640414.2020.1845439

Mok, N. W., Brauer, S. G., & Hodges, P. W. (2004). Hip strategy for balance control in quiet standing is reduced in people with low back pain. *Spine, 29*(6), E107–E112. https://doi.org/10.1097/01.brs.0000115134 .97854.c9

Nadler, S. F., Malanga, G. A., Bartoli, L. A., Feinberg, J. H., Prybicien, M., & Deprince, M. (2002). Hip muscle imbalance and low back pain in athletes: Influence of core strengthening. *Medicine & Science in Sports & Exercise, 34*(1), 9–16. https://doi.org/10.1097/00005768-200201000-00003

Nadler, S. F., Malanga, G. A., Feinberg, J. H., Rubanni, M., Moley, P., & Foye, P. (2002). Functional performance deficits in athletes with previous lower extremity injury. *Clinical Journal of Sport Medicine, 12*(2), 73–78. https://doi.org/10.1097/00042752-200203000-00002

Nadler, S. F., Moley, P., Malanga, G. A., Rubbani, M., Prybicien, M., & Feinberg, J. H. (2002). Functional deficits in athletes with a history of low back pain: A pilot study. *Archives of Physical Medicine and Rehabilitation, 83*(12), 1753–1758. https://doi.org/10.1053/apmr.2002.35659

Neumann, D. (2017). *Kinesiology of the musculoskeletal system: Foundations for physical rehabilitation* (3rd ed.). Mosby.

Noehren, B., Abraham, A., Curry, M., Johnson, D., & Ireland, M. L. (2014). Evaluation of proximal joint kinematics and muscle strength following ACL reconstruction surgery in female athletes. *Journal of Orthopaedic Research: Official Publication of the Orthopaedic Research Society, 32*(10), 1305–1310. https://doi.org/10.1002/jor.22678

O'Sullivan, P. B., Beales, D. J., Beetham, J. A., Cripps, J., Graf, F., Lin, I. B., Tucker, B., & Avery, A. (2002). Altered motor control strategies in subjects with sacroiliac joint pain during the active straight-leg-raise test. *Spine, 27*(1), E1–E8. https://doi.org/10.1097/00007632-200201010-00015

O'Sullivan, P. B., Phyty, G. D., Twomey, L. T., & Allison, G. T. (1997). Evaluation of specific stabilizing exercise in the treatment of chronic low back pain with radiologic diagnosis of spondylolysis or spondylolisthesis. *Spine, 22*(24), 2959–2967. https://doi.org/10.1097/00007632-199712150-00020

O'Sullivan, P. B., Twomey, L., & Allison, G. T. (1998). Altered abdominal muscle recruitment in patients with chronic back pain following a specific exercise intervention. *Journal of Orthopaedic and Sports Physical Therapy, 27*(2), 114–124. https://doi.org/10.2519/jospt.1998.27.2.114

Paillard, T. (2019). Relationship between sport expertise and postural skills. *Frontiers in Psychology, 10*, 1428. https://doi.org/10.3389/fpsyg.2019.01428

Paterno, M. V., Schmitt, L. C., Ford, K. R., Rauh, M. J., Myer, G. D., Huang, B., & Hewett, T. E. (2010). Biomechanical measures during landing and postural stability predict second anterior cruciate ligament injury after anterior cruciate ligament reconstruction and return to sport. *American Journal of Sports Medicine, 38*(10), 1968–1978. https://doi.org/10.1177/0363546510376053

Putnam, C. A. (1993). Sequential motions of body segments in striking and throwing skills: Descriptions and explanations. *Journal of Biomechanics, 26*(suppl 1), 125–135. https://doi.org/10.1016/0021-9290(93)90084-r

Rantanen, J., Hurme, M., Falck, B., Alaranta, H., Nykvist, F., Lehto, M., Einola, S., & Kalimo, H. (1993). The lumbar multifidus muscle five years after surgery for a lumbar intervertebral disc herniation. *Spine, 18*(5), 568–574. https://doi.org/10.1097/00007632-199304000-00008

Read, P. J., Oliver, J. L., De Ste Croix, M. B., Myer, G. D., & Lloyd, R. S. (2016). Neuromuscular risk factors for knee and ankle ligament injuries in male youth soccer players. *Sports Medicine (Auckland, NZ), 46*(8), 1059–1066. https://doi.org/10.1007/s40279-016-0479-z

Richardson, C. (Ed.). (1999). *Therapeutic exercise for spinal segmental stabilization in low back pain: Scientific basis and clinical approach.* Churchill Livingstone.

Richardson, C. A., Snijders, C. J., Hides, J. A., Damen, L., Pas, M. S., & Storm, J. (2002). The relation between the transversus abdominis muscles, sacroiliac joint mechanics, and low back pain. *Spine, 27*(4), 399–405. https://doi.org/10.1097/00007632-200202150-00015

Roussel, N. A., Nijs, J., Mottram, S., Van Moorsel, A., Truijen, S., & Stassijns, G. (2009). Altered lumbopelvic movement control but not generalized joint hypermobility is associated with increased injury in dancers: A prospective study. *Manual Therapy, 14*(6), 630–635. https://doi.org/10.1016/j.math.2008.12.004

Sahrmann, S. A. (2002). *Diagnosis and treatment of movement impairment syndromes.* Mosby.

Smart, J., McCurdy, K., Miller, B., & Pankey, R. (2011). The effect of core training on tennis serve velocity: *Journal of Strength and Conditioning Research, 25*, S103–S104. https://doi.org/10.1097/01.JSC.0000395743.57804.e8

Suehiro, T., Mizutani, M., Watanabe, S., Ishida, H., Kobara, K., & Osaka, H. (2014). Comparison of spine motion and trunk muscle activity between abdominal hollowing and abdominal bracing maneuvers during prone hip extension. *Journal of Bodywork & Movement Therapies, 18*(3), 482–488. https://doi.org/10.1016/j.jbmt .2014.04.012

Sung, D. J., Park, S. J., Kim, S., Kwon, M. S., & Lim, Y.-T. (2016). Effects of core and non-dominant arm strength training on drive distance in elite golfers. *Journal of Sport and Health Science*, *5*(2), 219–225. https://doi.org/10.1016/j.jshs.2014.12.006

Taylor, J. B., Ford, K. R., Schmitz, R. J., Ross, S. E., Ackerman, T. A., & Shultz, S. J. (2017). Biomechanical differences of multidirectional jump landings among female basketball and soccer players. *Journal of Strength and Conditioning Research*, *31*(11), 3034–3045. https://doi.org/10.1519/JSC.0000000000001785

Urquhart, D. M., Hodges, P. W., Allen, T. J., & Story, I. H. (2005). Abdominal muscle recruitment during a range of voluntary exercises. *Manual Therapy*, *10*(2), 144–153. https://doi.org/10.1016/j.math.2004.08.011

Vaičienė, G., Berškienė, K., Slapsinskaite, A., Mauricienė, V., & Razon, S. (2018). Not only static: Stabilization maneuvers in dynamic exercises: A pilot study. *PLoS One*, *13*(8), e0201017. https://doi.org/10.1371/journal.pone.0201017

Wilder, D. G., Aleksiev, A. R., Magnusson, M. L., Pope, M. H., Spratt, K. F., & Goel, V. K. (1996). Muscular response to sudden load: A tool to evaluate fatigue and rehabilitation. *Spine*, *21*(22), 2628–2639. https://doi.org/10.1097/00007632-199611150-00013

Williams, P. E., & Goldspink, G. (1978). Changes in sarcomere length and physiological properties in immobilized muscle. *Journal of Anatomy*, *127*(pt 3), 459–468.

Youdas, J. W., Hollman, J. H., & Krause, D. A. (2006). The effects of gender, age, and body mass index on standing lumbar curvature in persons without current low back pain. *Physiotherapy Theory and Practice*, *22*(5), 229–237. https://doi.org/10.1080/09593980600927864

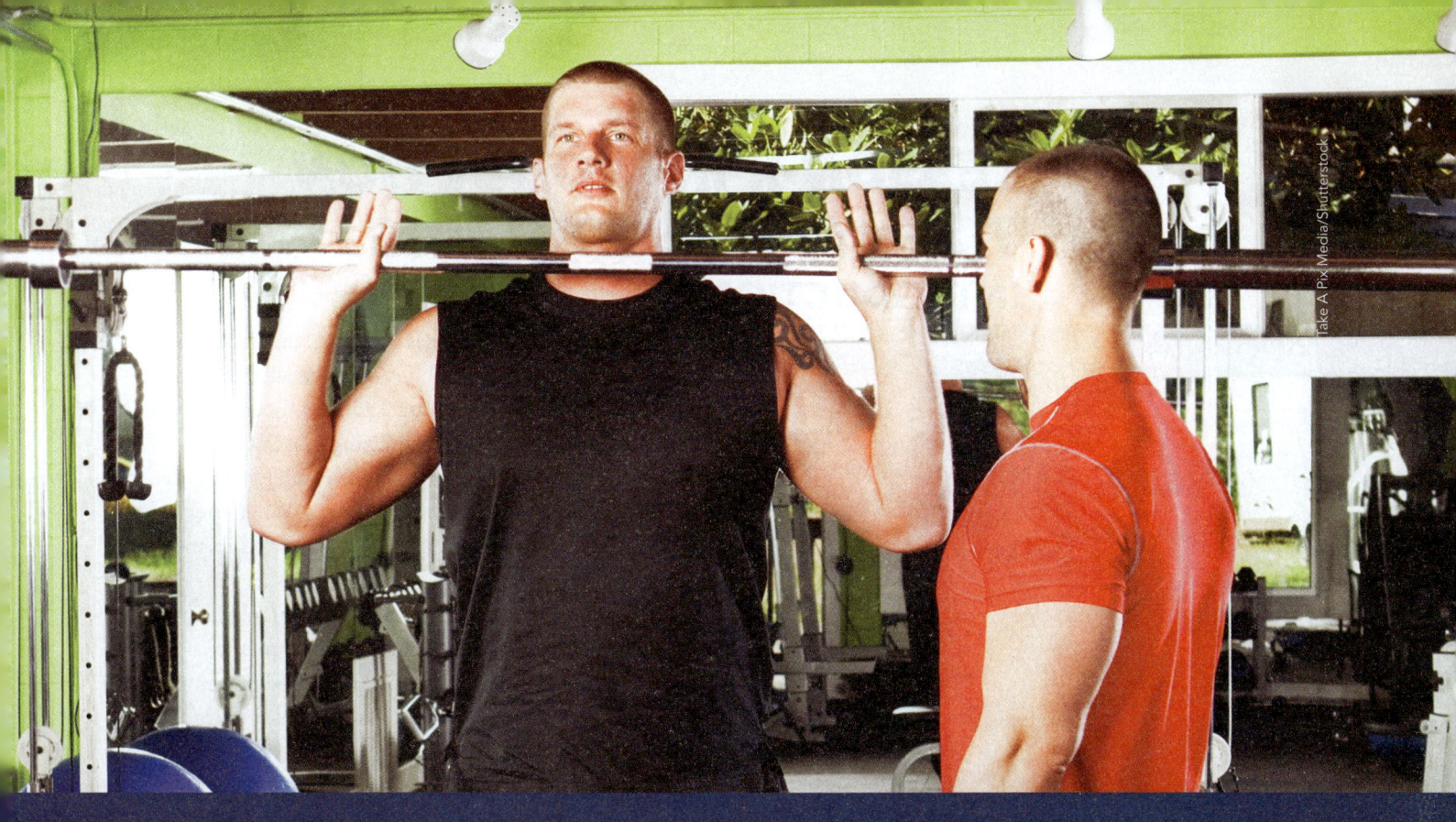

BALANCE TRAINING FOR SPORTS PERFORMANCE

LEARNING OBJECTIVES

Upon completion of this chapter, the Sports Performance Coach will be able to:

- **Summarize** the importance of balance training for athletes with differing performance-related goals.

- **Explain** the scientific rationale for balance training.

- **Describe** different balance training techniques used within performance training.

- **Identify** appropriate acute training variables for balance training.

- **Select** balance programs or techniques based on the athlete's needs.

LESSON 1: INTRODUCTION TO BALANCE TRAINING

INTRODUCTION

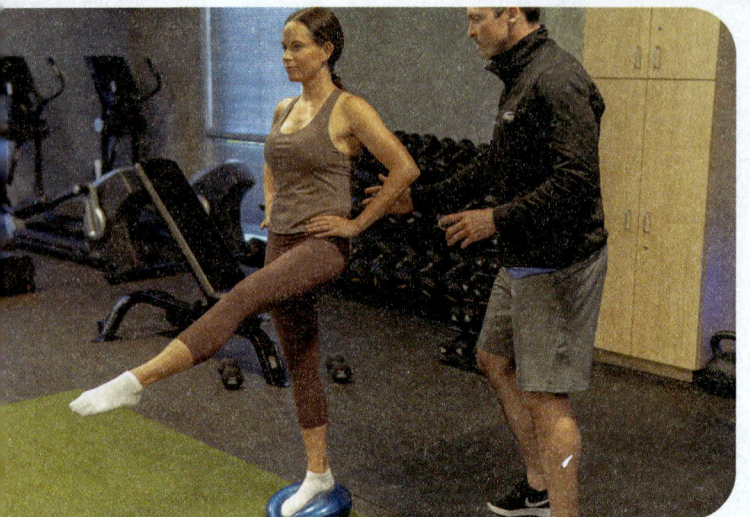

Balance training is vital for athletes because it enhances body awareness, coordination, and stability—critical elements in almost every sport. Balance training is inherently core-centric, as it targets many of the smaller, stabilizing muscles of the ankle, knee, and lumbo-pelvic-hip complex (LPHC) that are often neglected in standard training regimens. When they improve their balance, athletes can enhance their performance by increasing agility and reducing reaction times and the risk of injury. For instance, maintaining or quickly regaining balance during dynamic movements can prevent falls or missteps. Furthermore, better balance can lead to improved power and precision in movements, as many athletic actions require a stable base from which to generate force.

Balance is the complex integration of many systems to ensure the body's center of mass remains within its base of support to allow effective movements, both statically and dynamically (DiStefano et al., 2009; Sousa et al., 2012; Zech et al., 2010). Without ideal **sensorimotor input** from the balance system, the body loses fine-tuned control and movement efficiency.

Together, ideal sensorimotor input and movement efficiency provide the foundation for optimal performance attributes such as strength, power, speed, and agility (Brachman et al., 2017). In addition, the neuromuscular system constantly receives sensory feedback that it uses to modify motor outputs so as to meet the changing demands of a dynamic environment. This integration is necessary for postural control of the entire human movement system (HMS) and stability of the individual joints.

> **SENSORI-MOTOR INPUT** →
>
> Information received from the sensory system (vision, hearing, smell, taste, touch, vestibular, and proprioception).

📋 COACH'S CORNER

Balance training should be a part of a comprehensive neuromuscular training program that includes core, plyometrics, and resistance training. Integrating these training modalities optimizes the performance-related adaptations without eliminating certain neurological adaptations, which can occur when a program is too narrowly focused on a particular quality. In addition, the interrelationship among training variables presents ample overlap, requiring comprehensive programming instead of targeting skills such as balance in isolation.

As part of a comprehensive training model, balance training positively correlates with sports performance (Hrysomallis, 2011). Even in the absence of a targeted balance training program, sports participation stimulates balance adaptations commensurate with the demands of the sport. Athletes participating in a sport generally outperform non-athlete controls when assessing each for postural sway (a key indicator of balance ability). Nevertheless, a high degree of variability is observed when comparing the balance of athletes participating in different sports (Kiers et al., 2013).

For example, when athletes competing in the same sport at different levels were compared, national-level athletes had higher balance scores than regional athletes—a finding that suggests the importance of balance for more highly competitive performance (Paillard et al., 2006). Regardless of the exact stimulus, the proprioceptive control developed through balance training is strongly implicated in success for athletes. Hans and colleagues (2014) created a predictive model that showed 80% accuracy in classifying athletes as top-level or lower-level based on ankle proprioception and years of training. Thus, evaluating the balance abilities of athletes may provide an opportunity for practitioners to identify a weakness or help predict their future success in their sport.

In athletic movement, forces are transmitted from the ground up the kinetic chain through each joint by all the muscles involved. The more stably an athlete can maintain their position, the more coordinated the transmission of force is, and the more precise the expression of the skill will be. As the limbs change position during movement, the muscles adjust through increased force output and changing limb position to counteract the weight shift.

For example, when an athlete assumes the **universal athletic position**, their center of gravity is shifted down as their ankles, knees, and hips flex (**Figure 11.1**). This position is commonly used across many sports, as it allows for quick, agile movements in all directions. However, the lowered position with the hips back shifts the center of gravity posteriorly, so the athlete must learn to maintain equilibrium by shifting the torso forward. While this simple example may seem intuitive to most athletes, it is a clear demonstration of how the body meets the demands of a changing environment by maintaining equilibrium and postural control of the body's balance capacity.

> **UNIVERSAL ATHLETIC POSITION** →
>
> Standing in an approximate one-quarter squat, hips behind the center of gravity, back straight, and feet flat; also referred to as the "ready position."

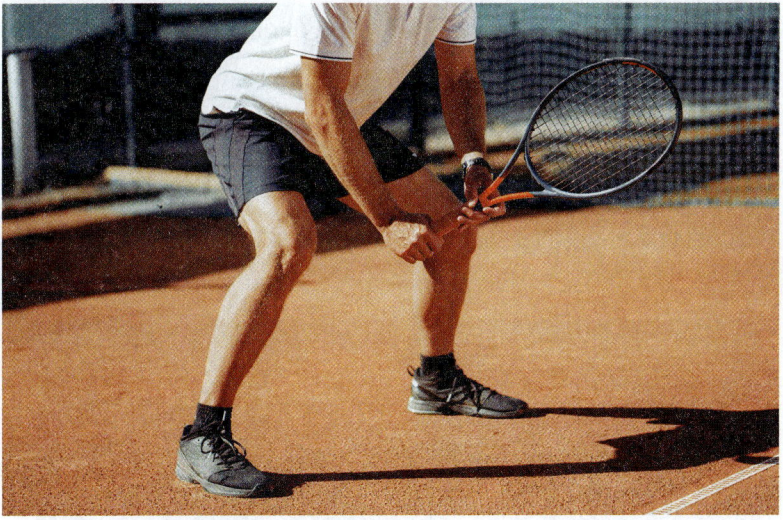

FIGURE 11.1 Universal Athletic Position
© FabrikaSimf/Shutterstock

✔ CHECK IT OUT

Consider the difference between an untrained adolescent and a competitive collegiate athlete. The child has all sorts of expressions of speed, agility, and raw athleticism in the presence of excessive limb and body movements. In contrast, the collegiate athlete has efficiency in their movements that comes with advanced physical development based on biological age and a robust training program.

SPORT-SPECIFIC BALANCE REQUIREMENTS

Every sport has unique balance applications that require specific training methods to mimic these demands. Given these variable demands, the concept of a universal balance training program should be avoided in favor of a more tailored approach (Hrysomallis, 2011; Kiers et al., 2013). Challenges to balance and postural control during gameplay should be evaluated to ensure performance conditions are replicated in training. However, the Sports Performance Coach should also recognize that different sports may have cross-over movement patterns.

For example, notice the similarities in the single-leg stabilization required when pitching in baseball (**Figure 11.2**) and shooting in lacrosse (**Figure 11.3**). Athletes participating in both of these sports will likely benefit from single-leg balance drills such as a single-leg Romanian deadlift. Similarly, a hockey player requires single-leg balance, but the skate's blade offers a much smaller base of support than the cleats of baseball or lacrosse shoes. Therefore, the hockey player may benefit from single-leg balance exercises using a wobble board in the frontal plane to replicate the balance requirements when on skates.

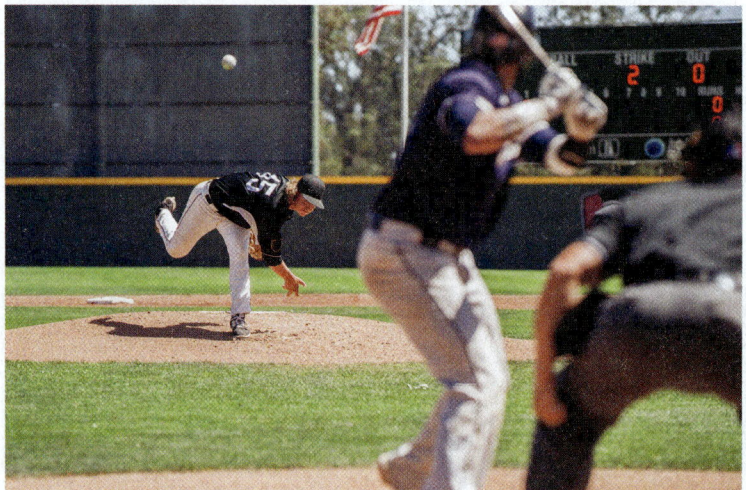

FIGURE 11.2 Single-Leg Stabilization During Baseball Pitch
© Jon Osumi/Shutterstock

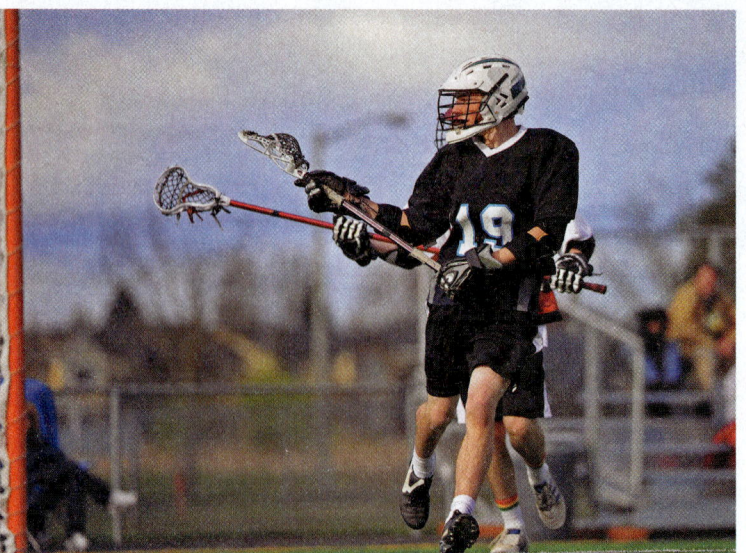

FIGURE 11.3 Single-Leg Stabilization During Lacrosse Shooting
© James A Boardman/Shutterstock

In contrast, wrestlers may find themselves performing single-leg stabilization combined with single-arm bracing. In this context, not only is joint stabilization required, but core control and coordination between the upper and lower limbs are also necessary, making an exercise like a single-leg/single-arm cable press relevant. Again, creativity is beneficial for a balance training program, but not at the expense of ignoring the athlete's needs. Alternatively, certain positions and challenges to balance may be relevant to other sports with similar movement patterns.

Just because a balance drill is challenging for an athlete does not mean it will improve performance (Kümmel et al., 2016). Unstable surface training is a method that athletes commonly use to increase the challenge of a balance drill, but the context of the implementation matters for its effectiveness. For example, a study of a group of collegiate soccer athletes used a program in which an intervention group completed various exercises on an unstable surface and a control group completed the same exercises on stable ground (Cressey et al., 2007). Interestingly, the unstable surface group did not outperform the stable surface group in jumping, sprinting, or agility post-intervention.

An important note regarding this study is that the participants were past the primary stages of development and participated at a high level of competition (NCAA Division I). Advanced athletes tend to have greater postural control than lower-level athletes (Paillard et al., 2006). With healthy advanced athletes, unstable surface training is generally not a primary factor in improving performance outcomes. However, unstable surface training can be integrated into rehabilitation and a holistic neuromuscular training program (Hrysomallis, 2011).

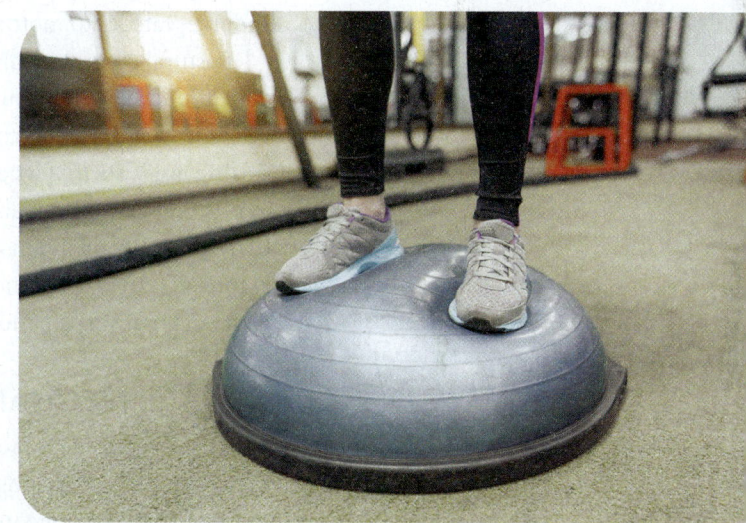

© VH-studio/Shutterstock

Balance training has tremendous benefits for improving proprioception and ankle stability, and it is a proven technique used within comprehensive injury prevention programs (Brachman et al., 2017; Hübscher et al., 2010). Consequently, Sports Performance Coaches should integrate balance training into the comprehensive training plan for athletes in conjunction with training techniques to increase strength, muscular hypertrophy, and power. In addition, balance training exercises can easily be implemented into the athlete's warm-up protocols and performed during active recovery sessions.

LESSON 2: BALANCE SYSTEMS
THE POSTURAL CONTROL SYSTEM

The **postural control system** is a vital mechanism in the human body that allows us to maintain balance and adjust our posture during different activities. It consists of several interconnected components, including sensory systems, the musculoskeletal system, the nervous system, and cognitive processes.

The underpinning characteristics of postural control stem from visual, vestibular, and somatosensory input (**Figure 11.4**) (Ivanko & Gurfinkel, 2018). The sensory information collected by these systems is combined in the central nervous system (CNS)—specifically within the brainstem, cerebellum, and basal ganglia—which processes the afferent signal to determine the nature of the peripheral motion and the position of the body in space (Sousa et al., 2012). The processed input is then converted into an appropriate efferent motor response that maintains equilibrium and efficiently controls movement (Ogard, 2011).

POSTURAL CONTROL SYSTEM →

The visual, vestibular, and somatosensory peripheral input that is processed by the central nervous system and integrated to create coordinated movement.

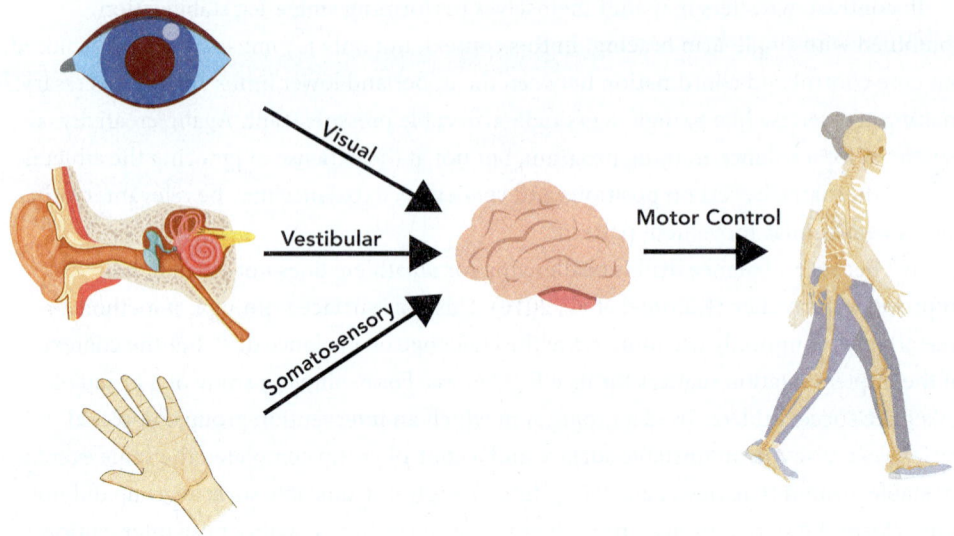

FIGURE 11.4 Postural Control System

Skill expression is a complex interaction between input and output interpreted by the brain and integrated into motor patterns.

Postural control involves a fine-tuned, constantly evolving interaction between the athlete and their environment (Sousa et al., 2012). For example, the field surface might be somewhat unpredictable for certain sports and require dynamic stabilization during cutting tasks, such as when a soccer athlete changes direction on a grass field. Challenges to postural control can also occur in contact sports—for example, when athletes have to dynamically maintain their balance while being checked, as in hockey. Meanwhile, gymnasts may require static postural control as they overcome or avoid limb movements while maintaining a handstand variation on the balance beam or parallel bars.

NEURAL MECHANISMS THAT REGULATE BALANCE

Balance is regulated by somatosensory input from the periphery that is processed and organized both consciously and subconsciously in the brain (Ogard, 2011). Many neural mechanisms simultaneously contribute to balance regulation.

One general term to describe peripheral sensory input is *proprioception*, which represents a subset of the somatosensory neural input from mechanoreceptors (Proske, 2006). A related term is **kinesthetic awareness**. Both proprioception and kinesthetic awareness collect input regarding spatial orientation and associated movements of those segments. The sensory receptors in and around joints are the primary mechanisms during dynamic balance activities (Ogard, 2011).

KINESTHETIC AWARENESS →

The awareness of the body's position as it moves through multiple planes of motion.

⚙ **PRACTICE THIS**

To understand the application of proprioception and kinesthetic awareness, stand with your eyes closed and your arms stretched to your sides. Then, touch your nose with one of your fingers. Not only can you complete the task without visual input, but you can also do it at a speed that offers precise control. Closing your eyes removes the visual input, which requires motor control from mechanoreceptor input. This is proprioception and kinesthesia at work!

VISION

Vision is an easily recognizable contributor to balance. One example of a training progression implemented in elite soccer players involved completing lateral hops with eyes open early and closed later in the program (Dello Iacono et al., 2016). Removing the visual input creates a deficit and requires the body to lean on other aspects of the postural control system. Further evidence supporting the importance of visual input for balance was found by comparing the balance of a group of subjects with normal vision and a group of subjects with vision impairment (Tomomitsu et al., 2013). The low-vision group had compromised performance on dynamic balance assessments on stable and unstable surfaces.

Vision provides valuable input that enables athletes to maintain postural control and respond accordingly to environmental changes. However, when visual tracking is a part of the technical aspects of the sport—such as when an athlete has to track a ball—the CNS may be forced to derive balance-related input from the vestibular and somatosensory systems to a greater degree (Hans et al., 2015). As a training tool, removing the visual input enhances the training effect on the other systems.

VESTIBULAR SYSTEM

The **vestibular system** is composed of small structures in the inner ear that send afferent signals to the brain based on the movement speed and direction of the head in space (Day & Fitzpatrick, 2005). When the head changes position, the sensory feedback from the vestibular system starts the process of motor unit activation to compensate for any vestibular alterations (Forbes et al., 2016). Under normal conditions, the vestibular system and visual input combine to yield motor output corresponding to the environmental demands (Ivanenko & Gurfinkel, 2018).

Following traumatic brain injuries, such as those sustained by fighters in combat sports, vestibular balance reflexes may decrease. It is hypothesized that this reduction in reflexes stems from accelerated vestibular hair cell loss after the shear forces experienced during rapid head rotation when receiving a punch to the face (Banman et al., 2021). In conditions where damage is not present, the vestibular system can be challenged by moving the head from side to side or up and down, as when responding "no" or "yes." Vestibular training helps to restore baseline function to athletes who experience head trauma, whether acute or chronic (Crampton et al., 2021). Regardless of the mechanism, a decrease in vestibular input compromises balance.

SOMATOSENSORY SYSTEM

The somatosensory system is a complex compilation of receptors throughout the body that communicate sensory information from the periphery to the brain for central interpretation and translation into appropriate motor output (Hendry & Hsiao, 2013). Multiple types of sensory receptors exist: mechanoreceptors, nociceptors, **chemoreceptors**, and **thermoreceptors** (Ten Donkelaar et al., 2020). The primary proprioceptive input for balance and performance comes from muscle spindles within the muscle belly, but many other mechanoreceptors play a role. Ultimately, the volume of sensory information derived from peripheral receptors provides the brain with ample information about the body's position in space, enabling fine-tuned movement control (i.e., balance and stability).

VESTIBULAR SYSTEM →

Provides information about the position of the body and head and spatial orientation relative to the surrounding environment; located in the inner ears and assists with balance.

CHEMO-RECEPTORS →

Specialized structures that respond to chemical stimuli, such as changes in carbon dioxide, oxygen, and pH levels.

THERMO-RECEPTORS →

Sensory organs that respond to changes in temperature, such as heat or cold.

MECHANORECEPTORS THAT AFFECT BALANCE

Balance in sports performance is frequently a dynamic interaction between the environment and the athlete. Fine-tuned adjustments are necessary for the body to respond to changes like limb position or external forces from an opponent. The somatosensory system is vital for relaying the sensory input from the periphery to the CNS for processing. Mechanoreceptors are sensitive to pressure, stretch, tension, or other mechanical input stimuli. This input is integrated in the brain to decide which movements or muscles are necessary to optimize body positioning and execute sports skills. Mechanoreceptors essential in maintaining balance include muscle spindles, Golgi tendon organs, Ruffini endings, **Pacinian corpuscles**, and nociceptors (**Figure 11.5**).

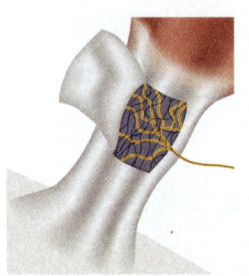 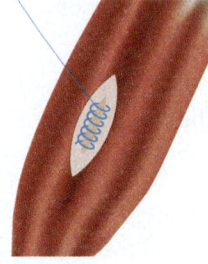 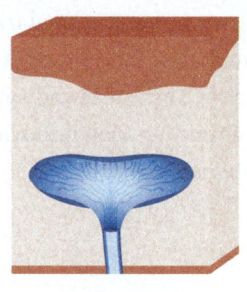 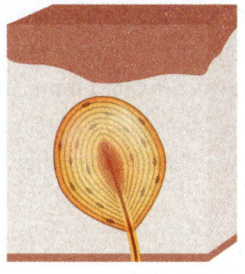 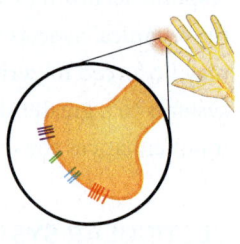

| Golgi Tendon Organ | Muscle Spindle | Ruffini Ending | Pacinian Corpuscle | Nociceptors |

FIGURE 11.5 Mechanoreceptors Involved in Balance

MUSCLE SPINDLES

Muscle spindles are specialized sensory receptors that play a crucial role in regulating balance by providing the CNS with continuous feedback on muscle length and rate of length change. They are located within the muscle belly. Thus, when a muscle stretches, the spindles are also stretched, and this information is then conveyed to the CNS. This sensory feedback is essential for maintaining posture and balance, enabling the nervous system to adjust to muscle tension and position. In addition to providing sensory input, muscle spindles contribute to the reflex arc, allowing for rapid and coordinated responses to changes in body position or external forces. By monitoring and responding to alterations in muscle length, muscle spindles help maintain stability and ensure proper body mechanics during movement.

GOLGI TENDON ORGANS

Combined with the length-sensing input of muscle spindles, Golgi tendon organs (GTOs) provide input about changes in muscular force to help control balance and movement (Kistemaker et al., 2013). Unlike muscle spindles, which are sensitive to changes in muscle length, GTOs respond to changes in muscle tension that occur as muscles contract or are passively stretched. In the context of balance, GTOs contribute to the fine-tuning of muscle tension during postural adjustments and movements. By continuously monitoring muscle tension, they help ensure that muscles generate just the right amount of force necessary for maintaining balance and performing coordinated movements, preventing both under- and over-activity of the muscles.

RUFFINI ENDINGS

Ruffini endings are similar in structure and function to GTOs and provide sensory input regarding joint position (Goodman & Bensmaia, 2021). As the joint moves or changes position due to shifts in the body's center of gravity, the Ruffini endings in the joint capsules respond to the changes in joint angle and send this information to the CNS. This allows the CNS to accurately track joint position and movement—information that is important to balance. Meanwhile, Ruffini endings in the skin provide information about pressure distribution on the soles of the feet, which is crucial for maintaining balance, especially during standing and walking.

By continuously monitoring joint position and skin stretch and pressure, Ruffini endings help generate a comprehensive internal model of the body's position and movement in space. The CNS continuously updates this model to coordinate muscle activity, maintain posture, and perform controlled movements, which are crucial for maintaining balance.

PACINIAN CORPUSCLES

Pacinian corpuscles are onion-like structures located in and around joints that are sensitive to high-frequency vibrations or sustained mechanical pressure, such as occurs in response to body and limb movements (Fleming & Luo, 2013; Quindlen et al., 2016). In addition to playing this role in joints, Pacinian corpuscles in the hand provide sensory feedback about handheld objects, which suggests their importance for athletes grasping objects like a lacrosse stick or a tennis racket (Goodman & Bensmaia, 2021).

Although not directly involved in regulating balance like muscle spindles or GTOs, Pacinian corpuscles play an indirect role in maintaining balance, particularly in situations where tactile feedback from the skin is important. For instance, when walking on an uneven surface or in a situation where visual feedback is limited, the Pacinian corpuscles in the soles of feet provide important information about the terrain and how the foot interacts with it. This feedback can inform the CNS about necessary adjustments to maintain balance.

NOCICEPTORS

Nociceptors (pain receptors) do not necessarily play a direct role in promoting balance, but they can impede balance if stimulated via **arthrogenic neuromuscular inhibition (ANI)** (Freeman et al., 2013). For example, in women with patellofemoral (kneecap) pain syndrome, the hip muscles are inhibited and demonstrate weakness (Glaviano et al., 2019). In this context, stimulation of nociceptors causes an inhibitory response leading to poor movement patterns, including diminished balance performance.

> **ARTHROGENIC →
> NEURO-
> MUSCULAR
> INHIBITION (ANI)**
>
> Inhibition of musculature surrounding a joint after damage to that joint.

> ### 🤖 GETTING TECHNICAL
>
> Arthrogenic neuromuscular inhibition is common after injury. In addition to muscular atrophy, neuromuscular inhibition is a prime contributor to muscular weakness. Instead of full activation, the CNS is inhibited by mechanisms like the disruption of sensory receptors at the location of injury from inflammation and swelling or from joint laxity and receptor damage (Rice & McNair, 2010). The effects of ANI may persist long after the initial trauma has healed.

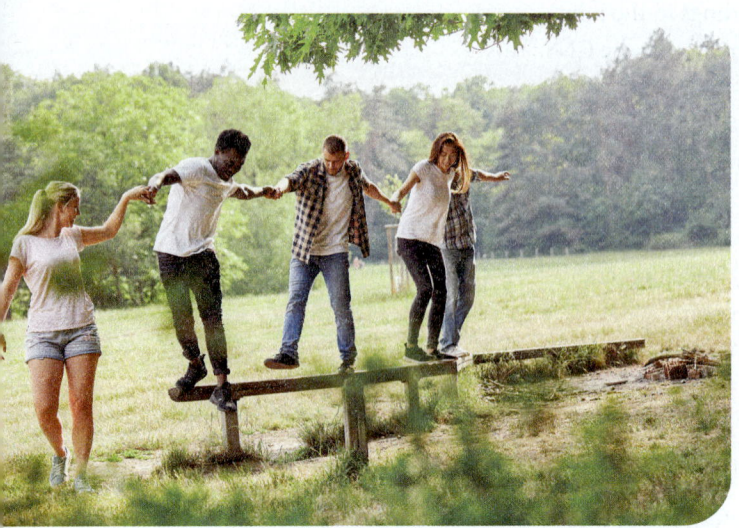

© Robert Kneschke/Shutterstock

CNS PROCESSING

For neural input to be applied to create motor output, the brain must process the incoming information, combine it, and collectively assign subsequent movements effectively and efficiently (Sousa et al., 2012). When challenges to postural control occur, balance is manifested as the CNS processes the collective neural input to provide intentional and practical skilled movements (Latash et al., 2010).

The role of the CNS is not simply to react to the environment. The recruitment of specific muscles precedes the voluntary activation of certain movement patterns. For example, anticipatory activation of the transverse abdominis has been observed during rapid limb movements (Massé-Alarie et al., 2015). The pre-activation (a feed-forward mechanism) of this muscle acts as a prerequisite stabilizer of the lumbopelvic structure, improving the efficiency of future limb movements.

Postural stabilization must be established before dynamic stabilization because a firm base of support needs to be created and maintained for neuromuscular efficiency to occur during skilled movements (Klous et al., 2011). Due to the complexity of sports skills, it is essential for the central processing of all sensory feedback from the periphery to be integrated with the voluntary motor control of prime movers without sacrificing postural control in a sport-specific application of balance ability.

LESSON 3: THE SCIENCE OF BALANCE TRAINING
SCIENTIFIC RATIONALE FOR BALANCE TRAINING

For balance training to be more than an isolated skill, there must be a scientific foundation that informs training decisions and implementation in programming. In addition, an athlete must target intermediate adaptations to influence sports performance, which must also be clearly defined to support their implementation. The neuromuscular developments derived from a comprehensive training program have a variety of benefits, including reduced risk of injury, more effective rehabilitation, and enhanced performance.

POSTURAL CONTROL

In sports performance, it is easy to become preoccupied with the expression of high-level skills rather than the underpinning fundamental movement competency that optimizes athleticism. Sport-specific skills are supported by neuromuscular developments that coordinate movement efficiency, which are commonly referred to as motor or postural control. **Postural control** is improved through neuromuscular training, as evidenced by improved functional movement patterns (Brachman et al., 2017; Moeskops et al., 2018). Neuromuscular training programs designed to improve motor control often include an integrated subset of training tactics, including dynamic stability, balance, strength, and power (Alonso-Aubin et al., 2021; Caldemeyer et al., 2020; Granacher et al., 2018).

> **POSTURAL CONTROL** →
>
> The ability of the body to maintain or change its position in space in a controlled and efficient manner.

Inefficient neuromuscular control and a lack of stabilization lead to abnormal stress throughout the HMS. Just as a lack of joint stabilization predisposes an athlete to functional instability, so a lack of postural control alters length–tension relationships, force–couple relationships, and joint kinematics, decreasing balance and performance and leading to tissue overload and possible injury (Myklebust et al., 2003). As the efficiency of the neuromuscular system decreases, the ability to maintain appropriate forces also decreases. This leads to altered movement patterns and subsequent excessive mechanical loading in both contractile and noncontractile tissues (Hewett et al., 2005).

The CNS allows recruitment of the prime movers only to the degree that the body maintains dynamic joint stabilization and postural control (Falla et al., 2003; Hungerford et al., 2003). After that point, the HMS may break down at the weak link or transfer forces elsewhere, which can lead to tissue overload, compensation, adaptation, and further altered patterns (Leetun et al., 2004). Each tissue located in the HMS breaks down at a different rate. For example, micro-failure occurs in collagen tissue when the tissue is deformed by as little as 6% to 8% (Zachazewski et al., 1996). Ultimately, with a lack of balance, movement will occur in an altered, less familiar motor pattern to maintain force production, which transfers forces to weaker links in the system.

Research has demonstrated that balance training restores dynamic stabilization mechanisms, improves neuromuscular efficiency, and stimulates joint and muscle receptors to encourage maximal sensory input into the CNS. Collectively, these factors improve proprioception, kinesthesia, and neuromuscular efficiency (central processing), which in turn can improve performance and decrease injury (Gioftsidou et al., 2006; Hewett et al., 2005; Kovacs et al., 2004; Padua & Marshall, 2006).

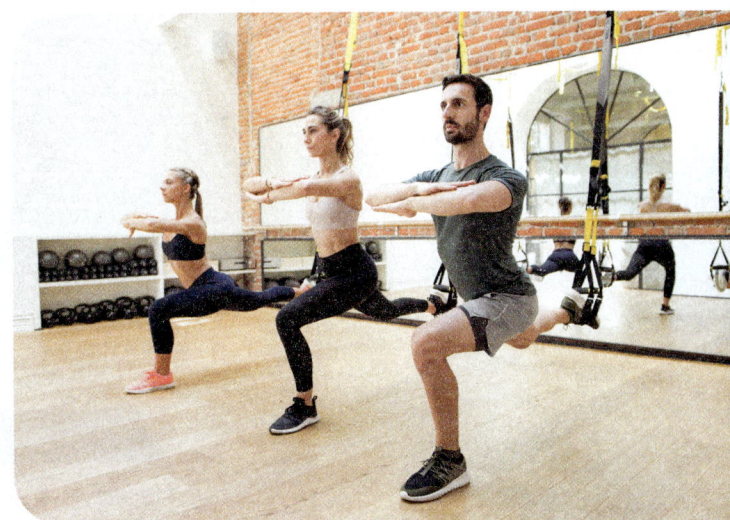

© Photology1971/Shutterstock

BALANCE TRAINING FOR INJURY RESISTANCE

Neuromuscular efficiency is not just about performance; it also has implications for injury risk reduction. The deficiencies in basic movement proficiency that can occur in the absence of a balance training program represent a movement liability that renders an athlete vulnerable to injury, particularly in regard to the lower body (Whittaker et al., 2017). This increased risk of injury can be reduced through a comprehensive neuromuscular training program that includes balance training (Caldemeyer et al., 2020; Riva et al., 2016). Key deficits that can precipitate injuries for athletes include strength deficits, neuromuscular imbalances between limbs, and deficits in postural stability (Brachman et al., 2017; Fort-Vanmeerhaeghe, Romero-Rodriguez, Montalvo, et al., 2016; Sugimoto et al., 2015). **Proprioceptive balance training**, however, can increase both postural stability (Paterno et al., 2004) and neuromuscular control (Fort-Vanmeerhaeghe, Romero-Rodriguez, Lloyd, et al., 2016). It appears to be a better option than sport-specific training alone (Tekin et al., 2018).

The more stable the body position, the less likely the joints are to deviate from the proper range of motion, thereby avoiding excessive compensatory forces outside the tolerance of what the joints are designed to handle (**Figure 11.6**) (Myer et al., 2006). Conversely, suppose neuromuscular efficiency is not present. In that case, the limbs and joints can deviate from the center of mass, increasing the **moment arm** at those joints

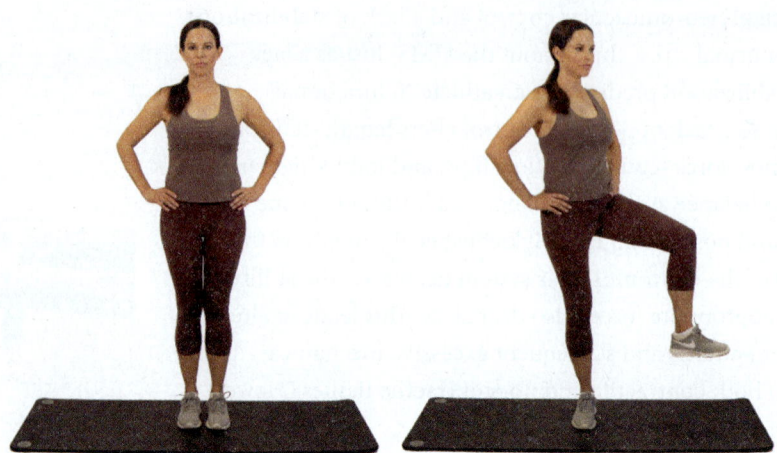

FIGURE 11.6 Stable Versus Unstable Body Position

and creating an opportunity for the extra forces to overcome the structural integrity of joint structures (Ogard, 2011). Beyond just functional instability, a lack of neuromuscular stabilization alters length–tension relationships, force–couple relationships, and joint kinematics, decreasing balance and performance and leading to tissue overload and possible injury (Mandelbaum et al., 2005; McGuine & Keene, 2006; Yoo et al., 2010).

🤖 GETTING TECHNICAL

A moment arm is the perpendicular distance from the axis of rotation (i.e., the joint) to the line of action (i.e., the load). The longer the moment arm of an external load, the more force that is required to stabilize the joint. Therefore, keeping a load close to the center of gravity is easier than holding it farther away. For example, when completing a squat, if the athlete demonstrates an excessive forward lean of the torso, it increases the moment arm of the load, simultaneously increasing the muscular force required by the lower back to keep the body from losing balance.

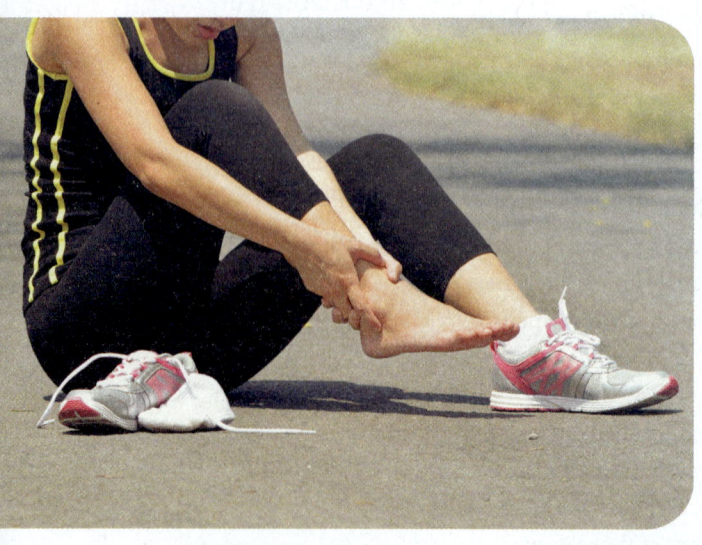

© Sawaddeebenz/Shutterstock

A preventive training program can reduce the risk of instability-related injuries, such as ankle sprains (Caldemeyer et al., 2020; McKeon & Hertel, 2008) and anterior cruciate ligament (ACL) injuries (Bellows & Wong, 2018; McGuine & Keene, 2006; Myklebust et al., 2003). One specific mechanism influencing injury risk reduction is a shortened latency period for muscle activation and improved coactivation of stabilizing muscles during dynamic efforts after a balance training program (Letafatkar et al., 2019).

Even if an injury does not occur immediately in the presence of instability, decreased neuromuscular control can lead to poor movement stabilization, setting an athlete up for an eventual injury because of chronic exposure to suboptimal loading patterns (Ogard, 2011). Therefore, alongside resistance, core, and plyometric training, balance training is an integral part of an overall neuromuscular training program to reduce injury risk (Sañudo et al., 2019).

ATHLETE REHABILITATION

Balance training plays a crucial role in athlete rehabilitation by helping to restore stability, coordination, and proprioception (the sense of body position) after an injury. For example, Di Stasi and Snyder-Mackler (2012) discovered that **perturbation balance training** (i.e., standing on a moving surface) reduced limb asymmetries and improved walking biomechanics in preoperative female athletes who sustained an ACL rupture. Similarly, neuromotor deficits during single-leg landing tasks were improved with neuromuscular training after ACL reconstruction (Nagelli et al., 2019; Nagelli et al., 2020). Proprioception is also reduced after injury, either because of the pain response or because of structural damage to the tissues responsible for sensory input (Ager et al., 2020).

Balance training can contribute to athlete rehabilitation in various ways:

1. Restoring proprioception: Following an injury, the body's ability to sense and respond to joint position and movement changes can be compromised. Balance training exercises help retrain the proprioceptive system, allowing athletes to regain their sense of body position and movement.

2. Strengthening stabilizing muscles: Balance training exercises typically engage the small stabilizing muscles, tendons, and ligaments that are often overlooked during traditional strength training. These exercises help to improve muscle strength, endurance, and stability around the injured area, promoting proper joint alignment and reducing the risk of future injuries.

3. Enhancing neuromuscular control: The communication between the brain and the muscles can be disrupted after an injury. Balance training helps to improve neuromuscular control, enhancing the coordination and timing of muscle activation. This, in turn, enhances joint stability, reduces compensatory movements, and improves overall movement efficiency.

4. Developing functional movement patterns: Athletes must regain their ability to perform sport-specific movements with proper form and technique. Balance training can be tailored to mimic the demands of their sport, focusing on exercises that challenge dynamic balance, agility, and coordination. Athletes can effectively bridge the gap between injury recovery and sport-specific performance by integrating these movements into their rehabilitation program.

5. Psychological benefits: Rehabilitation can be mentally challenging, and athletes may experience fear, loss of confidence, or decreased motivation after an injury. Balance training provides athletes with tangible proof of progress as they regain stability and control, boosting their confidence and motivation throughout rehabilitation.

Note that balance training should be implemented in tandem with other components of a comprehensive rehabilitation program, such as strength training, flexibility exercises, and cardiovascular conditioning. A multidisciplinary approach involving an athlete's sports training team is often necessary to develop an individualized rehabilitation plan tailored to the athlete's specific needs.

Balance training is beneficial for most injured athletes, but the benefits are more pronounced for those athletes with more severe deficits at the beginning of training (Hewett et al., 2017). In addition, athletes after an injury have varying levels of affected proprioception compared to noninjured athletes (Ghaderi et al., 2020; Ogard, 2011). This deficit can persist even after mechanical stability is restored post-surgery and post-rehabilitation, highlighting the importance of including proprioceptive balance training throughout the rehabilitation process (Courtney et al., 2019).

PERTURBATION →
BALANCE
TRAINING

A style of balance training that introduces external instability in a manner that is unpredictable to the athlete, requiring reflexive stabilization of the involved joints.

SPORTS PERFORMANCE ENHANCEMENT

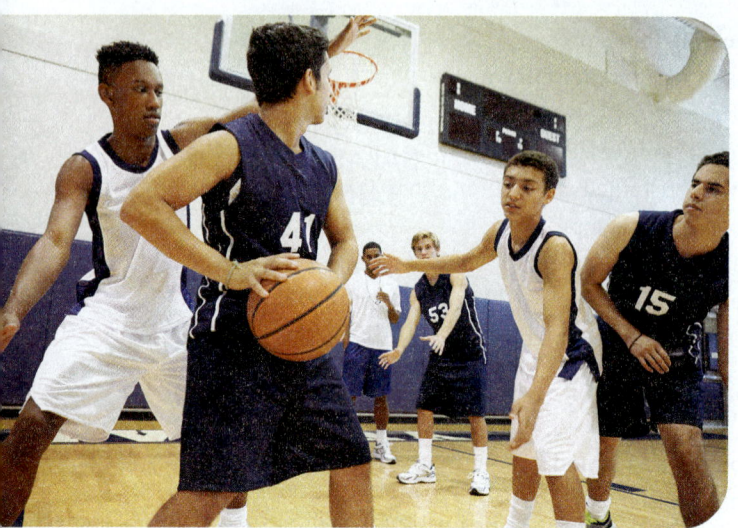

© Monkey Business Images/Shutterstock

Balance training can keep athletes healthy or help them return to play after injury, but it also influences sport-specific training metrics. Generally, the integration of balance exercises into a comprehensive program is associated with improvements in various sports disciplines (Brachman et al., 2017).

For example, Canli (2019) demonstrated a significant improvement in motoric fitness (agility, strength, power, flexibility, and balance) as well as sport-specific skills (shooting and dribbling) in young male basketball athletes who completed a comprehensive training program that included balance exercises, compared to a control group from the same team who did not participate in extra training with balance exercises. Both groups devoted the same practice time to skill development, but the experimental group demonstrated the most improvement in sport-specific skills. It is worth noting that the experimental group participated in a complete training program, with balance serving as only one component.

The findings of this study support the idea that balance training is likely most impactful when used within a comprehensive training program. Similar results have been found in women's basketball (Bouteraa et al., 2020), young elite soccer athletes (Hammami et al., 2016), young rugby athletes (Alonso-Aubin et al., 2021), Taekwondo (Ivanenko & Gurfinkel, 2018), and other sports (Brachman et al., 2017).

Some of the performance improvements can be attributed to correcting muscular asymmetries and imbalances with core stability and neuromuscular control training (Dello Iacono et al., 2016). Another moderating variable could be increased musculoskeletal fitness—a common adaptation to neuromuscular training programs (Ahmed & Ahmed, 2015). Additionally, the skilled application of basic adaptations has been observed in physical performance measures for speed, agility, and power (Sañudo et al., 2019; Trajković & Bogataj, 2020; Zech et al., 2010). These mechanisms are fundamental in youth athletes, helping them to develop these skills and laying a foundation for future performance (Williams et al., 2021). Interestingly, a neuromuscular training program that includes balance training may have an enduring influence on, for example, power output even after the training stimulus is removed during a period of detraining as long as 8 weeks (Nunes et al., 2021). When implemented as part of an integrated training program, balance training supports the development of fundamental movement competency and fitness that can enhance sports performance.

LESSON 4: PRINCIPLES OF BALANCE TRAINING
BALANCE TRAINING GUIDELINES

Balance exercises are a vital component of a sports training program, as they help to ensure optimal muscle recruitment and coordinated movement. Balance training exercises must be systematic and progressive. Sports Performance Coaches should follow specific program guidelines, including proper exercise selection criteria and milestones for progression. Balance is improved through repetitive exposure to a variety of proprioceptively enriched environments.

NEEDS ANALYSIS AND ASSESSMENT INFORMATION

As with any aspect of a sports performance program, an intentional and specific program needs to be developed for balance training per each athlete's needs. A needs analysis is the first step that allows the Sports Performance Coach to thoroughly understand the metabolic, mechanical, and injury potential for the athlete and the sport (**Figure 11.7**).

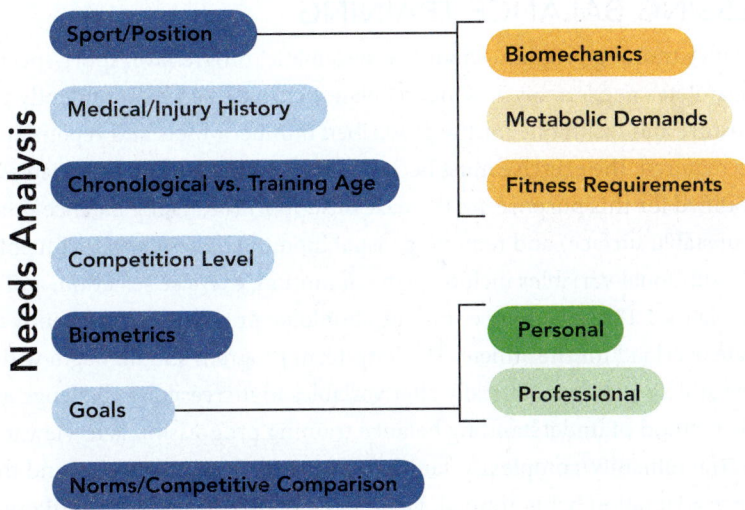

FIGURE 11.7 Needs Analysis

Balance training must be based on the needs analysis results and assessment information to ensure the exercises are tailored to the athlete's specific requirements, goals, and limitations. An individualized approach helps optimize the training process, improve balance capacities and overall performance, and reduce the likelihood of certain injuries.

The Sports Performance Coach should consider that metabolic demands depend on the pattern of play. For example, an endurance runner would have a more sustained, repeated effort balance requirement than an athlete performing a single anaerobic effort, such as an Olympic lifter completing a snatch.

A repeatable balance program could be created for the endurance runner to isolate and replicate the repeated single-leg requirements of running. A drill such as a step to balance can replicate and isolate the ankle, knee, and hip stabilization requirements during running in a position similar to running mechanics and could be focused more on volume.

In contrast, the weightlifter should consider hip stabilization in deeper hip flexion while still challenging the postural control of the hips. One method to challenge the hips in deep flexion is to target each leg individually using single-leg squats or pistol squats, which will have a greater load requirement than the balance exercises used for the endurance runner. These drills also replicate the emphasis on eccentric loading during the catch phase of the snatch. Furthermore, the snatch can be tough on the shoulders, so proper shoulder stabilization and core control with hip stabilization could be improved via a drill like a single-leg quarter squat with overhead stabilization.

Biomechanically, the balance training program should mimic the demands of the sport as closely as possible. In terms of injury, an athlete's injury history should be considered, as well as the types of injuries commonly associated with their sport. For example, if an athlete has a history of ankle sprain, balance drills should target ankle stability. In addition, using a drill like a single-leg hip opener on an unstable surface could be a way to overcome proprioceptive deficits and prepare the athlete for on-field efforts. On the preventive side, youth athletes are still developing the neuromuscular system and may have functional deficits similar to those observed after injury. Therefore, the balance training components of a program should be weighed against an athlete's age (Williams et al., 2021). Overall, the needs analysis provides a framework for developing a targeted program.

PROGRESSING BALANCE TRAINING

A proper balance training program should be systematic, progressive, sport-specific, and based on the athlete's needs analysis. Once a balance exercise can be confidently performed with ideal posture and technique for the prescribed number of sets and repetitions, and at the tempo required, the exercise must become more challenging. Two variables that are often modified for this purpose are the base of support (i.e., using balance modalities to create an unstable surface) and removing visual input (i.e., eyes closed) (Muehlbauer et al., 2012). Additional variables include plane of motion, exercise selection, and added resistance modalities. Finally, balance training should be progressed consistently to provide an appropriate overload for the athlete. The long-term program should begin with what is easiest for the athlete and systematically alter variables to increase the challenge gradually.

A holistic method of understanding balance training progression is to view it across multiple spectra: difficulty/complexity, familiarity/novelty, load/resistance, and the specific type of balance adaptation being trained. Depending on the athlete's needs, these spectra can be used as a roadmap and to facilitate a wide range of creativity in exercise selection. The needs of the athlete drive the choice of which progression ranges to consider. Each spectrum represents a progression methodology from which the next most difficult exercise can be identified, and rarely are they considered in isolation.

Table 11.1 identifies some example balance training variables.

SUMMARY OF BALANCE PROGRESSIONS

The preceding paragraphs described methods for progressing balance exercises by increasing demands on body position and limb movement. The following is a detailed summary:

- Progression 1: When introducing balance exercises into an exercise program, the exercises should initially involve little joint motion of the balance leg to focus on static balance adaptations. These entry-level balance exercises improve reflexive (automatic) joint stabilization contractions to increase joint stability. Using this protocol, the body is placed in an unstable environment, so it learns to react by contracting the right muscles at the right time to maintain balance. These exercises should be mastered before moving to more challenging forms of balance training.
  - Once these types of exercises have been mastered, the Sports Performance Coach can choose to make these exercises more challenging (if deemed appropriate) by integrating the following:
    - Balance modalities (e.g., balance beam, half foam roll, foam pad, balance disc, wobble board)
    - Cognitive, dual-task scenarios (e.g., naming the months of the year while balancing on one limb)
    - Closing eye tasks
    - Head or eye movement

TABLE 11.1   Example Balance Training Variables

Progression Spectrum	Example Progressions
Complexity/difficulty Simple to perform → Harder to perform **Associated variables:** • Exercise selection • Base of support • Plane of motion	Choose a new exercise with greater movement complexity. **Examples:** • A single-leg hop to balance is more complex than lifting a foot into a single-leg balance stance. • Standing on a balance modality (e.g., foam pad, balance disc) requires greater levels of motor control than standing on a solid floor. • A transverse plane lunge to balance has more combined movements than a forward lunge to balance.
Familiarity/novelty Known movements/positions → Unknown movements/positions **Associated variables:** • Exercise selection • Plane of motion • Visual input • Base of support	Choose a new exercise representing movement and body positions the athlete does not regularly perform. **Examples:** • Use a movement variation that the athlete has never done before. • Transverse and frontal plane movement is less familiar to most athletes than sagittal plane exercises. • Closing the eyes can make static balance positions more challenging. • Using a balance modality makes the base of support feel new and unknown at first.
Load/resistance No load → Increased load → Repositioned load **Associated variable:** Resistance modalities	Increase the amount and positioning of an external load progressively. **Example:** • Holding a sandbag during a single-leg balance, then holding it on the contralateral shoulder of the balance leg.
Balance adaptation type Static → Dynamic → Eccentric control **Associated variable:** Exercise selection	Changing the type of balance that is being trained. **Example:** • Use static balance exercises for the first several weeks, then switch to biomechanically similar dynamic exercises for the next mesocycle.

- Progression 2: The next progression involves dynamic eccentric and concentric movement of the balance leg through a full range of motion to emphasize dynamic balance adaptations. Movements require dynamic control in the mid-range of motion, with isometric stabilization at the end-range. The speed and neural demand of each exercise are progressed.
  - Once these types of exercises have been mastered, the Sports Performance Coach can again choose to make these exercises more challenging (if deemed appropriate) by integrating:
    - Planes of motion (sagittal, frontal, transverse)
    - Load (external resistance)
    - Balance modalities
    - Cognitive, dual-task scenarios
    - Closing eye tasks
    - Head or eye movement

- Progression 3: The last progression includes exercises designed to develop proper deceleration ability to move the body from a dynamic state to a controlled stationary position. This progression scheme places greater emphasis on eccentric control.
  - Once these types of exercises have been mastered, the Sports Performance Coach can again choose to make these exercises more challenging (if deemed appropriate) by integrating:
    - Planes of motion (sagittal, frontal, transverse)
    - Load (external resistance)
    - Balance modalities
    - Cognitive, dual-task scenarios
    - Closing eye tasks
    - Head or eye movement

Planning exercise progressions to challenge the balance system by manipulating one variable at a time is vital. The progressions implemented should be athlete-specific based on their unique physical capabilities and the needs of their sport.

How long an athlete spends on an exercise before progressing depends on individual skills and abilities. For example, whereas one individual may easily take to performing exercises with eyes closed, others may require a lot of practice spread out over multiple training sessions. Each individual has their entire lifetime of motor learning, and athletes will present in the gym with varying degrees of adaptability to novel experiences. Ultimately, progressions through added complexity and novelty will move at the pace at which the athlete can handle them. One method to simplify the progression process is to categorize balance training techniques as focusing on static, dynamic, or eccentric control.

STATIC BALANCE

Static balance is the ability to maintain a stable body position with complete postural control, keeping the center of mass within the base of support when minimal movement is present (Brachman et al., 2017; Çelenk et al., 2018) (**Figure 11.8**). Static balance is the foundation on which the rest of movement is built. If an athlete can stabilize a starting

**STATIC
BALANCE** →

The ability to maintain a stable body position with complete postural control, keeping the center of mass within the base of support when minimal movement is present.

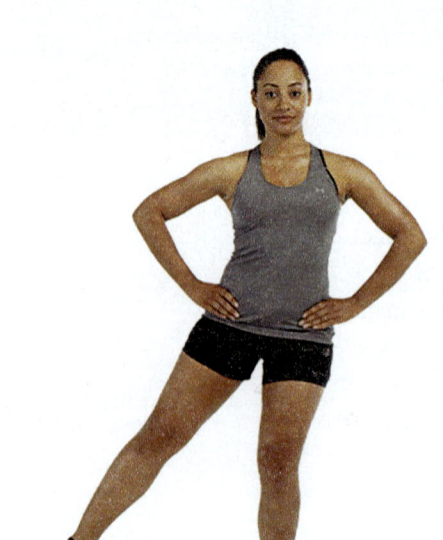
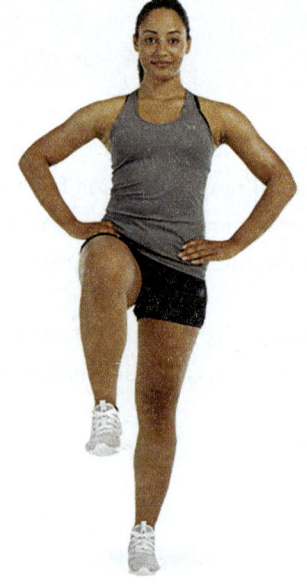
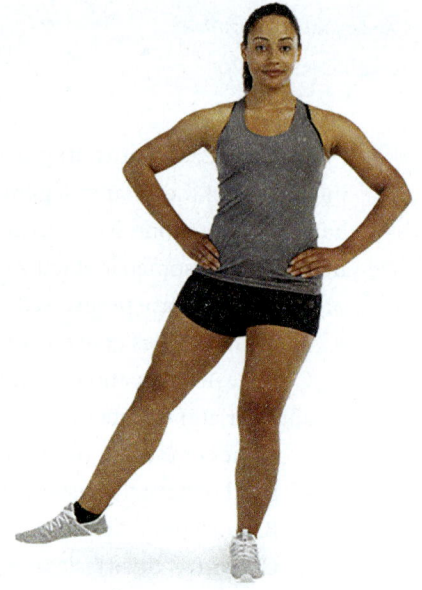

FIGURE 11.8 Static Balance

joint position, any subsequent application of force will be more efficient, with less misdirected effort. This is the difference between proactive and reactive stabilization.

DYNAMIC BALANCE

Dynamic balance is the ability to stabilize the body when there are perturbations to the system (Çelenk et al., 2018) (**Figure 11.9**). These perturbations often result in limb movements in response to an implement (e.g., ball, stick) or an opponent. However, the surface may also change for certain athletes, such as surfers or flyers in cheerleading. Sporting events require a large amount of dynamic stabilization due to the constantly changing conditions. Dynamic balance allows the athlete to control their movements in a coordinated way without overcompensating when changes—for example, in direction— are required.

**DYNAMIC   →
BALANCE**

The ability to maintain a stable body position with complete postural control, keeping the center of mass within the base of support when perturbations to the system are present.

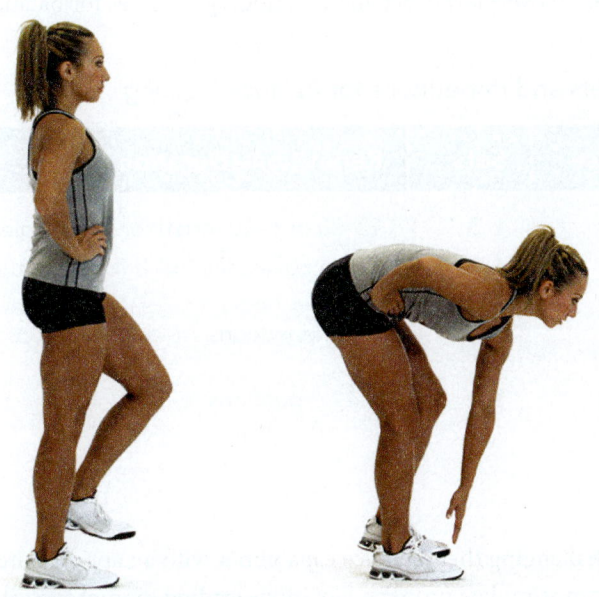

FIGURE 11.9 Dynamic Balance

👍 HELPFUL HINT

One way to remember the difference between static and dynamic balance is to recognize that they involve the same concepts as stretching. Like static stretching, static balance requires the athlete to hold a position for a specific time without moving. In terms of balance, this could be resisting unwanted movement (i.e., perturbations). In contrast, dynamic stretching and dynamic balance require movement and reactive stabilization.

ECCENTRIC CONTROL BALANCE

Eccentric control balance is a form of balance training that challenges the motor control present with a muscle-lengthening contraction. An example is landing a jump on a single leg. Due to differences in force fluctuation, motor unit recruitment, and cortical stimulation, eccentric contractions are more challenging to control than concentric activity (Perrey, 2018). Nevertheless, eccentric control is vital in maintaining proper positioning in skills such as deceleration or landing patterns.

**ECCENTRIC   →
CONTROL
BALANCE**

The ability to effectively maintain the center of mass over a reduced base of support during muscle-lengthening contractions, such as when landing a jump on a single leg.

ACUTE TRAINING VARIABLES FOR BALANCE TRAINING

The Sports Performance Coach must ensure that all programs follow the recommended acute training variables for balance training.

SETS AND REPETITIONS

Sets and repetitions are vital components of balance training for athletes, as they determine the volume and structure of the training session, directly impacting the development of strength, endurance, and overall performance. Adhering to appropriate sets and repetitions ensures that balance training remains challenging yet manageable, allowing for consistent progress while minimizing the risk of overtraining or injury. **Table 11.2** provides an overview of set and repetition guidelines for balance training.

TABLE 11.2   Sets and Repetitions for Balance Training

Type of Balance	Sets	Repetitions/Duration
Static	1–3	12–20 or 6–10 repetitions on single-leg exercises 30- to 60-second holds for isometrics
Dynamic	2–4	8–12 repetitions
Eccentric control	1–3	8–12 repetitions

INTENSITY

By progressively challenging their balance capabilities with an appropriate level of intensity, athletes can stimulate proper adaptations leading to improved stability and overall performance. Moreover, working at an optimal intensity helps to prevent plateaus in progress, ensuring continuous improvements in performance. However, it is essential to match intensity with the proper form and technique to minimize the risk of injury and maximize the effectiveness of each exercise. Recommended intensities will vary based on athlete experience, injury history, and assessment results. Balance exercises should be increased by adjusting the complexity of the exercise, neural demand, stance-leg range of motion (ROM), and tempo, rather than by increasing load. **Table 11.3** provides general recommendations.

TABLE 11.3   General Intensities for Balance Training

Type of Balance	Intensity
Static	Bodyweight
Dynamic	Bodyweight—moderate load. Intensity is increased by increasing complexity and/or difficulty.
Eccentric control	Bodyweight—moderate. Intensity is increased by increasing eccentric demand and/or complexity.

TRAINING FREQUENCY

A well-planned training schedule ensures that core muscles are consistently and progressively challenged, allowing for the necessary adaptations to occur, while also providing ample time for recovery and repair. By maintaining the optimal balance between training and recovery, athletes can prevent overtraining, reduce the risk of injuries, and maximize the benefits of balance training.

TRAINING VOLUME

The volume of balance training is critical for athletes, as it determines the overall workload. A well-calibrated training volume ensures that balance capabilities are sufficiently stimulated to trigger necessary adaptations while allowing for adequate recovery and repair. By finding the optimal pairing of training intensity and volume, athletes can experience continuous progress in their balance training, leading to improved performance across a wide range of sports. Moreover, appropriate training volume helps to prevent overtraining, reduces the risk of injuries, and contributes to a more sustainable and effective training program.

The Sports Performance Coach must recognize that balance training engages, to a large degree, the deep stabilization muscles surrounding joints. These muscles are subject to load and stress during the entire training session. For example, a traditional exercise, such as a lunge, requires significant activation of the hip stabilization muscles. Therefore, the general frequency and volume guidelines recommended in **Table 11.4** must be adjusted for each athlete to reflect the total training demand.

TABLE 11.4   Frequency and Volume for Balance Training

Type of Balance	Frequency	Volume
Static	4–6 sessions per week	20–48 repetitions/exercise
Dynamic	3–5 sessions per week	12–36 repetitions/exercise
Eccentric control	2–4 sessions per week	8–20 repetitions/exercise

LESSON 5: MODALITIES FOR BALANCE TRAINING
BALANCE TRAINING TECHNIQUES

Balance is a task-specific adaptation, so the exercise selection must mimic the demands of the sport as closely as possible. Static balance is the foundation for joint stabilization with minimal movement, but it can be progressed to dynamic stabilization, which emphasizes limb movement. Eccentric control is another aspect of balance that focuses on absorbing forces. An integrated program will emphasize these aspects of balance training in different ways but should always come back to the concept of sport-specificity. The purpose of balance training exercises for athletes is to enhance joint stabilization and proprioceptive control so that body positioning optimizes force expression.

STATIC BALANCE

Static balance training involves minimal movement of the distal joint but introduces perturbations to the system to necessitate a reflexive stabilization response. The control of the stance leg replicates sport-specific movements in which a plant leg facilitates ground reactive forces to allow throwing (e.g., baseball, javelin), receiving a check (e.g., hockey, lacrosse), or swinging an implement (e.g., tennis, golf). Any sports skill requiring an athlete to plant at least one leg while other movements occur around that stabilized limb or limbs may benefit from static balance training.

STATIC BALANCE EXERCISES

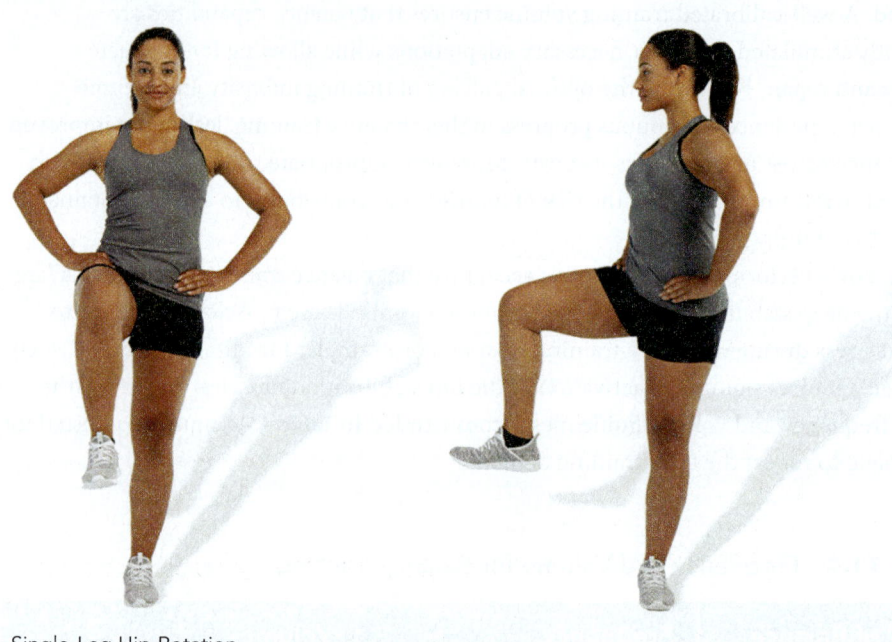

Single-Leg Hip Rotation

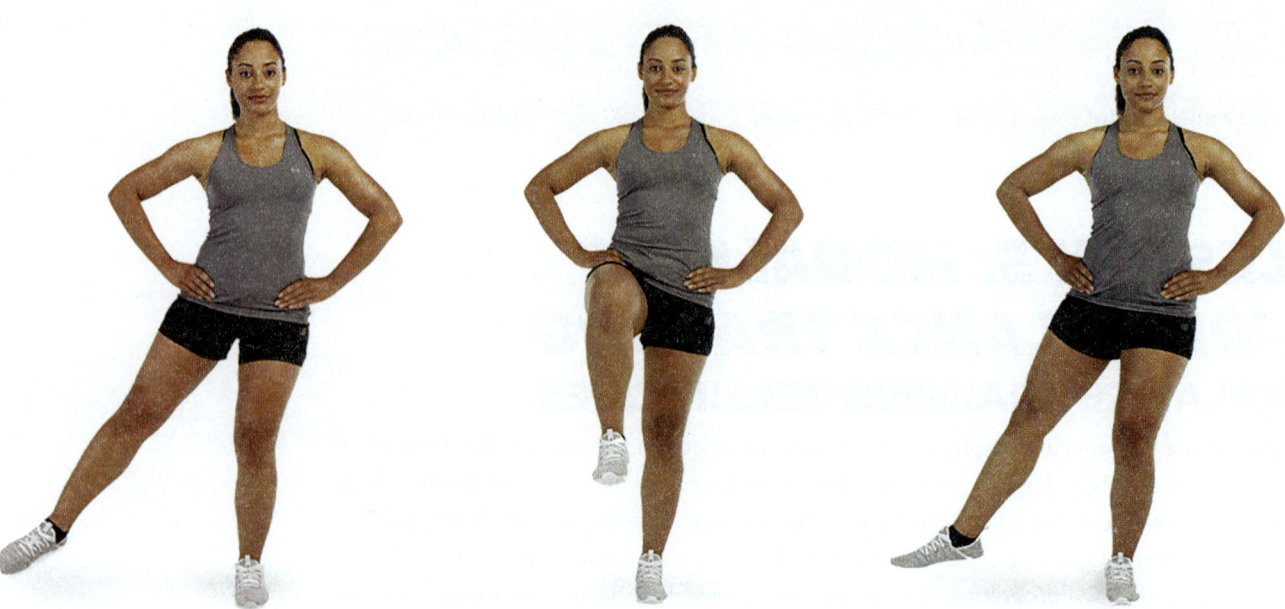

Single-Leg Balance Reach Progressions

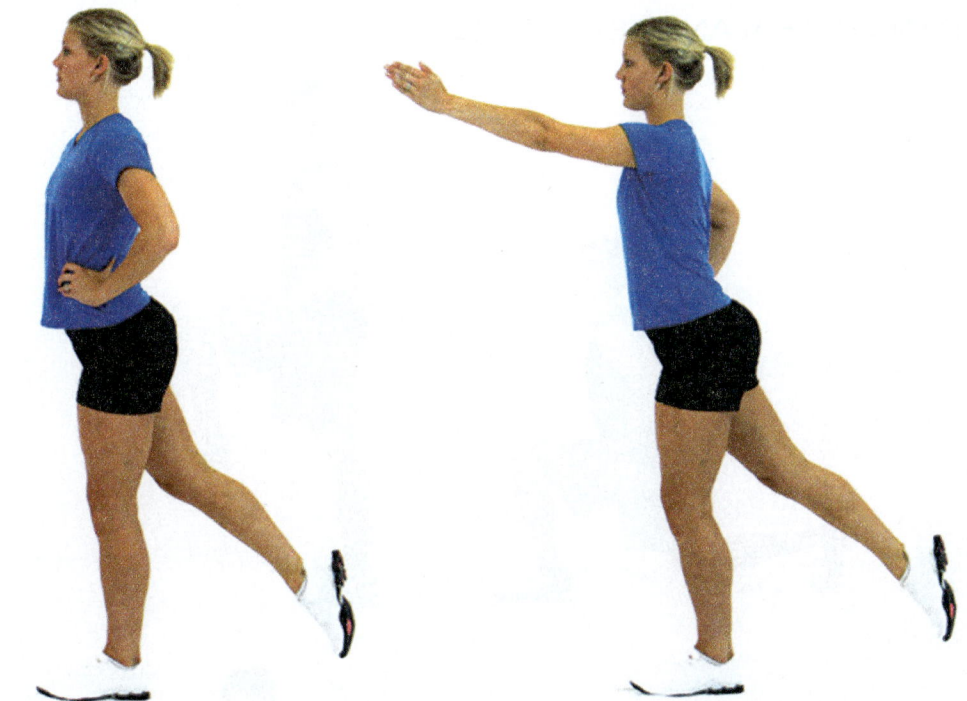

Single-Leg Balance Arm and Leg Motion

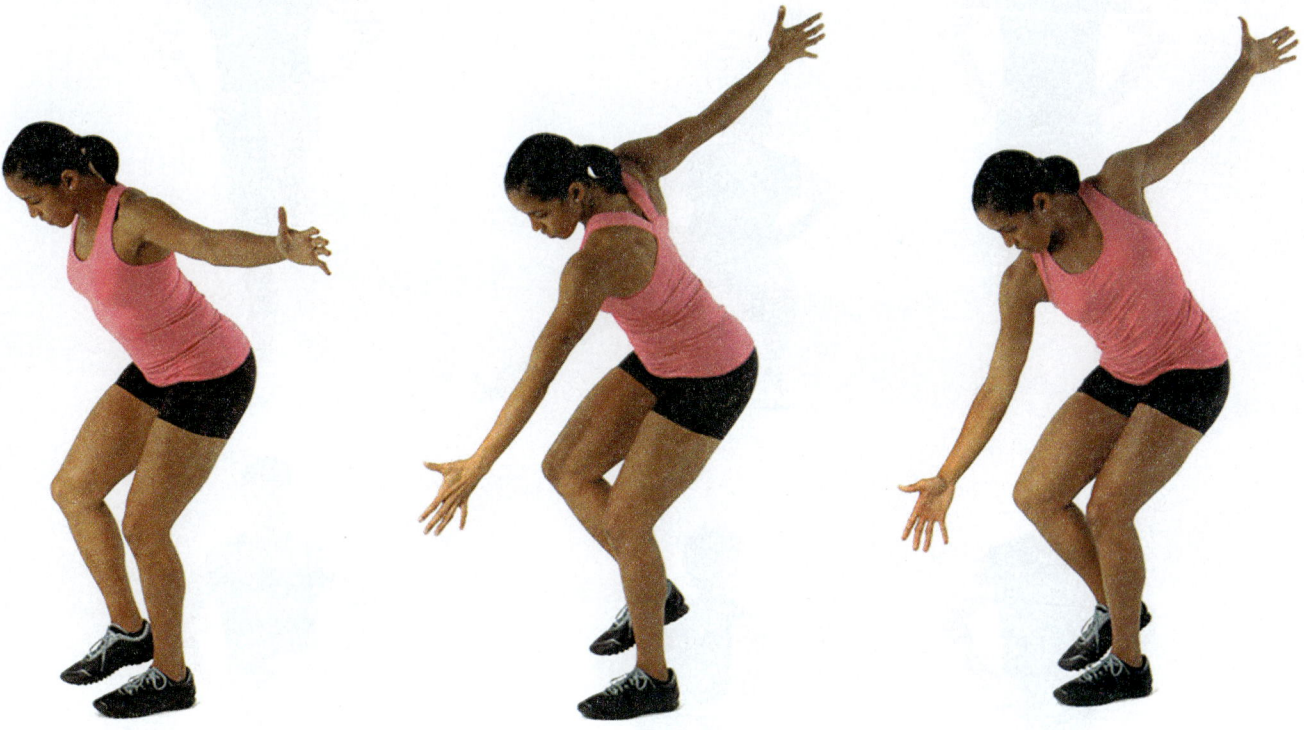

Single-Leg Windmill

DYNAMIC BALANCE

Dynamic balance training involves greater dynamic movements and perturbations to the system, requiring a greater reflexive stabilization response than static balance. The stance leg will be challenged due to the greater concentric and eccentric movement, requiring stronger neuromuscular control.

DYNAMIC BALANCE EXERCISES

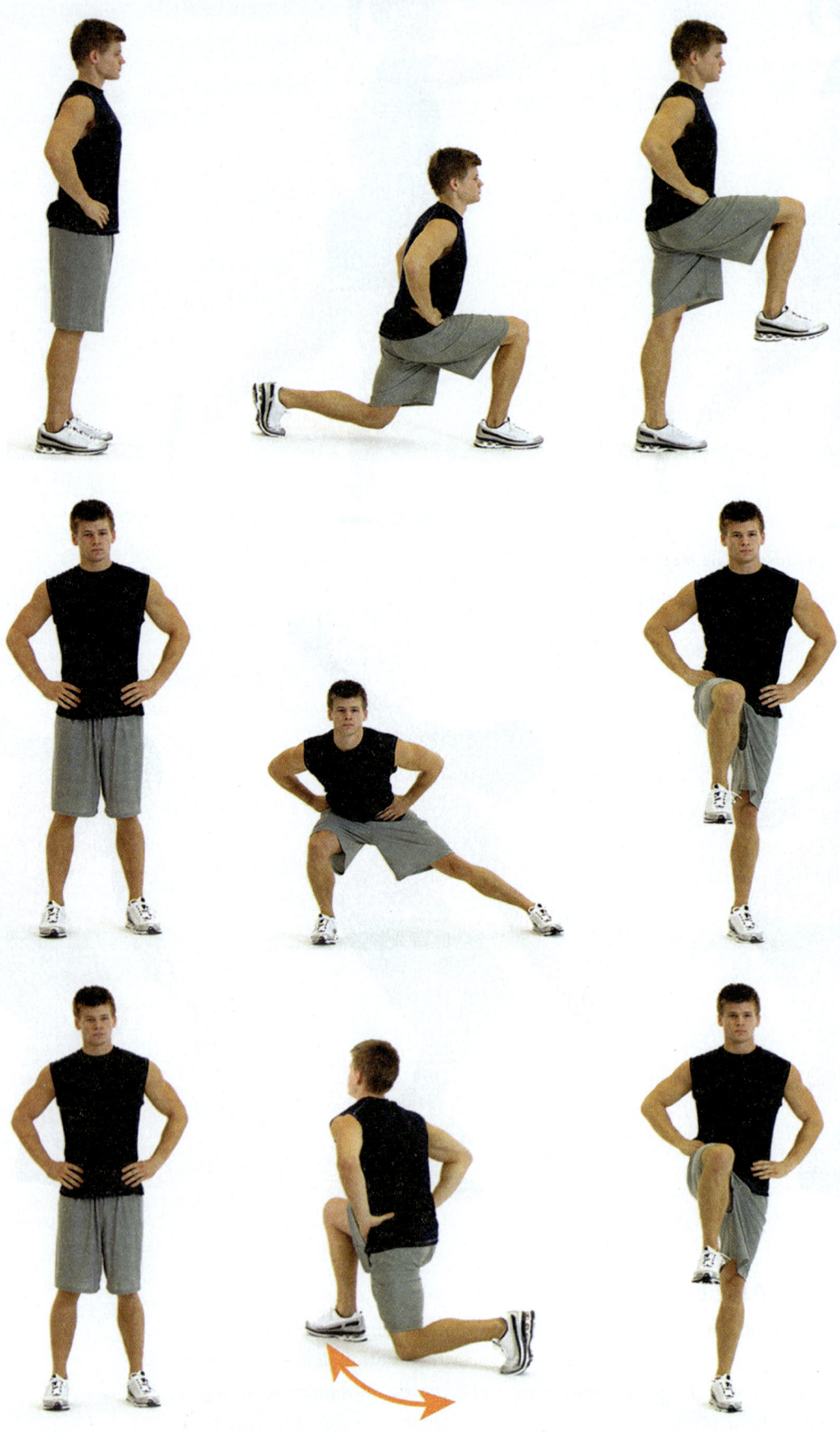

Multiplanar Lunge to Balance

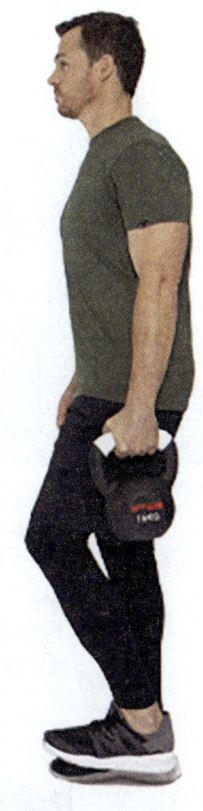
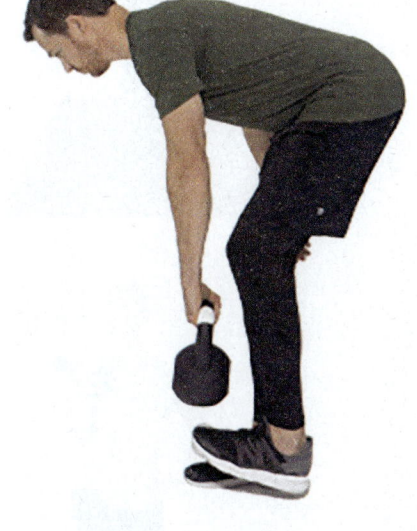

Single-Leg Romanian Deadlift

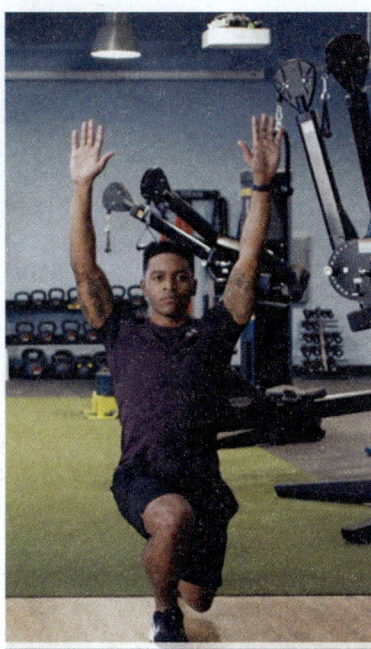
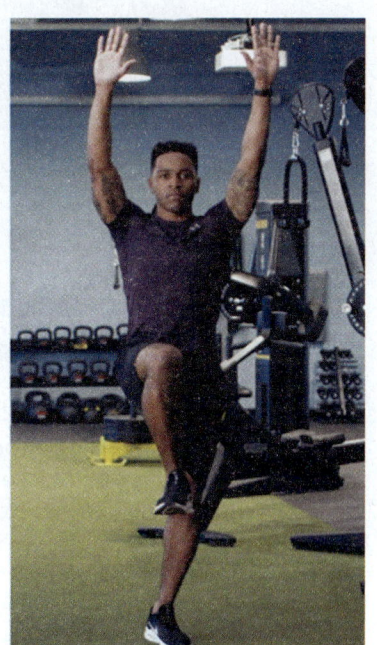

Overhead Lunge to Balance

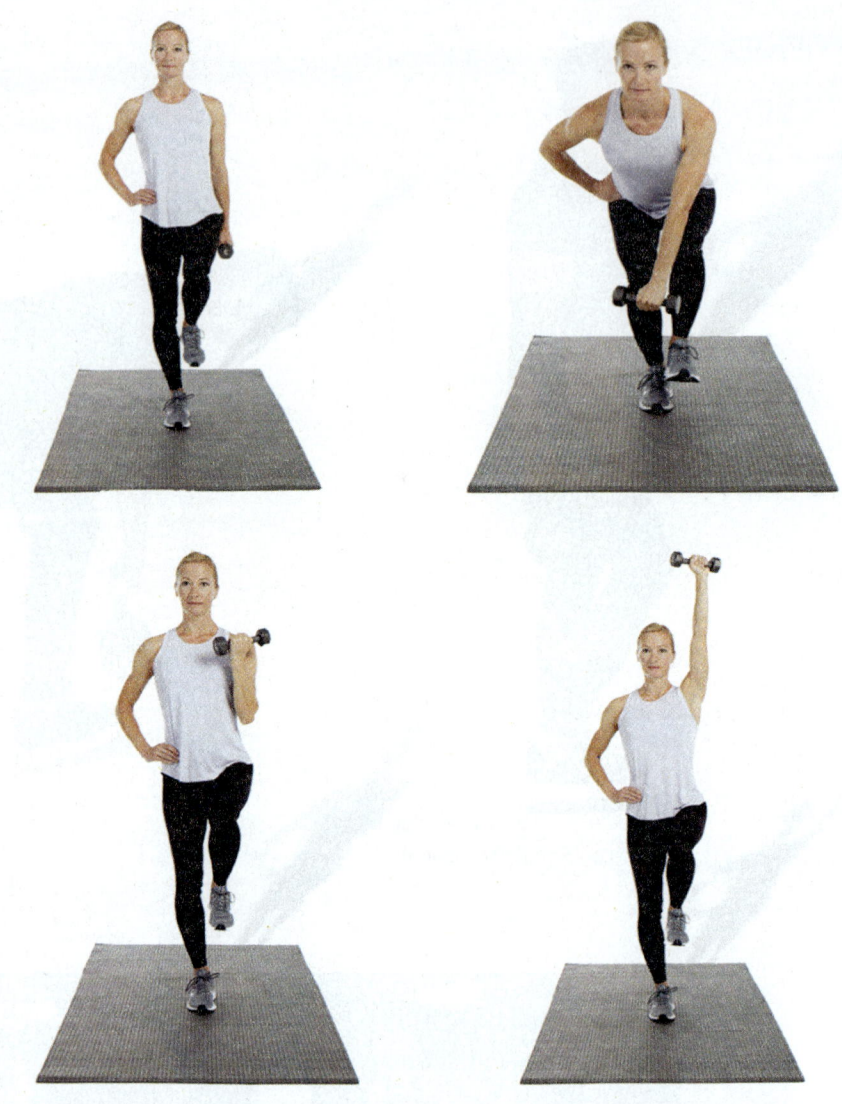

Single-Leg Squat, Curl to Overhead Press

ECCENTRIC CONTROL

Eccentric control exercises, like dynamic exercises, use concentric and eccentric movements but emphasize and challenge the eccentric contraction with a focus on stabilization and control. The motor control during the eccentric portion of a movement requires different patterns than the concentric portion and is often an area of weakness. Eccentric control is apparent in any landing technique after a jump (e.g., basketball, volleyball, gymnastics) and basic stance phase analysis for athletes sprinting or changing direction (e.g., soccer, lacrosse).

ECCENTRIC CONTROL EXERCISES

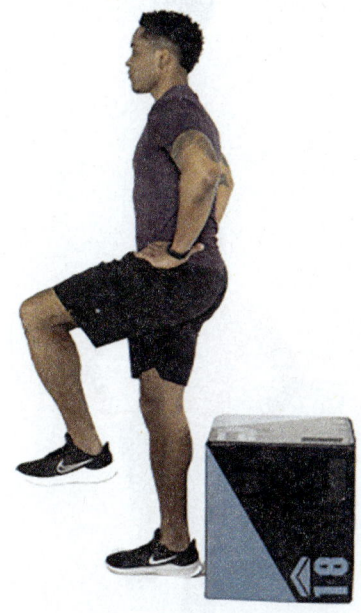
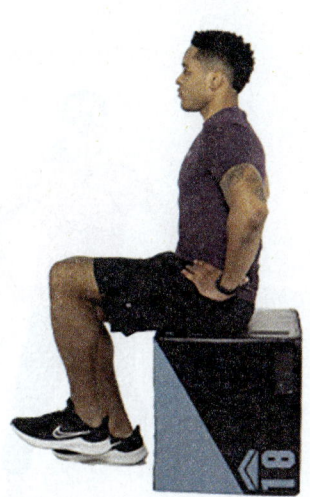

Single-Leg Box Squat

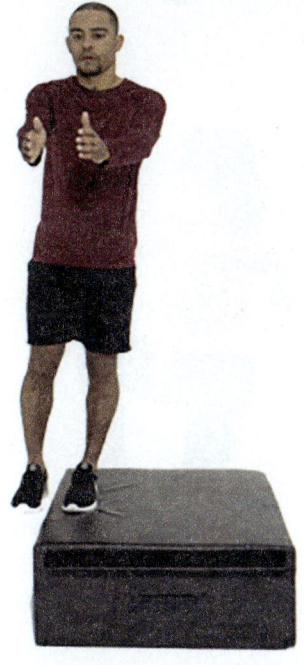
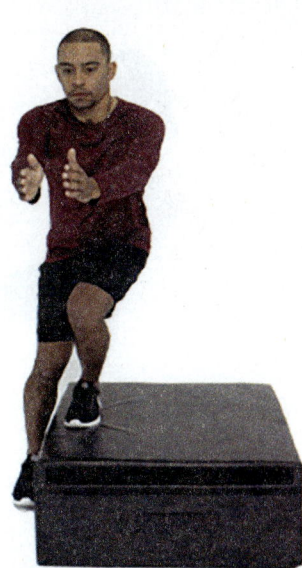

Single-Leg Lowering

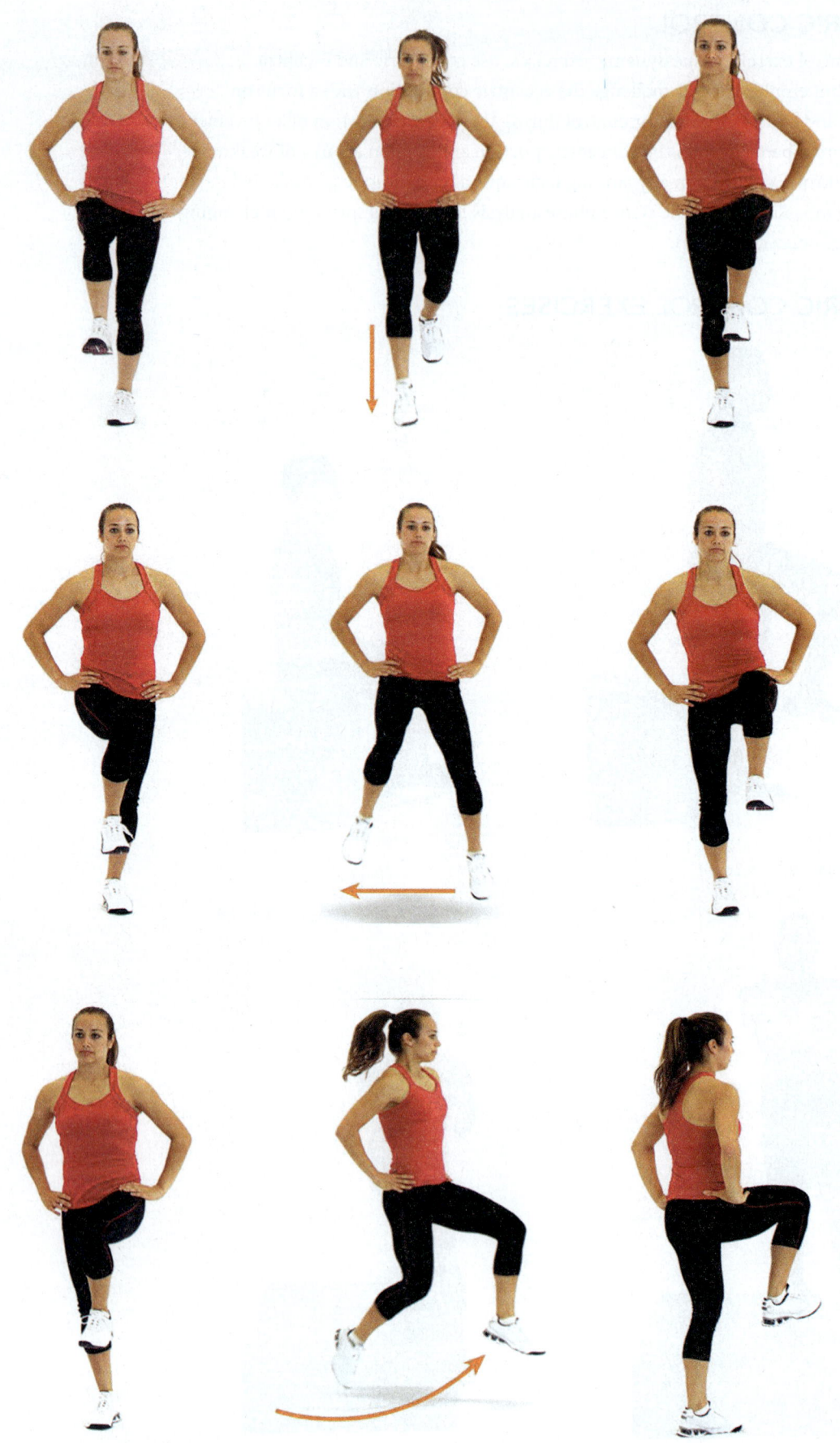

Multiplanar Hop with Stabilization

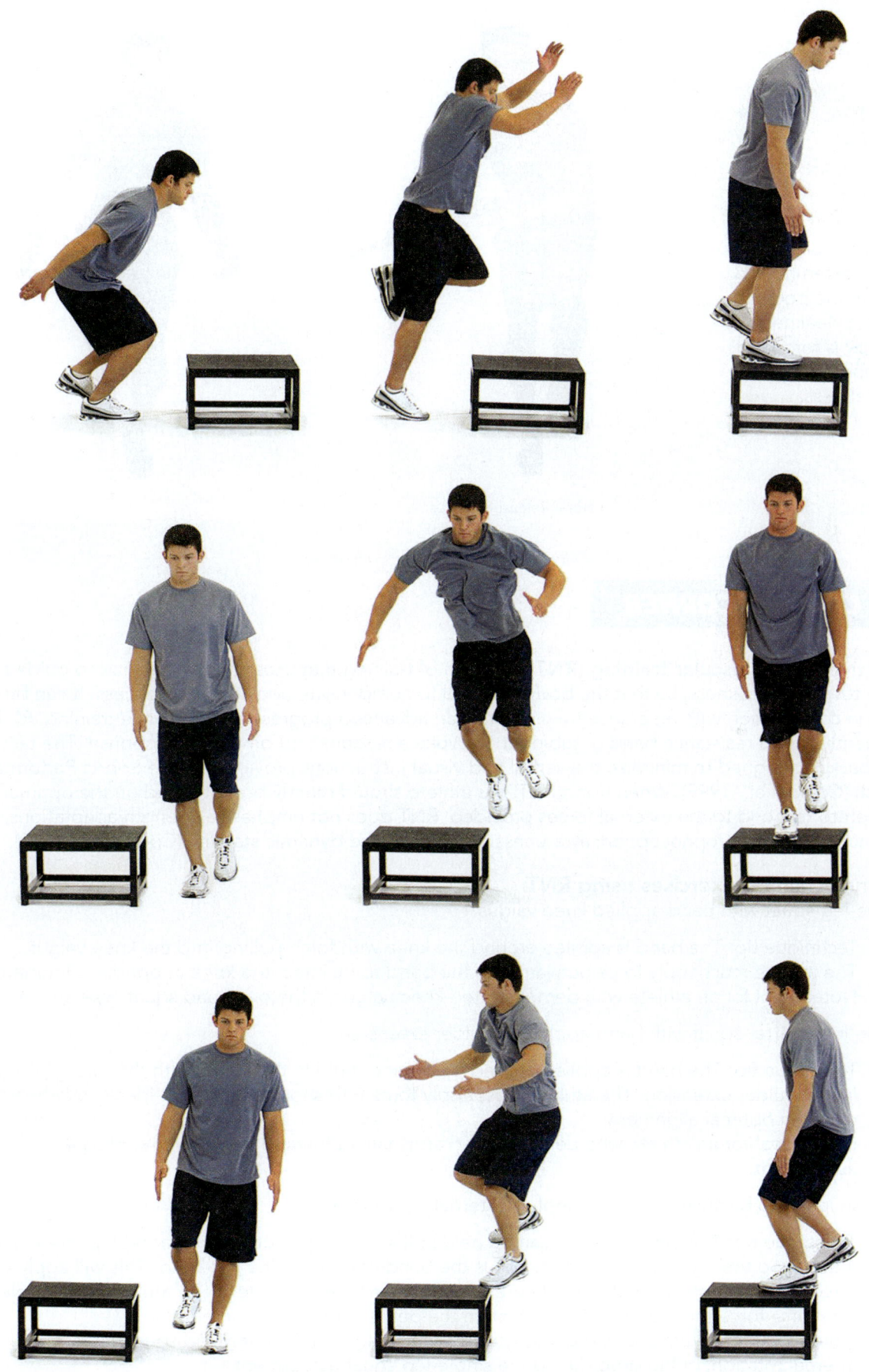

Multiplanar Hop-up with Stabilization

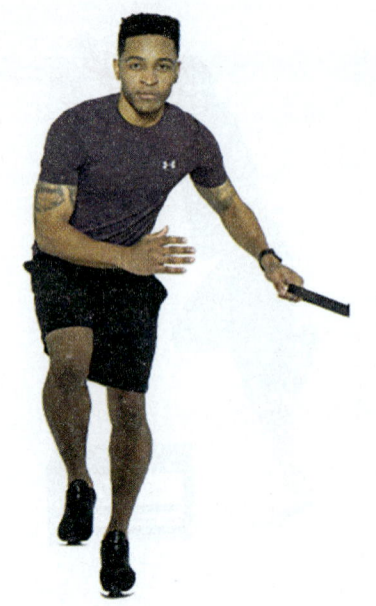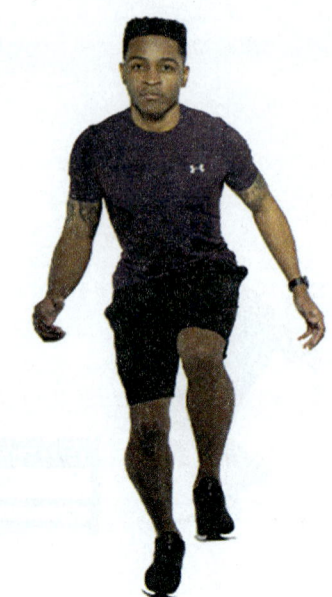

REACTIVE NEURO-MUSCULAR TRAINING (RNT) →
A form of training that uses an external load to guide the body toward a weakness, so the body is forced to compensate against the weakness.

Lateral Release Catches

📋 COACH'S CORNER

Reactive neuromuscular training (RNT) is a form of training that uses an external load to guide the body toward a weakness, so that the body is forced to compensate *against* the weakness. It can be used in combination with resistance training or as an advanced progression to balance training. RNT frequently uses a resistance band or tubing to provoke a reactive neuromuscular response. The tactile feedback is designed to minimize the verbal and visual instructions provided by the Sports Performance Coach (Cook et al., 1999). When using RNT, the athlete should merely be instructed on the optimal form and left to respond to the external forces provided. RNT does not emphasize strength adaptations, but instead focuses on proprioception, awareness of posture, and dynamic stability (Cook et al., 1999).

Balance training exercises using RNT:
Single-leg squat with band-applied knee valgus

- Technique tip: The band is applied around the knee with force pulling into the knee valgus. The athlete must apply force outward into the band to maintain the knee in optimal alignment.
- Note: Ideal for an athlete who demonstrated knee valgus in the overhead squat assessment.

Single-leg quarter squat with band-applied shoulder extension

- Technique tip: The band is applied around the wrist or held in the hands with the force pulling into shoulder extension. The athlete must apply force into shoulder flexion—ideally overhead—to maintain optimal alignment.
- Note: Ideal for an athlete who demonstrated arms falling forward in the overhead squat assessment.

Reverse lunge to balance with band-applied internal hip rotation

- Technique tip: The band or cable can be held in the hand opposite of the target hip. For example, if targeting the right hip, the athlete holds the band or cable in the left hand. This will apply a force that attempts to rotate the athlete's torso toward the stance leg. The athlete must apply rotational force through the hip to maintain the pelvis in optimal alignment.
- Note: Ideal for an athlete who demonstrated knee valgus in the overhead squat assessment, internal rotation, or hip drop during the single-leg squat assessment.

SUMMARY

Balance is an essential foundation for physical fitness and sports performance. The body's ability to maintain the center of mass within its base of support is critical for skill expression. The brain performs a complex integration by processing visual, vestibular, and sensorimotor input to create coordinated motor output. Balance training should mimic the biomechanical demands of the sport to promote optimal positive transfer. Various methods can be used to progressively overload the system, but any changes should occur with the intent to maintain optimal technique. With an intentional program, athletes can improve their balance function and create a better foundation for movement. A successful balance training program will improve sports performance and reduce the likelihood of injury, but can also be used as part of the rehabilitation process if an injury does occur. Although it does not replace other forms of training, balance training is an important aspect of a holistic performance model.

KEY TAKEAWAYS

- The combined effects of ideal sensorimotor input and movement efficiency on the neuromuscular system provide the necessary foundation for the optimal expression of performance attributes such as strength, power, speed, and agility.
- Neuromuscular training programs designed to improve motor control often include an integrated subset of training tactics, including dynamic stability, balance, strength, and power.
- Three key areas that precipitate injuries for athletes include strength deficits, neuromuscular imbalances between limbs, and deficits in postural stability. Proprioceptive balance training has been shown to increase postural stability and neuromuscular control for athletes and appears to be better at achieving these goals than sport-specific training alone.
- Post-injury athletes have varying levels of reduced proprioception at the affected joint compared to noninjured athletes. Furthermore, this deficit can persist after mechanical stability is restored post-surgery and post-rehabilitation, highlighting the importance of proprioceptive balance training throughout the rehabilitation process.
- The sensory information from vestibular systems is combined in the CNS, which processes the afferent signal to determine the nature of the peripheral motion and the body's position in space. The processed input is then converted into an appropriate efferent motor response that maintains equilibrium and efficiently controls movement.
- Every sport has unique balance applications that require specific training methods to mimic these demands. Therefore, the concept of a universal balance training program should be avoided in favor of a more tailored approach.
- Balance is a task-specific adaptation, so balance exercise selection must mimic the demands of the sport as closely as possible. Static balance is the foundation for joint stabilization with minimal movement; it can be progressed to dynamic stabilization, which emphasizes limb movement. Eccentric control is another aspect of balance that focuses on absorbing forces.
- An integrated program will emphasize these aspects of balance training in different ways but should always come back to the concept of sport-specificity.
- The purpose of balance training exercises for athletes is to enhance joint stabilization and proprioceptive control, so that body positioning optimizes the expression of force.

REFERENCES

Ager, A. L., Borms, D., Deschepper, L., Dhooghe, R., Dijkhuis, J., Roy, J. S., & Cools, A. (2020). Proprioception: How is it affected by shoulder pain? A systematic review. *Journal of Hand Therapy*, *33*(4), 507–516.

Ahmed, T., & Ahmed, E. (2015). Improving musculoskeletal fitness and the performance enhancement of basketball skills through neuromuscular training program. *Journal of Human Sport and Exercise*, *10*(3), 795–804.

Alonso-Aubin, D. A., Picón-Martínez, M., Rebullido, T. R., Faigenbaum, A. D., Cortell-Tormo, J. M., & Chulvi-Medrano, I. (2021). Integrative neuromuscular training enhances physical fitness in 6-to 14-year-old rugby players. *Journal of Strength and Conditioning Research, 35*(8), 2263–2271.

Banman, C. J., Schneider, K. J., Cluff, T., & Peters, R. M. (2021). Altered vestibular balance function in combat sport athletes. *Journal of Neurotrauma, 38*(16), 2291–2300.

Bellows, R., & Wong, C. K. (2018). The effect of bracing and balance training on ankle sprain incidence among athletes: A systematic review with meta-analysis. *International Journal of Sports Physical Therapy, 13*(3), 379.

Bouteraa, I., Negra, Y., Shephard, R. J., & Chelly, M. S. (2020). Effects of combined balance and plyometric training on athletic performance in female basketball players. *Journal of Strength and Conditioning Research, 34*(7), 1967–1973.

Brachman, A., Kamieniarz, A., Michalska, J., Pawłowski, M., Słomka, K. J., & Juras, G. (2017). Balance training programs in athletes: A systematic review. *Journal of Human Kinetics, 58*, 45.

Caldemeyer, L. E., Brown, S. M., & Mulcahey, M. K. (2020). Neuromuscular training for the prevention of ankle sprains in female athletes: A systematic review. *Physician and Sports Medicine, 48*(4), 363–369.

Canli, U. (2019). Effects of neuromuscular training on motoric and selected basketball skills in pre-pubescent basketball players. *Universal Journal of Educational Research, 7*(1), 16–23.

Çelenk, Ç., Arslan, H., Aktuğ, Z. B., & Şimşek, E. (2018). The comparison between static and dynamic balance performances of team and individual athletes. *European Journal of Physical Education and Sport Science, 4*(1), 28–34.

Cook, G., Burton, L., & Fields, K. (1999). Reactive neuromuscular training for the anterior cruciate ligament–deficient knee: A case report. *Journal of Athletic Training, 34*(2), 194–201.

Courtney, C. A., Atre, P., Foucher, K. C., & Alsouhibani, A. M. (2019). Hypoesthesia after anterior cruciate ligament reconstruction: The relationship between proprioception and vibration perception deficits in individuals greater than one year post-surgery. *The Knee, 26*(1), 194–200.

Crampton, A., Teel, E., Chevignard, M., & Gagnon, I. (2021). Vestibular–ocular reflex dysfunction following mild traumatic brain injury: A narrative review. *Neurochirurgie, 67*(3), 231–237.

Cressey, E. M., West, C. A., Tiberio, D. P., Kraemer, W. J., & Maresh, C. M. (2007). The effects of ten weeks of lower-body unstable surface training on markers of athletic performance. *Journal of Strength and Conditioning Research, 21*(2), 561–567.

Day, B. L., & Fitzpatrick, R. C. (2005). The vestibular system. *Current Biology, 15*(15), R583–R586.

Dello Iacono, A., Padulo, J., & Ayalon, M. (2016). Core stability training on lower limb balance strength. *Journal of Sports Sciences, 34*(7), 671–678.

Di Stasi, S. L., & Snyder-Mackler, L. (2012). The effects of neuromuscular training on the gait patterns of ACL-deficient men and women. *Clinical Biomechanics, 27*(4), 360–365.

DiStefano, L. J., Clark, M. A., & Padua, D. A. (2009). Evidence supporting balance training in healthy individuals: A systemic review. *Journal of Strength and Conditioning Research, 23*(9), 2718–2731.

Falla, D. L., Hess, S., & Richardson, C. (2003). Evaluation of shoulder internal rotator muscle strength in baseball players with physical signs of glenohumeral joint instability. *British Journal of Sports Medicine, 37*(5), 430–432. https://doi.org/10.1136/bjsm.37.5.430

Fleming, M. S., & Luo, W. (2013). The anatomy, function, and development of mammalian Aβ low-threshold mechanoreceptors. *Frontiers in biology, 8*(4), 408–420.

Forbes, P. A., Luu, B. L., Van der Loos, H. M., Croft, E. A., Inglis, J. T., & Blouin, J. S. (2016). Transformation of vestibular signals for the control of standing in humans. *Journal of Neuroscience, 36*(45), 11510–11520.

Fort-Vanmeerhaeghe, A., Romero-Rodriguez, D., Lloyd, R. S., Kushner, A., & Myer, G. D. (2016). Integrative neuromuscular training in youth athletes. Part II: Strategies to prevent injuries and improve performance. *Strength and Conditioning Journal, 38*(4), 9–27.

Fort-Vanmeerhaeghe, A., Romero-Rodriguez, D., Montalvo, A. M., Kiefer, A. W., Lloyd, R. S., & Myer, G. D. (2016). Integrative neuromuscular training and injury prevention in youth athletes. Part I: identifying risk factors. *Strength and Conditioning Journal, 38*(3), 36–48.

Freeman, S., Mascia, A., & McGill, S. (2013). Arthrogenic neuromusculature inhibition: A foundational investigation of existence in the hip joint. *Clinical Biomechanics, 28*(2), 171–177.

Ghaderi, M., Letafatkar, A., Almonroeder, T. G., & Keyhani, S. (2020). Neuromuscular training improves knee proprioception in athletes with a history of anterior cruciate ligament reconstruction: A randomized controlled trial. *Clinical Biomechanics, 80*, 105157.

Gioftsidou, A., Malliou, P., Pafis, G., Beneka, A., Godolias, G., & Maganaris, C. N. (2006). The effects of soccer training and timing of balance training on balance ability. *European Journal of Applied Physiology, 96*(6), 659–664. https://doi.org/10.1007/s00421-005-0123-3

Glaviano, N. R., Bazett-Jones, D. M., & Norte, G. (2019). Gluteal muscle inhibition: Consequences of patellofemoral pain? *Medical Hypotheses, 126*, 9–14.

Goodman, J. M., & Bensmaia, S. J. (2021). The neural mechanisms of touch and proprioception at the somatosensory periphery (pp. 2–27). In B. Fritzsch (Ed.), *The senses: A comprehensive reference* (2nd ed.). Elsevier.

Granacher, U., Puta, C., Gabriel, H. H., Behm, D. G., & Arampatzis, A. (2018). Neuromuscular training and adaptations in youth athletes. *Frontiers in Physiology, 9*, 1264.

Hammami, R., Granacher, U., Makhlouf, I., Behm, D. G., & Chaouachi, A. (2016). Sequencing effects of balance and plyometric training on physical performance in youth soccer athletes. *Journal of Strength and Conditioning Research, 30*(12), 3278–3289.

Hans, J., Anson, J., Waddington, G., & Adams, R. (2014). Sport attainment and proprioception. *International Journal of Sports Science & Coaching, 9*(1), 159–170.

Hans, J., Anson, J., Waddington, G., Adams, R., & Liu, Y. (2015). The role of ankle proprioception for balance control in relation to sports performance and injury. *BioMed Research International, 2015*, 1–8. https://doi.org/10.1155/2015/842804.

Hendry, S., & Hsiao, S. (2013). The somatosensory system. In *Fundamental neuroscience* (4th ed., pp. 531–551). Elsevier. https://doi.org/10.1016/B978-0-12-385870-2.00024-X

Hewett, T. E., Ford, K. R., Xu, Y. Y., Khoury, J., & Myer, G. D. (2017). Effectiveness of neuromuscular training based on the neuromuscular risk profile. *American Journal of Sports Medicine, 45*(9), 2142–2147.

Hewett, T. E., Myer, G. D., & Ford, K. R. (2005). Reducing knee and anterior cruciate ligament injuries among female athletes: A systematic review of neuromuscular training interventions. *Journal of Knee Surgery, 18*(1), 82–88. https://doi.org/10.1055/s-0030-1248163

Hrysomallis, C. (2011). Balance ability and athletic performance. *Sports Medicine, 41*, 221–232.

Hübscher, M., Zech, A., Pfeifer, K., Hänsel, F., Vogt, L., & Banzer, W. (2010). Neuromuscular training for sports injury prevention: A systematic review. *Medicine & Science in Sports & Exercise, 42*(3), 413–421. https://doi.org/10.1249/MSS.0b013e3181b88d37

Hungerford, B., Gilleard, W., & Hodges, P. (2003). Evidence of altered lumbopelvic muscle recruitment in the presence of sacroiliac joint pain. *Spine, 28*(14), 1593–1600.

Ivanenko, Y., & Gurfinkel, V. S. (2018). Human postural control. *Frontiers in Neuroscience, 12*, 171.

Kiers, H., van Dieën, J., Dekkers, H., Wittink, H., & Vanhees, L. (2013). A systematic review of the relationship between physical activities in sports or daily life and postural sway in upright stance. *Sports Medicine, 43*, 1171–1189.

Kistemaker, D. A., Van Soest, A. J. K., Wong, J. D., Kurtzer, I., & Gribble, P. L. (2013). Control of position and movement is simplified by combined muscle spindle and Golgi tendon organ feedback. *Journal of Neurophysiology, 109*(4), 1126–1139.

Klous, M., Mikulic, P., & Latash, M. L. (2011). Two aspects of feedforward postural control: Anticipatory postural adjustments and anticipatory synergy adjustments. *Journal of Neurophysiology, 105*(5), 2275–2288.

Kovacs, E. J., Birmingham, T. B., Forwell, L., & Litchfield, R. B. (2004). Effect of training on postural control in figure skaters: A randomized controlled trial of neuromuscular versus basic off-ice training programs. *Clinical Journal of Sport Medicine, 14*(4), 215–224. https://doi.org/10.1097/00042752-200407000-00004

Kümmel, J., Kramer, A., Giboin, L. S., & Gruber, M. (2016). Specificity of balance training in healthy individuals: A systematic review and meta-analysis. *Sports Medicine, 46*(9), 1261–1271.

Latash, M. L., Levin, M. F., Scholz, J. P., & Schöner, G. (2010). Motor control theories and their applications. *Medicina, 46*(6), 382.

Letafatkar, A., Rajabi, R., Minoonejad, H., & Rabiei, P. (2019). Efficacy of perturbation-enhanced neuromuscular training on hamstring and quadriceps onset time, activation and knee flexion during a tuck-jump task. *International Journal of Sports Physical Therapy, 14*(2), 214.

Mandelbaum, B. R., Silvers, H. J., Watanabe, D. S., Knarr, J. F., Thomas, S. D., Griffin, L. Y., Kirkendall, D. T., & Garrett, W. (2005). Effectiveness of a neuromuscular and proprioceptive training program in preventing anterior cruciate ligament injuries in female athletes: 2-year follow-up. *The American Journal of Sports Medicine, 33*(7), 1003–1010. https://doi.org/10.1177/0363546504272261

Massé-Alarie, H., Beaulieu, L. D., Preuss, R., & Schneider, C. (2015). Task-specificity of bilateral anticipatory activation of the deep abdominal muscles in healthy and chronic low back pain populations. *Gait & Posture, 41*(2), 440–447.

McGuine, T. A., & Keene, J. S. (2006). The effect of a balance training program on the risk of ankle sprains in high school athletes. *American Journal of Sports Medicine, 34*(7), 1103–1111.

McKeon, P. O., & Hertel, J. (2008). Systematic review of postural control and lateral ankle instability, part II: Is balance training clinically effective? *Journal of Athletic Training, 43*(3), 305–315.

Moeskops, S., Read, P. J., Oliver, J. L., & Lloyd, R. S. (2018). Individual responses to an 8-week neuromuscular training intervention in trained pre-pubescent female artistic gymnasts. *Sports, 6*(4), 128.

Muehlbauer, T., Roth, R., Bopp, M., & Granacher, U. (2012). An exercise sequence for progression in balance training. *Journal of Strength and Conditioning Research, 26*(2), 568–574.

Myer, G. D., Ford, K. R., McLean, S. G., & Hewett, T. E. (2006). The effects of plyometric versus dynamic stabilization and balance training on lower extremity biomechanics. *American Journal of Sports Medicine, 34*(3), 445–455.

Myklebust, G., Engebretsen, L., Braekken, I. H., Skjølberg, A., Olsen, O.-E., & Bahr, R. (2003). Prevention of anterior cruciate ligament injuries in female team handball players: A prospective intervention study over three seasons. *Clinical Journal of Sport Medicine, 13*(2), 71–78. https://doi.org/10.1097/00042752-200303000-00002

Nagelli, C., Di Stasi, S., Tatarski, R., Chen, A., Wordeman, S., Hoffman, J., & Hewett, T. E. (2020). Neuromuscular training improves self-reported function and single-leg landing hip biomechanics in athletes after anterior cruciate ligament reconstruction. *Orthopaedic Journal of Sports Medicine, 8*(10), 2325967120959347.

Nagelli, C. V., Di Stasi, S., Wordeman, S. C., Chen, A., Tatarski, R., Hoffman, J., & Hewett, T. E. (2019). Knee biomechanical deficits during a single-leg landing task are addressed with neuromuscular training in anterior cruciate ligament–reconstructed athletes. *Clinical Journal of Sport Medicine, 31*(6), e347–e353. https://doi.org/10.1097/jsm.0000000000000792

Nunes, A. C., Cattuzzo, M. T., Faigenbaum, A. D., & Mortatti, A. L. (2021). Effects of integrative neuromuscular training and detraining on countermovement jump performance in youth volleyball players. *Journal of Strength and Conditioning Research, 35*(8), 2242–2247.

Ogard, W. K. (2011). Proprioception in sports medicine and athletic conditioning. *Strength & Conditioning Journal, 33*(3), 111–118.

Padua, D. M., & Marshall, S. W. (2006). Evidence supporting ACL-injury-prevention exercise programs: A review of the literature. *Athletic Therapy Today, 11*, 11–23.

Paillard, T., Noe, F., Riviere, T., Marion, V., Montoya, R., & Dupui, P. (2006). Postural performance and strategy in the unipedal stance of soccer players at different levels of competition. *Journal of Athletic Training, 41*(2), 172.

Paterno, M. V., Myer, G. D., Ford, K. R., & Hewett, T. E. (2004). Neuromuscular training improves single-limb stability in young female athletes. *Journal of Orthopaedic & Sports Physical Therapy, 34*(6), 305–316.

Perrey, S. (2018). Brain activation associated with eccentric movement: A narrative review of the literature. *European Journal of Sport Science, 18*(1), 75–82.

Proske, U. (2006). Kinesthesia: The role of muscle receptors. *Muscle & Nerve: Official Journal of the American Association of Electrodiagnostic Medicine, 34*(5), 545–558.

Quindlen, J. C., Stolarski, H. K., Johnson, M. D., & Barocas, V. H. (2016). A multiphysics model of the Pacinian corpuscle. *Integrative Biology, 8*(11), 1111–1125.

Rice, D. A., & McNair, P. J. (2010, December). Quadriceps arthrogenic muscle inhibition: Neural mechanisms and treatment perspectives. *Seminars in Arthritis and Rheumatism, 40*(3), 250–266. https://doi.org/10.1016/j.semarthrit.2009.10.001

Riva, D., Bianchi, R., Rocca, F., & Mamo, C. (2016). Proprioceptive training and injury prevention in a professional men's basketball team: A six-year prospective study. *Journal of Strength and Conditioning Research, 30*(2), 461.

Sañudo, B., Sánchez-Hernández, J., Bernardo-Filho, M., Abdi, E., Taiar, R., & Núñez, J. (2019). Integrative neuromuscular training in young athletes, injury prevention, and performance optimization: A systematic review. *Applied Sciences, 9*(18), 3839.

Sousa, A. S., Silva, A., & Tavares, J. M. R. (2012). Biomechanical and neurophysiological mechanisms related to postural control and efficiency of movement: A review. *Somatosensory & Motor Research, 29*(4), 131–143.

Sugimoto, D., Myer, G. D., Foss, K. D. B., & Hewett, T. E. (2015). Specific exercise effects of preventive neuromuscular training intervention on anterior cruciate ligament injury risk reduction in young females: Meta-analysis and subgroup analysis. *British Journal of Sports Medicine, 49*(5), 282–289.

Tekin, D., Agopyan, A., & Baltaci, G. (2018). Balance training in modern dancers: Proprioceptive-neuromuscular training vs kinesio taping. *Medical Problems of Performing Artists, 33*(3), 156–165.

Ten Donkelaar, H. J., Broman, J., & van Domburg, P. (2020). The somatosensory system. In H. J. Ten Donkelaar, *Clinical neuroanatomy* (pp. 171–255). Springer International Publishing. https://doi.org/10.1007/978-3-030-41878-6_4

Tomomitsu, M. S., Alonso, A. C., Morimoto, E., Bobbio, T. G., & Greve, J. (2013). Static and dynamic postural control in low-vision and normal-vision adults. *Clinics, 68*, 517–521.

Trajković, N., & Bogataj, Š. (2020). Effects of neuromuscular training on motor competence and physical performance in young female volleyball players. *International Journal of Environmental Research and Public Health, 17*(5), 1755.

Whittaker, J. L., Booysen, N., de la Motte, S., Dennett, L., Lewis, C. L., Wilson, D., McKay, C., Warner, M., Padua, D., Emery, C. A., & Stokes, M. (2017). Predicting sport and occupational lower extremity injury risk through movement quality screening: A systematic review. *British Journal of Sports Medicine, 51*(7), 580–585. https://doi.org/10.1136/bjsports-2016-096760

Williams, M. D., Ramirez-Campillo, R., Chaabene, H., & Moran, J. (2021). Neuromuscular training and motor control in youth athletes: A meta-analysis. *Perceptual and Motor Skills*, 00315125211029006.

Yoo, J. H., Lim, B. O., Ha, M., Lee, S. W., Oh, S. J., Lee, Y. S., & Kim, J. G. (2010). A meta-analysis of the effect of neuromuscular training on the prevention of the anterior cruciate ligament injury in female athletes. *Knee Surgery, Sports Traumatology, Arthroscopy, 18*(6), 824–830.

Zachazewski, J. E., Magee, D. J., & Quillen, W. S. (Eds.). (1996). *Athletic injuries and rehabilitation*. Saunders.

Zech, A., Hübscher, M., Vogt, L., Banzer, W., Hänsel, F., & Pfeifer, K. (2010). Balance training for neuromuscular control and performance enhancement: A systematic review. *Journal of Athletic Training, 45*(4), 392–403.

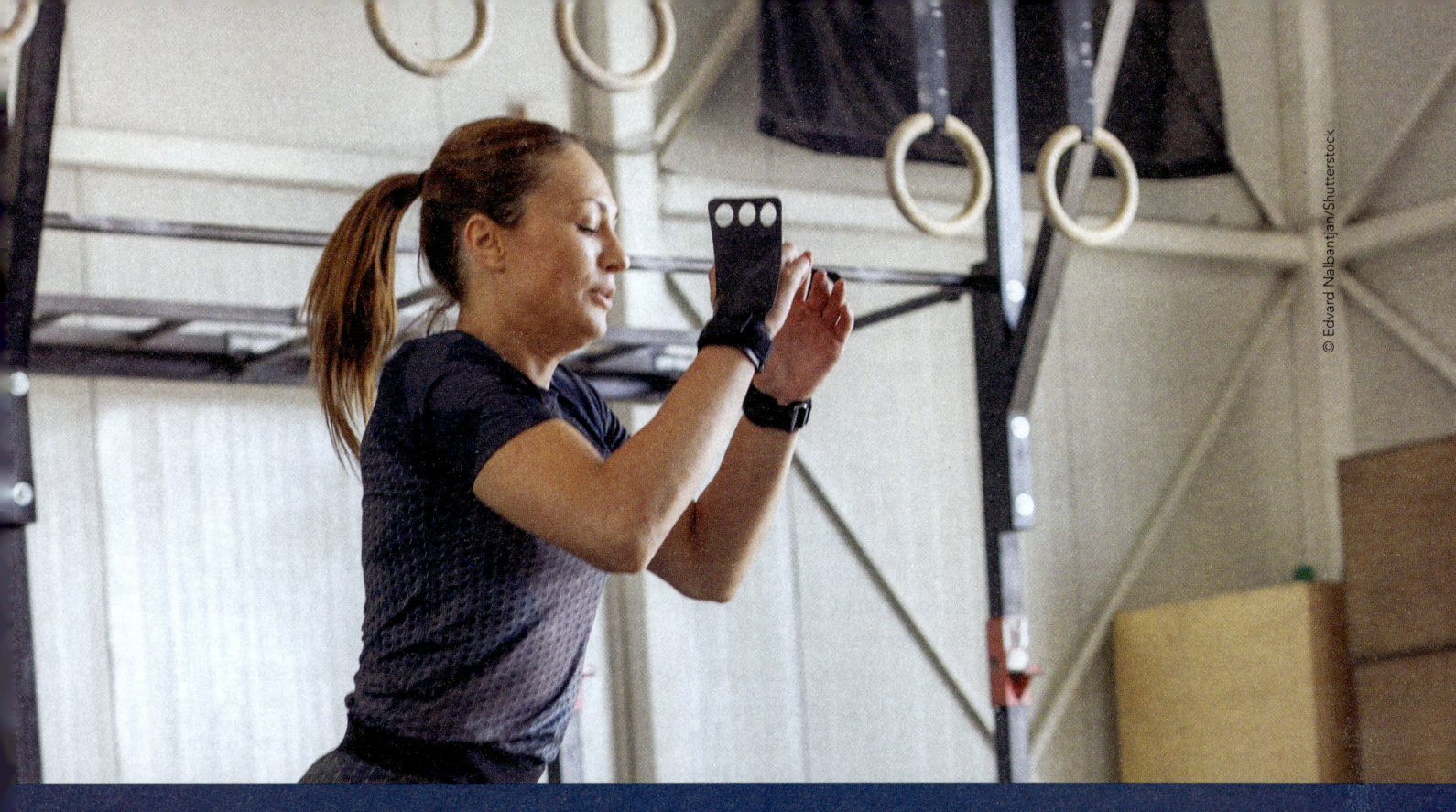

PLYOMETRIC TRAINING FOR SPORTS PERFORMANCE

CHAPTER TWELVE

LEARNING OBJECTIVES

Upon completion of this chapter, the Sports Performance Coach will be able to:

- **Summarize** the importance of plyometric training for athletes with differing performance-related goals.

- **Explain** the scientific rationale for plyometric training.

- **Describe** different plyometric training techniques used within performance training.

- **Identify** appropriate acute training variables for plyometric training.

- **Select** plyometric training programs or techniques based on athlete needs.

LESSON 1: INTRODUCTION TO PLYOMETRIC TRAINING

INTRODUCTION

Sports Performance Coaches must rely on various training methods and principles to optimally enhance athletic performance. As the speed and intensity of competition increase, the ability to display high levels of force in shorter periods of time should be prioritized in activities such as sprinting. Because of this, training methodologies such as **plyometrics** must be incorporated, rather than resorting only to traditional measures of strength, size, or speed (Healy et al., 2018).

Plyometric training is a specific method of training that can facilitate an improvement in **reactive strength**. A high degree of reactive strength helps bridge the gap between strength and speed by maximizing the highest amount of force produced in the shortest amount of time. Traditional plyometric movements, such as depth jumps or multiple response jumps, develop reactive strength by utilizing a concentric contraction following a rapid eccentric muscle action.

To properly prepare athletes for optimal performance, Sports Performance Coaches should utilize various training methods and strategies, such as plyometrics, to help make the connection between force and time. The time it takes for most athletes to express peak force (such as during a maximum-effort squat or bench press in powerlifting) is longer than the time available in most more reactive, elastic activities such as jumping, sprinting, cutting, and changing direction.

By utilizing a variety of training exercises, such as plyometrics, in addition to traditional strength-training methods, athletes can benefit from a more well-rounded and athlete-specific approach to their development. As such, Sports Performance Coaches should focus on a spectrum of lower-, upper-, and total-body exercises designed to improve athletes' reactive strength.

THE IMPORTANCE OF JOINT STABILITY

The value of plyometrics derives from its ability to address multiple qualities of performance enhancement, including improved sprinting (Abade et al., 2017; Lockie et al., 2014; Sáez de Villarreal et al., 2012), change of direction (Asadi et al., 2015), agility (Fischetti et al., 2019), and strength (al-Syurgawi & Shapie, 2019; Sáez de Villarreal et al., 2012). Furthermore, unlike traditional strength-training methods, which focus on increasing the size and strength of muscles directly, plyometric training emphasizes maximizing the neuromuscular system and enhancing the speed at which muscles contract (Davies et al., 2015), thereby enhancing joint stability.

Joint stability is of utmost importance for athletes because it supports the proper alignment and function of the body during movement. Stable joints can better handle the stress and strain of physical activity, which in turn reduces the risk of injury. Joint stability is achieved through a balance of strength, flexibility, and proprioception in the muscles and connective tissues surrounding a joint.

Plyometric training plays a significant role in enhancing joint stability. Plyometric exercises involve rapid stretching

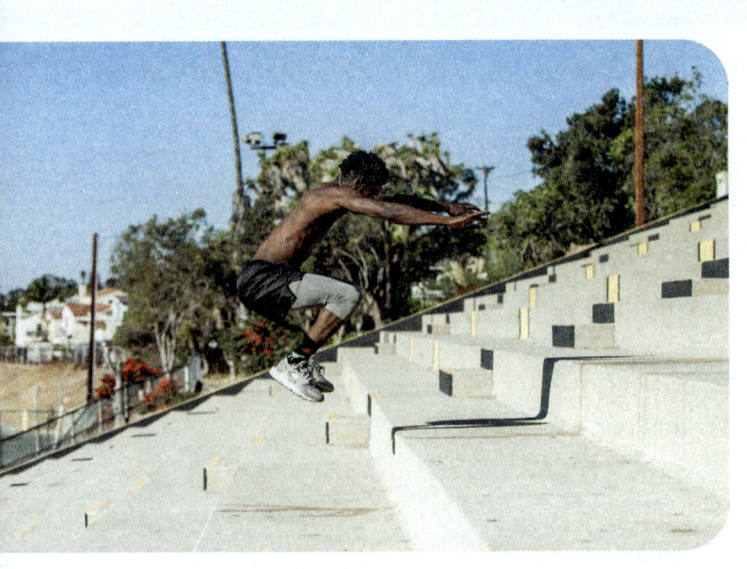

© Jon Osumi/Shutterstock

and contracting of the muscles around a joint, which helps strengthen these muscles and improve their elasticity. This, in turn, increases the joint's stability, allowing it to better absorb and distribute forces during high-impact activities.

Moreover, plyometric training also improves proprioception, the body's ability to perceive and understand its position and movement in space. Enhanced proprioception improves an athlete's balance and body control, further supporting joint stability.

Thus, plyometric training directly strengthens the muscles that provide joint stability and improves the body's overall control and balance, reducing the risk of misalignment or improper movements that could lead to joint injuries. Its multiple benefits support the need to take the necessary time to develop proper positioning and stabilization of athletes during early training phases, which will help with the transfer of power and elasticity during more intense and demanding training. To better understand this, the Sports Performance Coach should have detailed knowledge of the three phases of plyometric exercises.

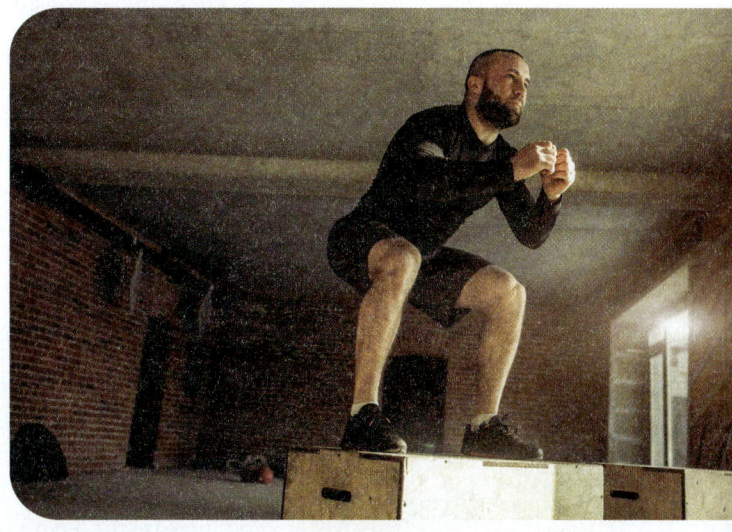
© UfaBizPhoto/Shutterstock

THREE PHASES OF PLYOMETRIC EXERCISE

Reactive strength is primarily developed from the rapid cyclical muscle action from eccentric to concentric contractions. This cyclical muscle action, called the **stretch–shortening cycle (SSC)**, includes the eccentric (or loading) phase, the amortization (or transition) phase, and the concentric (or unloading) phase (Davies et al., 2015; Turner & Jeffreys, 2010) (**Figure 12.1**). Athletes who utilize the SSC during movements such as jumping or throwing can stimulate a greater muscular contraction, resulting in a higher, faster, or longer display of force and power.

Plyometric Phases

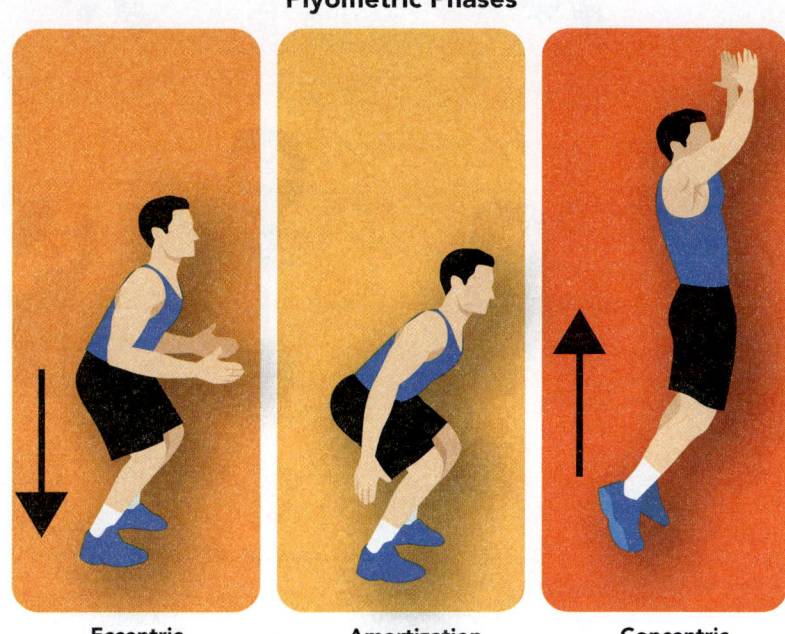

| Eccentric | Amortization | Concentric |

FIGURE 12.1 Plyometric Phases

For example, consider a famous track and field event, the triple jump. In the triple jump, the athlete sprints down the track into two consecutive jumps on the same limb and then alternates to the other limb for the final (third) jump. If you were to compare the triple jump to three consecutive jumps without the use of the SSC, you would notice a significant difference in the total distance covered. Thus, to maximize the expression of power in the shortest amount of time—an ability demonstrated in many sports and athletic activities—the use of activities involving the SSC is warranted.

ECCENTRIC PHASE

ECCENTRIC PHASE →

The phase in which muscle spindle activity is increased by pre-stretching the muscle prior to activation.

The first stage of a plyometric movement is known as the **eccentric phase**, but has also been called the loading or countermovement phase (Davies et al., 2015). This phase increases muscle spindle activity by pre-stretching the muscle prior to activation (Kubo et al., 2001). Potential energy is stored in the elastic components of the muscle during this loading phase. A slower eccentric phase has been shown to decrease overall jump height and increase the length of time during the amortization phase (Toumi et al., 2004).

To maximize the pre-stretch of the muscle, the eccentric phase should be completed quickly and aggressively (**Figure 12.2**). Individuals can achieve a higher jump height with the additional rapid eccentric in the countermovement jump.

AMORTIZATION PHASE

AMORTIZATION PHASE →

The transition from eccentric loading to concentric unloading during the stretch–shortening cycle.

The **amortization phase** involves dynamic stabilization and is the time between the end of the eccentric muscle action (the loading or deceleration phase) and the initiation of

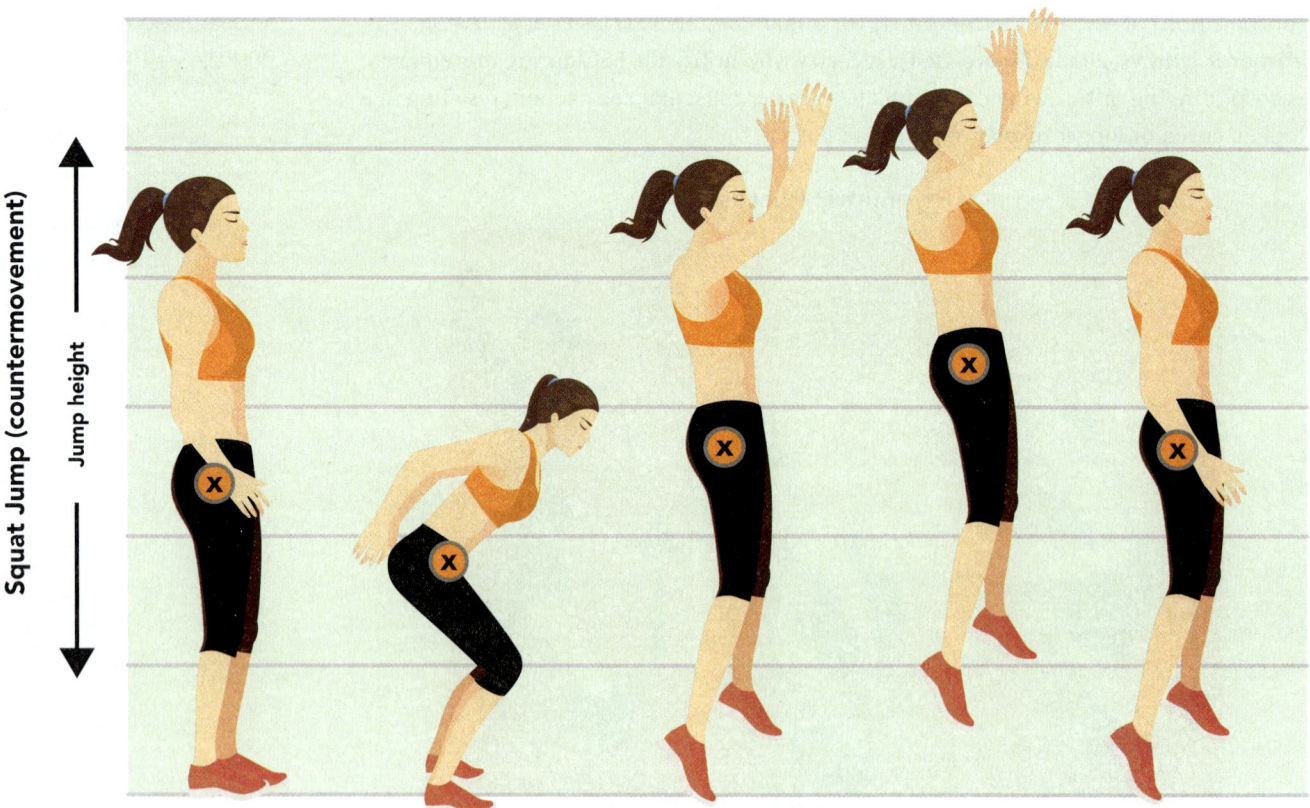

FIGURE 12.2 Impact of Eccentric-Phase Velocity

the concentric contraction (the unloading or force production phase) (Atanasković et al., 2015; Wilk et al., 1993). The length of the amortization phase (in milliseconds) is often used to categorize plyometrics as either fast (less than 250 milliseconds) or slow (more than 250 milliseconds) (Turner & Jeffreys, 2010).

A prolonged amortization phase results in less-than-optimal neuromuscular efficiency from a loss of elastic potential energy (Wilson et al., 1993). A rapid switch from an eccentric to a concentric contraction leads to a more powerful response. It can maximize transfer to sports performance by reducing elastic energy loss during the transition from eccentric to concentric muscle action.

For example, consider a triple-standing long jump test. Athlete 1 performs three long jumps, one at a time, by resetting each time. Athlete 2 performs three long jumps consecutively, jumping immediately after landing from the previous jump. By utilizing the fast eccentric muscle action and minimizing ground contact time, Athlete 2 would jump farther than Athlete 1 (**Figure 12.3**).

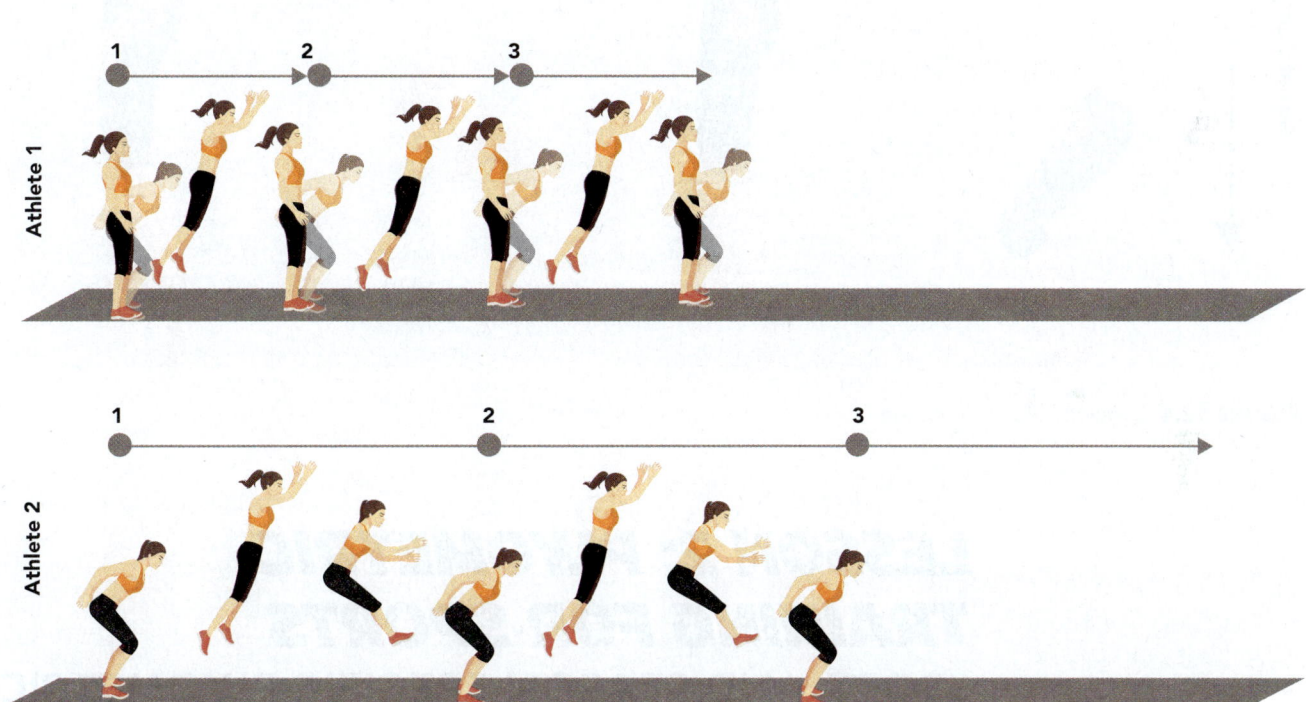

FIGURE 12.3 Amortization Phase: Example

CONCENTRIC PHASE

The **concentric phase** (or unloading phase) occurs immediately after the amortization phase and involves a concentric contraction; it results in enhanced muscular performance following the eccentric phase. This effect occurs secondary to enhanced summation and reutilization of elastic potential energy, muscle potentiation, and contribution of the myotatic stretch reflex (Fukunaga et al., 2002; Gollhofer et al., 1992; Rassier et al., 2005).

For most upper- and lower-body plyometrics, the concentric phase is the stage in which force and power are expressed in activity or sport. By initiating a fast eccentric muscle action and transitioning through a minimal amortization phase, the distance traveled, load lifted, or speed of concentric contraction can be enhanced (**Figure 12.4**).

CONCENTRIC → PHASE

The response to the eccentric and amortization phases, in which energy is released and directed toward athletic movement such as jumping or throwing.

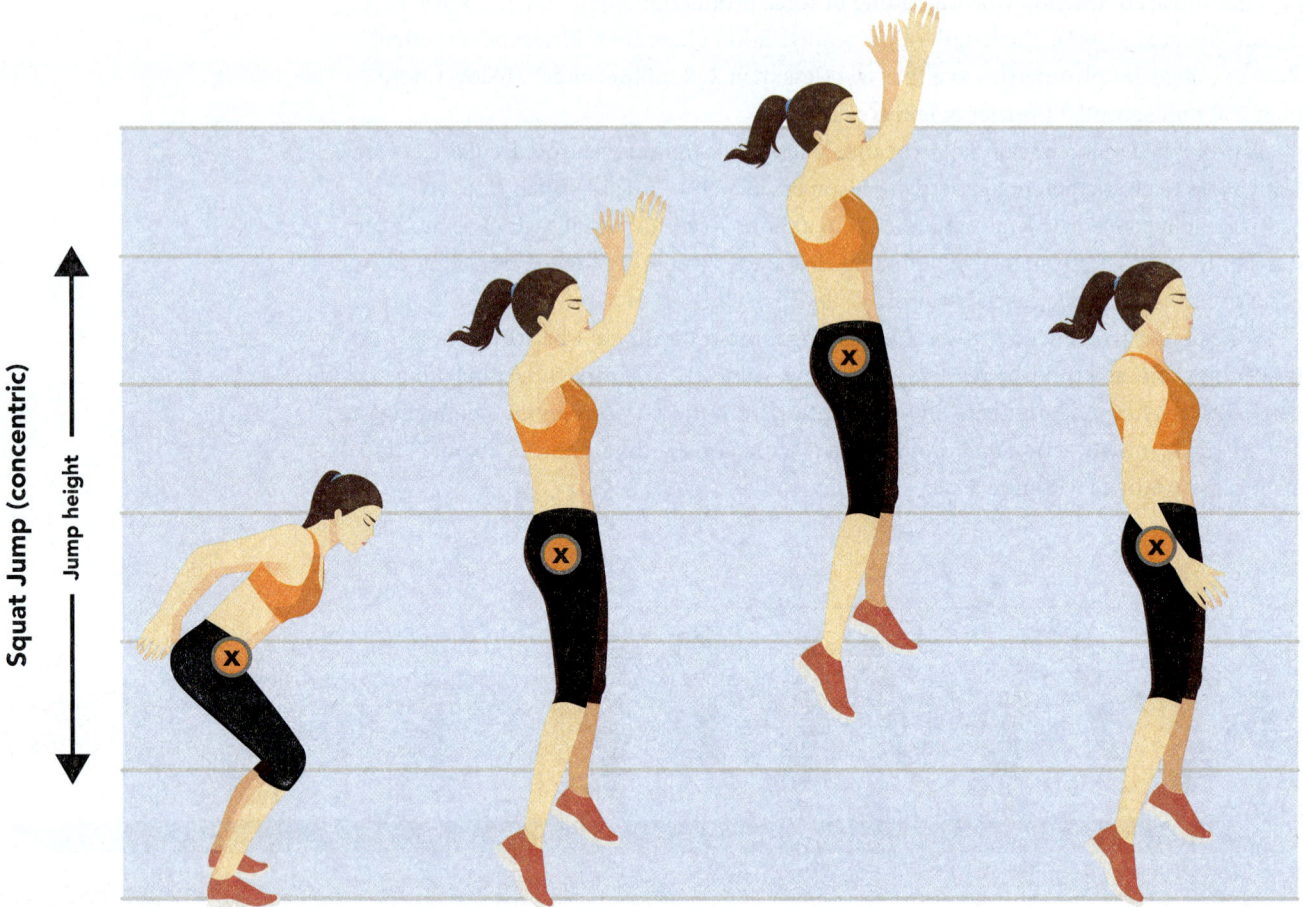

FIGURE 12.4 Concentric Force in Action

LESSON 2: PLYOMETRIC TRAINING FOR SPORTS
SPORT- AND SEASON-SPECIFIC PLYOMETRIC TRAINING

Sports Performance Coaches should consider how specific exercises can be best utilized in the overall seasonal or annual training plan. General exercises, such as jumping rope and skipping, might be an effective method to reintroduce plyometric training into a program after a long competitive season. As the athlete approaches the next competitive season, Sports Performance Coaches should progress from general to specific training modes to enhance sporting performance. For example, an offensive lineman might start with low box jumps after the season to reintroduce jump training and reinforce ideal form and control, and then progress to audible-reactive box jumps to stimulate game or practice-like conditions before the season. Sports Performance Coaches must periodize and plan exercise progressions appropriately over the season or year.

The differences in exercise choice may reflect **kinematic characteristics** specific to a sport. For example, non-field sports, including court and rink sports, have been reported to use more horizontal depth jumps, single-leg box jumps, and single-leg hurdle hops and bounds (Watkins, Gill, et al., 2021). Sports that involve frequent short sprints and direction

> **KINEMATIC CHARACTERISTICS** →
>
> How a body moves in space, including distance, speed, and velocity.

changes, such as hockey and basketball, may prioritize plyometric exercises that enhance eccentric force absorption and single-leg power during acceleration and reacceleration.

IN-SEASON PLYOMETRIC TRAINING

The use of plyometrics during specific periods of the training plan (e.g., in-season, off-season, or post-season) should be guided by a variety of factors that are heavily reliant on the metabolic and neurological demands of practice, competitions, and frequency of training:

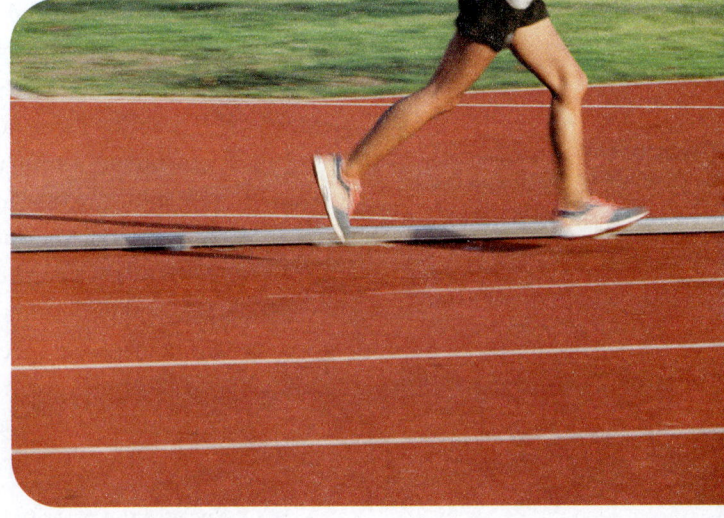

© Wattanawiboonkit Dew/Shutterstock

- Intensity: How difficult are the exercises? Are they primarily bilateral or unilateral? Stability-focused or explosive?
- Duration: How long are the plyometric sessions? How many contacts are being used?
- Frequency: How often are plyometrics being utilized? Every day? Alternating days? On speed and agility days or also on strength-training days?
- Length of recovery between bouts: Is adequate rest between jumps/throws being provided? Are the exercises grouped or separated by space and time?
- Amount of time before the next practice, training, session, or competition: Are certain exercises causing more muscle soreness than others? How does delayed-onset muscle soreness from other exercises affect overall plyometric programming?

As the athlete transitions into the in-season training period, Sports Performance Coaches naturally spend less time with athletes as they manage the varying demands of sports practice, competition, and training. Thus, an emphasis on plyometric training may be reduced. Additionally, athletes participating in sports like basketball, volleyball, and track and field may perform many plyometric-type jumps in practice or competitions. Thus, Sports Performance Coaches may consider decreasing the focus on plyometrics during the in-season period and instead emphasize establishing and maintaining adequate levels of stabilization and strength.

Research has shown that a low-intensity plyometric program that includes a higher number of foot contacts, rather than a high-intensity plyometric program that includes a smaller number of foot contacts, is more appropriate closer to competition performance (Lievens et al., 2021). This approach can help minimize acute performance decline and provide adequate stimuli to maintain and improve athleticism.

OFF-SEASON PLYOMETRIC TRAINING

As a period of time without daily practice and competition demands, the off-season offers an excellent opportunity to implement plyometrics as part of athletes' daily and weekly training. In the off-season, Sports Performance Coaches naturally have more time to develop athletes' abilities, such as by including higher volumes and intensities of plyometric exercises in their training programs. Additionally, Sports Performance Coaches may have more flexibility to design when and where to include upper- and lower-body plyometric exercises in the program, including the following timetables:

- During or directly after the warm-up
  - Low-intensity plyometric exercises are great options to help raise body temperature and prepare the muscular tissues for more intensive, explosive jumps, which can be done after a thorough warm-up.
- Within speed and agility training sessions
  - Plyometrics can be used as a primer to potentiate speed and agility movements or enhance power output during a contrast/complex resistance training session. Sports Performance Coaches could combine medicine ball throws or lateral bounding into direct sprint work application.
- Within strength-training sessions such as **complex training**
  - Examples include a squat paired with a vertical jump or a lateral lunge paired with a lateral bound. Complex training has been shown to enhance muscle force and power production due to post-activation potentiation (Iacono et al., 2019).
- On their own specific days as part of the training plan's focus.
  - If Sports Performance Coaches have an extended training plan organized over multiple days, athletes may find benefits in engaging in a directly targeted session solely for plyometric exercises and reactive strength development.

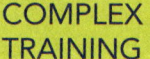

COMPLEX TRAINING →

Pairing a resistance training movement with a plyometric movement.

Because the priority in the off-season training period is developing specific sports performance qualities, the total volume (repetitions and sets) and exercise selection can be increased to higher levels than during the competitive season.

PLYOMETRIC BENEFITS FOR ALL ATHLETES AND SPORTS

Sports Performance Coaches and athletes may question the implementation of lower-body and upper-body plyometrics in a training plan if they cannot see a direct transfer to specific sporting actions such as jumping or throwing. However, the benefits of plyometric programming extend past simply higher vertical jumps or longer throws for both non-jumping and jumping sports.

NON-JUMPING SPORTS

Despite the lack of jumping in sports such as ice hockey, field hockey, and crew, the inclusion of plyometrics can still be beneficial to athletes who participate in them by improving their ability to change direction, speed, and power (Akdeniz & Sentürk, 2018;

Egan-Shuttler et al., 2017; Singh et al., 2018). Additionally, the use of upper-body-specific plyometrics such as medicine ball throws and push-up variations has been shown to improve measures of upper-body strength, ball speed, ball throwing distance, and power (Singla et al., 2018; Valadés Cerrato et al., 2018). Implementing plyometrics can also reinforce proper positions of stabilization to help absorb force and reduce the risk of future injury. For example, lateral bounds for hockey athletes can assist with the push phase when skating. Adding rotational medicine ball throws can help with the expression of rotational power for sports such as softball, golf, and baseball. Single-leg jumps and hops can enhance knee and ankle stabilization, benefiting field sport athletes such as those participating in lacrosse, field hockey, or soccer.

HIGH-VOLUME JUMPING SPORTS

When working with an athlete or team that spends a significant amount of time jumping, such as occurs in basketball, volleyball, and certain track and field events, Sports Performance Coaches should prioritize low-volume strength training in conjunction with a low-volume plyometric program to improve physical performance (Yáñez-García et al., 2022). In addition, coaches should closely monitor the total amount of ground contact experienced by athletes who participate in high-volume jumping sports to prevent overuse injuries such as shin splints, patellofemoral pain, and groin/hip pain (De Bleecker et al., 2020). To reduce the impact of jump training on an athlete's joints in the context of a high-volume jumping sport, Sports Performance Coaches can program jump training in water, which has been shown to improve athletes' strength, sprint speed, and power (Arazi & Asadi, 2011; Ploeg et al., 2010).

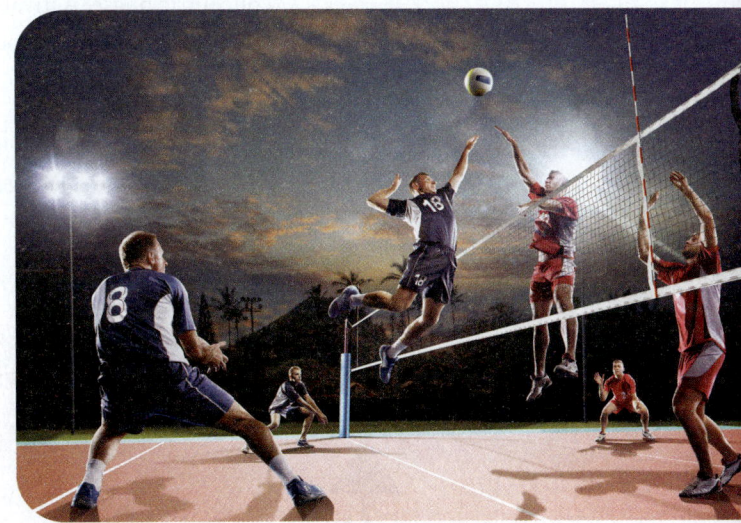

© Eugene Onischenko/Shutterstock

Along with monitoring the total amount of ground contacts or opting for plyometric sessions in the pool, Sports Performance Coaches should ensure their athletes display proper landing mechanics. During plyometric training, athletes must land on the midfoot (just behind the ball of the foot) to properly distribute the forces accrued during landing, with their knees tracking over the second and third toes (to avoid knee valgus). Likewise, athletes should avoid landing directly on their toes or heels to put them in a more favorable position for the next movement.

LESSON 3: THE SCIENCE OF PLYOMETRIC TRAINING
SCIENTIFIC RATIONALE FOR PLYOMETRIC TRAINING

Plyometric training is essential to maximize athlete performance. Sports Performance Coaches need to understand the scientific foundation for plyometric training to better explain the potential risks of this high-intensity training modality and promote safety among their athletes. This knowledge can guide coaches in program design by helping them determine which plyometric exercises are most beneficial for their athletes based on the sport's specific demands and movements.

Plyometric exercises utilize a muscle's elastic and proprioceptive properties to generate maximum force production by stimulating mechanoreceptors to facilitate an increase in muscle recruitment in a minimal amount of time (Wilk et al., 1993). Muscle spindles and Golgi tendon organs (GTOs) provide the proprioceptive basis for plyometric training.

The central nervous system (CNS) uses the sensory information from these mechanoreceptors to increase the set speed at which muscles can act (Davies et al., 2015). Stimulation of these receptors can cause facilitation, inhibition, and modulation of both agonist and antagonist muscle activity, enhancing neuromuscular efficiency and functional strength (Davies et al., 2015; Wathen, 1993). **Figure 12.5** provides an overview of this complex process. The eccentric phase stimulates receptors; this stimulation is then interpreted by the CNS, which responds with increased force production during the concentric phase. Activation of the stretch reflex works like any reflex, in that it does not include higher-order processing from the brain.

> ### CONTRACTILE → ELEMENT
>
> The muscle fibers that are capable of contracting and producing force.

Physiological Principles of Plyometric Training

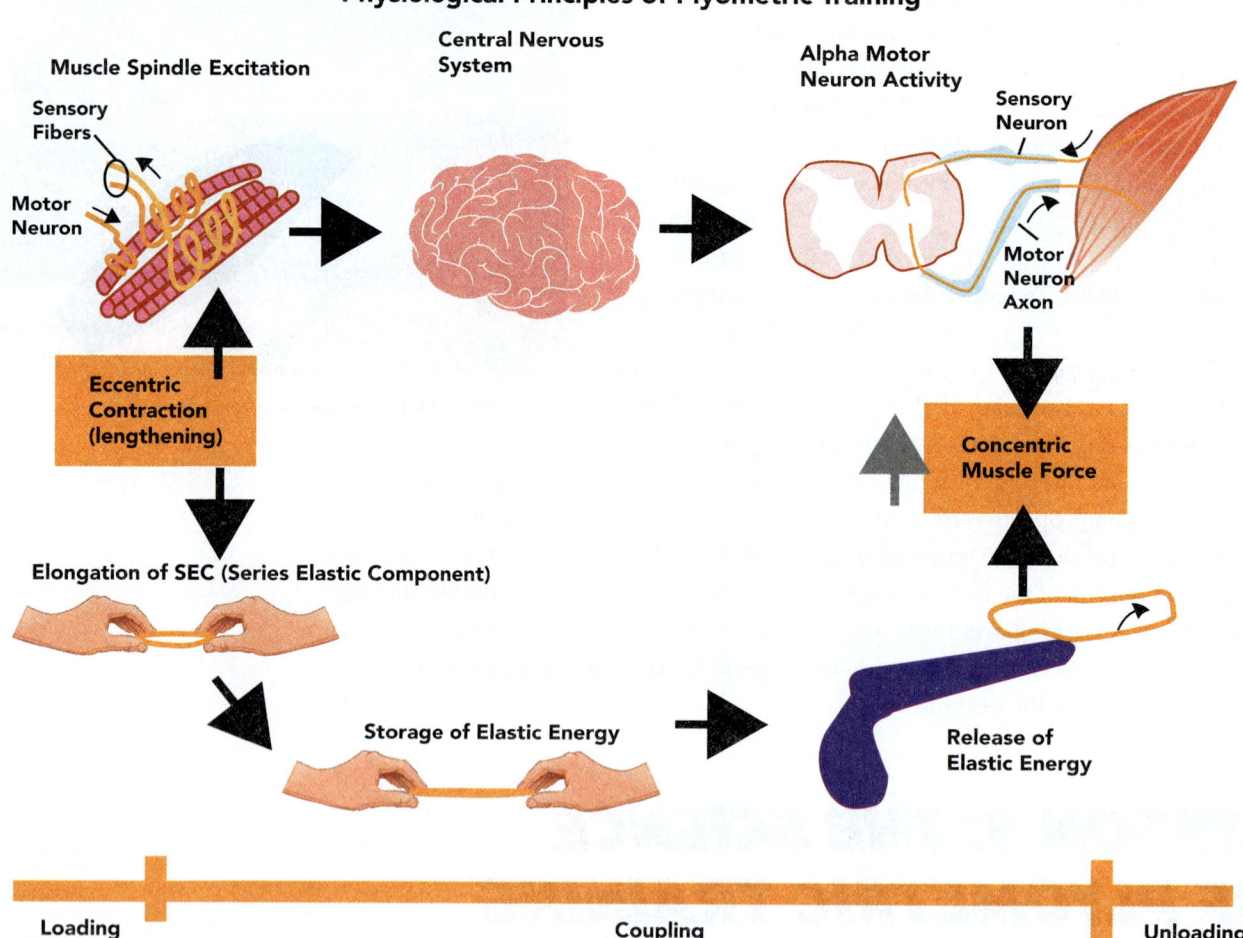

FIGURE 12.5 Physiological Principles of Plyometric Training

ELASTIC PROPERTIES OF MUSCLES

The concept of plyometrics is based on the three-component model of muscle. According to this model, muscle contains a **contractile element** and two elastic elements. The latter elements are named according to their relationship to the contractile component—one is in sequence with it (the series elastic element) and one is parallel to it (the parallel elastic component) (**Figure 12.6**).

Elastic Properties of Muscle

Parallel Elastic Component (PEC)

Series Elastic Component (SEC)

Contractile Component (CC)

FIGURE 12.6 Elastic Properties of Muscle

The **series elastic component (SEC)** lengthens and stores elastic energy like a spring when a musculotendinous unit is stretched through eccentric muscle action. When a muscle contracts, the SEC initially stores some of the energy of that contraction as it stretches, similar to how a spring stretches when a force is applied to it. During a rapid muscle action, such as in plyometric exercises, this stored energy in the SEC can be quickly released to aid in the subsequent muscle contraction. This release is a key component of the SSC. If a concentric muscle action occurs too long after the original stretch, energy is lost, and force and power are diminished.

The parallel elastic component (PEC) makes a more passive contribution when unstimulated muscle stretch occurs. PECs are called the "parallel" elastic component because these elements run parallel to the muscle fibers. During a passive stretch, or when a muscle is lengthened but not actively contracting, the resistance to stretch comes from both the muscle fibers and the connective tissues surrounding the muscle (the PEC). When the muscle contracts and shortens again, the energy stored in the PEC during the stretch can be released, contributing to the overall force of the muscle contraction.

Once sufficient tension has been generated, the tension at the ends of the muscle is sufficient to overcome the load, and the load is moved. For example, compare a traditional countermovement jump with a pogo jump. In the counter-movement jump, the athlete engages in a deeper stretch to move the center of mass as high as possible. In the pogo jump, the athlete takes a minimal eccentric stretch and aims to get their feet off the floor (**Figure 12.7**).

When a load is applied to a joint (eccentric phase), the elastic elements stretch and store potential energy (amortization phase) prior to the contractile element contracting (concentric phase) (**Figure 12.8**). During the loading of the muscle (e.g., when landing from a depth jump,

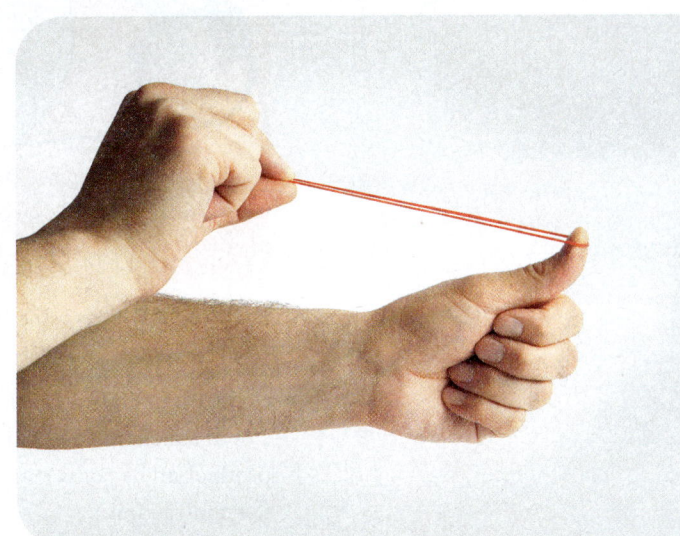

© Sharomka/Shutterstock

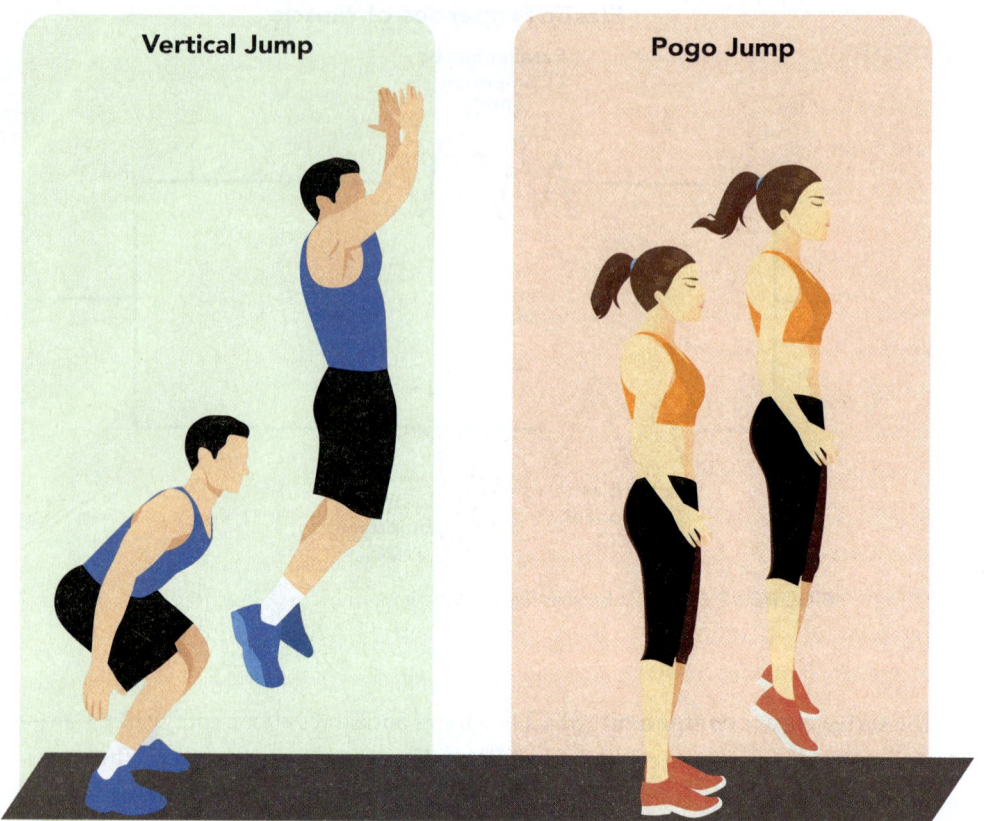

FIGURE 12.7 Vertical Jump Versus Pogo Jump

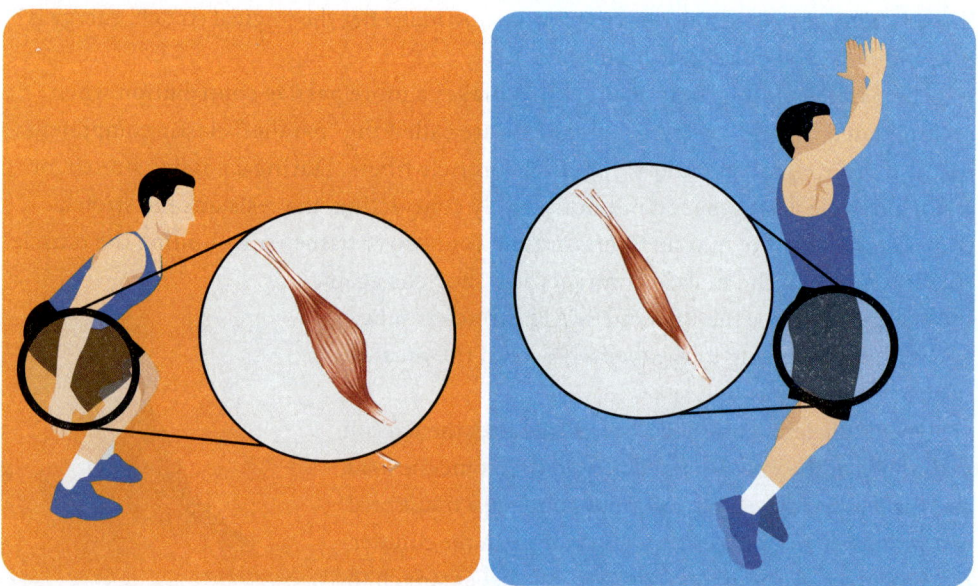

FIGURE 12.8 Plyometric Phases

as shown in **Figure 12.9**), the load is transferred to the series of elastic components and stored as elastic potential energy. The elastic elements then contribute to the overall force production by converting the stored elastic potential energy to kinetic energy, enhancing the contraction.

The improved muscular performance that occurs with the pre-stretch in a muscle results from the combined effects of both the storage of elastic potential energy and

Depth Jump Example

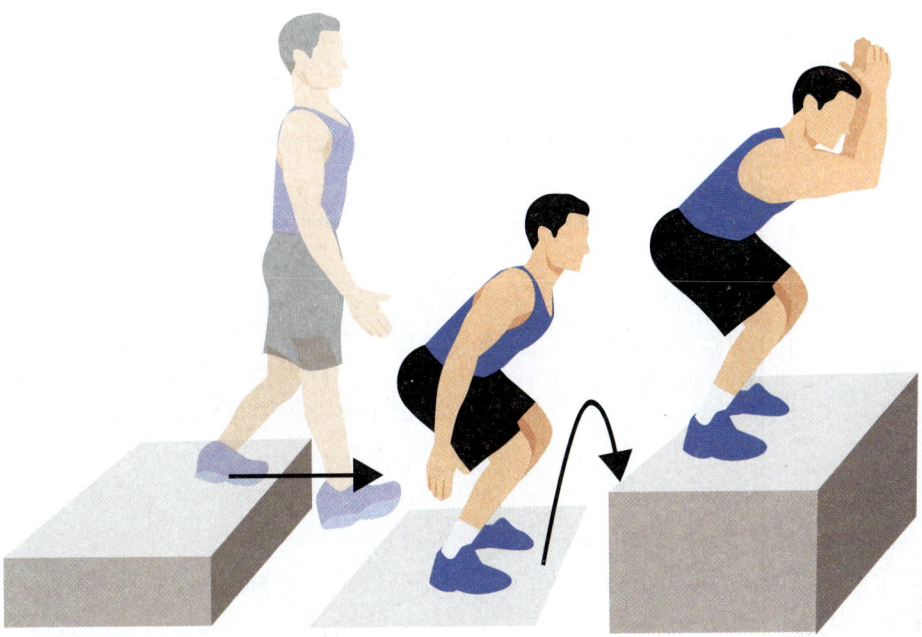

FIGURE 12.9 Depth Jump: Example

the proprioceptive properties of the muscle. Training that enhances neuromuscular efficiency decreases the time between the eccentric and concentric contraction, improving performance.

> ### ⚙ TRY THIS
>
> Take a rubber band and pull it back as if you were going to shoot it forward. Spend a few seconds aiming it before releasing it from your fingers. Note how far the rubber band went.
>
> Now, take the same rubber band and quickly pull it back and immediately release it. What do you notice? Assuming you did not hit anything, the second rubber band should go exponentially farther than the first.
>
> Our muscles are very similar to rubber bands in the conservation and expression of energy. As muscles stretch during eccentric muscle contraction, energy is stored within the bodily tissues to prepare for release. The longer we wait to jump, throw, or lift after a rapid pre-stretch, the more energy we lose, causing a reduction in total height, distance, and overall power. That is analogous to what happened with the first rubber band in the example.
>
> To maximize the SSC, consider minimizing the time between the eccentric and concentric phases. This will help improve plyometric performance and contribute to higher power and athletic performance outputs.

PLYOMETRIC TRAINING AND PERFORMANCE

Plyometric training variations serve as an integral method to enhance athletic performance, specifically by bridging heavier, slower strength-training exercises and high-velocity movements such as sprinting. A maximum-effort strength-training exercise sits on the higher-force, lower-velocity side when analyzing the force–velocity curve. Sprinting sits on the lower-force, higher-velocity end of this curve, and plyometrics sits directly in the middle (**Figure 12.10**). That bridging position explains why many Sports Performance Coaches utilize plyometrics in various manners inside their training plan.

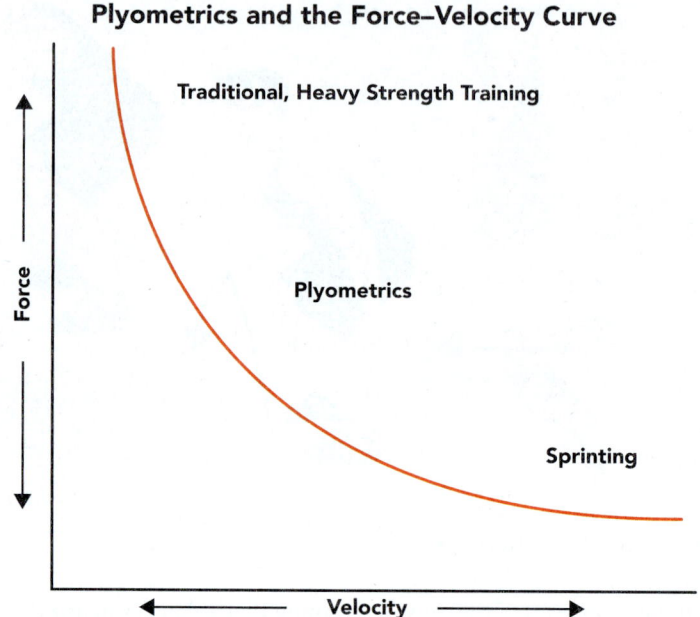

FIGURE 12.10 Plyometrics and the Force–Velocity Curve

In a recent study that interviewed Sports Performance Coaches worldwide (Weldon et al., 2022), most coaches reported using plyometrics in their training programs. The most frequently reported times for programming plyometrics are highlighted in **Figure 12.11**. The placement of plyometrics before weight training in a program most likely indicates that it was integrated into a comprehensive warm-up or movement preparation. When used in this manner, plyometric exercises allow athletes to prime the nervous system for enhanced neuromuscular efficiency during a weight training session.

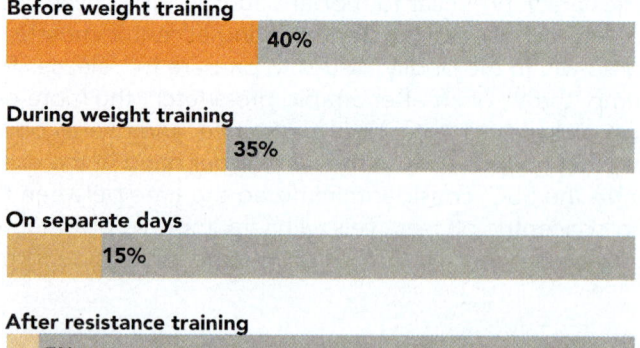

FIGURE 12.11 Reported Times for Prescribing Plyometrics

Data from Weldon, A., Duncan, M. J., Turner, A., LaPlaca, D., Sampaio, J., & Christie, C. J. (2022, May). Practices of strength and conditioning coaches: A snapshot from different sports, countries, and expertise levels. The Journal of Strength and Conditioning Research, 36(5): 1335–1344. https://doi.org/10.1519/jsc.0000000000003773

When properly utilized, plyometrics can also serve as an extension of a well-designed dynamic warm-up, preparing athletes for more intensive exercises such as speed drills or Olympic lifts. Sports Performance Coaches can take advantage of post-activation potentiation (PAP) by incorporating plyometrics into athletes' workouts. PAP allows athletes to express an enhanced level of force and power following a paired sequence of strength-training movements with plyometric or ballistic exercises (Iacono et al., 2019). Additionally, programming plyometrics on separate days, such as part of a speed, agility, or conditioning session, may be warranted to help with the organization and logistics of training due to space, time, or environment.

In the study cited earlier (Weldon et al., 2022), Sports Performance Coaches were also asked at what point in an athlete's season they integrated plyometric training (**Figure 12.12**). This training modality was implemented by most Sports Performance Coaches throughout most periods of the year (66%), suggesting it is viewed as a valuable component of an athletic performance training plan. By adjusting the intensity and volume of plyometric exercises, coaches can include additional alternatives for developing power and reducing the risk of injury during various points of the training year.

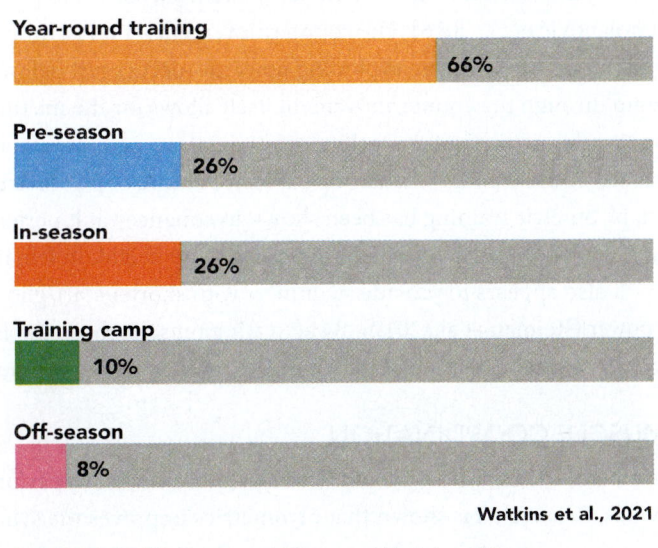

Reported Phase of Training When Implementing Plyometric Training

Year-round training — 66%
Pre-season — 26%
In-season — 26%
Training camp — 10%
Off-season — 8%

Watkins et al., 2021

FIGURE 12.12 Reported Phases of Training When Implementing Plyometric Training

Data from Watkins, C. M., Storey, A. G., McGuigan, M. R., & Gill, N. D. (2021, May). Implementation and efficacy of plyometric training: Bridging the gap between practice and research. The Journal of Strength and Conditioning Research, 35(5): 1244–1255. https://doi.org/10.1519/JSC.0000000000003985

For example, lower-body jumping exercises and upper-body throws may be safer alternatives for athletes in sports such as baseball or tennis during the in-season training period than other types of explosive lifts. Based on the training priorities set by the sports coach, the risks and benefits of specific exercises must be evaluated to maximize performance and decrease the risk of future injury. Research has consistently shown that athletes who utilize plyometrics and their variations as part of a well-rounded athletic enhancement program can improve their sports performance via means such as reducing injury rates, rehabilitating injuries, and enhancing speed, strength, and power (Alikhani et al., 2019; Asadi et al., 2015; Davies et al., 2015).

Whether the athlete engages in a collision sport (e.g., hockey or American football) or an individual skill sport (e.g., gymnastics or diving), the risk of injury is always present. An athlete's ability to control their body in chaotic and reactive environments can be a key determinant of their ability to stay healthy.

INCREASED STRENGTH

A meta-analysis conducted by Sáez de Villarreal et al. (2010) demonstrated that plyometric training has a positive effect on the development of strength. Plyometric exercises can assist both trained and untrained individuals to develop more strength. The integration of plyometric exercises has also been shown to increase lower-body strength, as measured by a one-repetition maximum (1RM) squat (al-Syurgawi & Shapie, 2019). Further, plyometric training has been used to improve jumping performance, linear sprint speed, change of direction, balance, and muscle strength in basketball players (Ramirez-Campillo et al., 2020). Of course, an athlete's training status should be considered when determining the overall volume of plyometrics, but supplementing strength training with plyometrics helps maximize strength gains for athletes. Additionally, there appears to be a maximum training threshold regarding volume that, once reached, will yield no further strength gains.

IMPROVED MUSCLE ACTIVATION

Compared to a squat jump, a countermovement jump has been shown to produce more explosive force (Stojanović et al., 2016). The countermovement—that is, dropping down into a deeper squat immediately before exploding upward—occurs just before the jump. The loading of the jump through the countermovement itself allows for the maximal activation of the concentric muscles, which in turn facilitates maximal strength development by activating all available muscle fibers—hence the explosive nature of plyometric exercises. In this same vein, plyometric training has been shown to enhance vault performance, including run-up/take-off velocity, post-flight time, and jump height, in female gymnasts (Hall et al., 2016). It also appears to provide swimmers with shorter start/glide times and greater take-off power (Rejman et al., 2017). By activating muscles through plyometric movements, more force can be developed to maximize the effectiveness of these techniques.

IMPROVED MUSCLE COORDINATION

As with any movement, the coordination of the musculature is vital to performing plyometric activities. Research has shown that plyometrics improves the synchronization of motor units and the ability of the athlete to perform the necessary movements (Issurin, 2013). This effect is believed to be caused by the forces developed through plyometric training and the recruitment of larger motor units through the myotatic reflex. Plyometric training is effective in developing coordination of muscle fiber recruitment, ultimately assisting with performance enhancement.

In the end, plyometric training has wide-ranging effects beyond power output. Indeed, moderately strong evidence indicates that when plyometric exercises are incorporated into an integrated training program, it leads to improvements in jumping ability, agility, power output, and rate of force development (Loturco et al., 2015; Ramachandran & Pradham, 2014; Sukamar, 2017). In one example, significant improvements in jump, sprint, and strength performance were achieved when plyometric training was combined with high-speed resistance training (Yáñez-García et al., 2022).

Additionally, plyometric training can serve as a complement to a comprehensive warm-up. Abade et al. (2017) found improved acute performance in both vertical jump and sprint performance when such exercises were used as part of a dynamic warm-up.

When such exercises are used in an isolated training program, however, plyometrics seems to have few positive benefits on performance (moderately strong evidence). Ideally, plyometric training should be undertaken as part of an integrated, holistic program.

PLYOMETRIC TRAINING FOR INJURY RESISTANCE

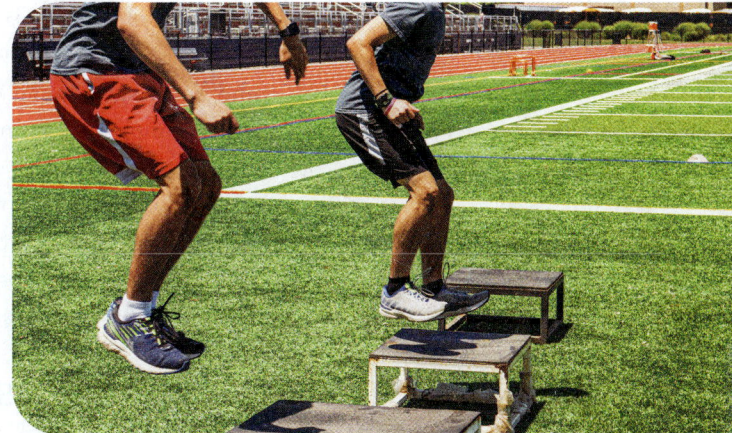

© WoodysPhotos/Shutterstock

Given that athletes may engage in chaotic and reactive situations in sport, the need to stabilize their bodies from both static and dynamic positions is essential. In many sports, athletes constantly sprint, jump, cut, and land in various positions. Athletes need to effectively control their body position during these movements to reduce the risk of certain injuries.

Plyometric training can enhance muscular strength, resulting in a greater ability to withstand the high forces and rapid changes in direction often encountered during athletic activities. This can reduce the risk of overuse injuries and acute musculoskeletal injuries, such as sprains and strains. Plyometric training can also improve joint stability by strengthening the muscles and connective tissues surrounding the joints. Stable joints are better equipped to handle the stress and strain of physical activity, reducing the risk of joint injuries.

In one study of the plyometrics–injury relationship, Enginsu et al. (2014) examined 36 female volleyball players who engaged in plyometric training for 12 weeks and a control group who did not engage in physical training. After 12 weeks, only the plyometric training group had significantly improved lower limb movement patterns. The researchers concluded that plyometric training improves lower limb kinematics and functional performance, and suggested that these exercises could offer benefits in programs to prevent anterior cruciate ligament (ACL) injuries.

In addition, plyometric training can improve neuromuscular control and proprioception, leading to better body control, balance, and coordination. These abilities can help athletes avoid falls and other injuries associated with poor movement control or balance.

The use of lower-body plyometrics has been shown to assist in the proper control of lower-body biomechanics and assist performance by promoting the following changes:

- Reducing lower-extremity valgus during both single- and double-leg movements (Myer et al., 2006)
- Improving dynamic balance, postural control, and knee proprioception (Alikhani et al., 2019; Asadi et al., 2015)
- Enhancing muscle activation and neurological efficiency (Chimera et al., 2004)

However, although plyometric training may be able to help with injury prevention, it must be properly implemented to avoid *causing* injuries. Plyometric exercises are high-intensity activities that can place significant stress on the musculoskeletal system, so they should be incorporated into training programs carefully. For this reason, Sports Performance Coaches should consider how plyometrics fit into their overall training plan. The specific intensity, volume, and exercise selection may change based on factors such as an athlete's specific training period or the equipment available. Nevertheless, plyometrics can provide Sports Performance Coaches with various unique exercises to improve athletic performance for an extensive range of athletes and sports.

LESSON 4: PRINCIPLES OF PLYOMETRIC TRAINING
PLYOMETRIC TRAINING GUIDELINES

Plyometric training is paramount for athletes because it enhances power, speed, and agility—all of which are critical components of high-level athletic performance. By engaging the SSC, plyometric exercises help athletes generate maximal force in minimal time, boosting their explosive power. This power is integral to many sports movements, such as jumping, sprinting, and changing direction quickly. In addition, plyometrics can improve neuromuscular control and proprioception, leading to better body control and coordination. This improves performance and aids in injury prevention, a key concern for any elite athlete. Moreover, the adaptability of plyometric training means that it can be tailored to mimic sport-specific movements, thereby enhancing its relevance and effectiveness in performance training.

NEEDS ANALYSIS AND ASSESSMENT INFORMATION

As with any aspect of a sports performance program, an intentional and specific program needs to be developed for plyometric training that is tailored to each athlete's needs. A needs analysis is the first step that allows the Sports Performance Coach to thoroughly understand the individual needs of the athlete and the sport.

Performing a needs analysis and gathering assessment information is crucial when designing plyometric training programs. It ensures the program is tailored to the individual athlete's requirements, abilities, and goals, thereby maximizing its effectiveness and minimizing the risk of injury. Information about the athlete's training age—that is, their experience with strength and conditioning exercises—is vital for selecting appropriate plyometric exercises and determining progression rates. For instance, a novice may need to start with low-intensity exercises and gradually progress to more complex movements. The exercise order should also be considered, as fatigue from previous exercises can affect performance and safety in subsequent plyometric drills.

Exercises should also be categorized based on their complexity and the specific muscles they target, with the goal of developing a balanced and comprehensive training program. Furthermore, attention must be given to exercises in different planes of motion (sagittal, frontal, and transverse), as sports often involve multidirectional movements. Finally, the number of sets and repetitions and the intensity of the exercises should be carefully determined based on the athlete's current fitness level, sport-specific demands, and training goals. Collectively, these factors underscore the importance of performing a thorough needs analysis and assessment for creating an effective, safe, and individualized plyometric training program.

> ✔ **CHECK IT OUT**
>
> More than 70% of Sports Performance Coaches use plyometric training regularly, and more than 96% use some type of periodization strategy when programming plyometrics into their sessions (Watkins, Storey, et al., 2021). The following section explores a variety of factors to consider when determining a plyometric program for the athlete.

PROGRESSING PLYOMETRIC TRAINING

As plyometric training is considered one of the more advanced training tools, athletes need proper levels of flexibility, core strength, and balance before they are progressed into plyometric training. Sports Performance Coaches must apply specific program guidelines, proper exercise selection criteria, and detailed program variables to achieve the best outcome and the lowest risk of injury. **Table 12.1** lists some of the variables to consider when designing a plyometric training program.

TABLE 12.1 Variables to Consider for Plyometric Training Programs

Variable	Explanation
Training age	More experienced athletes will be able to perform more challenging exercises such as weighted, band-resisted, and single-leg options.
Body mass	The total-body mass of the client or athlete can alter the difficulty of exercises such as depth jumps and multiple-plane hops.
Training surface	Softer surfaces such as grass and sand can minimize ground reaction forces from landing. Harder surfaces such as rubber floors and courts can maximize the elastic response in more advanced exercises.
Availability of equipment/space	Lack of plyometric equipment such as hurdles, boxes, or medicine balls will decrease the possible variation of exercises.
Time of training	Exercise selection can vary based on when training will occur, such as before, during, or after resistance training; between warm-ups; or on its own developmental session.
Seasonal priority	Frequency, intensity, and duration are dependent on which season the athlete is training in.
Planes of motion	Exercise selection varies based on which planes of motion need the most support or development. This can help maximize the transfer of training effects and/or reduce the risk of future injury.
Range of motion	Sport-specific joint angles and muscle actions take greater precedence as the athlete moves closer to competition.
Speed of drill	Greater speeds, especially during repeated or explosive tempos, will affect the difficulty of the drill.
Duration/frequency	Limited time during the sessions or the total number of sessions will influence the types of exercises selected.
Rest	The lengths of both intra- and inter-set rest periods can affect energy system utilization and primary goals.

Additionally, the systematic progression of plyometric training is key to promoting the body's gradual adaptation to the intense demands of these exercises. Plyometric exercises, which are characterized by rapid and explosive movements, can significantly stress muscles, tendons, and joints. Injury risk is minimized, and power, speed, and agility are optimized, by methodically escalating the intensity, volume, and complexity of plyometric workouts. Furthermore, proper progressions allow for a regulated improvement in neuromuscular efficiency, which is pivotal in sports. Finally, systematically advancing plyometric training nurtures consistent progress, empowering athletes to safely attain their athletic objectives.

Sports Performance Coaches should establish a spectrum of plyometric drills that can be progressively overloaded at appropriate time intervals once athletes have demonstrated mastery of the previous phase. Viewing the program exercises collectively, the Sports Performance Coach can divide ideal progressions into beginner, intermediate, and advanced levels. However, it is important to recognize that these categories are not based on an athlete's ability. Instead, they should be aligned with the overall training process. For example, even some of the most advanced athletes may need to perform *beginner* plyometric exercises to emphasize technique and coordination. **Table 12.2** provides an example of potential plyometric training progressions.

TABLE 12.2   Example Plyometric Training Progressions

Exercise Selection	Example
Simple to complex	Squat jump → depth jump→ depth jump to horizontal jump
Single to double	Vertical jump → vertical hop
General to specific	Squat jump → position-specific jump
Vertical to linear plane	Squat jump in place → forward squat jump
Uniplanar to multiplanar	Squat jump → lateral squat jump → rotational squat jump
Stable to continuous	Tuck jump with stabilization → repeat tuck jump
Programmed to reactive	Self-directed jump → jump based on audible or visual stimuli

BEGINNER PLYOMETRIC EXERCISES

When introducing plyometric exercises, especially to beginner athletes, the movements should initially involve small jumps (lower amplitude) to best learn the movement pattern. Such beginner exercises are designed to establish optimal landing mechanics, postural alignment, and eccentric strength (ability to decelerate). When an athlete lands during these exercises, they should hold the landing position (or stabilize) for 3 to 5 seconds. During this time, athletes should make any adjustments necessary to correct faulty postures before performing the next jump.

INTERMEDIATE PLYOMETRIC EXERCISES

The first progressions involve adding jumps with more amplitude and dynamic motion. The speed of the jumps can also be progressed. These exercises are intended to improve dynamic joint stabilization, eccentric strength, rate of force production, and coordination of the entire human body. They are performed in a repetitive fashion, with the athlete spending a relatively short amount of time on the ground before repeating the drill. In other words, the athlete no longer holds the landing position for 3 to 5 seconds, but instead initiates another jump upon landing using a moderate (repeating) tempo.

ADVANCED PLYOMETRIC EXERCISES

The last progression includes exercises that involve explosive, powerful movements. These exercises are designed to further improve the rate of force production, eccentric strength, and reactive joint stabilization. They are performed as fast and as explosively as possible.

> ### ✔ CHECK IT OUT
>
> Intensities can be highly variable during plyometric training based on the complexity and execution of each exercise. Although traditional plyometric training attempts to utilize and enhance the SSC, plyometric exercises can be regressed to reduce or eliminate impact and ground reaction forces if necessary. For example, beginner-level exercises focus on improving landing technique (i.e., landing softly with optimal form). Thus, an athlete can perform a small squat jump (minimal amplitude), landing on the reactive portion of the foot and focusing on absorbing the impact through the feet, ankle, knee, and hip. Or, if this is too much impact due to an injury, an athlete can work on reactive strength by simply driving up to triple extension (ankle plantar flexion, knee and hip extension) and then quickly returning to a loaded or ready position. Again, the athlete can work on force reduction and form with virtually no impact.

ACUTE TRAINING VARIABLES FOR PLYOMETRIC TRAINING

The Sports Performance Coach must ensure that all programs follow the recommended acute training variables for plyometric training.

SETS AND REPETITIONS

The total number of sets and repetitions that should be performed for each plyometric exercise depends on a variety of factors:

- Assessment results
- Training goals
- Amount of time allocated during training
- The overall stress of the athlete from practices, competitions, and other life stressors
- The intensity of the exercise itself
- How the exercise fits within the larger landscape of the training session

Although more volume leads to a higher training stimulus, *excessive* volume could lead to fatigue, which could hinder future sports performance. For example, sprinters may need a high volume of contacts because they use plyometrics as part of their practice plan, whereas an athlete in a field sport may benefit just as much from a lower volume of contacts. As exercises become more complex, the Sports Performance Coach should aim for fewer repetitions per set for proper instruction and management of fatigue.

In addition, as the intensity of the exercise increases, the overall total number of contacts (either by feet or by hands) should be decreased. The initial number of foot

contacts should be less than 60 per session (spread out over two to four different exercises) and no more than 80 to 120 foot contacts per session (Bedoya et al., 2015). However, most coaches continue to program plyometrics at even lower numbers of contacts (fewer than 30) per session, according to research on explosive strength development (Laputin & Oleshko, 1986).

Ideally, Sports Performance Coaches should aim for 5 to 12 repetitions of traditional plyometrics exercises performed for one to five sets to maximize power and minimize intra-set fatigue (**Table 12.3**).

TABLE 12.3 Sets and Repetitions for Plyometric Training

Level of Plyometric Training	Sets	Repetitions/ Duration	Volume
Beginner	1–3	5–8 repetitions	8–24 reps/exercise
Intermediate	2–4	8–12 repetitions	16–50 reps/exercise
Advanced	3–5	8–12 repetitions	16–50 reps/exercise

INTENSITY

Plyometric training is generally high intensity by nature. If the intensity is too low, the desired improvements in power, speed, and agility may not be achieved. Conversely, if the intensity is too high, it may lead to overtraining, diminishing returns, and a greater risk of injury. Multiple factors affect the intensity of plyometric exercises, such as the following:

- Complexity of the exercise (i.e., increased neural demand)
- Amplitude (e.g., jumping higher, height of implements)
- Speed of execution (tempo) (e.g., holding landing position versus repetitive)
- Landing and take-off positions (e.g., staggered, split stance, or single- or double-leg)
- Uniplanar or multiplanar (e.g., vertical jump or vertical jump to long jump)

The speed of execution (tempo) plays a crucial role in varying training intensity and optimizing training effects. Longer, more controlled tempos with a pause for stabilization are generally considered low intensity and are best used to teach jumping, throwing, landing, and catching mechanics in the correct positions. As athletes progress through the spectrum of general to more specific plyometric exercises, the tempo of each repetition increases to take advantage of the SSC (**Table 12.4**).

TABLE 12.4 Tempo Spectrum of Plyometric Exercises

Short Response	Medium Response	Long Response
Quick ground contact time (Example: Explosive hurdle jump)	Moderate ground contact time (Example: Hurdle jump with bounce)	Long ground contact time (Example: Hurdle jump with stabilization)

Sports Performance Coaches should use a program design progression that considers these and other factors when deciding how to progress an athlete in training. Research has shown that performance improvements occur whether there is an increase in volume, intensity, or both if the total load (volume × intensity × frequency) is matched (Lievens et al., 2021). **Table 12.5** provides some examples of basic progressions for plyometric exercises.

TABLE 12.5 General Intensities for Plyometric Training

Level of Plyometric Training	Intensity
Beginner	Simple; small amplitude; hold landing position for 3–5 seconds (long response)
Intermediate	Increase complexity, amplitude, and speed of execution (medium response)
Advanced	Increase complexity, amplitude, and speed of execution (short response); decrease base of support (e.g., single leg)

TRAINING FREQUENCY

Plyometric training is demanding and places significant stress on the musculoskeletal and nervous systems. Proper recovery time between sessions is critical to allow the body to repair itself and strengthen. If plyometric workouts are performed too frequently without enough recovery time, it can lead to overtraining, decreased performance, and increased risk of injury. Nevertheless, the body needs a certain frequency of training stimuli to adapt and improve. If plyometric workouts are too infrequent, the body may not receive enough stimulation to improve power, speed, and neuromuscular efficiency. Between 24 and 48 hours of rest between sessions is recommended to prevent overtraining and maintain training effectiveness (Radcliffe & Farentinos, 2015).

The training frequency largely depends on how many training sessions the athlete participates in during a weekly rotation. Implementing plyometrics one to three times per week is a realistic guideline for athletes who both compete in-season and train during the off-season. Sports Performance Coaches should consider front-loading the beginning of their training sessions and training weeks with more plyometric and power-focused exercises to minimize residual fatigue toward the end of the week. **Table 12.6** summarizes plyometric training frequency recommendations.

TABLE 12.6 Frequency for Plyometric Training

Level of Plyometric Training	Frequency
Beginner	2–4 sessions per week
Intermediate	2–4 sessions per week
Advanced	2–4 sessions per week

LESSON 5: MODALITIES FOR PLYOMETRIC TRAINING

PLYOMETRIC TRAINING TECHNIQUES

Implementing a plyometric training program requires that Sports Performance Coaches follow a systematic program strategy to ensure the safety and effectiveness of the program. When progressing plyometrics, the individual goals of athletes need to be considered. If plyometrics are being performed to complement agility training, higher volumes may not be necessary. However, if the goal of speed is important, more plyometric training should be considered, and it should be progressed according to the needs analysis of the athlete and sport.

EXERCISE CATEGORIES

Improper or unclear terminology can confuse Sports Performance Coaches and athletes. What may be considered as a double-leg jump by one coach may be interpreted as a single-leg jump by another coach. More precisely, when working in any system, keeping the entire staff on the same page regarding coaching terminology and technique is vital. There should be clarity regarding exercise naming and technique corrections. The naming conventions for lower-body plyometric training presented in **Table 12.7**, which were originally developed by Boyle (2016) and Feit and Smith (2016), have been widely adopted. A framework for upper-body plyometric training is also presented in Table 12.7.

TABLE 12.7 Lower-Body and Upper-Body Medicine Ball (MB) Exercise Naming Convention

Lower-Body and Upper-Body Medicine Ball Exercises	
Jump	A two-leg take-off with a two-leg landing (e.g., vertical jump)
Hop	A one-leg take-off with the same one-leg landing (e.g., vertical hop)
Bound	A one-leg take-off with an alternate one-leg landing (e.g., lateral bound)
Hybrid	A combination of any type of jump, hop, or bound with the possible addition of an MB for upper-body power development (e.g., lateral bound to double-leg landing or a hurdle jump to MB punch)
Upper-Body Medicine Ball Exercises	
Punch	An MB throw directed in the linear or rotational direction toward a wall or partner with hands positioned to push the ball (e.g., standing MB punch)
Slam	An MB throw directed in the vertical direction toward the floor with hands positioned on top of the ball (e.g., overhead MB slam)
Toss	An MB throw directed in the rotational direction toward a wall or partner with hands clasped underneath the MB (e.g., MB side toss)
Launch	An MB throw directed in the vertical or linear direction for maximum distance (e.g., MB vertical launch)

BEGINNER PLYOMETRIC EXERCISES

Initial plyometric exercises should focus on enhancing landing mechanics and control. Such movements should involve small jumps (lower amplitude), and the landing position should be held for 3 to 5 seconds. During this time, athletes should make any adjustments necessary to correct faulty postures before performing the next jump.

INTERMEDIATE PLYOMETRIC EXERCISES

The next level of plyometric exercises involves jumps with more amplitude and dynamic motion, with the execution speed being increased to a moderate response. These exercises are performed in a repetitive fashion and are intended to improve dynamic joint stabilization, eccentric strength, rate of force production, and coordination of the entire human body.

ADVANCED PLYOMETRIC EXERCISES

The last progression includes exercises that involve powerful short-response movements. These exercises are designed to further improve the rate of force production, eccentric strength, and reactive joint stabilization. They are performed as fast and as explosively as possible.

PLYOMETRIC TRAINING EXERCISES

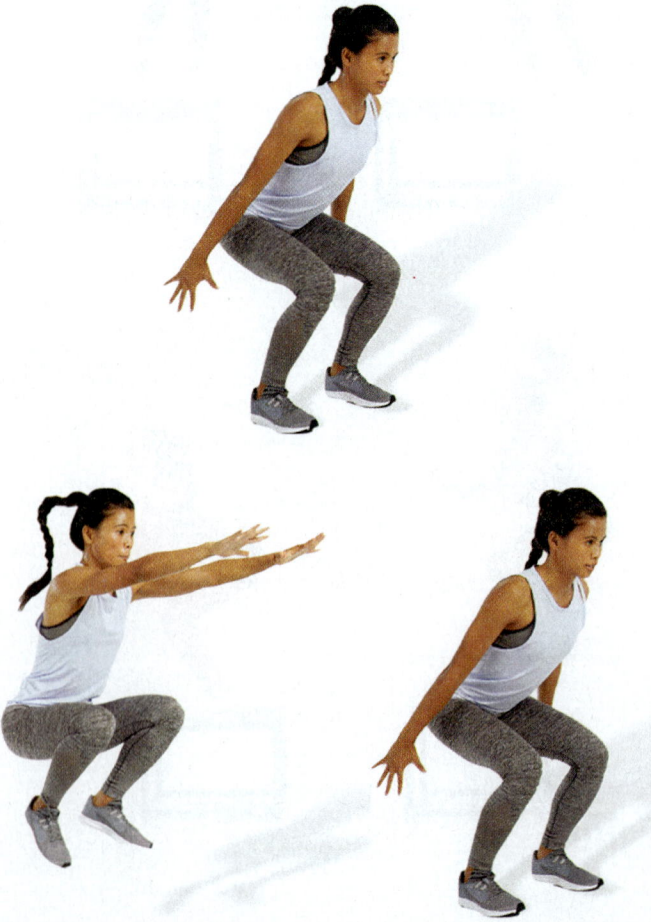

Squat Jump with Stabilization

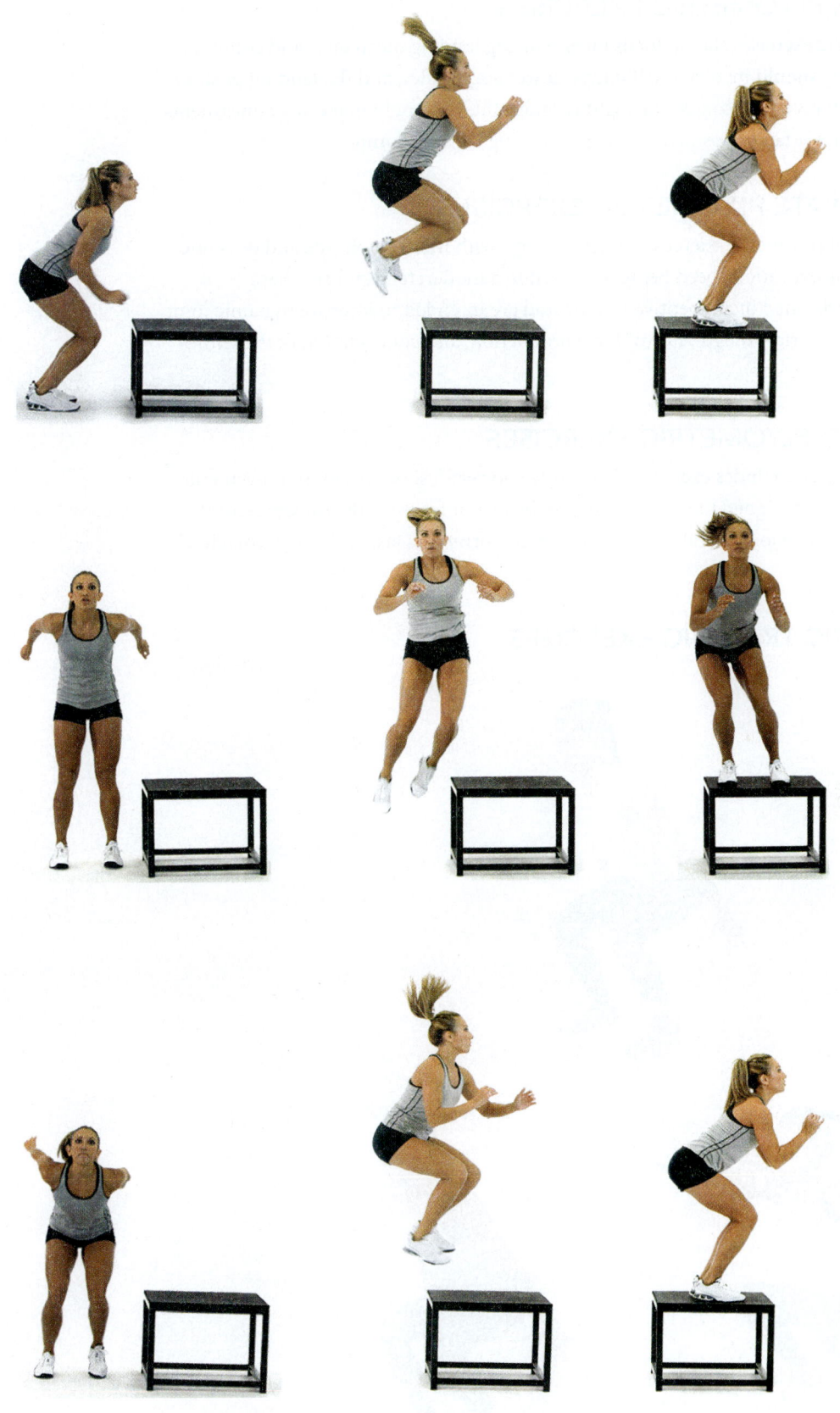

Multiplanar Jump-up with Stabilization

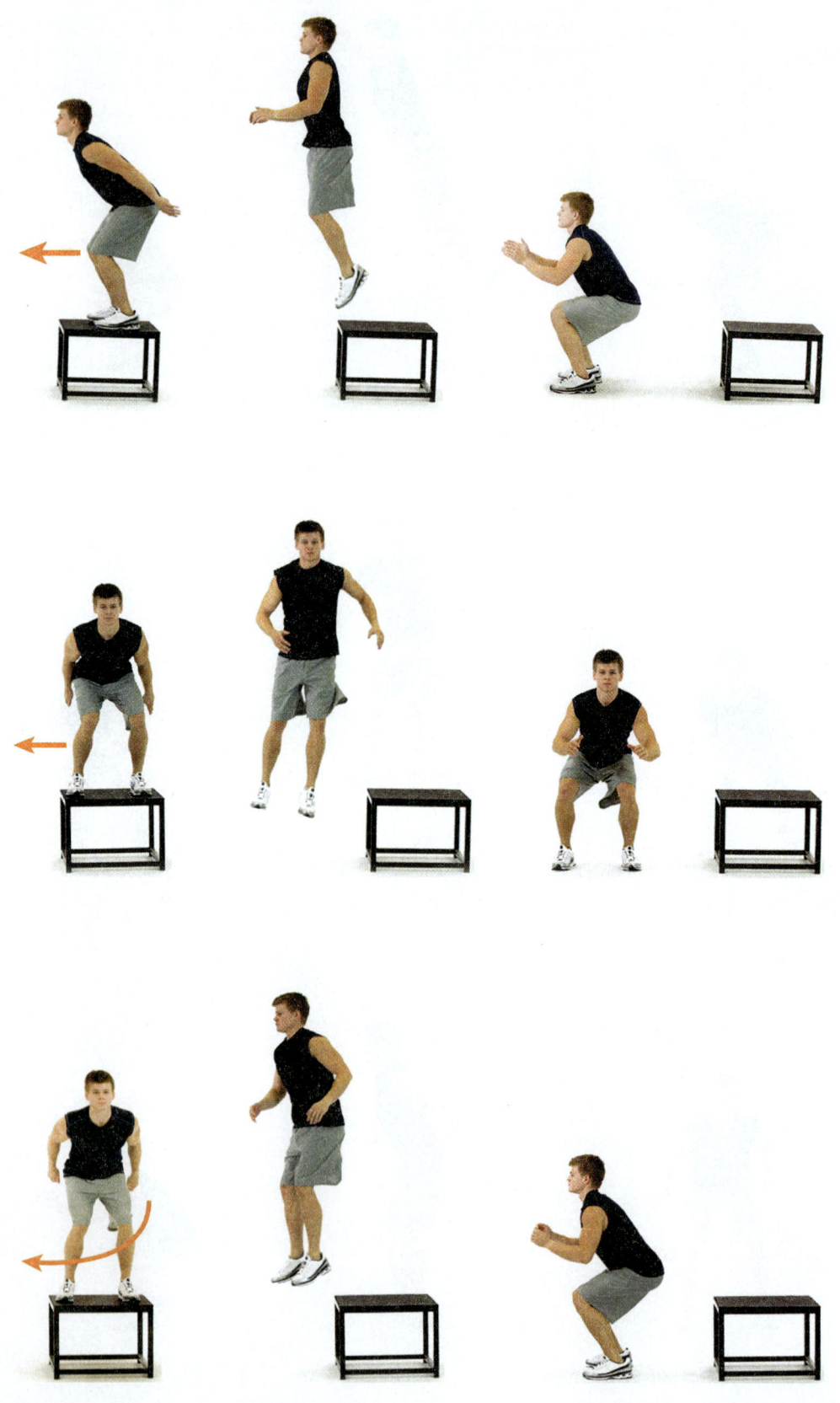

Multiplanar Box Jump-down with Stabilization

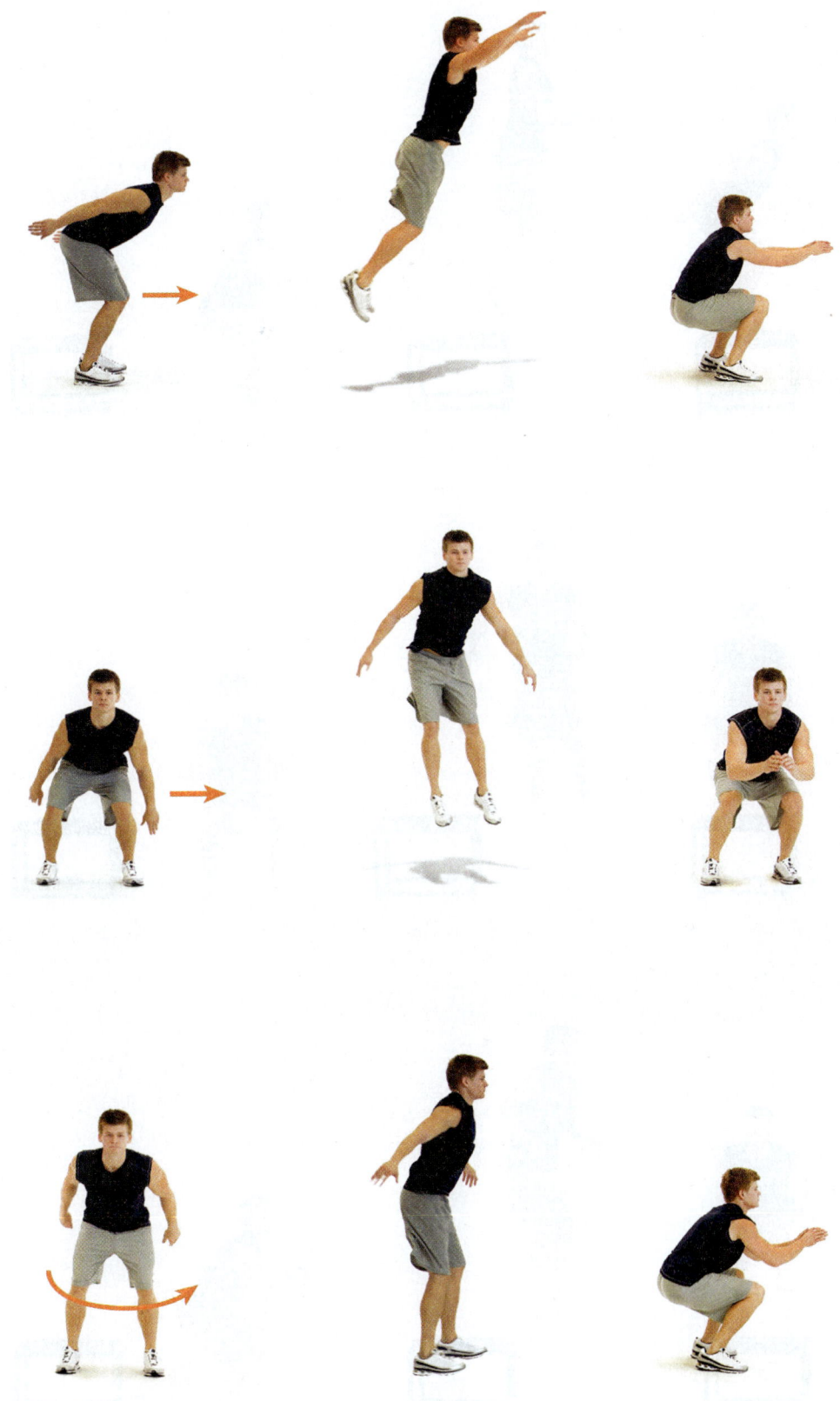

Multiplanar Jump with Stabilization

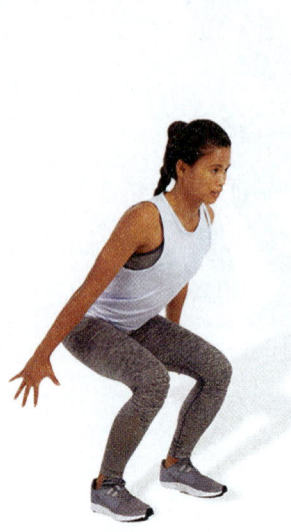
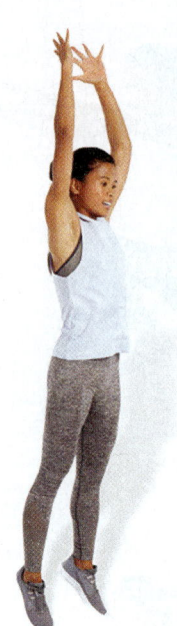
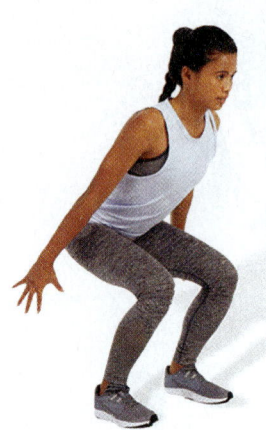

Plyometric Squat

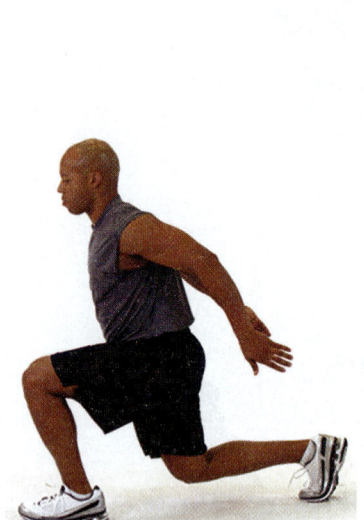
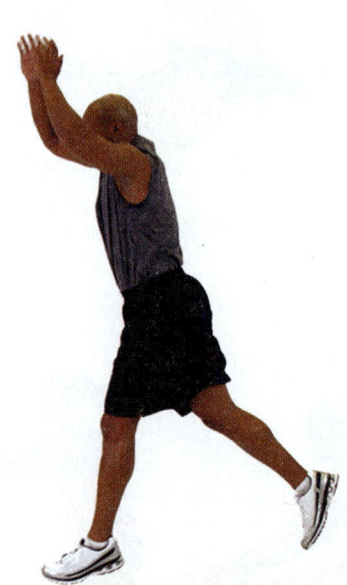
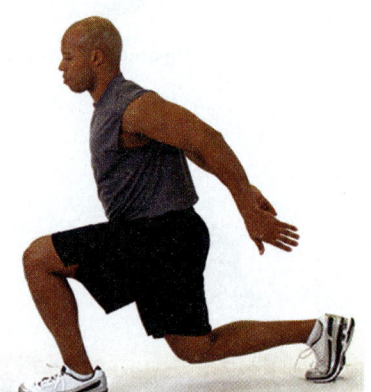

Plyometric Lunge Jumps

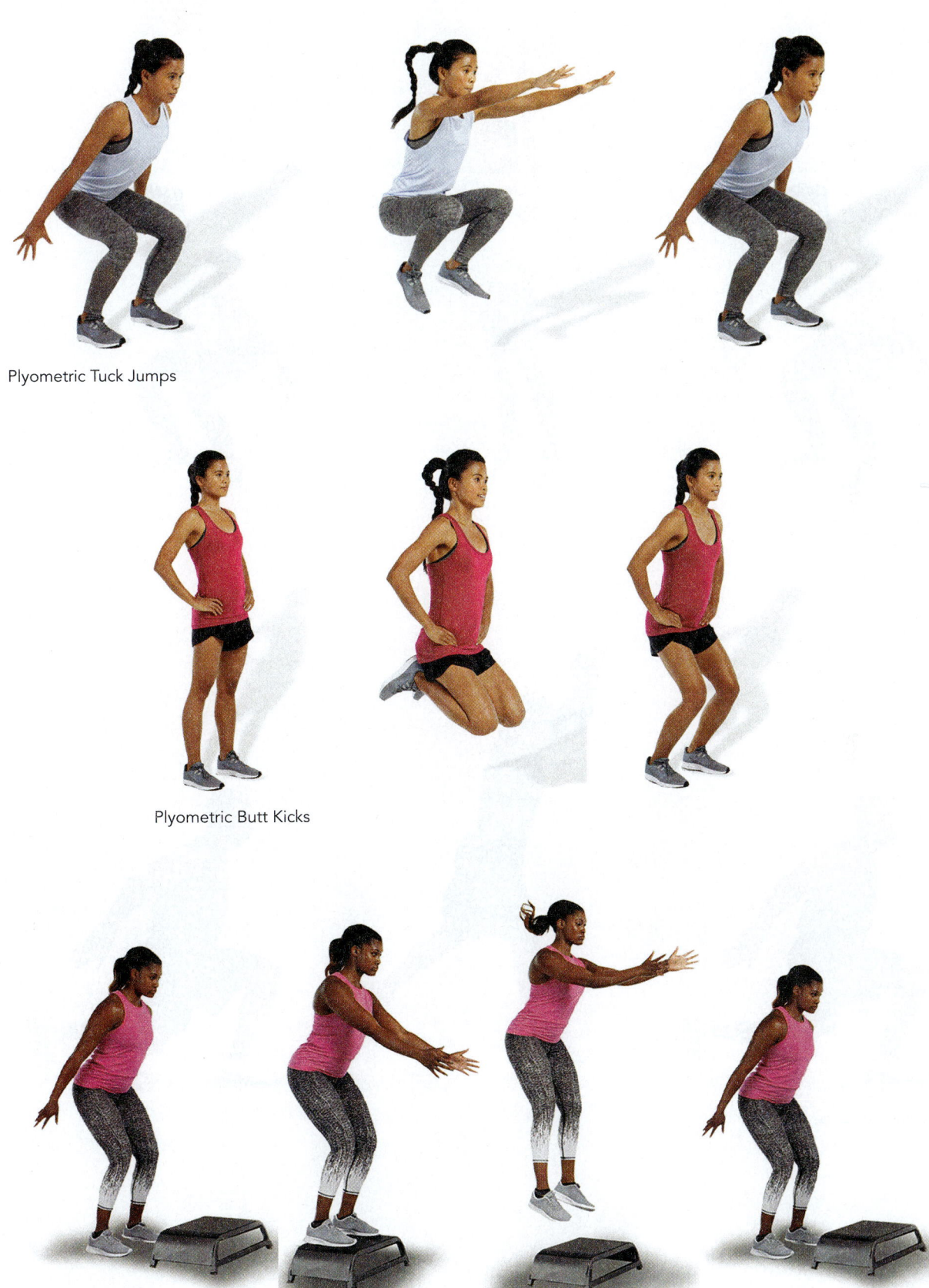

Plyometric Tuck Jumps

Plyometric Butt Kicks

Repeat Box Jumps

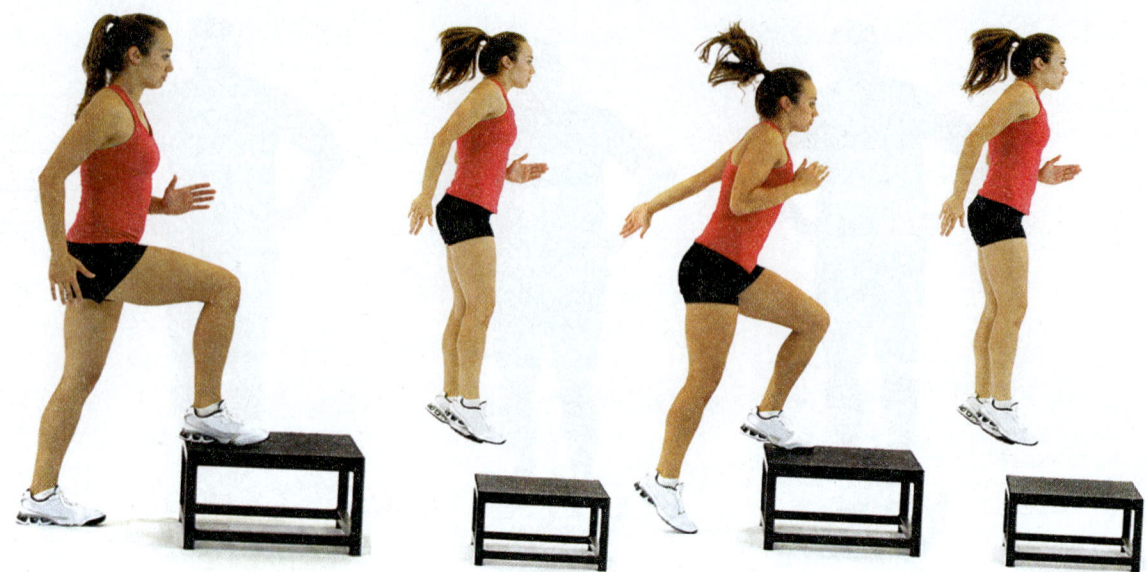

Plyometric Power Step-up

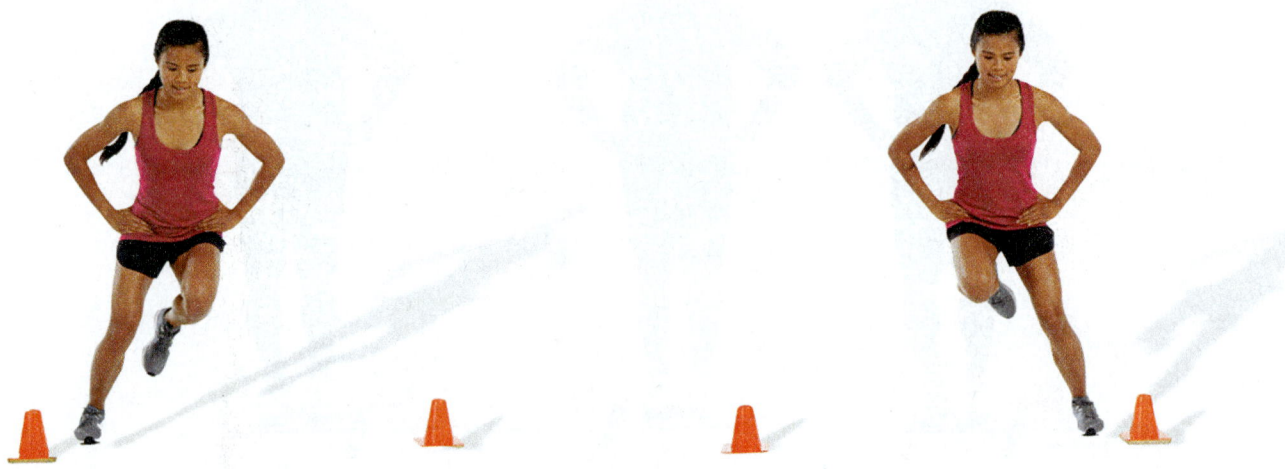

Ice Skaters

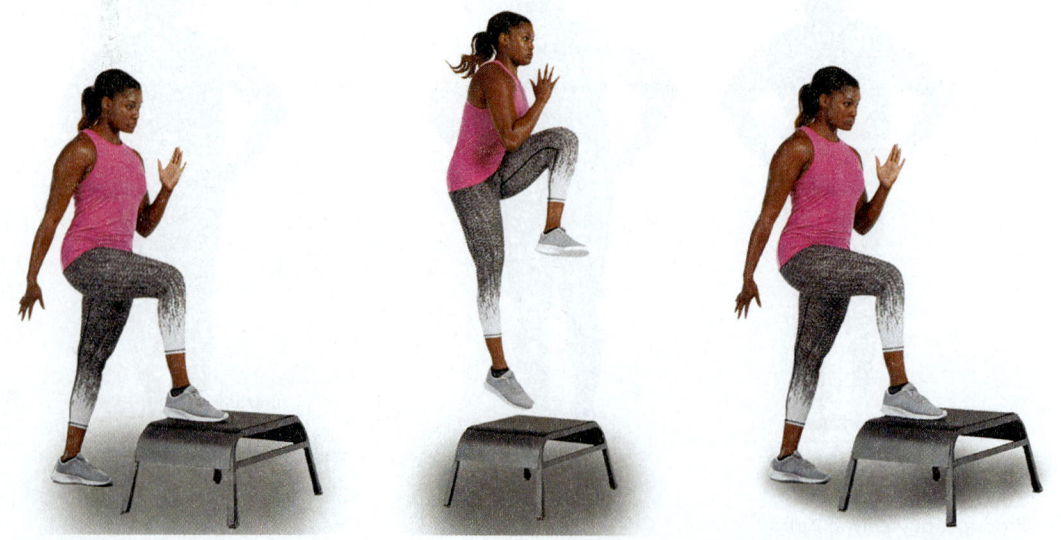

Multiplanar Power Step-up

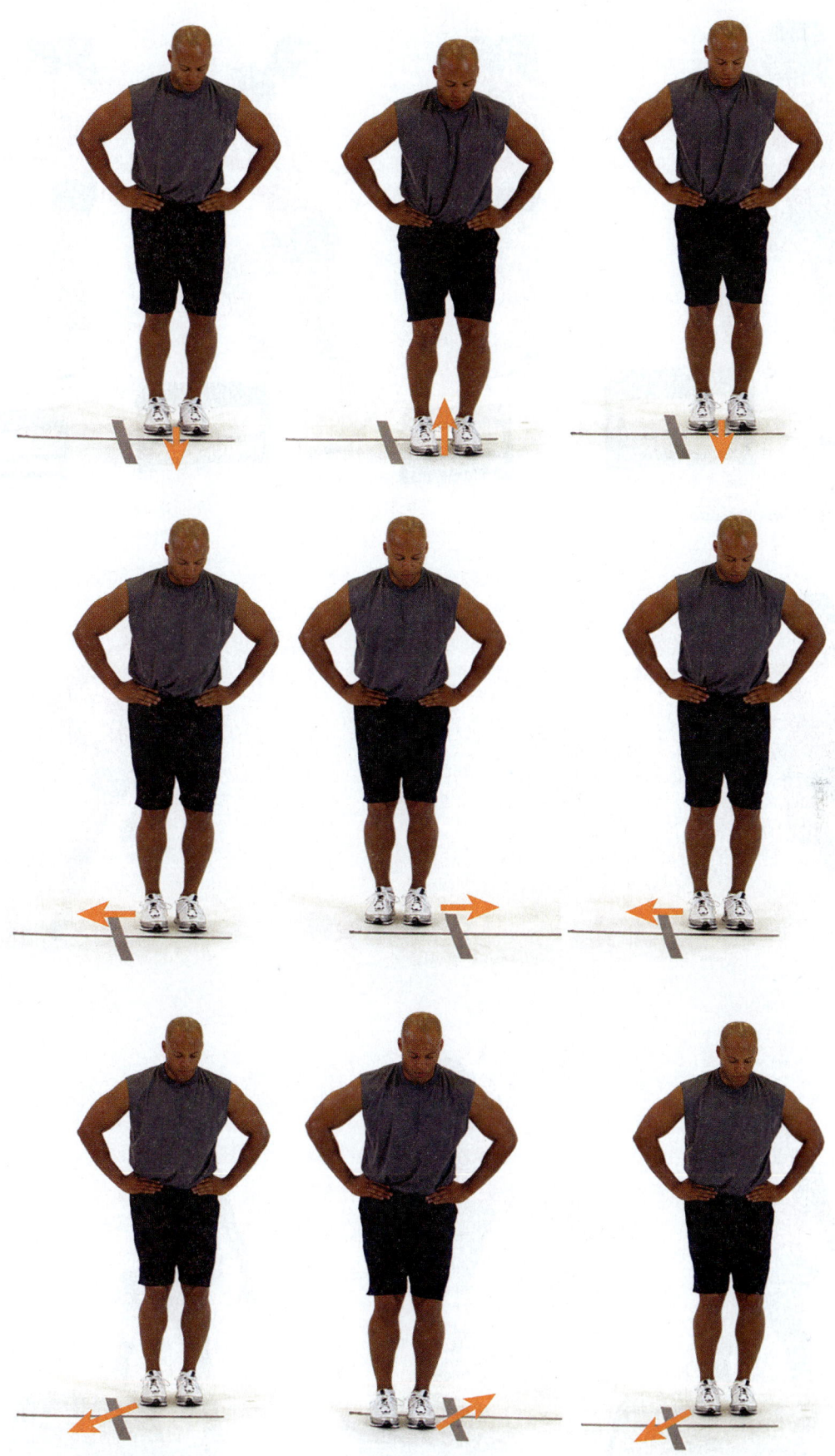

Proprioceptive Plyometrics

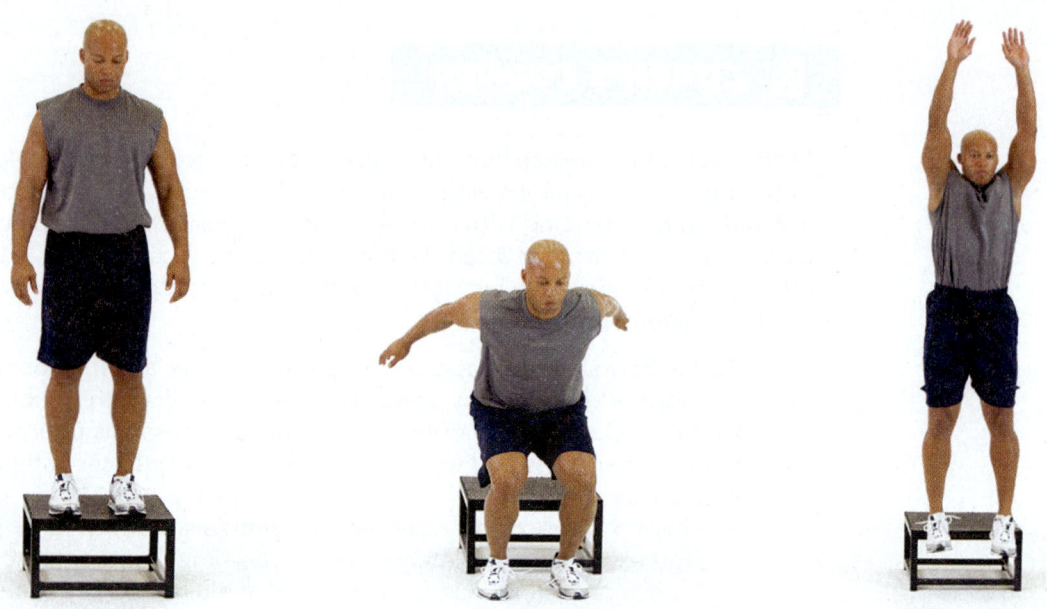

Plyometric Depth Jump

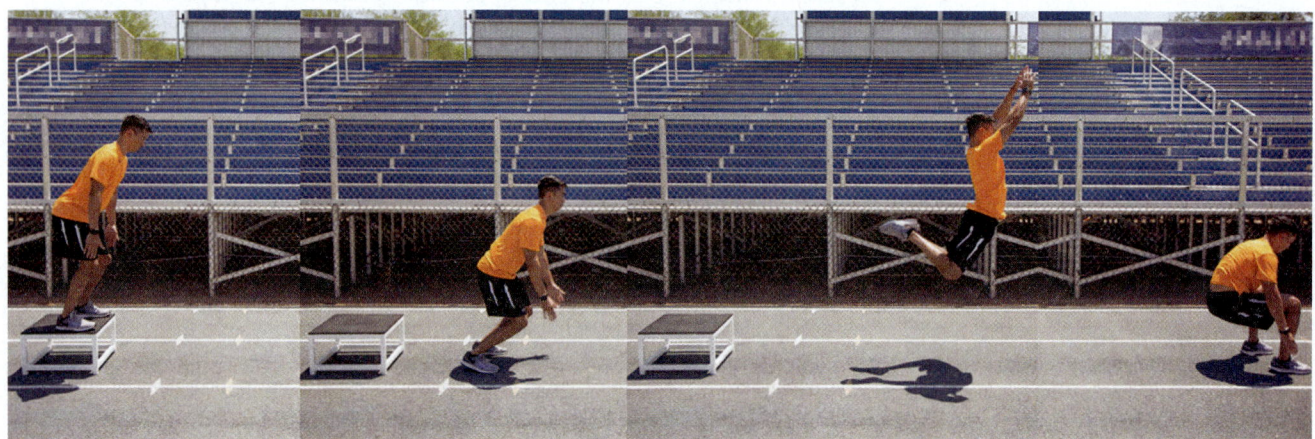

Depth Jump to Long Jump

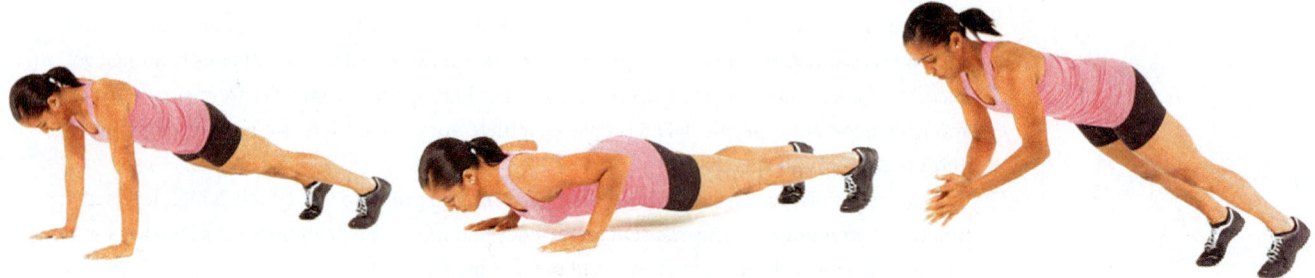

Plyometric Push-up

SUMMARY

Plyometric training is an essential component of all integrated performance training programs. All sporting activities require a unique approach to expressing various amounts of force at varying levels of speeds and directions. By using plyometrics, athletes can enhance their reactive strength and express a higher amount of force in a shorter period of time. In addition, plyometrics have been shown to improve sprinting, change of direction, agility, power, and strength, and to decrease the risk of future injury.

Programming plyometrics requires consideration of multiple factors and situations to optimize athletic performance. Plyometrics should be done in a variety of planes and angles, and should encompass a spectrum of jumps, hops, bounds, and throws specific to an athlete's training age, needs, and goals. Sports Performance Coaches should progress plyometrics from simple to complex, and from general to specific, when preparing athletes for competition that requires high force outputs at very high speeds.

The use of plyometrics in an integrated performance program can establish high levels of functional strength and neuromuscular efficiency and improve all components necessary for an athlete to perform at the highest level and prevent injury.

KEY TAKEAWAYS

- Plyometrics help develop reactive strength in athletes; improve sprinting, change of direction, agility, power, and strength; and decrease the risk of future injury.
- Not all jumps and throws are plyometric in nature. True plyometrics take advantage of the rapid pre-stretch of muscles prior to expressing force at high speeds in short amounts of time.

- Plyometrics can benefit a variety of athletes and sports, and can be utilized in all phases of athletic competition, including pre-season, in-season, and off-season.
- Sports Performance Coaches should consider a variety of factors when designing a plyometric program, including an athlete's training age, body mass, training surface, equipment/space availability, planes of motion, ranges of motion, needs assessment, and individual goals.

REFERENCES

Abade, E., Sampaio, J., Gonçalves, B., Baptista, J., Alves, A., & Viana, J. (2017). Effects of different re-warm up activities in football players' performance. *PLoS One, 12*(6), e0180152. https://doi.org/10.1371/journal .pone.0180152

Akdeniz, H., & Şentürk, A. (2018). Reviewing the effect of plyometrics training performed by icemen play in super league on quick power and maximal power. *European Journal of Physical Education and Sport Science, 4*(2), 37–51. https://doi.org/10.5281/ZENODO.1174547

Alikhani, R., Shahrjerdi, S., Golpaigany, M., & Kazemi, M. (2019). The effect of a six-week plyometric training on dynamic balance and knee proprioception in female badminton players. *Journal of the Canadian Chiropractic Association, 63*(3), 144–153.

al-Syurgawi, D., & Shapie, M. N. M. (2019). The effects of a 6-week plyometric training on muscular strength performance in silat athletes. *Revista de Artes Marciales Asiáticas, 14*(2s), 28–30. http://doi.org/10.18002 /rama.v14i2s.5976

Arazi, H., & Asadi, A. (2011). The effect of aquatic and land plyometric training on strength, sprint, and balance in young basketball players. *Journal of Human Sport and Exercise, 6*(1), 101–111. https://doi.org/10.4100 /jhse.2011.61.12

Asadi, A., Saez de Villarreal, E., & Arazi, H. (2015). The effects of plyometric type neuromuscular training on postural control performance of male team basketball players. *Journal of Strength and Conditioning Research, 29*(7), 1870–1875. https://doi.org/10.1519/JSC.0000000000000832

Atanasković, A., Georgiev, M., & Mutavdzić, V. (2015). The impact of plyometrics and aqua plyometrics on the lower extremities explosive strength in children aged 11–15. *Research in Kinesiology, 43*(1), 111–114.

Bedoya, A. A., Miltenberger, M. R., & Lopez, R. M. (2015). Plyometric training effects on athletic performance in youth soccer athletes: A systematic review. *Journal of Strength and Conditioning Research, 29*(8), 2351–2360. https://doi.org/10.1519/jsc.0000000000000877

Boyle, M. (2016). *New functional training for sports* (2nd ed.). Human Kinetics.

Chimera, N. J., Swanik, K. A., Swanik, C. B., & Straub, S. J. (2004). Effects of plyometric training on muscle-activation strategies and performance in female athletes. *Journal of Athletic Training, 39*(1), 24–31.

Davies, G., Riemann, B. L., & Manske, R. (2015). Current concepts of plyometric exercise. *International Journal of Sports Physical Therapy, 10*(6), 760–786.

De Bleecker, C., Vermeulen, S., De Blaiser, C., Willems, T., De Ridder, R., & Roosen, P. (2020). Relationship between jump-landing kinematics and lower extremity overuse injuries in physically active populations: A systematic review and meta-analysis. *Sports Medicine, 50*(8), 1515–1532. https://doi.org/10.1007/s40279-020-01296-7

Egan-Shuttler, J. D., Edmonds, R., Eddy, C., O'Neill, V., & Ives, S. J. (2017). The effect of concurrent plyometric training versus submaximal aerobic cycling on rowing economy, peak power, and performance in male high school rowers. *Sports Medicine Open, 3*(1), 7. https://doi.org/10.1186/s40798-017-0075-2

Enginsu, M., Lokmaoğlu, R., Korkmaz, E., Arıbaş, İ., & Selimoğlu, Ş. (2014). Effect of plyometric training on prevention of ACL injuries in females volleyball players. *Orthopaedic Journal of Sports Medicine, 2*(3 suppl), 2325967114S00220. https://doi.org/10.1177/2325967114S00220

Feit, A., & Smith, B. (2016). *Complete jumps training: Coaches guide to jump training.* Reach Your Potential Training.

Fischetti, F., Cataldi, S., & Greco, G. (2019, June). Lower-limb plyometric training improves vertical jump and agility abilities in adult female soccer players. *Journal of Physical Education and Sport, 19*(2), 1254–1261. http://doi.org/10.7752/jpes.2019.02182

Fukunaga, T., Kawakami, Y., Kubo, K., & Kanehisa, H. (2002, July). Muscle and tendon interaction during human movements. *Exercise and Sport Sciences Reviews, 30*(3), 106–110. https://doi.org/10.1097/00003677 -200207000-00003

Gollhofer, A., Strojnik, V., Rapp, W., & Schweizer, L. (1992). Behaviour of triceps surae muscle–tendon complex in different jump conditions. *European Journal of Applied Physiology and Occupational Physiology, 64*(4), 283–291. https://doi.org/10.1007/BF00636213

Hall, E., Bishop, D. C., & Gee, T. I. (2016). Effect of plyometric training on handspring vault performance and functional power in youth female gymnasts. *PLoS One, 11*(2), 1–10. https://doi.org/10.1371/journal.pone.0148790

Healy, R., Kenny, I. C., & Harrison, A. J. (2018). Reactive strength index: A poor indicator of reactive strength? *International Journal of Sports Physiology and Performance, 13*(6), 802–809. https://doi.org/10.1123/ijspp.2017-0511

Iacono, A. D., Beato, M., & Halperin, I. (2019). The effects of cluster-set and traditional-set postactivation potentiation protocols on vertical jump performance. *International Journal of Sports Physiology and Performance, 15*(4), 464–469. https://doi.org/10.1123/ijspp.2019-0186

Issurin, V. B. (2013). Training transfer: Scientific background and insights for practical application. *Sports Medicine, 43*(8), 675–694. https://doi.org/10.1007/s40279-013-0049-6

Kubo, K., Kanehisa, H., Ito, M., & Fukunaga, T. (2001). Effects of isometric training on the elasticity of human tendon structures in vivo. *Journal of Applied Physiology, 91*(1), 26–32. https://doi.org/10.1152/jappl.2001.91.1.26

Laputin, P., & Oleshko, V. (1986). *Managing the training of weightlifters.* Sportivny Press.

Lievens, M., Bourgois, J. G., & Boone, J. (2021). Periodization of plyometrics: Is there an optimal overload principle? *Journal of Strength and Conditioning Research, 35*(10), 2669–2676. https://doi.org/10.1519/JSC.0000000000003231

Lockie, R. G., Murphy, A. J., Callaghan, S. J., & Jeffriess, M. D. (2014). Effects of sprint and plyometrics training on field sport acceleration technique. *Journal of Strength and Conditioning Research, 28*(7), 1790–1801. https://doi.org/10.1519/JSC.0000000000000297

Loturco, I., Pereira, L. A., Kobal, R., Zanetti, V., Kitamura, K., Abad, C. C. C., & Nakamura, F. Y. (2015). Transference effect of vertical and horizontal plyometrics on sprint performance of high-level U-20 soccer players. *Journal of Sports Sciences, 33*(20), 2182–2191. https://doi.org/10.1080/02640414.2015.1081394

Myer, G. D., Ford, K. R., McLean, S. G., & Hewett, T. E. (2006). The effects of plyometric versus dynamic stabilization and balance training on lower extremity biomechanics. *American Journal of Sports Medicine, 34*(3), 445–455. https://doi.org/10.1177/0363546505281241

Ploeg, A. H., Miller, M. G., Holcomb, W. R., O'Donoghue, J., Berry, D., & Dibbet, T. J. (2010). The effects of high volume aquatic plyometric training on vertical jump, muscle power, and torque. *International Journal of Aquatic Research and Education, 4*(1), 6. https://doi.org/10.25035/ijare.04.01.06

Radcliffe, J., & Farentinos, R. (2015). *High-powered plyometrics* (2nd ed). Human Kinetics.

Ramachandran, S., & Pradhan, B. (2014). Effects of short-term two weeks low intensity plyometrics combined with dynamic stretching training in improving vertical jump height and agility on trained basketball players. *Indian Journal of Physiology and Pharmacology, 58*(2), 133–136.

Ramirez-Campillo, R., Garcia-Hermoso, A., Moran, J., Chaabene, H., Negra, Y., & Scanlan, A. T. (2020). The effects of plyometric jump training on physical fitness attributes in basketball players: A meta-analysis. *Journal of Sport and Health Science,* S2095-2546(20)30169-1. https://doi.org/10.1016/j.jshs.2020.12.005

Rassier, D. E., Lee, E.-J., & Herzog, W. (2005). Modulation of passive force in single skeletal muscle fibres. *Biology Letters, 1*(3), 342–345. https://doi.org/10.1098/rsbl.2005.0337

Rejman, M., Bilewski, M., Szczepan, S., Klarowicz, A., Rudnik, D., & Maćkała, K. (2017). Assessing the impact of a targeted plyometric training on changes in selected kinematic parameters of the swimming start. *Acta of Bioengineering and Biomechanics, 19*(2), 149–160. https://doi.org/10.5277/ABB-00627-2016-03

Sáez de Villarreal, E., Requena, B., & Cronin, J. B. (2012). The effects of plyometric training on sprint performance: A meta-analysis. *Journal of Strength and Conditioning Research, 26*(2), 575–584. https://doi.org/10.1519/JSC.0b013e318220fd03

Sáez de Villarreal, E., Requena, B., & Newton, R. U. (2010). Does plyometric training improve strength performance? A meta-analysis. *Journal of Science and Medicine in Sport, 13*(5), 513–522. https://doi.org/10.1016/j.jsams.2009.08.005

Singh, J., Appleby, B. B., & Lavender, A. P. (2018). Effect of plyometric training on speed and change of direction ability in elite field hockey players. *Sports, 6*(4), 144. https://doi.org/10.3390/sports6040144

Singla, D., Hussain, M. E., & Moiz, J. A. (2018). Effect of upper body plyometric training on physical performance in healthy individuals: A systematic review. *Physical Therapy in Sport, 29,* 51–60. https://doi.org/10.1016/j.ptsp.2017.11.005

Stojanović, N. M., Coh, M., & Bratić, M. (2016). The role of countermovement in the manifestation of explosive leg strength in vertical jumps. *Facta Universitatis: Series Physical Education and Sport,* 13–22.

Sukumar, B. (2017). Effect of plyometric exercises on agility among the netball players. *International Journal of Physical Education, Sports and Health, 4,* 277–279.

Toumi, H., Best, T. M., Martin, A., F'Guyer, S., & Poumarat, G. (2004). Effects of eccentric phase velocity of plyometric training on the vertical jump. *International Journal of Sports Medicine, 25*(5), 391–398. https://doi.org/10.1055/s-2004-815843

Turner, A. N., & Jeffreys, I. (2010). The stretch-shortening cycle: Proposed mechanisms and methods for enhancement. *Strength and Conditioning Journal, 32*(4), 87–99. https://doi.org/10.1519/SSC.0b013e3181e928f9

Valadés Cerrato, D., Palao, J. M., Femia, P., & Ureña, A. (2018, Oct.). Effect of eight weeks of upper-body plyometric training during the competitive season on professional female volleyball players. *The Journal of Sports Medicine and Physical Fitness, 58*(10), 1423–1431. https://doi.org/10.23736/S0022-4707.17.07527-2

Wathen, D. (1993). Literature review: Explosive/plyometric exercises. *National Strength and Conditioning Journal, 15*(3), 17–19.

Watkins, C. M., Gill, N. D., Maunder, E., Downes, P., Young, J. D., McGuigan, M. R., & Storey, A. G. (2021). The effect of low-volume preseason plyometric training on force-velocity profiles in semiprofessional rugby union players. *Journal of Strength and Conditioning Research, 35*(3), 604–615. https://doi.org/10.1519/JSC.0000000000003917

Watkins, C. M., Storey, A. G., McGuigan, M. R., & Gill, N. D. (2021). Implementation and efficacy of plyometric training: Bridging the gap between practice and research. *Journal of Strength and Conditioning Research, 35*(5), 1244–1255. https://doi.org/10.1519/JSC.0000000000003985

Weldon, A., Duncan, M. J., Turner, A., LaPlaca, D., Sampaio, J., & Christie, C. J. (2022). Practices of strength and conditioning coaches: A snapshot from different sports, countries, and expertise levels. *Journal of Strength and Conditioning Research, 36*(5), 1335–1344. https://doi.org/10.1519/jsc.0000000000003773

Wilk, K. E., Voight, M. L., Keirns, M. A., Gambetta, V., Andrews, J. R., & Dillman, C. J. (1993). Stretch-shortening drills for the upper extremities: Theory and clinical application. *Journal of Orthopaedic & Sports Physical Therapy, 17*(5), 225–239. https://doi.org/10.2519/jospt.1993.17.5.225

Wilson, G. J., Newton, R. U., Murphy, A. J., & Humphries, B. J. (1993). The optimal training load for the development of dynamic athletic performance. *Medicine & Science in Sports & Exercise, 25*(11), 1279–1286.

Yáñez-García, J. M., Rodríguez-Rosell, D., Mora-Custodio, R., & González-Badillo, J. J. (2022). Changes in muscle strength, jump, and sprint performance in young elite basketball players: The impact of combined high-speed resistance training and plyometrics. *Journal of Strength and Conditioning Research, 36*(2), 478-485. https://doi.org/10.1519/jsc.0000000000003472

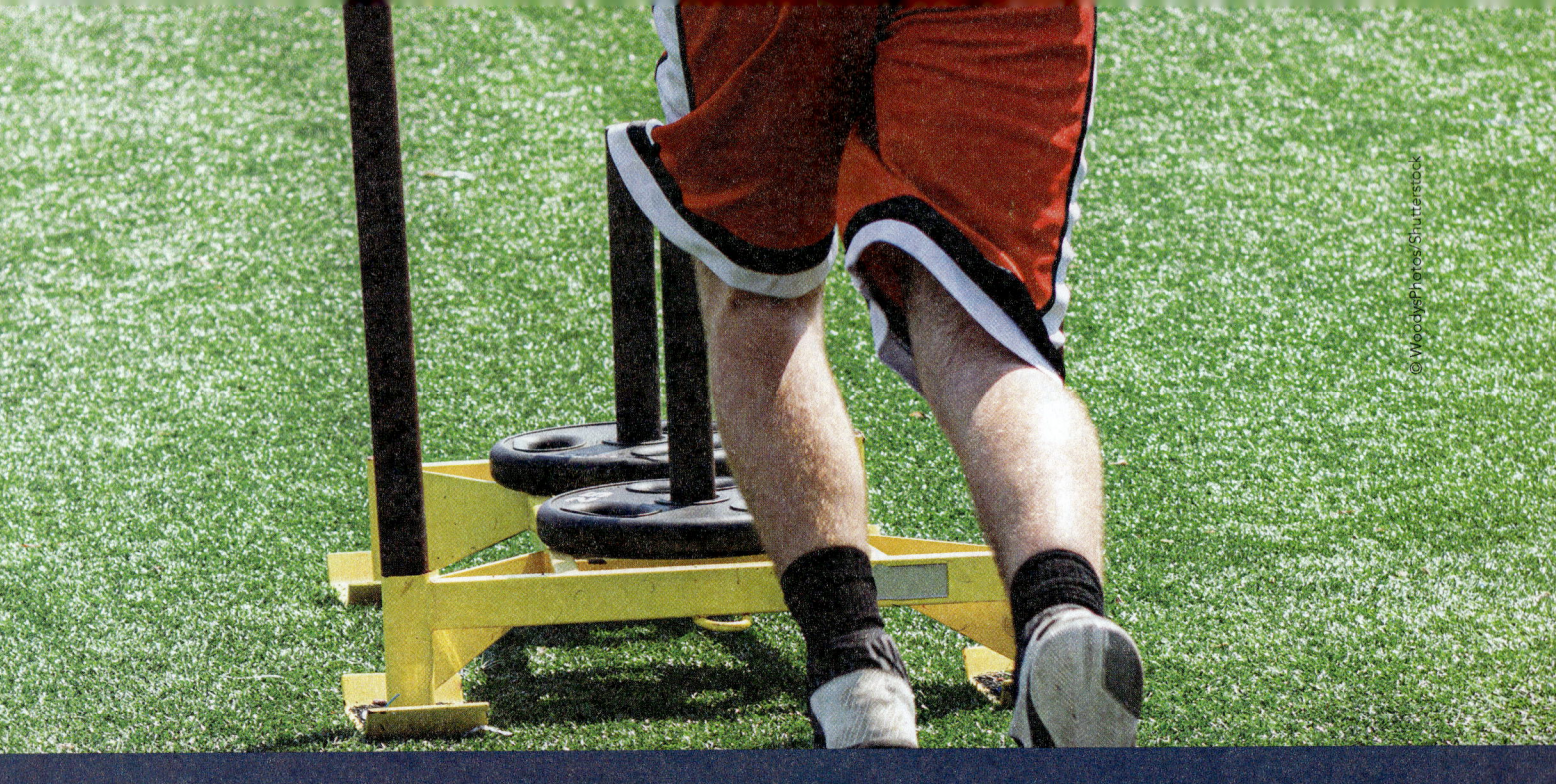

SPEED, AGILITY, AND QUICKNESS TRAINING FOR SPORTS PERFORMANCE

CHAPTER THIRTEEN

LEARNING OBJECTIVES

Upon completion of this chapter, the Sports Performance Coach will be able to:

- **Summarize** the importance of speed, agility, and quickness (SAQ) training for athletes with differing performance-related goals.

- **Explain** the scientific rationale for SAQ training.

- **Describe** different SAQ training techniques used within performance training.

- **Identify** appropriate acute training variables for SAQ training.

- **Select** SAQ programs or techniques based on the athlete's needs.

LESSON 1: INTRODUCTION TO SPEED, AGILITY, AND QUICKNESS TRAINING

INTRODUCTION

In sports performance training, proper development of certain biomotor abilities such as speed, agility, and quickness (SAQ) is necessary for athletic performance and longevity in team sports and, subsequently, athletic success (Bompa et al., 2019). **Biomotor abilities**, also referred to as motor abilities, are athletic capacities underpinning physical performance proficiency that can be developed and enhanced through various training methods (Bompa & Buzzichelli, 2018; Schmidt et al., 2019). Each sport and often different playing positions within a sport have a dominant biomotor ability of strength, speed, or endurance that must be enhanced for athletic success, especially in sports requiring fast linear speed and multidirectional movements.

A primary goal of any sports training program should be to improve the athlete's ability to anticipate an opponent's actions, react quickly, and apply substantial **ground reaction force (GRF)** in the appropriate direction and with the optimal force. This is the explicit purpose of SAQ training. Paszkewicz et al. (2012) demonstrated the feasibility and importance of addressing these factors of athleticism in methodologically sound SAQ training programs designed with careful attention to develop the primary biomotor ability of speed and the secondary skills of agility and quickness, reduce the risk of injuries, and improve overall athletic performance.

> 👍 **HELPFUL HINT**
>
> Examples of fundamental multidirectional movements include starting, stopping, cutting, feinting, and faking in a forward, backward, lateral, or diagonal direction.

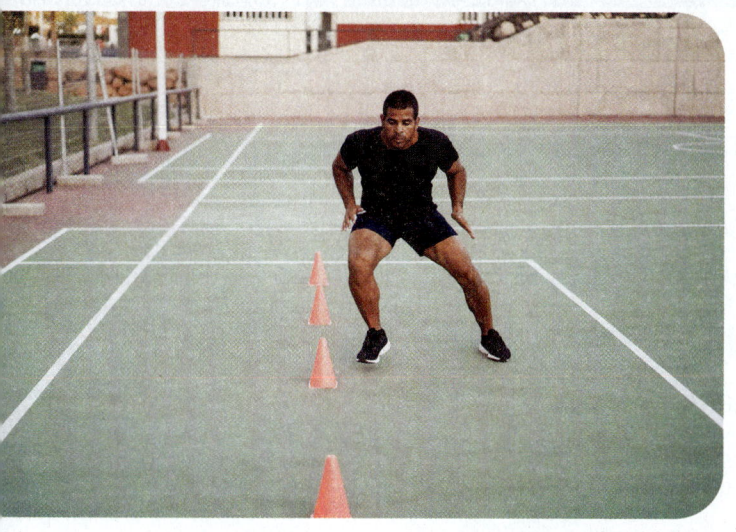

© Tint Media/Shutterstock

SAQ involves biomotor ability development, rapid force generation, and application of GRF quickly by the feet (Dintiman, 2020). Development of relative strength and power underlies SAQ improvements by increasing the athlete's capacity to exert greater force in less time during sports actions, which often require multidirectional speed and repetitive changes of direction (Bolger et al., 2015; Healy et al., 2021; Keiner et al., 2020; Keller et al., 2020; Komi, 2005, 2011; Styles et al., 2016). Although each athlete will vary in the magnitude and proficiency of their motor abilities and learning capacity, executing efficient functional movements initially in the motor learning process can improve overall athletic ability and enhance sports performance.

For multiple reasons, acquiring a comprehensive understanding of SAQ training methods is crucial for the

Sports Performance Coach. A key reason is to prevent injuries in athletes by mastering and applying the correct techniques in both non-fatigued and fatigued states where a certain amount of exhaustion is necessary for full development.

Another reason for gaining an in-depth understanding of SAQ training relates to the diverse clientele whom each Sports Performance Coach will encounter in practice. Regardless of the athlete, SAQ training concepts can enhance their performance in many different and often atypical sports and competitive events, depending on how the training program is designed. Without understanding of the concepts, methods, and techniques of SAQ training, however, injuries may occur, progress could wane or even regress, and athletes may be inadvertently set up for failure instead of success. To help avoid these negative outcomes, this chapter aims to introduce and define the most significant components of SAQ that can aid Sports Performance Coaches in creating effective real-world programs for various athletes.

DETERMINANTS OF SAQ

Before moving into the more detailed aspects of SAQ training, it is helpful to consider the conceptual basis of SAQ methods. SAQ training is a paradigm of sports science and sports performance training that utilizes specialized physical training with the following aims: (1) to facilitate motor learning, (2) to enhance motor neuron drive (Del Vecchio et al., 2019), (3) to capitalize on muscle reflex properties (Komi, 2011), and (4) to elicit necessary and sufficient stimuli for the adaption, development, and enhancement of sport-specific abilities. Each exercise, drill, or method should align with one or more of these aims. In this paradigm of sports performance training, speed, strength, and endurance are the dominant biomotor abilities that interact to form other sport-specific biomotor abilities, such as agility.

Agility, in turn, is a multifaceted combination of mutually dependent motor skills (i.e., speed, strength, and endurance) that enable an athlete to respond to a stimulus through fast acceleration, deceleration, and change of direction. Meanwhile, quickness represents an athlete's awareness, anticipation of opponents, cognitive recognition of patterns, and tactical knowledge of the sport (Bompa & Haff, 2009). With these definitions in mind, the following sections examine aspects of SAQ and detail the scientific rationale for SAQ training.

Although SAQ can seem complex, understanding how each component corresponds to training paints a more comprehensive picture of the processes required for practical and functional sports movements. The general determinants of SAQ include muscle strength, power, endurance, myofiber composition and contractility, neural motor unit recruitment ability, motor neuron drive, muscle stretch–shortening cycle (SSC) activities, visual processing speed, **reaction time**, and the integration of these components (Del Vecchio et al., 2019; Komi, 2011). In addition, movement speed is a function of strength, application of force, reactive capacity, quickness, and the ability to respond to environmental changes.

For these reasons, much of the research surrounding SAQ tends to focus on linear speed development. However, the Sports Performance Coach must recognize how SAQ abilities are separate but interrelated concepts.

FOUNDATION TRAINING

Developing a solid foundation for SAQ training requires optimal joint mobility, stability, and flexibility. During sprinting, the **stride rate** is affected by how easily the lower limbs travel through the full range of motion (ROM). Soft tissue will achieve efficient

REACTION TIME →

The interval of time between stimulus detection, pattern recognition, response selection, and initiation of an action.

STRIDE RATE →

The number of strides accomplished per second, ascertained by ground contact time and flight time.

extensibility only if optimal bodily control is maintained throughout the entire joint ROM. In addition, the integrity of the muscle tissue and its ability to relax and contract appropriately during movement can be a limiting factor in adequate joint mobility. For example, a sprinter needs proper ROM during hip extension, which in turn requires sufficient strength of the hip extensors and length of the hip flexors (**Figure 13.1**). When there is an imbalance of strength or flexibility around the hip, the ROM will be compromised, affecting force output and movement speed.

**Appropriate Flexibility
and Range of Motion**

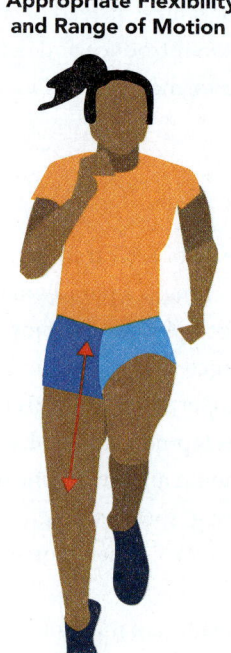

FIGURE 13.1 Appropriate Flexibility and Range of Motion

In addition, performance will be diminished if fatigue, injury, stiffness, adhesions, or other hindering factors are present. Based on the assessment and athlete data results, proper flexibility training should be designed to improve joint mobility and flexibility.

Stability training is a crucial aspect of enhancing SAQ. Such training develops the appropriate dynamic balance needed for effective strength and power training that will enhance the athlete's ability to create and reduce the time required to generate force. Without dynamic balance, the capacity to generate force diminishes quickly. For this reason, exercises for more unstable areas—for example, the foot and ankle, knee, and lumbo-pelvic-hip complex (LPHC)—should be prioritized when performing stability drills specific to speed development. Along with stability training, core training is one of the most vital program components for developing efficient sports movements, especially speed improvement.

Training of the core is intended to integrate the flexibility, stability, strength, and power of the torso and hips, representing the center of body mass and juncture of overall stability for sports performance. Well-functioning muscles of the LPHC (**Figure 13.2**) enhance sprinting mechanics and form the foundation for force production by transferring energy to ensure an athlete's center of mass remains stable under conditions of a dynamic support base (i.e., achieving dynamic balance) (Sado et al., 2020).

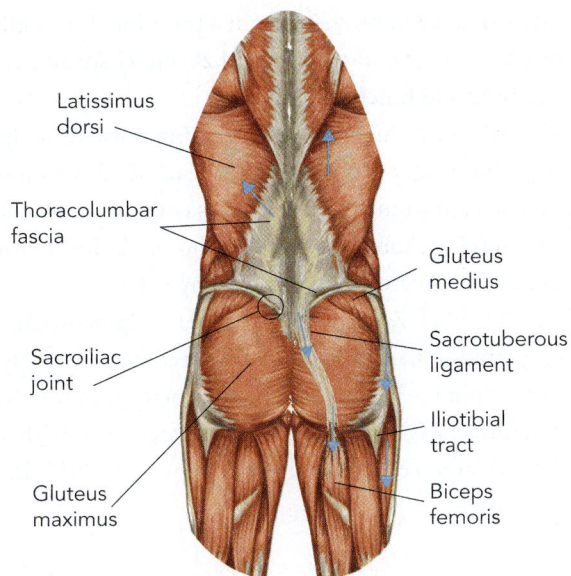

FIGURE 13.2 The Lumbo-Pelvic-Hip Complex

Dynamic balance occurs when an athlete can maintain optimal posture and high levels of force production under conditions of a moving or dynamic base of support. When dynamic balance is achieved along with stability and mobility, greater and faster application of force can be developed, which is an essential prerequisite for linear speed. Sports Performance Coaches should view stability, flexibility, mobility, dynamic balance, and the resulting force application as the foundation for the development of linear speed performance. Facilitating this development also requires ingraining effective sprinting form, movement technique, and posture in clients and athletes through proper motor learning.

STRENGTH AND POWER TRAINING

Strength and power training increases an athlete's ability to produce high levels of force at high rates of speed while maintaining stability (Komi, 2005, 2011). Although stability and core training develop the appropriate foundation to achieve dynamic balance, strength training improves the body's ability to generate force.

Further, power training decreases the time needed to generate that force, which improves linear speed. As part of strength and power training to develop speed, exercises emphasizing powerful plantar flexion and dorsiflexion of the ankles and extension and flexion of the knees, hips, and core are essential components. Resistance training for strength has been shown in several studies to improve speed—primarily through exercises such as the squat and variations of the deadlift—because they target the prime movers of a sprint (i.e., quadriceps, gluteals, and hamstrings).

For example, Styles et al. (2016) demonstrated that a 6-week strength training intervention for professional soccer players implemented in the competitive season twice per week significantly increased absolute strength, relative strength, and sprint execution spanning 5, 10, and 20 meters. In addition, in a study of elite youth soccer athletes, Keiner et al. (2020)

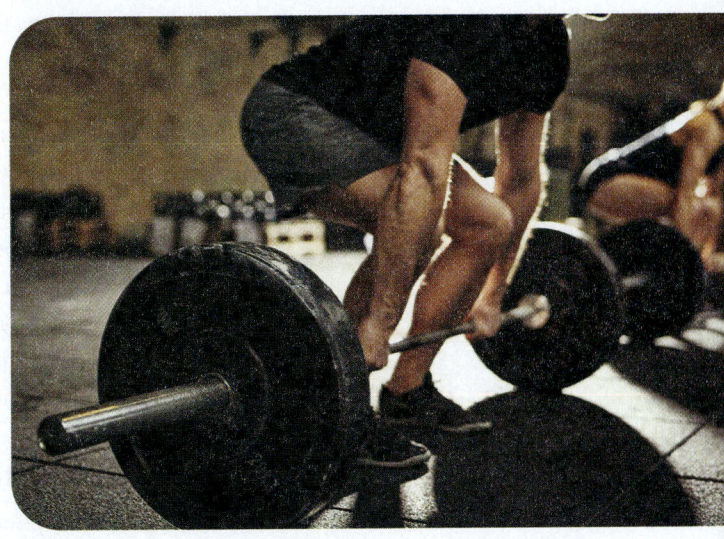

© Ground Picture/Shutterstock

UNI-
DIRECTIONAL
TRAINING →

Use of a single mode
of training (i.e.,
traditional strength
training) to improve
one biomotor ability
during a training
session or at the
micro-cycle level
to enhance sport
performance.

observed significant performance improvements in a traditional strength training group in terms of maximal strength, change of direction, and 20-meter sprint execution, compared to plyometric-sprint training and functional training.

In **unidirectional training**, a single mode of training is used to improve one biomotor ability during a training session (Bompa & Haff, 2009; Verkhoshansky & Siff, 2009). In contrast, in complex training (also known as concurrent training), two or more training modalities for improving more than one biomotor ability are used simultaneously in the training session or at the micro-cycle level (Bompa et al., 2019; Bompa & Haff, 2009; Verkhoshansky & Siff, 2009; Zatsiorsky et al., 2021) (**Figure 13.3**). The combination of complex training (e.g., traditional resistance training coupled with plyometrics) and several modes of power training (e.g., contrast, high velocity, or moderate velocity) with traditional resistance training has also been shown to increase strength and power, as well as to improve linear SAQ (Cavaco et al., 2014; Hammami et al., 2017; Rhea et al., 2016; Rodríguez-Rosell et al., 2017).

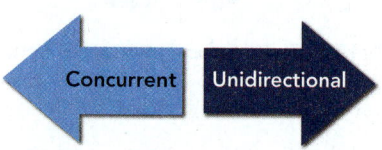

FIGURE 13.3 Unidirectional Versus Concurrent Training

When a resistance training program is well planned, the resulting improvements in strength increase force production and rate of force development during linear sprinting, jumping, cutting, acceleration, and deceleration, thereby enhancing SAQ performance. However, force production is often a limiting factor of SAQ for younger and older athletes lacking overall strength; hence, strength development should be a primary focus of their training. As strength levels increase, the rate of force development must also increase for the athlete to show improvement in SAQ. Plyometric training can be integrated to improve the rate of force production. SAQ drills do not specifically address underlying strength or power deficits. Nevertheless, when used along with strength and power training, SAQ training refines motor coordination and improves the way strength and power are applied by the athlete throughout sporting activities.

Increasing SAQ requires laying a solid foundation of the optimal technique alongside adequate joint mobility, flexibility, and stability to maintain dynamic balance. Once this solid foundation is in place, strength and power training can help the athlete quickly generate greater levels of force. The effectiveness of various strength and power training modalities in increasing force production and rate of force production and improving linear speed is well documented. Even so, Sports Performance Coaches should understand that strength and power training must be planned and used judiciously, given the athlete's background. For instance, a novice athlete who has just initiated speed training would benefit more from unidirectional strength training than from concurrent resistance and power training. The novice athlete should also focus on core strength, stability, and sprinting technique and increase overall strength before moving on to the more advanced speed development methods outlined in the next section.

ADVANCED NEUROMUSCULAR TRAINING METHODS

The neuromuscular system of an athlete is expected to respond rapidly and efficiently, with succeeding eccentric muscle actions used to generate concentric contractions with the required force in the appropriate direction (Oden et al., 2014). Preparing for sport-specific demands requires well-designed exercises, emphasizing unidirectional or complex training to exploit muscle reflexes and other neuromuscular properties. Training the neuromuscular system improves performance by enhancing maximal force production and the rate of force development to improve linear speed, maintain movement velocity during rapid direction changes, and improve coordination and balance. Training to improve linear speed primarily involves resistance, power, and plyometric exercises to enhance sport-specific performance (Zemková & Hamar, 2018).

Ballistic movement is created by a rapid stretching (e.g., eccentric phase) of a preactivated muscle (e.g., isometric phase) when the ground is encountered, followed immediately by a shortening of the muscle (e.g., concentric phase), creating an elastic energy recoil effect, above and beyond the organically produced force of the muscle (Komi, 2011). Muscle and joint elasticity is the most critical aspect of ballistic training and enhances the SSC (Komi, 2011; Seiberl et al., 2021). The SSC is mediated by the nervous system through neurological control, intrinsic qualities of the muscle, and musculotendinous junctions involved with a specific sporting movement (Komi, 2011).

The action of the SSC is reflexive. Training it enhances the ability of the muscle and tendon to load eccentrically and rapidly release elastic energy concentrically, improving the magnitude and effectiveness of the SSC (Komi, 2011). Plyometric training capitalizes on the SSC to improve explosive force during sports actions such as sprinting, jumping, hitting, and throwing (Chaabene et al., 2021; King & Cipriani, 2010; Nicol, 2009; Ramirez-Campillo et al., 2020; Salonikidis & Zafeiridis, 2008).

> **BALLISTIC MOVEMENT** →
>
> A movement that includes a rapid stretching of a muscle, followed immediately by a shortening of the muscle, creating an elastic energy recoil effect, above and beyond the organically produced force of the muscle.

> 👍 **HELPFUL HINT**
>
> A simple way to consider the SSC while sprinting is to imagine the muscle as a spring that compresses and releases. In this case, the muscles are stretched when the foot contacts the ground, which immediately stores elastic energy and creates greater muscular efficiency to propel the body forward.

Another concept is post-activation potentiation (PAP), which refers to the increased muscle twitch torque that occurs after a conditioning muscle contraction (Bergmann et al., 2013). PAP represents increased muscle force and rate of force development from prior muscle activation. Complex training that alternates high-load resistance training and plyometric exercises with similar biomechanical profiles for each set of a single training session can exploit the PAP phenomenon to increase power and rate of force production.

In a more general sense, complex training refers to coupling a high-power exercise with a high-force movement to take advantage of the enhanced force production produced by PAP. Training methods that capitalize on PAP or SSC are considered more advanced speed training programs, which put considerable stress on the neuromuscular system. Therefore, the Sports Performance Coach must take a cautious approach toward including these methods in the program, and ensure that athletes have first developed a sufficient foundation of core strength and dynamic balance and learned proper sprinting form and technique. Once athletes have established a solid foundation, other methods can be used to improve SAQ, such as specialized drills, which are detailed in a later section of this chapter.

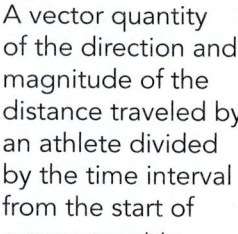

📋 COACH'S CORNER

Combining a set of high-load resistance exercises with a set of plyometrics (and vice versa) increases the rate of force development and power-generating capacity. Common examples of such combinations include the following supersets:

- Heavy barbell squat → Explosive squat jump
- Heavy barbell deadlift → Explosive tuck jump
- Heavy barbell bench press → Explosive medicine ball chest pass
- Heavy bent-over barbell row → Speed tubing row

LESSON 2: PRINCIPLES OF SAQ TRAINING
PRINCIPLES OF SPEED, AGILITY, AND QUICKNESS

SAQ training is a cornerstone of many sports performance programs due to its importance in a wide range of athletic activities. The multidirectional nature of many sports requires the development of speed, a key component, but also includes the concept of velocity, which combines the direction of movement with the rate of motion. Agility extends the concept of speed by adding the ability to change direction quickly and effectively, often in response to a stimulus. Quickness, or reaction time, reflects an athlete's ability to respond to that stimulus and initiate movement. Underpinning all these abilities is the importance of correct form and technique. Proper form not only optimizes performance, but also reduces the risk of injury. It ensures efficient movement patterns, allowing athletes to fully harness their power and speed while maintaining control and balance during rapid, complex movements.

SPEED AND VELOCITY

Training athletes for success in most sports requires the Sports Performance Coach to comprehend and understand linear speed and velocity. **Linear speed** is best defined as a scalar quantity (rate)—that is, the distance traveled by the athlete divided by the time taken to travel the distance, measured only in magnitude (Hamill et al., 2015). A more straightforward way to think of speed is the "rate of performance" of a sporting activity or movement. A somewhat different measurement is **movement velocity**, a vector quantity of the direction and magnitude of the distance traveled by an athlete divided by the time interval from the start of a movement to completion. Sport movement **velocity** is defined as the change in displacement from one position to another divided by the change in time elapsing to move among the positions (Hamill et al., 2015).

LINEAR SPEED →

A scalar quantity (rate) of the distance traveled by the athlete divided by time taken to travel the distance, measured only in magnitude.

MOVEMENT VELOCITY →

A vector quantity of the direction and magnitude of the distance traveled by an athlete divided by the time interval from the start of a movement to completion.

VELOCITY →

A vector quantity of the direction and magnitude of the distance traveled by an object or athlete divided by the time interval from the start of a movement to completion; the speed at which an object is traveling.

This distinction is important because the velocity at which an athlete executes a movement can mean the difference between success and failure and between elite and sub-elite performance. The movement velocity differences between elite and sub-elite performances have been documented for soccer (Trecroci et al., 2018), sprinting (Bayne, 2018), and swimming (Gonjo & Olstad, 2021), among other sports. Notably, less than 1 second often separates an elite and sub-elite classification in sprinting (Bayne, 2018). With this distinction in mind, the terms *speed* and *velocity* are often used interchangeably to simplify the understanding of SAQ (**Figure 13.4**).

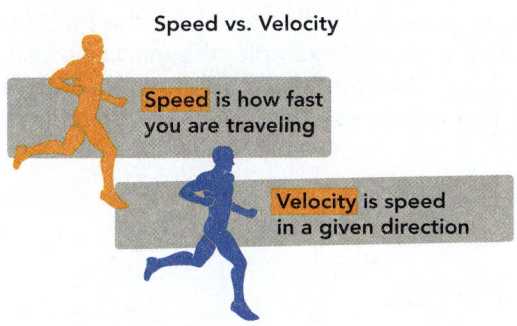

FIGURE 13.4 Speed Versus Velocity

Linear speed culminates in reactive ability, rapid force development, quick force application, and effective movement technique. According to the force–velocity curve (**Figure 13.5**), the movement's velocity output decreases when an activity's force demands increase (Komi, 2005, 2011). Because the velocity of movement is inversely proportional to the external resistance (force or load), the highest velocities occur under circumstances of low external resistance. The lowest velocities are achieved in conditions of high external resistance, whereas medium velocities occur with intermediate external resistance (Hamill et al., 2015; Komi, 2011; Özkaya et al., 2017; Verkhoshansky & Siff, 2009).

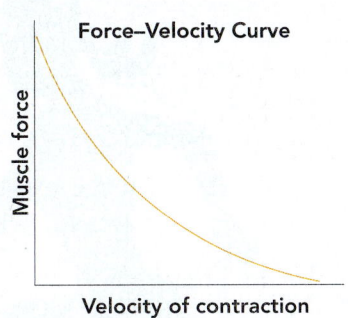

FIGURE 13.5 Force–Velocity Curve

Sports movements occur under various velocities and loads; hence, a fundamental goal of speed training is to shift the force–velocity curve up and to the right, meaning that the athlete develops the ability to generate greater force at higher movement velocities. An athlete's capacity to increase the rate of sport-specific movements results from shifting the curve up and to the right and learning to maintain proper posture and optimal body and limb positioning.

An athlete lifting a heavy object, such as a loaded barbell, requires massive force. However, the velocity at which the barbell travels is relatively slow. Conversely, throwing a light medicine ball requires less force, but the rate at which the medicine ball travels is much faster than the barbell. This analogy is the essence of the force–velocity curve.

Power is defined as force × velocity. Both of the preceding examples provide an expression of power. However, the total power output may not be much different because, in the first example, the barbell moves at a slow velocity, whereas, in the second example, the medicine ball throw requires less force. The goal is to train athletes to improve their ability to apply greater force at higher velocities, which shifts the force–velocity curve up and to the right.

DETERMINANTS OF SPEED

The three main determinants of speed are force generation capacity, stride rate, and stride length, with the ability to generate force serving as the basis for attaining the ideal stride rate, stride length, and top speed (Jeffreys, 2013). Linear speed is a function of both stride rate (stride cadence) and stride length; specifically, it is the product of these two factors (Dintiman, 2020; Young, 2021). Stride rate is the number of strides accomplished per second, which is ascertained by **ground contact time (GCT)** and flight time. In contrast, **stride length** (**Figure 13.6**) comprises the interval of distance completed with each stride, which is determined by flight time and speed (Brown & Ferrigno, 2015; Dintiman, 2020; Jeffreys, 2013).

**GROUND →
CONTACT TIME
(GCT)**

The time interval during which the foot is in contact with the ground throughout each force application of a stride.

**STRIDE →
LENGTH**

The interval of distance completed with each stride, determined by flight time and flight speed.

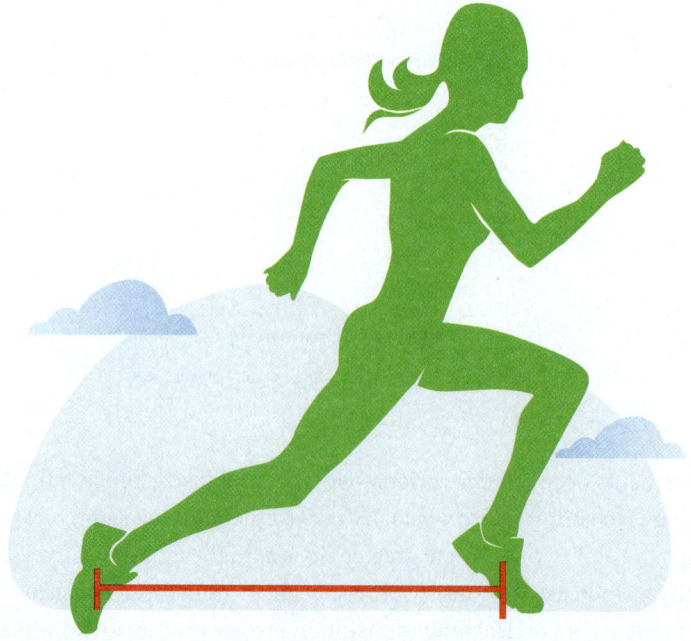

Stride Length

FIGURE 13.6 Stride Length

To develop linear speed in athletes, Dintiman (2020) and Gambetta (2007) recommend placing the primary emphasis on sprinting form and technique. This involves using motor learning principles to teach correct sprinting mechanics, which will enable the athlete to have an efficient start, rapidly generate the maximum force during acceleration, and maintain the optimal stride rate and length to reach maximum speed while eliminating unwanted movements.

> **⚠ CRITICAL**
>
> Attempting to force faster foot contact to increase stride frequency results in a significantly shorter stride length, which subsequently creates an inefficient running motion. It is also sometimes a factor contributing to hamstring strains.

IMPROVING STRIDE RATE

Improving stride rate and frequency by enhancing mechanics and force production can increase overall speed because linear speed is a function of stride rate and length (Young, 2021). Enhancing the force applied with each stride increases stride length, whereas improving the movement efficiency and rate of force development increases stride frequency. Both factors should occur in a coordinated manner to foster optimal performance. Simply attempting to improve stride rate at the expense of stride length, or vice versa, is counterproductive and may lead to motor learning of improper sprint mechanics. For instance, attempting to increase stride length by reaching for greater distance with each stride often results in over striding, as the foot contacts the ground well in front of the athlete's **center of mass (CoM)**, which creates a braking force. In contrast, achieving the maximal linear speed results from an optimal relationship between stride length and stride rate.

Considering all of these aspects, speed training aims to develop proper form, technique, and sprinting mechanics through various training methods to achieve the following goals:

- Improve the first two steps of a sprint (e.g., the start).
- Develop the ability to apply maximum GRF.
- Reduce GCT in the briefest time achievable.
- Increase propulsive force vertically.
- Remove noncontributing forward momentum movements during acceleration.
- Develop **repeated-sprint ability (RSA)**. RSA training can also counter the effects of fatigue, which often result in premature deceleration and reduced GRF.

Programs designed to enhance linear speed typically include five components (**Figure 13.7**). Building a solid foundation to maintain joint mobility through a full ROM with flexibility training is essential for fast sports movements. Stability training is needed to develop balance. In contrast, core training focuses on integrating flexibility, strength, power, and coordination to express the use of dynamic balance in sport. Other components that help build the foundation for speed training programs and other movement skills include sprinting technique and form, and arm and leg movement posture.

CENTER OF MASS (CoM) →

The point at which the mass or weight (the product of mass and acceleration due to gravity) of the body is evenly distributed.

REPEATED-SPRINT ABILITY (RSA) →

The ability to execute optimal sprint mechanics in sequential sprints lasting less than or equal to 10 seconds, intermingled with short and infrequent recovery periods.

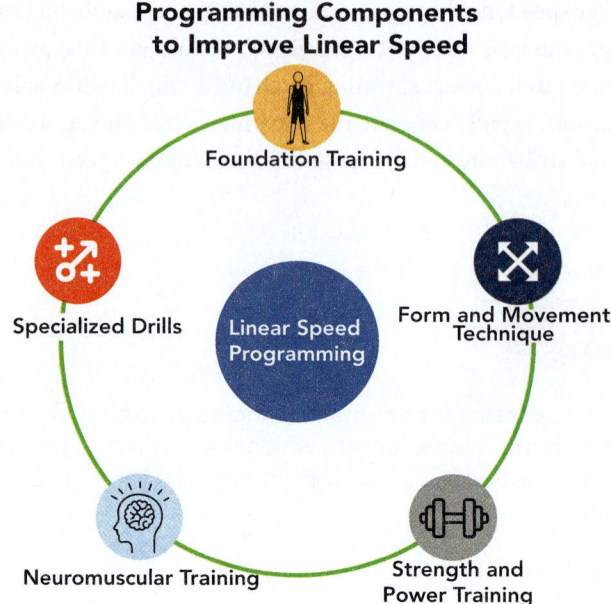

FIGURE 13.7 Components to Improve Speed

In addition, strength and power training is used to improve the ability to generate force rapidly, which contributes significantly to enhancing linear speed. Neuromuscular training is another component of linear speed programs that capitalizes on muscle reflexes and properties known to improve force production and speed. The final pieces of linear speed programs include specialized drills, consisting of over-speed and assisted drills to add heightened demands to the neuromuscular system and develop dominant biomotor abilities.

FORM AND MOVEMENT TECHNIQUES

Proper form and technique must be learned in key areas to develop optimal speed (**Figure 13.8**). Improving speed depends on correct motor learning and mastery of sprinting techniques. The optimal sprinting technique includes applying proper biomechanics, ensuring correct posture, and enabling the athlete to execute movements as fast and efficiently as possible. Proper movement technique allows the body and limbs to achieve biomechanically advantageous positions for optimal force production, increasing movement speed. Movement efficiency then becomes an essential differentiator between levels of sports performance, with high levels characterized by little wasted movement and optimal movement coordination.

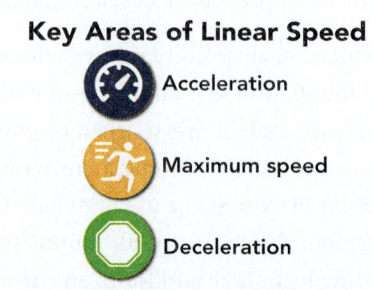

FIGURE 13.8 Key Areas of Linear Speed

According to Dintiman (2020), the ideal sprinting technique reduces energetic constraints, delays peripheral fatigue, and enhances sports performance. In addition, when the ideal position for ground contact is maintained, the vertical propulsive force increases, **negative foot speed** reduces, and leg stiffness improves to apply greater GRF.

Learning the correct technique is vital to achieving optimal front-side mechanics (dorsiflexion, knee flexion, and hip flexion) and back-side mechanics (plantar flexion, knee extension, and hip extension) while maintaining a neutral pelvis (**Figure 13.9**) (Dintiman, 2020; Gambetta, 2007). Many of these concepts also apply to multidirectional speed training.

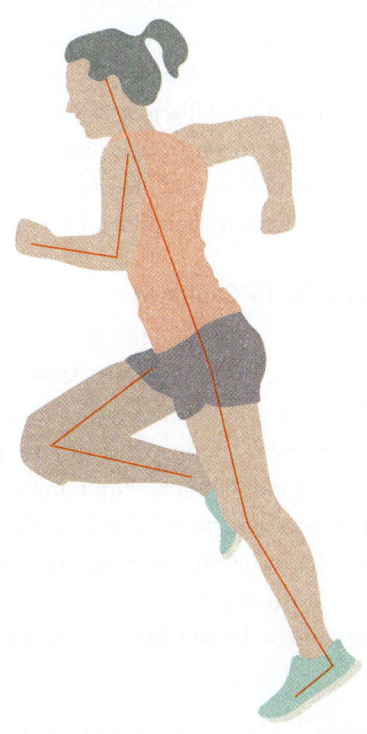

FIGURE 13.9 Front-Side and Back-Side Mechanics

Dintiman (2020) noted that the sprint stride cycle includes three distinct phases:

1. **Drive phase**: The foot is in contact with the ground.
2. **Recovery phase**: The leg swings from the hip while the foot clears the ground.
3. **Support phase**: The mass of the sprinter is loaded onto or carried by the entire foot.

📋 COACH'S CORNER

The sprint stride cycle phases are fundamental to identify when teaching sprinting mechanics so athletes can receive feedback when problems are evident.

NEGATIVE FOOT SPEED

The rate at which the foot moves backward as it strikes the ground.

DRIVE PHASE →

Sprint phase that includes the start (first two steps) and acceleration in the first 10 yards; the sprint stride cycle phase in which the foot is in contact with the ground.

RECOVERY PHASE

Sprint stride cycle phase in which the leg swings from the hip while the foot clears the ground.

SUPPORT PHASE

Sprint stride cycle phase in which the mass of the sprinter is loaded onto or carried by the entire foot.

Linear Speed Mechanics

Proper linear sprint mechanics cover many body parts and movements, and problems can occur in many areas of the stride cycle. However, identifying the problem and understanding the cause can enable the Sports Performance Coach to determine the correct drills or methods to rectify the issue. Proper Linear Sprint Mechanics (**Appendix E**) details proper linear sprint mechanics focusing on essential body parts, a summary of the movement, problems, causes, and corrective drills.

The ideal technique for effective and efficient linear speed depends on the dominant biomotor ability aligning with the specific needs of the desired task in the sport. For most sports, improving acceleration and maximal sprinting speed is a necessity. Furthermore, athletic proficiency in sports demands effective mechanical execution of acceleration and linear speed, although top speed is rarely achieved in a competition. The Sports Performance Coach should understand that the proper execution of the sprinting technique (i.e., skilled movement mechanics) is essential for improving linear speed. Further, this forms the foundation for other movement skills, just as joint mobility, flexibility, stability, and core training provide the essentials to perform accurate sprint mechanics. Thus, training programs should aim to establish sound linear speed mechanics before progressing to more advanced skills developed through strength and power training methods.

FUNDAMENTALS OF A SPEED PROGRAM

The Sports Performance Coach must understand the fundamental components of a linear speed development program for several reasons (**Table 13.1**). The first component is a foundational requirement—that the athlete establish the core strength and stability needed for dynamic balance while maintaining sufficient joint mobility and flexibility to help prevent injuries. The second foundational requirement for linear speed is proper motor learning of sprinting form, movement technique, and maintenance of posture. This ensures that the athlete can establish accurate sprinting mechanics, apply force efficiently, and eliminate faulty movements impeding forward momentum. The third component of strength and power training can also be considered a foundational aspect of speed; it

TABLE 13.1 Components of Linear Speed Development

Component	Importance
Joint mobility, flexibility, stability, and core training	A foundational requirement for linear speed; establish the core strength and stability needed for dynamic balance while maintaining sufficient joint mobility and flexibility to help prevent injuries.
Motor learning of sprinting form, movement technique, and maintenance of posture	Establish accurate sprinting mechanics to apply force efficiently and eliminate faulty movements impeding forward momentum.
Strength and power training	Develop force production capability and the rate of force development during sprinting.
Advanced neuromuscular speed training	An advanced form of training that capitalizes on muscle-reflexive properties, including plyometric training, complex training, and PAP.
Specialized drills	An advanced form of training that transfers gains in force production capacity to apply force to the ground.

is used to develop force production capability and the rate of force development during sprinting. Advanced neuromuscular speed training (i.e., the fourth component) and specialized drills (i.e., the fifth component) are more advanced aspects of linear speed. Advanced neuromuscular speed training capitalizes on muscle-reflexive properties, whereas specialized drills transfer gains in force production capacity to apply force to the ground. Many of the skills developed by these components have direct application to agility and multidirectional speed.

AGILITY AND MULTIDIRECTIONAL SPEED

The ability to quickly change movement velocity by redirecting speed in response to changing demands of the sport is a fundamental factor for successful sports performance. **Agility** can be defined as the ability to change direction or body orientation with rapid and accurate cognitive processing of external and internal information without a substantive loss of movement speed (Brown & Ferrigno, 2015; Komi, 2011). Galpin et al. (2008) and Dintiman (2020) characterize agility as including the expression of cognitive actions (e.g., awareness, perception, anticipation, deciding, and reading the opponent's actions), physical demands of the start or first two steps (e.g., movement speed and strength), change of direction (e.g., forward, backward, lateral, or diagonal), and technical skills (e.g., movement technique or footwork). In contrast, other researchers have suggested that agility refers to situations involving rapid directional changes and decisions regardless of the quality and magnitude of the athlete's perceptive and reactive abilities (Young et al., 2002). Agility is expressed predominantly as the interaction of power, muscular strength, and speed (Bompa et al., 2019; Bompa & Buzzichelli, 2018; Bompa & Haff, 2009). Thus, although agility has been formally defined in many ways, Galpin et al. (2008) and Dintiman (2020) provide the most thorough characterization that encompasses cognitive actions, physical demands of the first two steps, change of direction, and technical skills.

Perhaps the most critical aspect of SAQ training for success in random, intermittent sports performance is acceleration out of a change of direction (COD). COD, a defining feature of agility, involves an important capacity referred to as **multidirectional speed (MDS)**. MDS is the ability to propel the body at high speed in many directions (e.g., starting, stopping, and cutting) and to achieve high-speed directional changes rapidly (e.g., forward, backward, lateral, or diagonal) (**Figure 13.10**) (Brown & Ferrigno, 2015; Chaouachi et al., 2014; Dintiman, 2020; Lockie et al., 2014).

AGILITY →

The ability to change direction or body orientation with rapid and accurate cognitive processing of external and internal information without a substantive loss of movement speed.

MULTI-DIRECTIONAL → SPEED (MDS)

The ability to propel or move the body at high speed in many directions (e.g., starting, stopping, cutting, feinting, or faking) and to achieve high-speed directional changes rapidly.

Agility and Multidirectional Speed

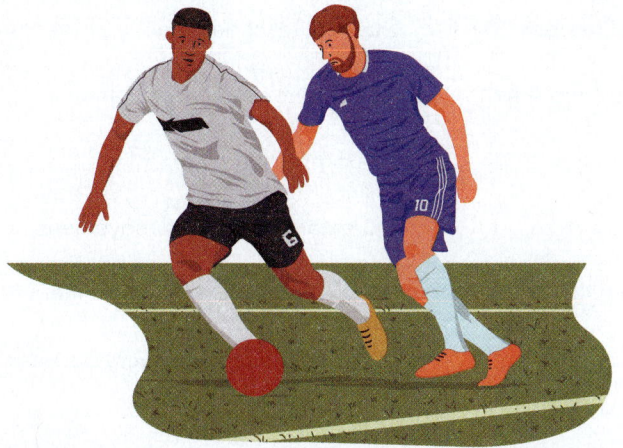

FIGURE 13.10 Agility and Multidirectional Speed

Agile athletes proficient with COD, MDS, power, and linear speed effectively achieve and control speed in any direction. Research suggests that agility and MDS training are more effective than traditional methods in developing SAQ (Azmi & Kusnanik, 2018; Bloomfield et al., 2007; Chaouachi et al., 2014; Jovanovic et al., 2011; Lennemann et al., 2013; Miller et al., 2006; Zago et al., 2016). Specifically, the findings of these studies demonstrated that agility and MDS training can improve the functional, coordinative, and fundamental elements of athleticism. As a whole, this research implies the high practical value of agility and MDS training as a central element of athletic performance and development.

Moreover, other studies have determined that agility and MDS training improve proprioception, spatial anticipation, kinesthetic awareness, reaction time, movement time, and **total response time** (Brewer, 2017; Brown & Ferrigno, 2015; Levin, 2014; Schmidt et al., 2019). These improvements aid in heightening overall athleticism, which enhances proficiency in nearly every athletic activity.

FUNDAMENTALS OF AGILITY AND MDS PROGRAMS

Agility and MDS training often resembles the actual activities of a given sport and may, therefore, be the most effective way to address the neuromuscular and metabolic demands required to perform sport-specific skills (Cissik & Barnes, 2011; Dintiman, 2020; Uthoff et al., 2020; Zago et al., 2016). General skills and concepts learned during linear speed training also apply to agility and MDS training. These skills include acceleration after the start, optimal footwork, deceleration capabilities, maximizing force production and rate of force development, ideal posture, and proper lower- and upper-body orientation and biomechanics during movement. However, agility and MDS training also include many specific skill demands that must be addressed in developing training programs to improve the key components of athleticism. Dintiman (2020) and Gambetta (2007) suggest the vital components of agility and MDS training include those listed in **Table 13.2**.

> **TOTAL RESPONSE TIME** →
>
> The summation of reaction time and movement time.

TABLE 13.2 Key Components of Agility and Multidirectional Speed Development

Component	Importance
Body control and awareness	More efficiency of movement
Recognition and reaction	Lowers reaction time
The start: the first two steps	Sets up for ideal acceleration
Acceleration	Faster movements
Footwork	Greater efficiency of movement
Change of direction	More stability while transitioning to acceleration
Speed endurance	Less fatigue and recovery between movement bouts
Stopping	More efficient deceleration

The component of **speed endurance** should be further elaborated upon. Speed endurance is essential for sports performance because fatigue accumulation results in a reduction in sprint capacity. As fatigue continues to accumulate, the extent of the ground support phase increases, as the stride length is increased concurrently with a decrease in the stride rate (DeWeese & Nimphius, 2016) (**Figure 13.11**).

SPEED ENDURANCE →

The ability to perform both repetitive short sprints and long sprints greater than 100 yards with minor deceleration due to fatigue.

Fatigue and Sprinting Capacity

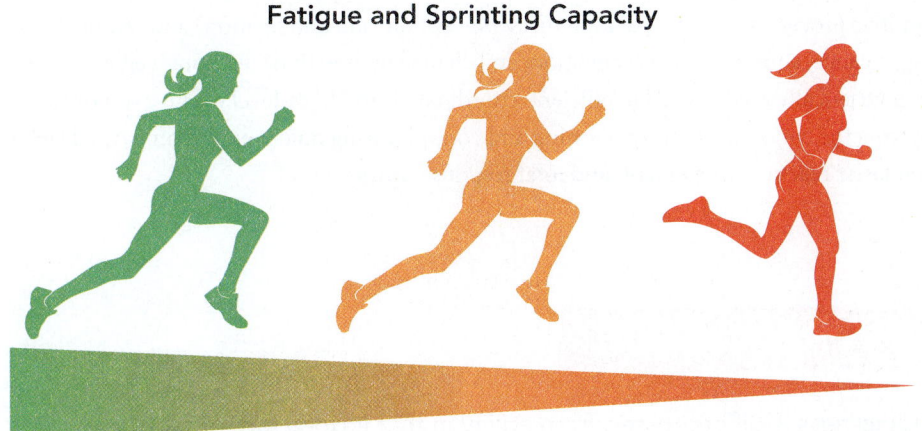

FIGURE 13.11 Fatigue and Sprinting Capacity

The components of agility and MDS training proposed by Dintiman (2020) and Gambetta (2007) involve developing biomotor skills and can, therefore, be trained. Effective movement for these components is a culmination of agility, MDS skills, and the biomotor abilities required for sprinting. Because these skills must be highly integrated during game performance, they are often trained simultaneously during agility and MDS drills. For athletes at any level of athleticism wishing to work on sport-specific aspects of agility and MDS, drills can be broken into individual segments or phases that are specific to the sport and the preparedness of the athlete.

QUICKNESS

As a vital component of both speed and agility, quickness addresses the quality and magnitude of the athlete's perceptive and reactive abilities, which may be one of the most significant components contributing to athletic success (Brewer, 2017; Gambetta, 2007). A quick athlete can assess or read a game situation and react at a very high speed. Although many athletes may possess a high level of performance for other biomotor abilities and game skills such as power, agility, strength, speed, and MDS, those who can apply the appropriate skills at the right time and at the fastest rate will be the most successful (Bompa et al., 2019).

Quickness refers to the combination of power, agility, and reactive ability that enables the athlete to respond to and change the position and direction of the body at maximum velocity under conditions of low external resistance ($\leq$ 15% of maximal strength). The primary role of quickness is to generate high-velocity movement that does not require high external resistance, power, strength, or energy expenditure. Quickness

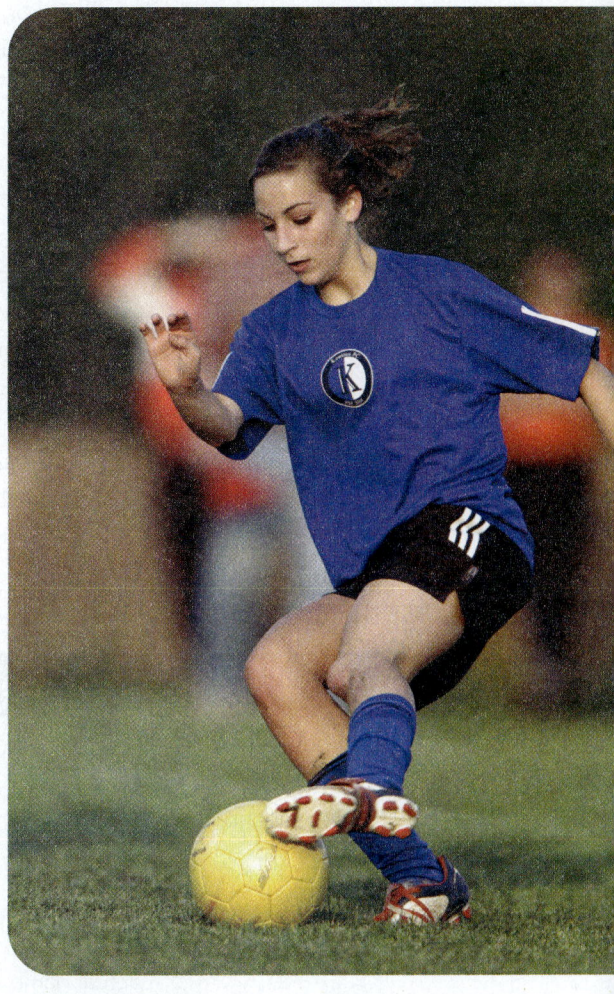

© Shawn Pecor/Shutterstock

training involves developing the biomotor skills of power and agility while decreasing reaction time to environmental stimuli (Schmidt et al., 2019). Reaction time—defined as the interval between stimulus detection, pattern recognition, response selection, and the initiation of an action (Levin, 2014)—is directly dependent on **response programming**.

Along with the time it takes to initiate an appropriate response, the time it takes to execute the reactionary movement (i.e., movement time) is another concern. Quickness training aims to address each mechanism involved with total response time, thereby improving the related cognitive processes (e.g., spatial awareness, perception, and anticipation) and motor skills (e.g., balance, coordination, acceleration, and change of direction). Although elite athletes are often genetically predisposed to efficient, coordinated, and high-level reactive motor skills, applying the concepts of motor learning and control during quickness training can develop an even faster reaction, movement, and total response times.

✔ CHECK IT OUT

Quickness is differentiated from agility in that it does the following:

- Quickness appears only when external resistance is at or below 15% of maximal strength.
- Training for quickness involves reducing reaction time.
- Quickness is a reactive ability.
- Quickness can be expressed as nonambulatory movements such as hitting a baseball, returning a tennis serve, or swerving a car to avoid an accident.

Training for quickness entails taking all the skills required for effective speed and agility plus the specific skills needed in a sport and applying them to the reactionary demands of that sport (Bompa & Haff, 2009; Schmidt et al., 2019). This process begins with general coordination and teaching effective, biomechanically efficient, sport-specific movement patterns; once proficiency is established, movement speed is then addressed (Schmidt et al., 2019). Next, efficient movement in quickness drills is paired with specific reactionary demands that the athlete will encounter during an athletic competition (Bompa & Haff, 2009). Finally, a large amount of competitive game experience allows for the accurate, sport-specific application of these skills. These components are summarized in **Table 13.3**.

TABLE 13.3 Components of Quickness Development

Component	Importance
General coordination	Coordination forms the basis for learning and mastering new motor skills.
Specific reactionary demands	Mimics the specific scenarios that an athlete may encounter in their sport, enhancing their ability to respond rapidly and effectively.
Competitive game experience	A real-world platform to apply training under conditions that closely replicate those of actual competitions. This helps athletes translate the quickness developed in training to actual game scenarios.

Soccer requires effective acceleration, top-end speed, deceleration, and multidirectional speed changes. In the initial training phases for a soccer player, the program focuses on teaching the technique drills for the required skills and movements. Once these are mastered, the soccer athlete can practice the movements in planned drills that mimic sports competition. Execution of these drills is often timed to monitor speed and proficiency. Once an established time criterion is met, the soccer ball is added to make the drills sport- and position-specific. In addition, reactionary demands replace the practiced, predictable patterns of planned drills, such as cone drills. For example, cones can be removed, and the athlete must respond to a coach's whistle or visual cue. Finally, scrimmages and game scenarios are added to training, keeping proper movement skills in mind but adding the sport-specific neuromuscular and metabolic demands of actual competition. The practice of this process results in quick athletes conditioned to the rigors of competition, increasing the likelihood of successful sports performance during actual competitions.

Quickness is demonstrated by effectively assessing the environment and competition and reacting at high speed. Athletes who can apply the biomotor abilities of power, strength, speed, and agility at the correct time and at the fastest rate will be the most successful in sports performance. Linear speed and agility-MDS training alone are not enough to improve performance—optimal performance on the field or court also requires quickness training. At this example suggests, it is critical that Sports Performance Coaches understand and implement quickness training with each athlete.

LESSON 3: THE SCIENCE OF SAQ TRAINING

SCIENTIFIC RATIONALE FOR SAQ TRAINING

The use of SAQ training to improve performance in most sports is generally accepted by experienced coaches, sports scientists, and sports performance specialists. However, the scientific basis for SAQ and the mechanisms by which it enhances performance are not well understood among training professionals. As with other aspects of SAQ, the underlying science can be divided into the individual components of speed, agility, and quickness.

Speed training is about improving the maximum rate at which an athlete can move from one point to another. It involves the neuromuscular system, biomechanics, and energy systems. The science behind speed training involves principles of force production, stride length, frequency, and energy system conditioning.

Agility is the ability to change direction quickly and efficiently while maintaining control. It involves aspects of balance, coordination, spatial awareness, and reaction to stimuli. The science of agility training is tied to neuromuscular adaptation, proprioception, and decision making under physical stress.

Quickness refers to the ability to react and get moving quickly. It involves the neuromuscular system's response to a need for sudden movement, often as a reaction to an external stimulus. The science of quickness training involves understanding reaction times, muscle fiber types, and neural pathways.

Collectively, the scientific rationale for SAQ as a component of integrated sports performance training is outlined and explained in terms of postural control, injury risk reduction, athlete rehabilitation, and six key factors of sports performance enhancement:

- Vertical jump
- Linear speed
- Multidirectional speed
- Hand–eye coordination
- Reaction time
- Dynamic balance

POSTURAL CONTROL

SAQ training can play a significant role in enhancing postural control. One of the key ways this is achieved is through the improvement of proprioception, the body's inherent ability to sense its position, movements, and actions. By constantly engaging in SAQ exercises that demand swift reactions and balance maintenance, athletes can significantly enhance their proprioceptive abilities.

Engineering kinematics applied to human movement patterns and the interdependence of different body regions when executing complex motor movements have been recognized for almost a century, as evidenced by the identification of distinct human kinetic chains (Karandikar & Ortiz Vargas, 2011). As a dictating quality of dynamic balance, posture represents the positioning of the vertebral segments of the spine and predominately regulates the proficiency and stress of movement imposed on the spine during movement of the kinetic chain (Hamill et al., 2015) (**Figure 13.12**). In standing, working, or modified postures, the spine is stabilized mainly by proprioceptive feedback

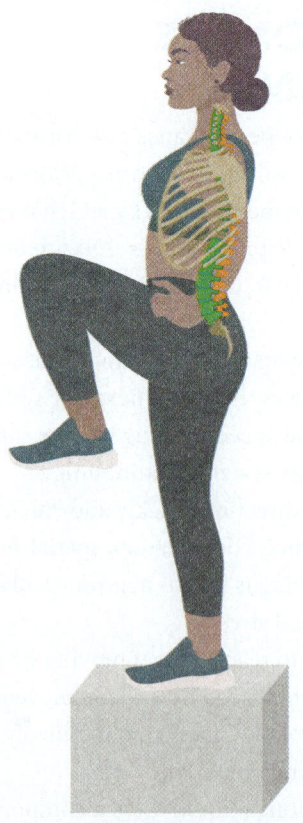

FIGURE 13.12 Postural Control

from mechanoreceptors of the spinal joints, tendons, and specific core muscles (Powers & Howley, 2018).

An experiment by Zemková et al. (2007) examined the effect of maximal anaerobic exercise on postural sway underpinning static and dynamic balance in athletes and non-athletes. These researchers had participants perform a yaw head movement and observed that equilibrium was significantly lower in non-athletes than in athletes. Zemková et al. (2007) suggested that physical performance from previous maximal anaerobic training, such as multidirectional sprinting, in which head position changes, enabled the athletes to better maintain their postural control.

Paillard (2014) notes that repetitive techniques (e.g., linear sprinting, multidirectional speed, and change of direction) can improve sport-specific and position-specific posture directly related to enhancing specific motor abilities. Subsequently, repetitive SAQ drills evoke specific visual, somatosensory, and vestibular motor chains that enable the activation of optimal posture maintenance strategies under different sporting situations.

Studies have also demonstrated that agility-based exercises work as well as traditional strength and balance training for improving explosive power in trunk musculature (Lichtenstein et al., 2020). These findings suggest that SAQ-type training might positively impact core strength and postural control in populations of various ages.

INJURY RISK REDUCTION

It is common for athletes to incur an injury in competition or in their training history due to improper positioning during training or sports movements. When any of the five kinetic chain checkpoints (**Figure 13.13**) falls out of alignment during dynamic motion, it sets the stage for injuries that could otherwise be avoided. Because sports movements result from a reaction to the environment and include all planes of motion at different velocities, an inability or decreased efficiency to respond rapidly to stimuli by altering movement velocity may be considered a primary risk factor for injury. Therefore, athletes' injury prevention and risk reduction can be accomplished through carefully planned SAQ training programs.

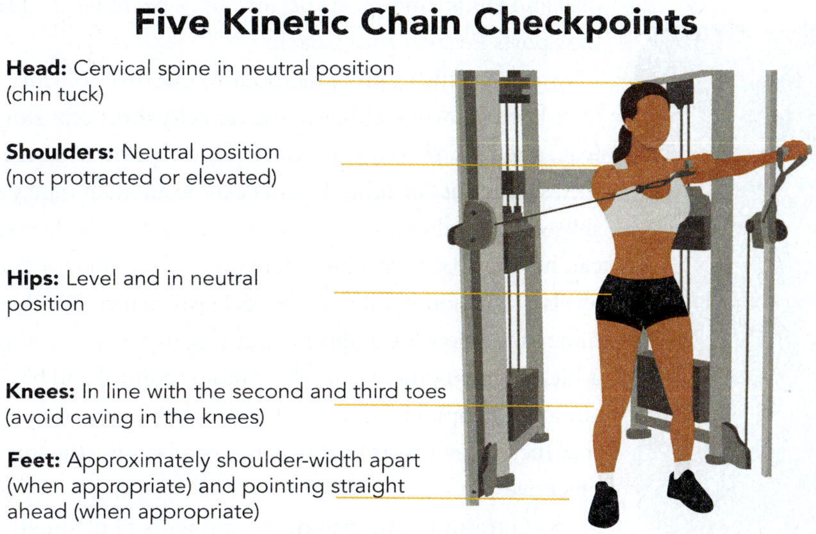

Five Kinetic Chain Checkpoints

Head: Cervical spine in neutral position (chin tuck)

Shoulders: Neutral position (not protracted or elevated)

Hips: Level and in neutral position

Knees: In line with the second and third toes (avoid caving in the knees)

Feet: Approximately shoulder-width apart (when appropriate) and pointing straight ahead (when appropriate)

FIGURE 13.13 Five Kinetic Chain Checkpoints

SAQ training programs should be progressive, beginning with more basic drills performed with optimal form and control before progressing to advanced exercises. Taking additional time to plan thoughtful SAQ training will reduce the risk of injuries and time spent in athlete rehabilitation efforts.

SAQ training can help reduce injury risk in several ways:

- SAQ training often includes resistance and plyometric exercises, which can improve muscle strength and joint stability.
- SAQ training helps to improve an athlete's balance and body awareness (proprioception), reducing the likelihood of falls and missteps, which can lead to injury.
- The rapid, variable movements involved in SAQ training enhance neuromuscular coordination and responsiveness, enabling athletes to more effectively and safely respond to the unpredictable movements inherent in many sports, and thereby reducing the risk of certain injuries.
- SAQ training tailored to mimic the demands of specific sports helps athletes prepare more effectively for the particular stresses faced during those sports, which can also reduce the risk of injury.

In their study, Dijksma et al. (2019) incorporated speed and agility drills into the training of military recruits. These exercises resulted in faster T-test and Illinois Agility Test times, enhanced motor control and change of direction speed, and a dramatic drop in the relative risk of attrition from injuries.

ATHLETE REHABILITATION

SAQ training plays a significant role in the rehabilitation process for athletes, providing multiple benefits that help them return to their sports. First, SAQ training is integral in helping athletes regain their pre-injury levels of speed, agility, and quickness, all of which are fundamental to athletic performance. By integrating sports-specific movements into the regimen, SAQ training can assist athletes in returning to their sports more rapidly and efficiently. SAQ training also improves neuromuscular control, allowing for safer and more effective movement, which helps athletes avoid compensatory patterns that could lead to new injuries. Once an athlete reaches the last phases of formal rehabilitation, returning to play and enhancing sports performance becomes the priority of the Sports Performance Coach.

SAQ-specific training methods to improve control have been shown to enhance the capacity for motor skills (e.g., strength, power, and agility) following injuries. Adhesions (i.e., scar tissue) or other trauma can occur at an injury site and subsequently alter motor recruitment patterns. SAQ training can help restore neuromuscular control and improve previous levels of biomotor abilities. Sports Performance Coaches should understand how SAQ-specific training methods work to help athletes regain previous levels of motor control and biomotor ability development and to enhance rehabilitation efforts so that increasing sports performance can become the top training objective.

SAQ training can include components of plyometrics that utilize PAP. This form of training is commonly incorporated

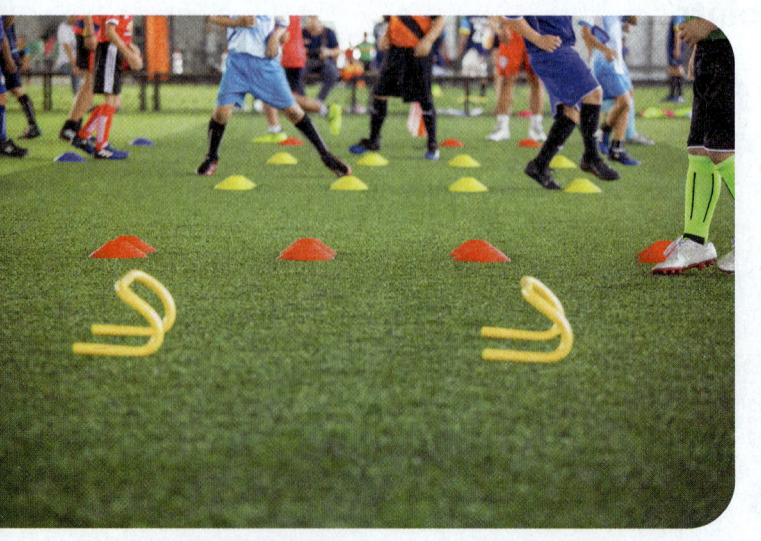
© Noomcpk/Shutterstock

into training programs initiated immediately following terminal rehabilitation phases and is predominantly dictated by the healing phase of the injury (Beam, 2002; Lorenz, 2011). The effectiveness of incorporating SAQ training methods promptly after rehabilitation was demonstrated by Mehran et al. (2016). These researchers found that high-level basketball players who returned to SAQ and sport-specific training after surgical repair and formal rehabilitation of anterior cruciate ligament (ACL) injuries performed almost identically on measures of speed, acceleration, quickness, agility, and vertical jump compared to age-, position-, skill-, and size-matched basketball players without ACL injuries.

SPORTS PERFORMANCE ENHANCEMENT

One body of evidence focuses on the mechanisms by which SAQ training functions to elicit neuromuscular adaptation and to develop, refine, and enhance motor skills. This line of research suggests that SAQ training is an effective modality for improving performance across various disciplines and biomotor abilities essential to sports. Specifically, evidence supports its ability to improve athletes' vertical jump, linear speed performance, multidirectional speed, hand–eye coordination, reaction time, and dynamic balance.

VERTICAL JUMP

As a frequently used component of SAQ training, plyometrics to exploit the reflexive actions of the muscle has consistently been shown to improve vertical jump performance and force applied to the ground (Harry et al., 2018; King & Cipriani, 2010; Maloney et al., 2019; Ramirez-Campillo et al., 2020; Rodríguez-Rosell et al., 2017). Moreover, Ramirez-Campillo et al. (2020) observed that sequencing of plyometric training before regular soccer practice significantly enhanced vertical jump and soccer performance compared to plyometric methods performed after other training or game practice. Beyond plyometric training, spinal stabilization and stiffness training are also known to enhance vertical jumps (Maloney et al., 2019; Mills & Taunton, 2003). In particular, enhanced vertical jump performance can be augmented with PAP (Bergmann et al., 2013), contrast training of power (Hammami et al., 2017), and agility-specific tests (Sassi et al., 2009).

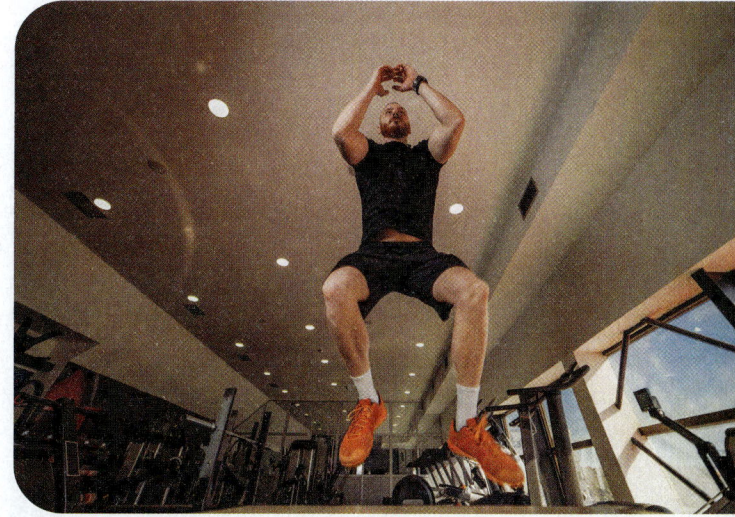

© Vladimir Borovic/Shutterstock

Although resisted jump training can increase vertical jump height, plyometric depth jump training is equally effective in achieving this outcome (Hrysomallis, 2012).

LINEAR SPEED PERFORMANCE

Additional studies support the use of SAQ training to enhance athletic performance in terms of linear speed. For example, Bloomfield et al. (2007) conducted experiments to determine an effective speed and agility conditioning methodology for random intermittent dynamic sports. The researchers divided participants into three groups: (1) a programmed SAQ conditioning group, whose members learned and practiced specific SAQ drills to correct movement mechanics before the drills increased in complexity; (2) a random conditioning group, whose members participated in two, three, and four small-sided games; and (3) a control group. Bloomfield et al. (2007) observed significant improvements in acceleration, deceleration, dynamic balance, leg power, and percentage increases in all parameters in the programmed SAQ conditioning group compared to the random conditioning and control groups, demonstrating the importance of the principles of specificity, overload, and adaptation.

Other research has suggested that resisted speed training boosts linear speed performance more than unresisted speed training (Hrysomallis, 2012; Panascì et al., 2023).

MULTIDIRECTIONAL SPEED PERFORMANCE

Maintaining multidirectional speed performance during repetitive and prolonged athletic activity is essential to random, dynamic intermittent sports and is an important aspect of speed development. Although there is considerable debate over the best methods to enhance qualities related to MDS, Keller et al. (2020) demonstrated the importance of resistance training methods to develop strength and power, thereby improving COD and MDS performance. SAQ training incorporating resistance training to enhance MDS performance increases lean body mass and strength (i.e., relative strength) and leads to greater hip abduction and knee flexion when COD and MDS movements occur (Keller et al., 2020). Subsequently, these improvements enhance MDS performance by increasing an athlete's ability to decelerate, reduce GCT, and generate more power vertically and horizontally during acceleration out of a change of direction.

HAND–EYE COORDINATION

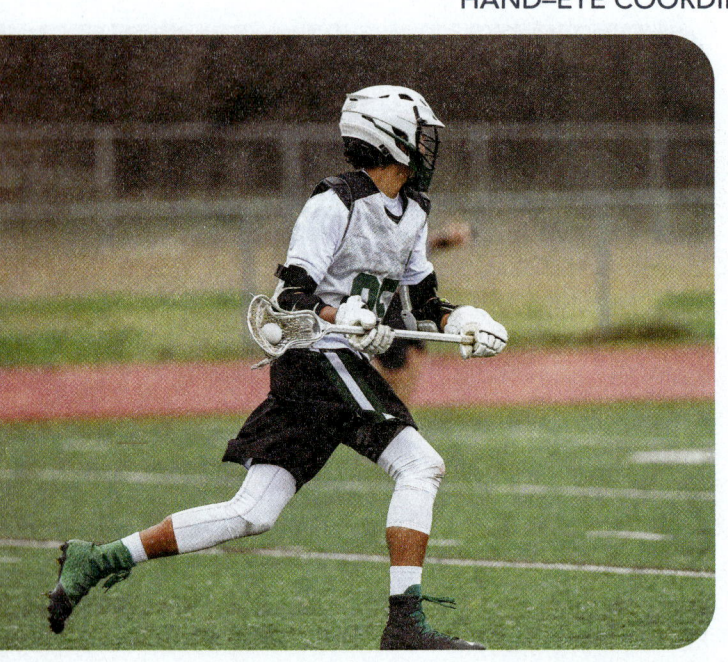

© JoeSAPhotos/Shutterstock

Hand–eye coordination is the ability to process information visually and to guide hand movement to complete a task. Most sports movements rely on hand–eye coordination for planning or reflexively initiating an action in response to visual stimuli through visual processing. Visual processing represents the critical input of vision that is processed through cognitive and perceptual skills to interpret or perceive stimuli within the competition environment.

Hand–eye coordination is innate to each athlete, although it can be developed through SAQ training. This coordination requires an athlete not only to sustain focus on sports implements such as a ball or bat, but also to track movements with the eyes and maintain a spatial awareness of teammates and opponents concurrently. Without proficiently developed hand–eye coordination, visually locating and tracking an object (i.e., a ball), processing the information, and initiating a movement to intercept the object's trajectory takes longer and is associated with more movement errors. These factors are often the difference between successful and unsuccessful sporting attempts. Sport-specific SAQ training develops the cognitive performance (e.g., total reaction time, speed of perception, and neuromuscular control) needed to enhance hand–eye coordination (Formenti et al., 2019). One experimental study of young students demonstrated that a 6-week SAQ intervention resulted in significant improvements in pre- and post-test hand–eye coordination measures in an experimental SAQ training group compared to a control group with no SAQ training (Shapie & Rohizam, 2018).

REACTION TIME

SAQ training aims to shorten total reaction time throughout the continuum of muscle action (e.g., isometric stabilization, concentric acceleration, and eccentric deceleration) and transfer an increased reactive ability to develop agility and quickness further. Reaction time is limited by how fast visual and proprioceptive stimuli can be perceived and processed and by the speed of neuromuscular coordination. Research has shown that SAQ training improves sprinting, reactive agility, and other SAQ skills' reaction time.

Trecroci et al. (2016) observed that speed, agility, and quickness training positively enhance the cognitive skills underpinning improved reaction time.

DYNAMIC BALANCE

Dynamic balance occurs when the kinetic chain's muscles, joints, and ligaments can stabilize the pelvis, spine, and distal limbs to maintain posture. Dynamic balance forms the basis from which to apply force in multiple directions effectively. One example of a dynamic balance is the dominance of the leg extensors, lumbopelvic extensors, lateral flexors, and hip abductors, which perform the primary mechanical work during block starts of a sprint (Sado et al., 2020). Stability imparts the balance required to develop the strength and power to improve athletic ability and create and reduce the time to apply force, without which the capacity to generate force rapidly is lessened.

The effectiveness of SAQ training to enhance dynamic balance depends on several sport-specific factors. Zemková et al. (2007) demonstrated that (1) stability of posture is dependent on somatosensory, visual, and vestibular feedback systems; (2) sensory modality compensation works to maintain posture stability under maximal exercise; and (3) the vestibular system is more adversely influenced by the metabolic response to maximal anaerobic exercise than the somatosensory system during conditions of dynamic balance. In other words, posture stability is maintained by multiple sensory systems that work together, which compensate for changes in movement. The vestibular system that works predominately to maintain balance and a sense of equilibrium is most affected during maximal anaerobic exercise.

Given the complexity of the interplay of these sensory systems to maintain posture and dynamic balance under sport-specific demands, the ability to maintain posture across different sports conditions arises from the development of dynamic sport-specific balance achieved through SAQ training.

- Tanir (2018) observed that balance and stability drills as a part of SAQ training for young soccer players significantly improved their static and dynamic balance.
- Shapie and Rohizam (2018) showed significant improvements in 13 out of 16 dynamic balance measures in an experimental SAQ training group, compared to controls, after a 6-week SAQ training intervention.

LESSON 4: SAQ TRAINING GUIDELINES
PRINCIPLES OF SAQ TRAINING

The overarching goal when creating and implementing an SAQ performance program for most athletes is continual improvement geared toward optimizing performance during competition. A successful program is carefully designed to leverage various methods to impart the ability to produce a high force quickly, at the correct time, with proper

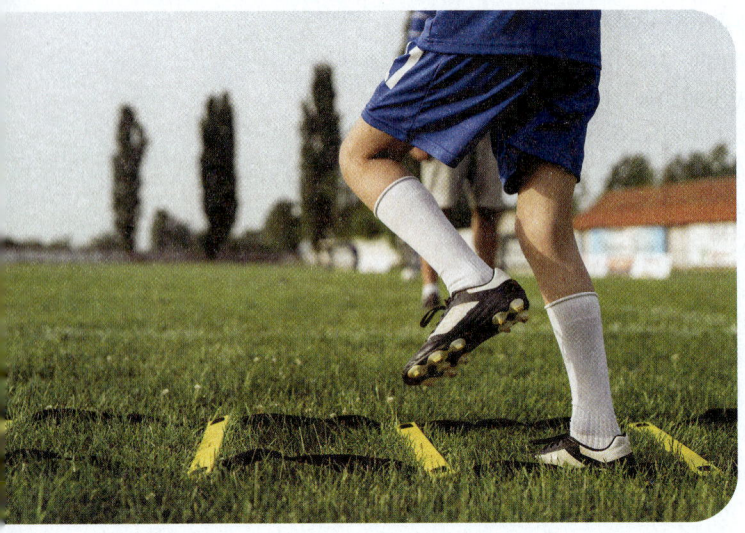

© Miljan Zivkovic/Shutterstock

mechanics for efficient movement. The SAQ training guidelines discussed here are important for the Sports Performance Coach for several reasons:

1. Information from the needs analysis of the athlete and the sport play an essential role in tailoring speed training to meet the athlete's goals.
2. Acute training variables should be manipulated to condition the energy systems, provide sufficient stimulus for adaptation, and, subsequently, manage fatigue to improve performance.
3. Exercise or drill selection and loading of drills must follow a logical progression over time to ensure there are sufficient stimuli for adaptation.
4. The training can be planned effectively and easily implemented.

Much of athletic development focuses on developing linear speed. However, because most movements in team sports rely on linear acceleration and multidirectional speed, the Sports Performance Coach needs to understand that agility and MDS training are essential to optimize athletic performance. The creation and implementation of the agility and MDS aspects of a performance program aims to refine and improve linear speed and transfer these gains to agility and multidirectional speed. Practically, this means using drills that revolve around linear speed to increase the force production capacity and rate of force development, while maintaining proper movement mechanics and adding directional components to the sprinting movements. Predictable and unpredictable drills are used when multiple directional components are added to movement patterns.

Agility and MDS training, however, address just one aspect of the athlete's overall training goals. To further refine acceleration and multidirectional speed, quickness training is essential. Creating and implementing a quickness aspect of a performance program is important to develop reactive ability. Practically, this involves using drills that mimic the fluid environment of competition.

NEEDS ANALYSIS AND ASSESSMENT INFORMATION

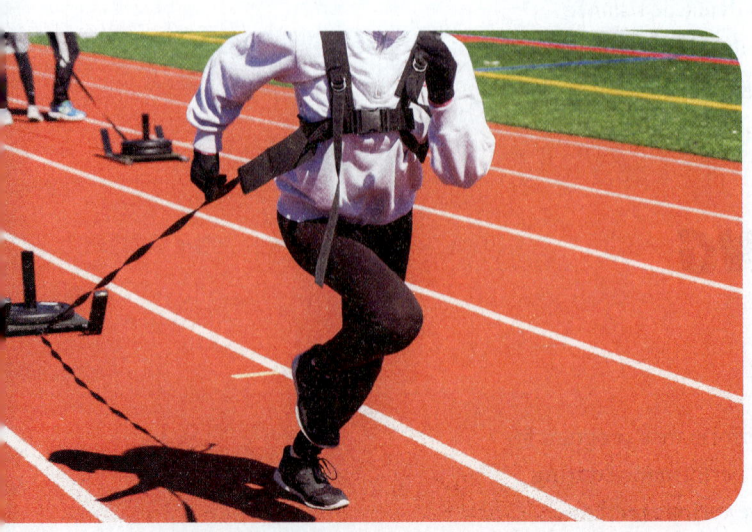

© WoodysPhotos/Shutterstock

The information gathered during the needs analysis of the athlete and the sport is needed for Sports Performance Coaches to plan and program acute training variables properly. Key aspects of the needs analysis related to SAQ training include training history, injuries, sprinting form, technique, performance assessment, reactive abilities, posture and movement assessments, and the metabolic demands and typical movement patterns of the sport and playing position. When it takes this information into account, the SAQ training program can facilitate learning optimal techniques, addressing deficiencies, and tailoring the athlete's training based on the metabolic demands specific to the sport and playing position. In addition, knowing the metabolic demands of the sport and position is crucial to organizing training with the proper work-to-rest ratios.

Form, technique, and skill development should progress based on the athlete's proficiency during training sessions. Although certain techniques can vary from athlete to athlete, serious deviations should be addressed as soon as possible by modifying the training plan to break up the training into separate areas of focus and devoting more training time to the deficient areas with submaximal intensity. This allows the athlete to assess each component separately throughout several training sessions with feedback from the coach before implementing maximal-intensity workouts. Evidence of proficiency can be seen daily, monthly, and sometimes yearly. However, the Sports Performance Coach must use insight and objectivity to determine whether the training proficiency observed in practice necessitates progressing an athlete to higher loading as an intermediate- or advanced-level athlete. In all aspects of SAQ training, mechanics should be mastered before progressing training.

When an athlete returns to training following an injury, the volume and intensity of the program should be lowered. The volume can be reduced to 50% of the guideline values and incrementally increased by 5% to 10% in each micro-cycle (i.e., week). Submaximal intensity should be maintained until the athlete reaches the guideline values for volume. Once the volume is achieved, shorter distances (repetitions) are used while returning to maximal intensity. Then, distances can increase while adhering to the work-to-rest ratios for a full recovery. Because athlete responses may vary, the Sports Performance Coach must constantly monitor program effectiveness through observation, assessments, data collection, and open communication with each athlete to manage fatigue when greater volume loads are used.

PROGRESSING SAQ TRAINING

Carefully planned progressions are crucial during SAQ training to ensure optimal development and minimize the risk of injury. A progressive approach gives the body adequate time to adapt to the physical demands of the training, thereby promoting gradual improvements in strength, speed, and agility. It also enables the continuous refinement of movement skills, as each phase of progression allows athletes to master the technique at one level before moving on to more challenging exercises. This mastery is crucial for transferring these skills effectively to sport-specific movements.

SAQ exercises should be carefully integrated into an athlete's overall training program. As the demands for movement speed and reactivity increase, so do the risks of injury. The safety and success of an SAQ program depend on the athlete's physical capabilities and fitness level. When the Sports Performance Coach better matches drills to an athlete's capabilities, the program will be safer and more effective. All exercises should be performed with precise techniques to minimize the risk of injury.

Sports Performance Coaches should establish a spectrum of SAQ exercises and drills that can be progressively overloaded at appropriate time intervals once athletes have demonstrated mastery of the previous phase. They can divide ideal progressions into beginner, intermediate, and advanced levels. However, it is important to recognize that these categories are not based on an athlete's ability. Instead, they should be aligned with the overall training process. For example, even some of the most advanced athletes may need to perform *beginner* SAQ exercises to emphasize technique and movement efficiency.

Due to the complexity of SAQ training, basic progressions between levels will be discussed independently in this section.

PROGRESSIONS FOR SPEED

Figure 13.14 shows a general progression model for speed in a basic performance program. For beginners, the training session aims to master proper sprint mechanics. In contrast, intermediate-level athletes focus on increasing linear speed, while more advanced athletes must develop repeated sprint ability, a part of speed endurance.

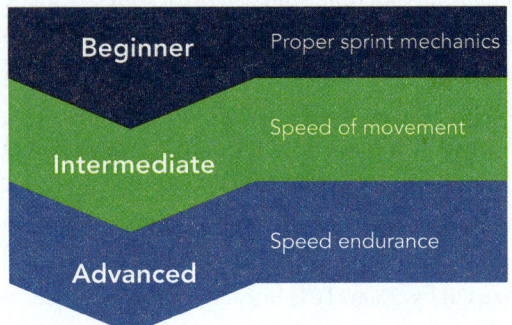

FIGURE 13.14 Speed Progression Model

The Sports Performance Coach should focus on improving playing speed or addressing the specific skills identified by the needs assessment. When designing speed training programs, the goal is to increase the GRF and the speed with which it is applied with each step. The improvements in speed from creating more GRF positively affect stride rate and stride length, targeting all areas in the phases of a sprint. Depending on the athlete's skill, the programmed progression would occur after an active dynamic warm-up involving sprint technique work, speed of movement drills, or both.

Sprints are the mainstay of linear speed training for maximal speed training, with variations resulting from changes in repetitions (i.e., distance), sets, and rest intervals. Therefore, when designing a speed component of SAQ training, it is important to understand that either maximal linear speed or linear acceleration is chosen as the training session focus.

PROGRESSIONS FOR AGILITY AND MDS

Figure 13.15 shows a general progression model for agility-MDS in a basic performance program. Depending on the athlete's skill, the training session would occur after an active dynamic warm-up focusing on agility-MDS technique work, speed of movement drills, or both. The progression of agility training is paramount for the development of an athlete, particularly because it involves different targeted areas at various stages of proficiency.

Agility-MDS Progression Model

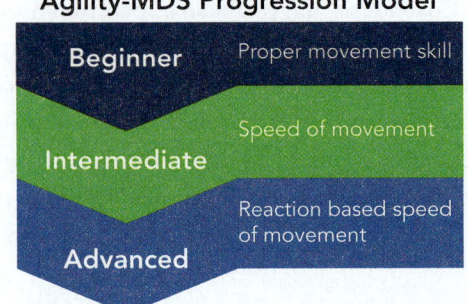

FIGURE 13.15 Agility-MDS Progression Model

For beginners, the primary emphasis should be on proper movement skills. Mastery of correct form, body mechanics, and technique is foundational and will set the stage for future training success while minimizing injury risk. As the athlete moves to an intermediate level, the focus shifts to the speed of movement. At this stage, athletes work to increase their quickness and efficiency while still maintaining correct technique. This helps develop the ability to change direction swiftly, a crucial component of agility in many sports.

Finally, for advanced athletes, the emphasis is on reaction-based speed of movement. The goal here is to simulate the unpredictable nature of sports, where athletes must rapidly respond to external stimuli. This highest level of training pushes athletes to apply their agility under sport-specific conditions, enhancing their performance during competition. This progressive approach ensures that athletes develop solid fundamental movement skills, increase their speed, and enhance their reactive agility as they advance, resulting in overall improved agility performance.

PROGRESSIONS FOR QUICKNESS

Figure 13.16 shows a general progression model for quickness training in a basic performance program. Depending on the athlete's skill, the training session would occur after an active dynamic warm-up involving agility and MDS movements, movement speed drills, or both.

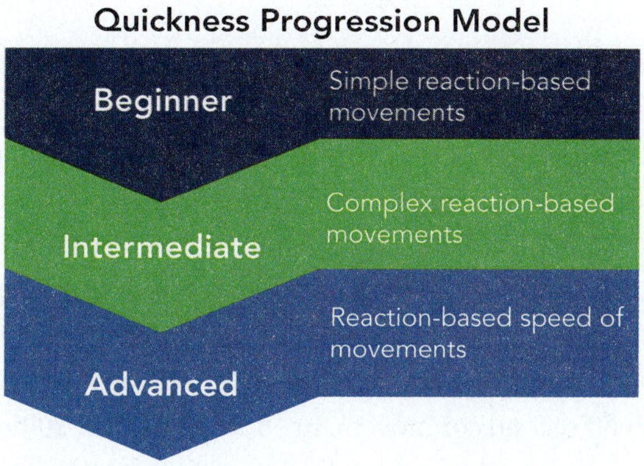

Quickness Progression Model

Beginner — Simple reaction-based movements

Intermediate — Complex reaction-based movements

Advanced — Reaction-based speed of movements

FIGURE 13.16 Quickness Progression Model

For beginners, the initial focus should be on simple reaction-based movements. This level emphasizes mastering the basics of movement in response to a single, predictable stimulus, building a foundation for reaction speed. Training incorporates more complex reaction-based movements as athletes advance to an intermediate level. This stage often introduces multiple stimuli or less predictable cues, requiring athletes to process information and respond quickly, improving their cognitive speed, decision-making capabilities, and physical quickness.

Finally, at an advanced level, athletes must focus on reaction-based speed of movements. This phase incorporates all the skills developed in the previous stages but at a faster pace and under more challenging conditions, closely mirroring the dynamics of actual competition.

These progressions ensure that athletes gradually develop their quickness while improving their cognitive processing, decision-making, and sport-specific skills, enhancing performance in their respective sports.

ACUTE TRAINING VARIABLES FOR SAQ TRAINING

Successful SAQ programs manipulate acute training variables to improve movement speed and athlete ability by creating high-force production at the correct time in the right direction for efficient movement. Due to the high demands of many SAQ exercises, the intent when selecting acute training variables should be well understood before designing comprehensive programs. In addition, some acute variables depend on other variables (e.g., energy systems, fatigue, level of athleticism) that must be addressed early in program design. The following sections describe the proper inclusion of some acute training variables for SAQ programs.

EXERCISE SELECTION

Training for SAQ should revolve around linear speed as the dominant ability and target of all training sessions because it is the most important underlying factor for sports performance in most game situations. Maximal linear sprinting requires athletes to execute movements at high speeds by generating significant force during foot contact in the stride cycle with a high rate-of-force development, which heavily taxes the neuromuscular system. This degree of neural drive necessitates the selection of exercises, sprinting drills, and variations of sprinting drills that increase neural drive by loading the muscles of the knees and hips, which are involved with the SSC.

If speed development is the aim of a training session, the Sports Performance Coach can dedicate a single training session to either maximum linear speed drills or linear acceleration drills, and variations of these drills that include plyometrics. Exercise and drill selection partly influences how energy systems are taxed. For example, when maximum speed drills are performed, the athlete's force generation capacity starts to decrease as fatigue begins to accumulate. More specifically, the adenosine triphosphate-creatine phosphate (ATP-CP) energy pathway can provide energy for only approximately 10 seconds of the sprint; fatigue metabolites from the breakdown of glycogen then start to accumulate at 40 to 60 seconds of movement (Bompa & Haff, 2009). Therefore, fatigue must be managed using sufficient rest periods during the training session to fully recover and counter this phenomenon.

Fatigue is also a concern when acceleration and COD drills are used. Agility and multidirectional speed drills are highly taxing neuromuscular activities. For this reason, multidirectional speed and agility drills should be prioritized for exercise selection on days when maximal linear speed or acceleration drills are used.

When selecting quickness drills, the Sports Performance Coach should choose drills that most closely resemble the demands of the sport. Although quickness drills do not produce the same impact on energy systems as maximal speed training does, they require the athlete to be in a fresh state to be effective. Therefore, quickness drills should ideally be selected for days without maximal speed, acceleration, or MDS training.

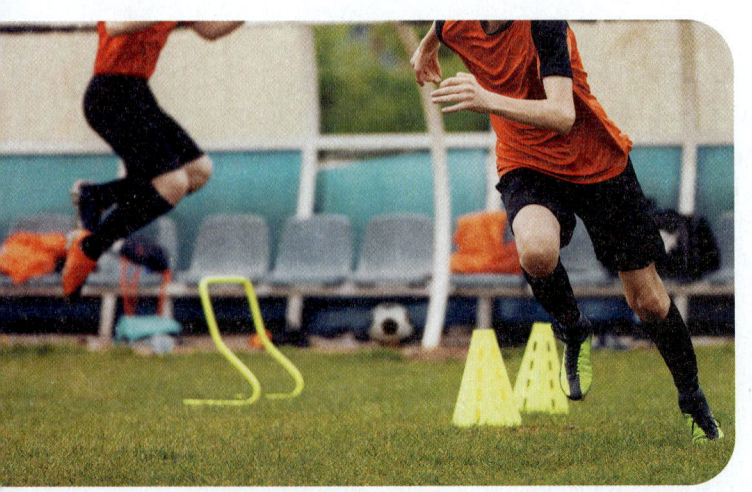

© Matimix/Shutterstock

INTENSITY

The following equation is used to calculate the intensity of SAQ training:

$$\text{Intensity} = (\text{m-s}^{-1}) = \text{distance (m) / time (s)}$$

where distance is measured in meters, time in seconds, and intensity as the product of meters and seconds raised to the power of negative 1 (i.e., m-s^{-1} or m/s) (Bompa & Haff, 2009). According to this equation, an athlete who sprints 100 m in 25 s would have an intensity of 4.0 m/s. With this formula for intensity, as the time to cover the distance decreases, the magnitude of intensity increases, and the volume load (meters × intensity) decreases (**Table 13.4**).

TABLE 13.4 Estimation of Average Sprinting Intensity and Volume Load

Distance (m)	Time (s)	Intensity (m/s)	Volume Load
250	60	4.17	15,000
250	45	5.56	11,250
250	47	5.32	11,750
250	49	5.10	12,250
250	44	5.68	11,000
Average sprinting intensity = (m/s) =		5.17	
Average sprinting volume load = (m × s) =			12,250

Data from Bompa, T. O., & Haff, G. G. (2009). Periodization: Theory and methodology of training (5th ed.). Champaign, IL: Human Kinetics.

One caveat with this intensity estimation method is that it does not account for sprinting at very fast velocities over short distances. This aspect must be considered when using this method to guide intensity levels for sprinting, agility, and MDS drills. The intensity estimation method can be used for speed and MDS drills for maximal linear speed training and longer distance multidirectional speed training. However, it is impractical if the training distances are less than 50 to 75 meters.

Most Sports Performance Coaches working with athletes do not need intensity estimations; instead, they train athletes for maximum effort and focus once the athletes learn proper form and technique. Young (2017) refers to maximum effort and intent as maximum intensity and suggests that all linear speed work, multidirectional speed, and agility training should be executed under the most significant effort and focus that the athlete can produce. This type of maximum effort and focus is required to increase the neural drive so as to enhance performance and continually increase motor skills' speed. An intensity method like this is very demanding, so special attention should be paid to warm-up, rest, and recovery procedures.

TRAINING VOLUME

Training volume for SAQ comprises the quantity of work for a given training bout (i.e., one 100-m sprint) or task and the total work prescribed for an individual training session or cycle. One notable method to assess the volume of work completed in a training session is volume load. Training volume is similar to intensity in that volume load (distance × intensity) can be estimated after intensity is established, although a simpler, more straightforward approach is equally effective. When programming volume for sprinting, the Sports Performance Coach should time the athlete, record the data, and average the volume and intensity over more than two sprinting sessions. The training bout volume for an SAQ drill is simply the volume load, and its formula is also part of the intensity equation:

$$\text{Volume load} = \text{distance (m)} \times \text{intensity (m/s)}$$

Thus, volume load is the product of the distance completed per sprint bout and intensity (Bompa & Haff, 2009).

Current best practices in SAQ training suggest that maximal intensity for each training bout should be maintained. Therefore, when considering an athlete's sprinting, MDS, and agility drill volume, **Table 13.5** summarizes the distances covered in the prescribed work, assuming maximal intensity (i.e., maximal effort and focus).

TABLE 13.5 SAQ Training Volume

Linear speed	• Maximal linear speed: volume (200–350 m) • Linear acceleration: volume (150–200 m)
Agility and MDS	• Agility and MDS (predictable: linear speed + COD): volume (150–300 m) • Agility and MDS (unpredictable: linear speed + COD): volume (150–300 m)
Quickness	• Quickness (predictable drills): volume (200–300 m) • Quickness (unpredictable drills): volume (200–300 m)

Total volume for a training session represents the sum of the volume load (i.e., the work for each training bout). Total volume can also be expressed as the product of the number of drills, sets, and repetitions (Volume_{Tot} = number of drills $\times$ number of sets $\times$ number of repetitions). In contrast, training bout volume is expressed as simply the product of the number of sets and repetitions of a single drill (Volume_{Bout} = number of sets $\times$ number of repetitions). Considering only training session volume, as each work bout for a specific task is completed, ATP-CP turnover slows, and glycogen becomes depleted even after recovery due to peripheral fatigue, reduced phosphagen availability, and exhaustion of glycogen. Ultimately, performance will begin to decline after the athlete completes a certain amount of work during the training session.

📋 COACH'S CORNER

When using this progression for linear speed and acceleration, the Sports Performance Coach must consider the volume for all other types of training outside of SAQ. A judgment call must then be made on whether the volume, intensity, or rest interval should be adjusted to align with the specific athlete or training volume added from other training modes.

TRAINING FREQUENCY

Training frequency for SAQ refers to the number of training sessions performed over a certain period or cycle. Intermediate- and advanced-level athletes are more resilient to increases in training frequency. Hence, when determining the training frequency for an athlete, the level of athleticism and fitness should be considered. However, improvements in SAQ are observed mainly when training frequency remains at two to three training sessions per week. This is primarily because of the amount of work required for other activities such as strength, core, and cardiorespiratory training, which must be considered global training stressors; the programming training frequency for SAQ drills and exercises that have high neuromuscular demands must be considered as well. **Table 13.6** shows reasonable starting frequencies when programming training frequency at the training session level.

TABLE 13.6 SAQ Training Frequency

Linear speed	• Maximal linear speed: 1–3 training sessions per week • Linear acceleration: 1–3 training sessions per week
Agility and MDS	• Agility and MDS (predictable: linear speed + COD): 1–3 training sessions per week • Agility and MDS (unpredictable: linear speed + COD): 1–3 training sessions per week
Quickness	• Quickness (predictable drills): 1–3 training sessions per week • Quickness (unpredictable drills): 1–3 training sessions per week

When SAQ training is performed too frequently, it can result in peripheral fatigue, which reduces muscle function and neural drive due to insufficient replenishment of energy substrates, electrolytes, or repair of cells within muscles. In addition, over repeated sessions, central fatigue can occur; this lowered ability to stimulate motor neurons effectively leads to a reduction in neural drive and force generation ability. Both consequences primarily depend on athleticism and can be resolved by decreasing the frequency of training sessions over a week.

EXERCISE ORDER

Exercise order is important for improving SAQ given the large effort imposed on the neuromuscular system during challenging, maximal linear speed training. Quickness drills are designed to mimic the reactive demands of a sport to decrease total reaction time. Because reactive ability is sensitive to fatigue, quickness drills are best implemented when the athlete is in a fresh state and no residual fatigue will inhibit the rapid performance of reactionary movements. Current best practices indicate that an integrated warm-up should be performed, using various modalities, including a dynamic warm-up. The dynamic warm-up should increase in difficulty from general to more complex movement patterns. Afterward, drills can be progressed based on demand and predictability. **Table 13.7** summarizes the recommended SAQ exercise order.

TABLE 13.7 SAQ Exercise Order

1. Quickness drills (first training session or on a different training day)
2. Maximum linear speed or acceleration (after quickness drills: second training session)
3. Agility and MDS (predictable: linear speed + COD)
4. Agility and MDS (unpredictable: linear speed + COD)

The order of exercises and drills may impact the athlete's energy systems and, in turn, their performance. For example, programming repeated bouts of maximal linear sprints before quickness drills will likely induce fatigue, resulting in impaired reactive ability and a lack of the stimulus necessary to improve reaction times.

REST PERIODS

Rest periods or intervals for SAQ training consist of a period of recovery following a drill or exercise set. Except for tempo work, the work-to-rest ratio is used to assign rest intervals for SAQ training based on the number of repetitions (i.e., the time taken to execute a drill over a certain distance in meters). For example, if a speed drill for 1 set of 30 meters is performed with a work-to-rest ratio of 1:6, the athlete will have a recovery period of 3 times the duration of work recorded to execute the technique drill. If the duration of the set is 30 seconds to perform the drill, the athlete will rest for 180 seconds. In practice, the performance professional will prescribe the **work-to-rest ratio** based on published times, experience with the athlete, or the specific aim of the training session.

Table 13.8 shows that a work-to-rest interval of 1:6 maintains the primary contribution of the ATP-CP and fast anaerobic systems (i.e., fast glycolysis) for maximal linear speed training. In contrast, the intervals of 1:3 and 1:2 maintain the main contributions of the anaerobic system (i.e., fast and slow glycolysis) and the aerobic (i.e., oxidative) system, respectively (Bompa & Haff, 2009).

> **WORK-TO-REST RATIO** →
>
> The proportion of sport activity to the proportion of rest, which is used to assign rest intervals that are specific to a sport, sport position, or sporting movement.

TABLE 13.8 Bioenergetics and Work-to-Rest Ratios

Training Type	Energy System	Aim	Distance	Work-to-Rest Ratio	Rest Interval
Speed	ATP-CP	Acceleration	20–30 m	1:6	2–3 minutes
	Glycolytic	Speed	30–80 m	1:6	3–8 minutes
Speed endurance	ATP-CP	Short	60–90 m	1:3	3–4.5 minutes
	Glycolytic	Short	< 90 m	1:3	< 3 minutes
	ATP-CP + glycolytic	Medium	60–150 m	1:3	3–7.5 minutes
	Oxidative	Long	150–300 m	1:2	5–10 minutes

Data from Bompa, T. O., & Haff, G. G. (2009). Periodization: Theory and methodology of training (5th ed.). Champaign, IL: Human Kinetics.

LESSON 5: MODALITIES FOR SPEED TRAINING
SPEED TRAINING TECHNIQUES

A fundamental principle in developing SAQ is the involvement of linear speed in each training session. Each training session for novice, intermediate, or advanced athletes must include some aspect of linear speed. Two basic avenues to incorporate linear speed in training sessions include the following:

- Maximal linear speed
- Maximal linear acceleration

The foundational exercise (i.e., drill) for speed development is the linear sprint for maximal linear speed and acceleration. Each training session should use either maximal speed or acceleration work. Sprinting progressions for three combinations of sets and repetitions while holding volume constant for either maximal linear speed or maximal linear acceleration are included in **Table 13.9**.

An integrated dynamic warm-up is used to prepare the athlete for maximal-intensity sprint work for each maximal linear speed or acceleration training session. In addition, specialized resistance training exercises can be implemented as warranted on separate training days that focus on developing the hamstrings, glute muscles, and quadriceps. External resistance for linear sprints can also be incorporated at the intermediate level to include the following:

- 30- to 40-meter assisted sprints using a towing apparatus for maximal linear speed
- 10- to 20-meter resisted sprints using an apparatus for acceleration
- 30- to 60-meter resisted sprints using an apparatus for maximal linear speed

Linear speed is best accomplished by focusing on the start, acceleration, maximum speed, and deceleration—that is, the phases of sprinting. For an athlete to run fast,

TABLE 13.9 Sprinting Progressions

Linear speed	1. Maximal linear speed: sprint drill volume (200–350 m); sets (4–7); repetitions (50 m); work-to-rest ratio (1:5)
	2. Maximal linear speed: sprint drill volume (200–350 m); sets (3–5); repetitions (75 m); work-to-rest ratio (1:5)
	3. Maximal linear speed: sprint drill volume (200–350 m); sets (2–3); repetitions (100 m); work-to-rest ratio (1:5)
Linear acceleration	1. Linear acceleration: acceleration drill volume (150–200 m); sets (15–20); repetitions (10 m); work-to-rest ratio (1:5)
	2. Linear acceleration: acceleration drill volume (150–200 m); sets (8–10); repetitions (20 m); work-to-rest ratio (1:5)
	3. Linear acceleration: acceleration drill volume (150–200 m); sets (5–7); repetitions (30 m); work-to-rest ratio (1:5)

they must be able to generate optimal ground contact force to increase the velocity of the body's center of mass during flight and other phases of a sprint (Dintiman, 2020). Elite sprinters do not reach a maximum speed until 55 to 60 meters, and most team sport athletes possess a lower maximum velocity (mph speed) than elite sprinters and may attain top speed in distances as short as 40 yards or less. Nevertheless, studies show that most sprints during team sports competitions are less than 30 yards (Dintiman, 2020). The phases of linear speed, as seen in sports, resemble the phases of the sprint, and can be described as the drive, **transition phase**, and top speed (**Figure 13.17**).

> **TRANSITION PHASE** →
>
> (sprinting) Sprint phase in which back-side mechanics transition to front-side mechanics, moving from the acceleration angle to a more upright stance, preparing for top speed.

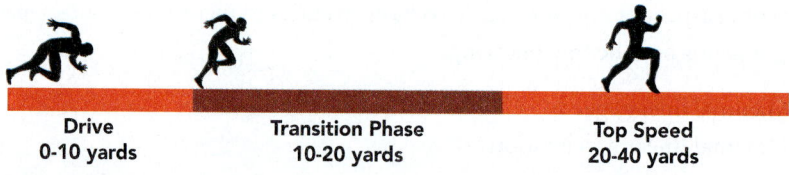

| Drive | Transition Phase | Top Speed |
| 0-10 yards | 10-20 yards | 20-40 yards |

FIGURE 13.17 Linear Speed Phases

The Sports Performance Coach must identify appropriate progressions and loading parameters within an entire SAQ development plan consisting of core, balance, plyometrics, and resistance training, rather than solely focusing on speed, agility, and quickness as separate skills. This requires the Sports Performance Coach to consistently instruct the athlete in quality repetitions. The prescription of linear speed parameters should begin with setting the volume of the training session and using shorter distances (i.e., 50 meters or repetitions) and enough sets to meet the volume requirements. In addition, sprinting movements should be controlled, focusing on proper technique, then progressing to longer distances (i.e., 75 to 100 meters or repetitions) for intermediate and advanced levels, and encouraging maximum effort (i.e., maximal intensity) for each set of sprints. Utilizing the correct active, dynamic warm-up is essential, as is progressing from basic movement patterns to more complex patterns to prepare the athlete for maximal-intensity training to enhance performance during the speed training session.

SPECIALIZED RESISTANCE TRAINING FOR SPEED

Specialized resistance training exercises are vital to developing linear speed and acceleration. However, the Sports Performance Coach must consider the total volume of the session and not load the athlete past the maximum volume if implementing specialized resistance training exercises and external resistance for linear sprints. Supplemental external resistance often is not warranted to develop maximal linear speed. When resistance exercises for strength are implemented, they should follow traditional acute training variables (**Table 13.10**).

TABLE 13.10 Acute Training Variables for Specialized Strength Exercises

Training Focus	Beginner	Intermediate	Advanced
Endurance	1–3 sets 12–20 reps 50–70% intensity Slow tempo 2–4 times per week		
Strength development		2–4 sets 8–12 reps 70–80% intensity Medium tempo 2–4 times per week	
Power			3–5 sets 8–10 reps 30–45% intensity Fast tempo 2–4 times per week

SPECIALIZED STRENGTH EXERCISES FOR SPEED

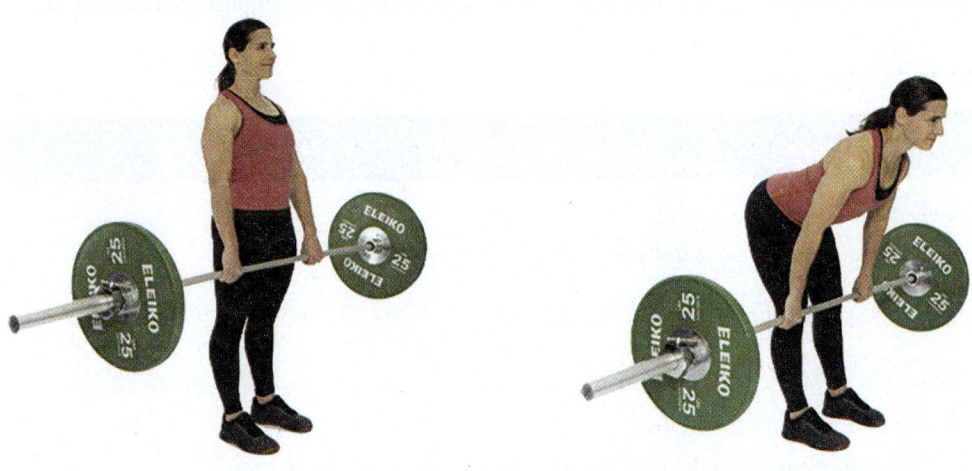

Romanian Deadlift

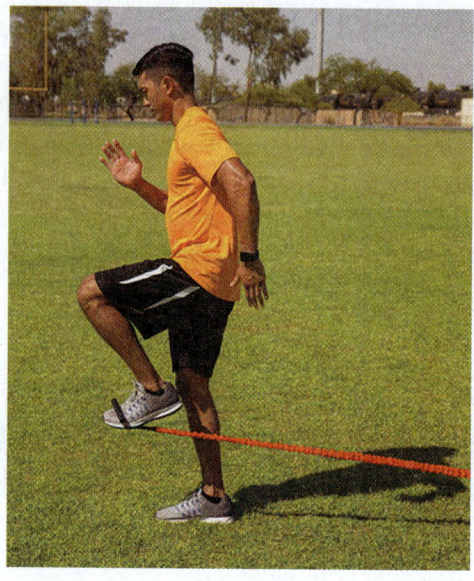

Band Knee Drive

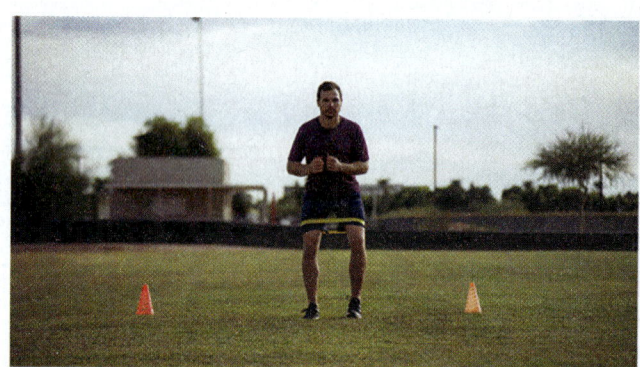

Lateral Band Walk

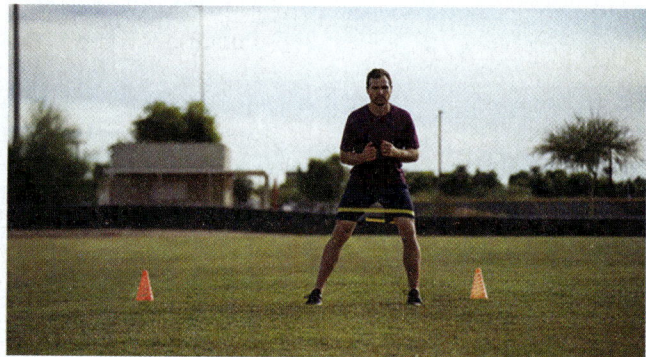

DRILLS FOR LINEAR SPEED

Regarding other speed drills, progressions may vary based on the athlete's level of conditioning and needs. However, as noted earlier in the chapter, most athletes begin by focusing on improving technique and linear speed, with the goal of mastering mechanics. They then reduce the emphasis on the foundational techniques and increase the emphasis on speed of movement. The last progressions may include increased complexity (**Table 13.11**).

TABLE 13.11   Summary of Speed Progressions

Level of Athlete	SAQ Exercises
Beginner	3–4 technique drills (simple) 3–5 speed of movement drills (linear)
Intermediate	2–3 technique drills (increasing complexity) 5–7 speed of movement drills (predictable, linear)
Advanced	1–2 technique drills (complex) 7–10 speed of movement drills (unpredictable, reaction-based, linear)

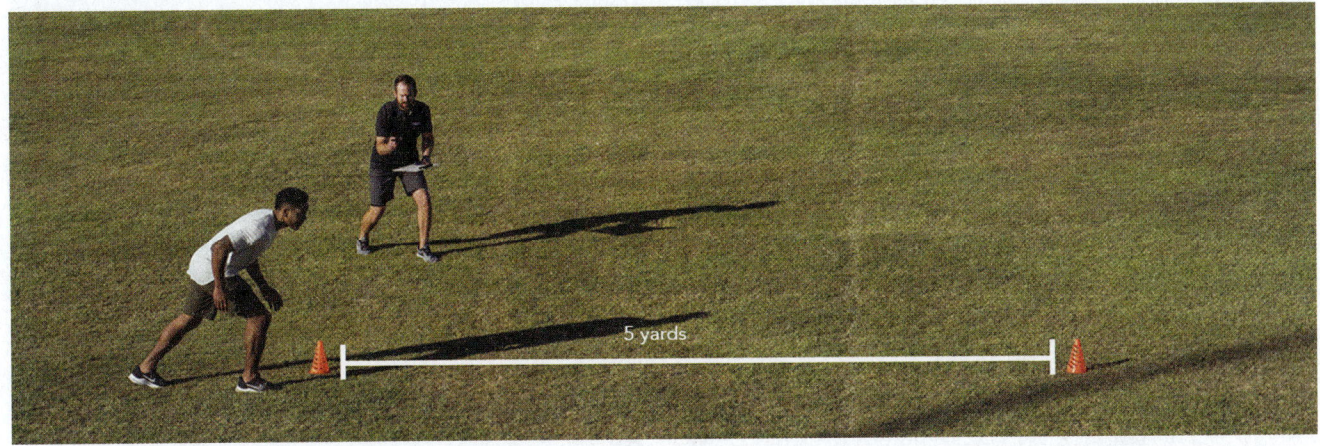

5-Yard Dash

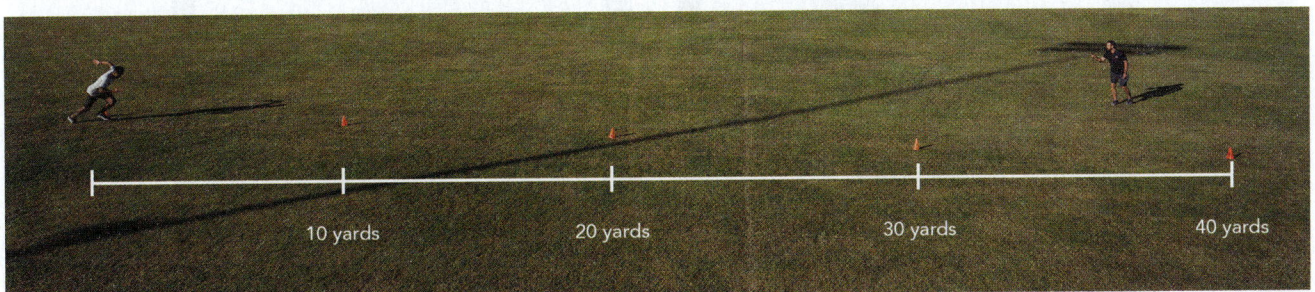

Flying 40-Yard Dash

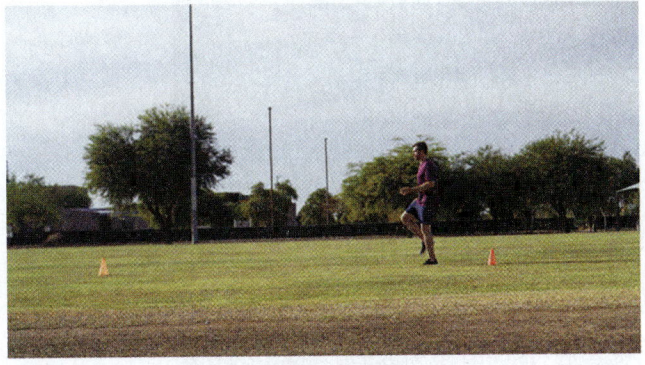

Marches

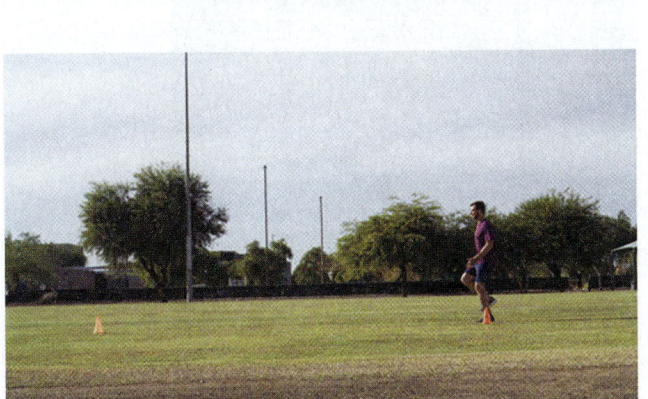

A-Skips

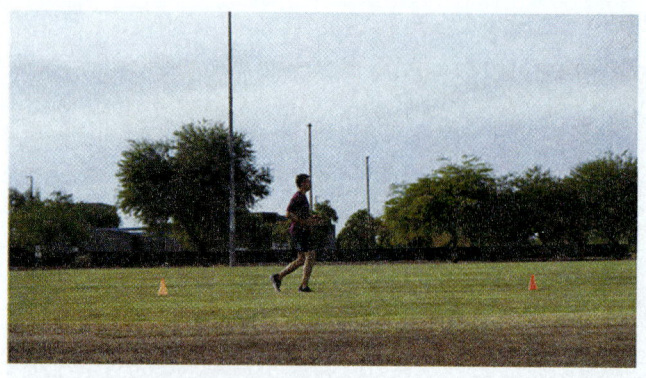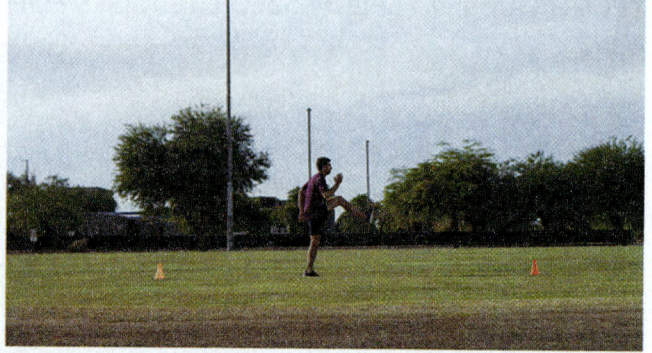

Cycling B-Skips

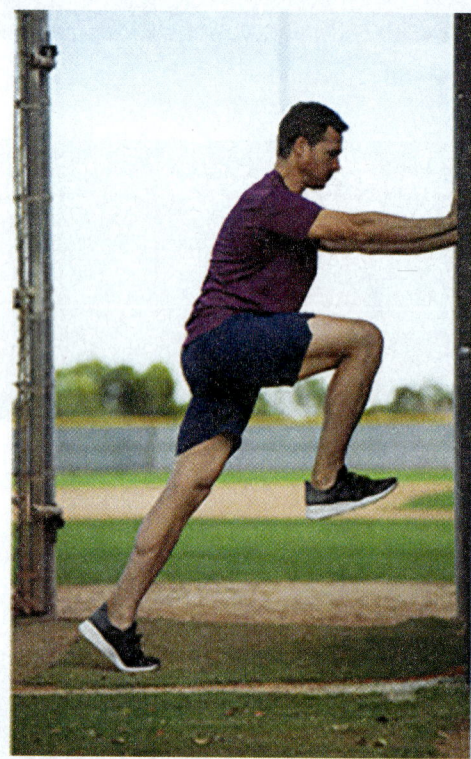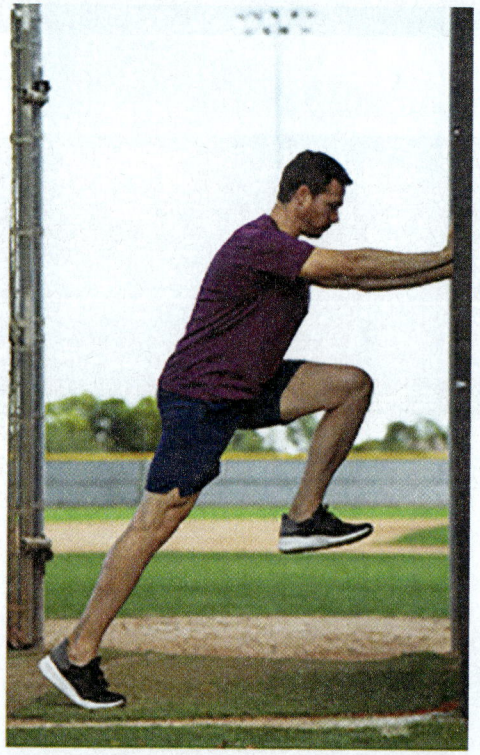

1/3/5 Wall Drill

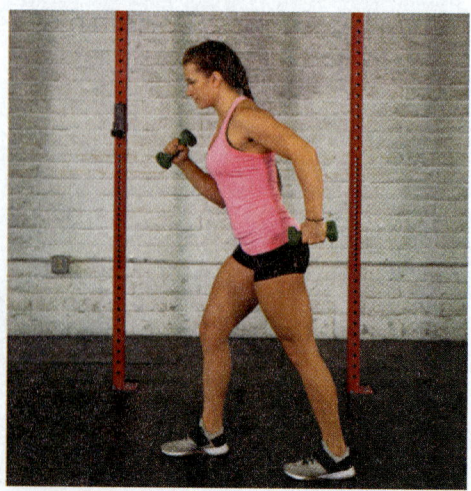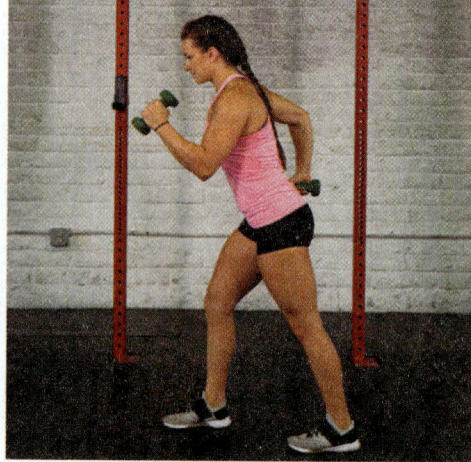

Standing Arm Swings

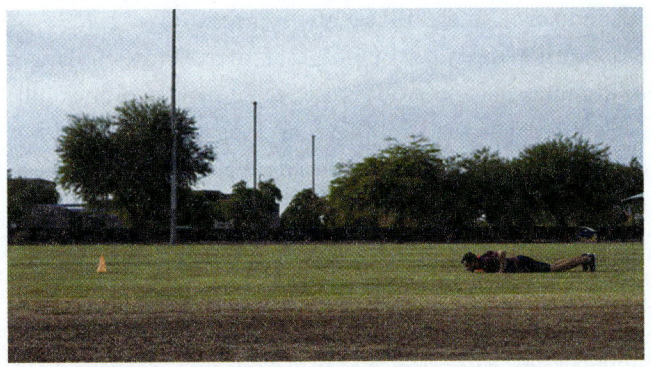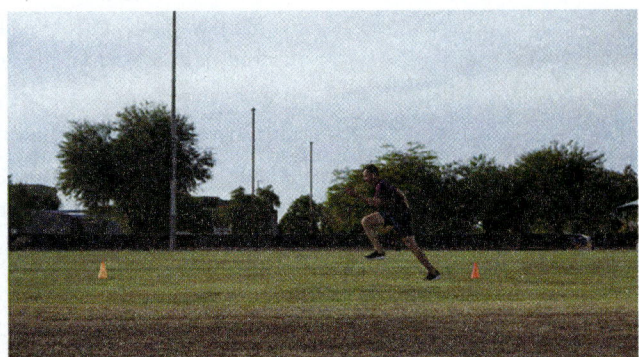

Push-up Sprints

SPECIALIZED SPEED DRILLS

If force (or rate of force development) is a limiting factor of SAQ and general stabilization, strength and power training can enhance performance by altering the force–velocity curve. The point at which strength is sufficient to achieve maximal speed during sports activities varies from athlete to athlete. Therefore, building a solid foundation of stabilization, strength, and power is appropriate, along with mastering basic movement patterns in the early phases of athletic development. After sound mechanical proficiency is established, specialized drills are effective in facilitating higher levels of performance specific to the demands of an athlete's sport. Specialized drills reinforce proper movement patterns in a sport-specific environment while adding heightened demands to the neuromuscular system. These drills often imitate sports scenarios, adding additional reactionary, force, or other neuromuscular demands. However, they do not have to mimic a specific sport to enhance performance in that sport. A common means of adding neuromuscular stimuli to movement drills is by applying the concepts of resisted and assisted speed (**Table 13.12**).

TABLE 13.12   Over-speed and Assisted Drills

Drill Type	Drills
Over-speed drills	Downhill running
	Band-assisted sprinting
Resisted speed drills	Uphill running
	Sled pushes
	Band-resisted sprinting
	Parachute sprinting

OVER-SPEED (ASSISTED DRILLS)

Over-speed or assisted running drills involve an apparatus or changes to the grade of running surfaces that aid in accelerating an athlete's movement. Moderate-grade (5% to 6%) downhill running, assisted bungee cord movement, and other towing mechanisms are used for this type of training. Accelerating at a rate to which the athlete is usually unaccustomed forces the neuromuscular system to adapt to the higher speeds. Assisted speed drills are also effective for improving stride frequency, a key component of running speed.

Sports Performance Coaches should avoid these drills with beginners and use discretion in applying safe amounts of assistance that will not result in overstress or danger to more experienced athletes. For example, 5% to 6% slopes are recommended if downhill running is used, but only if the athlete can perform sprints at that slope without falling. Because this type of training is done at speeds beyond the normal capabilities of an athlete, it is important to have a sound foundation of strength and mechanics to attain maximal effectiveness and prevent injury.

RESISTED SPEED DRILLS

Resisted speed drills require an athlete to move against increased horizontal or vertical loads, which aids in improving force production during the drive phase of the running stride and improves stride length. Weight vests, sled pushes and pulls, uphill running, and partner-resisted drills are all types of resisted speed drills. Light loads (7% to 20% of body weight) are generally recommended for maximal skill carryover because they allow for technique, joint velocities, and loads like those experienced in competition. However, many coaches and trainers use much higher loads to further overload to develop leg strength specific to speed skills such as acceleration.

As with any load-intensive resistance program, proper progression of exercises must be observed. Variation in methods and loads may be the preferred approach to stimulate and develop the many different aspects of speed production.

SPECIALIZED DRILLS FOR SPEED

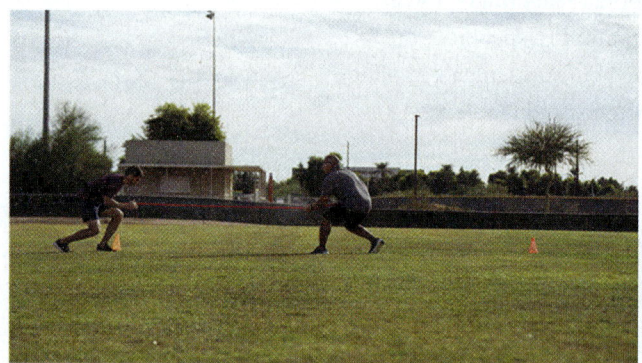
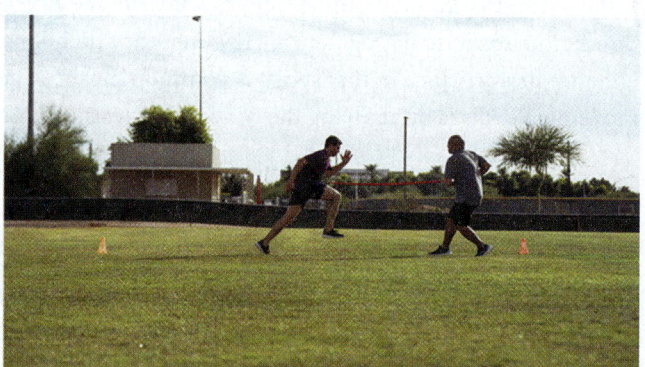

Band-Assisted Sprints

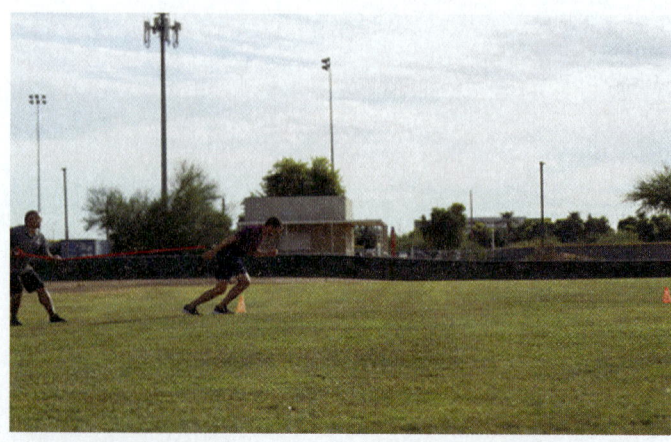

Band-Resisted Sprints

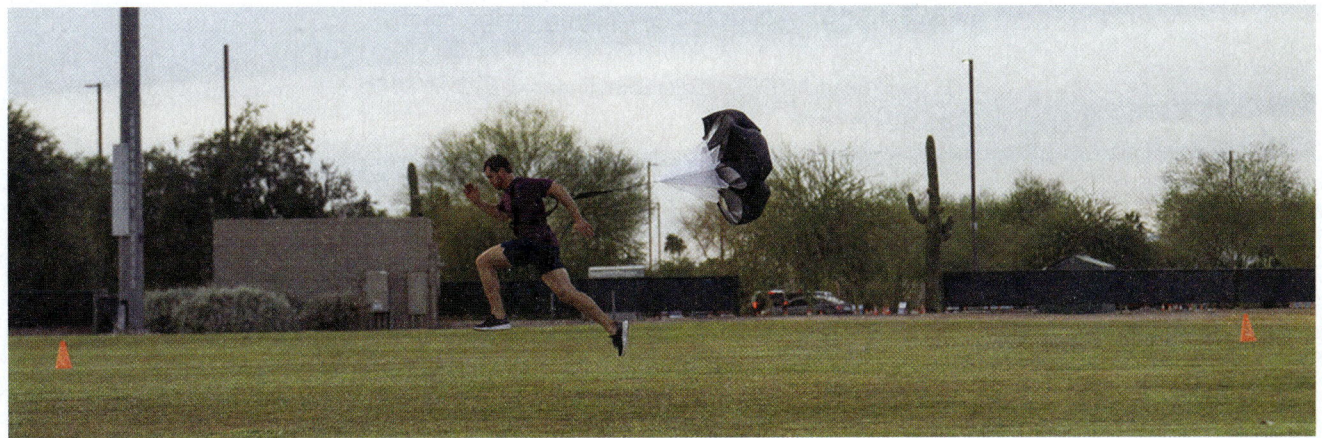

Parachute-Resisted Sprints

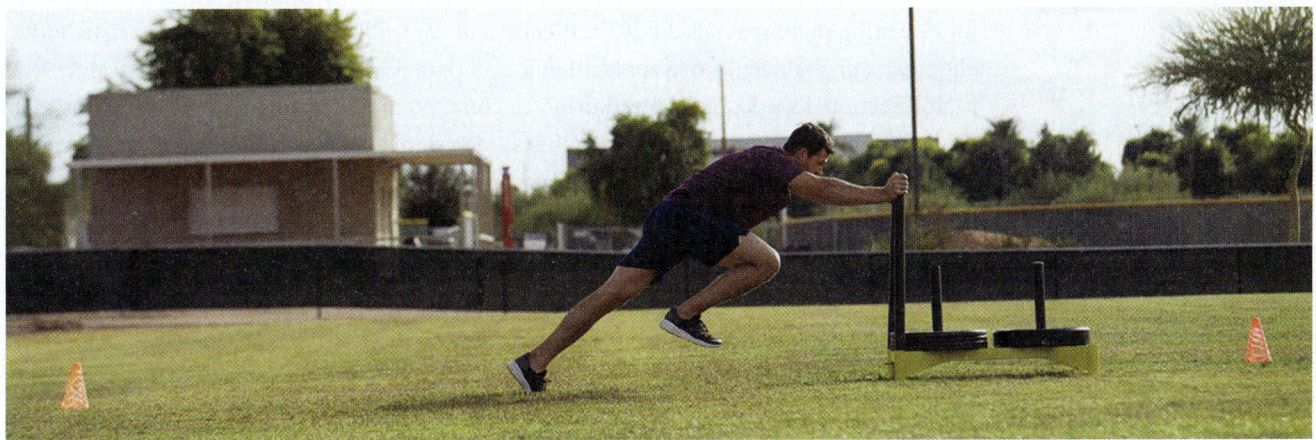

Sled Push

LESSON 6: MODALITIES FOR AGILITY, MDS, AND QUICKNESS TRAINING
AGILITY AND MDS TRAINING TECHNIQUES

When developing SAQ programs, the fundamental guiding principle for acute training variables and progressions is to center the training on maximal linear speed. Therefore, the agility and MDS training sessions for beginning, intermediate, and advanced athletes must incorporate linear speed. There are two basic ways in which linear speed is implemented into agility and MDS training using the established volume parameters:

- Agility and MDS (predictable: linear speed + COD): volume (150–300 m)
- Agility and MDS (unpredictable: linear speed + COD): volume (150–300 m)

The foundational exercise for agility and MDS development is a sprint drill that incorporates directional movement patterns and changes of direction with linear sprinting and acceleration work. Progressions of agility and MDS for three combinations of sets and repetitions while holding the volume constant are identified in **Table 13.13**.

TABLE 13.13   Agility/MDS Training Progressions

1. Agility and MDS (predictable: linear speed + COD): drill volume (150–300 m)
   Sets (3–6); repetitions (50 m); work-to-rest ratio (1:5)
   Sets (2–4); repetitions (75 m); work-to-rest ratio (1:5)
   Sets (1–3); repetitions (100 m); work-to-rest ratio (1:5)

2. Agility and MDS (unpredictable: linear speed + COD): drill volume (150–300 m)
   Sets (3–6); repetitions (50 m); work-to-rest ratio (1:5)
   Sets (2–4); repetitions (75 m); work-to-rest ratio (1:5)
   Sets (1–3); repetitions (100 m); work-to-rest ratio (1:5)

DRILLS FOR AGILITY AND MDS

Mastery of technique forms the foundation of effective agility training and is a prerequisite for executing more specialized drills. Precise and controlled movement, appropriate body alignment, and efficient force application are all paramount for improving agility and multidirectional speed. Specialized drills, in contrast, provide sport-specific scenarios that challenge and enhance an athlete's quickness, decision-making, and adaptability. These drills often simulate sports' dynamic, unpredictable nature and highlight the importance of training athletes to rapidly and accurately change direction in response to varying stimuli. This blend of technique and specialized drills ensures athletes have the necessary skills to excel in their respective sports.

TECHNIQUE AND SPECIALIZED EXERCISES FOR AGILITY AND MDS

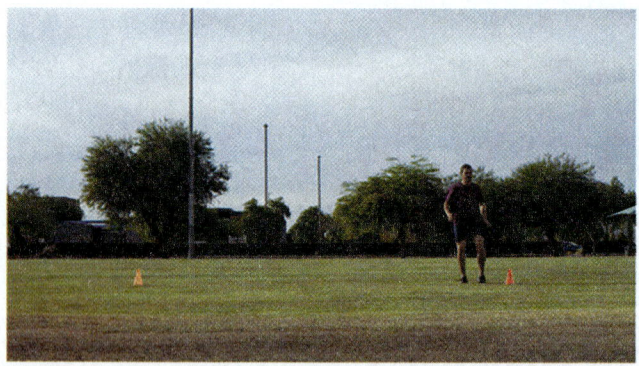 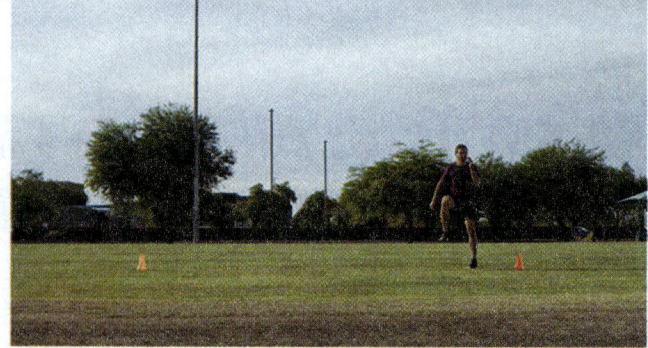

Lateral A-Skips

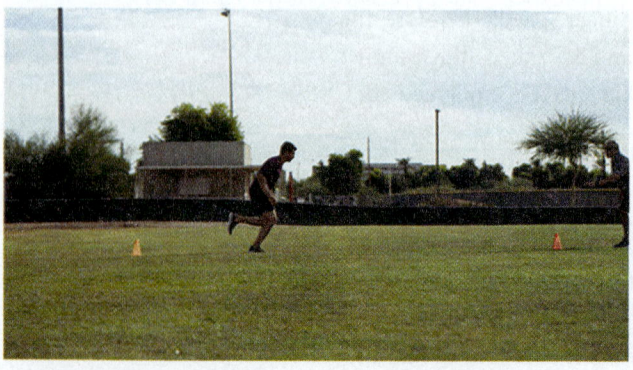 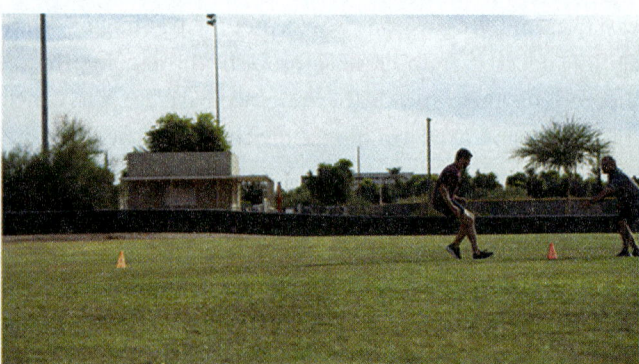

Line-Stop Deceleration Drill (Linear and Lateral)

AGILITY LADDER DRILLS

One current controversy regarding agility training methods involves ladder drills. For Sports Performance Coaches, staying abreast of research can help them to develop a thorough understanding of what is known and cultivate a curious but skeptical approach when examining the efficacy of exercises and drills they use with athletes. The agility ladder is a very common, inexpensive, and easy-to-use training implement that allows trainees and Sports Performance Coaches to create novel constraints during drills to mimic patterns of movement coordination inherent to a specific sport. Unfortunately, despite its widespread popularity and the generally accepted hypothetical benefits of agility ladder use as a training method, there is little research evidence demonstrating the unequivocal validity of this training method to enhance SAQ.

In response to this lack of evidence, recent research has called into question the effectiveness of agility ladders in enhancing SAQ skills. In any case, agility ladders can be a good tool to include during a warm-up and can be used as a novel modality within the athlete's training plan if warranted.

LADDER EXERCISES FOR AGILITY

Jumping Jacks

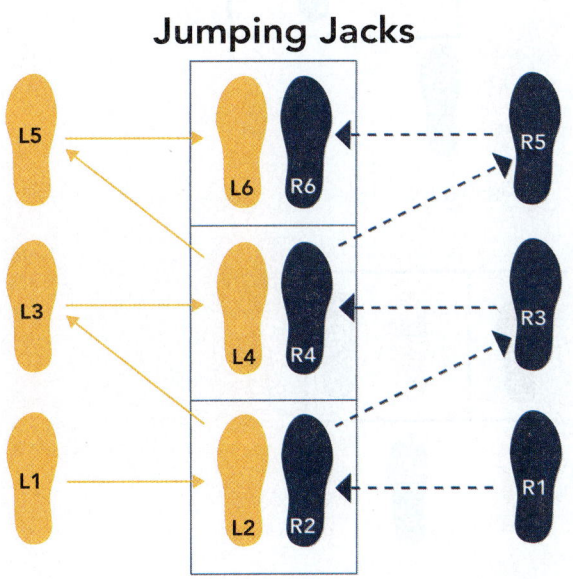

Jumping Jacks

1-In's

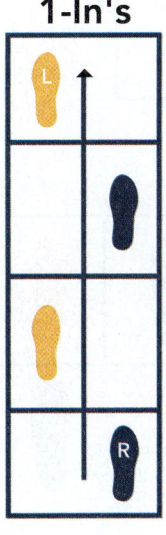

1-In's

2-In's

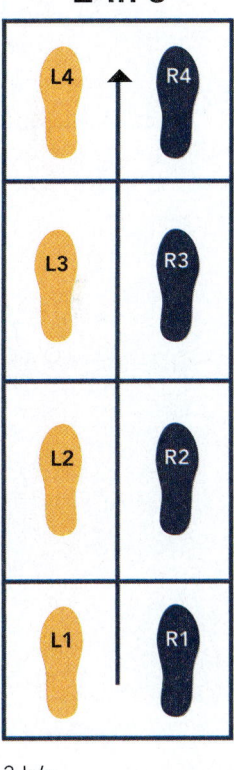

2-In's

Side Shuffle

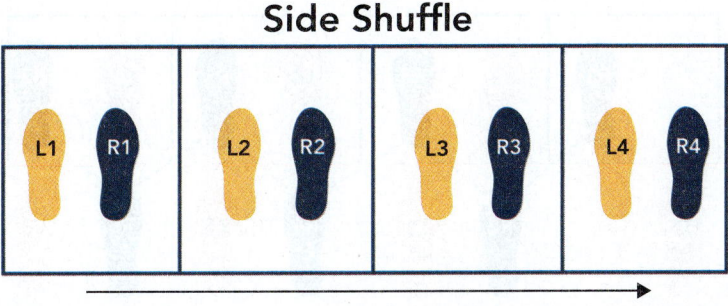

Side Shuffle

Out-Out-In-In

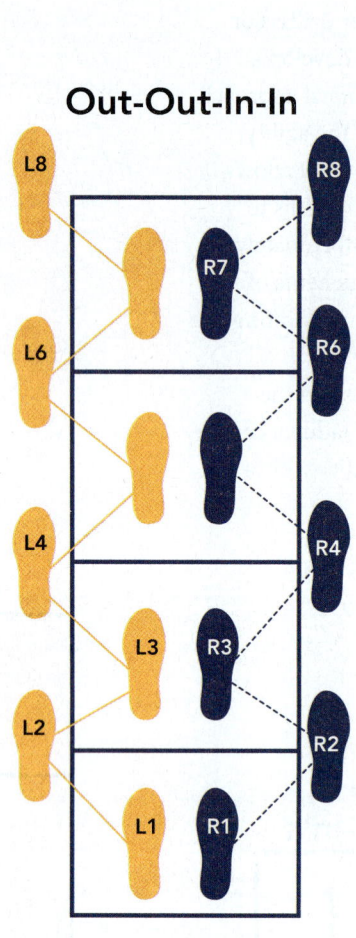

Out-Out-In-In

Zig-Zag

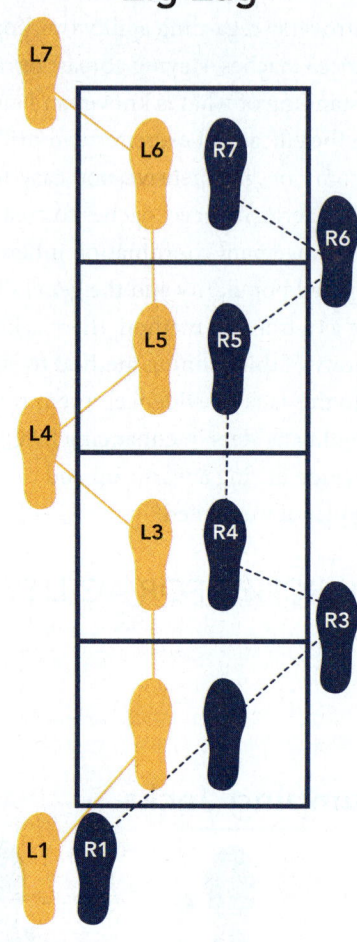

Zig-Zag

Ali Shuffle

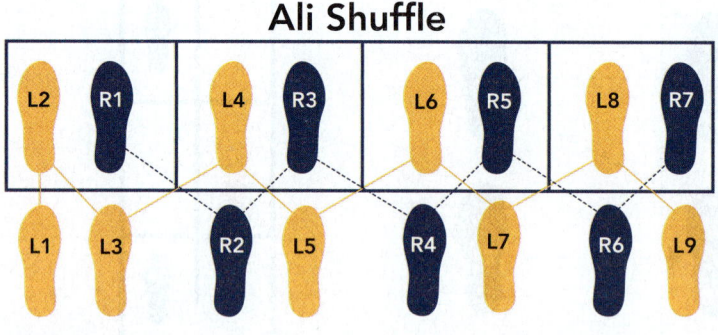

Ali Shuffle

Ali Crossover

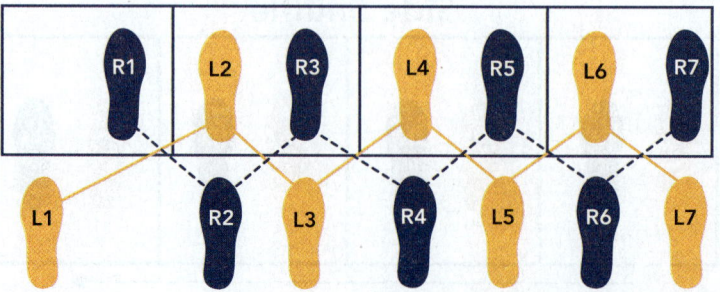

Ali Crossover

W-Weave

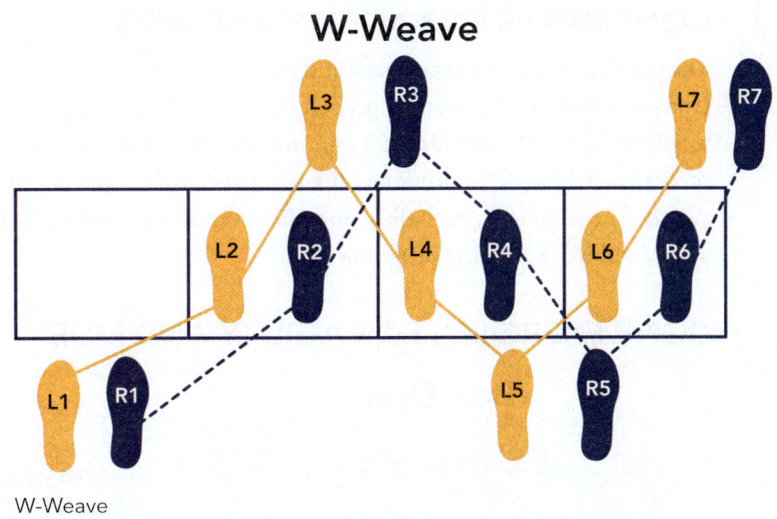

W-Weave

Upper-Body Agility Drill

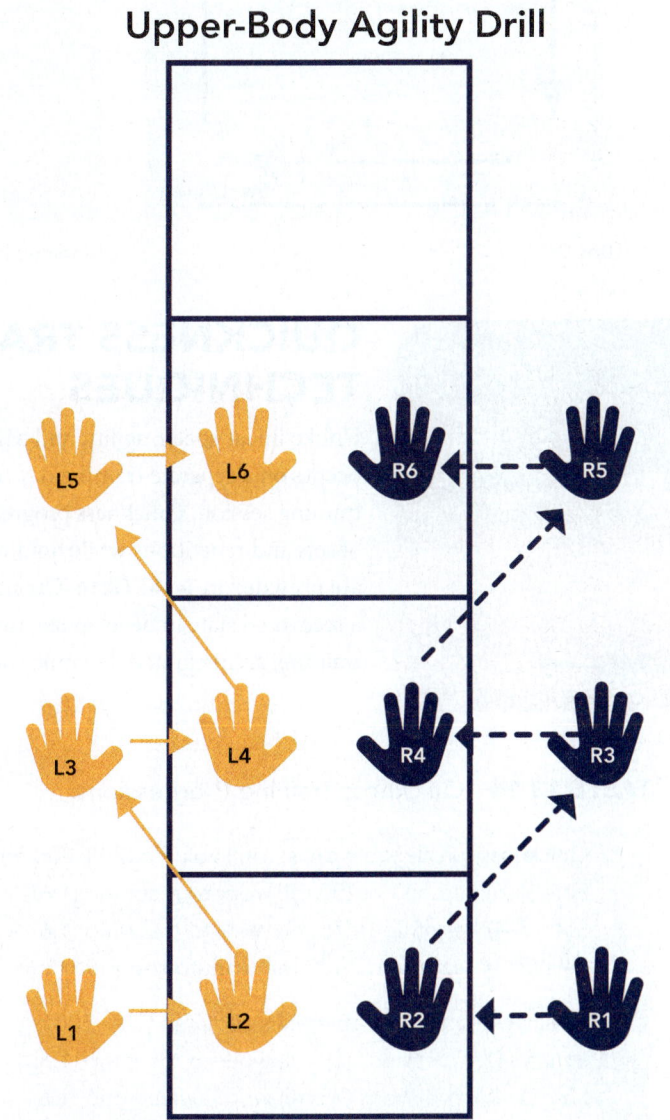

Upper-Body Agility Drill

CONE DRILLS FOR AGILITY AND MDS

The use of cones is both prevalent and an effective tool for developing agility and MDS. Cones are employed to outline predetermined paths, creating clear visual cues for athletes to follow. They can be arranged in numerous configurations to simulate various game-like scenarios, helping to improve an athlete's speed, agility, and ability to change direction swiftly. The simplicity, versatility, and effectiveness of cones make them a cornerstone in agility and MDS training programs.

CONE EXERCISES FOR AGILITY AND MDS

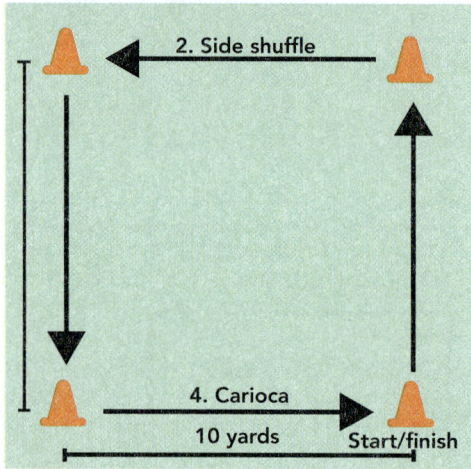

Box Drill

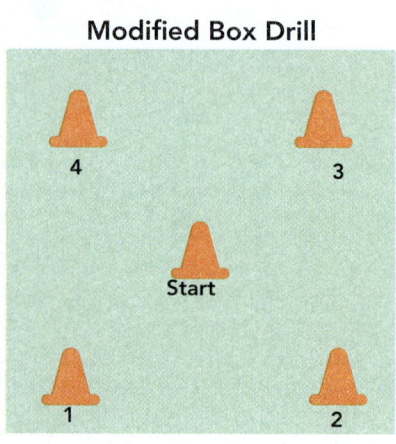

Modified Box Drill

QUICKNESS TRAINING TECHNIQUES

Unlike linear speed, agility, and MDS training, quickness training occurs on a separate training day or at the beginning of an SAQ training session. Quickness progressions for three combinations of sets and repetitions while holding the volume constant are provided in **Table 13.14**. Quickness is best developed in a recovered state to develop reactive ability. Like linear speed training, an integrated dynamic warm-up is recommended.

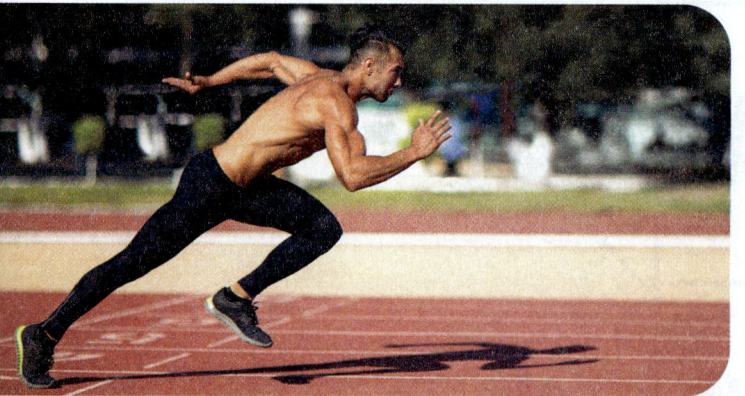

© Jesus Cervantes/Shutterstock

TABLE 13.14 Quickness Training Progressions

1. Quickness (predictable drills): drill volume (200–300 m)
   Sets (4–6); repetitions (50 m); work-to-rest ratio (1:6)
   Sets (3–4); repetitions (75 m); work-to-rest ratio (1:6)
   Sets (2–3); repetitions (100 m); work-to-rest ratio (1:6)

2. Quickness (unpredictable drills): volume (200–300 m)
   Sets (4–6); repetitions (50 m); work-to-rest ratio (1:6)
   Sets (3–4); repetitions (75 m); work-to-rest ratio (1:6)
   Sets (2–3); repetitions (100 m); work-to-rest ratio (1:6)

SPECIALIZED DRILLS FOR QUICKNESS

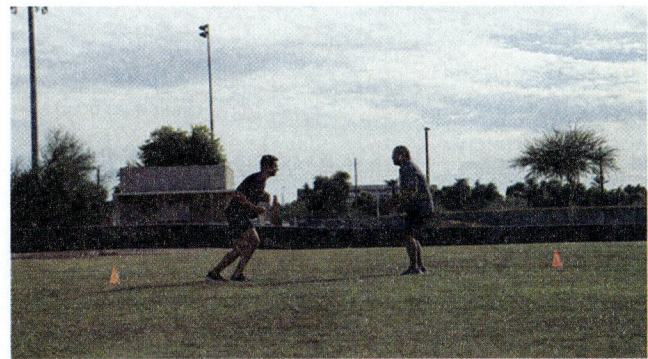
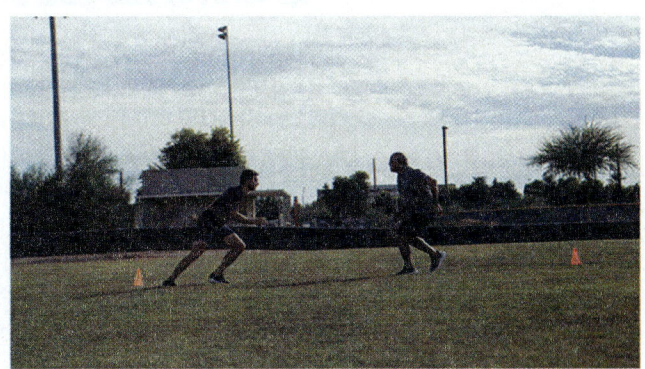

Partner Mirror Drills

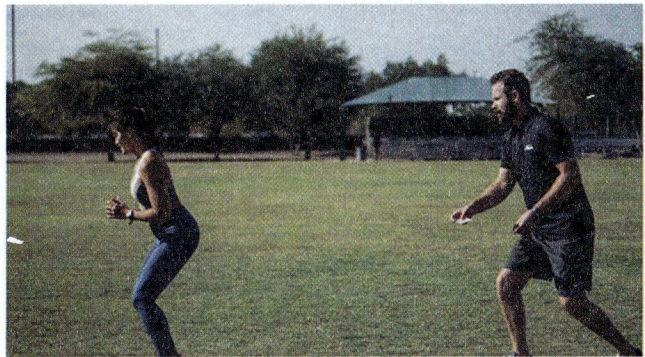
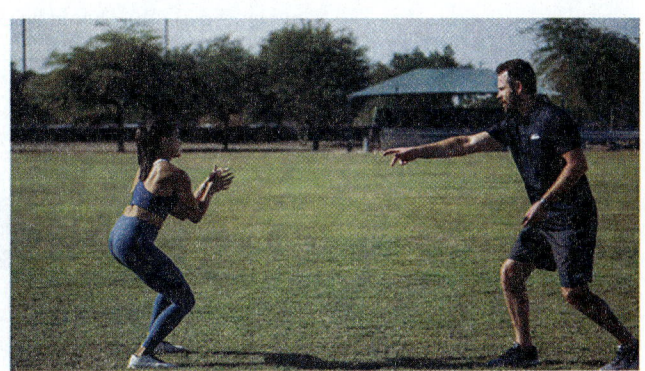

Turn and Grab

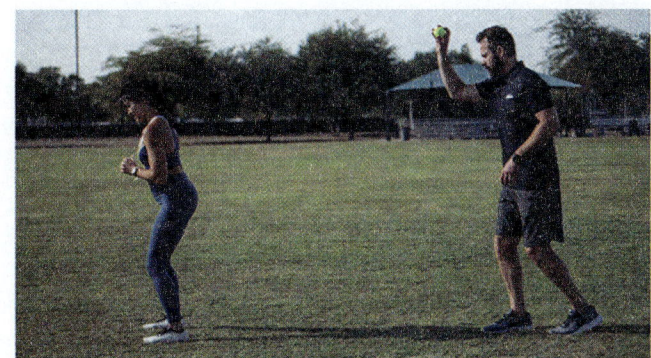
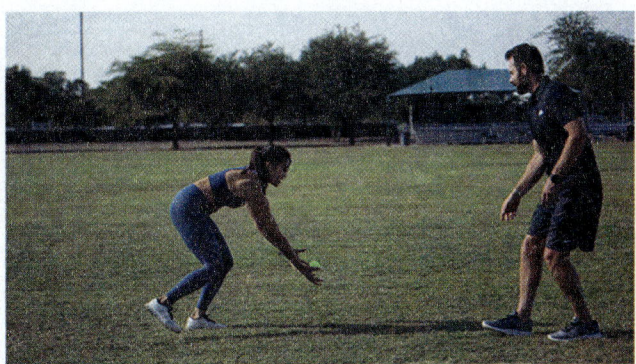

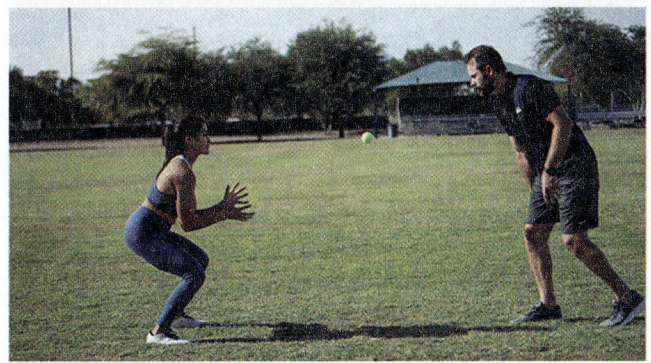
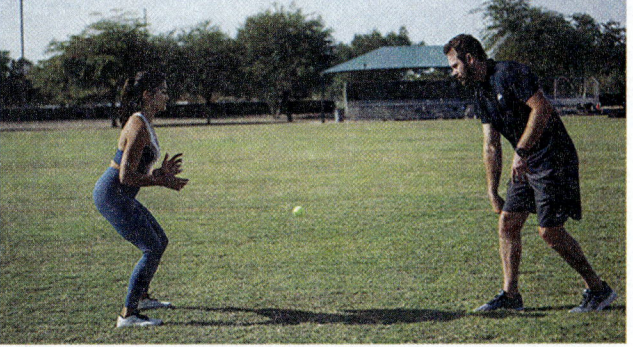

Ball Drill

SUMMARY

This chapter presented the scientific evidence and concepts supporting speed, agility-MDS, and quickness training to promote postural control, reduce injury risk, and facilitate athlete rehabilitation while enhancing sports performance. Further, the acute training variables for SAQ training programs were discussed, with close attention given to the influence of SAQ-specific variables on athletes' energy systems and other acute training variables. Practical information was presented and discussed for each SAQ training guideline, and a systematic approach using a formal needs analysis was recommended to determine the acute training variables needed to develop proper exercise progressions. In addition, SAQ training exercises for speed, agility-MDS, and quickness were identified to allow proper selection of technique drills and exercises by the Sports Performance Coach. The Sports Performance Coach must systematically develop SAQ training programs and thoroughly understand the science regarding SAQ concepts to improve sports performance effectively for athletes.

Table 13.15 illustrates drills for improving the components of linear speed, agility-MDS, and quickness. This should be used as a resource and can be used to determine which drills apply specifically to individual sports.

TABLE 13.15 Summary of Sport Specific Drills

	Football	Basketball	Soccer	Baseball	Hockey	Volleyball
Resisted Knee Drives	x	x	x	x	x	x
Supine Heel Pushes	x		x	x	x	x
Lateral Tube Walking	x	x	x	x	x	x
Reverse Calf Raises	x	x	x	x		x
Superman	x	x	x	x	x	x
Weighted Arm Swings	x		x	x		
Towel Pulls	x	x	x	x		x
Marches	x		x	x		
A-Skips	x		x	x		
Cycling B-Skips	x		x	x		
1/3/5 Wall Drill	x	x	x	x		x
Standing Arm Swings	x		x	x		
Push-Up Sprints	x	x	x	x	x	x

	Football	Basketball	Soccer	Baseball	Hockey	Volleyball
Resisted Sprints	X	X	X	X	X	X
Assisted Sprints	X		X			
Lateral A-Skips	X	X	X	X	X	X
Line-Stop Deceleration	X	X	X			X
Jumping Jacks	X	X	X	X	X	X
In and Out	X	X	X	X		X
Upper-Body Agility	X	X		X	X	X
5–10–5 Drill	X	X	X	X	X	X
T-Drill	X	X	X	X	X	X
Box Drill	X	X	X	X	X	X
Modified Box Drill	X	X	X	X	X	X
W-Drill	X	X	X		X	
Partner Mirror Drill	X	X	X		X	
Turn and Grab Card Drill	X	X		X		X
Agility Ball Drills	X	X	X	X		X

KEY TAKEAWAYS

- SAQ capacities are biomotor skills that can be trained.
- Speed of movement is a determinant of success or failure in many sports.
- Acceleration out of a change of direction is the most important aspect of SAQ training and success in most sports.
- Agility is a biomotor ability that enables the athlete to rapidly change direction and accurately process game stimuli without substantial loss of speed.
- Quickness is a neuromuscular ability that enables the athlete to react, change body position, and perform fast movements without engaging a preceding muscle stretch when external resistance remains at or below 15% of maximal strength.
- A vast body of scientific evidence supports SAQ capacities and concepts.
- Effective SAQ training programs require the judicious application of SAQ concepts, including the following:
  - Athlete needs analysis: strengths and weaknesses of the athlete
  - Sport demands: SAQ training must mimic sport-specific demands

- Acute training variables: exercise selection, sets, repetitions, work-to-rest ratios, and interactive effects on energy systems and substrate usage
- SAQ training variables must be integrated systematically into the OPT Model in the correct levels and phases to develop effective SAQ training programs for clients and athletes.

REFERENCES

Azmi, K., & Kusnanik, N. W. (2018). Effect of exercise program speed, agility, and quickness (SAQ) in improving speed, agility, and acceleration. *Journal of Physics: Conference Series, 947*(012043), 1–6. https://doi.org /10.1088/1742-6596/947/1/012043

Bayne, H. (2018). Force–velocity–power profiles of elite sprinters: Inter-and intra-individual determinants of performance. *ISBS Proceedings Archive, 36*(1), 245.

Beam, J. W. (2002). Rehabilitation including sport-specific functional progression for the competitive athlete. *Journal of Bodywork and Movement Therapies, 6*(4), 205–219. https://doi.org/10.1054/jbmt.2002.0291

Bergmann, J., Kramer, A., & Gruber, M. (2013). Repetitive hops induce postactivation potentiation in triceps surae as well as an increase in the jump height of subsequent maximal drop jumps. *PLoS One, 8*(10), e77705. https://doi.org/10.1371/journal.pone.0077705

Bloomfield, J., Polman, R., O'Donoghue, P., & McNaughton, L. (2007). Effective speed and agility conditioning methodology for random intermittent dynamic type sports. *Journal of Strength and Conditioning Research, 21*(4), 1093–1100. https://pubmed.ncbi.nlm.nih.gov/18076227

Bolger, R., Lyons, M., Harrison, A. J., & Kenny, I. C. (2015). Sprinting performance and resistance-based training interventions: A systematic review. *Journal of Strength and Conditioning Research, 29*(4), 1146–1156. https:// doi.org/10.1519/jsc.0000000000000720

Bompa, T. O., Blumenstein, B., Hoffman, J., Howell, S., & Orbach, I. (2019). *Integrated periodization in sports training and athletic development: Combining training methodology, sports psychology, and nutrition to optimize performance.* AGA Press.

Bompa, T. O., & Buzzichelli, C. A. (2018). *Periodization: Theory and methodology of training* (6th ed.). Human Kinetics.

Bompa, T. O., & Haff, G. G. (2009). Periodization: *Theory and methodology of training* (5th ed.). Human Kinetics.

Brewer, C. (2017). *Athletic movement skills: Training for sports performance.* Human Kinetics.

Brown, L. E., & Ferrigno, V. A. (Eds.). (2015). *Training for speed, agility, and quickness* (3rd ed.) Human Kinetics.

Cavaco, B., Sousa, N., Dos Reis, V. M., Garrido, N., Saavedra, F., Mendes, R., & Vilaça-Alves, J. (2014). Short-term effects of complex training on agility with the ball, speed, efficiency of crossing and shooting in youth soccer players. *Journal of Human Kinetics, 43,* 105–112. https://www.ncbi.nlm.nih.gov/pmc/articles/PMC4332169

Chaabene, H., Negra, Y., Moran, J., Prieske, O., Sammoud, S., Ramirez-Campillo, R., & Granacher, U. (2021). Plyometric training improves not only measures of linear speed, power, and change-of-direction speed but also repeated sprint ability in young female handball players. *Journal of Strength and Conditioning Research, 35*(8), 2230–2235. https://doi.org/10.1519/jsc.0000000000003128

Chaouachi, A., Chtara, M., Hammami, R., Chtara, H., Turki, O., & Castagna, C. (2014). Multidirectional sprints and small-sided games training effect on agility and change of direction abilities in youth soccer. *Journal of Strength & Conditioning Research, 28*(11), 3121–3127. https://doi.org/10.1519/jsc.0000000000000505

Cissik, J. M., & Barnes, M. (2011). *Sport speed and agility training* (2nd ed.). Coaches Choice.

Del Vecchio, A., Negro, F., Holobar, A., Casolo, A., Folland, J. P., Felici, F., & Farina, D. (2019). You are as fast as your motor neurons: Speed of recruitment and maximal discharge of motor neurons determine the maximal rate of force development in humans. *Journal of Physiology, 597*(9), 2445–2456. https://doi.org/https://doi .org/10.1113/JP277396

DeWeese, B. H., & Nimphius, S. (2016). Program design and technique for speed and agility training. In G. G. Haff & N. T. Triplett (Eds.), *Essentials of strength training and conditioning* (4th ed., pp. 521–558). Human Kinetics.

Dijksma, I., Perry, S. I. B., Zimmermann, W. O., Lucas, C., & Stuiver, M. M. (2019). Effects of agility training on body control, change of direction speed and injury attrition rates in Dutch recruits: A pilot study. *Journal of Military and Veterans' Health, 27*(2), 28–40.

Dintiman, G. B. (2020). *NASE essentials of next-generation sports speed training.* Healthy Learning.

Formenti, D., Duca, M., Trecroci, A., Ansaldi, L., Bonfanti, L., Alberti, G., & Iodice, P. (2019). Perceptual vision training in non-sport-specific context: Effect on performance skills and cognition in young females. *Scientific Reports, 9*(18671), 1–13. https://doi.org/10.1038/s41598-019-55252-1

Galpin, A. J., Li, Y., Lohnes, C. A., & Schilling, B. K. (2008). A 4-week choice foot speed and choice reaction training program improves agility in previously non-agility trained, but active men and women. *Journal of Strength and Conditioning Research, 22*(6), 1901–1907. https://doi.org/10.1519/JSC.0b013e3181887e3f

Gambetta, V. (2007). *Athletic development: The art and science of functional sports conditioning.* Human Kinetics.

Gonjo, T., & Olstad, B. H. (2021). Differences between elite and sub-elite swimmers in a 100 m breaststroke: A new race analysis approach with time-series velocity data. *Sports Biomechanics,* 1–12. https://doi.org /10.1080/14763141.2021.1954238

Hamill, J., Knutzen, K. M., & Derrick, T. R. (2015). *Biomechanical basis of human movement* (4th ed.). Wolters Kluwer.

Hammami, M., Negra, Y., Shephard, R. J., & Chelly, M. S. (2017). The effect of standard strength vs. contrast strength training on the development of sprint, agility, repeated change of direction, and jump in junior male soccer players. *Journal of Strength and Conditioning Research, 31*(4), 901–912. https://doi.org/10.1519 /jsc.0000000000001815

Harry, J. R., Barker, L. A., James, R., & Dufek, J. S. (2018). Performance differences among skilled soccer players of different playing positions during vertical jumping and landing. *Journal of Strength and Conditioning Research, 32*(2), 304–312. https://doi.org/10.1519/jsc.0000000000002343

Healy, R., Kenny, I. C., & Harrison, A. J. (2021). Resistance training practices of sprint coaches. *Journal of Strength and Conditioning Research, 35*(7), 1939–1948. https://doi.org/10.1519/jsc.0000000000002992

Hrysomallis, C. (2012). The effectiveness of resisted movement training on sprinting and jumping performance. *Journal of Strength and Conditioning Research, 26*(1), 299–306. https://doi.org/10.1519/JSC .0b013e3182185186

Jeffreys, I. (2013). *Developing speed.* Human Kinetics.

Jovanovic, M., Sporis, G., Omrcen, D., & Fiorentini, F. (2011). Effects of speed, agility, quickness training method on power performance in elite soccer players. *Journal of Strength and Conditioning Research, 25*(5), 1285–1292. https://doi.org/10.1519/JSC.0b013e3181d67c65

Karandikar, N., & Ortiz Vargas, O. O. (2011). Kinetic chains: A review of the concept and its clinical applications. *PM&R, 3*(8), 739–745. https://doi.org/10.1016/j.pmrj.2011.02.021

Keiner, M., Kadlubowski, B., Sander, A., Hartmann, H., & Wirth, K. (2020). Effects of 10 months of speed, functional, and traditional strength training on strength, linear sprint, change of direction, and jump performance in trained adolescent soccer players. *Journal of Strength and Conditioning Research, 36*(8), 2236–2246. https://doi.org/10.1519/JSC.0000000000003807

Keller, S., Koob, A., Corak, D., von Schöning, V., & Born, D.-P. (2020). How to improve change-of-direction speed in junior team sport athletes—horizontal, vertical, maximal, or explosive strength training? *Journal of Strength and Conditioning Research, 34*(2), 473–482. https://doi.org/10.1519/jsc.0000000000002814

King, J. A., & Cipriani, D. J. (2010). Comparing preseason frontal and sagittal plane plyometric programs on vertical jump height in high-school basketball players. *Journal of Strength and Conditioning Research, 24*(8), 2109–2114. https://doi.org/10.1519/JSC.0b013e3181e347d1

Komi, P. V. (Ed.). (2005). *Strength and power in sport: Volume III of the encyclopaedia of sports medicine* (2nd ed.). Wiley-Blackwell Science.

Komi, P. V. (Ed.). (2011). *Neuromuscular aspects of sport performance: Volume XVII of the encyclopedia of sports medicine.* Wiley-Blackwell.

Lennemann, L. M., Sidrow, K. M., Johnson, E. M., Harrison, C. R., Vojta, C. N., & Walker, T. B. (2013). The influence of agility training on physiological and cognitive performance. *Journal of Strength and Conditioning Research, 27*(12), 3300–3309. https://doi.org/10.1519/JSC.0b013e31828ddf06

Levin, M. F. (2014). *Progress in motor control: Skill learning, performance, health, and injury* (Vol. 826). Springer. https://doi.org/10.1007/978-1-4939-1338-1

Lichtenstein, E., Morat, M., Roth, R., Donath, L., & Faude, O. (2020). Agility-based exercise training compared to traditional strength and balance training in older adults: A pilot randomized trial. *PeerJ, 8,* e8781. https:// doi.org/10.7717/peerj.8781

Lockie, R. G., Schultz, A. B., Callaghan, S. J., & Jeffriess, M. D. (2014). The effects of traditional and enforced stopping speed and agility training on multidirectional speed and athletic function. *Journal of Strength & Conditioning Research, 28*(6), 1538–1551. https://doi.org/10.1519/jsc.0000000000000309

Lorenz, D. (2011). Postactivation potentiation: An introduction. *International Journal of Sports Physical Therapy, 6*(3), 234–240.

Maloney, S. J., Richards, J., Jelly, L., & Fletcher, I. M. (2019). Unilateral stiffness interventions augment vertical stiffness and change of direction speed. *Journal of Strength and Conditioning Research, 33*(2), 372–379. https://doi.org/10.1519/jsc.0000000000002006

Mehran, N., Williams, P. N., Keller, R. A., Khalil, L. S., Lombardo, S. J., & Kharrazi, F. D. (2016). Athletic performance at the National Basketball Association combine after anterior cruciate ligament reconstruction. *Orthopaedic Journal of Sports Medicine, 4*(5), 2325967116648083. https://doi.org/10.1177/2325967116648083

Miller, M. G., Herniman, J. J., Ricard, M. D., Cheatham, C. C., & Michael, T. J. (2006). The effects of a 6-week plyometric training program on agility. *Journal of Sports Science & Medicine, 5*(3), 459–465.

Mills, J. D., & Taunton, J. E. (2003). The effect of spinal stabilisation training on spinal mobility, vertical jump, agility, and balance. *Medicine & Science in Sports & Exercise, 35*(5), S323. http://doi.org/10.1097/00005768-200305001-01791

Nicol, C. (2009). The stretch–shortening cycle as a model to study compensatory mechanisms of muscle-tendon deficits. *Biomechanics.* Université de la Méditerranée - Aix-Marseille II. https://hal-amu.archives-ouvertes.fr/tel-01644913

Oden, G. L., Wagner, M. C., & Glave, A. P. (2014). Development of agility utilizing a multidimensional modality of plyometrics. *Journal of Fitness Research, 3,* 51–59.

Özkaya, N., Leger, D., Goldsheyder, D., & Nordin, M. (2017). *Fundamentals of biomechanics: Equilibrium, motion, and deformation* (4th ed.). Springer International. https://doi.org/10.1007/978-3-319-44738-4

Paillard, T. (2014). Sport-specific balance develops specific postural skills. *Sports Medicine, 44*(7), 1019–1020. https://doi.org/10.1007/s40279-014-0174-x

Panascì, M., Di Gennaro, S., Ferrando, V., Filipas, L., Ruggeri, P., & Faelli, E. (2023). Efficacy of resisted sled sprint training compared with unresisted sprint training on acceleration and sprint performance in rugby players: An 8-week randomized controlled trial. *International Journal of Sports Physiology and Performance, 18*(10), 1189–1195. https://doi.org/10.1123/ijspp.2023-0103

Paszkewicz, J., Webb, T., Waters, B., Welch McCarty, C., & Van Lunen, B. (2012). The effectiveness of injury-prevention programs in reducing the incidence of anterior cruciate ligament sprains in adolescent athletes. *Journal of Sport Rehabilitation, 21*(4), 371–377. https://doi.org/10.1123/jsr.21.4.371

Powers, S. K., & Howley, E. T. (2018). *Exercise physiology: Theory and application to fitness and performance* (10th ed.). McGraw-Hill.

Ramirez-Campillo, R., Alvarez, C., Gentil, P., Loturco, I., Sanchez-Sanchez, J., Izquierdo, M., Moran, J., Nakamura, F., Chaabene, H., Granacher, U. (2020). Sequencing effects of plyometric training applied before or after regular soccer training on measures of physical fitness in young players. *Journal of Strength and Conditioning Research, 34*(7), 1959–1966. https://doi.org/10.1519/jsc.0000000000002525

Rhea, M. R., Kenn, J. G., Peterson, M. D., Massey, D., Simão, R., Marín, P., Favero, M., Cardozo, D., & Krein, D. (2016). Joint-angle specific strength adaptations influence improvements in power in highly trained athletes. *Human Movement, 17*(1), 43–49. https://doi.org/10.1515/humo-2016-0006

Rodríguez-Rosell, D., Franco-Márquez, F., Mora-Custodio, R., & González-Badillo, J. J. (2017). Effect of high-speed strength training on physical performance in young soccer players of different ages. *Journal of Strength and Conditioning Research, 31*(9), 2498–2508. https://doi.org/10.1519/jsc.0000000000001706

Sado, N., Yoshioka, S., & Fukashiro, S. (2020). Three-dimensional kinetic function of the lumbo-pelvic-hip complex during block start. *PLoS One, 15*(3), e0230145. https://doi.org/10.1371/journal.pone.0230145

Salonikidis, K., & Zafeiridis, A. (2008). The effects of plyometric, tennis-drills, and combined training on reaction, lateral and linear speed, power, and strength in novice tennis players. *Journal of Strength and Conditioning Research, 22*(1), 182–191. https://doi.org/10.1519/JSC.0b013e31815f57ad

Sassi, R. H., Dardouri, W., Yahmed, M. H., Gmada, N., Mahfoudhi, M. E., & Gharbi, Z. (2009). Relative and absolute reliability of a modified agility T-test and its relationship with vertical jump and straight sprint. *Journal of Strength and Conditioning Research, 23*(6), 1644–1651. https://doi.org/10.1519/JSC.0b013e3181b425d2

Schmidt, R. A., Lee, T. D., Winstein, C. J., Wulf, G., & Zelaznik, H. N. (2019). *Motor control and learning: A behavioral emphasis* (6th ed.). Human Kinetics.

Seiberl, W., Hahn, D., Power, G. A., Fletcher, J. R., & Siebert, T. (2021). The stretch–shortening cycle of active muscle and muscle-tendon complex: What, why and how it increases muscle performance? *Frontiers in Physiology, 12,* 693141. https://doi.org/10.3389/fphys.2021.693141

Shapie, M. N. M., & Rohizam, R. N. F. R. (2018). A case study: The effects of speed, agility and quickness (SAQ) training program on hand-eye coordination and dynamic balance among children. *Journal of Physical Fitness, Medicine & Treatment in Sports, 2*(4), 1–6. https://doi.org/10.19080/JPFMTS.2018.02.555591

Styles, W. J., Matthews, M. J., & Comfort, P. (2016). Effects of strength training on squat and sprint performance in soccer players. *Journal of Strength and Conditioning Research, 30*(6), 1534–1539. https://doi.org/10.1519/jsc.0000000000001243

Tanir, H. (2018). The effect of balance and stability workouts on the development of static and dynamic balance in 10–12-year-old soccer players. *Journal of Education and Training Studies, 6*(9), 132–135. https://doi.org/10.11114/jets.v6i9.3499

Trecroci, A., Milanović, Z., Frontini, M., Iaia, F. M., & Alberti, G. (2018). Physical performance comparison between under 15 elite and sub-elite soccer players. *Journal of Human Kinetics, 61,* 209–216. https://www.ncbi.nlm.nih.gov/pmc/articles/PMC5873350

Trecroci, A., Milanović, Z., Rossi, A., Broggi, M., Formenti, D., & Alberti, G. (2016). Agility profile in sub-elite under-11 soccer players: Is SAQ training adequate to improve sprint, change of direction speed and reactive agility performance? *Research in Sports Medicine, 24*(4), 331–340. https://doi.org/10.1080/15438627.2016.1228063

Uthoff, A., Oliver, J., Cronin, J., Harrison, C., & Winwood, P. (2020). Sprint-specific training in youth: Backward running vs. forward running training on speed and power measures in adolescent male athletes. *Journal of Strength and Conditioning Research, 34*(4), 1113–1122. https://doi.org/10.1519/jsc.0000000000002914

Verkhoshansky, Y. V., & Siff, M. C. (2009). *Supertraining* (6th ed.). Ultimate Athlete Concepts.

Young, M. (2017). *Smart speed and power training with Mike Young: Episode 1* [Video]. Fusion Sport. https://www.youtube.com/watch?v=CogtRux-5t0

Young, M. (2021). Maximal velocity sprint mechanics. *Human Performance Consulting, 1–14.*

Young, W., James, R., & Montgomery, I. (2002). Is muscle power related to running speed with changes of direction? *Journal of Sports Medicine and Physical Fitness, 42*(3), 282–288.

Zago, M., Giuriola, M., & Sforza, C. (2016). Effects of a combined technique and agility program on youth soccer players' skills. *International Journal of Sports Science & Coaching, 11*(5), 710–720. https://doi.org/10.1177/1747954116667109

Zatsiorsky, V. M., Kraemer, W. J., & Fry, A. C. (2021). *Science and practice of strength training* (3rd ed.). Human Kinetics.

Zemková, E., & Hamar, D. (2018). Sport-specific assessment of the effectiveness of neuromuscular training in young athletes. *Frontiers in Physiology, 9,* 264. https://doi.org/10.3389/fphys.2018.00264

Zemková, E., Viitasalo, J., Hannola, H., Blomqvist, M., Konttine-N, N., & Mononen, K. (2007). The effect of maximal exercise on static and dynamic balance in athletes and non-athletes. *Medicina Sportiva, 11*(3), 70–77. https://www.researchgate.net/publication/245342164_The_Effect_of_Maximal_Exercise_on_Static_and_Dynamic_Balance_in_Athletes_and_Non-Athletes

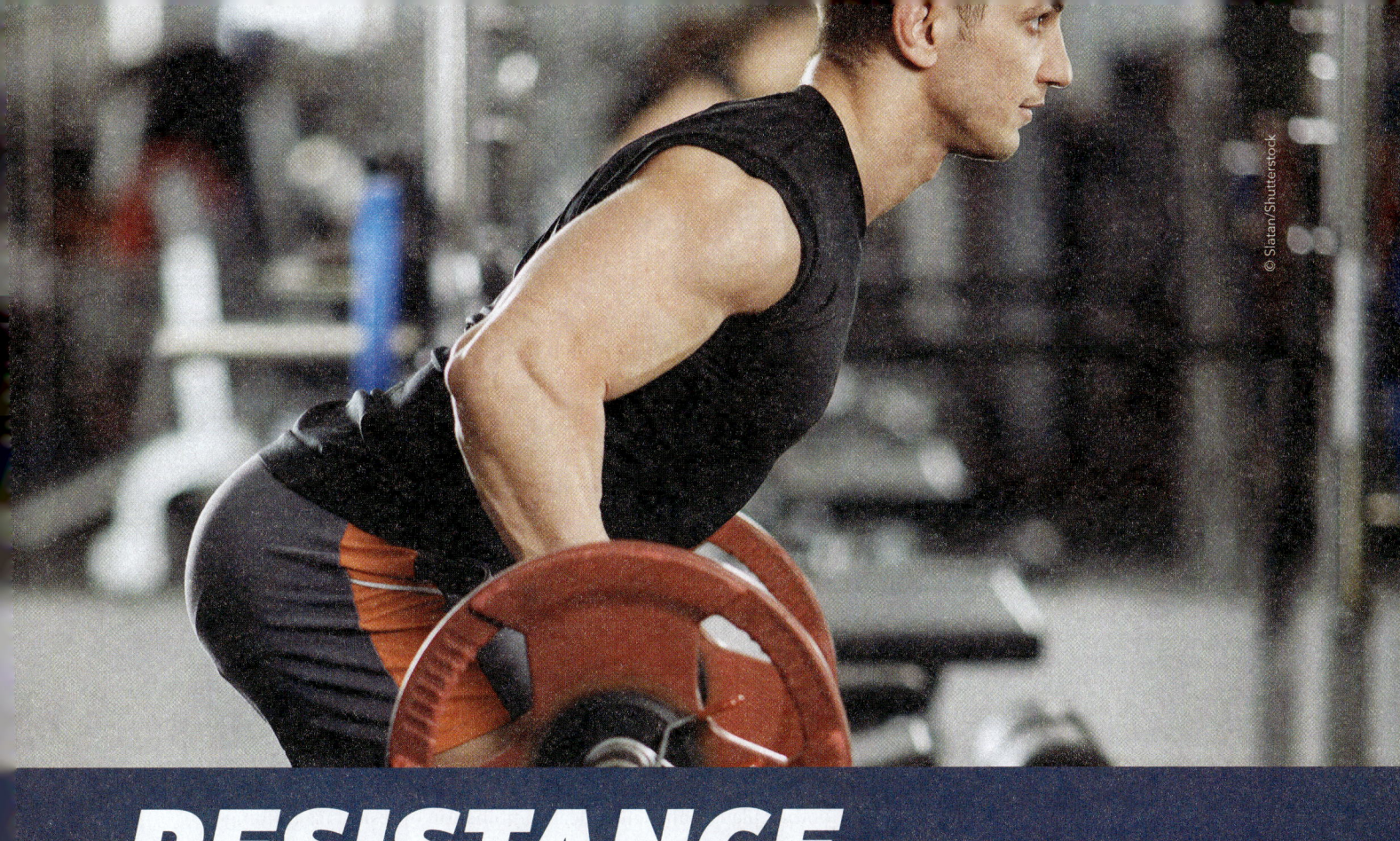

RESISTANCE TRAINING FOR SPORTS PERFORMANCE

LEARNING OBJECTIVES

Upon completion of this chapter, the Sports Performance Coach will be able to:

- **Summarize** the importance of resistance training for athletes with differing performance-related goals.

- **Explain** the scientific rationale for resistance training.

- **Describe** different resistance training techniques used within performance training.

- **Identify** appropriate acute training variables for resistance training.

- **Select** resistance training programs or techniques based on athlete needs.

LESSON 1: INTRODUCTION TO RESISTANCE TRAINING

INTRODUCTION

Resistance training develops a wide range of strength capacities and is a cornerstone in the physical preparation for athletes of all levels (Suchomel et al., 2016). **Strength capacity** is the maximal output of the neuromuscular system. Resistance training leads to improvements in muscular endurance, maximal strength, power, and speed, all of which underpin performance in a myriad of sports. It can also reduce the risk of acute sports injuries like anterior cruciate ligament (ACL) ruptures and chronic injuries like tendinopathies (Lauersen et al., 2018).

However, there is more to resistance training than just lifting heavy barbells or dumbbells. In fact, Sports Performance Coaches can utilize a wide variety of loading parameters when designing individualized, sport-specific, and progressive resistance training programs to improve sports performance and build resilience against injury. Every aspect of a resistance training program—such as exercise selection, exercise order, intensity, speed of movement (i.e., tempo), and rest periods—deserves careful thought to optimize physical and physiological adaptations.

For example, while maximal strength and power are essential for ice hockey players and American football players alike, the ideal combination of resistance training methodologies and the prioritization of exercises will differ depending on the context. Sports Performance Coaches can develop more effective resistance training programs by understanding how the neuromuscular system adapts to resistance training, analyzing sport-specific demands, applying the most suitable loading parameters, and monitoring how athletes respond and improve over time. These skills are core requirements for all Sports Performance Coaches to maximize athletes' success.

Resistance training plays a crucial role in enhancing sport performance across a broad spectrum of disciplines, where each requires different focus areas. For endurance sports such as marathon running or long-distance cycling, resistance training can help improve muscular endurance and strength, reducing the risk of injury and enhancing performance efficiency. For strength sports such as powerlifting or weightlifting, resistance training is the core of the training program, aiming to maximize muscle mass, absolute strength, and neuromuscular coordination. Power sports such as sprinting or jumping necessitate resistance training to enhance explosive force and speed. In these disciplines, athletes often employ plyometric or high-intensity resistance training to optimize power output. Thus, resistance training, when tailored appropriately, can help athletes meet and surpass their sport-specific performance requirements.

RESISTANCE TRAINING FOR ENDURANCE SPORTS

Endurance athletes can benefit from strength training, as it contributes directly to increased movement economy—a key factor for endurance sport performance. Here are a few tips and considerations for training the endurance athlete.

First, many endurance athletes are unaccustomed to resistance training. Just as with youth athletes, a training period that focuses on technical competencies for squatting, hip hinging, pushing, pulling, and overhead pressing is essential. Additionally, acquiring a solid foundation of stability and muscular endurance is recommended before progressing

---

> **STRENGTH CAPACITY** →
>
> The maximal output of the neuromuscular system; can be classified in different ways such as maximal strength, stabilization, muscle hypertrophy, and power.

to more advanced forms of resistance exercise. Research shows that improper stabilization can negatively affect a muscle's force production (Behm et al., 2010; Brachman et al., 2017; Rivera et al., 2017). Resistance training exercises that concentrate on increased connective tissue strength, neuromuscular coordination, joint stability and mobility, and movement quality are crucial for reducing injury risk and building resilience.

Second, progressive overload is critical. Endurance athletes are used to pushing their bodies. But in the case of resistance training, it is not a matter of pushing through the proverbial wall. Instead, a slow and progressive resistance training program is key.

Third, to avoid unwanted muscle hypertrophy, focus on loading parameters that minimize time under tension—less than 15 seconds per set. Movement economy can be best addressed by increasing maximal strength and explosive strength using heavy resistance training (i.e., 85% to 100% 1RM) and power training (i.e., 30% to 45% of 1RM with high movement velocity). Sports Performance Coaches can also limit unwanted neuromuscular fatigue that could impair other forms of training by avoiding momentary failure, keeping a couple of repetitions in reserve, and using short, intense sessions. Do not forget that the endurance athlete should also focus on maintaining a healthy kinetic chain.

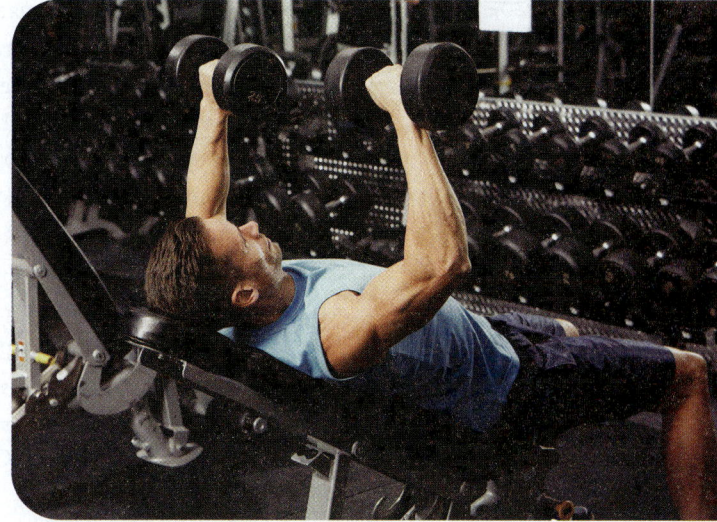

© Kurhan/Shutterstock

RESISTANCE TRAINING FOR STRENGTH AND POWER SPORTS

Resistance training programs have traditionally focused on developing maximal strength in individual muscles, emphasizing one plane of motion, typically the sagittal plane. Because all muscles function eccentrically, isometrically, and concentrically in all three planes of motion (sagittal, frontal, and transverse) and at different speeds, sports conditioning programs should be designed using a progressive overload approach emphasizing appropriate exercise selection in all planes of motion.

Each muscle operates under the control of the central nervous system. In consequence, strength needs to be considered not as a function of muscle, but rather as the result of activating the neuromuscular (muscular + nervous) system. Resistance training increases the neural demand and recruitment of muscle fibers until a recruitment plateau is reached. Further increases in strength then result from muscle fiber hypertrophy (Evans, 2019; Lasevicius et al., 2018; Schoenfeld, 2010).

© Real Sports Photos/Shutterstock

The majority of strength increases will occur during the first 12 weeks of resistance training from increased neural recruitment and muscle hypertrophy (Duchateau et al., 2006; Evans, 2019; Schoenfeld, 2010; Schoenfeld et al., 2015). Intermediate and advanced athletes will find it necessary to carry out a more demanding program in terms of training volume and intensity by following a sound periodized schedule.

Power training focuses on getting the neuromuscular system to generate force as quickly as possible. An increase in either force or velocity will produce an increase in power. Training for power can be achieved by increasing the weight (force), as seen in the strength adaptations, or by increasing the speed with which the weight is moved (velocity). Power training allows for an increased rate of force production by increasing the number of motor units activated, the synchronization between them, and the speed at which they are activated (Maffiuletti et al., 2016; Tredrea, 2017). The principle of specificity dictates that to maximize training for this type of adaptation, both heavy and light loads must be moved as fast as possible. Thus, using both training methods in a superset fashion can create the necessary adaptations to enhance the body's ability to recruit many motor units and increase the rate (speed) of activation (Hermassi et al., 2019; Maffiuletti et al., 2016; Pichardo et al., 2019; Rhea & Alderman, 2004).

Sports Performance Coaches can help the strength and power athletes by doing the following:

- Focusing on technical capacities (i.e., sprinting mechanics and proper exercise technique)
- Training with a strong emphasis on quality to optimize neural adaptations to resistance training
- Selecting high-intensity efforts using the principle of specificity
- Following a systematic and progressive approach to avoid training plateaus

UNILATERAL VERSUS BILATERAL RESISTANCE TRAINING EXERCISES

Bilateral exercises use both limbs in unison to create force and movement. Examples of bilateral exercises include the back squat, front squat, and barbell bench press. In contrast, unilateral exercises involve each limb working independently. Examples of unilateral exercises include single-leg squats, Bulgarian split squats, and single-arm dumbbell overhead presses.

The bilateral deficit is a unique feature of unilateral versus bilateral exercises (Škarabot et al., 2016). The bilateral deficit states that the sum (i.e., right + left) strength or power of the right and left limbs when a movement is performed with just one side is greater than the sum when both limbs perform the movement together at the same time. For example, an athlete's right-leg jump might be 20 cm, and their left-leg jump might be 21 cm (20 cm +21 cm = 41 cm), but they may reach only 36 cm in a bilateral jump.

Better intramuscular coordination (i.e., increased neural drive) coming from the motor cortex (i.e., the brain) during unilateral exercises compared to bilateral exercises underpins the bilateral deficit (Bobbert et al., 2006; Škarabot et al., 2016). Additionally, in jumping, a unilateral single-leg jump shifts the athlete higher on the force–velocity relationship of the leg extensor muscles, meaning that more force can be generated (Bobbert et al., 2006). A cross-education effect has also been observed during unilateral training. In this phenomenon, training the right limb contributes to left limb strength without any additional training of the left limb (Manca et al., 2017).

Additionally, most sports skills require the expression of muscle force and power with one limb. Running, skating, off-set lunge stance positions (like those found in American football and wrestling), striking in combative sports, throwing, and swimming all involve unilateral movements.

Including unilateral training as a part of a resistance training program appears to offer distinct advantages because of the potential for a better training effect and the capacity to develop the motor control for unilateral sports skills. Research suggests that unilateral training is as effective as bilateral training for developing maximal strength, power, and speed (Appleby et al., 2019; Liao et al., 2021; McCurdy et al., 2005; Moran et al., 2021; Speirs et al., 2016; Stern et al., 2020), and they have a similar neuromuscular demand (Costa et al., 2015).

Finally, the notion of limb symmetry appears frequently in the literature. Sports Performance Coaches should focus on ensuring athletes have two strong limbs that are relatively symmetrical in their strength and power capacity to reduce the risk of sports injuries like ACL tears (Ryman Augustsson & Ageberg, 2017; Steidl-Müller et al., 2018). In this setting, unilateral training appears to be necessary to increase lower limb strength symmetry and elicits a better effect than bilateral training (Gonzalo-Skok et al., 2017).

Here are some recommendations for the programming of bilateral versus unilateral exercises:

- Test limb symmetry in regard to strength and power capacity. The increased availability of dual force plate systems can enable Sports Performance Coaches to more accurately identify between-limb deficits.
- Aim to achieve strong and symmetrical limbs in terms of strength and power. The difference between limbs should be less than 10%.
- Program bilateral and unilateral exercises on a 1:1 basis when athletes have two strong and symmetrical limbs.
- Increase the volume of unilateral training to 60% to 70% when higher asymmetries have been found.
- Unilateral training appears to be as effective as bilateral training for increasing maximal strength and power, but do not let the pendulum swing too far. Increasing muscle strength and power on a global basis with bilateral exercises can still transfer very well to improving unilateral sports skills like change-of-direction maneuvers (Appleby et al., 2020).

ROTATIONAL STRENGTH AND POWER

Just like unilateral strength capacity, rotational strength and power are essential for a multitude of sports skills, such as throwing a football, hitting a baseball or tennis ball, or striking a boxing opponent. Rotational power arises from a complex interaction of the kinetic chain, whereby the proximal muscles of the trunk and hips form a mechanical engine that drives high movement velocities of the limbs in combination with the distal musculature of the extremities (Lee & McGill, 2015, 2017; McGill & Cholewicki, 2001; McGill et al., 2010). The capacity to generate spinal stiffness and spinal rotational energy is a requirement for effective sports skills that rely on high rotational strength and power (McGill et al., 2010).

The first focus is spinal stability. The architecture of the adult spine permits a large range of motion (ROM). Just like a flexible rod that is in a vertical position with guy wires tensioned equally around its base to create stability, the spine muscles coordinate to create spinal stiffness (McGill & Cholewicki, 2001) (**Figure 14.1**).

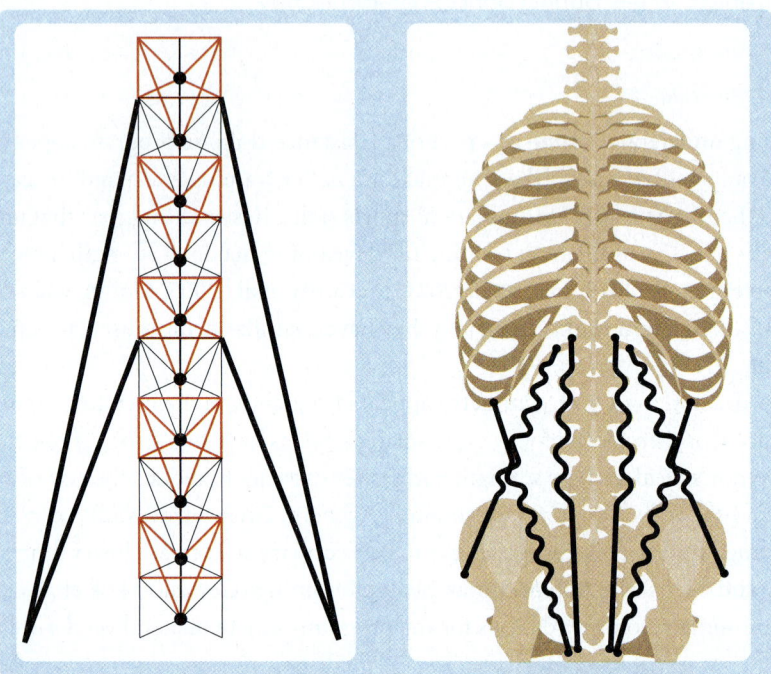

FIGURE 14.1 Spinal Stiffness Analogy

Now, consider how rotational power is generated. In addition to maintaining a strong core pillar from the rib cage down to the pelvis through effective co-contraction of the spinal muscles, rotational energy is generated by muscles such as the external/internal obliques, the latissimus dorsi, and the erector spinae muscles (Vera Garcia et al., 2014).

These observations lay a foundation for training for rotational power and strength. First, isometric core exercises and rotational exercises appear necessary to maximize movement velocity and force in rotational movements (Lee & McGill, 2017). Second, as with all sports skills discussed throughout this chapter, lots of practice and coaching while doing the sports skill itself are necessary to achieve optimal intermuscular coordination and enhance the transfer-of-training effect.

> ✔ **CHECK IT OUT**
>
> Increased spine stiffness developed from isometric core training and rotational power developed through exercises such as medicine ball throws are necessary to maximize the rotational strength and power for sports skills such as striking, throwing, and swinging a bat.

LINEAR STRENGTH AND POWER

Linear strength and power are vital abilities behind maximal acceleration capacity and speed in movements like running and skating. Linear strength and power are also necessary for sports skills like blocking in American football, gymnastics, the start in swimming, and weightlifting.

The maximum velocity in sprinting is characterized by short ground contact times (less than 100 ms in elite sprinters), high lower limb stiffness and rate of force development (RFD), and high movement velocity of the lower limbs. The movement velocity of the lower limbs is best trained by sprinting. Sports Performance Coaches should be cautious about devising resistance training exercises that mimic sprinting movements, as they can disrupt movement patterns.

However, resistance training can help athletes achieve high RFD and lower limb stiffness for maximum velocity in sprinting. Sports Performance Coaches can maximize the transfer between resistance training and maximum velocity sprinting by focusing on the following aspects:

- Heavy resistance training with intensities of 85% to 100% 1RM (i.e., 1 to 5 repetitions)
- Combining heavy resistance training with plyometric exercises
- Combining heavy resistance training with speed, agility, and quickness drills

---

📋 COACH'S CORNER

The Sports Performance Coach must be mindful of certain considerations before beginning a resistance training program:

- Perform a needs analysis and comprehensive assessment of the athlete.
- Review the athlete's prior conditioning programs.
- Determine the athlete's primary and secondary training objectives.
- Identify the athlete's training, practice, and competition schedule.
- Select the appropriate loading parameters and acute training variables.
- Select appropriate primary and secondary exercises based on the athlete's assessment results, training objectives, and technical competency.
- Adjust the exercise program as needed.

LESSON 2: DEFINING STRENGTH CAPACITIES
STRENGTH CAPACITIES

Sports Performance Coaches may be most familiar with maximal strength capacity, but it is just one of the many capacities targeted with resistance training. Certain capacities (e.g., stabilization or muscle hypertrophy) underpin other capacities (e.g., power) dictated by muscle physiology. For example, the bigger a muscle, the more force and power it can generate. Here, the engine capacity supports the horsepower of muscle. These different aspects of strength capacity can be developed through targeted training, and the specific capacities that an athlete focuses on will depend on the requirements of their sport or activity. This section focuses on crucial neuromuscular strength capacities and their relationship to sports performance.

STABILIZATION AND INTERMUSCULAR COORDINATION

Intermuscular coordination is the ability of the neuromuscular system to allow all muscles to work together to facilitate fluid, effective, and coordinated movement. Imagine an orchestra conductor who carefully coordinates the various instruments to make beautiful music. In this analogy, the musical instruments are the muscles, and the conductor— the neuromuscular system—works synergistically to generate the appropriate level of neuromuscular activity to maximize sports performance and protect the musculoskeletal system from injury.

Intermuscular coordination is a critical factor supporting long-term adaptations to resistance training (Balshaw et al., 2019). It is also a focus of stabilization or balance training. In this type of training, unstable surfaces, single-stance positions, and limb dissociation patterns are used to challenge an athlete's ability to maintain a stable posture and withstand unexpected perturbations (Anderson & Behm, 2005) (**Figure 14.2**). Stabilization training is a critical component of a resistance training program, especially for youth athletes and after injury (Behm et al., 2017; Granacher et al., 2016; Hall et al., 2018; Lauber et al., 2021).

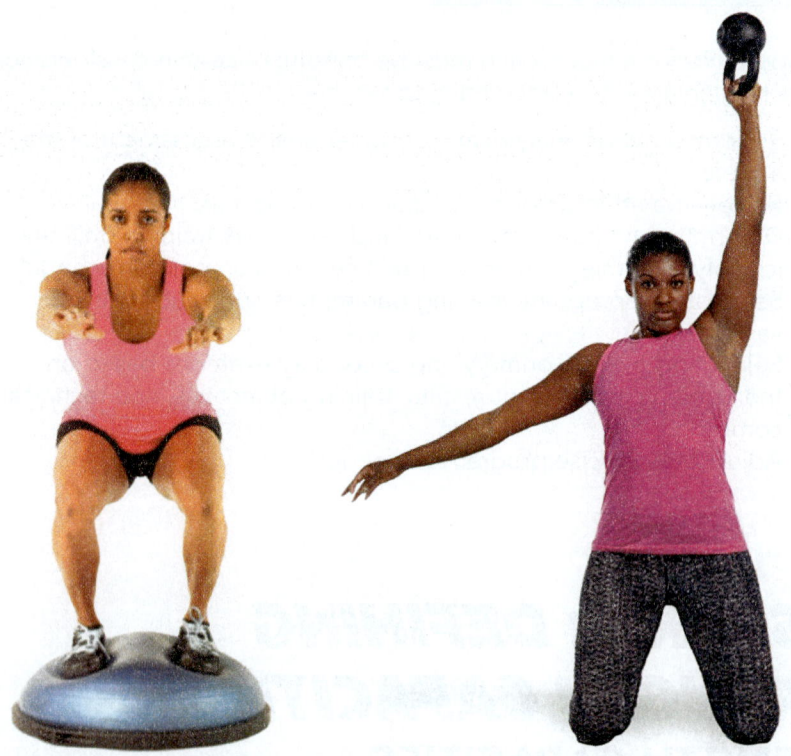

FIGURE 14.2 Stabilization-Focused Exercises

However, stabilization training does not replace the need for maximal strength or power training, but rather works to complement such training as part of an integrated training system. Whereas balance training improves postural stability and muscular endurance in athletes, heavy resistance training remains superior for increasing explosive strength, power, and maximal strength (Zech et al., 2010). Therefore, Sports Performance

Coaches should integrate all forms of exercise into a systematic and progressive system that aims to simultaneously improve critical physical abilities, such as flexibility, muscular and aerobic endurance, core stabilization, balance, maximal strength, and power.

MUSCULAR DEVELOPMENT

Muscular development (**hypertrophy**) can take one of two primary forms: in series or in parallel. In-series hypertrophy is achieved by increasing the number of sarcomeres—the basic functional unit of a muscle—along the length of the fiber, akin to adding segments to a rope. However, the primary mechanism for hypertrophy associated with resistance training is an increase in the number of sarcomeres in parallel. As the term implies, in-parallel hypertrophy is achieved when sarcomeres are added next to each other, much like adding sardines in a tin can. In this way, the muscle cross-sectional area increases, producing a thicker, fuller muscle.

Muscular development can be compared to the size of an engine in a race car. The bigger the muscular engine, the more force and power it can generate. In other words, the capacity of a muscle to generate force is proportional to its physiological cross-sectional area. Very few sports demand muscular hypertrophy in and of themselves, unless it is a bodybuilder or an athlete moving up a weight class. However, developing muscle hypertrophy can be a foundational performance factor that increases an athlete's maximal power capacity.

Muscles are always in a state of renewing their protein structures (Damas et al., 2015). Muscle proteins turn over every single day. This process requires energy: The more muscle mass an athlete has, the higher their basal metabolic rate. Muscle hypertrophy occurs when the net protein synthesis balance is positive, meaning the muscle creates more protein than it is breaking down.

When protein breakdown exceeds protein synthesis, atrophy occurs. A common strategy to promote protein synthesis is to eat adequate protein with a target of 1.6 to 2.2 grams/kilograms of bodyweight (0.7 to 1.0 gram/pound). This ratio assumes that the athlete also performs a structured and progressive resistance training routine.

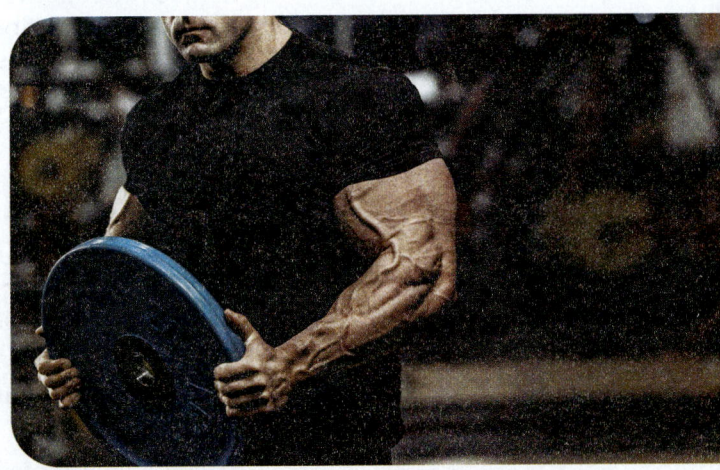
© Fotokvadrat/Shutterstock

Regarding resistance training, the loading parameters that elicit muscle hypertrophy have recently been revised (Schmidtbleicher & Buehrle, 1987; Schoenfeld et al., 2017; Schoenfeld et al., 2019; Schoenfeld et al., 2021). Whereas moderate load resistance training in the range of 8 to 12 RM was typically recommended, evidence now highlights the benefit of various loading schemes, depending on the athlete's goals and training status. In other words, the ideal loading scheme depends on the context.

MAXIMAL STRENGTH

Maximal strength is the maximum force, torque, or tension a muscle can generate, irrespective of time. Maximal strength is often discussed with respect to the maximum voluntary contraction (MVC). This relationship is important because involuntary contraction strength can be quantified under certain conditions, such as during electrical muscle stimulation. In sports performance, however, the voluntary contraction strength is most important.

> **HYPERTROPHY →**
>
> Enlargement of an organ or tissue; in the context of fitness, the enlargement of skeletal muscle.

> **MAXIMAL STRENGTH →**
>
> The maximal force or torque generated by a muscle or muscles in a single maximum voluntary contraction, which is specific to each type of muscle action.

Maximal strength is specific to the three types of muscle actions: eccentric, isometric, and concentric. Muscles can generate as much as 40% more force in an eccentric muscle action, though this occurs under involuntary muscle activation. When it comes to an athlete trying to tap into the full potential of their muscles, heavy resistance training can remove the inhibition in the system and maximize the neural drive of the working muscles to reach their full force-generating potential.

A range of loading schemes can increase maximal strength. Importantly, the volume and intensity required to achieve improvements with elite athletes must be higher than that for youth, adolescent, or less well-trained athletes.

✔ CHECK IT OUT

Maximal strength should not be thought of in isolation. Strength is built on the foundation of stabilization, requiring muscles, tendons, and ligaments to be prepared for the load required to increase strength beyond the initial stages of training. Whereas stabilization-focused resistance training is designed to capitalize on the characteristics of type I, slow-twitch muscle fibers (slow-contracting, low-tension output, and resistant to fatigue), strength-focused resistance training matches the characteristics of type II muscle fibers (quick-contracting, high-tension output, prone to fatigue). Thus, resistance training variables (sets, reps, and intensities) are manipulated to take advantage of the specific characteristics of each fiber type.

MAXIMAL POWER

Maximal power plays a significant role in sports that require explosive movements, such as sprinting, jumping, or throwing. By understanding an athlete's maximal power, a coach can develop targeted training programs to enhance this capacity, ultimately improving athletic performance.

Power is properly defined as the muscle work rate. The formulas for power are shown here:

$$\text{Work} = \text{force} \times \text{distance}$$

$$\text{Power} = \frac{\text{work}}{\text{time}}$$

The formula for velocity is as follows:

$$\text{Velocity} = \frac{\text{distance}}{\text{time}}$$

Using the previous formulas, the formula for power can be rewritten as follows:

$$\text{Power} = \frac{\text{force} \times \text{distance}}{\text{time}}$$

$$\text{Power} = \text{force} \times \frac{\text{distance}}{\text{time}}$$

$$\text{Power} = \text{force} \times \text{velocity}$$

The last formula, power = force × velocity, provides vital information for training maximal power for sports performance. As power is a function of force and velocity, both the force and velocity components of the equation must be trained (Cormie et al., 2011b). An increase in either force or velocity will produce an increase in power. Training for power can be achieved by increasing the weight (force), as seen in heavy resistance training, or by increasing the speed with which weight is moved (velocity), as seen in explosive plyometrics and speed drills.

EXPLOSIVE STRENGTH

Explosive strength (quantified as the RFD) is the time frame for applying force in competitive skills and is a vital component of athleticism. For example, it can take more than 2 seconds (2000 ms) for an athlete to reach maximum voluntary contraction strength (maximal strength). In contrast, the ground contact time in sprinting is less than 100 ms for elite sprinters, and the skating stride for an ice hockey player is between 150 and 200 ms. A boxer releases a jab in 50 to 100 ms, and the downward pedal stroke of an elite sprint cyclist is 100 to 150 ms. The key here is not how much force the athlete can generate, but rather how fast the athlete can generate force given the time constraints of the competitive skill. Explosive strength is a critically important capacity, yet very few Sports Performance Coaches measure it or train it properly (Aagaard et al., 2002; Blazevich et al., 2020; Maffiuletti et al., 2016). Additionally, it is clear that after sports injuries, such as an ACL rupture, explosive strength can remain impaired for up to two years, which may place the athlete at future risk for ACL injury (Turpeinen et al., 2020)

Observational studies indicate that a noncontact ACL injury occurs in a fraction of a second—specifically, in 30 to 50 ms (Krosshaug et al., 2007). In fact, such injuries appear in time frames that are even shorter than the sports skills listed previously. In other words, muscles must contract fast to protect the knee against external forces that cause ACL injury (**Figure 14.3**).

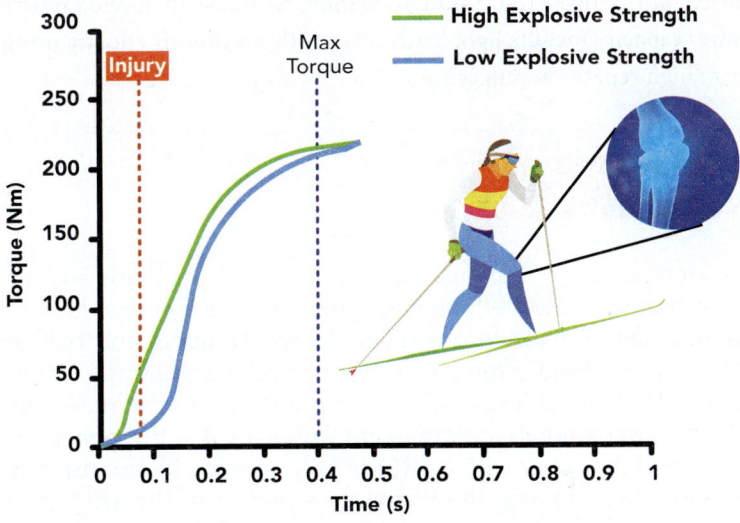

FIGURE 14.3 Importance of Rate of Force Development (RFD) for Protecting the Knee

Understanding how to train explosive strength is essential for the contexts of sports performance and sports injury. Different neuromuscular control factors underpin explosive strength compared to maximal strength. In this setting, the fiber type, the ability to make motor units fire quickly at the onset of muscle action, and tendon stiffness help to increase explosive strength (Aagaard et al., 2002). The intentional application of rapid force development during resistance training is key for training explosive strength (Blazevich et al., 2020).

Providing this occurs, both heavy resistance training and power training methods can effectively increase explosive strength. Additionally, given the high neural demands of explosive strength training, choosing exercises with as much specificity as possible to the competitive skill is important to transfer exercise training to sports performance.

MUSCULAR AND POWER ENDURANCE

Developing and improving muscular endurance is an integral component of a sports performance program. It helps increase core and joint stabilization, the foundation on which hypertrophy, strength, and power are built. Moreover, training muscular endurance of the core (lumbo-pelvic-hip complex) focuses on the recruitment of muscles responsible for postural stability—namely, type I muscle fibers.

Research has shown that resistance training protocols using high repetitions are the most effective means of improving muscular endurance. In addition, a periodization training program can enhance local muscular endurance. After an initial training effect occurs in previously untrained individuals, multiple sets of periodized training may prove superior to single-set training for improving muscle endurance (Evans, 2019). Previous position statements by Ratamess et al. (2009) noted the existence of a relationship between increases in strength and local muscular endurance, indicating that strength training alone may improve endurance to a certain extent. Training to increase muscular endurance implies performing lots of repetitions, increasing a muscle's time under tension, and/or minimizing rest periods between sets (Evans, 2019; Schoenfeld et al., 2021).

In contrast to muscular endurance, **power endurance** is the capacity to maintain mechanical power in a sports skill or task. It is often tested using repeated vertical jump tests (Jordan et al., 2017) or during various types of cycle ergometry assessments such as the 30- to 60-second Wingate test. Standard loading protocols to develop power endurance or repeat power capacity include light loads lifted with maximum velocity using a variety of moderate to high repetition ranges.

> **POWER ENDURANCE** →
>
> The capacity to maintain mechanical power in a sports skill or task.

✔ CHECK IT OUT

Protocols for muscular endurance typically involve light loads and high repetition schemes. However, the strength reserve is a critical factor that supports muscular endurance. For example, the National Football League (NFL) Scouting Combine often includes a muscular endurance test in which athletes perform a bench press with 225 pounds for a maximum number of repetitions. Imagine two athletes, one with a 1RM in the bench press of 275 pounds and the other with a 1RM of 500 pounds. No matter how much muscular endurance training the first athlete performs, the 1RM continuum shows that the ability to improve on this test would be impossible without increasing their strength reserve. By comparison, the bench press test is less than 50% of the second athlete's 1RM, enabling them to perform many repetitions because the relative intensity is lower. This example highlights that improving muscular endurance and maximal strength must go hand in hand.

FORCE–VELOCITY RELATIONSHIP

The final strength capacities can be illustrated using the force–velocity relationship (**Figure 14.4**). The force–velocity relationship is not just a theoretical training consideration, given that it is a fundamental property of skeletal muscle; it is also a trainable and testable capacity in the sports performance realm. For example, a loaded vertical jump test is often used to create a whole-body force–velocity profile. The profile characteristics can then help Sports Performance Coaches program resistance training exercises (Jiménez-Reyes et al., 2017; Samozino et al., 2012).

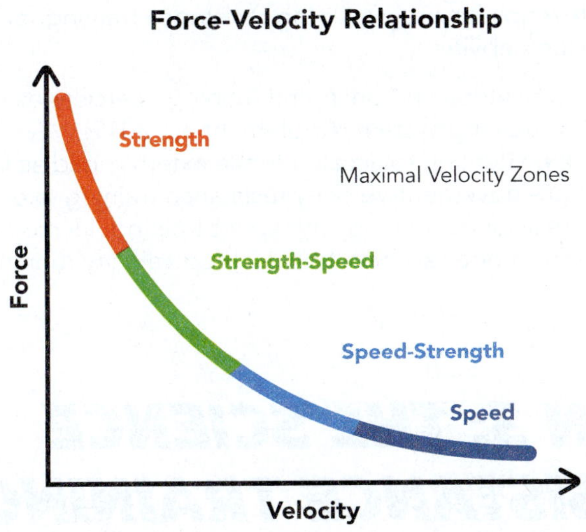

Force-Velocity Relationship

FIGURE 14.4 Force–Velocity Relationship and Maximal Velocity Zones

Long-term resistance training aims to shift the force–velocity profile up and to the right. However, specific adaptations occur by training at different regions of the force–velocity curve (Moritani, 1993). Notably, high-force training increases the maximum force region of the relationship, moderate load ballistic training improves the **strength-speed** and **speed-strength** regions, and plyometric training and speed training increases the maximum velocity region (Jiménez-Reyes et al., 2017; Moritani, 1993).

> ⚙ **TRY THIS**
>
> Try performing three vertical jumps with three different loading conditions: 0% of body mass, 30% of body mass, and 60% of body mass. The slope of the line and the jump performance at each load can help describe an athlete's strength-speed, speed-strength, and maximal velocity capacities.

STRENGTH-SPEED →

Moving relatively heavy loads as fast as possible.

SPEED-STRENGTH →

Moving at high speed with the maximum load possible.

Whether an optimal profile exists is unclear. However, a good rule for Sports Performance Coaches is to *surf* the curve. The best method to bring about long-term adaptations in strength capacities across the force–velocity continuum is to use a combination of loading parameters that address the maximal strength, strength-speed, speed-strength, and maximal velocity regions.

Heavy resistance training, accentuated eccentric exercise, and ballistic training transfer positively to improve speed and change-of-direction maneuvers (Blazevich et al., 2020; Chaabene et al., 2020; Lum & Barbosa, 2019; Seitz et al., 2014; Spiteri et al., 2014). Resistance training contributes to speed and change-of-direction capacity by increasing neural drive to the working muscles and tendon stiffness, increasing the neuromuscular system's capacity for RFD and stretch–shorten cycle movements.

Here are a few tips for programming resistance training for speed and change-of-direction ability:

- Utilize both bilateral and unilateral training exercises as part of a progressive training system (Appleby et al., 2019).
- Focus on the intention to accelerate the external load as fast as possible.
- Include high-movement-velocity resistance training exercises.
- Combine resistance training with sprint training, including a strong emphasis on proper acceleration and top velocity running mechanics.

LESSON 3: THE SCIENCE OF RESISTANCE TRAINING

SCIENTIFIC RATIONALE FOR RESISTANCE TRAINING

A substantial body of scientific evidence explains how the neuromuscular system adapts to resistance training and the ensuing effects on sports performance. Unlike general physical activity, sports-specific resistance training must consider the desired athletic results and the understanding that adaptations are specific to the imposed demand.

SPORT PERFORMANCE

When it comes to sports performance, context is everything, and the selected resistance training loading parameters depend heavily on the context. Research strongly supports including resistance training for athletes in all sports and across all ages (Behm et al., 2017; Lum & Barbosa, 2019; Suchomel et al., 2016).

When applying resistance training, a key consideration for Sports Performance Coaches is the principle of transfer effect, or how well the training transfers to sporting-related activities (Young, 2006).

Warren Young (2006) introduced an analogy to help Sports Performance Coaches grasp where and how resistance training fits into an athlete's training regime: Compare the athlete's neuromuscular system to a race car. The size of the race car's engine, or, in the case of the athlete, the size of their muscles, reflects the capacity to generate power. The bigger the engine, the more power it can generate. This basic physiological property of muscle shows that a muscle's force- and power-generating capacity is proportional to its size. For this reason, muscular development training is often a key focus for an athletic population. It is not that increasing muscle size is important in and of itself. Instead, it is important because it increases the muscle's force- and power-generating capacity (**Figure 14.5**).

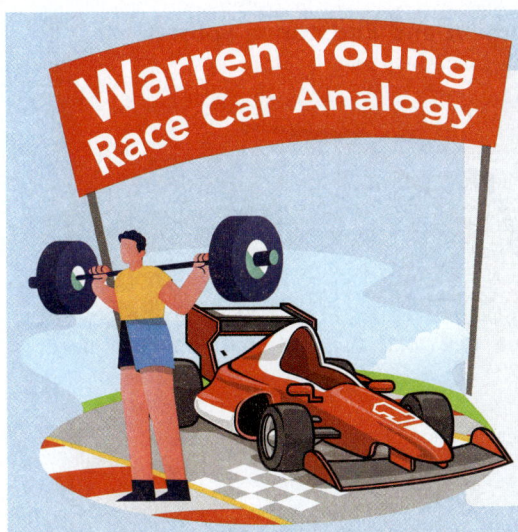

FIGURE 14.5 Warren Young Race Car Analogy

Data from Young, W. B. (2006, June). Transfer of strength and power training to sports performance. *International Journal of Sports Physiology and Performance*, 1(2): 74–83. https://doi.org/10.1123/ijspp.1.2.74

But just as a race car needs more than just a big engine, so the athlete requires more than large muscles to perform. The engine must be tuned appropriately to transfer power into the drive shaft. Likewise, the electrical signal that fires down from the athlete's brain through their nerves to their working muscles must be "tuned." The stronger the neural signal, the more force the working muscles can generate.

Two factors influence neural signaling: **motor unit recruitment** and rate coding. These factors impact the capacity for intramuscular coordination. Resistance training increases intramuscular coordination, which is comparable to bringing the race car to a mechanic to get an engine tune-up. After the tune-up, the engine's full capacity can be accessed.

> 👍 **HELPFUL HINT**
>
> A motor unit consists of the motor nerve and the bundle of muscle fibers it innervates. It is the functional unit of the neuromuscular system.

MOTOR UNIT RECRUITMENT →

The physiological process by which motor units are activated to produce muscle contraction.

One other key factor (target capacity) reinforces how resistance training can help augment sports performance—intermuscular coordination. Think about the race car: Now that the engine size is maximized and tuned correctly, the engine power must be transferred through the tires onto the road. From a sports performance perspective, resistance training should address the appropriate coordination between muscles, including the optimal activation of synergists, antagonists, and stabilizer muscles and the direction of the force application.

Sports Performance Coaches should also consider the movement velocity and the time frame for force application. For example, consider an elite cross-country skier. Cross-country skiers often employ a double-poling technique to maximize propulsion. A double-poling cycle lasts approximately 200 ms, and peak pole forces are attained in less than 100 ms. The latter is the same time frame in which the foot is in contact with the ground for elite track and field sprinters. In this setting, the key is to maximize how fast force is applied to the ground—that is, the RFD (**Figure 14.6**).

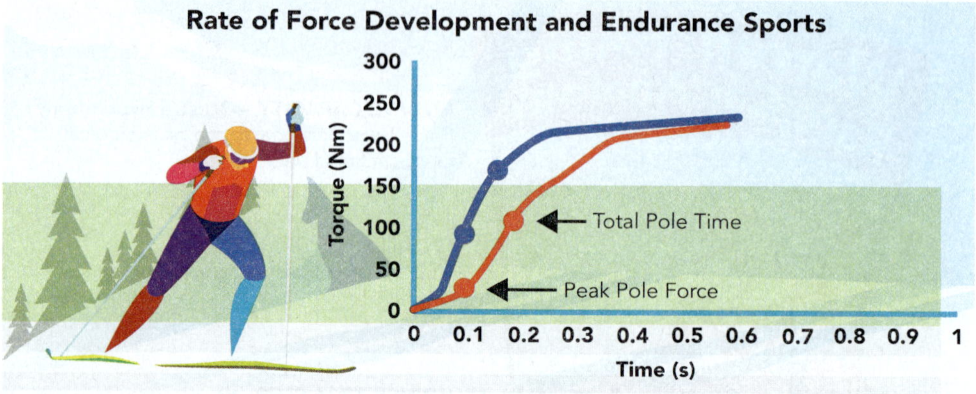

FIGURE 14.6 Rate of Force Development in Endurance Sports

STRENGTH RESERVE →

The difference between an individual's maximal strength capacity and the strength requirement of the competitive skill or sport movement. A higher strength reserve acts as a buffer between what is needed to play the sport and the strength required to meet unforeseen demands.

TENDINOPATHY →

Overuse injuries of the tendon characterized by pain, inflammation, tissue structure change, decreased exercise tolerance, and movement dysfunction.

GOLDILOCKS EFFECT →

Finding the "just right" balance in workout intensity and volume to optimize muscle growth and strength gains while minimizing the risk of injury and overtraining.

Young's (2006) race car provides a compelling analogy for how Sports Performance Coaches can think about various neuromuscular adaptations to resistance training, including the importance of sport specificity and the transfer-of-training effect to optimize program design for sports performance. The challenge for the Sports Performance Coach is to first understand the *why* behind adaptations to resistance training; then undertake an evaluation of the context and the athlete; and, finally, select the appropriate sequence of training objectives to achieve the desired outcome. One thing is certain: There are many resistance training modalities and techniques available that can help fine-tune an athlete's neuromuscular system and uplift their sports performance.

REDUCING THE RISK OF SPORT INJURY

Resistance training is a potent stimulus to build resilience against sports injury (Lauersen et al., 2018; Ryman Augustsson & Ageberg, 2017). One contributing factor is the **strength reserve**. The strength reserve is like a buffer between an athlete's maximal strength capacity and the forces and energies encountered on the field of play, including unexpectedly high-energy events that often lead to sports injuries like ACL ruptures. Research suggests that the strength reserve has diminished for young athletes today compared to a few decades ago; however, the strength reserve remains important for athletes of all ages (Faigenbaum et al., 2019).

Resistance training has also been proposed to have protective effects for tendon health for endurance athletes (Aagaard & Andersen, 2010). For example, heavy resistance training stimulates muscle growth (hypertrophy) and tendon growth (Kongsgaard et al., 2007). Increasing the cross-sectional area of a tendon distributes forces through a larger area, thereby increasing its stress capacity and reducing the risk of **tendinopathy**.

✔ CHECK IT OUT

An athlete trains not only to perform optimally in their sport, but also to meet unforeseen physical demands and stay healthy and safe. Resistance training can be a protective training stimulus that fends off sport-related injury.

As endurance athletes often perform exceptionally high training volumes to promote cardiovascular fitness, a heavy resistance training cycle focused on tendon hypertrophy may increase the structural tolerance of the endurance athlete's connective tissues (Aagaard & Andersen, 2010). This adaptation is another excellent example of how resistance training has many profound effects beyond increases in strength and power.

Finally, neuromuscular training programs that include stabilization-focused resistance exercises in a warm-up before training or games substantially reduce the risk of sports injury (Emery & Pasanen, 2019). Research suggests that neuromuscular injury prevention programs done as part of a warm-up can reduce the risk of sports injuries by at least 35% (Emery & Pasanen, 2019).

There are many well-documented neuromuscular injury prevention programs. They are typically 10 to 15 minutes in duration, and include stabilization-focused exercises targeting the spinal musculature, hip rotators and abductors, the rotator cuff, and the hamstrings. However, the **Goldilocks effect** must be considered: To use resistance training in this context, the intensity and volume are reduced to capitalize on the injury prevention effects while not causing undue neuromuscular fatigue that might impair sports performance.

REHABILITATION

Sports injuries, such as ACL ruptures and muscle strains, often lead to a multitude of neuromuscular impairments that cause decreased muscle strength and **power**, muscle atrophy, and altered neuromuscular control (Hewett et al., 2013; Hiemstra et al., 2000; Jordan et al., 2015a, 2015b, 2017; King et al., 2021; Morris et al., 2020; Read et al., 2020; Turpeinen et al., 2020). These impairments elevate the risk for a subsequent reinjury, and many athletes never return to their pre-injury performance level (Ardern et al., 2014). Consequently, resistance training is a critical component of the long-term rehabilitation plan to support athletes transitioning back to their sport.

Resistance training after an injury often focuses on restoring strength and between-limb symmetry (i.e., the athlete returns to the sport with two relatively symmetrical and strong limbs). Various techniques have been highlighted in the scientific literature that support the retraining of neuromuscular function and neuromuscular control after sports injuries. For example, a substantial body of scientific evidence supports the application of **blood flow restriction (BFR)** alongside light load resistance training to increase muscle hypertrophy and strength after musculoskeletal injuries and orthopedic surgeries (Hughes et al., 2017; Tennent et al., 2018; Wengle et al., 2021).

In addition to novel techniques like BFR, resistance training with a unilateral focus, including methods to restore the neural drive to the working muscle, can help Sports Performance Coaches address persistent neuromuscular deficits after injury once the athlete has been given medical clearance. Restoring the neural drive must be prioritized alongside remedying injury-induced muscle atrophy. A reduced neural drive can diminish the strength and power necessary for sports performance, but serves to safeguard passive tissues such as ligaments against reinjury (Turpeinen et al., 2020).

POWER →

The amount of work that can be completed in a fixed amount of time.

BLOOD FLOW RESTRICTION (BFR) →

The application of a pressurized cuff that restricts the venous return of blood from working muscles; often used in conjunction with light resistance training to stimulate muscle hypertrophy.

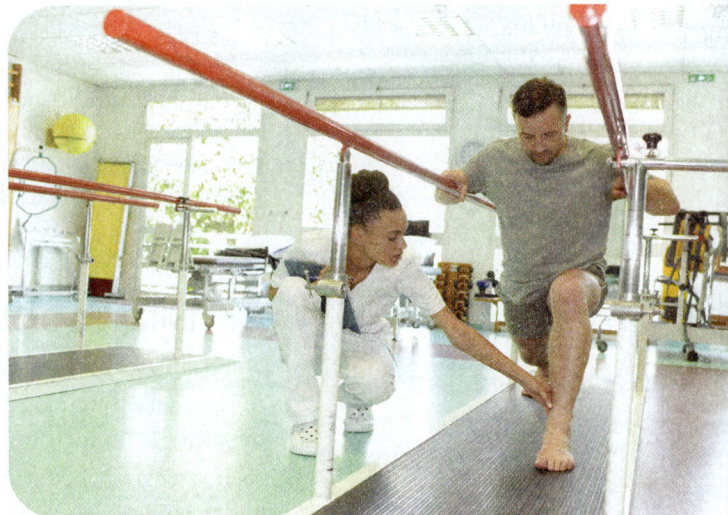
© ALPA PROD/Shutterstock

Returning to Young's (2006) analogy, a race car needs a big engine alongside a tuned engine to maximally transfer its power into the road. Similarly, an injured athlete must restore their muscular engine (i.e., combat muscle atrophy) and increase their neural drive (i.e., reduce neuromuscular inhibition) to regain strength and power after injury. A seminal paper by Schmidtbleicher and Buehrle (1987) provides a framework for how resistance training methods can be organized to optimize long-term adaptations for injured and noninjured athletes alike. This paper evaluated the neuromuscular adaptations of three repetition and intensity schemes, including high-load/low-repetition resistance training (targeting maximal strength), moderate-load/low-repetition ballistic resistance training (targeting maximal power), and moderate-load/high-repetition exhaustive resistance training (targeting muscular hypertrophy). While the moderate-load/high-repetition scheme favored muscle hypertrophy development, the high-load/low-repetition scheme promoted neural adaptations. Schmidtbleicher and Buehrle (1987) concluded that both methods should be alternated over time to promote long-term adaptations to resistance training, also called **undulation**.

The periodization scheme of alternating between periods of moderate load and high load in resistance training ensures that both hypertrophic and neural adaptations are addressed in the injured athlete as they transition back to sport and competition. It also highlights how Young's (2006) analogy can be employed in general, alongside the appropriate selection of loading parameters to fine-tune a resistance training program design in a precise and individualized manner.

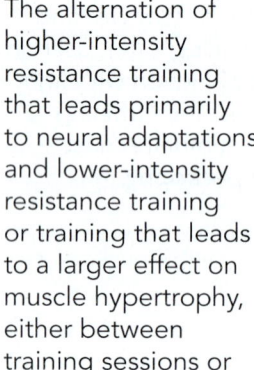

UNDULATION →

The alternation of higher-intensity resistance training that leads primarily to neural adaptations and lower-intensity resistance training or training that leads to a larger effect on muscle hypertrophy, either between training sessions or between training cycles.

> ### 👍 HELPFUL HINT
>
> As previously discussed, athletes need to exert maximal force quickly (bigger car engine). However, they must also be able to decelerate, like a race car using a proficient braking system. Neuromuscular (stabilization-focused) exercises and practicing ideal movement patterns help develop the required neuromuscular control to decelerate and change direction in an optimal manner (Zebis et al., 2016).

OPTIMIZING BODY COMPOSITION

Some athletes may be restricted by a weight class and feel limited when it comes to resistance training. Sports Performance Coaches may prevent unwanted muscle hypertrophy in such athletes who must optimize their body composition and maximize their strength by reducing the training volume (Schoenfeld et al., 2019). Both the science and practice support the contention that very short, high-intensity resistance training sessions can help trained individuals increase their maximal strength, supported by the increased neural drive to the working muscles (Aagaard et al., 2002).

Power training methods also elicit neuromuscular adaptations without stimulating muscle hypertrophy (Cormie et al., 2011a). A few standard methods fall under the umbrella of power training:

**COMPEN- →
SATORY
ACCELERATION**

The maximal intentional acceleration of an external load to develop the internal muscular rate of force development capacity and maximal neuromuscular activation.

1. Heavy strength training: high-load, low-repetition training focusing on **compensatory acceleration** (i.e., maximal acceleration of the heavy external load).
2. Power (ballistic) training: light-load, moderate-repetition training focusing on compensatory acceleration.

3. Plyometric training: fast stretch–shortening cycle (SSC) movements less than 200 ms with little to no external load.
4. Combined training: the combined use of heavy strength training and ballistic training or heavy strength training and plyometric training.
5. Contrast training: The alternating combination of moderate to heavy strength training and ballistic or plyometric training to capitalize on post-activation potentiation (PAP).

All five of these methods are suitable for athletes who must maximize their strength and power while minimizing gains in lean body mass to optimize their body composition.

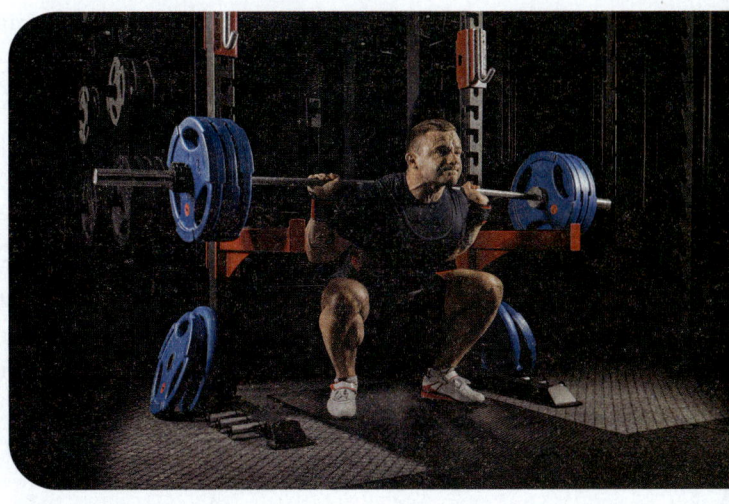

© Andy Gin/Shutterstock

LESSON 4: PRINCIPLES OF RESISTANCE TRAINING
RESISTANCE TRAINING GUIDELINES

Resistance training guidelines are vital because they provide structure, direction, and safety during workouts. They include elements such as a needs analysis, comprehensive assessments, and safety measures to ensure effective and injury-free training. A needs analysis is a fundamental first step in identifying an athlete's current athletic condition, goals, and training history. Comprehensive assessments must also be completed, as they provide a realistic starting point and valuable insights into the progress and effectiveness of the training program. This allows the Sports Performance Coach to adjust and adapt the program based on the athlete's evolving levels and goals. Additionally, implementing safety measures during resistance training is essential to prevent injuries, which can cause setbacks or long-term health problems. These guidelines should cover correct lifting techniques, appropriate use of equipment, the importance of warm-ups and cool-downs, and rest periods to ensure overall well-being and the sustainability of the training program.

NEEDS ANALYSIS AND ASSESSMENT INFORMATION

Resistance training is the focus of many sports-specific training programs due to the foundational role that muscular strength and endurance play in performance. A needs analysis is the first step that allows the Sports Performance Coach to thoroughly understand the metabolic, mechanical, and injury potential for the athlete and the sport.

Resistance training must be based on the needs analysis results and assessment information to ensure the exercises are tailored to the athlete's specific requirements, goals, and limitations. An individualized approach helps optimize the training process, improving strength capacities and overall performance and reducing the likelihood of certain injuries.

Comprehensive assessments are vital tools for Sports Performance Coaches to design effective and safe resistance training programs for athletes. These assessments help to identify the athlete's strength, flexibility, balance, and neuromuscular control, as well as any muscle imbalances or movement dysfunctions that may increase the risk of injury or hinder performance.

Based on the information gathered from the assessments, a coach can design a resistance training program that addresses the athlete's individual needs and goals. This might include exercises to improve mobility in restricted areas, strengthen underactive muscles, correct imbalances, improve neuromuscular control, or enhance performance in specific movements relevant to the athlete's sport.

PROGRESSING RESISTANCE TRAINING

Resistance training progressions are at the center of NASM's OPT™ Model (**Figure 14.7**). The OPT Model involves three levels: stabilization, strength, and power. Each level is progressively more challenging and builds on the skills developed in the previous stage.

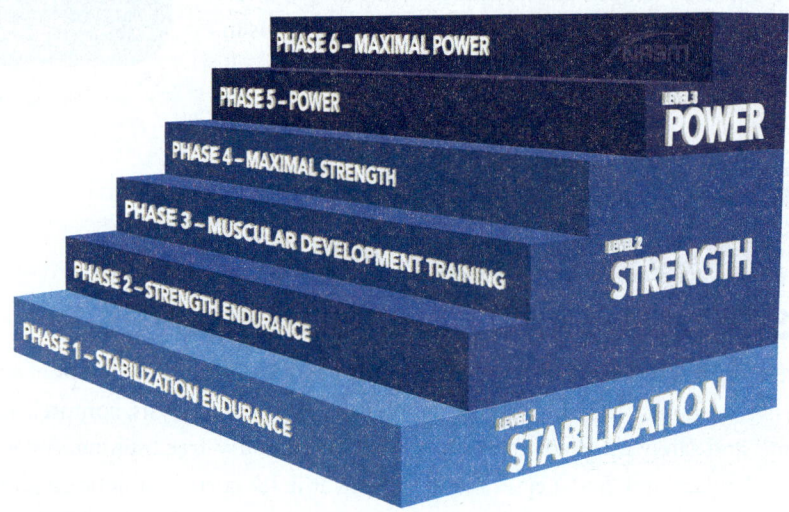

FIGURE 14.7 The OPT Model

In the stabilization level, the focus is on improving muscular endurance, enhancing joint stability, increasing flexibility, and developing proper movement patterns. After mastery of this phase, an athlete progresses to the strength level, which targets the development of lean body mass and overall strength. The strength level is further divided into three phases: strength endurance, muscular development, and maximal strength. Finally, in the power level, the focus shifts to enhancing the speed of muscle contraction and developing power. The OPT Model allows for systematic progression of resistance training, ensuring a balanced development of strength, power, endurance, stability, and flexibility, while minimizing the risk of injury.

Progressions can be categorized as the adaptations sought within the OPT Model, such as stabilization, muscular endurance, strength, hypertrophy, or power. Each level of the model features more detailed and specific progressions that are based on the athlete's abilities, goals, and sport.

ACUTE TRAINING VARIABLES

Acute training variables determine the amount of stress placed on the body and, ultimately, the physical adaptations that occur. Acute variables include repetitions, training intensity, sets, training volume, training frequency, repetition tempo, training duration, rest intervals, exercise selection, and exercise order. Each of these variables can significantly influence the overall training stimulus and, consequently, the adaptations achieved through the training program.

For instance, intensity (often defined as a percentage of the athlete's maximum lift) and volume are key determinants of muscular development, strength, and endurance responses to resistance training. Rest periods between sets can influence the metabolic and hormonal response to exercise and impact recovery and performance in subsequent sets. Tempo dictates the speed of each repetition, affecting time under tension—a critical component for muscular development.

Proper manipulation of these acute variables allows for training specificity, helping athletes meet their individual performance goals and requirements of their sport. Ultimately, a well-rounded understanding of these variables is essential for any coach or trainer hoping to design effective resistance training programs.

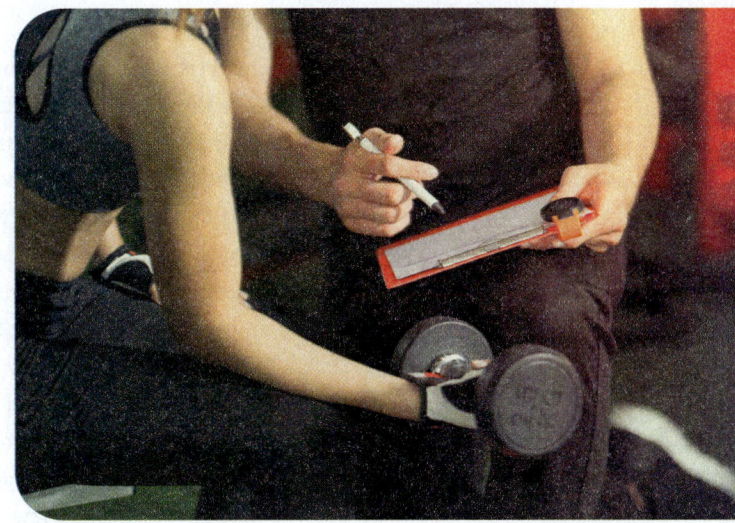

© TWStock/Shutterstock

REPETITIONS

The repetition range and the corresponding load are the key variables dictating the physiological response to the resistance training exercise. Repetitions are inversely related to the load lifted. In other words, the heavier the load, the lower the number of repetitions that can be achieved. Repetitions can be categorized as low (1 to 5), moderate (6 to 12), and high (13+). The repetition versus load relationship is often described using the **repetition maximum (RM) continuum** (**Figure 14.8**).

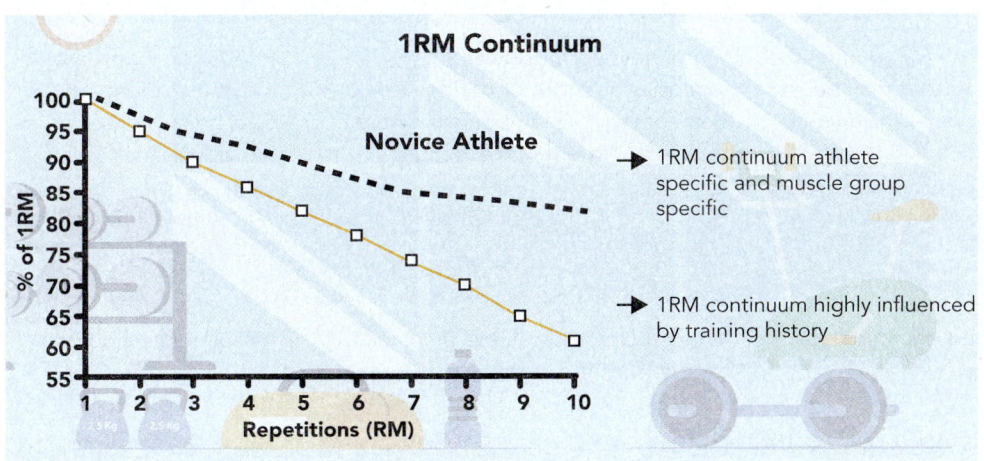

FIGURE 14.8 Repetition Maximum Continuum

A novice athlete can typically perform more repetitions at any given percentage of the one-repetition maximum (1RM) than can the elite athlete. This phenomenon has to do with the well-held notion that strength is a skill. The novice athlete does not have the skill to push their neuromuscular system to its full potential against the heaviest loads. Consequently, the 1RM may be underestimated for an untrained athlete. Evidence that novice untrained individuals are unable to recruit their muscles during maximum voluntary contractions optimally can be observed indirectly by the rapid improvement in strength that is often seen at the start of resistance training in the absence of muscle hypertrophy (Sale, 1988).

INTENSITY

The resistance training intensity typically corresponds to the lifted external load and how close the athlete is to reaching their momentary voluntary failure point (Suchomel et al., 2021; Thompson et al., 2020). Recall that RM is the maximum number of repetitions that can be performed at a given load—so an athlete could not perform 9 repetitions at their 8RM load. **Momentary failure** occurs when the athlete cannot lift the external load for another repetition on their own. Repetitions that exceed the RM require a spotter or external assistance. However, when researchers investigated whether athletes must hit the momentary failure point to optimize their resistance training adaptations, they found this failure was not necessary (Davies et al., 2016). In fact, avoiding momentary failure might provide superior gains in power and maximal strength.

Thus, resistance training intensity must be programmed carefully, along with the corresponding external load and repetition range (Suchomel et al., 2021; Thompson et al., 2020). **Table 14.1** identifies a few methods for programming intensity (it is not an exhaustive list).

TABLE 14.1 Programming Intensity

Method	Description	When to Use It	Cons
Repetition maximum	The maximum number of repetitions that can be performed at a given load	When momentary failure is important for training outcomes	Momentary failure can be taxing.
Percentage of 1RM	Programming a load at a certain percentage of an athlete's 1RM	When the 1RM is known and can be easily tracked	Most athletes do not know their 1RM.
Repetition in reserve	The number of additional repetitions that may be performed at a given load	When training for power and explosive strength or during demanding training periods where the risk for interference is high	Repetition in reserve may be challenging to estimate for some individuals.
Rating of perceived exertion	The athlete's subjective rating of intensity	When monitoring intensity is challenging	This may change with training age and injury.
Velocity-based training	The speed of movement	When technology allows the coach to monitor the speed of movement	It requires technology.

The ideal method for programming intensity depends on the context (Suchomel et al., 2021). For example, the percentage of 1RM method requires routine testing and monitoring of the athlete's 1RM. This method is feasible in only a few sports performance contexts, as 1RM testing requires experience and sound lifting technique. The rating of perceived exertion (RPE) provides a valid appraisal of resistance training exercise intensity, but, in novice athletes, it may be biased. The **velocity-based training (VBT)** method has the advantage of using a quantifiable outcome measure (bar speed or center of mass velocity), but Sports Performance Coaches require special equipment to make these measurements.

In combination, repetitions and intensity are the main variables dictating the physiological response to resistance training. However, as athletes gain more experience (i.e., training age), the corresponding intensity required to stimulate adaptation also increases (Peterson et al., 2005).

COACH'S CORNER

VBT has become more popular as wearable technology and linear position transducers have been introduced. These tools can help Sports Performance Coaches monitor velocity over time, which is a key outcome measure related to the development of power, performance fatigability, tapering, and peaking for competition.

SETS

Sets are groups of repetitions separated by a rest interval. The quantities of the other acute training variables (i.e., training frequency and intensity), the fitness level of the athlete, and training goals determine the number of sets that an individual will perform.

There is an inverse relationship between sets, repetitions, and intensity. The athlete usually performs fewer sets when performing higher repetitions at a lower intensity (lighter weight) and more sets when performing lower repetitions at a higher intensity (heavier weight).

As a rule, the greater the athlete's training age, the more sets that are required to elicit the desired training effect (Peterson et al., 2005). For example, the elite athlete may require numerous sets per exercise to achieve the desired training effect, whereas the novice or youth athlete may require only a few sets. An athlete's physical capabilities, fitness level, nutritional status, and goals determine the quantity of repetitions, sets, and training intensity (**Table 14.2**).

TABLE 14.2 Suggested Repetitions, Sets, and Training Intensity

Training Adaptation	Suggested Acute Variables*
Stabilization and muscular endurance	• Moderate to high repetitions: 12–20 or more • Low to moderate sets: 1–3 sets • Low to moderate training intensities: 50%–70% 1RM
Muscular hypertrophy[†]	• Low to moderate repetitions: 6–12 or more • Moderate to high sets: 3–6 sets • Moderate to high training intensities: 75%–85% 1RM
Maximal strength	• Low repetitions: 1–5 • High sets: 4–6 sets • High training intensities: 85%–100% 1RM
Power	• Low to moderate repetitions: 1–10 • Moderate to high sets: 3–6 sets • Low training intensities: about 10% of bodyweight (when using a medicine ball) or about 30%–45% (when using weights)

*The acute variables listed in this table are not absolutes. An athlete's training program, goals, and fitness level dictate appropriate acute variable selection.

[†]Muscle hypertrophy adaptations can be attained with various repetition, set, and intensity schemes depending on the total volume of training and the athlete's fitness level.

TRAINING VOLUME AND TRAINING FREQUENCY

Training volume is the product of total repetitions, sets, and loads performed in a training session (Schoenfeld et al., 2019). A simple formula exists for measuring it: Training volume = reps × sets × weight. Recent scientific evidence supports a dose-dependent relationship between the set number and muscular hypertrophy (Schoenfeld et al., 2017). To this end, 10 sets per muscle group per week can maximize muscle hypertrophy; however, individual responses are highly variable.

High-volume power training has been shown to positively affect maximal power and repeat power ability (Natera et al., 2020). A higher training volume measured by a greater number of sets has previously been considered necessary to maximize strength gains in well-trained athletes compared to untrained individuals (Peterson et al., 2005), but more recent evidence suggests that maximum strength can be developed using high-volume and low-volume schemes alike (Schoenfeld et al., 2019) (**Table 14.3**).

TABLE 14.3   Recommended Training Volume

Training Adaptation	Recommended Volume* (repetitions/exercise)	Training Frequency (sessions per week)
Stabilization and muscular endurance	36–75	• 2–3 for strength improvements
Muscular hypertrophy	27–36	• At least 1–2 to maintain physical, physiological, and performance improvements
Maximal strength	18–24	

*The acute variables listed in this table are not absolutes. An athlete's training program, goals, and fitness level dictate the appropriate total volume.

Recent expert opinion indicates that the training frequency may be a more important variable for increasing resistance training volume than increasing the number of sets, especially for the development of muscle hypertrophy (Dankel et al., 2017). But there is a caveat: Increasing the training frequency per week requires a decrease in the volume of any given training session. Thus, shorter, more intense training sessions are used to achieve the training effect, and because the impact of each resistance training session is lower, recovery between sessions occurs more quickly.

Collectively, these findings offer the following message regarding training volume and frequency:

- They can increase with an athlete's training age and when muscle hypertrophy is the primary training goal.
- Lower volumes can still elicit substantial improvements in maximal strength in trained individuals.
- Lower volume may allow prioritization of other physical capacities, especially during in-season training.
- There is no single best training volume or frequency. Adjusting training volume and training frequency as a source of variation and to fit within the context of the athlete's schedule and goals is encouraged.

TEMPO

Tempo refers to the movement speed for a given repetition (Wilk et al., 2021). There are four components to the exercise tempo: **eccentric**, **isometric**, **concentric**, and **isometric**. For example, a squat using a **4-2-1-1** tempo involves the following components:

- Lowering the body into the squat position for 4 seconds (**eccentric action**)
- Pausing in the squat position for 2 seconds (**isometric contraction**)
- Returning to the top position in 1 second (**concentric contraction**)
- Pausing at the top position for 1 second before repeating the next repetition (**isometric contraction**)

A dumbbell shoulder press using a **3-0-1-1** tempo involves the following components:

- Pressing the dumbbells overhead for 1 second (**concentric contraction**)
- Pausing at the top for 1 second (**isometric contraction**)
- Lowering the dumbbells for 3 seconds (**eccentric action**)
- Pausing at the bottom position for 0 seconds before repeating the next repetition (**isometric contraction**)

The tempo serves many important purposes. First, it allows the Sports Performance Coach to calculate and control the **time under tension**. A time under tension of 30 to 60 seconds generally promotes muscle hypertrophy, whereas a time under tension less than 15 seconds is typically used to stimulate neural adaptations to resistance training (Wilk et al., 2021). Second, repetition tempo is a source of program variation when training muscle hypertrophy, as both fast and slow tempos can effectively stimulate muscle growth (Wilk et al., 2021). Third, Sports Performance Coaches may maximize neural adaptations to resistance training that promote maximal strength and power by employing a technique known as compensatory acceleration. In this scenario, the athlete applies maximal effort to accelerate a heavy external load in the concentric movement phase; this technique maximizes intramuscular coordination. Finally, slow eccentric movement tempos may be employed to develop eccentric strength and eccentric control. **Table 14.4** provides a general overview of repetition tempos.

> **TIME UNDER TENSION** →
>
> The number of seconds the muscle is under tension in a single set; calculated by adding the tempo for the speed of movement and multiplying by the number of repetitions.

TABLE 14.4 Repetition Tempos

Training Adaptation	Recommended Tempo*
Muscular endurance and stability	Slow and controlled
Muscular hypertrophy	Moderate to fast
Maximal strength and power	Explosive

*The acute variables listed in this table are not absolutes.

TRAINING DURATION

Training duration has two prominent meanings: (1) the time frame from the start of the workout to the finish of the workout, not including the warm-up or cool-down, and (2) the amount of time (number of weeks) spent in one phase (or period) of training. The training duration for a workout is a function of the number of repetitions, number of sets, number of exercises, and length of the rest intervals. The training duration for an entire training phase is dictated by the athlete's level of physical ability, goal, and compliance with the program.

Typically, a training phase will last 4 weeks, as this is the amount of time it generally takes for the body to adapt to a given stimulus. Most adaptations to a stimulus will be realized within 4 weeks. Afterward, the training stimulus must be raised to promote further adaptations (Bompa, 1993).

Depending on the athlete's training status, training durations that exceed 60 to 90 minutes (excluding warm-up/cool-down) may be associated with rapidly declining energy levels for training. This causes alterations in hormonal and immune system responses that can hurt a training program and raise the risk of minor infections, especially upper respiratory infections (Kraemer & Ratamess, 2000).

REST

The inter-set rest interval is measured in seconds or minutes, and the inter-session rest interval is measured in days (Bird et al., 2005). As the intensity of resistance training exercise increases, the inter-set intervals typically increase (**Table 14.5**). This is especially critical when considering the overall training objective of the resistance training program. For example, if maximal strength is the primary training priority, then longer rest intervals that promote recovery of the ATP-CP energy pathway and limit the accumulation of metabolites that could impair the central nervous system (CNS) drive are paramount. However, in other instances, increasing the overall training intensity with short inter-set rest intervals may be desirable. For example, short inter-set rest intervals are sometimes used to increase the intensity when targeting muscle hypertrophy via metabolic pathways (Bird et al., 2005).

TABLE 14.5 Rest Intervals

Training Adaptation	Recommended Rest Periods*
Stabilization and muscular endurance	Short rest periods: 0–90 seconds
Muscular hypertrophy[†]	Short to moderately long rest periods: 0–180 seconds
Maximal strength	Long rest periods: 3–5 minutes
Power	Long rest periods: 3–5 minutes

*The acute variables listed in this table are not absolutes. An athlete's training program, goals, and fitness level dictate appropriate rest intervals.

[†]Muscle hypertrophy adaptations can be attained with various rest interval schemes depending on the total training volume and the athlete's fitness level.

EXERCISE SELECTION

The principle of exercise selection for sports performance is based on a few significant factors. First, each resistance training exercise elicits a specific neuromuscular response. For example, the incline bench press emphasizes the clavicular region of the pectoralis major, whereas the flat bench press emphasizes the sternal region pectoralis major. Additionally, exercise selection can affect the regional activation of the hamstring muscles (Bourne et al., 2017). The Nordic hamstring exercise, the Romanian deadlift, an isometric hamstring bridge, and a leg curl elicit different medial hamstrings (semitendinosus or semimembranosus) versus lateral hamstring (biceps femoris) muscle activity patterns.

Second, the ROM of an exercise (e.g., a full squat versus a half squat) can be manipulated to optimize adaptations for a given strength capacity. For example, a full ROM may be superior for increasing maximal strength and hypertrophy (Bird et al., 2005). In contrast, partial ROM and full ROM resistance training exercises may be equally effective for developing power and speed (Blazevich et al., 2020; Werkhausen et al., 2021).

Third, exercise selection should consider the movement velocity and time frames for force application, especially when training to improve power output (Blazevich et al., 2020). Additionally, when the training movement is more like the testing or competition movement, there is the potential

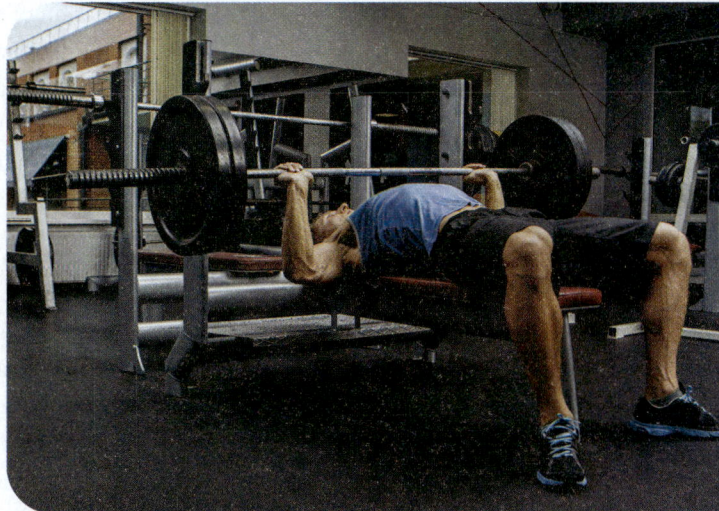

© BLACKDAY/Shutterstock

for a greater transfer of power (Blazevich et al., 2020). In support of this notion, and as previously discussed, exercise selection should reflect the positions and postures required for the sports performance skill.

Finally, whereas multi-joint movements are often preferred for developing maximal strength and power, combining multi-joint and single-joint exercises may best stimulate muscle hypertrophy (Bird et al., 2005). Single-joint movements may provide better isolation when addressing stabilizing muscles like the rotator cuff or hip rotators. These movements are often referred to as assistant or accessory exercises, and they are selected to complement the primary exercises of the program that target the primary training effect.

EXERCISE ORDER

The exercise order is the final loading parameter that can affect the efficacy of a resistance training program for sports performance (Bird et al., 2005). In this context, the principle of exercise order follows a few rules:

- Fast exercises before slower exercises (after a comprehensive warm-up)
- Multi-joint exercises before single-joint exercises
- Primary training goals before secondary or tertiary training goals

The arrangement of exercise order describes how exercises are performed during the workout and is influenced by factors including the athlete's goals, the fatigue response of the activity, and the specific type of exercise, such as multi-joint or single-joint. The primary method of exercise order is to first arrange exercises in order of priority. Specifically, the athlete will first perform those exercises that emphasize their specific goals in the workout, and then implement the less specific exercises toward the end of the training session. Reducing the element of fatigue is the primary justification for placing the priority exercise first.

The other method of exercise order is based on the type of exercise: multi-joint versus single-joint. Multi-joint (compound) exercises engage a large muscle mass that affects two or more primary joints. Single-joint exercises (e.g., bicep curls or triceps extensions) typically recruit a smaller muscle mass and use a single joint. The Sports Performance Coach should have the ability to choose from a multitude of options for both multi-joint and single-joint exercises.

This organization of exercise order allows the athlete to perform compound exercises under low fatigue while also maximizing excellent technique. To this end, the Sports Performance Coach should be able to optimize the training loads and tolerance levels for all athletes by arranging them in an ideal way to best reduce fatigue.

The Sports Performance Coach is encouraged to develop a checklist that covers nine specific aspects of performance training that should be included in each training session:

1. Athlete history and assessment
2. Review the previous program
3. Determine the primary and secondary training objectives of the current program
4. Determine the available training days, equipment, and training split if applicable
5. Select appropriate loading variables/parameters
6. Select the appropriate exercises
7. Write down primary and secondary exercises and corresponding loading variables
8. Write down additional accessory and supplementary exercises
9. Print and review the program

LESSON 5: REDUCING INJURY RISKS IN RESISTANCE TRAINING
RESISTANCE TRAINING SAFETY

The most important objective and goal for the Sports Performance Coach is to commit to doing no harm to the athlete. As in all athletic activities, the potential for injury is ever present during resistance training. However, the Sports Performance Coach should use all risk management measures to keep the injury risk to a minimum while maximizing athlete results. When the Sports Performance Coach increases knowledge through science and application, awareness is enhanced, and the risk of client injury due to poor judgment and negligence is decreased.

MAINTAINING A SAFE ENVIRONMENT

The Sports Performance Coach's scope of practice involves interviewing athletes to gather relevant information regarding their personal health and injury history, lifestyle, and sport-specific goals. This coach's care centers on instructing, demonstrating, teaching, evaluating, and providing extensive education and motivation to athletes. The Sports Performance Coach must effectively create and endorse the use of safe and efficient exercise programming through appropriate screening and comprehensive evaluations. They should also be able to respond appropriately to any emergencies that arise.

PROPER EQUIPMENT SETUP

Equipment should be grouped according to specific categories, including free weights, resistance training machines, plyometrics, and warm-up areas. A proper setup ensures adequate flow throughout the weight room, reducing congestion and maximizing the use of space. Sports Performance Coaches should be cognizant of the specific equipment used during their sessions and return all equipment to its original place. This helps maintain the condition of equipment and potentially reduces the risk of injury because unkempt or untidy equipment can become a tripping hazard. Sports Performance Coaches should never use damaged equipment in the facility, such as equipment with frayed cables or missing/unstable pieces. All equipment should be repaired or replaced if broken. Current and existing equipment should be cleaned regularly and upgraded over time.

FIVE KINETIC CHAIN CHECKPOINTS

Sports Performance Coaches must be diligent and meticulous when monitoring athletes' movements, and provide the appropriate corrections and cueing to ensure optimal form is maintained. This minimizes injury risk and maximizes muscle recruitment. As with all exercises, quality should always come before quantity or weight progression, and the five kinetic chain checkpoints should continuously be monitored (**Figure 14.9**). Although some variation might be allowed depending on the specific exercise (e.g., some powerlifting movements can be performed with the feet wider than neutral stance), most exercises should be performed with neutral alignment:

1. **Feet:** approximately shoulder-width apart and pointing straight ahead (unless the exercise requires a different foot position)
2. **Knees:** in line with the second and third toes (Avoid allowing knees to cave inward.)
3. **Hips:** level and in a neutral position
4. **Shoulders:** in a neutral position (Avoid protracting or elevating the shoulders unless the exercise requires these positions.)
5. **Head:** cervical spine in a neutral position

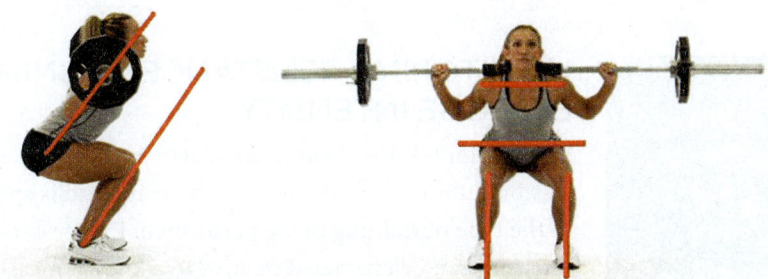

FIGURE 14.9 Five Kinetic Chain Checkpoints

📋 COACH'S CORNER

Additional checkpoints may need to be monitored during exercise to ensure proper form and technique. These checkpoints may include elbow, wrist, and grip position. Moreover, the velocity of movement, landing and sprinting mechanics, and heart rate responses or ratings of perceived exertion during exercise are important when evaluating athletes' performance.

PROPER BREATHING TECHNIQUE

Breathing mechanics influence muscular function and posture because the habitual use of breathing muscles during respiration affects how these muscles are used during exercise (Courtney, 2009). Especially during resistance training, Sports Performance Coaches need to teach athletes proper breathing techniques to maximize performance and minimize

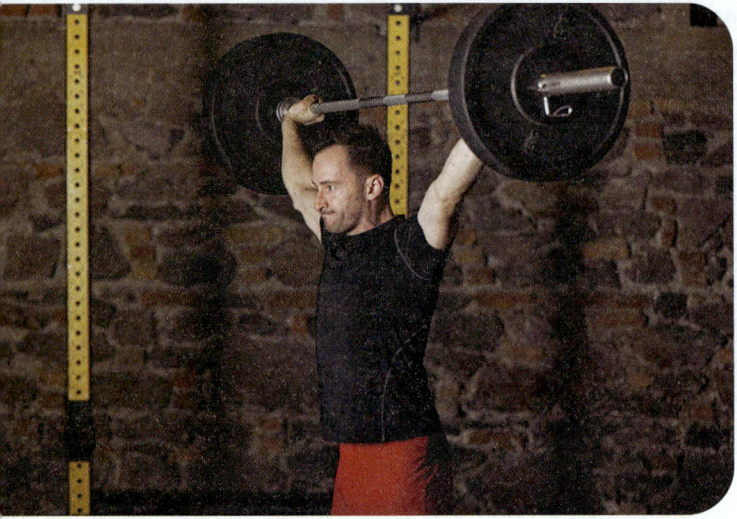

© Berkomaster/Shutterstock

injury risk. Except during special circumstances (i.e., power lifting), the athlete should breathe out (exhalation) during the concentric phase and breathe in (inhalation) during the eccentric phase.

The Valsalva maneuver can be a helpful breathing strategy when performing maximal or near-maximal lifts to ensure spinal stability (Hackett & Chow, 2013). This process involves expiring against a closed glottis, which creates additional intra-abdominal pressure and spinal stability, and reduces the associative compressive forces on the spinal discs during lifting. Keeping the spine stable requires individuals to brace the trunk, using many abdominal muscles and therefore generating large amounts of intra-abdominal pressure—a critically important factor when lifting heavy loads (Kroell & Mike, 2017).

However, the Valsalva maneuver is also potentially dangerous because it can cause lightheadedness and dizziness, impede the return of venous blood to the heart, and raise an individual's heart rate and blood pressure. Using the Valsalva maneuver is generally not recommended for athletes presenting with hypertension and other forms of heart disease (Looga, 2005). If an athlete is not training for maximal strength development, the Valsalva maneuver is usually not recommended.

MONITORING RESISTANCE TRAINING EXERCISE INTENSITY

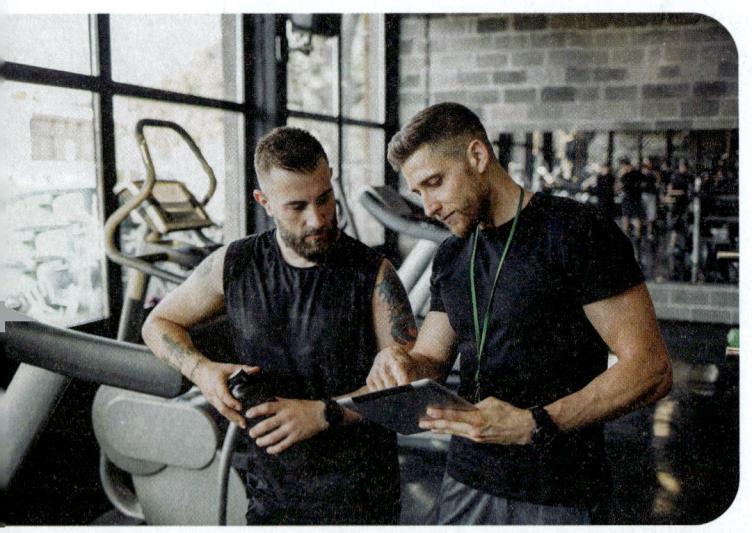

© Gardinovachki/Shutterstock

The session training load is calculated as the product of the session duration and the session intensity, and is specific to the type of training being performed. Exercise training intensity can be estimated relative to a known measure. For example, suppose an athlete performs an incremental exercise test on a cycle ergometer. In this example, the athlete's maximal aerobic power can easily be determined alongside their maximal heart rate. Sports Performance Coaches can monitor training intensity using these measures, particularly when athletes engage in cardiorespiratory exercise. However, when it comes to resistance training, the Sports Performance Coach may not know the 1RM strength or maximum speed of movement for a given exercise at a given load. Training intensity can also be viewed according to the internal physiological intensity that is incurred by the athlete, which further complicates the process of quantifying resistance training intensity.

The process of tracking training load (i.e., number of lb/kg lifted) is frequently used but is limited in its application. Imagine two athletes performing a 100-lb back squat. The first athlete has a 1RM in the back squat of 200 lb; therefore, they are lifting 50% of their 1RM. The second athlete has a 1RM of 120 lb; consequently, they are lifting 83% of their 1RM. While the resistance training intensity may be measured as the external load lifted (i.e., 100 lb), the second athlete's relative intensity is higher.

PERCENTAGE OF 1RM

There are a few scientifically validated methods to quantify resistance training intensity (Suchomel et al., 2021). Approaches to tracking the training load and its components (volume and intensity) are essential for a more deliberate and scientific approach to resistance training.

The notion of progressive resistance training targeted to the individual's strength capacity was first introduced by Captain Thomas Delorme (1945) with the term *repetition maximum* (RM). RM is the maximum number of repetitions that can be performed at a given external load (Delorme, 1945; Delorme & Watkins, 1948). Delorme (1945) applied the concept of progressive resistance training in a rehabilitation setting to help injured soldiers returning from war. The concept of RM entails achieving momentary failure (i.e., the athlete cannot complete another repetition without compensating with their technique or getting the assistance of a spotter) (Suchomel et al., 2021). A sequence of progressive loading is typically done in the first training session to determine an athlete's RM load (**Table 14.6**).

TABLE 14.6 Determining RM Load

Set Number	Repetitions	Load
Warm-up	5	135 lb
Set 1	8	175 lb
Set 2	8	185 lb
Set 3	8	200 lb
Set 4	8	205 lb

The percentage of 1RM method is one of the most commonly used approaches for identifying resistance training intensity (Suchomel et al., 2021). The athlete's 1RM is determined either through 1RM testing or predicted 1RM testing. A range of percentages is then used to target strength endurance, hypertrophy, and maximal strength training. This method does have some drawbacks, however. For example, the 1RM value will change with training age, muscle group, exercise, and fatigue/readiness. It also requires ongoing assessment of the 1RM load, which can be time-consuming.

📋 COACH'S CORNER

An athlete's 1RM must be determined for a given exercise to use the percentage of 1RM method. For example, if 70% intensity is programmed for a resistance training exercise, then the Sports Performance Coach will multiply the athlete's 1RM by 0.7. However, this method may be impractical because it requires consistent testing and tracking of the athlete's 1RM.

An alternative to the percentage of 1RM method is based on the progressive resistance training concept. This method typically uses a three-repetition bracket (e.g., 6 to 8 RM). When the athlete can complete the upper end of the repetition bracket for their working set, it is appropriate to increase the load in the subsequent training session (**Table 14.7**).

TABLE 14.7 Progressive Resistance Training Sets of 6 to 8 RM Example

Set Number	Repetitions	Load
Warm-up	5	135 lb
Set 1	8	175 lb
Set 2	8	185 lb
Set 3	8	200 lb
Set 4	8	205 lb
Next session		Working set = 210 lb

RATINGS OF PERCEIVED EXERTION

To address the limitations of the percentage of 1RM method, resistance training intensity may be prescribed using ratings of perceived exertion (RPE). RPE is a subjective rating scale from 1 to 10 in which athletes subjectively rate their level of effort during exercise based on physical markers, such as breathlessness, fatigue, sweat rate, and muscle soreness (Muyor, 2013) (**Table 14.8**). A lower score indicates light effort, whereas scores closer to 10 indicate intense effort.

TABLE 14.8 Ratings of Perceived Exertion

Rating	Perceived Exertion Level
0	No exertion, at rest
1	Very light
2–3	Light
4–5	Moderate, somewhat hard
6–7	High, vigorous
8–9	Very hard
10	Maximum effort, highest possible

VELOCITY-BASED TRAINING

Measuring and monitoring the movement or barbell velocity is the final method for programming resistance training intensity. This method has been called velocity-based training (VBT). The increasing availability of technology that measures bar or movement velocity has made it easier for Sports Performance Coaches to use this method. It can be done using inertial measurement unit (IMU) technology, accelerometers, and linear position transducers (LPT). The advantage of the VBT method is the ability to quantify resistance training intensity across all loading zones, especially when the goal is to maximize the movement speed, as in the case of power training.

 COACH'S CORNER

Resistance training intensity may be quantified and managed most effectively using a combination of methods under the umbrella of autoregulation (Suchomel et al., 2021). Coaches may want to adjust the program's intensity because athletes' readiness to train may vary due to poor sleep, muscle soreness, and psychological factors. In such a case, a coach could prescribe an intensity with the percentage of 1RM method (e.g., 85% of 1RM) along with RPE (e.g., RPE = 8) that allows the athlete to adjust the intensity if needed.

SPOTTING TECHNIQUES

Spotting is the process of assisting a lifter during a set of an exercises either as a safety measure or to slightly lessen the resistance so the lifter can perform the requisite number of repetitions. The Sports Performance Coach must teach and model proper technique during exercise, perform proper spotting, and monitor all exercise movements to ensure safe execution. It is critical for Sports Performance Coaches to exhibit large degrees of confidence and experience concerning spotting techniques to provide maximum safety and high-quality coaching for every session. Compound exercises, such as a barbell back squat, bench press, or dumbbell shoulder press, require a spotter to reduce injury risk, especially when using heavier loads. Research has indicated that a decrease in injuries occurs through proper spotting techniques (Lombardi & Troxel, 2003).

The Sports Performance Coach should use the following checklist during spotting activities. The spotter should:

- Identify the number of total repetitions before the beginning of each set.
- Stand and maintain a stable, wide-stance body position.
- Deliver adequate and ample support for the successful execution of the lift, especially through the sticking point (the range of greatest mechanical disadvantage).
- Spot at the client's wrists instead of the elbows when using dumbbells (i.e., in a dumbbell shoulder press) to prevent the arms from caving inward.
- Be positioned behind the lifter during a squat and place their upper arms underneath the lifter's armpits. If the athlete is uncomfortable with this procedure, employ the use of two spotters positioned at both ends of the barbell (**Figure 14.10**).
- Use an additional spotter for exercises when the load surpasses what a single spotter can successfully manage on their own.
- Not spot machine-based or cable-based exercises by placing their hands underneath the weight stack.

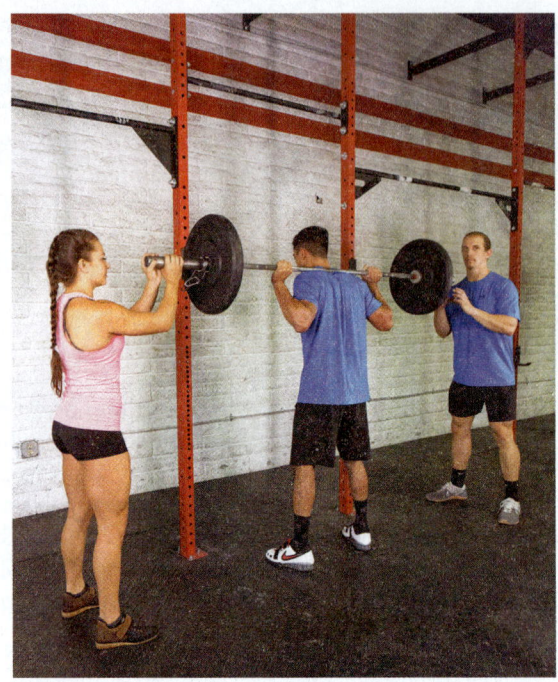

FIGURE 14.10 Two People Spotting a Barbell Squat

LESSON 6: RESISTANCE TRAINING MISCONCEPTIONS
COUNTERING MISCONCEPTIONS ABOUT RESISTANCE TRAINING

Resistance training has been used for more than 3,000 years to help athletes augment sports performance and build resilience against injury. Even with the long history of resistance training, the debate about whether resistance training is good or bad for all athletes continues.

There can be several reasons why some athletes are hesitant to engage in resistance training. One common misconception is the fear of gaining too much muscle mass, which they believe could affect their mobility, agility, or speed, especially in sports where a lean physique is beneficial. Other athletes may be concerned about the risk of injury from lifting heavy weights, particularly if they have previously experienced injuries or have a limited understanding of proper lifting techniques. Some athletes may prioritize sport-specific skills training over resistance training, viewing it as secondary or less important to their performance. Lastly, some athletes might not have access to appropriate training facilities or might lack the knowledge about how to effectively and safely incorporate resistance training into their training regimen. It is essential for coaches and trainers to address these concerns and misconceptions and to educate athletes about the significant benefits that resistance training can offer in terms of strength, injury prevention, and overall performance.

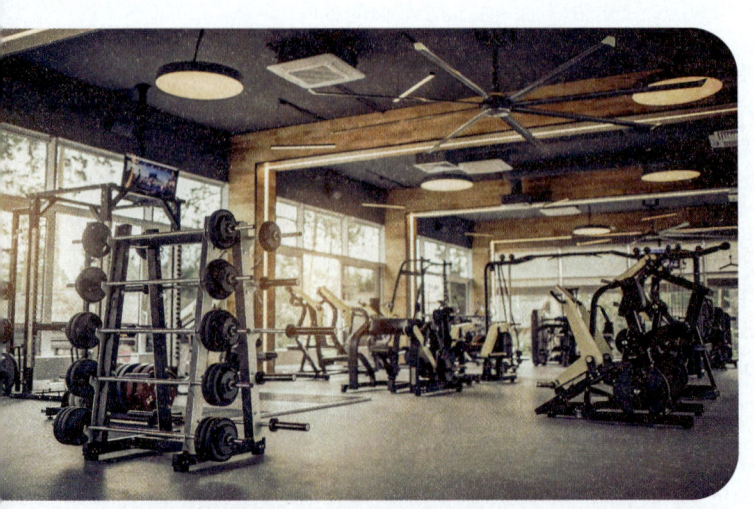

YOUTH ATHLETE AND PARENT MISCONCEPTIONS

There is a widely held misconception that resistance training may harm the physical development of adolescent athletes and children, increasing their risk for injury. However, experts strongly disagree with this notion. Scientific evidence suggests that children and adolescents need resistance training today more than ever (Behm et al., 2017; Faigenbaum et al., 2016; Faigenbaum et al., 2019; Granacher et al., 2016; Laurson et al., 2017; Lesinski et al., 2016; Ryman Augustsson & Ageberg, 2017).

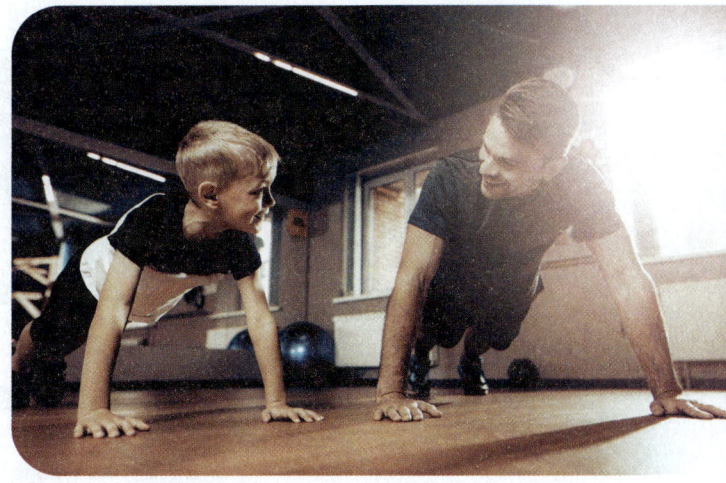

© VGstockstudio/Shutterstock

Today's adolescents are substantially less strong than their counterparts from three decades ago (Laurson et al., 2017). The term **pediatric dynapenia** is used to describe the widespread loss of muscle strength and power that was once thought to impact only elderly individuals (Faigenbaum et al., 2016; Faigenbaum et al., 2019). Today's youth athletes have lower muscle strength than a few generations ago, which negatively impacts their sports performance. There are several factors underpinning this reality.

First, there is increasing pressure on youth athletes to specialize in just a few sports and to place less emphasis on strength and conditioning (Granacher et al., 2016). This phenomenon has reduced children's and adolescents' strength reserve (Behm et al., 2017; Faigenbaum et al., 2016; Faigenbaum et al., 2019). The strength reserve is a safety buffer between the physical limits of the athlete and the unforeseen high-force and high-energy events that occur quite routinely in all kinds of sports. The strength reserve and higher levels of maximal strength positively impact sports performance and capacities such as speed and change-of-direction maneuvers (Behm et al., 2017; Chaabene et al., 2020; Faigenbaum et al., 2016; Granacher et al., 2016). They also decrease the risk of lower-extremity injuries like noncontact ACL rupture (Ryman Augustsson & Ageberg, 2017; Steidl-Müller et al., 2018).

Moreover, when it comes to adolescents and children, power training does not substitute for traditional strength training for increasing speed and lower-body strength (Behm et al., 2017).

The belief that resistance training will cause harm to children and adolescents' growth plates has been refuted. Even so, children and adolescents should not be regarded as simply "small adults." Consequently, Sports Performance Coaches are encouraged to think carefully about long-term athlete development, conduct a proper needs analysis and initial assessment, and then apply the principles of progressive resistance training discussed throughout this chapter (Granacher et al., 2016). They should also consider the chronological (biological) age and the athlete's training age.

The starting point in the journey to sports performance begins with acquiring basic physical literacy skills such as running, jumping, throwing, and tumbling. Next, athletes should engage in a progressive increase in training, including resistance training. Resistance training requires technical competencies alongside the biological milieu to promote positive adaptations (e.g., sufficient endocrinological development, motor control, and executive function).

Biological maturation and readiness to train with higher intensities may unfold differently for individual athletes. Thus, Sports Performance Coaches should monitor progress throughout adolescence to ensure the training methods align with the athlete's biological development and training age (**Figure 14.11**).

PEDIATRIC DYNAPENIA →

The medical term for loss of muscle strength and power that impacts function in children.

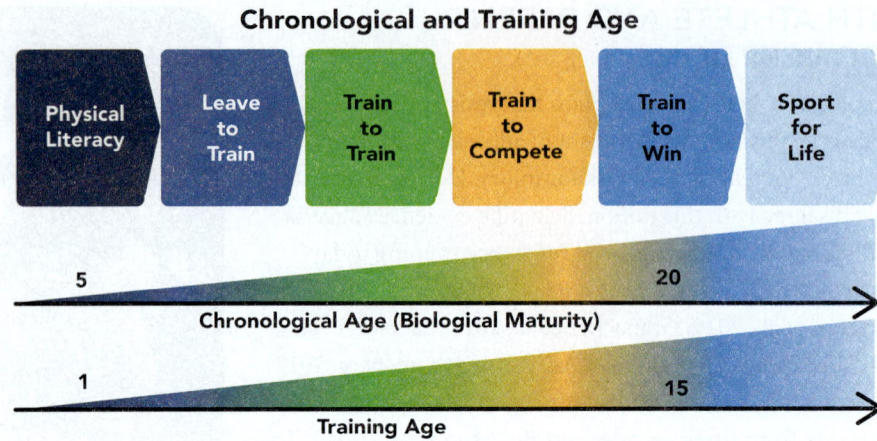

FIGURE 14.11 Long-Term Athlete Development Model

ENDURANCE SPORTS MISCONCEPTIONS

Endurance athletes (e.g., marathon runners, cross-country skiers, cyclists, and triathletes) are often concerned that resistance training will be counterproductive for their performance due to unwanted muscle hypertrophy and impairment of the physiological contributors to endurance performance, such as movement economy, maximal oxygen consumption (VO_2 max), and the lactate threshold. However, the scientific evidence is unequivocal: The correct type of resistance training has a highly beneficial effect on endurance performance (Aagaard & Andersen, 2010; Häkkinen et al., 2003; Peterson et al., 2005; Rønnestad & Mujika, 2014; Wilson et al., 2012). In fact, research demonstrates that heavy resistance training positively affects performance in **time-based Olympic sports** independent of age and the sport (Lum & Barbosa, 2019). The primary mechanisms by which resistance training augments endurance performance are by increasing neuromuscular drive, tendon stiffness, and plyometric ability, leading to improved movement economy (Heggelund et al., 2013; Li et al., 2021; Rønnestad et al., 2015). These physiological adaptations are a massive advantage for endurance athletes.

Focusing on heavy resistance training and plyometric training for the endurance athlete might seem contrary to intuition. If they do not consider the science that shows how resistance training should be applied to endurance athletes, Sports Performance Coaches may erroneously believe that muscular endurance training should be the primary focus for endurance athletes. However, muscular endurance training may be ineffective for improving movement economy in endurance athletes. Also, experts have recently revisited the loading parameters that cause muscle hypertrophy. Light-load, high-repetition resistance training schemes are now well known to elicit muscle hypertrophy in certain populations (Schoenfeld et al., 2021). Resistance training—specifically heavy strength training and plyometric training—can profoundly affect endurance performance, and the best athletes routinely employ these methods to increase their movement economy.

INTERFERENCE EFFECT MISCONCEPTIONS

Recall that the interference effect occurs when two or more competing molecular pathways arise from training, and one pathway consumes the energy required by the second pathway, thereby blunting the desired training effect (Fyfe et al., 2014). In simpler terms, the body's energy resources are limited, and adaptations to all forms of training require energy.

> **TIME-BASED OLYMPIC SPORTS** →
>
> Events raced against the clock, where the fastest time wins the race; also known as cyclical sports.

Now consider a training program targeting aerobic capacity alongside muscle hypertrophy. The aerobic training involves continuous, long-duration, low-intensity cycling, whereas the hypertrophy training involves whole-body exercises, multiple sets and repetitions, and high time under tension. In this case, the two training stimuli (aerobic and hypertrophy training) stimulate the muscle differently.

The training stimulus signals the neuromuscular system how to adapt. An interference effect means that one type of training gets in the way of the other by impairing the signal and the energy reserve, so that the muscle cannot adapt properly. In the example, interference might occur within the same training session due to the sheer existence of both training stimuli, due to the order within the session (i.e., whether resistance training comes first or aerobic training), or because of the order between sessions.

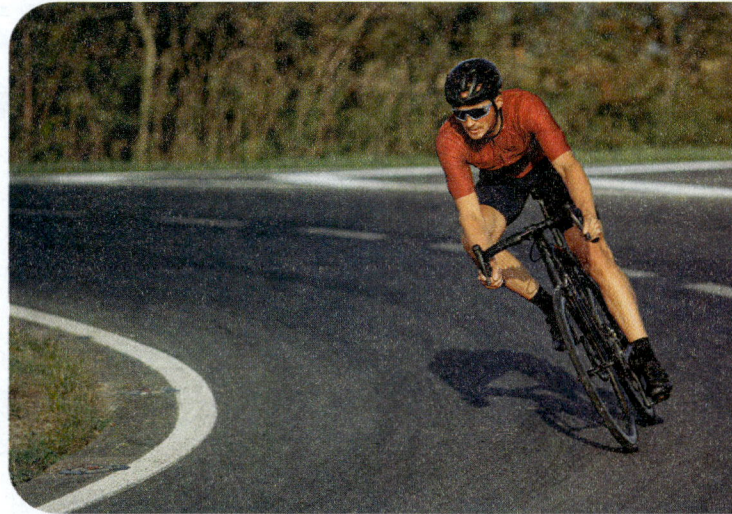

© LovetheLifeyouLive/Shutterstock

Resistance training is often thought to interfere with speed development, adaptations to endurance exercise, change-of-direction ability, and quickness. On all accounts, science paints a very different picture than these myths. First, heavy strength training and the combination of heavy strength training with plyometric training are associated with improvements in running speed (Seitz et al., 2014; Spiteri et al., 2014). Moreover, maximal strength can almost be viewed as a prerequisite for muscle power and speed in youth athletes (Behm et al., 2017). In other words, resistance training is synergistic with speed, quickness, and change-of-direction ability.

Interestingly, in regard to resistance training and endurance training, the interference effect happens in one direction but not the other. That is, endurance training may blunt resistance training adaptations such as improvements in explosive strength and maximal power (Wilson et al., 2012). In contrast,

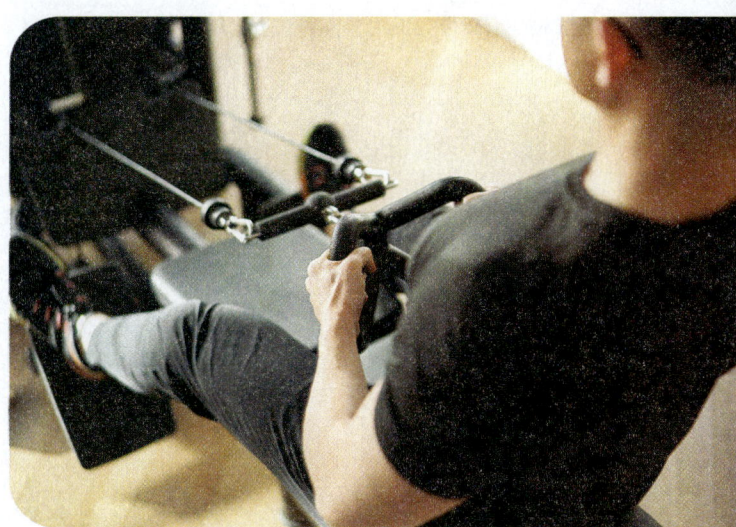

© Mapo_Japan/Shutterstock

resistance training does not have any adverse effects on endurance training adaptations such as muscle capillarization (i.e., increased muscle capillaries) and improvements in VO_2 max. Further, while the training order endurance training + resistance training may impair strength and hypertrophy adaptations, the training order resistance training + endurance training may elicit a synergistic effect provided that the endurance training exercise is at a moderate level (Eddens et al., 2018; Fernandez-Gonzalo et al., 2013; Lundberg et al., 2013).

Acute exposure to heavy resistance training has also been shown to increase RFD and maximal power due to PAP (Blazevich & Babault, 2019; Cuenca-Fernández et al., 2017; Prieske et al., 2020). This adaption is the opposite of an interference effect. Imagine increasing an athlete's explosive strength or maximal power just by doing a little heavy resistance training before a competition or a race. This is what PAP entails, and it even occurs remotely—for example, intense resistance training for the upper body can increase lower-body maximal power and explosive strength (Cuenca-Fernández et al., 2017).

The notion that resistance training interferes with other sports performance capacities such as speed, change-of-direction capacity, and endurance is unfounded. However, Sports Performance Coaches are encouraged to consider that too little or too much of any good thing might be a problem; a middle ground exists for the synergistic effects of resistance training.

LESSON 7: RESISTANCE TRAINING EXERCISES

Table 14.9 lists some commonly used stabilization-focused, strength-focused, and power-focused resistance training exercises, though this is not an exhaustive list. When designing resistance training programs, the Sports Performance Coach should consider specific acute training variables for each focus.

TABLE 14.9 Common Acute Training Variables for Resistance Training

Focus of Exercise	Primary Goal	Training Variables
Stabilization	Joint stabilization and muscular endurance	• Repetitions: 12–20 or more • Sets: 1–3 • Intensity: 50%–70% of 1RM
Strength	Prime mover strength	Muscular development • Repetitions: 6–12 or more • Sets: 3–6 • Intensity: 75%–85% of 1RM Maximal strength • Repetitions: 1–5 • Sets: 4–6 • Intensity: 85%–100% of 1RM
Power	Rate of force production	• Repetitions: 1–10 • Sets: 3–6 • Intensity: approximately 10% of bodyweight with medicine ball training and 30%–45% of 1RM with weight training

TOTAL-BODY EXERCISES

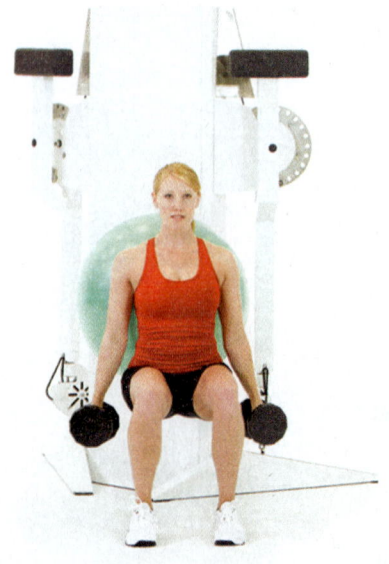 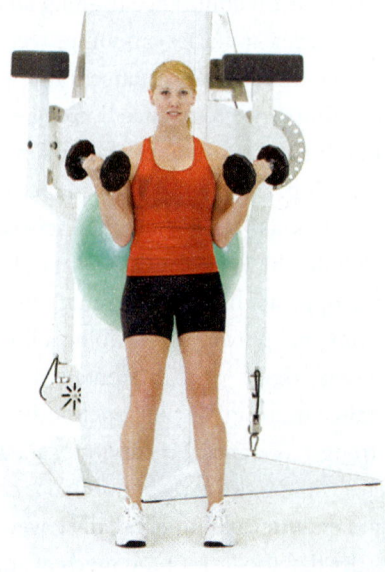 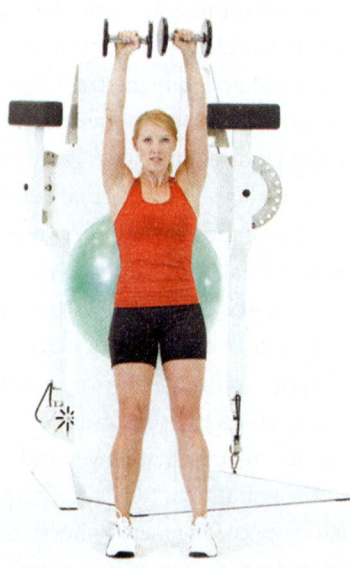

Ball Squat, Curl to Press

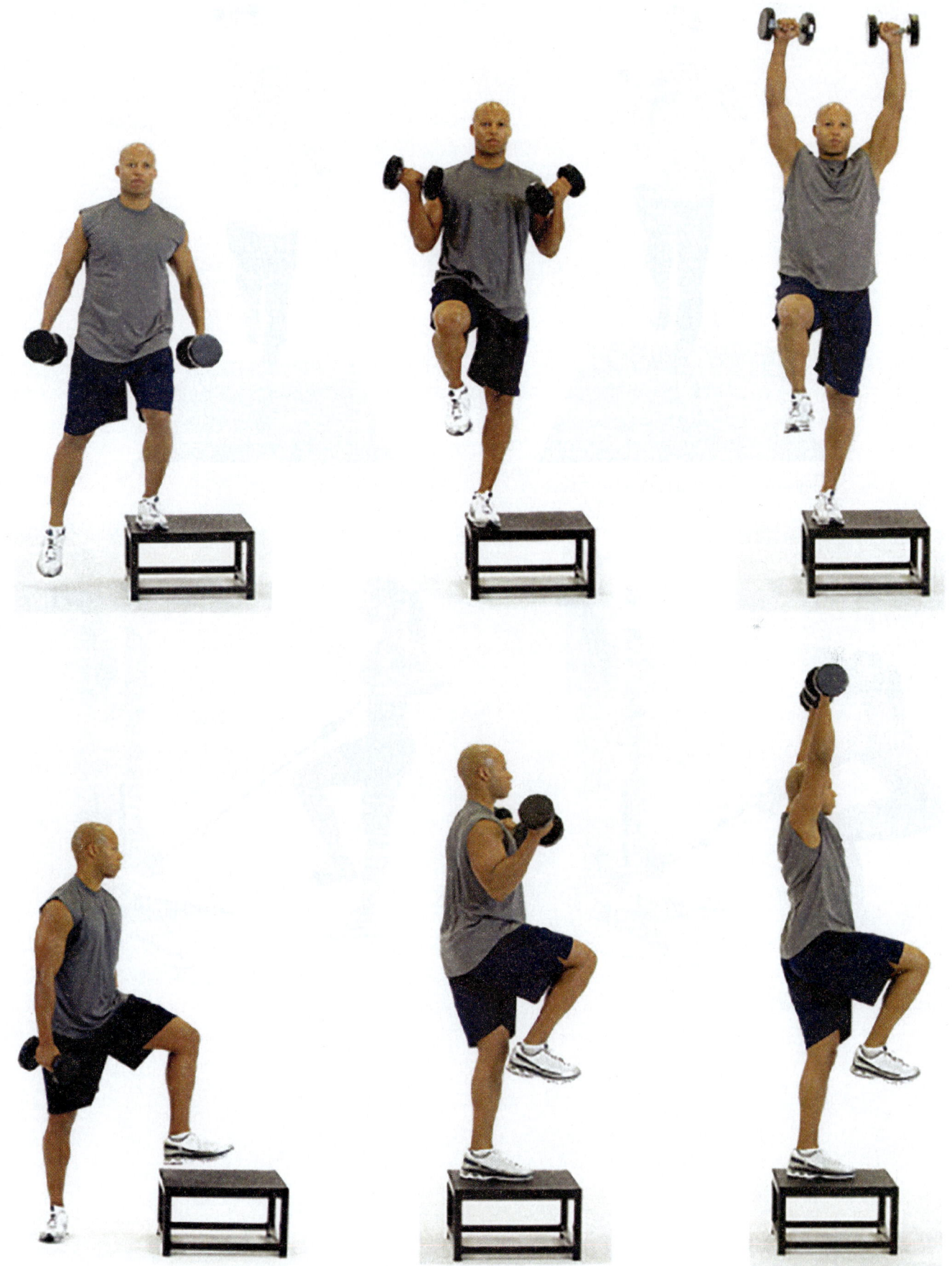

Multiplanar Step-up, Balance, Overhead Press

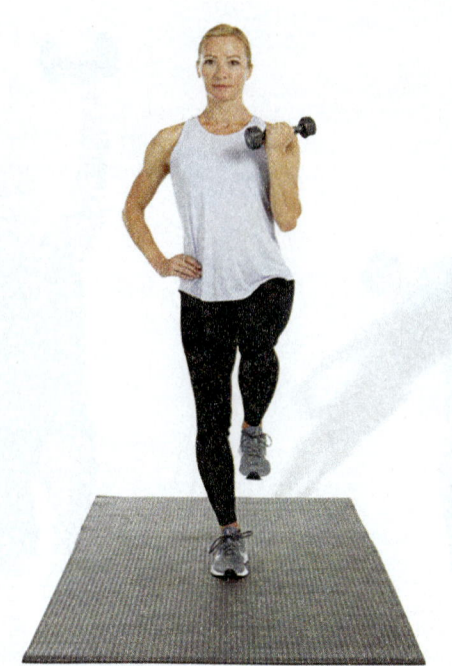 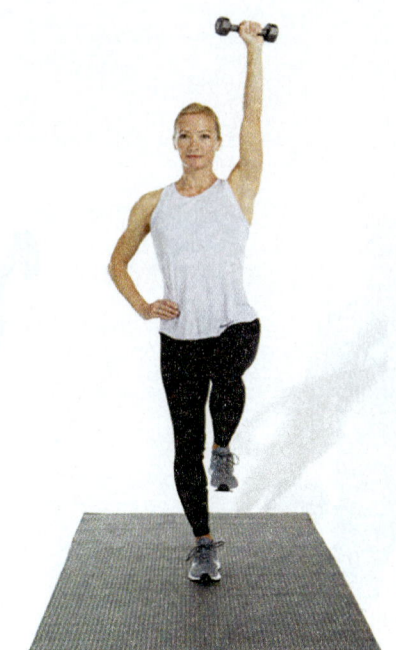

Single-Leg Squat, Curl to Overhead Press

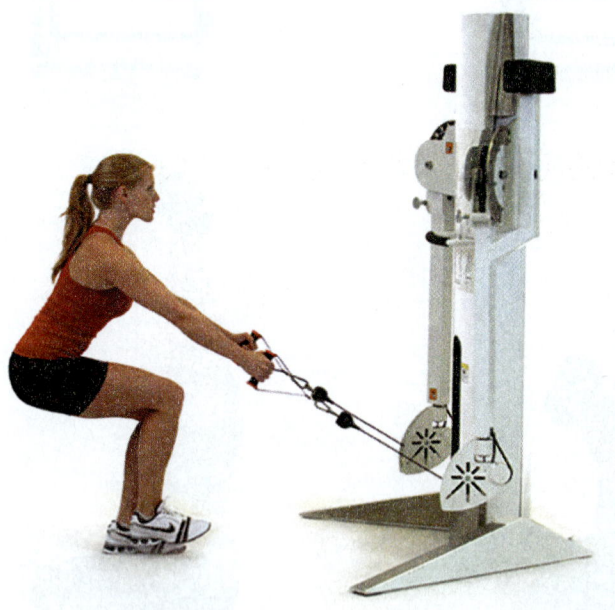 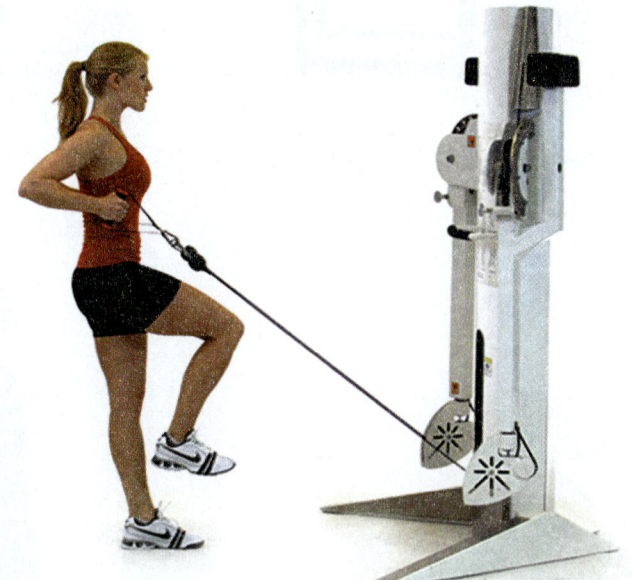

Single-Leg Squat to Row

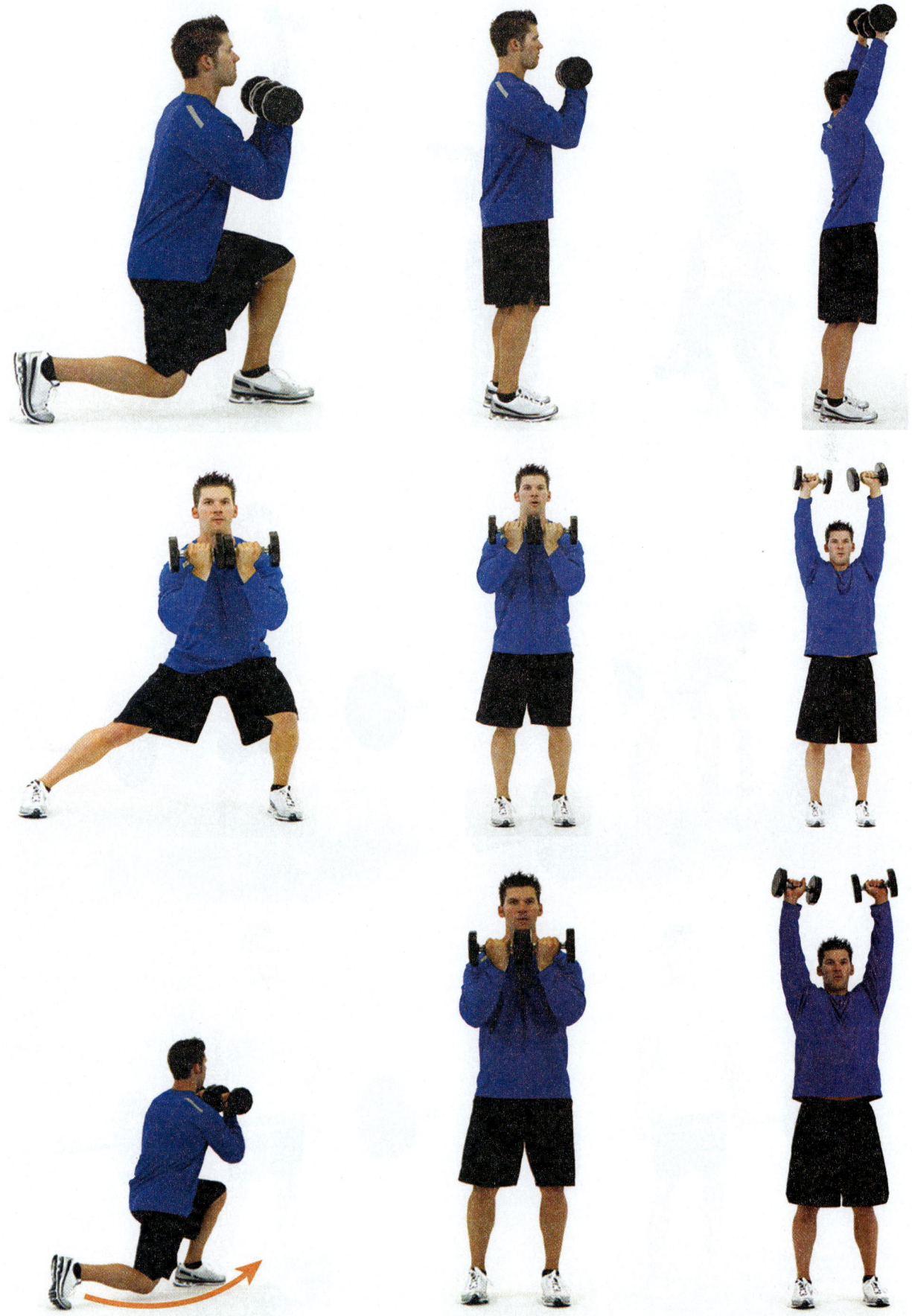

Multiplanar Lunge to Two-Arm Dumbbell Press

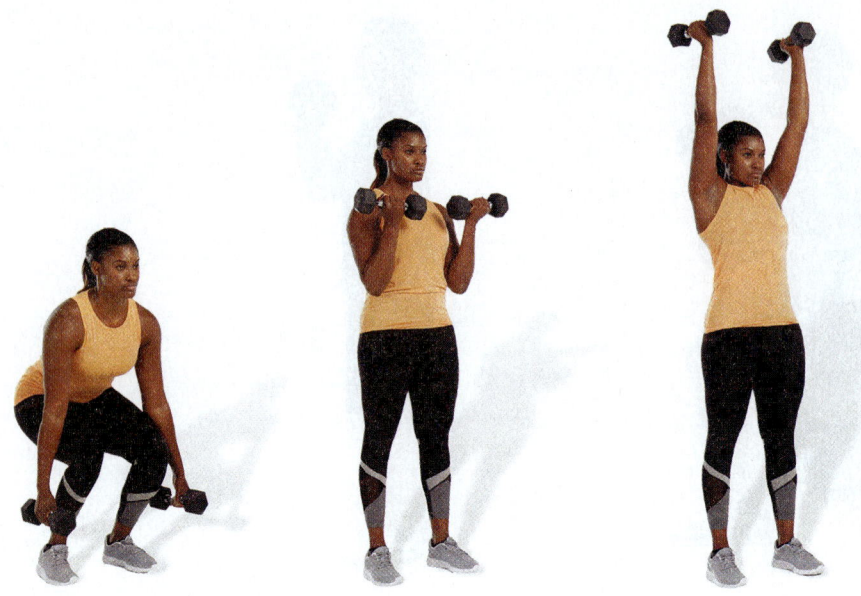

Squat, Curl to Two-Arm Press

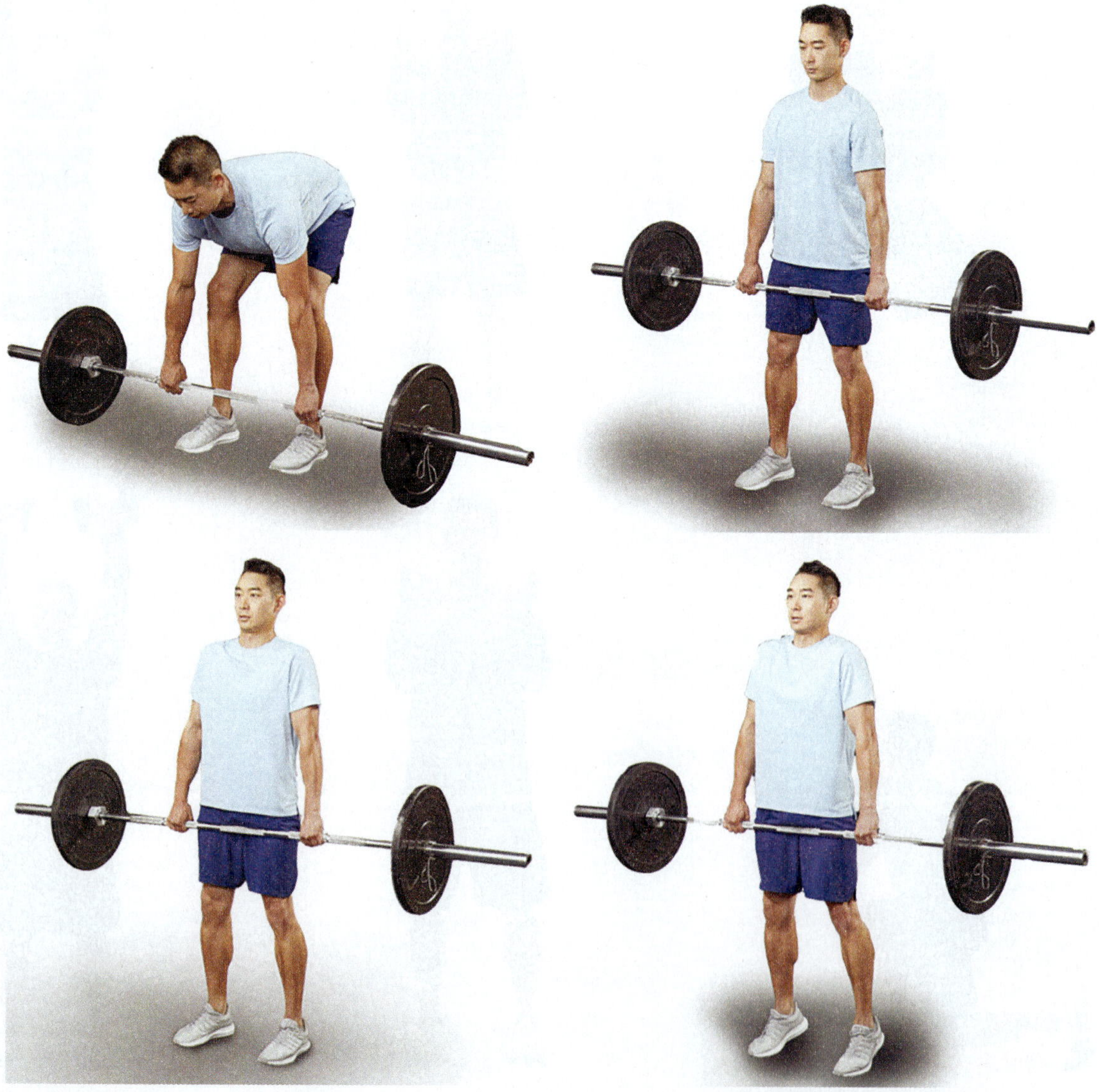

Barbell Deadlift, Shrug to Calf Raise

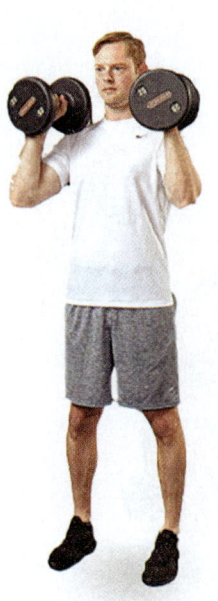
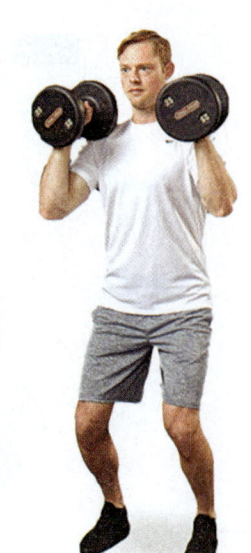
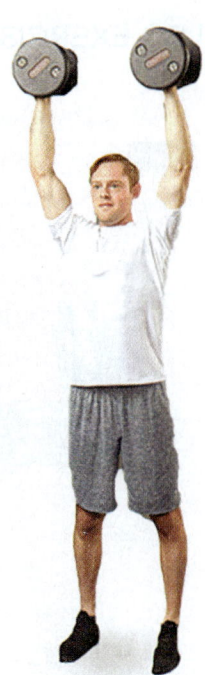

Two-Arm Push Press

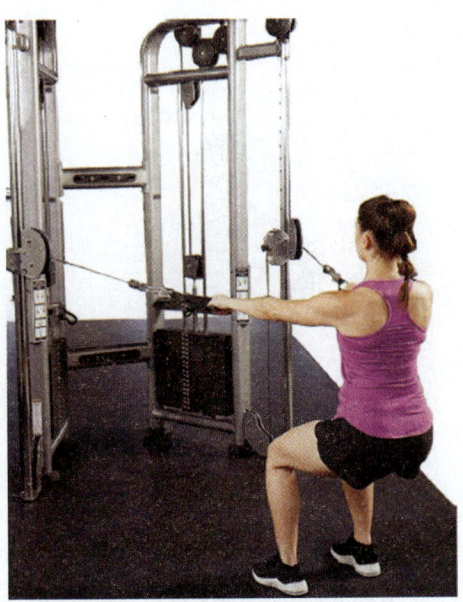
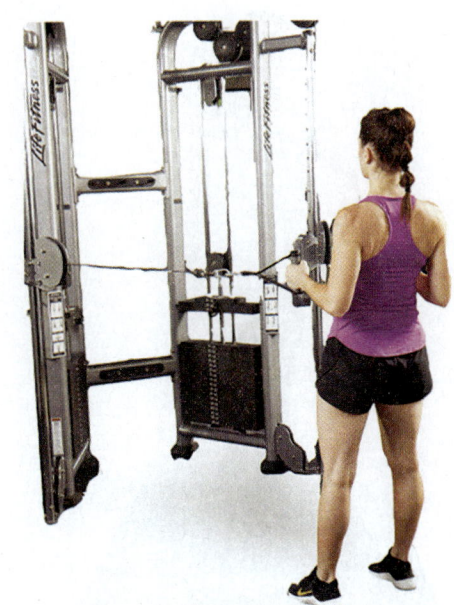

Squat to Row

LEG EXERCISES

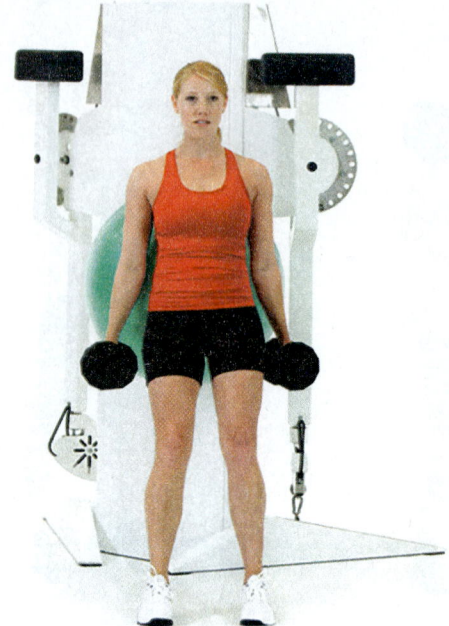 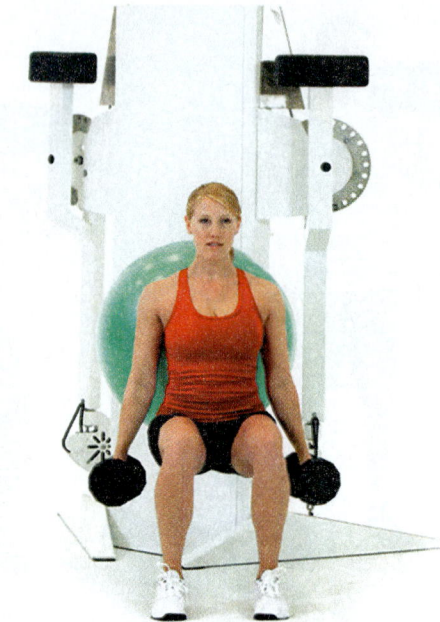

Ball Squat

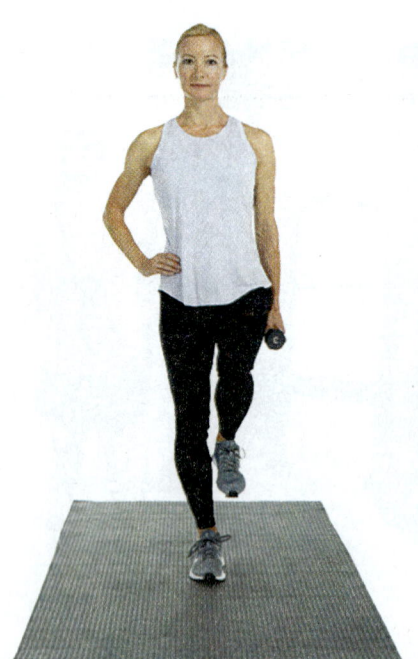 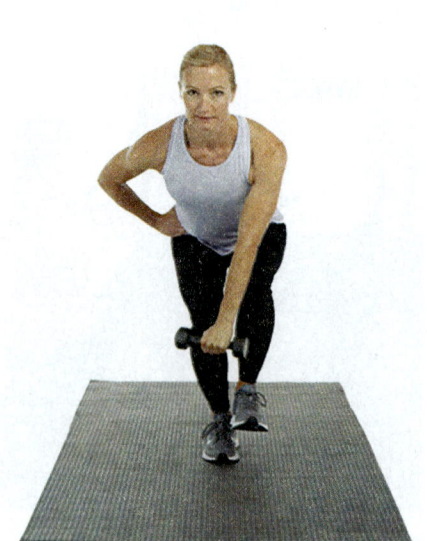

Single-Leg Squat

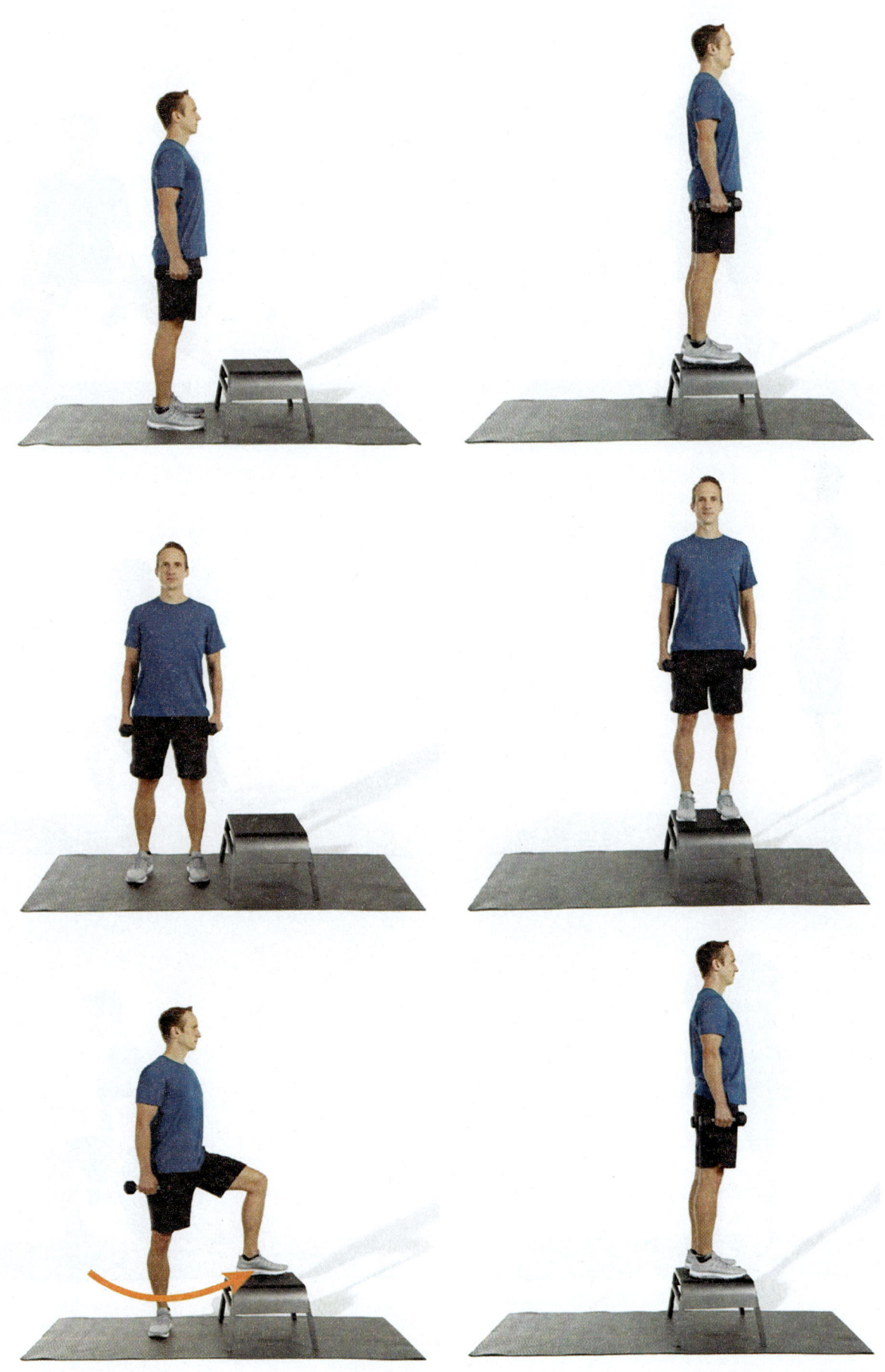

Multiplanar Step-up

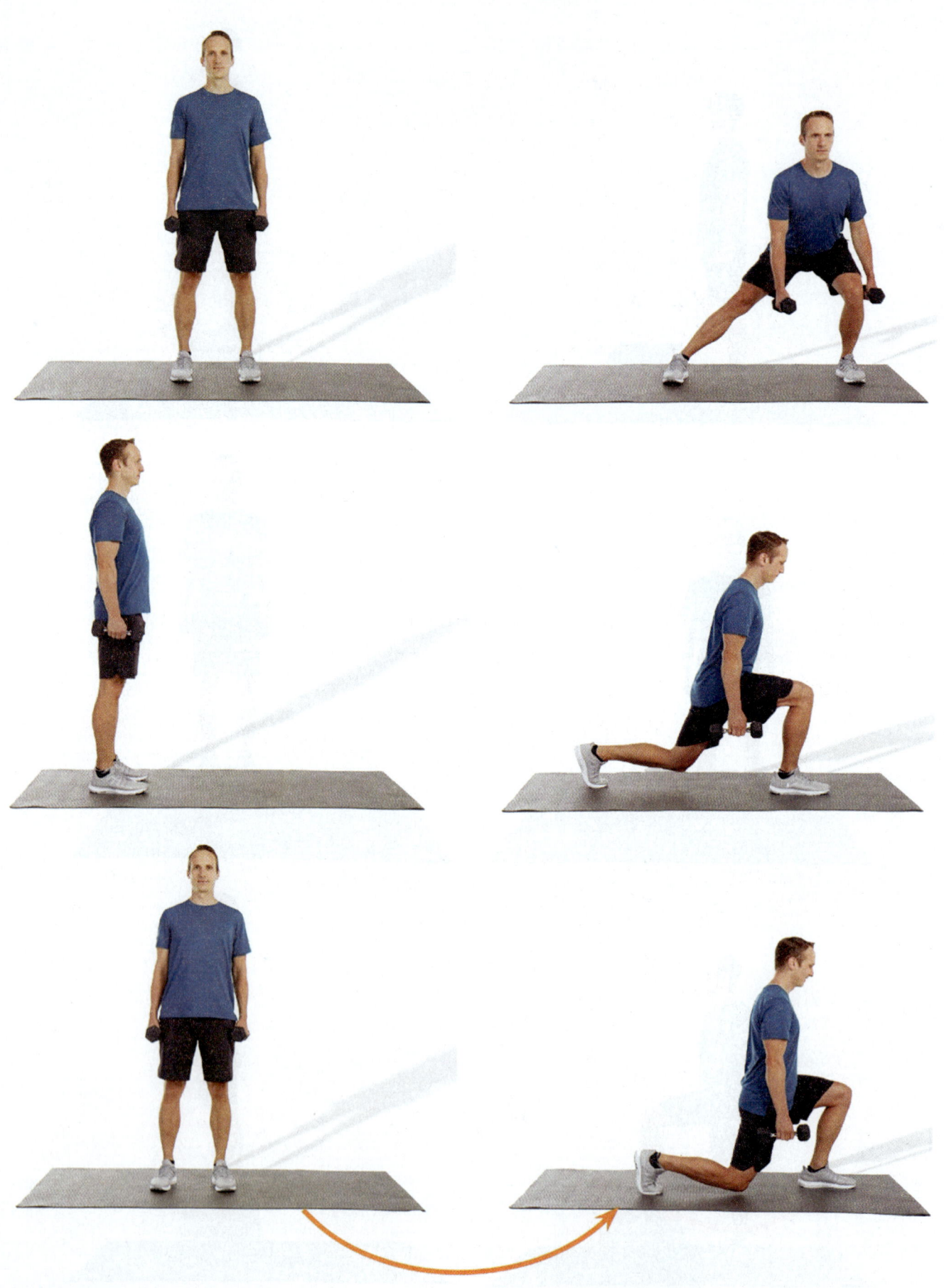

Multiplanar Lunge

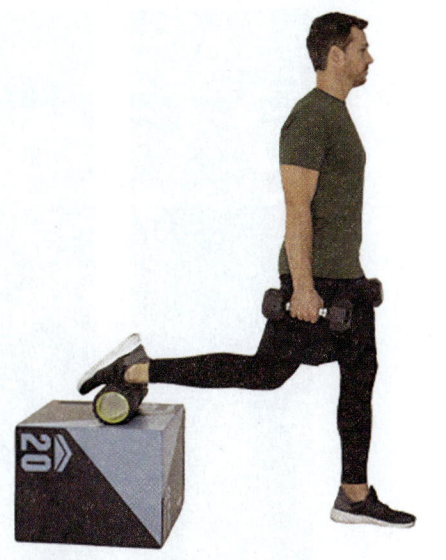 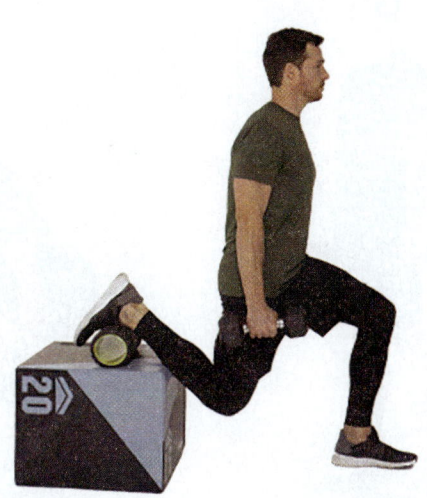

Bulgarian Split Squat

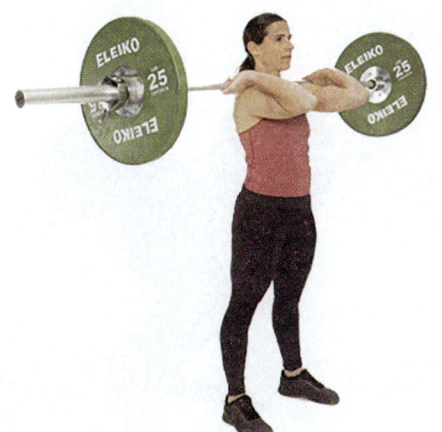 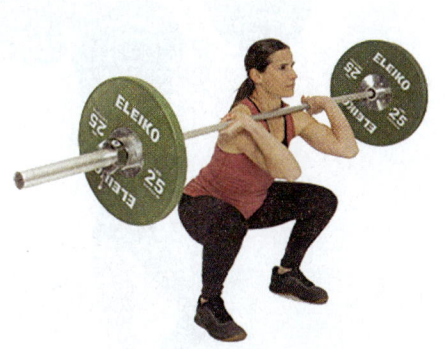

Front Squat

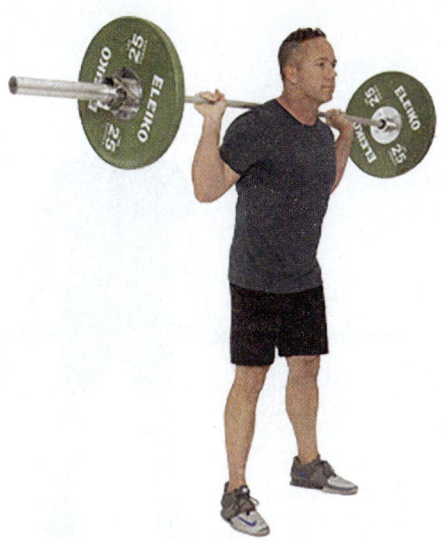

Barbell Squat

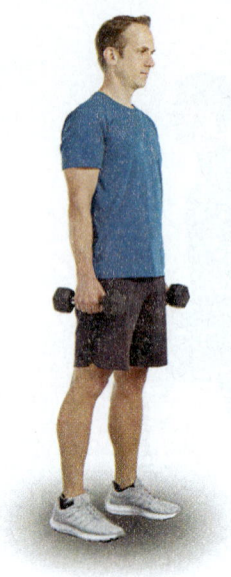

Dumbbell Squat

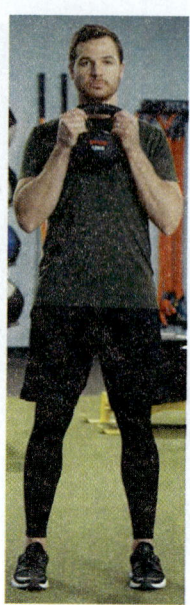

Goblet Squat

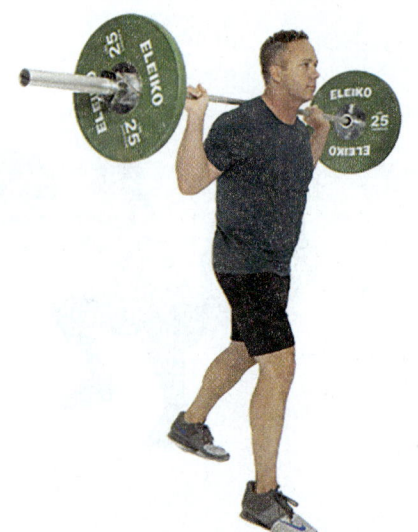

Barbell Split Squat

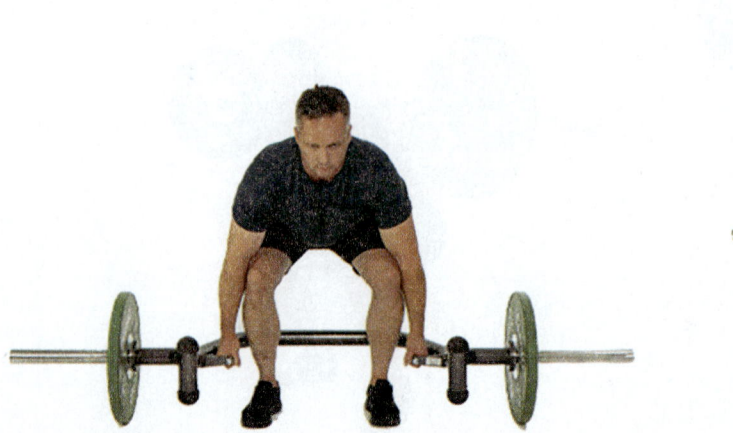

Trap Bar Deadlift

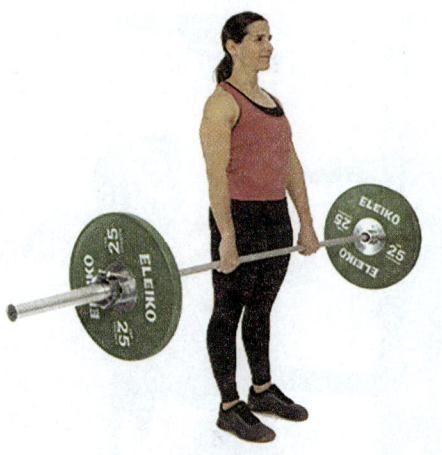

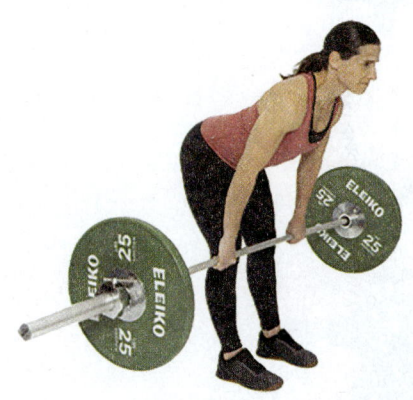

Barbell Romanian Deadlift

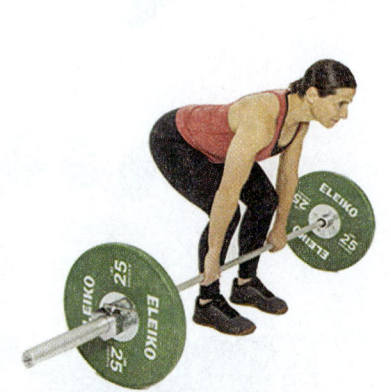

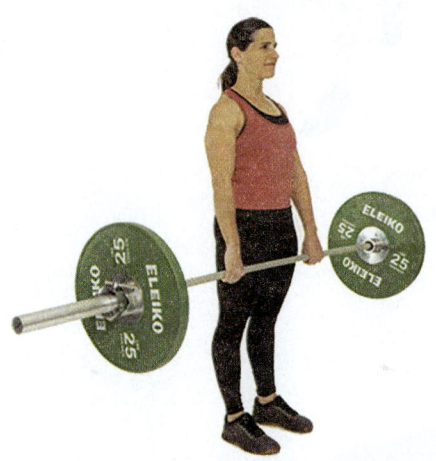

Barbell Deadlift

UPPER-BODY PUSHING EXERCISES

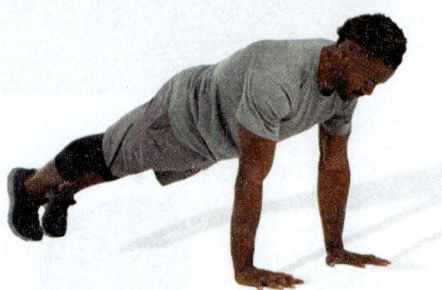

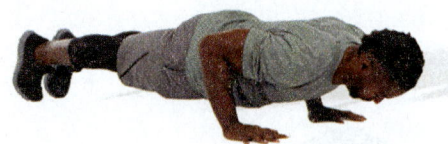

Push-up

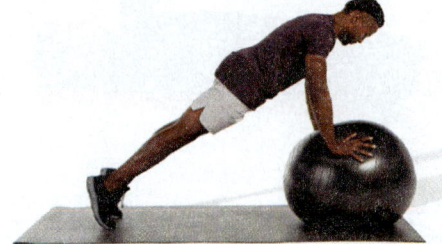

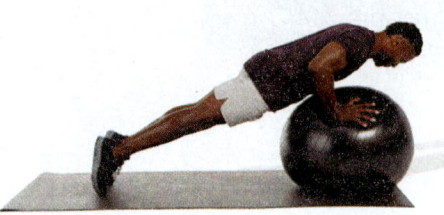

Push-up: Hands on Stability Ball

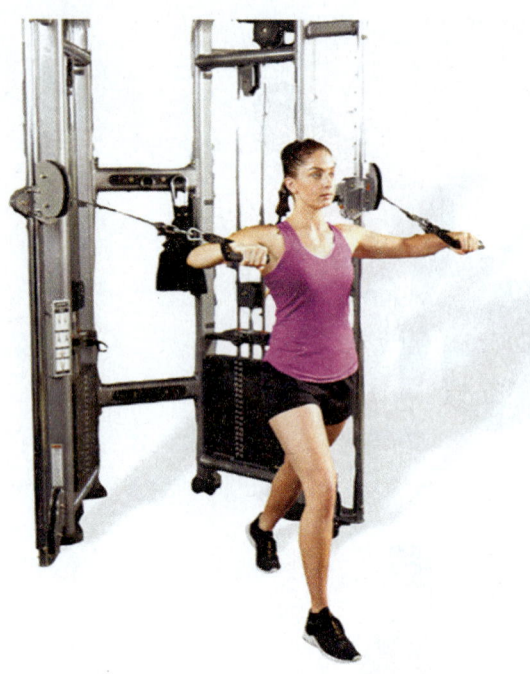
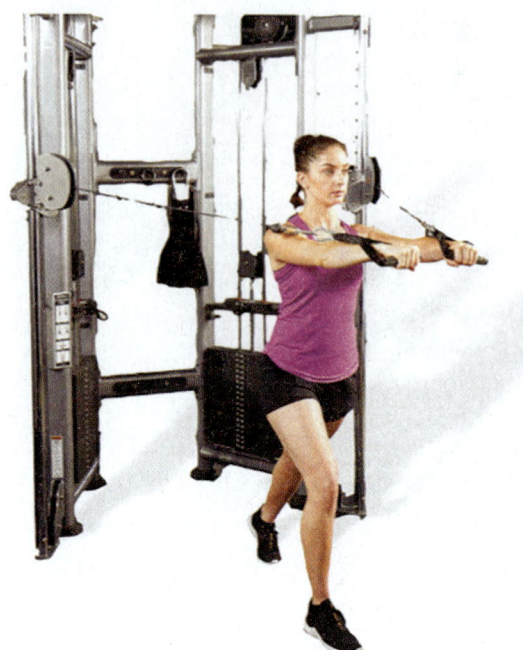

Standing Cable Chest Press

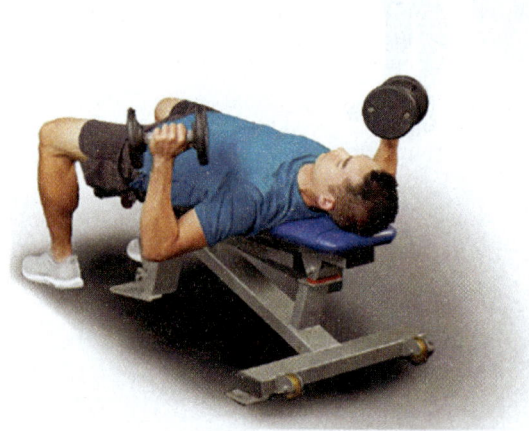
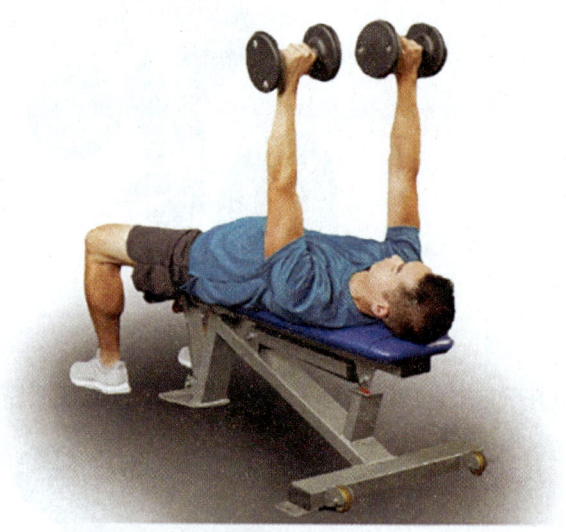

Flat Dumbbell Chest Press

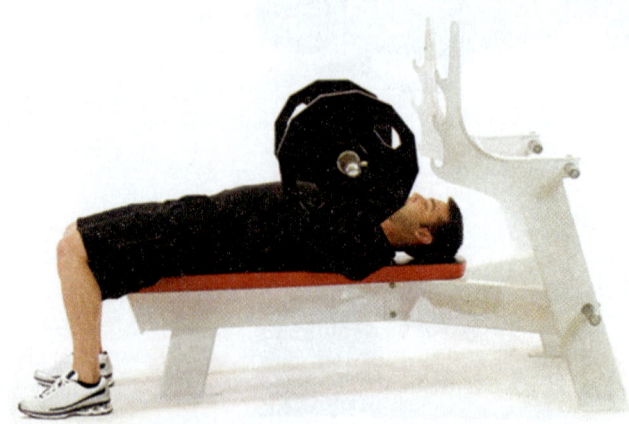
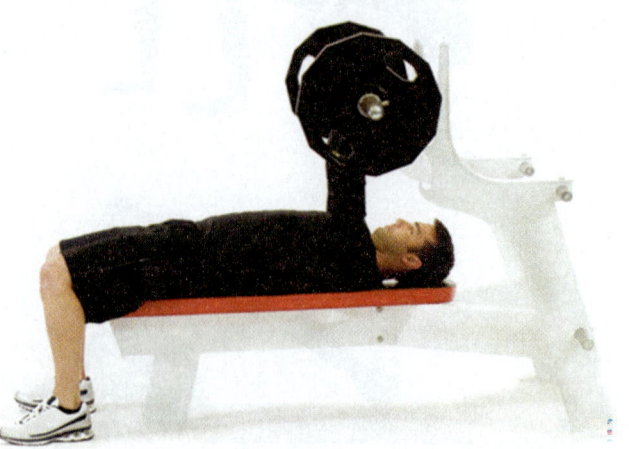

Barbell Bench Press

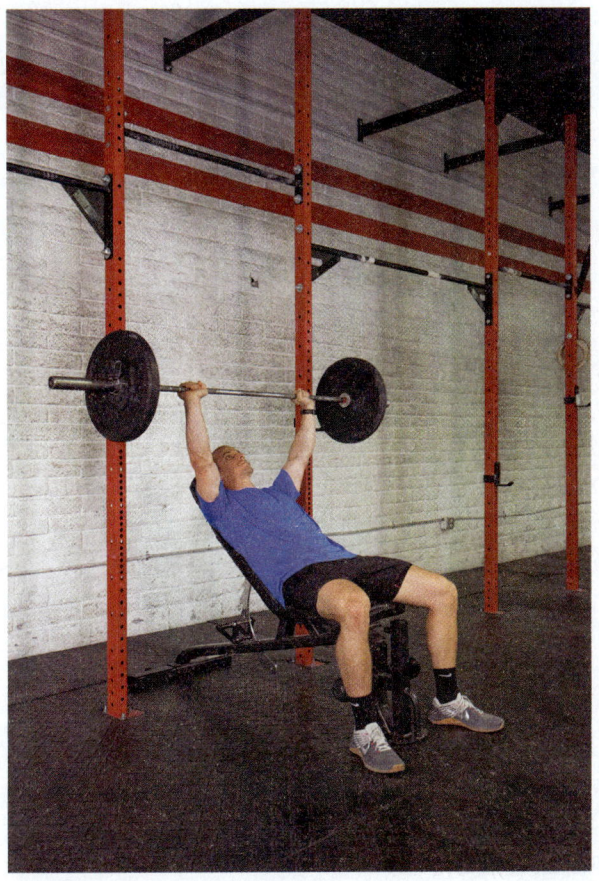
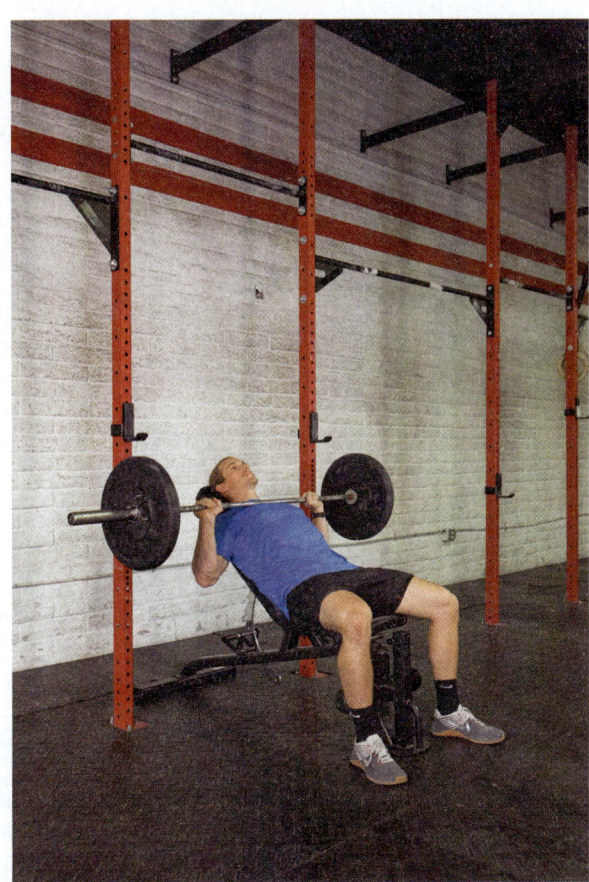

Incline Barbell Bench Press

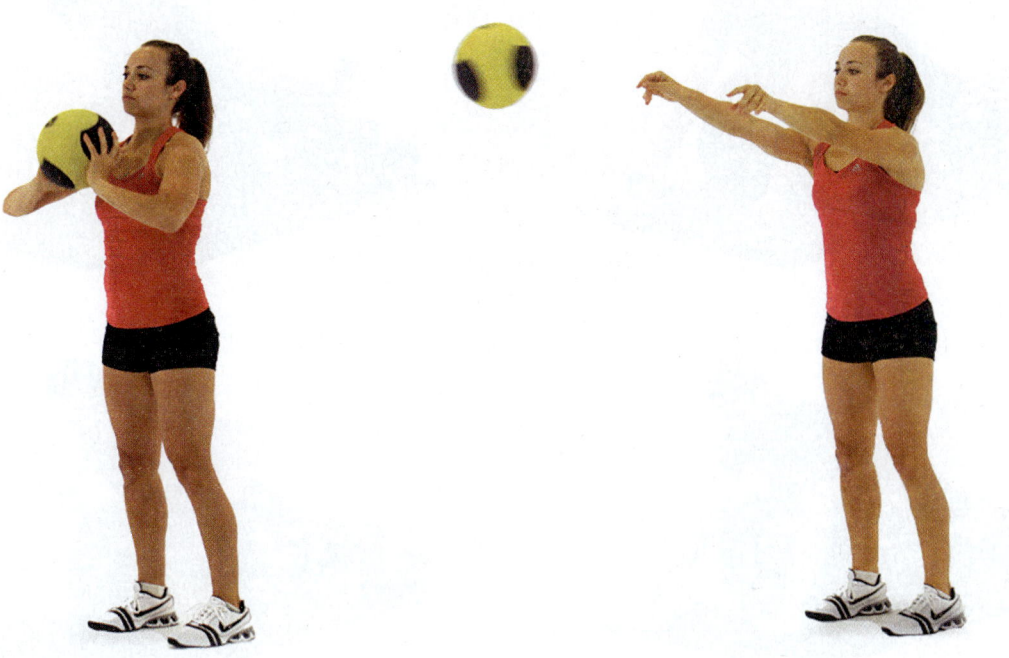

Medicine Ball Chest Pass

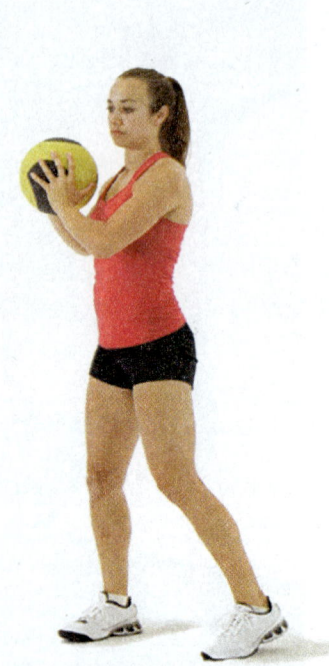
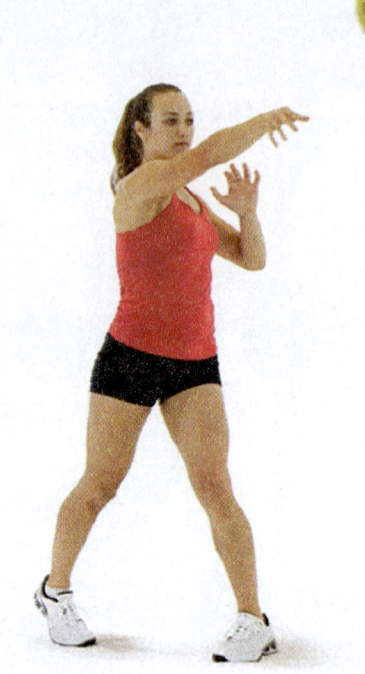

Medicine Ball Rotation Chest Pass

UPPER-BODY PULLING EXERCISES

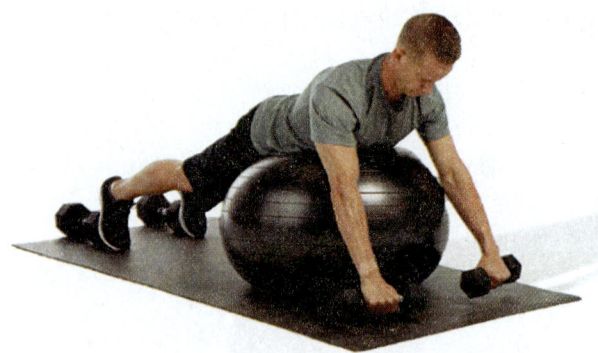
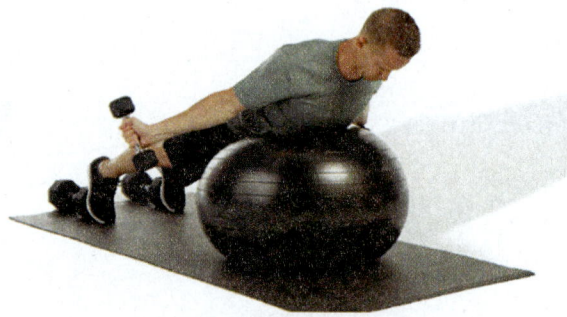

Ball Cobra

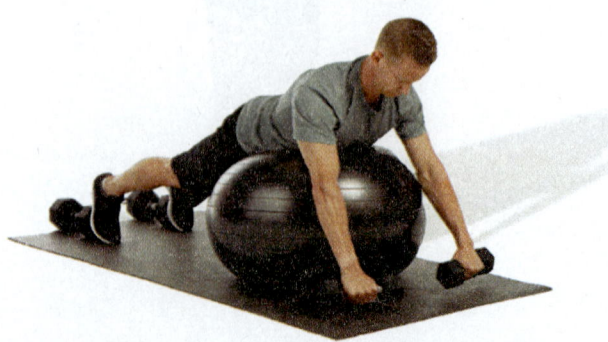
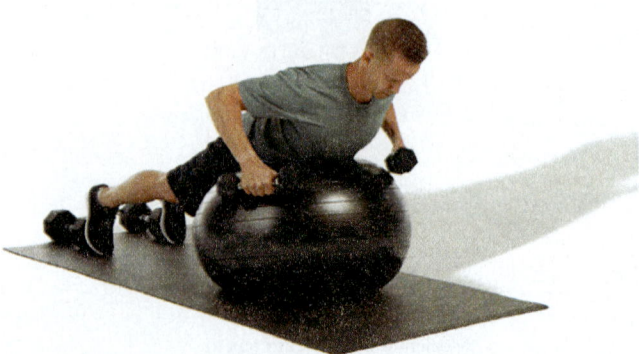

Ball Dumbbell Row

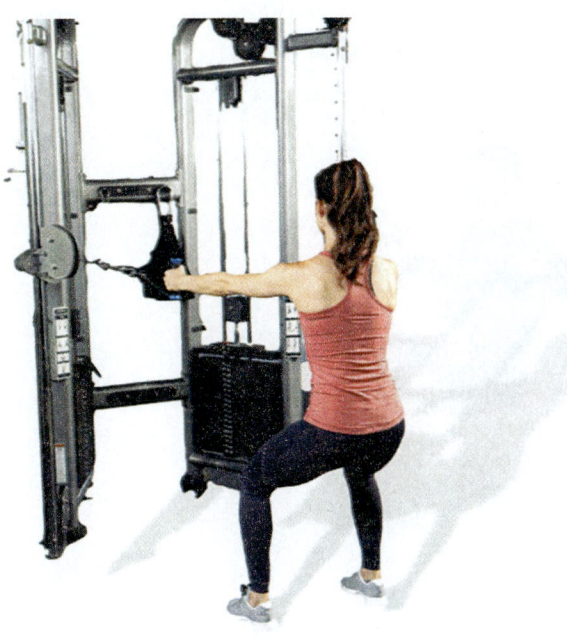 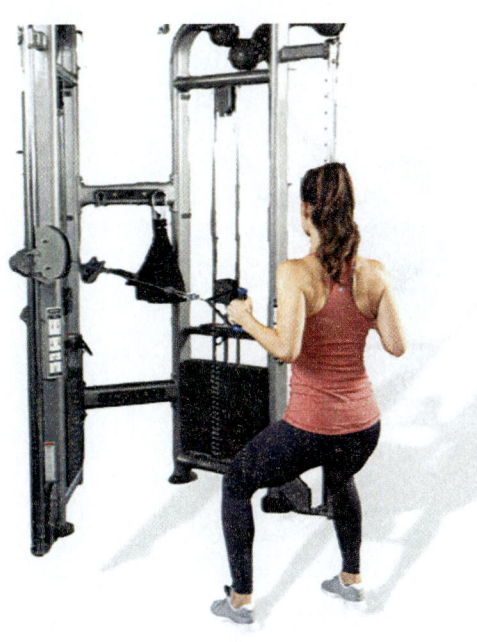

Standing Cable Row

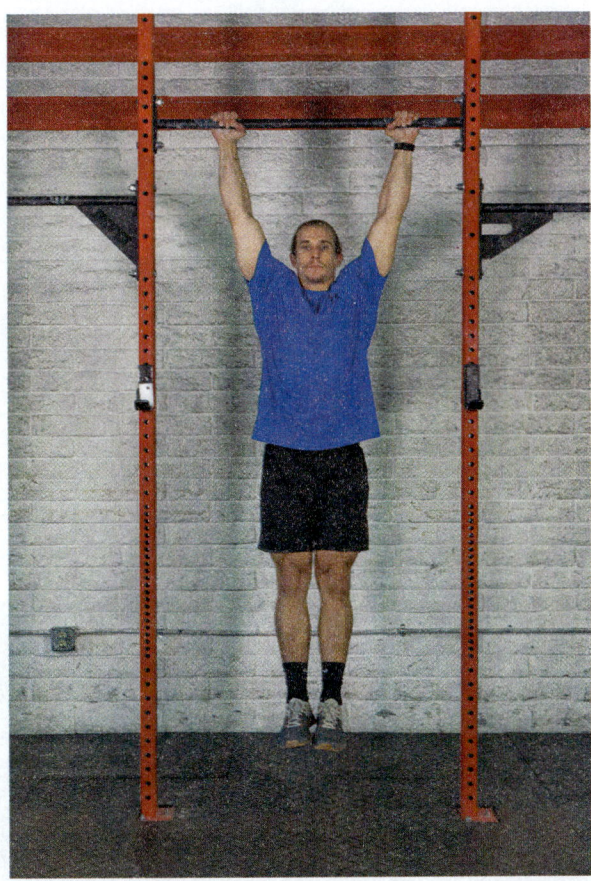 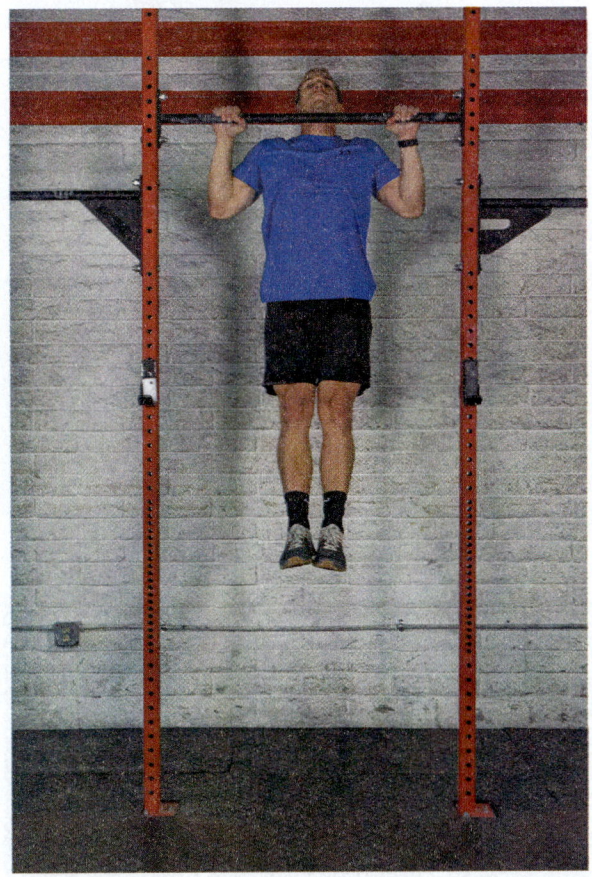

Pull-up/Chin-up

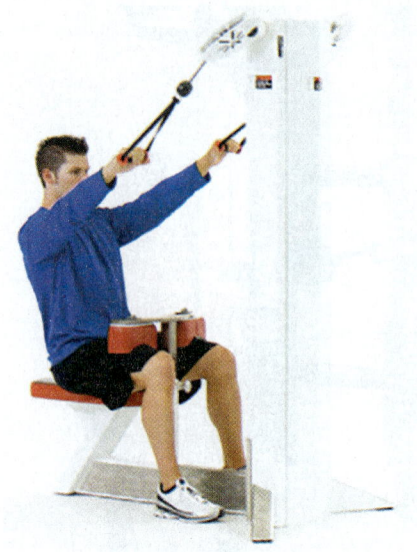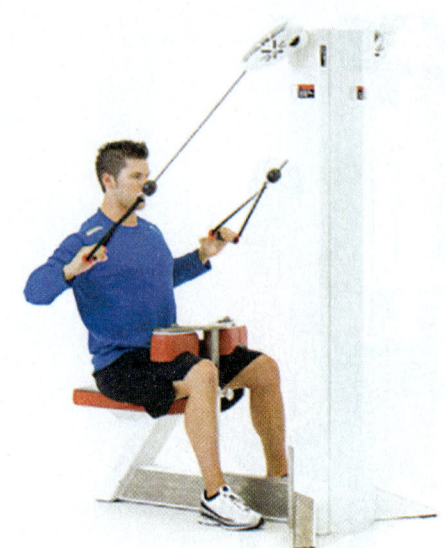

Seated Cable Row

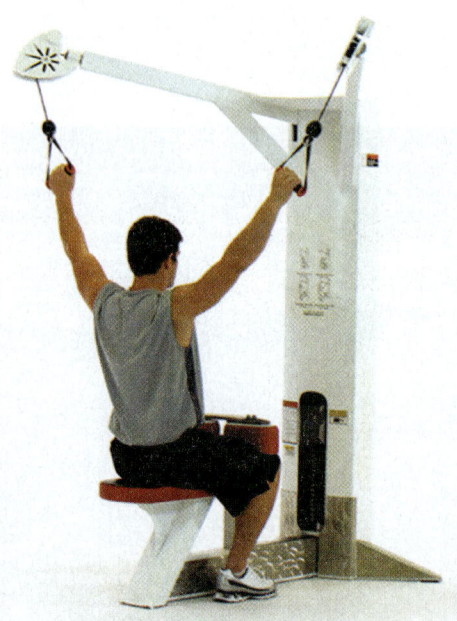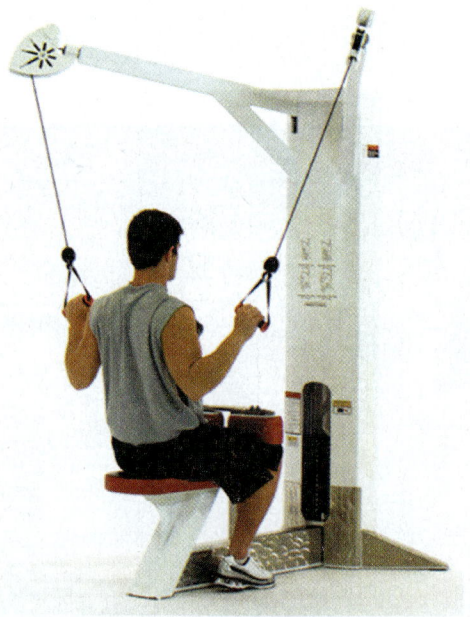

Seated Latissimus Pulldown

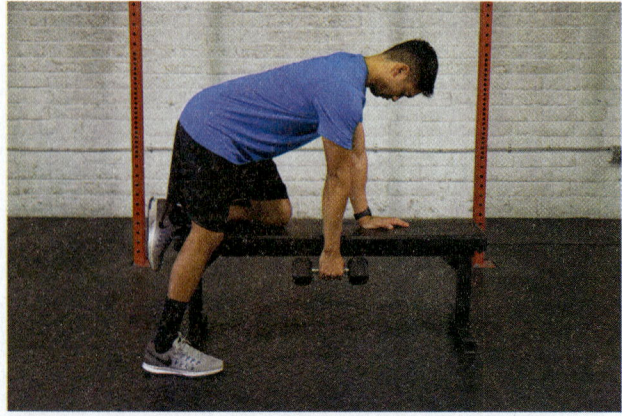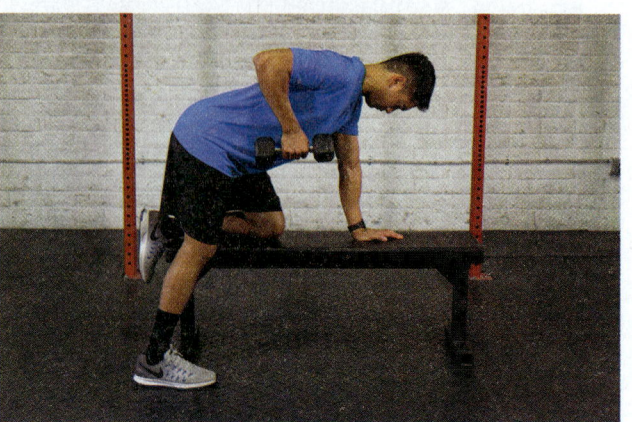

Bent-Over Single-Arm Dumbbell Row

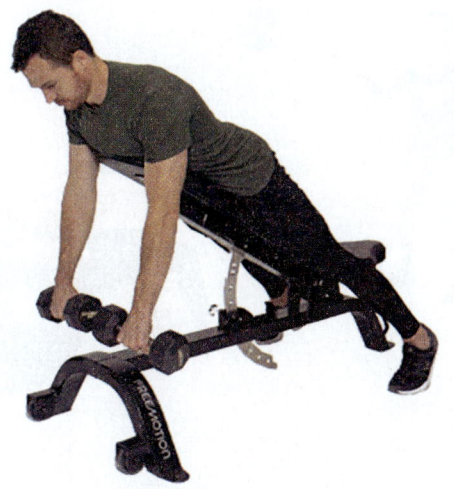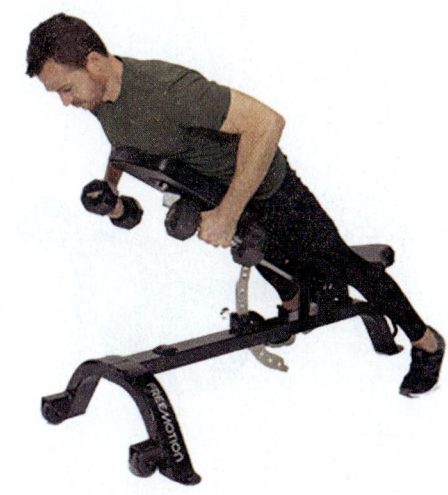

Incline Bench Dumbbell Row

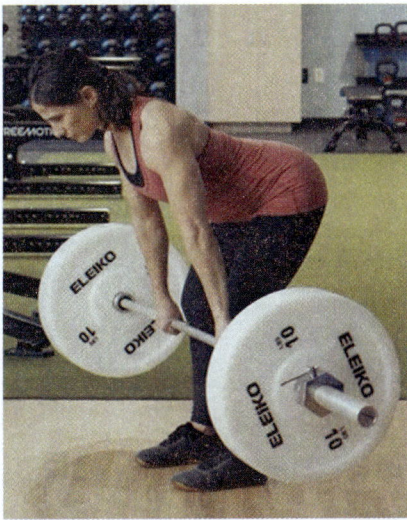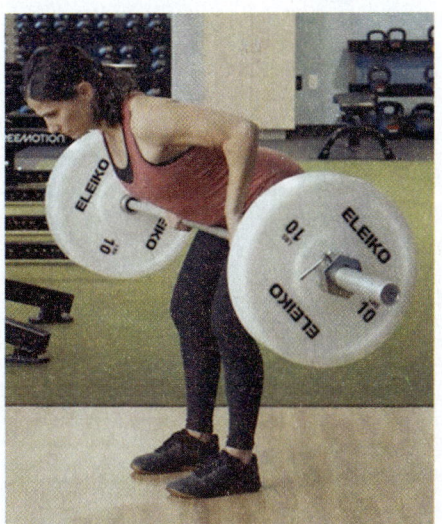

Bent-Over Barbell Row

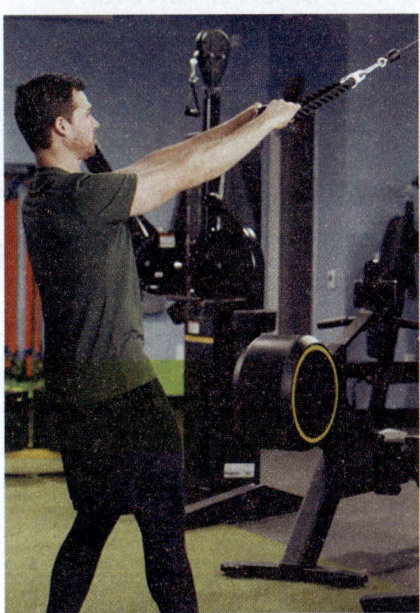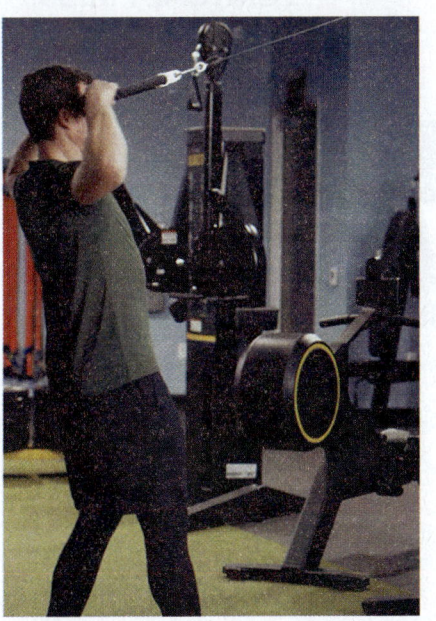

Face Pull

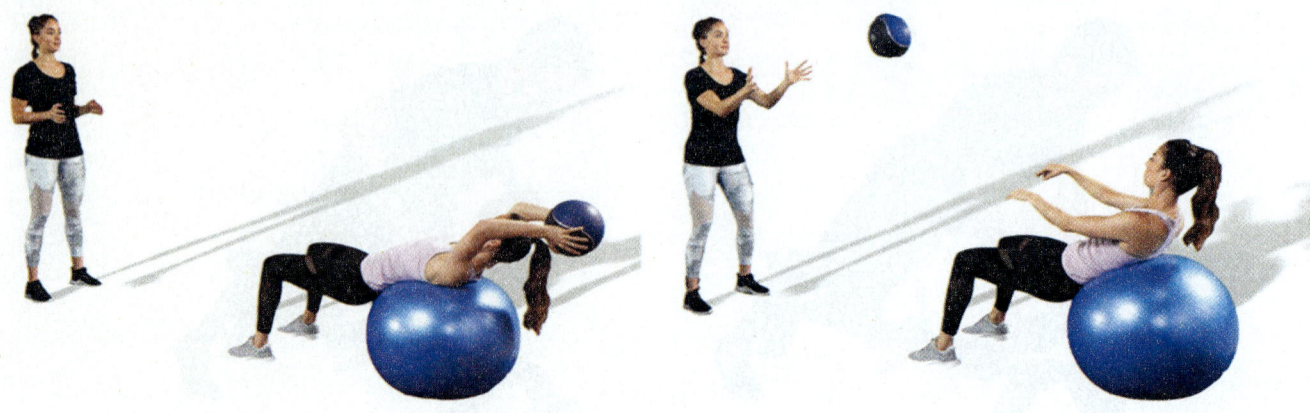

Medicine Ball Pullover Throw

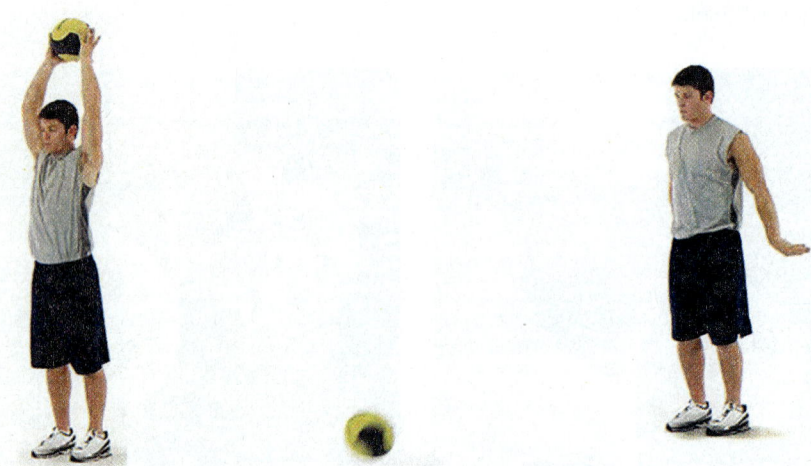

Medicine Ball Soccer Throw

VERTICAL PRESSING/SHOULDER EXERCISES

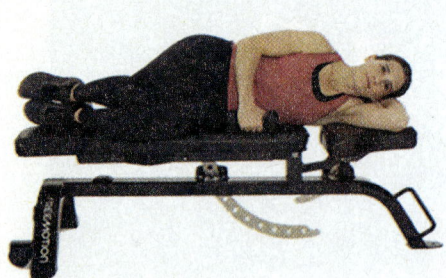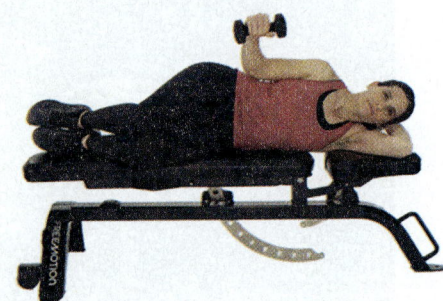

Side-Lying External Rotation

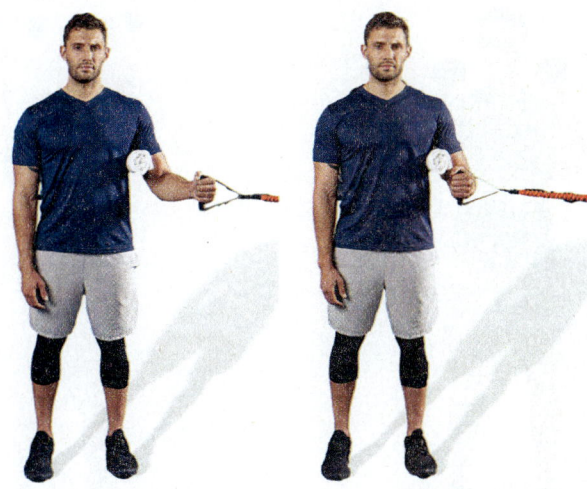

Tubing Internal Rotation

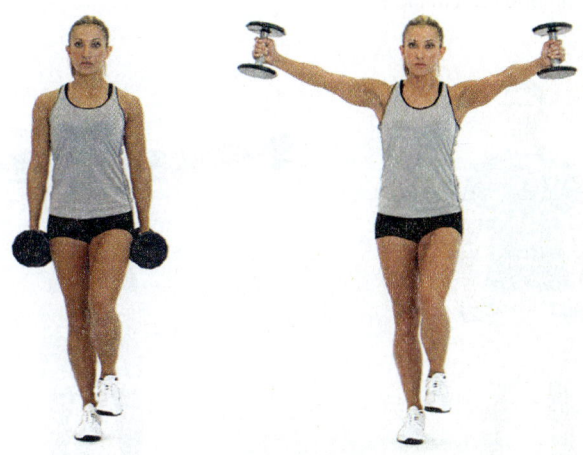

Single-Leg Dumbbell Scaption

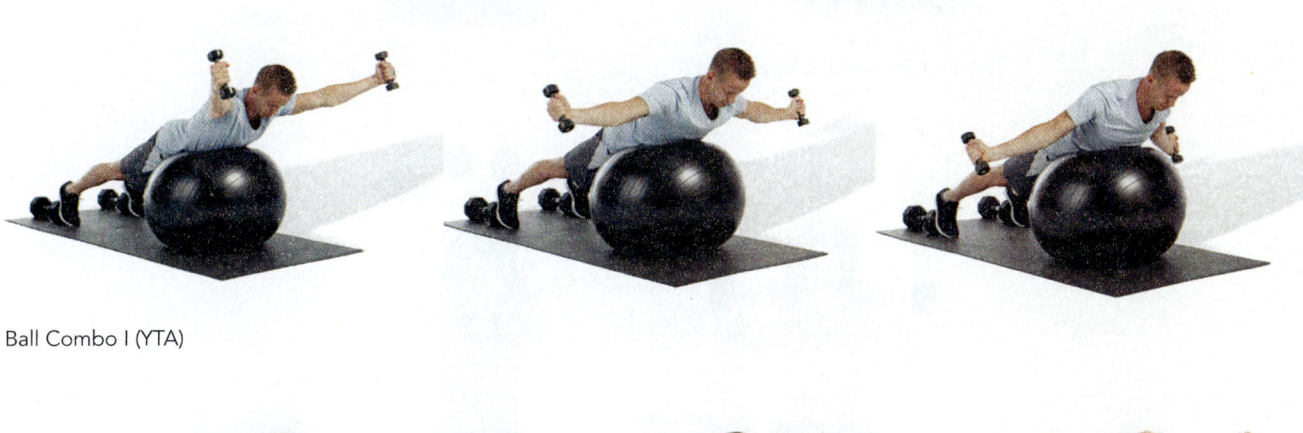

Ball Combo I (YTA)

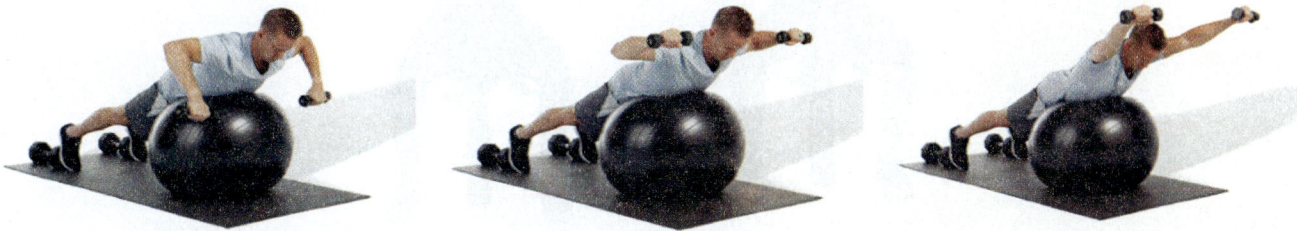

Ball Combo II (Row, External Rotation, Overhead Press)

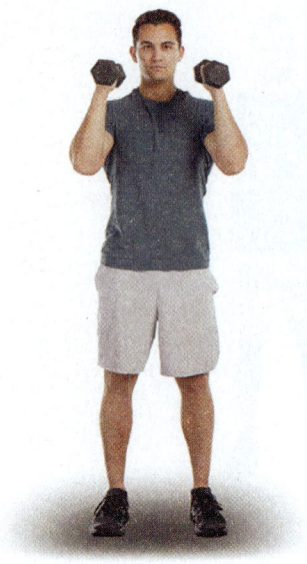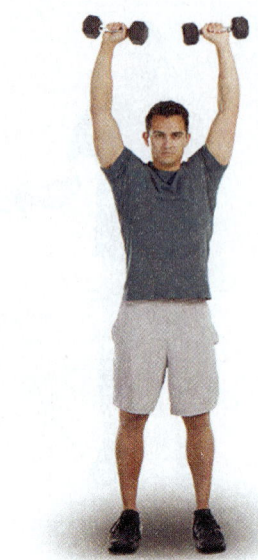

Standing Dumbbell Overhead Press

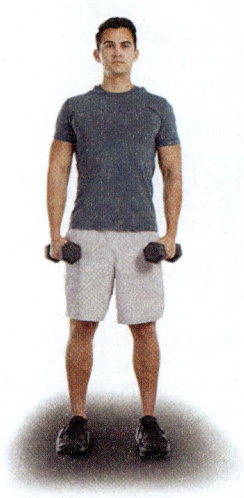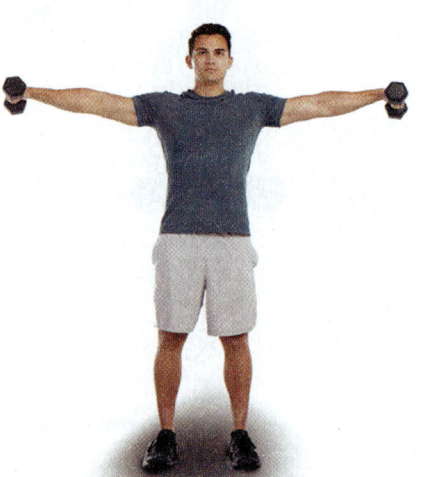

Standing Dumbbell Lateral Raise

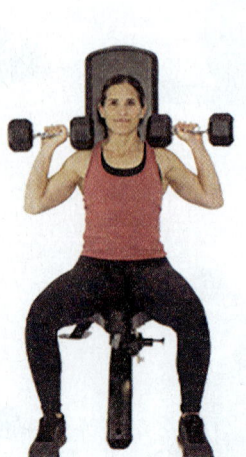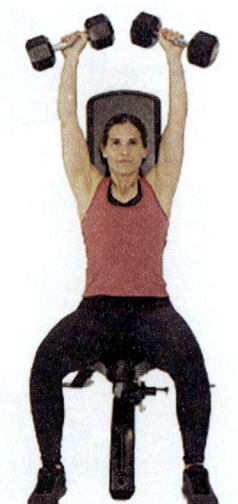

Seated Dumbbell Shoulder Press

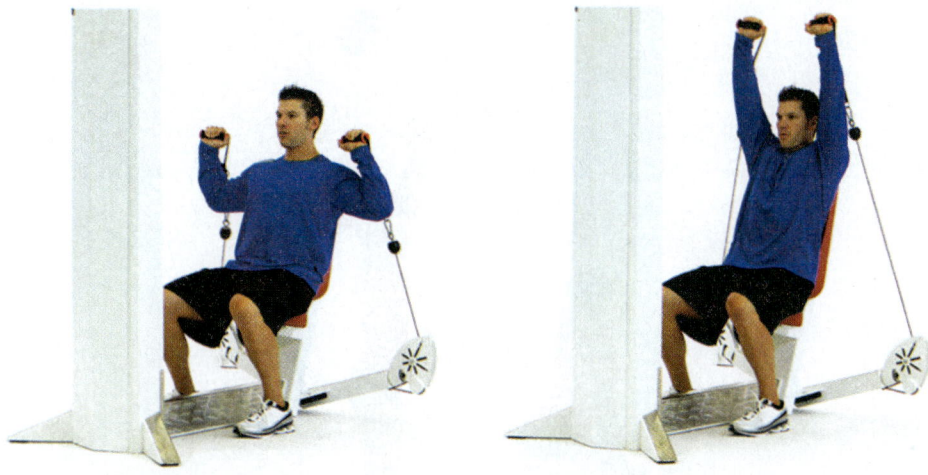

Seated Shoulder Press Machine

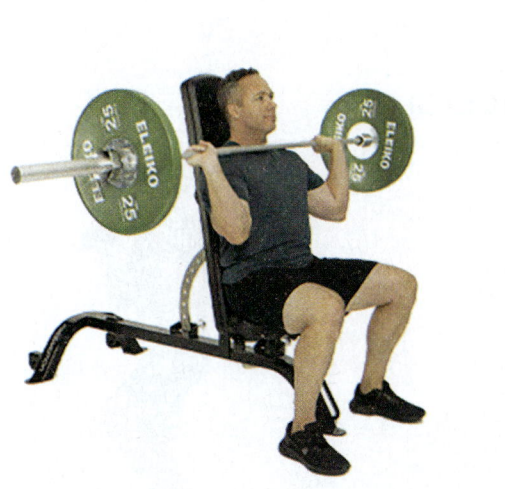
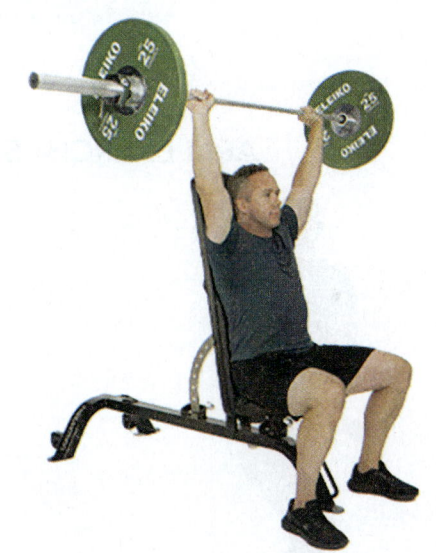

Barbell Military Press

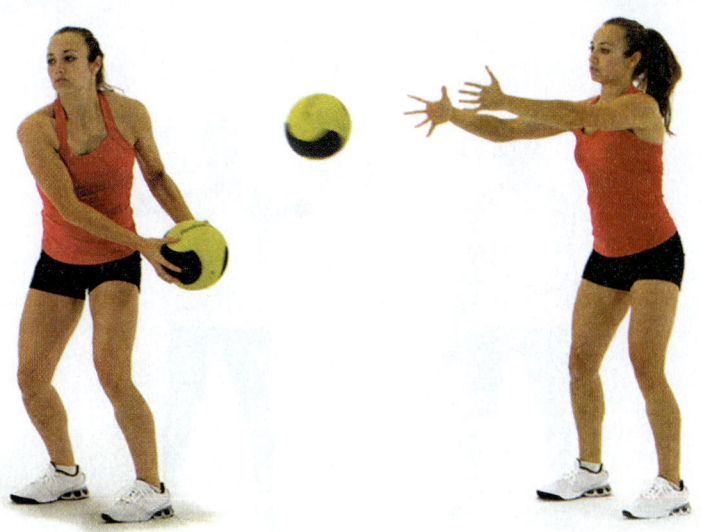

Front Medicine Ball Oblique Throw

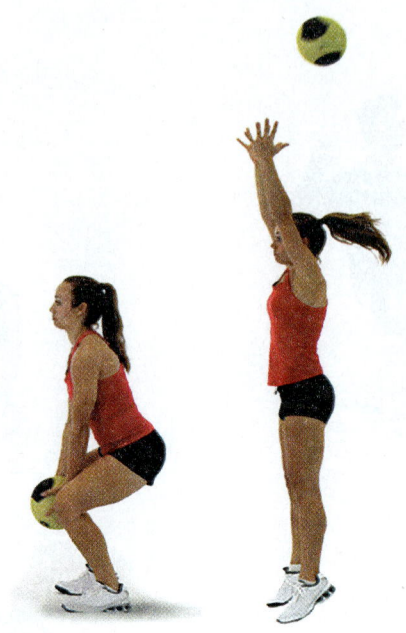

Overhead Medicine Ball Throw

ARM EXERCISES (BICEPS)

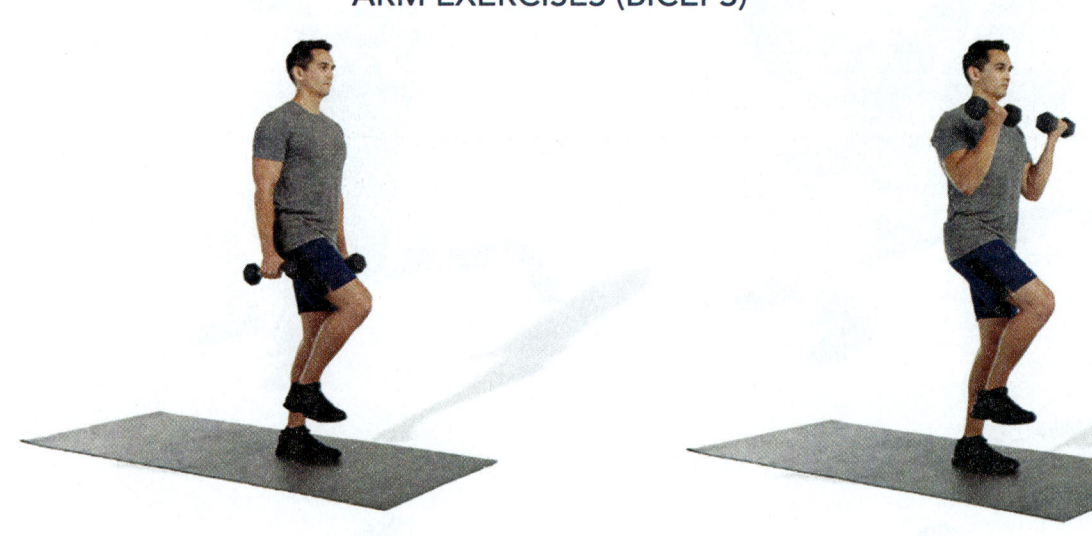

Single-Leg Dumbbell Curl

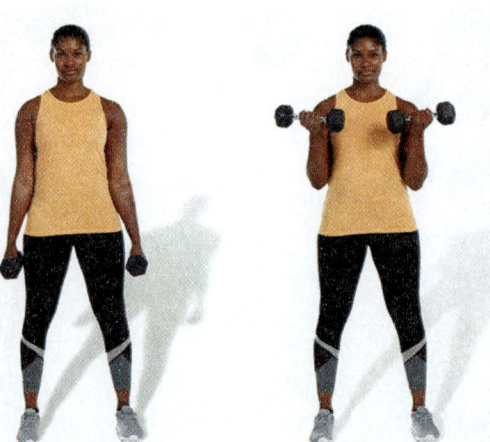

Standing Dumbbell Curl

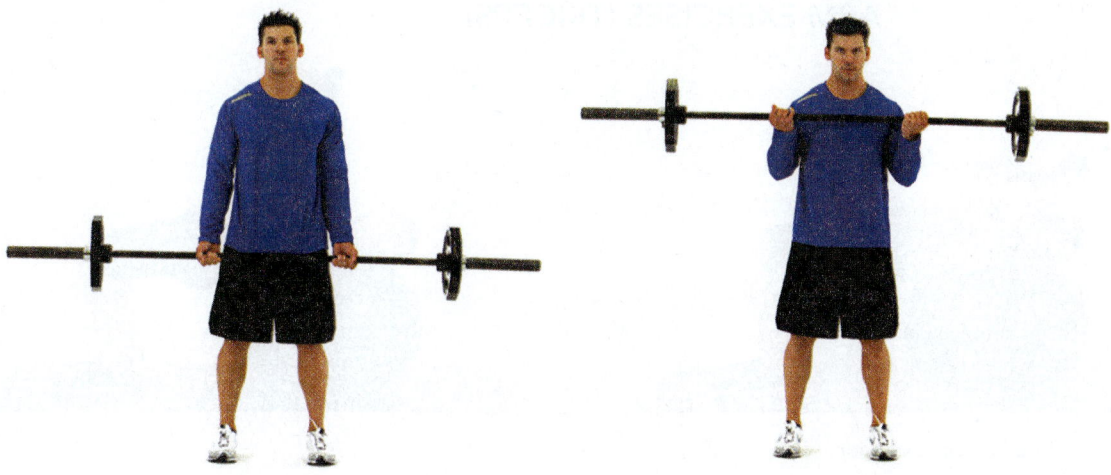

Standing Barbell Curl

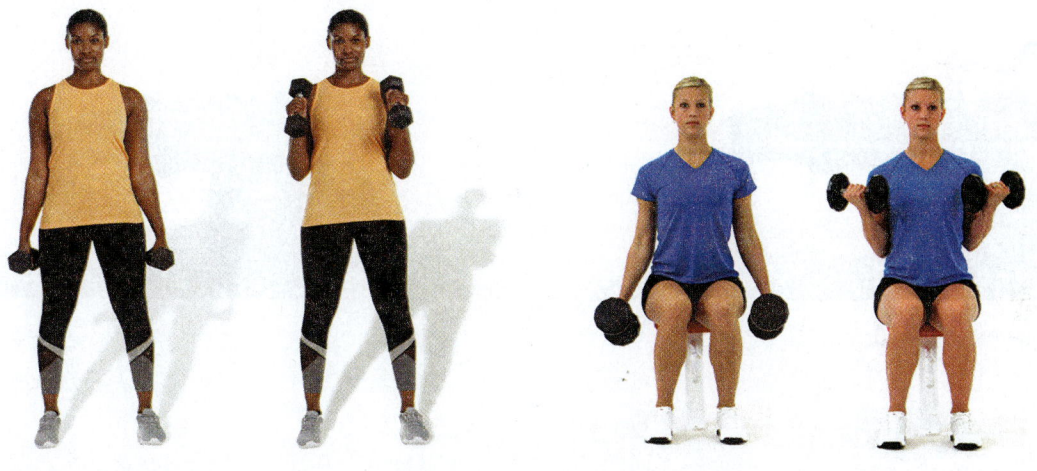

Standing Hammer Curl

Seated Two-Arm Dumbbell Biceps Curl

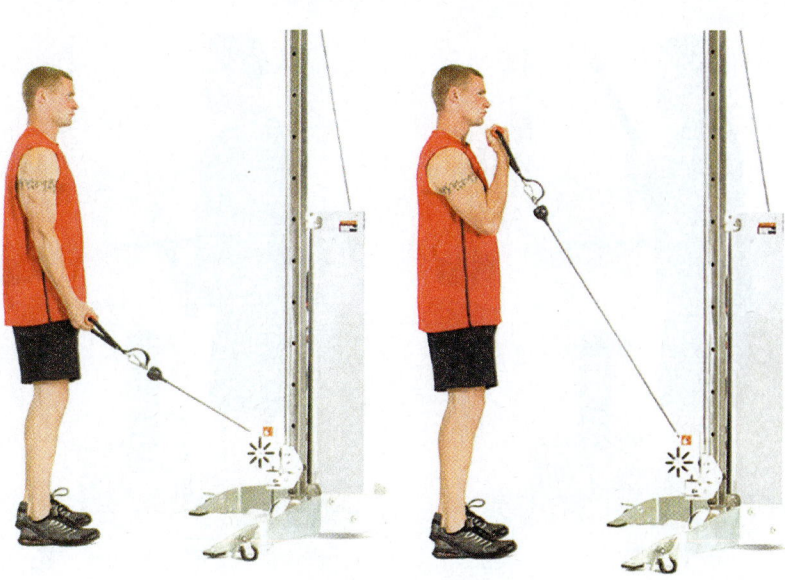

Biceps Curl Machine

ARM EXERCISES (TRICEPS)

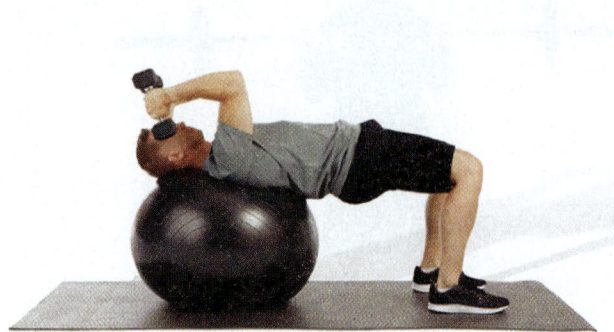
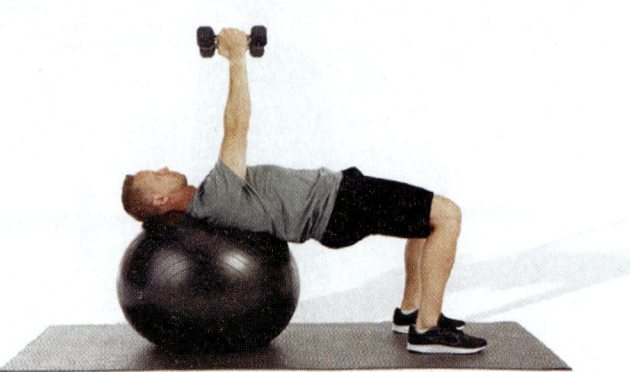

Supine Ball Dumbbell Triceps Extension

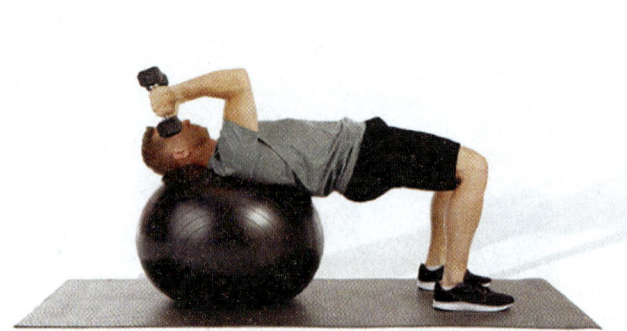
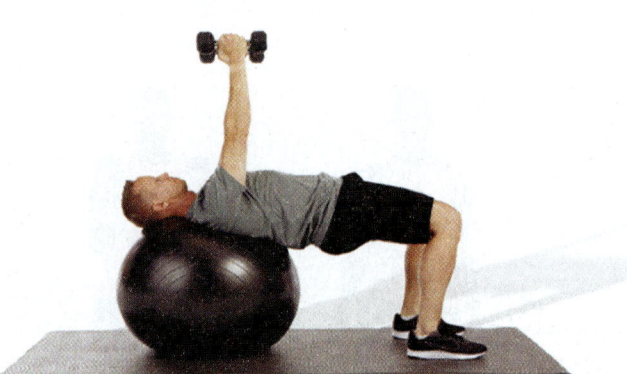

Prone Ball Triceps Extension

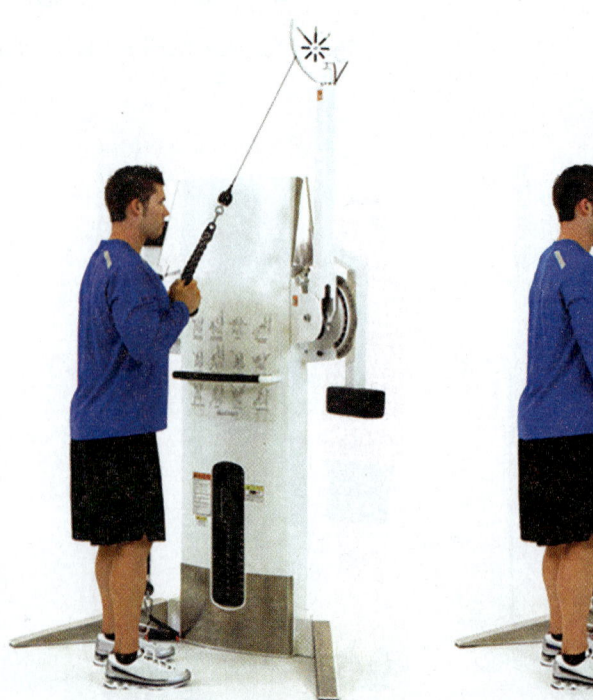

Cable Pushdown

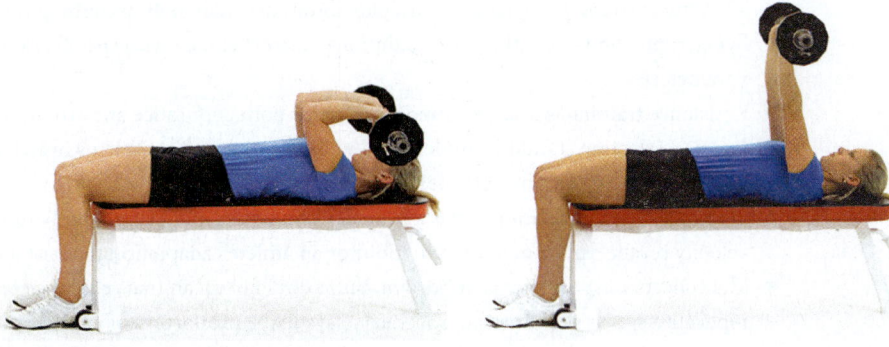

Supine Bench Barbell Triceps Extension

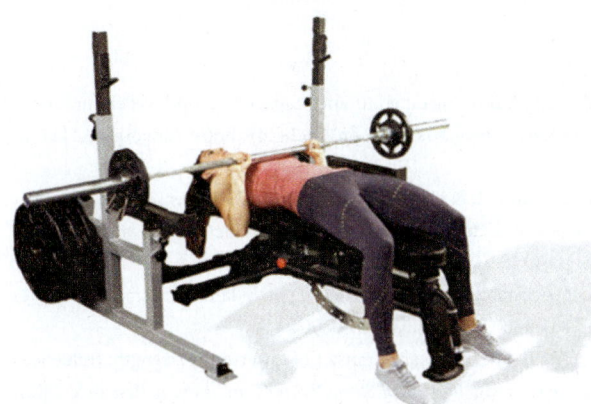
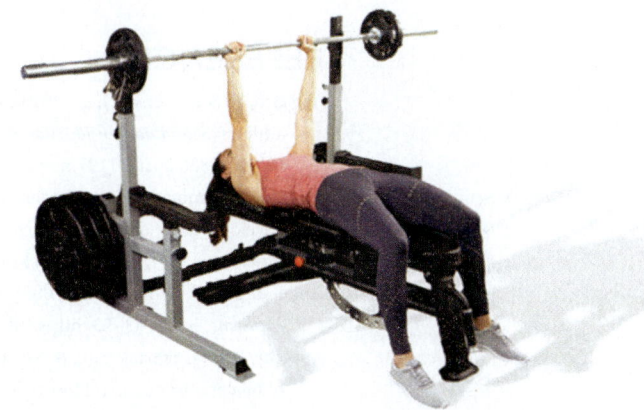

Close Grip Bench Press

SUMMARY

Resistance training is a cornerstone for sports performance. It directly impacts speed, change-of-direction ability, physical performance, and resilience against injury. Sports Performance Coaches must have a deep understanding of the physiology, biomechanics, and training science that underpin how the human body adapts to resistance training. They must also carry out a carefully thought-out plan with specific objectives that reflect the needs of the individual and the sport as well as knowledge of how to apply loading parameters and exercise selection to accomplish the training objectives.

The loading parameters (repetitions, sets, tempo, rest, intensity, load, and exercise selection) represent the levers a coach can pull to improve sports performance with resistance training. Although repetition and intensity are the primary variables dictating the training response, all of the loading parameters must be chosen carefully. There is no perfect program; however, there are inferior programs for the context. Consequently, the only way a Sports Performance Coach can increase the chance of success is to analyze the individual's needs and the demands of the sport to prioritize the training needs.

KEY TAKEAWAYS

- Repetition and intensity are the primary variables dictating the training response.
- The loading parameters (repetitions, sets, tempo, rest, intensity, load, and exercise selection) represent the levers a Sports Performance Coach can pull to improve sports performance with resistance training.
- Every resistance training program should start with a careful assessment of the individual athlete's needs and the sport-specific demands.

- The critical strength capacities (muscular endurance, maximal strength, power, muscle hypertrophy, and strength/power endurance) are developed with specific ranges and loading parameters.
- Resistance training is a key training method for both endurance and strength-based athletes.
- Exercise selection should be undertaken with attention to the athlete's individual needs, injury history, and, most importantly, technical competency.
- The force–velocity relationship is a property of muscle, and a whole-body functional force–velocity profile can be measured to monitor an athlete's adaptation to resistance training.
- The concept of specificity is important, but it does not mean that resistance training should replicate a sports skill. Instead, specificity says that a proportion of exercises should reflect the postures, positions, speed of movement, and contraction time of the competitive skill.

REFERENCES

Aagaard, P., & Andersen, J. L. (2010). Effects of strength training on endurance capacity in top-level endurance athletes. *Scandinavian Journal of Medicine & Science in Sports*, *20*(suppl 2), 39–47. https://doi.org/10.1111/j.1600-0838.2010.01197.x

Aagaard, P., Simonsen, E. B., Andersen, J. L., Magnusson, P., & Dyhre-Poulsen, P. (2002). Increased rate of force development and neural drive of human skeletal muscle following resistance training. *Journal of Applied Physiology, 93*(4), 1318–1326. https://doi.org/10.1152/japplphysiol.00283.2002

Anderson, K., & Behm, D. G. (2005). The impact of instability resistance training on balance and stability. *Sports Medicine, 35*(1), 43–53. https://doi.org/10.2165/00007256-200535010-00004

Appleby, B. B., Cormack, S. J., & Newton, R. U. (2019). Specificity and transfer of lower-body strength: Influence of bilateral or unilateral lower-body resistance training. *Journal of Strength and Conditioning Research, 33*(2), 318–326. https://doi.org/10.1519/JSC.0000000000002923

Appleby, B. B., Cormack, S. J., & Newton, R. U. (2020). Unilateral and bilateral lower-body resistance training does not transfer equally to sprint and change of direction performance. *Journal of Strength and Conditioning Research, 34*(1), 54–64. https://doi.org/10.1519/JSC.0000000000003035

Ardern, C. L., Taylor, N. F., Feller, J. A., & Webster, K. E. (2014). Fifty-five per cent return to competitive sport following anterior cruciate ligament reconstruction surgery: An updated systematic review and meta-analysis including aspects of physical functioning and contextual factors. *British Journal of Sports Medicine, 48*(21), 1543–1552. https://doi.org/10.1136/bjsports-2013-093398

Balshaw, T. G., Massey, G. J., Maden-Wilkinson, T. M., Lanza, M. B., & Folland, J. P. (2019). Neural adaptations after 4 years vs 12 weeks of resistance training vs untrained. *Scandinavian Journal of Medicine & Science in Sports, 29*(3), 348–359. https://doi.org/10.1111/sms.13331

Behm, D. G., Drinkwater, E. J., Willardson, J. M., & Cowley, P. M. (2010). Canadian Society for Exercise Physiology position stand: The use of instability to train the core in athletic and nonathletic conditioning. *Applied Physiology, Nutrition, and Metabolism, 35*(1), 109–112. https://doi.org/10.1139/H09-128

Behm, D. G., Young, J. D., Whitten, J. H. D., Reid, J. C., Quigley, P. J., Low, J., Li, Y., Lima, C. D., Hodgson, D. D., Chaouachi, A., Prieske, O., & Granacher, U. (2017). Effectiveness of traditional strength vs. power training on muscle strength, power and speed with youth: A systematic review and meta-analysis. *Frontiers in Physiology, 8*, 423. https://doi.org/10.3389/fphys.2017.00423

Bird, S. P., Tarpenning, K. M., & Marino, F. E. (2005). Designing resistance training programmes to enhance fitness: A review of the acute programme. *Sports Medicine, 35*(10), 841–851. https://doi.org/10.2165/00007256-200535100-00002

Blazevich, A. J., & Babault, N. (2019). Post-activation potentiation versus post-activation performance enhancement in humans: Historical perspective, underlying mechanisms, and current issues. *Frontiers in Physiology, 10,* 1359. https://doi.org/10.3389/fphys.2019.01359

Blazevich, A. J., Wilson, C. J., Alcaraz, P. E., & Rubio-Arias, J. A. (2020). Effects of resistance training movement pattern and velocity on isometric muscular rate of force development: A systematic review with meta-analysis and meta-regression. *Sports Medicine, 50*(5), 943–963. https://doi.org/10.1007/s40279-019-01239-x

Bobbert, M. F., de Graaf, W. W., Jonk, J. N., & Casius, L. J. R. (2006). Explanation of the bilateral deficit in human vertical squat jumping. *Journal of Applied Physiology, 100*(2), 493–499. https://doi.org/10.1152/japplphysiol.00637.2005

Bompa, T. O. (1993). *Periodization of strength: The new wave in strength training.* Verita Publishing.

Bourne, M. N., Williams, M. D., Opar, D. A., Al Najjar, A., Kerr, G. K., & Shield, A. J. (2017). Impact of exercise selection on hamstring muscle activation. *British Journal of Sports Medicine, 51*(13), 1021–1028. https://doi.org/10.1136/bjsports-2015-095739

Brachman, A., Kamieniarz, A., Michalska, J., Pawłowski, M., Słomka, K. J., & Juras, G. (2017). Balance training programs in athletes: A systematic review. *Journal of Human Kinetics, 58,* 45–64. https://www.ncbi.nlm.nih.gov/pmc/articles/PMC5548154

Chaabene, H., Prieske, O., Moran, J., Negra, Y., Attia, A., & Granacher, U. (2020). Effects of resistance training on change-of-direction speed in youth and young physically active and athletic adults: A systematic review with meta-analysis. *Sports Medicine, 50*(8), 1483–1499. https://doi.org/10.1007/s40279-020-01293-w

Cormie, P., McGuigan, M. R., & Newton, R. U. (2011a). Developing maximal neuromuscular power: Part 1: Biological basis of maximal power production. *Sports Medicine, 41*(1), 17–38. https://doi.org/10.2165/11537690-000000000-00000

Cormie, P., McGuigan, M. R., & Newton, R. U. (2011b). Developing maximal neuromuscular power: Part 2: Training considerations for improving maximal power production. *Sports Medicine, 41*(2), 125–146. https://doi.org/10.2165/11538500-000000000-00000

Costa, E. C., Moreira, A., Cavalcanti, B., Krinski, K., & Aoki, M. S. (2015). Effect of unilateral and bilateral resistance exercise on maximal voluntary strength, total volume of load lifted, and perceptual and metabolic responses. *Biology of Sport, 32*(1), 35–40. https://www.ncbi.nlm.nih.gov/pmc/articles/PMC4314602

Courtney, R. (2009). The function of breathing and its dysfunctions and their relationship to breathing therapy. *International Journal of Osteopathic Medicine, 12*(3), 78–85. https://doi.org/10.1016/j.ijosm.2009.04.002

Cuenca-Fernández, F., Smith, I. C., Jordan, M. J., MacIntosh, B. R., López-Contreras, G., Arellano, R., & Herzog, W. (2017). Nonlocalized postactivation performance enhancement (PAPE) effects in trained athletes: A pilot study. *Applied Physiology, Nutrition, and Metabolism, 42*(10), 1122–1125. https://doi.org/10.1139/apnm-2017-0217

Damas, F., Phillips, S., Vechin, F. C., & Ugrinowitsch, C. (2015). A review of resistance training–induced changes in skeletal muscle protein synthesis and their contribution to hypertrophy. *Sports Medicine, 45*(6), 801–807. https://doi.org/10.1007/s40279-015-0320-0

Dankel, S. J., Mattocks, K. T., Jessee, M. B., Buckner, S. L., Mouser, J. G., Counts, B. R., Laurentino, G. C., & Loenneke, J. P. (2017). Frequency: The overlooked resistance training variable for inducing muscle hypertrophy? *Sports Medicine, 47*(5), 799–805. https://doi.org/10.1007/s40279-016-0640-8

Davies, T., Orr, R., Halaki, M., & Hackett, D. (2016). Effect of training leading to repetition failure on muscular strength: A systematic review and meta-analysis. *Sports Medicine, 46*(4), 487–502. https://doi.org/10.1007/s40279-015-0451-3

Delorme, T. L. (1945). Restoration of muscle power by heavy resistance exercises. *Journal of Bone & Joint Surgery, 27*(4), 645–667.

Delorme, T. L., & Watkins, A. L. (1948). Techniques of progressive resistance exercise. *Archives of Physical Medicine and Rehabilitation, 29*(5), 263–273.

Duchateau, J., Semmler, J. G., & Enoka, R. M. (2006). Training adaptations in the behavior of human motor units. *Journal of Applied Physiology, 101*(6), 1766–1775. https://doi.org/10.1152/japplphysiol.00543.2006

Eddens, L., van Someren, K., & Howatson, G. (2018). The role of intra-session exercise sequence in the interference effect: A systematic review with meta-analysis. *Sports Medicine, 48*(1), 177–188. https://doi.org/10.1007/s40279-017-0784-1

Emery, C. A., & Pasanen, K. (2019). Current trends in sport injury prevention. *Best Practice & Research. Clinical Rheumatology, 33*(1), 3–15. https://doi.org/10.1016/j.berh.2019.02.009

Evans, J. W. (2019). Periodized resistance training for enhancing skeletal muscle hypertrophy and strength: A mini-review. *Frontiers in Physiology, 10,* 13. https://doi.org/10.3389/fphys.2019.00013

Faigenbaum, A. D., Lloyd, R. S., MacDonald, J., & Myer, G. D. (2016). Citius, altius, fortius: Beneficial effects of resistance training for young athletes: Narrative review. *British Journal of Sports Medicine, 50*(1), 3–7. https://doi.org/10.1136/bjsports-2015-094621

Faigenbaum, A. D., MacDonald, J. P., & Haff, G. G. (2019). Are young athletes strong enough for sport? DREAM on. *Current Sports Medicine Reports, 18*(1), 6–8. https://doi.org/10.1249/JSR.0000000000000554

Fernandez-Gonzalo, R., Lundberg, T. R., & Tesch, P. A. (2013). Acute molecular responses in untrained and trained muscle subjected to aerobic and resistance exercise training versus resistance training alone. *Acta Physiologica, 209*(4), 283–294. https://doi.org/10.1111/apha.12174

Fyfe, J. J., Bishop, D. J., & Stepto, N. K. (2014). Interference between concurrent resistance and endurance exercise: molecular bases and the role of individual training variables. *Sports Medicine, 44*(6), 743–762. https://doi.org/10.1007/s40279-014-0162-1

Gonzalo-Skok, O., Tous-Fajardo, J., Suarez-Arrones, L., Arjol-Serrano, J. L., Casajús, J. A., & Mendez-Villanueva, A. (2017). Single-leg power output and between-limbs imbalances in team-sport players: Unilateral versus bilateral combined resistance training. *International Journal of Sports Physiology and Performance, 12*(1), 106–114. https://doi.org/10.1123/ijspp.2015-0743

Granacher, U., Lesinski, M., Büsch, D., Muehlbauer, T., Prieske, O., Puta, C., Gollhofer, A., & Behm, D. G. (2016). Effects of resistance training in youth athletes on muscular fitness and athletic performance: A conceptual model for long-term athlete development. *Frontiers in Physiology, 7*. https://doi.org/10.3389/fphys.2016.00164

Hackett, D. A., & Chow, C.-M. (2013). The Valsalva maneuver: Its effect on intra-abdominal pressure and safety issues during resistance exercise. *Journal of Strength and Conditioning Research, 27*(8), 2338–2345. https://doi.org/10.1519/JSC.0b013e31827de07d

Häkkinen, K., Alen, M., Kraemer, W. J., Gorostiaga, E., Izquierdo, M., Rusko, H., Mikkola, J., Häkkinen, A., Valkeinen, H., Kaarakainen, E., Romu, S., Erola, V., Ahtiainen, J., & Paavolainen, L. (2003). Neuromuscular adaptations during concurrent strength and endurance training versus strength training. *European Journal of Applied Physiology, 89*(1), 42–52. https://doi.org/10.1007/s00421-002-0751-9

Hall, E. A., Chomistek, A. K., Kingma, J. K., & Docherty, C. L. (2018). Balance- and strength-training protocols to improve chronic ankle instability deficits, part I: Assessing clinical outcome measures. *Journal of Athletic Training, 53*(8), 568–577. https://doi.org/10.4085/1062-6050-385-16

Heggelund, J., Fimland, M. S., Helgerud, J., & Hoff, J. (2013). Maximal strength training improves work economy, rate of force development and maximal strength more than conventional strength training. *European Journal of Applied Physiology, 113*(6), 1565–1573. https://doi.org/10.1007/s00421-013-2586-y

Hermassi, S., Ghaith, A., Schwesig, R., Shephard, R. J., & Souhaiel Chelly, M. (2019). Effects of short-term resistance training and tapering on maximal strength, peak power, throwing ball velocity, and sprint performance in handball players. *PLoS One, 14*(7), e0214827. https://doi.org/10.1371/journal.pone.0214827

Hewett, T. E., Di Stasi, S. L., & Myer, G. D. (2013). Current concepts for injury prevention in athletes after anterior cruciate ligament reconstruction. *American Journal of Sports Medicine, 41*(1), 216–224. https://doi.org/10.1177/0363546512459638

Hiemstra, L. A., Webber, S., MacDonald, P. B., & Kriellaars, D. J. (2000). Knee strength deficits after hamstring tendon and patellar tendon anterior cruciate ligament reconstruction. *Medicine & Science in Sports & Exercise, 32*(8), 1472–1479. https://doi.org/10.1097/00005768-200008000-00016

Hughes, L., Paton, B., Rosenblatt, B., Gissane, C., & Patterson, S. D. (2017). Blood flow restriction training in clinical musculoskeletal rehabilitation: A systematic review and meta-analysis. *British Journal of Sports Medicine, 51*(13), 1003–1011. https://doi.org/10.1136/bjsports-2016-097071

Jiménez-Reyes, P., Samozino, P., Brughelli, M., & Morin, J.-B. (2017). Effectiveness of an individualized training based on force-velocity profiling during jumping. *Frontiers in Physiology, 7,* 677. https://doi.org/10.3389/fphys.2016.00677

Jordan, M. J., Aagaard, P., & Herzog, W. (2015a). Lower limb asymmetry in mechanical muscle function: A comparison between ski racers with and without ACL reconstruction. *Scandinavian Journal of Medicine & Science in Sports, 25*(3), e301–e309. https://doi.org/10.1111/sms.12314

Jordan, M. J., Aagaard, P., & Herzog, W. (2015b). Rapid hamstrings/quadriceps strength in ACL-reconstructed elite alpine ski racers. *Medicine & Science in Sports & Exercise, 47*(1), 109–119. https://doi.org/10.1249/MSS.0000000000000375

Jordan, M. J., Aagaard, P., & Herzog, W. (2017). Asymmetry and thigh muscle coactivity in fatigued ACL-reconstructed elite skiers. *Medicine & Science in Sports & Exercise, 49*(1), 11–20. https://doi.org/10.1249/MSS.0000000000001076

King, E., Richter, C., Daniels, K. A. J., Franklyn-Miller, A., Falvey, E., Myer, G. D., Jackson, M., Moran, R., & Strike, S. (2021). Can biomechanical testing after anterior cruciate ligament reconstruction identify athletes at risk for subsequent ACL injury to the contralateral uninjured limb? *American Journal of Sports Medicine, 49*(3), 609–619. https://doi.org/10.1177/0363546520985283

Kongsgaard, M., Reitelseder, S., Pedersen, T. G., Holm, L., Aagaard, P., Kjaer, M., & Magnusson, S. P. (2007). Region specific patellar tendon hypertrophy in humans following resistance training. *Acta Physiologica, 191*(2), 111–121. https://doi.org/10.1111/j.1748-1716.2007.01714.x

Kraemer, W. J., & Ratamess, N. A. (2000). Physiology of resistance training. *Orthopedic Clinics of North America, 9,* 467–513.

Kroell, J., &, Mike, J. N. (2017). Exploring the standard barbell overhead press. *Strength and Conditioning Journal, 39*(6), 70–75. https://doi.org/10.1519/SSC.0000000000000324

Krosshaug, T., Nakamae, A., Boden, B. P., Engebretsen, L., Smith, G., Slauterbeck, J. R., Hewett, T. E., & Bahr, R. (2007). Mechanisms of anterior cruciate ligament injury in basketball: Video analysis of 39 cases. *American Journal of Sports Medicine, 35*(3), 359–367. https://doi.org/10.1177/0363546506293899

Lasevicius, T., Ugrinowitsch, C., Schoenfeld, B. J., Roschel, H., Tavares, L. D., De Souza, E. O., Laurentino, G., & Tricoli, V. (2018). Effects of different intensities of resistance training with equated volume load on muscle strength and hypertrophy. *European Journal of Sport Science, 18*(6), 772–780. https://doi.org/10.1080/17461391.2018.1450898

Lauber, B., Gollhofer, A., & Taube, W. (2021). What to train first: Balance or explosive strength? Impact on performance and intracortical inhibition. *Scandinavian Journal of Medicine & Science in Sports, 31*(6), 1301–1312. https://doi.org/10.1111/sms.13939

Lauersen, J. B., Andersen, T. E., & Andersen, L. B. (2018). Strength training as superior, dose-dependent and safe prevention of acute and overuse sports injuries: A systematic review, qualitative analysis and meta-analysis. *British Journal of Sports Medicine, 52*(24), 1557–1563. https://doi.org/10.1136/bjsports-2018-099078

Laurson, K. R., Saint-Maurice, P. F., Welk, G. J., & Eisenmann, J. C. (2017). Reference curves for field tests of musculoskeletal fitness in U.S. children and adolescents: The 2012 NHANES national youth fitness survey. *Journal of Strength and Conditioning Research, 31*(8), 2075–2082. https://doi.org/10.1519/JSC.0000000000001678

Lee, B. C. Y., & McGill, S. M. (2015). Effect of long-term isometric training on core/torso stiffness. *Journal of Strength and Conditioning Research, 29*(6), 1515–1526. https://doi.org/10.1519/JSC.0000000000000740

Lee, B. C. Y., & McGill, S. M. (2017). The effect of core training on distal limb performance during ballistic strike manoeuvres. *Journal of Sports Sciences, 35*(18), 1–13. https://doi.org/10.1080/02640414.2016.1236207

Lesinski, M., Prieske, O., & Granacher, U. (2016). Effects and dose–response relationships of resistance training on physical performance in youth athletes: A systematic review and meta-analysis. *British Journal of Sports Medicine, 50*(13), 781–795. https://doi.org/10.1136/bjsports-2015-095497

Li, F., Newton, R. U., Shi, Y., Sutton, D., & Ding, H. (2021). Correlation of eccentric strength, reactive strength, and leg stiffness with running economy in well-trained distance runners. *Journal of Strength and Conditioning Research, 35*(6), 1491–1499. https://doi.org/10.1519/jsc.0000000000003446

Liao, K.-F., Nassis, G., Bishop, C., Yang, W., Bian, C., & Li, Y.-M. (2021). Effects of unilateral vs. bilateral resistance training interventions on measures of strength, jump, linear and change of direction speed: A systematic review and meta-analysis. *Biology of Sport, 39*(3), 485–497. https://doi.org/10.5114/biolsport.2022.107024

Lombardi, V. P., & Troxel, R. K. (2003). U.S. injuries and deaths associated with weight training. *Medicine & Science in Sports & Exercise, 35*(5 suppl), S203.

Looga, R. (2005). The Valsalva manoeuvre: Cardiovascular effects and performance technique: A critical review. *Respiratory Physiology & Neurobiology, 147*(1), 39–49. https://doi.org/10.1016/j.resp.2005.01.003

Lum, D., & Barbosa, T. M. (2019). Effects of strength training on Olympic time-based sport performance: A systematic review and meta-analysis of randomized controlled trials. *International Journal of Sports Physiology and Performance, 14*(10), 1–13. https://doi.org/10.1123/ijspp.2019-0329

Lundberg, T. R., Fernandez-Gonzalo, R., Gustafsson, T., & Tesch, P. A. (2013). Aerobic exercise does not compromise muscle hypertrophy response to short-term resistance training. *Journal of Applied Physiology, 114*(1), 81–89. https://doi.org/10.1152/japplphysiol.01013.2012

Maffiuletti, N. A., Aagaard, P., Blazevich, A. J., Folland, J., Tillin, N., & Duchateau, J. (2016). Rate of force development: Physiological and methodological considerations. *European Journal of Applied Physiology, 116*(6), 1091–1116. https://doi.org/10.1007/s00421-016-3346-6

Manca, A., Dragone, D., Dvir, Z., & Deriu, F. (2017). Cross-education of muscular strength following unilateral resistance training: a meta-analysis. *European Journal of Applied Physiology, 117*(11), 2335–2354. https://doi.org/10.1007/s00421-017-3720-z

McCurdy, K. W., Langford, G. A., Doscher, M. W., Wiley, L. P., & Mallard, K. G. (2005). The effects of short-term unilateral and bilateral lower-body resistance training on measures of strength and power. *Journal of Strength and Conditioning Research, 19*(1), 9–15. https://pubmed.ncbi.nlm.nih.gov/15705051

McGill, S. M, Chaimberg, J. D., Frost, D. M., & Fenwick, C. M. J. (2010). Evidence of a double peak in muscle activation to enhance strike speed and force: An example with elite mixed martial arts fighters. *Journal of Strength and Conditioning Research, 24*(2), 348–357. https://doi.org/10.1519/JSC.0b013e3181cc23d5

McGill, S. M., & Cholewicki, J. (2001). Biomechanical basis for stability: An explanation to enhance clinical utility. *Journal of Orthopaedic and Sports Physical Therapy, 31*(2), 96–100. https://doi.org/10.2519/jospt.2001.31.2.96

Moran, J., Ramirez-Campillo, R., Liew, B., Chaabene, H., Behm, D. G., García-Hermoso, A., Izquierdo, M., & Granacher, U. (2021). Effects of bilateral and unilateral resistance training on horizontally orientated movement performance: A systematic review and meta-analysis. *Sports Medicine, 51*(2), 225–242. https://doi.org/10.1007/s40279-020-01367-9

Moritani, T. (1993). Neuromuscular adaptations during the acquisition of muscle strength, power and motor tasks. *Journal of Biomechanics, 26*(suppl 1), 95–107. https://pubmed.ncbi.nlm.nih.gov/8505356

Morris, N., Jordan, M. J., Sumar, S., van Adrichem, B., Heard, M., & Herzog, W. (2020). Joint angle-specific impairments in rate of force development, strength, and muscle morphology after hamstring autograft. *Translational Sports Medicine, 4*(1), 104–114. https://doi.org/10.1002/tsm2.189

Muyor, J. M. (2013). Exercise intensity and validity of the ratings of perceived exertion (Borg and OMNI scales) in an indoor cycling session. *Journal of Human Kinetics, 39*, 93–101. https://www.ncbi.nlm.nih.gov/pmc/articles/PMC3916918

Natera, A. O., Cardinale, M., & Keogh, J. W. L. (2020). The effect of high volume power training on repeated high-intensity performance and the assessment of repeat power ability: A systematic review. *Sports Medicine, 50*(7), 1317–1339. https://doi.org/10.1007/s40279-020-01273-0

Peterson, M. D., Rhea, M. R., & Alvar, B. A. (2005). Applications of the dose–response for muscular strength development: A review of meta-analytic efficacy and reliability for designing training prescription. *Journal of Strength and Conditioning Research, 19*(4), 950–958. https://pubmed.ncbi.nlm.nih.gov/16287373

Pichardo, A. W., Oliver, J. L., Harrison, C. B., Maulder, P. S., Lloyd, R. S., & Kandoi, R. (2019). Effects of combined resistance training and weightlifting on motor skill performance of adolescent male athletes. *Journal of Strength and Conditioning Research, 33*(12), 3226–3235. https://doi.org/10.1519/JSC.0000000000003108

Prieske, O., Behrens, M., Chaabene, H., Granacher, U., & Maffiuletti, N. A. (2020). Time to differentiate postactivation "potentiation" from "performance enhancement" in the strength and conditioning community. *Sports Medicine, 50*(9), 1559–1565. https://doi.org/10.1007/s40279-020-01300-0

Ratamess, N., Alvar, B. A., Evetoch, T. K., Housh, T. J., Kibler, W. B., Kraemer, W. J., & Triplett, N. T. (2009). American College of Sports Medicine position stand: Progression models in resistance training for healthy adults. *Medicine & Science in Sports & Exercise, 41*(3), 687–708. https://doi.org/10.1249/MSS.0b013e3181915670

Read, P. J., Auliffe, S. M., Wilson, M. G., & Graham-Smith, P. (2020). Lower limb kinetic asymmetries in professional soccer players with and without anterior cruciate ligament reconstruction: Nine months is not enough time to restore "functional" symmetry or return to performance. *American Journal of Sports Medicine, 48*(6), 1365–1373. https://doi.org/10.1177/0363546520912218

Rhea, M. R., & Alderman, B. L. (2004). A meta-analysis of periodized versus nonperiodized strength and power training programs. *Research Quarterly for Exercise and Sport, 75*(4), 413–422. https://doi.org/10.1080/02701367.2004.10609174

Rivera, M. J., Winkelmann, Z. K., Powden, C. J., & Games, K. E. (2017). Proprioceptive training for the prevention of ankle sprains: An evidence-based review. *Journal of Athletic Training, 52*(11), 1065–1067. https://doi.org/10.4085/1062-6050-52.11.16

Rønnestad, B. R., Hansen, J., Hollan, I., & Ellefsen, S. (2015). Strength training improves performance and pedaling characteristics in elite cyclists. *Scandinavian Journal of Medicine & Science in Sports, 25*(1), e89–e98. https://doi.org/10.1111/sms.12257

Rønnestad, B. R., & Mujika, I. (2014). Optimizing strength training for running and cycling endurance performance: A review. *Scandinavian Journal of Medicine & Science in Sports, 24*(4), 603–612. https://doi.org/10.1111/sms.12104

Ryman Augustsson, S., & Ageberg, E. (2017). Weaker lower extremity muscle strength predicts traumatic knee injury in youth female but not male athletes. *BMJ Open Sport and Exercise Medicine, 3*(1), e000222. https://doi.org/10.1136/bmjsem-2017-000222

Sale, D. G. (1988). Neural adaptation to resistance training. *Medicine & Science in Sports & Exercise, 20*(5), S135–S145. https://doi.org/10.1249/00005768-198810001-00009

Samozino, P., Rejc, E., Di Prampero, P. E., Belli, A., & Morin, J. B. (2012). Optimal force-velocity profile in ballistic movements: Altius. *Medicine & Science in Sports & Exercise, 44*(2), 313–322. https://doi.org/10.1249/MSS.0b013e31822d757a

Schmidtbleicher, D., & Buehrle, M. (1987). Neuronal adaptation and increase of cross-sectional area studying different strength training. In B. Johnson (Ed.), *Biomechanics X-B: International series on biomechanics* (Vol. 6B, pp. 615–620). Human Kinetics.

Schoenfeld, B. J. (2010). The mechanisms of muscle hypertrophy and their application to resistance training. *Journal of Strength and Conditioning Research, 24*(10), 2857–2872. https://doi.org/10.1519/jsc.0b013e3181e840f3

Schoenfeld, B. J., Contreras, B., Krieger, J., Grgic, J., Delcastillo, K., Belliard, R., & Alto, A. (2019). Resistance training volume enhances muscle hypertrophy but not strength in trained men. *Medicine & Science in Sports & Exercise, 51*(1), 94–103. https://doi.org/10.1249/MSS.0000000000001764

Schoenfeld, B. J., Grgic, J., Van Every, D. W., & Plotkin, D. L. (2021). Loading recommendations for muscle strength, hypertrophy, and local endurance: A re-examination of the repetition continuum. *Sports, 9*(2), 32. https://doi.org/10.3390/sports9020032

Schoenfeld, B. J., Ogborn, D., & Krieger, J. W. (2017). Dose–response relationship between weekly resistance training volume and increases in muscle mass: A systematic review and meta-analysis. *Journal of Sports Sciences, 35*(11), 1073–1082. https://doi.org/10.1080/02640414.2016.1210197

Schoenfeld, B. J., Ratamess, N. A., Peterson, M. D., Contreras, B., & Tiryaki-Sonmez, G. (2015). Influence of resistance training frequency on muscular adaptations in well-trained men. *Journal of Strength and Conditioning Research, 29*(7), 1829–1829. https://doi.org/10.1519/JSC.0000000000000970

Seitz, L. B., Reyes, A., Tran, T. T., de Villarreal, E. S., & Haff, G. G. (2014). Increases in lower-body strength transfer positively to sprint performance: A systematic review with meta-analysis. *Sports Medicine, 44*(12), 1693–1702. https://doi.org/10.1007/s40279-014-0227-1

Škarabot, J., Cronin, N., Strojnik, V., & Avela, J. (2016). Bilateral deficit in maximal force production. *European Journal of Applied Physiology, 116*(11–12), 2057–2084. https://doi.org/10.1007/s00421-016-3458-z

Speirs, D. E., Bennett, M. A., Finn, C. V., & Turner, A. P. (2016). Unilateral vs. bilateral squat training for strength, sprints, and agility in academy rugby players. *Journal of Strength and Conditioning Research, 30*(2), 386–392. https://doi.org/10.1519/JSC.0000000000001096

Spiteri, T., Nimphius, S., Hart, N. H., Specos, C., Sheppard, J. M., & Newton, R. U. (2014). Contribution of strength characteristics to change of direction and agility performance in female basketball athletes. *Journal of Strength and Conditioning Research, 28*(9), 2415–2423. https://doi.org/10.1519/JSC.0000000000000547

Steidl-Müller, L., Hildebrandt, C., Müller, E., Fink, C., & Raschner, C. (2018). Limb symmetry index in competitive alpine ski racers: Reference values and injury risk identification according to age-related performance levels. *Journal of Sport and Health Science, 7*(4), 405–415. https://doi.org/10.1016/j.jshs.2018.09.002

Stern, D., Gonzalo-Skok, O., Loturco, I., Turner, A., & Bishop, C. (2020). A comparison of bilateral vs. unilateral-biased strength and power training interventions on measures of physical performance in elite youth soccer players. *Journal of Strength and Conditioning Research, 34*(8), 2105–2111. https://doi.org/10.1519/JSC.0000000000003659

Suchomel, T. J., Nimphius, S., Bellon, C. R., Hornsby, W. G., & Stone, M. H. (2021). Training for muscular strength: Methods for monitoring and adjusting training intensity. *Sports Medicine, 51*(10), 2051–2066. https://doi.org/10.1007/s40279-021-01488-9

Suchomel, T. J., Nimphius, S., & Stone, M. H. (2016). The importance of muscular strength in athletic performance. *Sports Medicine, 46*(10), 1419–1449. https://doi.org/10.1007/s40279-016-0486-0

Tennent, D. J., Burns, T. C., Johnson, A. E., Owens, J. G., & Hylden, C. M. (2018). Blood flow restriction training for postoperative lower-extremity weakness: A report of three cases. *Current Sports Medicine Reports, 17*(4), 119–122. https://doi.org/10.1249/jsr.0000000000000470

Thompson, S. W., Rogerson, D., Ruddock, A., & Barnes, A. (2020). The effectiveness of two methods of prescribing load on maximal strength development: A systematic review. *Sports Medicine, 50*(5), 919–938. https://doi.org/10.1007/s40279-019-01241-3

Tredrea, M. S. J. (2017). Applied complex training: An updated review and practical applications. *Journal of Australian Strength and Conditioning, 25*(3), 15.

Turpeinen, J.-T., Freitas, T. T., Rubio-Arias, J. Á., Jordan, M. J., & Aagaard, P. (2020). Contractile rate of force development after anterior cruciate ligament reconstruction: A comprehensive review and meta-analysis. *Scandinavian Journal of Medicine and Science in Sports, 30*(9), 1572–1585. https://doi.org/10.1111/sms.13733

Vera Garcia, F. J., Ruiz Pérez, I., Barbado, D., Juan-Recio, C., & McGill, S. M. (2014). Trunk and shoulder EMG and lumbar kinematics of medicine-ball side throw and side catch and throw. *European Journal of Human Movement, 33*(2014), 93–109.

Wengle, L., Migliorini, F., Leroux, T., Chahal, J., Theodoropoulos, J., & Betsch, M. (2021, August). The effects of blood flow restriction in patients undergoing knee surgery: A systematic review and meta-analysis. *American Journal of Sports Medicine,* 3635465211027296. https://doi.org/10.1177/03635465211027296

Werkhausen, A., Solberg, C. E., Paulsen, G., Bojsen-Møller, J., & Seynnes, O. R. (2021). Adaptations to explosive resistance training with partial range of motion are not inferior to full range of motion. *Scandinavian Journal of Medicine & Science in Sports, 31*(5), 1026–1035. https://doi.org/10.1111/sms.13921

Wilk, M., Zajac, A., & Tufano, J. J. (2021). The influence of movement tempo during resistance training on muscular strength and hypertrophy responses: A review. *Sports Medicine, 51*(8), 1629–1650. https://doi.org/10.1007/s40279-021-01465-2

Wilson, J. M., Marin, P. J., Rhea, M. R., Wilson, S. M. C., Loenneke, J. P., & Anderson, J. C. (2012). Concurrent training: A meta-analysis examining interference of aerobic and resistance exercise. *Journal of Strength and Conditioning Research, 26*(8), 2293–2307. https://doi.org/10.1519/jsc.0b013e31823a3e2d

Young, W. B. (2006). Transfer of strength and power training to sports performance. *International Journal of Sports Physiology and Performance, 1*(2), 74–83. https://doi.org/10.1123/ijspp.1.2.74

Zebis, M. K., Andersen, L. L., Brandt, M., Myklebust, G., Bencke, J., Lauridsen, H. B., Bandholm, T., Thorborg, K., Hölmich, P., & Aagaard, P. (2016). Effects of evidence-based prevention training on neuromuscular and biomechanical risk factors for ACL injury in adolescent female athletes: A randomised controlled trial. *British Journal of Sports Medicine, 50*(9), 552–557. https://doi.org/10.1136/bjsports-2015-094776

Zech, A., Hübscher, M., Vogt, L., Banzer, W., Hänsel, F., & Pfeifer, K. (2010). Balance training for neuromuscular control and performance enhancement: A systematic review. *Journal of Athletic Training, 45*(4), 392–403. https://doi.org/10.4085/1062-6050-45.4.392

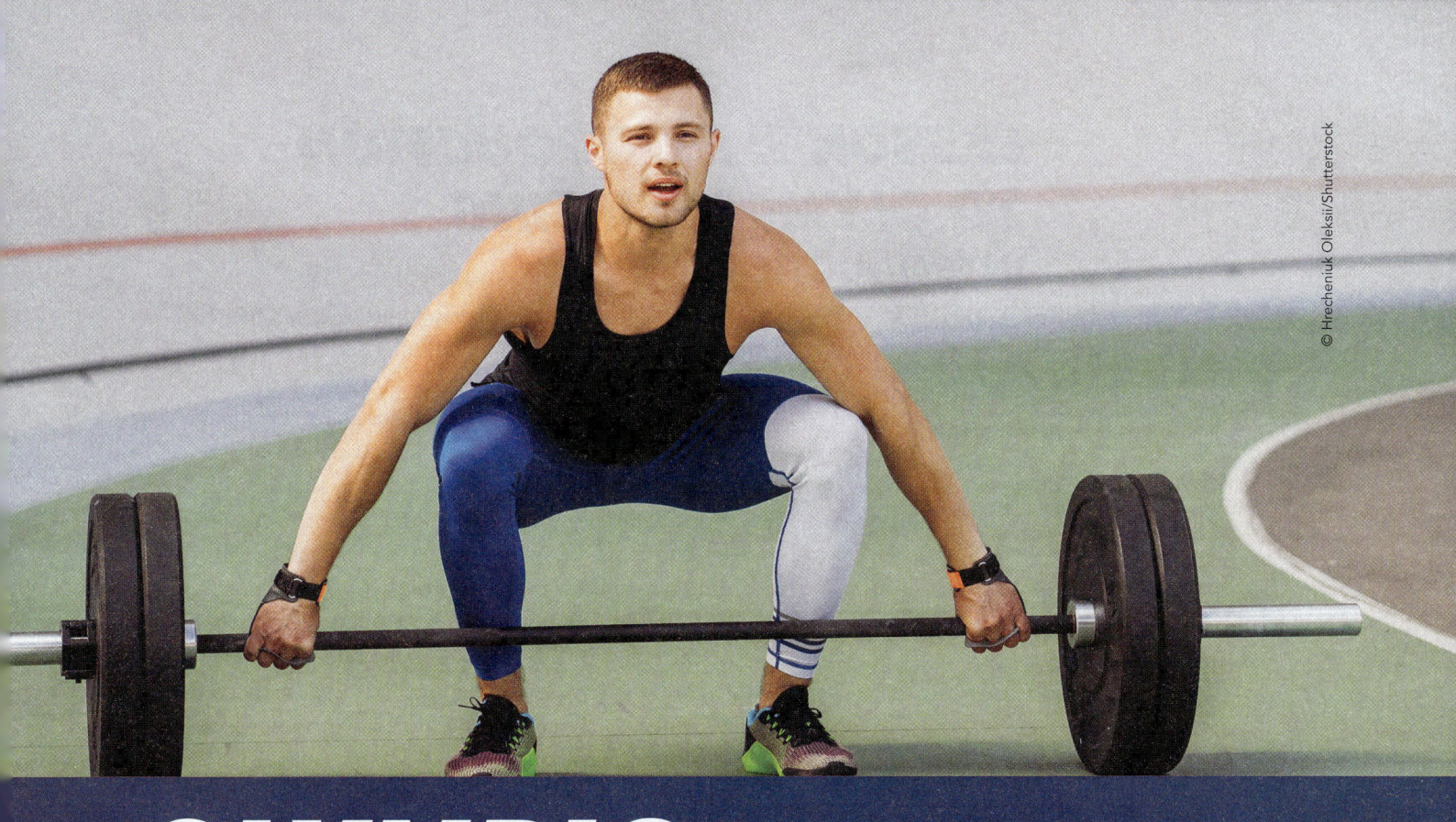

OLYMPIC WEIGHTLIFTING FOR SPORTS PERFORMANCE

CHAPTER FIFTEEN

LEARNING OBJECTIVES

Upon completion of this chapter, the Sports Performance Coach will be able to:

- **Summarize** the importance of Olympic lifting for athletes with differing performance-related goals.

- **Explain** the scientific rationale for Olympic lifting improving sports performance.

- **Identify** prerequisites for the addition of Olympic lifting to a program.

- **Evaluate** Olympic lifting technique, including common compensations.

- **Explain** safe and appropriate use of Olympic lifting following the OPT™ Model.

LESSON 1: INTRODUCTION TO OLYMPIC LIFTING
INTRODUCTION

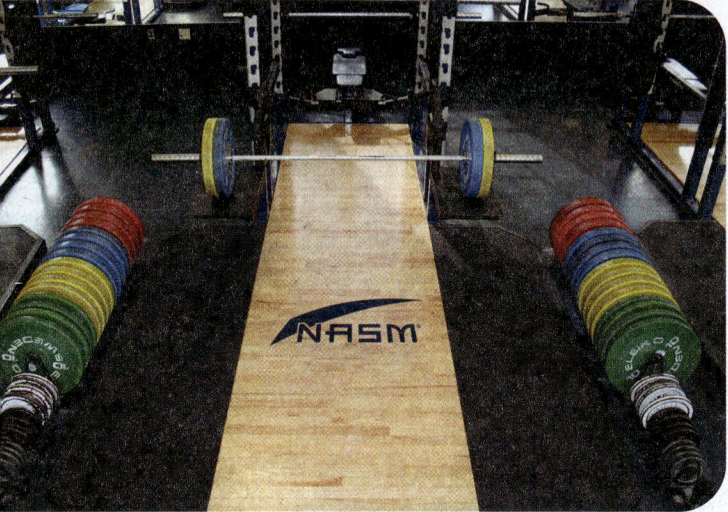

In the world of sports performance improvement, the incorporation of Olympic weightlifting holds paramount importance.

Traditionally regarded as an elite discipline, Olympic weightlifting is now recognized as a fundamental component in enhancing athletic performance across a broad spectrum of sports. It fosters critical attributes such as strength, power, speed, coordination, agility, balance, and flexibility, which are all indispensable to an athlete's proficiency. Integrating Olympic weightlifting techniques into athletes' training can profoundly affect their performance. These exercises are not merely about lifting heavy weights, but rather involve complex, functional movements that simultaneously stimulate various muscle groups. Such holistic stimulation leads to an overall increase in physical capacity, enabling athletes to perform better in their respective sports. This introduction aims to underscore the significance of Olympic weightlifting in sports performance improvement programs, illuminating how it can cultivate athletes' physical skills and abilities, improve injury resilience, and ultimately elevate their competitive edge.

HISTORY OF OLYMPIC WEIGHTLIFTING

Modern-day weightlifting practices first became noticeable in Europe during the mid-1800s. Many weightlifting and strength training clubs emerged during this era, predominantly in Austria and Germany (Stone et al., 2006). During the late 1800s, "lifting" became a basic exercise. This form of training produced the strongmen seen in many circuses worldwide. These strongmen would perform various one-handed and two-handed lifts, which were the basis of the modern-day Olympic lifts (Stojiljkovic et al., 2013). Weightlifting made its first appearance in the 1896 Olympics (Stojiljkovic et al., 2013), and in 1891 the first Weightlifting World Championships were held in London (Stone et al., 2006). However, Olympic-style lifting at that time looked nothing like it does today.

After appearing in the Olympics only one more time (in 1904) over the next 24 years, the sport of weightlifting formed its federation in 1905. This federation was recognized by the International Olympic Committee (IOC) in 1914 (Stone et al., 2006). Finally, in 1920, weightlifting formally became an Olympic sport. By the 1928 Olympics, the lifts had become standardized and consisted of only three two-handed lifts: the snatch, the clean and jerk, and the clean and press.

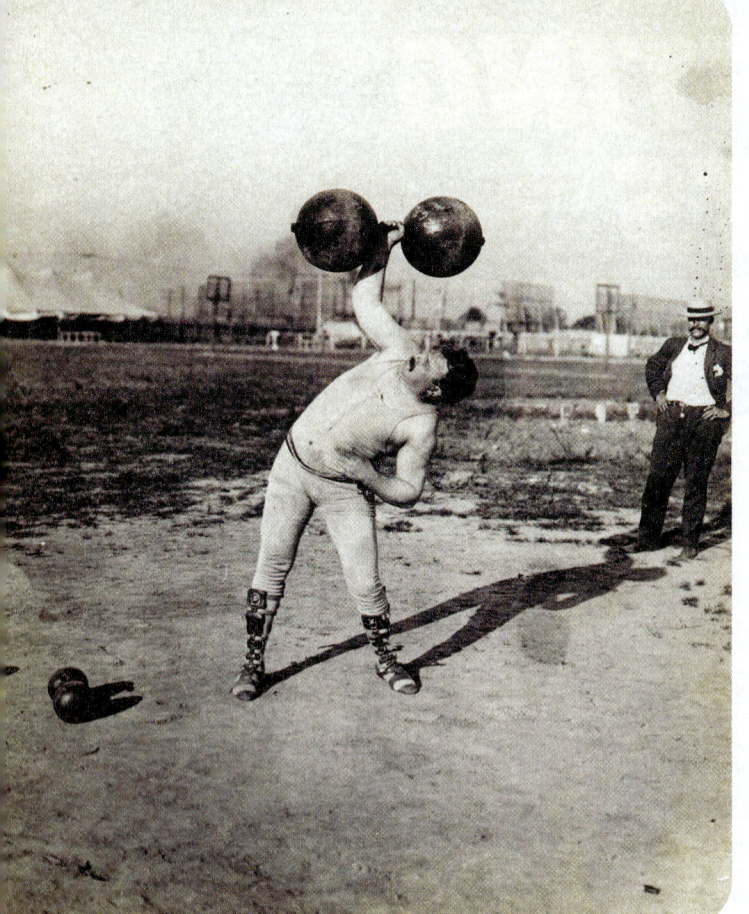

Courtesy of Jessie Tarbox Beals/Missouri History Museum

Weightlifting caught on quickly in the United States. From the 1930s through the 1960s, the United States was one of the world's most dominant nations in this sport, producing numerous Olympic champions (Stone et al., 2006). In 1972, the clean and press was removed from competition due to difficulties in judging, leaving the snatch and the clean and jerk as the two Olympics lifts used today.

Many elite Sports Performance Coaches use these two lifts and several variations, or **derivatives**, to augment their athletes' training programs. In the 1980s, women's weightlifting began to draw increasing interest and exposure, especially in the United States and China. The first Women's World Championships were held in 1987, and the women's sport was finally included in the 2000 Olympic Games (Stone et al., 2006).

Historically, male and female elite weightlifters tend to have physical characteristics that may provide good leverage and force production. For example, successful weightlifters typically have shorter limbs and longer torsos, have higher lean body mass to body fat ratios, and are generally shorter than other athletes with the same body mass. The combination of these attributes can be ideal for lifting larger amounts of weight from the floor to overhead, as it favors a greater cross-sectional area of muscle, associated with better force production and better overall leverage (Stone et al., 2006).

THE OLYMPIC LIFTS

Olympic weightlifting is a competitive sport requiring great technical skill to lift a barbell from the ground to an overhead position. Two lifts are used in competition, the **snatch** and the **clean and jerk**. The snatch has a wider grip and requires moving the bar from the ground to overhead in one motion (**Figure 15.1**). The clean and jerk has a narrower grip and requires moving the bar from the ground to overhead in two motions (**Figure 15.2**).

The Snatch Olympic Lift

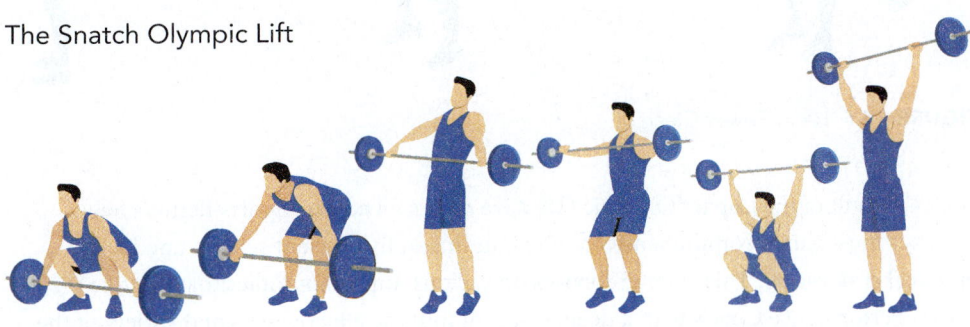

FIGURE 15.1 Snatch

The Clean and Jerk Olympic Lift

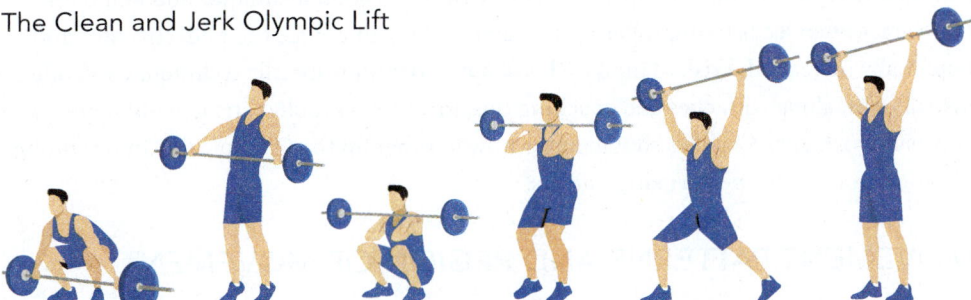

FIGURE 15.2 Clean and Jerk

DERIVATIVES →

Lifts that emphasize a specific phase found within the two competition Olympic lifts (e.g., snatch pull) and/or are modified versions of them (e.g., hang power clean).

SNATCH →

An Olympic lift involving the lifting of a barbell from a stationary position on the ground to directly overhead in multiple phases using a fairly wide grip.

CLEAN AND JERK →

An Olympic lift involving the lifting of a barbell from a stationary position on the ground to the chest and then directly overhead in multiple phases using a fairly narrow grip.

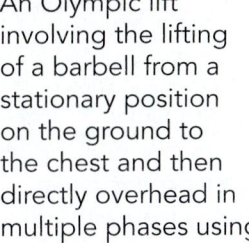

The snatch and the clean and jerk are considered competition or full lifts. Beyond those full lifts, Olympic weightlifting is highly diversified, including several derivative lifts used outside competition. These emphasize specific phases of the two competition lifts and modified versions of the full lifts. Examples of these derivatives include the **hang power snatch** (**Figure 15.3**) and the **hang power clean** (**Figure 15.4**).

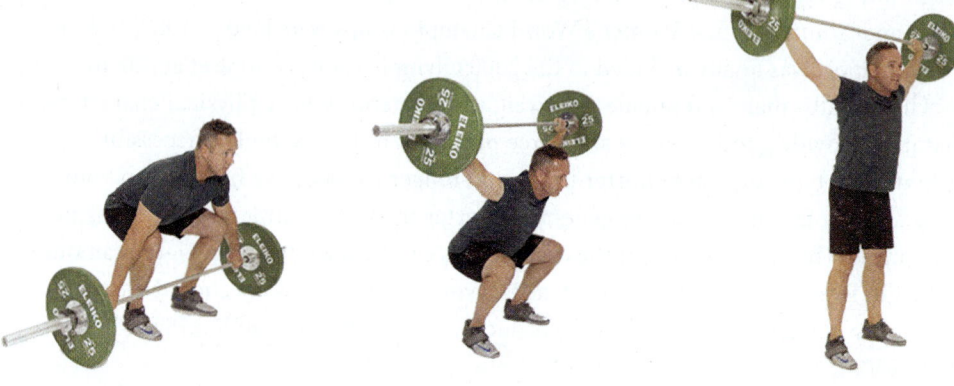

FIGURE 15.3 Hang Power Snatch

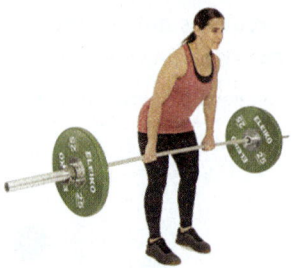 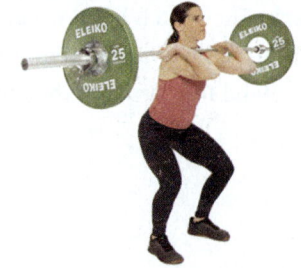 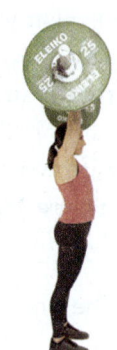

FIGURE 15.4 Hang Power Clean

> **HANG POWER →**
> **SNATCH**
>
> Catching derivative of the snatch with a starting position at the knee, mid-thigh, or hip and finishing in a half squat position.

> **HANG POWER →**
> **CLEAN**
>
> Catching derivative of the clean with a starting position at the knee, mid-thigh, or hip and finishing in a half squat position.

> **HANG CLEAN →**
>
> Catching derivative of the clean with a starting position at the knee, mid-thigh, or hip and finishing in a full or deep squat position.

As a result of the impact Olympic lifts have on performance, Sports Performance Coaches must gain a comprehensive understanding of the present science and its practical application. This chapter focuses on various important topics that provide the Sports Performance Coach with a deeper insight into the effectiveness and variety of the Olympic lifts. First, it is essential to understand how flexibility, mobility, stability, posture, neuromuscular control, and strength affect athletes' ability to execute the Olympic lifts and their derivatives. The Olympic lifts require skill and good technique, and failure in these areas often leads to improper performance. This can reduce their effectiveness and potentially increase the risk of injury. This chapter identifies specific techniques and offers instructions, along with cues and coaching tips, to address problematic issues. Finally, Sports Performance Coaches should know how to program the Olympic lifts into training programs for various performance clients.

MOVEMENT PATTERNS AND REGION OF MOVEMENT

Biomechanically, some of the most common positions and movement patterns across sports utilize the universal athletic position, hip hinge, triple flexion, and triple extension.

Likewise, these positions and movement patterns are necessary for the Olympic lifts. When seen side-by-side, the biomechanical similarities between sporting movements and the Olympic lifts are readily evident. However, as a Sports Performance Coach, it is important to understand that specificity in one area (e.g., a similar movement pattern only) does not necessarily determine a successful outcome (Arabatzi & Kellis, 2012; MacKenzie et al., 2014). Performance enhancement may come through force, velocity, power, metabolic, and a combination of these attributes (Arabatzi & Kellis, 2012; Haugen et al., 2019; Hori et al., 2005; James et al., 2018; James et al., 2019; MacKenzie et al., 2014; Suchomel et al., 2017).

UNIVERSAL ATHLETIC POSITION

The universal athletic position is like the half squat position commonly seen with linebackers in American football, infielders and outfielders in baseball waiting for the ball, and a defensive position in basketball. Similarly, both Olympic lifts require the ability to utilize the universal athletic position (**Figure 15.5**). The ability to react explosively from this position can determine a successful versus unsuccessful performance outcome.

HANG SNATCH →

Catching derivative of the snatch with a starting position at the knee, mid-thigh, or hip and finishing in a full or deep squat position.

POWER CLEAN →

Catching derivative of the clean with a starting position at the floor and finishing in a half squat position.

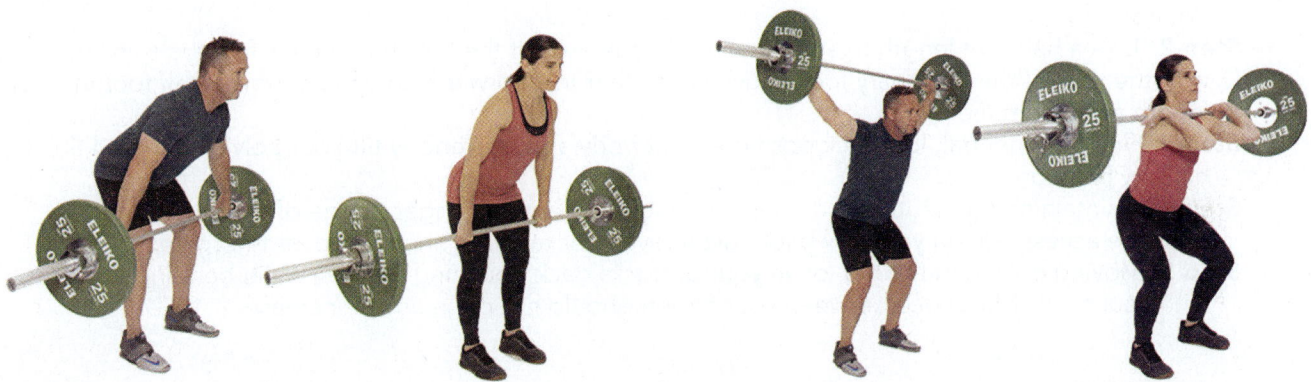

FIGURE 15.5 Universal Athletic Position and the Olympic Lifts

Depending on the lift, or the derivative used, the arrival at the universal athletic position may occur at different times within the lift. For example, the athlete will start in the universal athletic position when using the **hang clean** or **hang snatch**. In the **power clean** or **power snatch**, the athlete will finish in the universal athletic position with the barbell (load) in a different position relative to the body. Using different derivatives can alter the challenge placed on the athlete, who has to move or control the barbell through varying motions. This topic will be discussed in more detail in the section on specific Olympic lifting derivatives.

HIP HINGE

A hip hinge is a hip-dominant flexion/extension motion commonly seen in the stance of a lineman in American football, when fielding a ground ball in baseball, and when a goalie fields the ball from the ground in soccer. Both of the Olympic lifts and their derivatives also require the athlete to be able to perform a hip hinge. More specifically, the hip hinge is used when lifting from the floor and **hang** positions to different degrees (**Figure 15.6**).

POWER SNATCH →

Catching derivative of the snatch with a starting position at the floor and finishing in a half squat position.

HANG →

Starting position for an Olympic lift that is from a hanging position at the knee, mid-thigh, or hip.

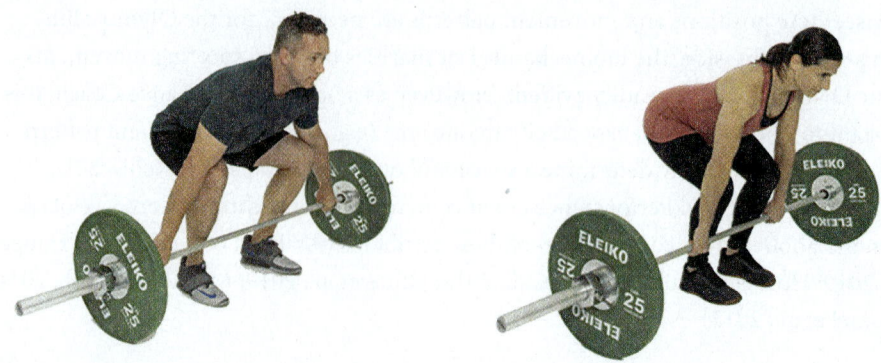

FIGURE 15.6 Hip Hinge and the Olympic Lifts

TRIPLE FLEXION

Triple flexion is the concurrent flexing of the hip, knee, and ankle joints commonly seen in actions such as a catcher's stance in baseball, the front leg of a sprinter, and the start position in swimming. For both of the Olympic lifts and most derivatives, the starting position will be from a triple flexion position. In addition, the catch phase for both lifts and the return to the starting position for most derivatives also involve the use and control of triple flexion (**Figure 15.7**).

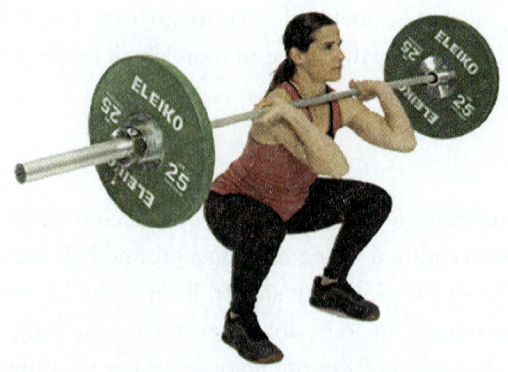

FIGURE 15.7 Triple Flexion

TRIPLE EXTENSION

Triple extension is the concurrent extending of the hip, knee, and ankle joints that can be seen in jumping up for a rebound or layup in basketball, the rear leg of a sprinter, and pushing off from the start and the wall in swimming. One of the primary purposes when using the Olympic lifts is to maximize power production during triple extension, whether the full lift from the floor or any other derivative (**Figure 15.8**).

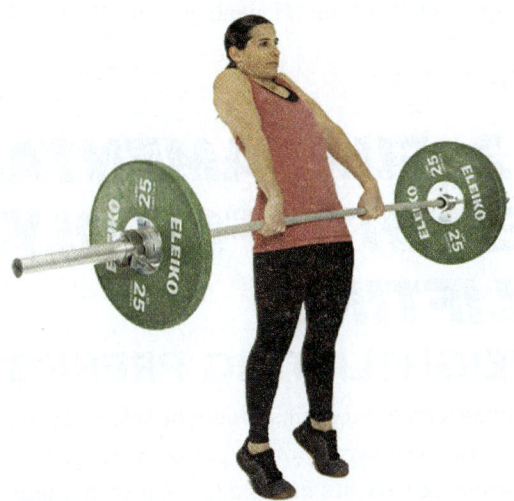

FIGURE 15.8 Triple Extension and the Olympic Lifts

OVERHEAD LIFTING

Achieving an overhead lift (**Figure 15.9**), whether an overhead press, jerk, or snatch, requires up to 180 degrees of shoulder flexion, with concurrent abduction and external rotation for the snatch (Howe & Blagrove, 2015). The total amount of motion can be broken down to about 120 degrees for the glenohumeral (GH) joint and 60 degrees of

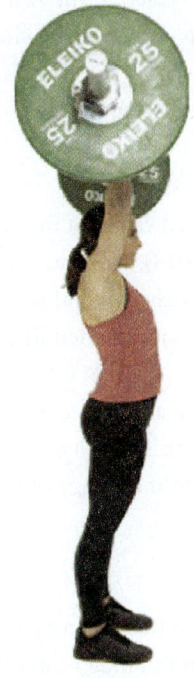

FIGURE 15.9 Overhead Lift

upward rotation of the scapulothoracic (ST) joint (Howe & Blagrove, 2015). The total shoulder movement includes the sternoclavicular (SC) and acromioclavicular (AC) joint motion. Whenever the shoulder moves, there must also be concurrent motion in the thoracic spine (TS) (Crosbie et al., 2008; Heneghan et al., 2019; Heneghan et al., 2020; Webb et al., 2017). Bilateral shoulder flexion, performed during the overhead lifts, requires the TS to move into approximately 12 to 15 degrees of spinal extension (Heneghan et al., 2019; Heneghan et al., 2020; Webb et al., 2017). For shoulder abduction, the TS produces approximately 9 to 15 degrees of extension (Heneghan et al., 2019; Webb et al., 2017).

LESSON 2: FUNDAMENTAL REQUIREMENTS FOR OLYMPIC WEIGHTLIFTING

OLYMPIC WEIGHTLIFTING PREREQUISITES

Effective performance enhancement programs should be safe and progressive to reduce the risk of injury and increase the longevity of the performance gains for the client. To achieve this, Sports Performance Coaches must be familiar with important prerequisite information regarding the athlete and the weightlifting environment.

PERFORMANCE PREREQUISITES

The Olympic lifts require more complex neural activation strategies and motor skills to enhance performance. Therefore, understanding the prerequisite neuromuscular abilities needed for performing Olympic lifting safely and effectively is critical. In addition, identifying and addressing the neuromuscular efficiency of a performance client allows for better planning, programming, and progression toward a successful outcome. Sports Performance Coaches should be well versed in the assessment procedures discussed in Chapters 7 and 8 so that they can help performance clients overcome barriers that may hinder them from optimal performance. Key prerequisites for Olympic weightlifting include mobility, stability, posture, and strength.

MOBILITY

Currently, there is a lack of standardized range of motion (ROM) requirements for Olympic lifting (Bousquet & Olson, 2018). However, it is well known that Olympic weightlifting (and its derivatives) comprise several total-body lifts, usually performed under loaded conditions. Using multi-joint loaded lifts necessitates good mobility to ensure safe and effective outcomes (Bousquet & Olson, 2018). For Olympic lifting, mobility can be thought of as achieving as close to an optimal ROM as possible at each involved joint with good control (or stability). In other words, it requires being able to move the joints of the body with the right amount of ROM, at the right time, and in the right direction.

Ankles

The forces produced at the ankles make the highest contributions to the acceleration and velocity of the barbell (Kipp, 2020). Thus, ankle mobility is crucial to attain an efficient setup position and move explosively from dorsiflexion to plantarflexion. Good ankle dorsiflexion is potentially the most critical position to obtain. It allows optimal kinetic chain alignment during the squatting motions required when performing the Olympic lifts (Kim et al., 2015) (**Table 15.1**). More specifically, it aids in preventing the knees, hips, and lower back from experiencing too much stress during the squatting aspects of the Olympic lifts (Bousquet & Olson, 2018). Dorsiflexion ROM should be between 12 and 20 degrees to ensure optimal foot placement, stance width, and safe and effective outcomes are maintained (Bousquet & Olson, 2018; Kusuma et al., 2018; Liu et al., 2018; Winwood et al., 2015) (**Figure 15.10**).

TABLE 15.1 Ankle Range of Motion Prerequisites for Olympic Lifting

Ankle Motion	ROM	Purpose of Motion
Dorsiflexion	12–20 degrees	• Provides optimal kinetic chain alignment during setup and catch phases • Aids in proper foot placement and stance width • Reduces stress on the knees, hips, and low back

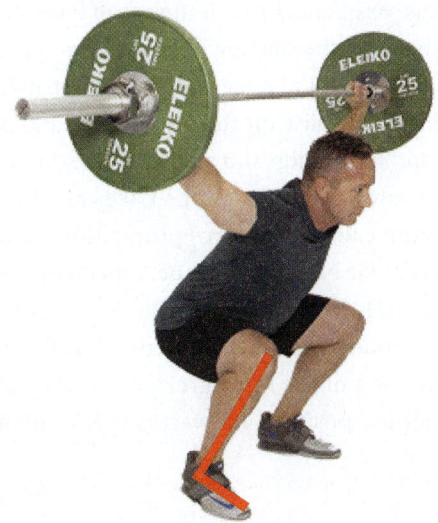

FIGURE 15.10 Ankle Dorsiflexion Prerequisite

Plantar flexion of the ankle is a vital part of the triple extension needed during the Olympic lifts. As the ankle joint is a primary contributor to the overall power output of the Olympic lifts, the ability to extend through the ankles is also important (Kipp, 2020). The amount of plantar flexion ROM needed during a lift can fluctuate depending on the load used and the amount of knee flexion at the top of the second pull.

Knees and Hips

Mobility in the knee and hip flexion is also essential for a proper setup and catch position. This is necessary when performing the Olympic lifts from the floor and a catch phase in a deep squat position, especially with heavier loads (Hadi et al., 2012; Werner et al., 2021). Knee flexion requirements can be as much as 145 to 150 degrees, with hip flexion being upward of 95 to 135 degrees (Bousquet & Olson, 2018; Kusuma et al., 2018; Liu et al., 2018; Winwood et al., 2015) (**Figure 15.11**). Although the stated ROM might appear greater than orthopedic measurements, this results from load and how angles are measured. The most important takeaway is that knee and hip flexion can be maximal.

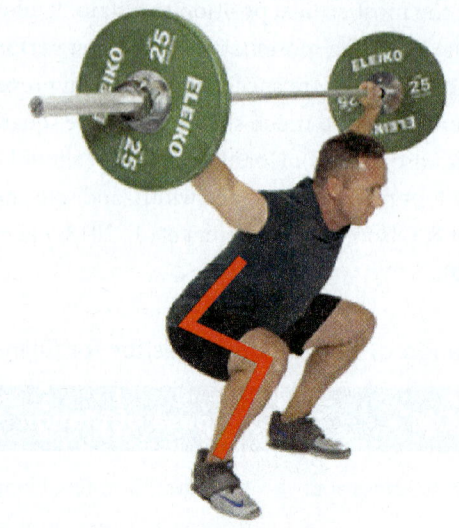

FIGURE 15.11 Knee and Hip Flexion Prerequisites

Flexion values can change dramatically with the use of lower loads and in other derivatives. For example, changing the starting position from the floor to the knee position will immediately decrease the amount of knee and hip flexion and ankle dorsiflexion. Also, there is no deep squat in the catch phase for the power clean and power snatch lifts. This will further decrease knee and hip flexion and ankle dorsiflexion requirements.

Optimizing mobility in extension through the knees and hips is also very important. Optimal extension can impact force production, as well as the positioning of the bar relative to the body for better technique, especially when loads increase (Kipp, 2020; Werner et al., 2021; Winwood et al., 2015). The knees may not fully extend, dependent on the amount of load and extension at the hip and ankle (plantar flexion). However, full extension of the hips (greater than 0 degrees from vertical) may be advantageous for a better bar position and vertical movement of the body and bar (**Figure 15.12**).

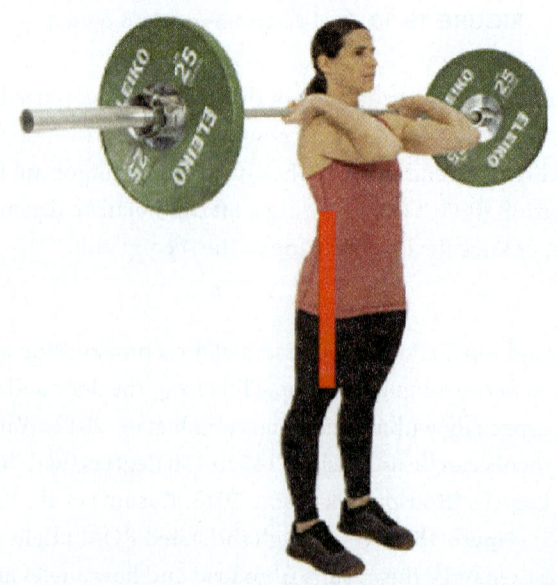

FIGURE 15.12 Hip Extension Prerequisite

Looking at the combined requirements for the ankles, knees, and hips (**Table 15.2**), the importance of mobility through triple flexion and triple extension during the Olympic lifts becomes clear. Other essential mobility requirements that aid in triple flexion and extension include internal and external rotation of the hip. Lack of hip internal rotation, asymmetrical hip rotation, and total hip rotation (internal + external rotation) have been correlated with decreased performance and low back pain (Ibrahim et al., 2007; Sadeghisani et al., 2015). Total hip rotation should be greater than 50 degrees (Ibrahim et al., 2007), with internal and external rotation greater than 25 degrees. Good mobility in hip rotation can also allow for greater depth during squatting and help maintain knee alignment throughout the lifts (Todoroff, 2017). Collectively, these characteristics will translate to better sports performance measures (Berton et al., 2018; Chaouachi et al., 2014; Hackett et al., 2016; Hoffman et al., 2004; MacKenzie et al., 2014; Markström & Olsson, 2013; Mujika et al., 2009; Teo et al., 2016; Ziv & Lidor, 2010) and reduce the risk of injury (Bousquet & Olson, 2018).

TABLE 15.2 Hip and Knee Range of Motion Prerequisites for Olympic Lifting

Knee/Hip Flexion	ROM	Purpose of Motion
Knee	Up to 150 degrees	• Provides optimal kinetic chain alignment during setup and catch phases
Hip	95–135 degrees	• Aids in proper foot placement and stance width
Knee/Hip Extension	**ROM**	**Purpose of Motion**
Knee	May not fully extend	• Allows optimal triple extension for maximal force production
Hip	> 0 degrees (from vertical)	• Aids in proper body–bar alignment
Hip Rotation	**ROM**	**Purpose of Motion**
Internal	> 25 degrees	• Decreases lower back stress
External	> 50 degrees total rotation	• Decreases the risk of certain injuries • Increases squat depth and knee alignment

Observe whether the athlete can reach the optimal ROM before compensation at the pelvis or lumbar spine.

Shoulders, Spine, and Arms

Overhead lifting is part of both Olympic lifts and their derivatives. This action demands prerequisite mobility of the entire shoulder complex, trunk, and upper extremities, including 180 degrees of shoulder flexion (**Figure 15.13**). The shoulder has a large capacity for motion, which comes from a multitude of joints, including the sternoclavicular (SC) and acromioclavicular (AC), glenohumeral (GH), scapulothoracic (ST), and thoracic spine (TS) joints. Each is intimately linked to shoulder movement (Crosbie et al., 2008; Heneghan et al., 2020; Howe & Blagrove, 2015).

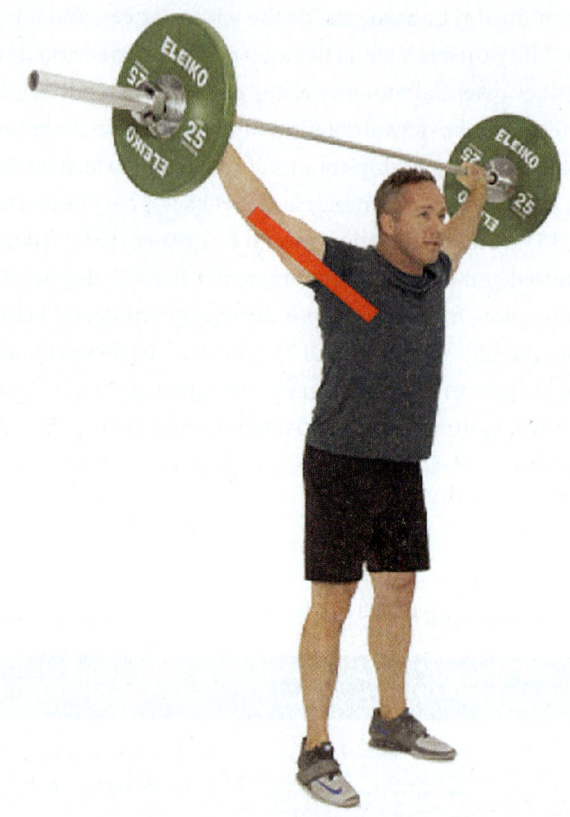

FIGURE 15.13 Shoulder Flexion Prerequisite

The cervical spine (CS), TS, and lumbar spine (LS) are also intimately linked together. Movement in one of these areas can influence the others (Endo et al., 2016), impacting the shoulder motions involved in the Olympic lifts. Thus, spinal mobility in the CS, TS, and LS is important for safe and effective overhead lifting to reduce the risk of injury (Crosbie et al., 2008; Endo et al., 2016; Heneghan et al., 2020). This can further help increase the proficiency of the technique.

Good mobility in the shoulder's internal and external rotation is also paramount. These motions are necessary for the safe and effective transitioning of the barbell from the second pull to a proper catch phase. Lack of ROM in either internal or external shoulder rotation has been shown to increase the risk of shoulder injury in overhead athletes (Clarsen et al., 2014; Cools et al., 2015; de Oliveira et al., 2019). Therefore, although specific ROM data are unavailable, it is advised that near-full mobility, as determined by the suggested mobility tests, should be attained.

Lastly, the elbows and wrists have an often-overlooked impact on lifting ability and technique when performing the Olympic lifts. Poor ROM in elbow flexion and wrist extension can lead to improper positioning of the bar relative to the body. This can increase the amount of stress on the spine and low back, and even the lifter's balance. Similarly, elbow extension and maintaining an extended elbow are critical when performing the snatch and the jerk. Inability to fully extend the elbow and maintain this extension can result in poor positioning of the bar; increased stress on the shoulder, spine, and low back; and alteration of the lifter's technique and balance. Ultimately, this can increase the risk of injury.

The shoulder is an important component of the Olympic lifts and many derivatives. For shoulder movement to occur in the Olympic lifts, the performance client should be assessed for mobility in various motions. These include shoulder flexion; internal and external rotation; CS, TS, and LS extension; elbow flexion and extension; and wrist extension (**Table 15.3**).

TABLE 15.3 Shoulder, Spine, and Arm Range of Motion Prerequisites for Olympic Lifting

Upper-Extremity Motion	ROM	Purpose of Motion
Shoulder flexion	Up to 180 degrees	• Decreased risk of shoulder impingement and injury • Aids in the proper overhead placement of the bar
Shoulder internal rotation	>30 degrees	• Decreased risk of shoulder impingement and injury • Provides for an optimal transition from second pull to catch phase
Shoulder external rotation	>70 degrees	
Thoracic extension	9–15 degrees	• Decreases stress placed on shoulder (glenohumeral) joint and rotator cuff • Aids in proper overhead placement of the bar
Lumbar extension	Close to full	

The entire kinetic chain must have a good amount of mobility to ensure the performance client can perform the Olympic lifts safely and effectively. Therefore, each joint must individually have sufficient ROM with good control. Furthermore, each joint must be able to move synergistically in a coordinated manner with the other joints to provide the total-body mobility necessary for optimal performance. However, mobility is only one part of the prerequisite abilities an athlete will need. Stability, posture, and strength prerequisites are also important for success in the Olympic lifts.

📋 COACH'S CORNER

The preceding mobility prerequisites are valuable for discerning how each joint should move. Movement assessment and testing should begin with the overhead squat assessment (OHSA) and then progress to mobility testing if necessary. Remember, squatting with the barbell overhead is an important component of the snatch. By using the OHSA, you can gain a good insight into the overall mobility of the athlete, as necessary for the snatch and the clean and jerk. This will help determine how prepared the athlete is for the Olympic lifts and which specific areas need to be addressed.

STABILITY

Stability goes together with mobility, posture, and strength. In essence, stability is the foundation for these other prerequisites, which is why it is an essential prerequisite for the Olympic lifts. Stability provides the structural integrity of soft tissue necessary for joint motion efficiency to occur throughout a ROM. It also provides dynamic anti-flexion, anti-extension, and anti-rotation, which are sometimes necessary to prevent motion from occurring at specific joints.

While stability is an essential part of efficient motion, much of Olympic lifting requires dynamic "anti-motion," which can be seen at the spine. Therefore, a stable, neutral spine from neck to low back is essential during the Olympic lifts. This positioning allows the trunk to act as an efficient third-class lever that enables the athlete to hinge at the hip and explode through the legs and shoulders to lift the barbell to the desired position. Conversely, too much flexion in the spine, especially the CS and TS, during the Olympic lifts when moving the bar overhead can cause unwanted stresses to the low back and shoulders as well as potentially alter force production, mechanics, and technique (Bousquet & Olson, 2018; Kim & Hwang, 2019; Schoenfeld, 2010; Thigpen et al., 2010).

Muscles can be classified as local (stability) or global (mobility), with the local muscles being unique to the global muscles in their makeup and function (Agten et al., 2020; Richardson, 2004). As both muscle groups must work together to ensure optimal performance, each must be trained to optimize its functional capacity. Olympic weightlifting consists of dynamic and explosive lifts, often under moderate to heavy loads, so it is important to follow systematic training progressions. This will help to ensure the stabilizing muscles of the ankle, knee, lumbo-pelvic-hip complex (LPHC), spine, and shoulders are well prepared for the tasks ahead.

Core Stability

The core has a significant role in transferring forces between the lower and upper extremities, which enhances the performance of various dynamic actions (Sato & Mokha, 2009; Shinkle et al., 2012). In fact, core stability throughout the spine and pelvis may be one of the most important stability factors for enhancing performance in Olympic lifts. Transference of force is a vital aspect of the Olympic lifts, and the ability to transfer force from the ground up is where the performance-enhancing attributes of the Olympic lifts are derived. As previously discussed, maintaining a more isometric positioning of the spine and pelvis is vital for creating the leverage necessary to generate higher levels of force and power in the Olympic lifts.

Two primary ways to enhance the stability of the core have been studied—namely, the drawing-in maneuver (also called abdominal hollowing) and abdominal bracing. Both are effective in enhancing the stabilizing mechanism of the spine and may operate as a continuum of core stabilization (Campbell et al., 2016; Kim & Kim, 2018; Linde et al., 2018; Muramoto & Kuruma, 2020; Norrie & Brown, 2020; Vaičienė et al., 2018). They collectively allow for a progressive increase in spine and trunk stability to address the increased force and load demands in Olympic weightlifting. From one perspective, an athlete demonstrating movement compensation at the LPHC may benefit from performing abdominal hollowing in the earlier phases of training to enhance segmental spinal stability. However, it is also recommended that abdominal bracing progress to the more demanding phases requiring increased strength and power.

A good abdominal activation strategy combining both the drawing-in maneuver and abdominal bracing is important for the enhanced core stability needed for Olympic weightlifting. However, it can be challenging to perform and coach. Here is a simple process to help you do both:

Step 1: Find a neutral spine.
- Cervical: Flex your neck all the way; then extend your neck all the way; now place it in between the two extremes.
- Thoracic: Slouch your shoulders all the way; then stick your chest out and pull your shoulders back as far; now position yourself in between the two extremes.
- Lumbar: Place hands on hips. Then tilt your tailbone up so the fingers are lower in front and the thumbs raise in the back; now do the opposite and tuck your tailbone under; now position yourself in between the two extremes.

Step 2: Exhale.

Step 3: Pretend you just realized you're going to the bathroom, and try to stop yourself (don't stop breathing).

Step 4: Slightly draw in your lower abdominal region (keep breathing normally).

Step 5: Maintain the drawn-in position and now inhale.

Step 6: Hold your breath and tighten (brace) your trunk for a punch without moving the spine. Maintaining this position and tension in your trunk, now breathe. You should be able to breathe and move without altering your lower abdominal or trunk positions and tensions.

POSTURE AND NEUROMUSCULAR CONTROL

Some postures promote better kinetic chain function, whereas others can decrease its functional capacity (Barrett et al., 2016; Endo et al., 2016; Moon et al., 2018). In addition, altered positioning of one joint or region of the body can alter others, influencing their function (Barrett et al., 2016; Endo et al., 2016; Moon et al., 2018). Attaining postures that promote better function requires neuromuscular control. **Neuromuscular control** provides the ability for the kinetic chain to move through a necessary ROM with control (Hoffman & Gabel, 2013).

In movement, sports, and Olympic weightlifting, posture must be dynamic, meaning it must constantly change to produce motion. For optimal performance to occur, an athlete must be able to transition from one optimal posture into another. This requires constant neuromuscular control. The ability to effectively and efficiently transition from one optimal posture to another is a technique. Thus, posture and neuromuscular control are the building blocks of the technique. This concept highlights the importance of understanding and using the kinetic chain checkpoints (feet/ankles, knees, LPHC, shoulders, and cervical spine/head) to assess and observe athletes before and during training sessions.

Posture and neuromuscular control, which make up technique, are especially vital for the Olympic lifts because these lifts combine multiple movements that require synchronization to achieve optimal outcomes. For example, both the snatch and the clean and jerk involve a deadlift, an explosive shrug to high-pull, and an overhead squat (for the snatch) or front squat (for the clean and jerk). Each of these movements within their respective Olympic lift requires rapidly changing postures with elevated levels of neuromuscular control to achieve an optimal outcome. Therefore, knowing which

NEURO-MUSCULAR CONTROL →

The response (conscious or unconscious) of the muscles within the body to control purposeful movement.

postures an athlete will need to move from and transition into is important. Progressively training these postures and transitions and focusing on technique with appropriate loads will be crucial for Sports Performance Coaches to provide safe and effective coaching and program design.

> ### ⚠ CRITICAL
>
> The importance of knowing the posture a lifter must be in during each phase of the Olympic lift or derivative, whether you are performing or coaching, cannot be overstated. Being in as optimal a posture as possible in each phase of the lift will help you develop good neuromuscular control. This is how you develop and improve technique and ultimately enhance the power with a decreased risk of injury.

STRENGTH

The last major prerequisite for performing the Olympic lifts is strength. The Olympic lifts are used because they allow athletes to generate higher levels of power. Recall from the force–velocity curve that power is the product of force × velocity, with force being the weight, or load, lifted. Moderate-to-heavy loads may eventually be used to generate the higher levels of power produced with Olympic lifts. This being the case, most researchers suggest that performance clients have a "good" level of strength before performing these lifts for higher power outputs (Bosquet & Olson, 2018; Carlock et al., 2004; Faigenbaum et al., 2009; Haff & Nimphius, 2012; Hori & Stone, 2005; Lloyd et al., 2014; Suchomel et al., 2017), and strength in the lower body has been the predominant area of study for the Olympic lifts.

Lower Body

A standard assessment used to determine lower-body prerequisite strength is relative squat strength. This assesses an athlete's one repetition maximum (1RM) relative to their body weight. For example, both a male athlete with a squat two times their bodyweight and a female athlete with a squat one and a half times their bodyweight are said to have good strength and are considered stronger performance clients (Case et al., 2020; McMaster et al., 2014). These guidelines are helpful for those using Olympic lifts with heavier loads. Nevertheless, the Olympic lifts, when used and coached correctly, have produced similar results in males considered "weaker," with a relative squat value of just over one times their bodyweight (James et al., 2018). Lastly, to learn and work on technique, low loads can be used by incorporating PVC pipes, wooden dowel rods, training bars (a 10-lb weighted bar that looks like an Olympic bar used for teaching Olympic lifts), or any weighted bar ranging from 5 to 20 lb. Progression in load usually entails increasing the weight by small increments over time. Thus, Olympic lifts can be practiced by all populations. Still, as more power is desired and load demands increase, the athlete should also attain higher levels of strength through traditional strength training.

Upper Body

From an upper-body perspective, there is no specific evidence of correlation between upper-body assessments (i.e., bench press) and Olympic lifting. However, research does support the use of a progressive sequence of overhead presses (Kroell & Mike, 2017) (**Table 15.4**). Using organized progressions can help ensure mobility, stability, and control are maintained

TABLE 15.4 Overhead Pressing Progression for Olympic Lifting

Equipment Progression	Position Progression	Movement Progression
Weighted bar (WB)	Seated with arms anterior (front loaded)	Strict press
Dumbbells (DB)	Seated with arms abducted (beside or behind head)	Push press
Kettlebells (KB)	Kneeling with arms anterior (front loaded)	Push jerk
Landmine (LM)	Kneeling with arms abducted (beside or behind head)	Split jerk
Barbells (BB)	Standing with arms anterior (front loaded)	
	Standing with arms abducted (beside or behind head; change hand width)	

Strict press: Overhead press using no lower-body motion.

Push press: Overhead press using a knee bend (dip), then driving upward into triple extension with legs, locking knees and pressing weight overhead.

Push jerk: Overhead press using a knee bend (dip), then driving upward into triple extension with legs, pushing body under bar, catching the weight overhead in a half squat position, and standing up.

Split jerk: Overhead press using a knee bend (dip), then driving upward into triple extension with legs, pushing body under bar, catching the weight overhead in a split-stance position, and standing up.

throughout the kinetic chain when performed in a standing position (Kroell & Mike, 2017; Soriano et al., 2019; Waller et al., 2009), which is essential for the overhead aspects of the Olympic lifting. Proper progressions are explicitly suggested for female lifters, as research has shown increased trunk and spinal motion in women during overhead lifts, especially with increased loads, compared to men (McKean & Burkett, 2015). Various types of equipment can also facilitate the progression and add variety. The use of training bars, standard barbells, dumbbells, kettlebells, and landmines can provide practical variation.

In addition, researchers have indicated that Olympic lifts and their derivatives can be used with beginners and children. As previously mentioned, some researchers suggest childhood may be an ideal time to begin training movements (Faigenbaum et al., 2009; Lloyd et al., 2014; McQuilliam et al., 2020). In addition, practicing techniques with lower weight loads, derivative lifts, and alternative equipment (e.g., dumbbells, kettlebells) can be a valuable way to increase core, balance, and reactive neuromuscular control.

ENVIRONMENT PREREQUISITES

The environment in which Olympic lifts are being performed plays an important part in safety and coaching (**Table 15.5**). The weightlifting area should be an open space of

TABLE 15.5 Summary of Environment Prerequisites

Lifting Space	Surrounding Area
• Approximately a 10 × 10 feet open space	• Clear of unnecessary items—personal items, extra bars, collars, or weights
• If using multiple platforms, have at least 2 feet between them	• All bars, collars, and weights should be kept in appropriate storage racks
• If not using a platform, have nonslip, shock-absorbing flooring (e.g., rubber)	• The ceiling should be approximately 12 feet high and clear of light fixtures and fans
• The floor of a lifting area must be solid to withstand the force of weights dropping	

approximately 10 × 10 feet. The floor underneath this entire area should be solid enough (e.g., concrete) to withstand the force of weights that could potentially drop during lifts. Platforms may be beneficial in designating the lifting area, with the surrounding space free of unnecessary items (e.g., personal items, extra bars, collars, or weights). If a platform is not used, it is necessary to have nonslip, shock-absorbing flooring (e.g., rubber) approximately 1 inch thick. The ceiling should be high enough to allow taller people to perform overhead lifts and be clear of ceiling fans and light fixtures. For example, a 6-foot-tall person holding a bar overhead loaded with plates will require approximately a 9-foot ceiling with no fans or lights. A safe height that accommodates most lifters is approximately 12 feet.

LESSON 3: SCIENTIFIC RATIONALE FOR OLYMPIC LIFTING TO IMPROVE SPORTS PERFORMANCE

SCIENTIFIC RATIONALE FOR OLYMPIC WEIGHTLIFTING

To be an informed and effective Sports Performance Coach, it is imperative to have a solid understanding of the scientific rationale behind the use of Olympic weightlifting. For any scientific rationale to provide value, it should address key elements and answer important questions related to the topic. Three key elements of the scientific rationale for using Olympic weightlifting as an effective training modality for performance enhancement are outlined in **Table 15.6**.

TABLE 15.6 Scientific Rationale for Olympic Weightlifting

Element	Question
Longevity	How long and how frequently has it been used?
Safety	Is it safe for all desired populations?
Efficacy	Does it work effectively for all desired populations?

LONGEVITY

From a historical standpoint, Olympic weightlifting and its associated movements and training methods have been performed for the last century. More specifically, Sports Performance Coaches from the high school, collegiate, and professional ranks have been using the Olympic lifts as a staple component of their performance enhancement programs for decades. In surveys conducted across major professional sports, researchers have found that 85% to 100% of those coaches who responded to surveys used Olympic lifts as a primary aspect of their programming (Ebben & Blackard, 2001; Ebben et al., 2004; Simenz et al., 2005). The exception was Major League Baseball, for which the proportion was less than 25% (Ebben et al., 2005). The same percentages hold for collegiate and high school Sports Performance Coaches in the United States (Duehring et al., 2009; Durell et al., 2003), with high school Sports Performance Coaches being closer to 100% (Duehring et al., 2009). Olympic weightlifting has also been shown to be a priority internationally in strength programs across various sports for male and female athletes of various age groups (Gee et al., 2011; Jones et al., 2016; Nicholson et al., 2021; Weldon et al., 2022).

SAFETY

Building on the premise that Olympic weightlifting has been used extensively for performance enhancement over many decades, it has also been shown to be safe for all populations. Several factors contribute to the determination of the safety of Olympic weightlifting, including injury rates, supervision, education, and equipment.

INJURY RATES

Injury rates associated with Olympic weightlifting have been studied across various populations for years. Research investigating the injury rates for weightlifting among youth has shown that it is noticeably safer than many other sports and activities. For example, the overall injury rate per 100 hours of weightlifting was shown to be 0.0013, compared to 0.8000 per 100 hours for rugby and 0.0120 per 100 hours for resistance training in general, as shown in **Table 15.7** (Faigenbaum et al., 2009).

TABLE 15.7 Injury Rates for Weightlifting Versus Other Sports/Activities

Sport	Bodybuilding/ Resistance Training	Weight-lifting	Power-lifting	Wrestling	Strong-man	High-land Games	Football/ Rugby
Older/ higher-level lifters (per 1,000 hours)	0.24	2.4–3.3	1.0–4.4	5.7	4.5–6.1	7.5	9.6
Youth (per 100 hours)	0.012	0.0013					0.8

Relative to higher-level lifters (national-level and Olympic athletes), weightlifting has also been shown to have a low injury rate of 2.4 to 3.3 injuries per 1,000 hours, compared to 9.6 per 1,000 hours for American football and 5.7 per 1,000 hours for wrestling (Aasa et al., 2017). Likewise, weightlifting compares favorably to other resistance training applications. It is positioned just above bodybuilding, which is shown to have the lowest injury rate at 0.24 per 1,000 hours, but well under Strongman and Highland games athletes, who have the highest injury rates—4.5 to 6.1 injuries and 7.5 injuries per 1,000 hours, respectively (Keogh & Winwood, 2017).

SUPERVISION

Researchers have proposed some important factors that contribute to weightlifting's safety, especially in the youth population. One such factor is the supervision that usually accompanies weightlifting. Due to the skill required to perform the Olympic lifts, coaches of competitive athletes are often well informed and qualified in the instruction and coaching aspects of these lifts. Another important factor contributing to the safety of weightlifting is the gradual and sensible load progressions used. As the technique used is vital for success in the Olympic lifts, the weight used is incrementally progressed to enable the athlete to maintain the proper technique. As weightlifting movements are more complex regarding neural activation and motor skill, researchers agree that childhood may be an ideal time to begin training these movements (Faigenbaum et al., 2009; Lloyd et al., 2014; McQuilliam et al., 2020).

EDUCATION

Another factor proposed as contributing to the safety of Olympic lifting is education. It is strongly suggested that individuals responsible for overseeing, teaching, and coaching the Olympic lifts be credentialed through an appropriate weightlifting coaching program (Lloyd et al., 2014). Organizations with an extended legacy in Olympic weightlifting, such as Eleiko and USA Weightlifting, provide courses specific to instruction and technique. The importance of being adequately trained with proven education cannot be overstated due to the technicality of these lifts and the variety of derivatives that can be used. Thus, education is necessary for Sports Performance Coaches to safely and effectively teach, train, and coach athletes on the Olympic lifts.

EQUIPMENT

Proper equipment designed for Olympic weightlifting contributes to safe and effective outcomes (Hori & Stone, 2005). Proper weightlifting equipment typically includes bars,

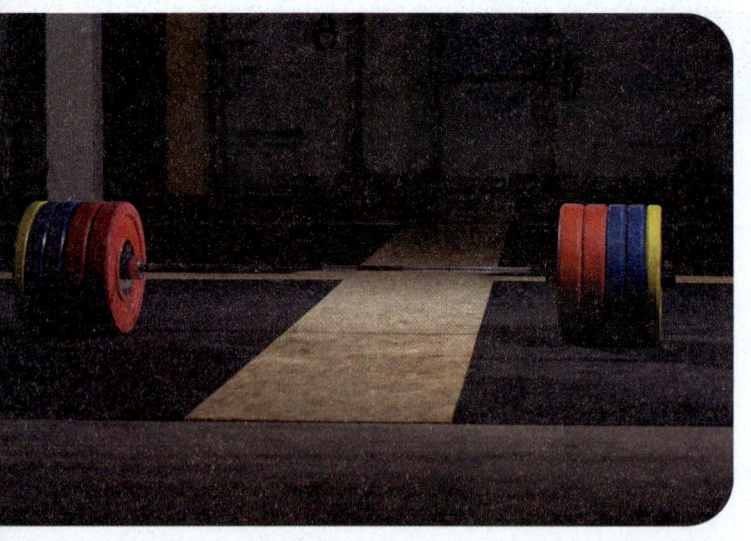

© Jasminko Ibrakovic/Shutterstock

bumper plates, collars, and platforms. The combination of a bar and bumper plates makes up what is referred to as a barbell. Bumper plates should fit securely with minimal space between the plate's center and the bar. The secure fit reduces the slack, or "play," that can be experienced when the barbell is lifted. Using collars ensures that the bumper plates remain securely fixed while the lift is being performed. Any slack, extra space, or unwanted movement between the bar and bumper plates can affect the timing and technique of the lifts, which can lead to unwanted compensation.

Proper sleeve rotation helps ensure the bar moves independently of the bumper plates during the lifts, reducing the risk of injury to the wrists, elbows, and shoulders. This will also help the athlete's timing and balance during the lift and translate into potentially better technique and less compensation (Hori & Stone, 2005).

📋 COACH'S CORNER

It is important to note that variations of the Olympic lifts can be performed with alternative equipment such as training bars, weighted bars, dumbbells, kettlebells, landmines, and other weighted objects. This can also introduce the lifts to athletes using lighter loads to help emphasize technique while building confidence.

EFFICACY

Aside from safety, the most practically important rationale for using Olympic weightlifting is its effectiveness in enhancing athletic performance. Over the last few decades, many studies have investigated the influence that weightlifting has on various performance assessments compared to other resistance training applications. Two specific performance assessments include jumping and sprinting.

VERTICAL JUMP

The vertical jump is a common sport-related assessment used by most Sports Performance Coaches. Research has correlated vertical jumps with successful sports performance across various skills (LaPlaca & McCullick, 2020; Markström & Olsson, 2013; Mujika et al., 2009; Ziv & Lidor, 2010). When compared to other forms of resistance training, weightlifting is as effective, and often more so, for improving vertical jump height in individuals with various ages, levels of ability, and genders (Ayers et al., 2016; Berton et al., 2018; Chaouachi et al., 2014; Hackett et al., 2016; Hoffman et al., 2004; MacKenzie et al., 2014; Mujika et al., 2009; Teo et al., 2016; Ziv & Lidor, 2010).

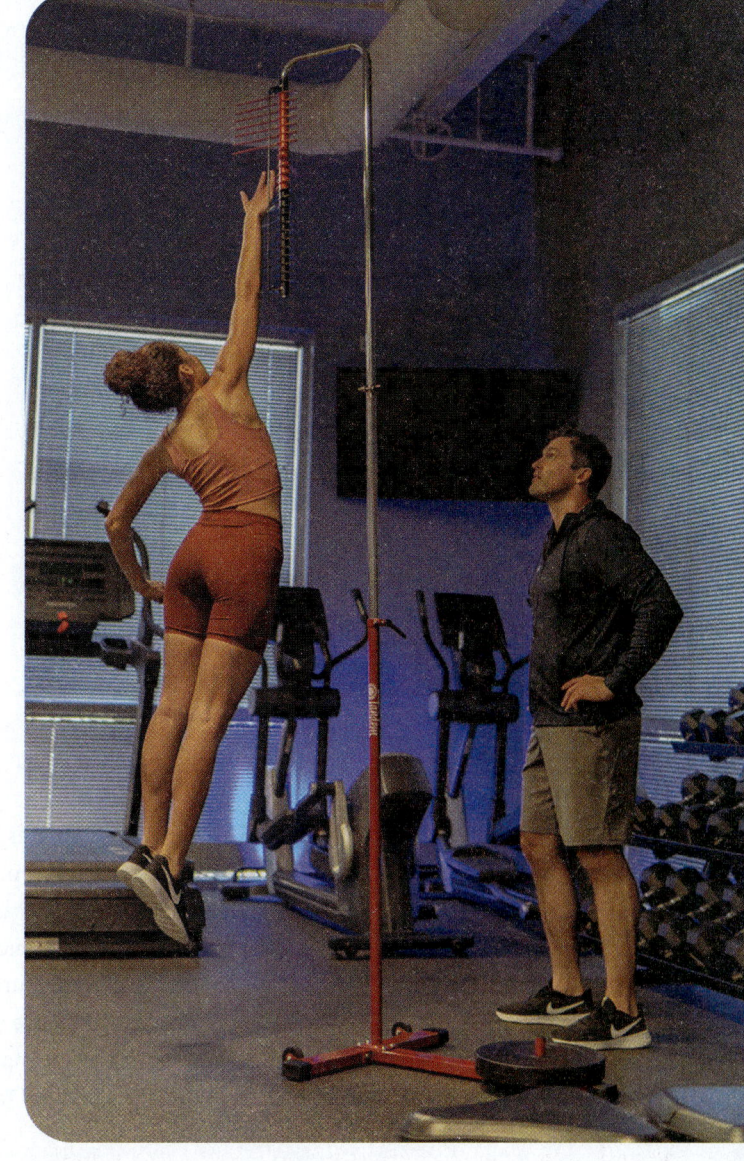

Research has shown that the power clean, a derivative of the clean and jerk, produces a greater rate of force development and force output than traditional forms of resistance training and jump training (MacKenzie et al., 2014). Even when the same load was used for both the power cleans and jump squats, the group performing the power cleans produced five times the force output with a better rate of force production—simply put, they demonstrated more power (MacKenzie et al., 2014). Higher amounts of force produced at a faster rate (power) are believed to be an important factor that weightlifting provides to help athletes increase athletic performance.

Weightlifting also appears to modify the coordination strategies of muscles around the knee differently than traditional forms of resistance training and jump training (Arabatzi & Kellis, 2012). When the power clean was compared to a squat jump and bodyweight jumping, the power clean was shown to produce better vertical stiffness (a measure of the body's ability to control the eccentric loading phase of a jump) and jump height. In addition, it produced a more favorable quadriceps-to-hamstring activation strategy around the knee. More specifically, the strategy showed a reduction of antagonistic hamstring coactivation, which increased the knee extension forces needed for optimal vertical propulsion (Arabatzi & Kellis, 2012).

Research looking specifically at weightlifters provides further support for the value of weightlifting in improving vertical jump performance. One study showed that weightlifters have greater isometric peak force and rate of force development than other strength and power athletes (Storey & Smith, 2012). In another study, weightlifters of all ages, levels, and genders were assessed on their vertical jump ability (Carlock et al., 2004). These researchers further correlated their vertical jump height with their weightlifting ability, which was measured by the weight they could successfully lift. They found that vertical jump height was significantly correlated with the lifter's ability level, implying that the better they were at weightlifting, the better their jump height was (Carlock et al., 2004) (**Table 15.8**).

TABLE 15.8 Effect of Weightlifting on Vertical Jump

1. Correlated to increased sports performance
2. Frequently more effective for improving vertical jump height in individuals of various ages, levels of ability, and genders
3. Greater rate of force development and force output than other forms of training
4. Greater vertical stiffness (body's ability to resist uncontrolled collapsing during the eccentric loading phase)
5. Greater jump height
6. More favorable quadriceps-to-hamstring activation strategy
7. Better weightlifters have better jump height

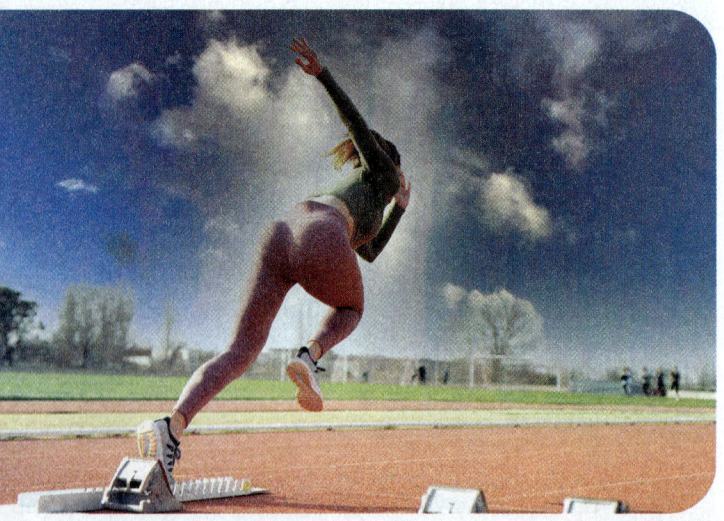
© Antonio Suarez Vega/Shutterstock

SPRINTING

Similarly, sprinting is another sport-related assessment used by most Sports Performance Coaches. Sprinting in its various forms, ranging from 5 yards to the 40-yard dash, has also been correlated with successful athletic performance (Martins et al., 2021; Mujika et al., 2009; Vincent et al., 2019). Several researchers have compared weightlifting with traditional resistance training for enhancing sprint velocity and time (Ayers et al., 2016; Chaouachi et al., 2014; Teo et al., 2016; Tricoli et al., 2005). The use of Olympic lifts has been shown to be as good, if not better, for the improvement in sprinting performance for individuals of different genders and ages (Ayers et al., 2016; Chaouachi et al., 2014; Haugen et al., 2019; Teo et al., 2016; Tricoli et al., 2005).

Relating the vertical jump to sprinting, there is a practical link between the two. Research has shown that vertical jump peak-force output and height significantly predict sprinting time (Markström & Olsson, 2013). In other words, athletes' vertical jumping ability can predict how fast they will run, as both of these actions rely on similar qualities for successful outcomes. The same researchers also highlighted the importance of training an athlete's jumping ability when designing program strategies. As the Olympic lifts have been demonstrated to be effective for enhancing both vertical jump and sprint performance in various populations, claims about the efficacy of their use appear to be warranted (**Table 15.9**).

TABLE 15.9 Effect of Weightlifting on Sprinting

1. Correlated to increased sports performance
2. Frequently more effective for improving sprint performance than other forms of training in individuals of various ages
3. Sprint speed is correlated to vertical jump height

UNDERSTANDING STRENGTH AND POWER

Olympic weightlifting enhances performance through a variety of critical factors, including (1) optimizing motor unit recruitment and control and (2) maximizing the rate of force development (Hackett et al., 2106; Haff & Nimphius, 2012; Haugen et al., 2019; Hoffman et al., 2004; Hori & Stone, 2005; James et al., 2018; Suchomel et al., 2017; Tricoli et al., 2005). In other words, the athlete can use the most efficient number and size of motor units at the right time (motor unit recruitment and control) and activate them as fast and intensely as possible (rate of force development) relative to the desired movement. This concept is vital to understand because this relates to power. The expression of power is commonly accepted as a key physical component of sports performance (Hackett et al., 2106; Haff & Nimphius, 2012; Haugen et al., 2019; Hoffman et al., 2004; Hori & Stone, 2005; James et al., 2018; Suchomel et al., 2017; Tricoli et al., 2005).

The basic equation for power is power = force × velocity. Looking at this equation relative to strength training, force essentially refers to the load being used, and the strength to the effort required to move it. (More formally, strength is the ability to overcome an external load.) Therefore, the stronger an athlete is, the more likely they are to potentially produce higher levels of power (Haff & Nimphius, 2012; Hori & Stone, 2005). Conversely, velocity refers to the speed of motion relative to the specific movement being performed.

👍 HELPFUL HINT

Think of power as a simple math equation. Power is usually measured in watts, but this example will not use a unit of measure. Instead, it is simply a way of demonstrating how a Sports Performance Coach could quantify power.

Power = how much weight you are lifting × how fast you are lifting it

So, if you are lifting a heavy weight, say 200 lb, but only at about 30 mph (13.4 m/s), as often seen in powerlifting, you are producing power (i.e., 200 × 30 = 6,000) even though you may be moving slower than possible. If you lift 150 lb at a speed of 40 mph, you are producing the same amount of power (i.e., 150 × 40 = 6,000) even though you lift less weight. As power is the combined outcome of both weight and speed, using only heavy loads or fast speeds of motion is not always necessary. It just depends on your desired outcome.

Based on the power equation, it is evident that different forms of power can exist. Practically speaking, power can come through use of a low load with high-velocity training, a moderate load with moderate-velocity training, or a high load with low-velocity training (Haff & Nimphius, 2012; Hori & Stone, 2005; Suchomel et al., 2017). This ties explicitly into understanding the application of the force–velocity curve (**Figure 15.14**).

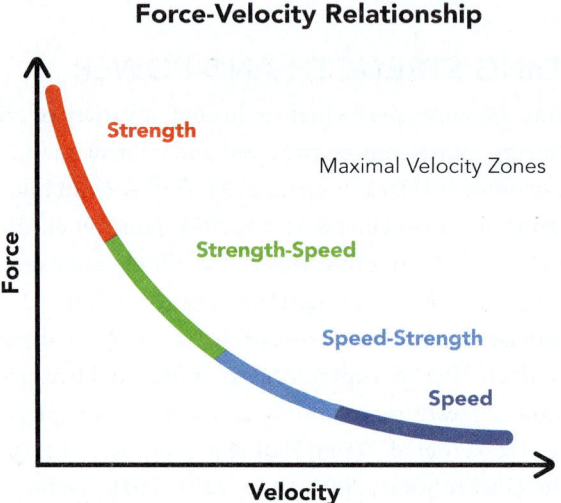

FIGURE 15.14 Force–Velocity Relationship

The Olympic lifts and their derivatives are often considered specialized training targeting only one primary adaptation. However, for the Sports Performance Coach, it is important to understand that these lifts are highly versatile, fitting into all categories of the force–velocity curve.

The force–velocity curve shows an inverse relationship between force and velocity, meaning that concentric muscle contractions will be slower with a higher load and faster with a lower load. Relating the force–velocity curve to strength training, research has shown that to attain the highest contraction velocities (maximal velocity or speed), athletes should use 45% or less of their 1RM—that is, low-load, high-velocity training. Getting stronger while maintaining high velocities (i.e., speed-strength) requires lower loads (Haff & Nimphius, 2012; Suchomel et al., 2017).

Athletes should use between 45% and 85% of 1RM if they want to attain maximal power. Getting faster with heavier loads (i.e., strength-speed) requires a moderate enough load where a relatively high movement velocity can still be achieved (Haff & Nimphius, 2012; Suchomel et al., 2017)—that is, moderate-load, moderate-velocity training.

Athletes should use loads of 85% of 1RM or greater to attain maximal strength—that is, high-load, low-velocity training. Maximal strength has been suggested to be one of the most important factors for athletes to progressively enhance power (Carlock et al., 2004; Haff & Nimphius, 2012; Suchomel et al., 2017). In addition, as strength increases, the ability to move lighter loads faster can increase power.

SCIENTIFIC RATIONALE KEY POINTS

From a practical standpoint, it is important to remember that power is achieved through strength (force) and speed of motion (velocity) (**Table 15.10**). Even though the region of

TABLE 15.10 Summary of Power Related to the Force–Velocity Curve

Type of Power	Training Variables	Adaptation
Speed-strength	40% or less of 1RM using maximal effort and velocity	Maximal velocity
Strength-speed	40%–85% of 1RM using maximal effort and velocity	Maximal power
Maximal strength	85% or more of 1RM using maximal effort and velocity	Maximal strength

the force–velocity curve that represents the greatest power output (maximal power) is essentially in the middle of the curve designated by training intensities of between 45% and 85% of 1RM, this does not mean that performance training should occur only in this region. Furthermore, it does not mean that this is the primary region or intensity within which the Olympic lifts must be used. Given that power is the combination of force and velocity, for an athlete to increase their maximal power successfully and continually, they must be able to produce and apply high levels of force as well as be accustomed to moving with high contraction velocities (Carlock et al., 2004; Haff & Nimphius, 2012; Suchomel et al., 2017). This requires using the entire force–velocity curve.

LESSON 4: THE OLYMPIC LIFTS
LEARNING THE OLYMPIC LIFTS

As noted earlier, there are two primary full Olympic lifts: the snatch and the clean and jerk. Both lifts involve lifting a barbell from its starting position on the floor to standing with the barbell overhead. Both lifts possess similarities, yet each is uniquely different, with minor nuances that Sports Performance Coaches must be aware of and understand if they are to coach athletes safely and effectively.

Both lifts have multiple phases that the lifter will progress through, moving the barbell from the floor to overhead to complete the entire lift. These phases require the changing postures discussed in the "Olympic Weightlifting Prerequisites" section. Maintaining proper posture with neuromuscular control throughout the lift will help ensure the efficient execution of motions and maximization of the technique. In addition, using the kinetic chain checkpoints will be instrumental in coaching and learning the Olympic lifts.

Lastly, the Sports Performance Coach must understand that the Olympic lifts are not just about coordinating body movements to lift a barbell overhead. They are also about coordinating the movement of the bar with the body. In other words, Olympic lifting is much like an orchestrated dance between the body and the bar, whereby the specific movements of the body control the bar, and the body moves around the bar. First, the body generates the movement of the bar, controlling where it goes and how fast. Then, the body must be appropriately positioned relative to the bar for a successful lift to occur to reap the numerous benefits from these lifts.

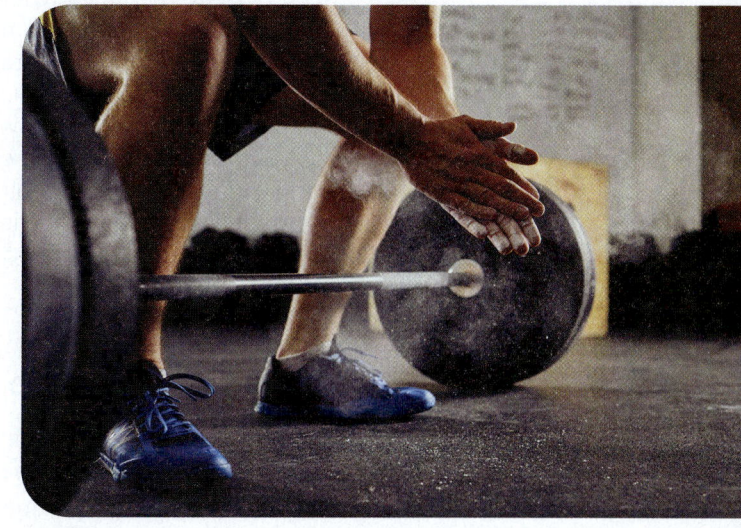
© Baranq/Shutterstock

THE SNATCH

The snatch can be described in many ways, with various phases and names used throughout the literature and in coaching circles. For ease of teaching and coaching in this section, the snatch will be described as the lifter moving through six primary phases after the initial setup: first pull, transition, second pull, pull-under, catch, and stand (**Figure 15.15**). Hand placement for the snatch is key to ensuring proper technique and will be wider than that for the clean and jerk. Specifically, the hands should be wide enough to allow the bar to rest in the crease of the hips around the level of the pubic bone.

The Snatch Olympic Lift

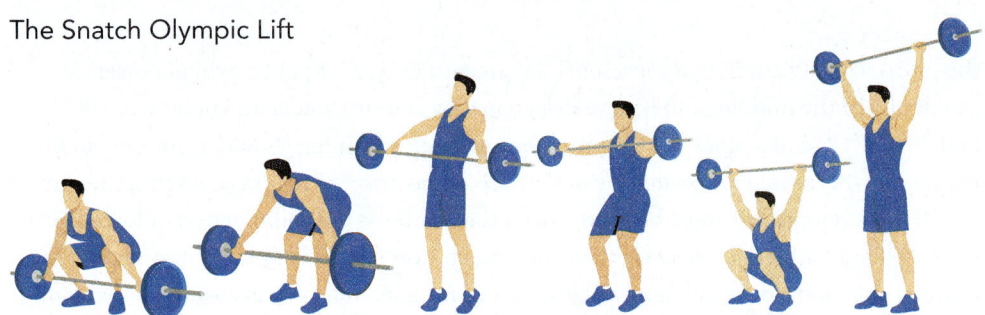

FIGURE 15.15 The Snatch Olympic Lift

The knees will be tracking over the toes. Viewed from the side, the LPHC will be in a neutral position and slightly higher than the knees, with the shoulders slightly higher than the LPHC. The gaze of the eyes should be at a point on the floor, approximately 3 to 5 feet in front of the bar, allowing the nose and sternum to point in the same direction. In the setup position, the shoulders should be over the bar, with the bar close to the shins and over the shoelaces. Key form considerations during the phases of the snatch are detailed in Appendix E.

> ⚠ **CRITICAL**
>
> **Bailing on the Catch**
> There are times when the catch phase may not go as planned. In these situations, the lifter may have to release the barbell. This is often called "bailing" on the catch. Should this happen, the weight will determine how the lifter should bail. If the lifter does not get under the barbell and the weight is too far forward, the lifter should let go of the barbell in front of them. If the barbell gets too far behind the lifter, the lifter should let go of and push the barbell behind them and move or fall forward away from the falling weight. This is also why it is important to have platforms or rubber covering over a solid floor with a clear area around the lifter.

THE CLEAN AND JERK

The clean and jerk Olympic lift is a compound movement of two separate stages, the clean and the jerk. Whereas the snatch takes the bar from the floor to overhead in one fluid motion, the clean portion gets the bar from the floor to rest on the chest, and then the jerk is a powerful overhead press with dynamic lower-body activity time. The clean will follow the same phases as the basic description for the snatch. The jerk component has its own phases that follow the completion of the clean (**Figure 15.16**). Other differences between the snatch and the clean and jerk are typically the grip width, setup position, and catch phase of the clean.

The Clean and Jerk Olympic Lift

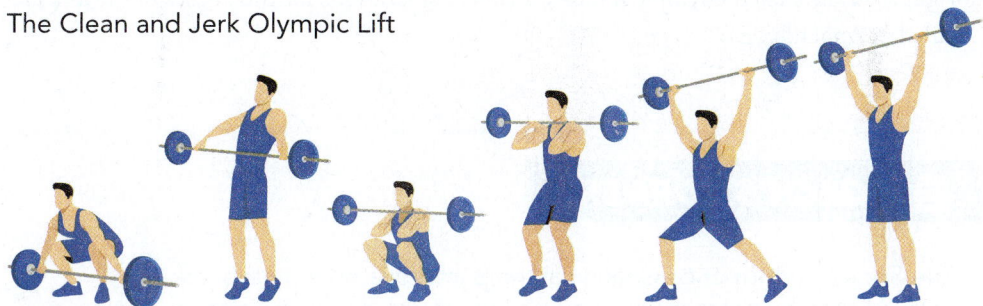

FIGURE 15.16 The Clean and Jerk Olympic Lift

THE CLEAN

The setup for the clean is like the snatch. However, during the clean and jerk, it is common for lifters to have a slightly narrower stance and grip. The general width of the grip is a thumb's distance from the outside of the thigh. Due to the closer grip, the most significant difference between the clean setup position and the snatch is a more upright trunk position with the knees potentially a little more forward. The first pull, transition, and second pull in the clean are all almost identical to those phases in the snatch, just with a narrower grip. However, the end of the transition phase in the clean is lower on the thigh than the snatch due to the narrower grip width. The pull-under is also like the snatch, except the elbows swing forward in a bent position instead of upward into a locked position.

The catch for the clean is characterized by the lifter "landing" in a deep squat position (triple flexion) and simultaneously punching the elbows forward with the wrists fully extended and the bar resting on the upper chest–shoulder region. The feet should be hitting the ground with a downward force while the elbows are punching forward. The same repositioning of the feet to a wider stance discussed in the snatch may also occur in the clean. From the deep catch position, the lifter then presses back up to standing with the bar resting on the upper chest and shoulders. Key form considerations for the phases of the clean are detailed in Appendix E.

THE JERK

The jerk immediately follows the clean. Therefore, the setup for the jerk will start with completing the standing phase of the clean. Lifters may readjust the bar, ensuring it rests on the upper chest and across the shoulder, their grip and elbow positions are proper, and their stance is more hip width. The dip phase of the jerk is a quick knee bend used to eccentrically load the lower body. The purpose of the dip is to activate the stretch–shortening cycle in preparation for the drive phase, much as in a vertical jump (Soriano et al., 2019). The upper body should remain vertical in the dip to ensure the barbell does not move from its position.

The drive phase is the rapid rebound upward that immediately follows the dip. This explosive vertical "drive" takes advantage of the stretch–shortening cycle's effect (Soriano et al., 2019). The completion of the drive phase should result in full triple extension, with the barbell elevating off the chest toward the chin/head. In the push-under phase, the lifter will be dynamically moving their body around the bar, requiring a quick dropping under the bar, as if landing from a jump into either a split stance (split jerk) or a wider athletic position stance (push jerk). The movements in the jerk catch are accomplished simultaneously, including the push-under, stabilizing the bar overhead, and standing fully upright as in the snatch Olympic lift. Key form considerations for the phases of the jerk are detailed in Appendix E.

> 📋 **COACH'S CORNER**
>
> The Sports Performance Coach can help improve an athlete's jerk performance by programming overhead lunges during resistance training. However, recall that the athlete must demonstrate optimal shoulder and thoracic spine ROM to perform any overhead exercise appropriately.

LESSON 5: OLYMPIC LIFT DERIVATIVES TO IMPROVE SPORTS PERFORMANCE

OLYMPIC LIFT DERIVATIVES

Olympic lifts are a composite of a multitude of movements linked together in an orchestrated sequence that provides athletes with numerous performance-enhancing benefits. In addition, beyond the two primary Olympic lifts are a vast array of derivative lifts that are extremely valuable for training athletes. Derivatives are lifts that emphasize a specific phase of the competition lifts in their modified versions. Most derivatives have been shown to help athletes both learn the two competition lifts and gain the performance-enhancing benefits without having to learn or master the full competition lifts (Berton et al., 2018; Bousquet & Olson, 2018; DeWeese et al., 2016; Hermassi et al., 2019; James et al., 2018; James et al., 2019; Jones et al., 2016; Soriano et al., 2019; Suchomel et al., 2017; Suchomel et al., 2019; Suchomel & Sole, 2017; Teo et al., 2016).

SNATCH/CLEAN DEADLIFT

The snatch deadlift and clean deadlift (**Figure 15.17**) are pulling derivatives typically performed from the floor. They can consist of the first pull only (from floor to knees) or a combination of the first pull plus the transition phase, ending with full hip extension. Performing the snatch/clean deadlift pull derivative from the knee or hip position can be a valuable way for Sports Performance Coaches to introduce or work on loaded hinging with a performance client. These positions can also be good options for starting and working with a performance client with limited ankle or hip mobility. The primary differences between these two lifts are the foot and grip setup positions, as the snatch setup requires a wider stance and grip than the clean, as previously discussed.

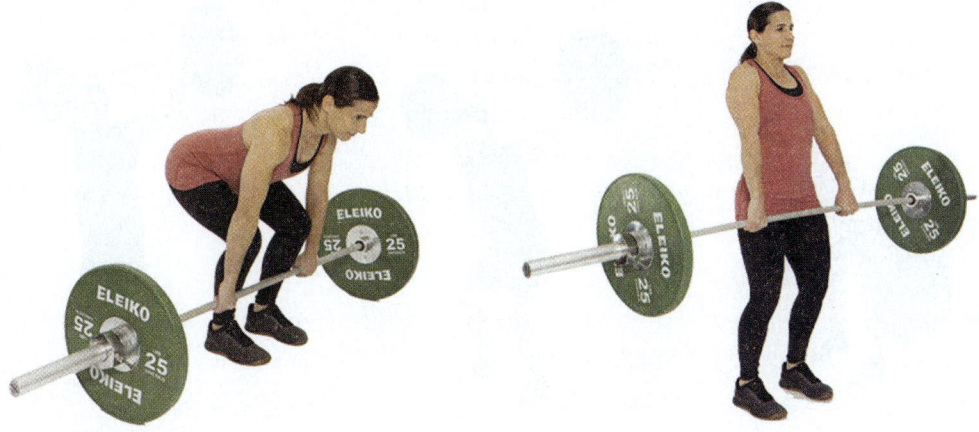

FIGURE 15.17 Clean Deadlift

SNATCH/CLEAN PULL

Like the snatch deadlift and clean deadlift, the snatch pull and clean pull (**Figure 15.18**) are typically performed from the floor. They include the shrug of the second pull only or both the shrug and high pull of the second pull. Snatch and clean pull derivatives can start from the knee or hip positions.

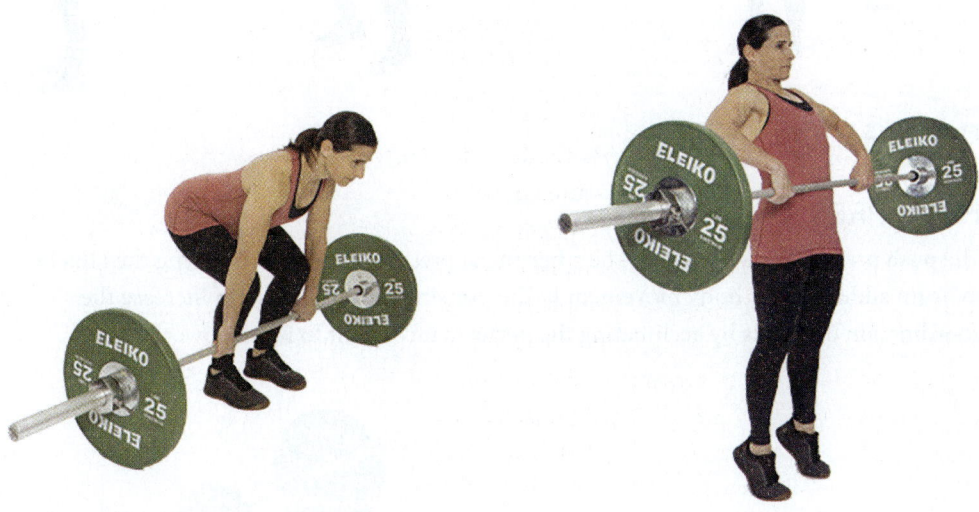

FIGURE 15.18 Clean Pull

HANG POWER SNATCH/CLEAN

The hang power snatch (**Figure 15.19**) and hang power clean (**Figure 15.20**) start from a hang position at knee, mid-thigh, or hip levels. They involve the second pull, pull-under, catch, and stand phases. The hang power snatch/clean is a good derivative for triple extension and catching motions while minimizing the ankle and hip ROM requirement that many performance clients initially lack (Ayers et al., 2016). If the hang position is not desired or preferred for the performance client, blocks or safety arms can be used to support the weight in the starting position.

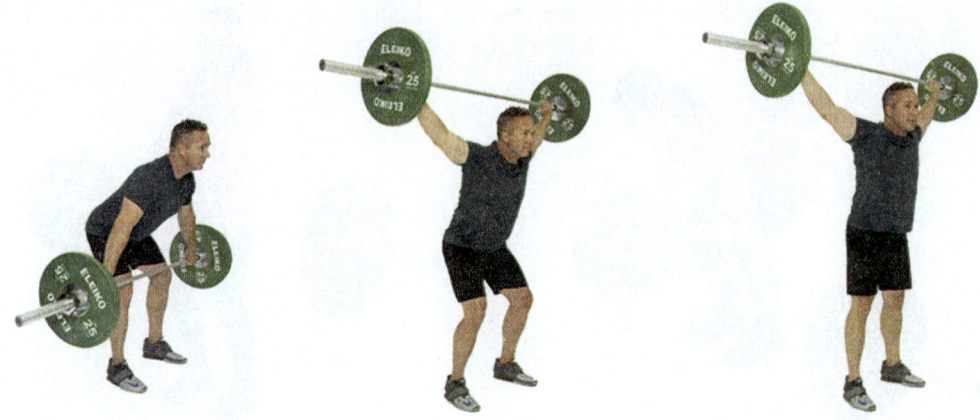

FIGURE 15.19 Hang Power Snatch

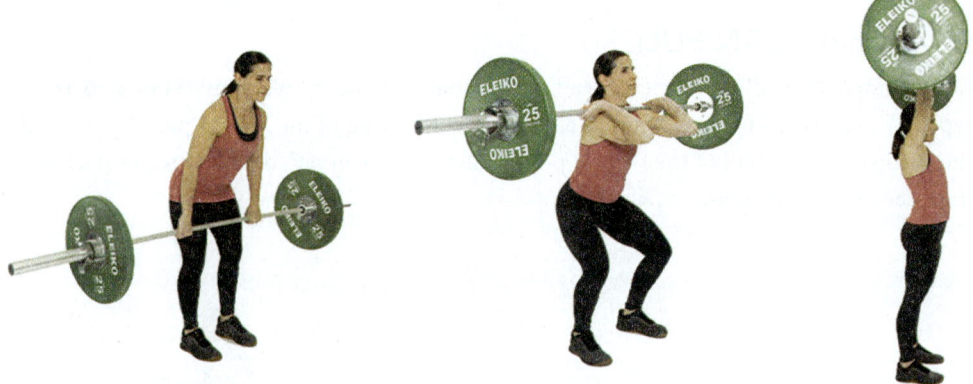

FIGURE 15.20 Hang Power Clean

PUSH PRESS

The push press (**Figure 15.21**) can be a beneficial pressing derivative allowing the athlete to begin adding lower-body movement to the pressing motion. This can increase the coordination demands by acclimating the performance client to more power-based

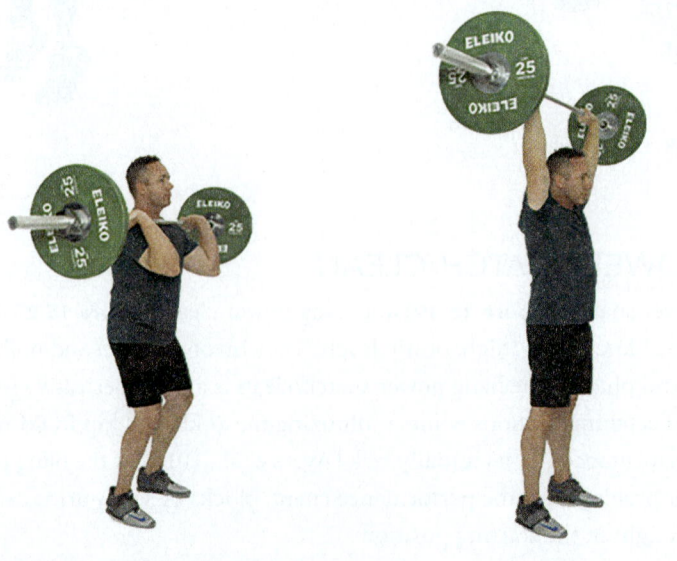

FIGURE 15.21 Push Press

pressing movements and preparing them for the push and split jerks (Soriano et al., 2019). This derivative can be performed from both the front- and back-loaded positions.

OVERHEAD SQUAT

The overhead squat (OHS) (**Figure 15.22**) is a vital component of the snatch, specifically in the catch and stand phases. Performing the OHS as a derivative can be a productive way to increase core, shoulder, and leg strength, balance, and coordination (Aspe & Swinton, 2014; Bautista et al., 2020), as well as help improve the snatch. Progressing by adding a barbell will increase the athlete's ability to position themselves for and perform an OHS and increase their shoulder strength through the various overhead pressing movements.

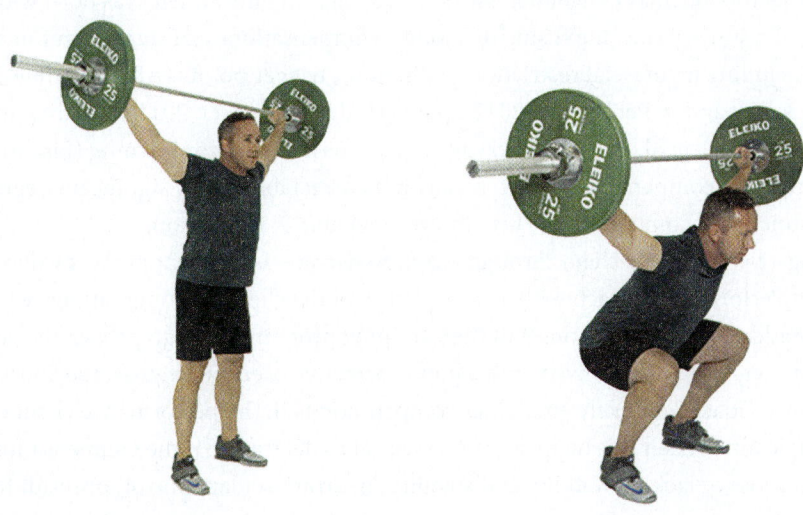

FIGURE 15.22 Overhead Squat

FRONT SQUAT

Front squats (**Figure 15.23**) are an important part of the clean explicitly used in the catch phase and are an excellent exercise for enhancing performance. Performing front squats is also an effective way to improve shoulder, core, and leg strength and stabilization (Bautista et al., 2020; Gullett et al., 2009; Yavuz et al., 2015). The use of front squats can also be helpful to enhance wrist and elbow alignment for the catch and stand phases of the clean as well as the setup and dip phases for the jerk.

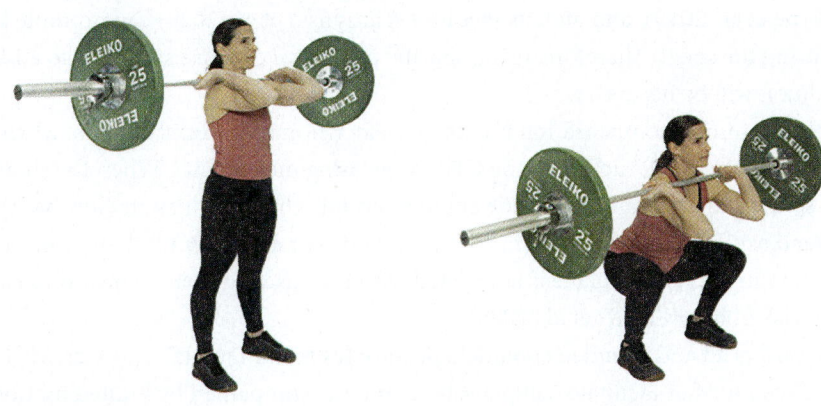

FIGURE 15.23 Front Squat

CORRECTING COMMON MOVEMENT IMPAIRMENTS

With any movement, there is the opportunity for movement compensation to occur. The most important thing for Sports Performance Coaches is to recognize and practically address them to ensure safe and effective lifting practices. Several compensations and ways to correct them have been mentioned in previous sections. This section focuses on understanding compensations, taking a deeper look into specific compensations and strategies to help correct them. These compensations include knee valgus (knees collapsing inward) during squatting motions, excessive lumbar extension with weight in the overhead position, and excessive trunk flexion in the clean catch and stand phases, which include front squats.

Compensations seen during movement can occur for a variety of reasons. Aside from structural factors, such as congenital issues (i.e., something the athlete was born with) or the result of a surgery (i.e., the fusing of a joint), compensations can stem from functional sources, including myofascial restrictions, adhesions, trigger points (Alburquerque-Sendín et al., 2013; Fernández-Pérez et al., 2012), pain (Hodges & Tucker, 2011), mindset and emotion (Michalak et al., 2009; Oosterwijk et al., 2009), and motor learning (Fischman, 2007). Structural compensations are typically not correctable to any significant degree, whereas functional compensations usually are amenable to correction.

Taking a performance client through a comprehensive assessment process will provide the Sports Performance Coach with a clear picture of the client's compensations, which should be addressed from the onset of their training program through proper corrective exercise strategies. However, even with a good corrective exercise strategy, the Sports Performance Coach will likely encounter compensations in the performance client during the Olympic lifts. When this happens, it is essential to determine if the compensations are due to a loss or lack of mobility and stability (neuromuscular control) or result from motor learning, meaning the performance client does not yet understand how the body or joints should be positioned and moved. Using suggestions from the Coach's Corner and Critical boxes in the snatch and the clean and jerk sections can be an excellent way for Sports Performance Coaches to address many of the issues discussed in this section. Impairments, considerations, and corrections for motor learning and neuromuscular control impairments are described in Appendix E.

COMMON COMPENSATIONS

One of the most prevalent compensations seen during squatting motions is knee valgus—that is, the knees collapsing inward. In addition, a lack of flexibility in the calf complex and weakness in the anterior tibialis (Kim et al., 2015; Schoenfeld, 2010), gluteus maximus (Buckthorpe et al., 2019), and gluteus medius (Wilczyński et al., 2020) can promote knee valgus during the squat. Therefore, using specific corrective exercise strategies to address this condition will be necessary.

Another common compensation is excessive extension in the lumbar spine when weight is lifted overhead, such as in the OHS or pressing movements. When the shoulders, thoracic spine, and hips cannot provide enough motion, the lumbar spine (low back) will often extend excessively during overhead movements. For example, a lack of thoracic spine motion in the sagittal plane is associated with increased lumbar spine motion and an increased risk of injury (Ruiz et al., 2020).

A forward head and rounded shoulders posture (as seen in Janda's upper crossed syndrome) can further facilitate compensation and is accompanied by limited motion of the pectorals and latissimus dorsi and weakness of the serratus anterior (Thigpen et al., 2010). When this occurs, the scapula (shoulder blade) and shoulder joint movement is decreased during overhead lifts. With less motion available at the shoulder and thoracic spine, the lumbar spine must extend to a greater extent. Using specific corrective exercise strategies to address this compensation is important.

During the catch phase of the clean and its derivatives, a common compensation is excessive trunk flexion. As the catch for the clean involves shoulder flexion and protraction, any limitation in the posterior shoulder muscles (i.e., latissimus) can affect shoulder position and influence the thoracic spine to flex. Also, wrist mobility and shoulder strength can play crucial roles. Cleans require considerable amounts of wrist mobility in extension and shoulder activation in flexion. Trunk flexion may be caused by an inability to keep the elbows up, which is the product of wrist mobility and shoulder strength. If the client will be performing clean movements, especially with barbells, it is suggested that front squats be implemented as part of their training programs. This will help work on the shoulder and wrist mobility and the core strength they will need to perform the clean movements safely.

LESSON 6: OLYMPIC WEIGHTLIFTING AND THE OPT MODEL
INTEGRATING OLYMPIC LIFTS INTO THE OPT MODEL

Olympic lifts are highly adaptable and consist of many variations. Typically, Olympic lifts are considered power movements, which is the correct interpretation. However, depending on the load and speed of movement used, the Olympic lifts and their derivatives can be used in all phases of the OPT Model.

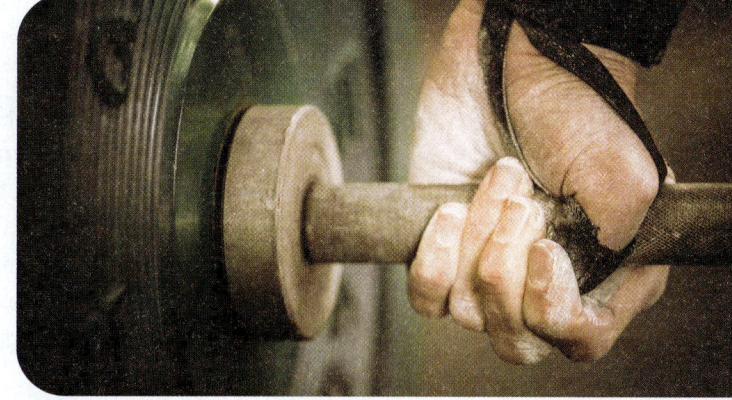

© Toby Grayson/Shutterstock

The widespread applicability of these lifts underlines the importance of understanding the concepts of periodization. Periodization is about progressively manipulating the acute variables of training to promote ongoing adaptations. While the movements used have influence, how they are used (i.e., repetitions, set, load, tempo, rest) ultimately promotes the desired adaptation. This is the whole purpose of having acute variables.

The derivatives of the Olympic lifts are excellent movements to use throughout the warm-up, activation, skill development, and resistance training sections of an OPT program. In addition, as each phase of the OPT Model has designated acute variables, the Sports Performance Coach can easily plug various lifts into each training phase. This section outlines example programs for each training phase to show how the Olympic lifts can be spread across all components of an OPT program and in each phase within the OPT Model.

PHASE 1: STABILIZATION ENDURANCE TRAINING

Phase 1, stabilization endurance training, focuses on maximizing stabilization and postural control to increase proprioception. As such, this is a perfect point for introducing aspects of the Olympic lifts. Working on the mobility and stability in the ankles, hips, core, thoracic spine and shoulders, and wrists is needed to progress and perform the Olympic lifts while moving forward safely. Sports Performance Coaches also need to help athletes become accustomed to the different positions and motions found in the Olympic lifts, such as triple extension with balance, a wider stance with squatting, performing front squats, and practicing drop-downs. Phase 1 also suggests slower tempos. This can be beneficial to work on technique in many derivative lifts—for example, to become more precise with the hinge in deadlifting, work on triple extension with a shrugging motion, and focus on posture during front squats. The lifts in Phase 1 use lighter loads with various types of equipment, which will help performance clients gain confidence in the movement patterns. **Table 15.11** provides an example of appropriate Phase 1 Olympic lifts along with a rationale for their use.

TABLE 15.11 Example Phase 1 Olympic Lifts

OPT Model Phase	Olympic Lifts	Rationale
Stabilization endurance	1. Clean deadlifts (knee) 2. Shrug pulls to balance (knee) 3. Split jerk foot footwork squats (1/4–1/2)	1. Hip motion and core stability with decreased hip ROM 2. Triple extension with shoulder extension 3. Foot speed and hip flexion of front leg 4. Leg and core strength with decreased hip ROM

PHASE 2: STRENGTH ENDURANCE TRAINING

In Phase 2, strength endurance training, the focus is on increasing stability under load and strength. The Sports Performance Coach can increase the load and speed of motion and add more of the derivatives in this phase. In addition, Phase 2 is an excellent place to introduce more barbell movements and overall volume to help condition the athlete and acclimate them to the movement patterns. However, if the barbell, even unloaded, is too heavy for an athlete, the Sports Performance Coach should use dowel rods, PVC pipes, or weighted bars.

Key areas to focus on in Phase 2 include increasing core strength and the ROM of the lifts used. For example, athletes can work on moving from the knee to the floor in some of the deadlifting and pulling derivatives and promoting a full squat with the front and OHS movements. This can help athletes gain confidence in their lifting ability and may contribute to increased strength and power over time, especially in less experienced lifters (Waller & Townsend, 2007; Wirth et al., 2017; Munger et al., 2017). This ties back into the importance of improving mobility and stability and ensuring the athlete is comfortable in the proper stance width to allow them to move into a full squat position safely and effectively. **Table 15.12** provides an example of appropriate Phase 2 Olympic lifts along with a rationale for their use.

TABLE 15.12 Example Phase 2 Olympic Lifts

OPT Model Phase	Olympic Lifts	Rationale
Strength endurance	1. Push press 2. Clean and snatch deadlifts 3. High-pulls 4. Split jerk footwork 5. Front and overhead squats	1. Shoulder flexion, overhead, and total-body strength 2. Hip strength and core stability 3. Triple extension with shoulder work 4. Foot speed 5. Leg, core, shoulder, and overhead strength

PHASE 3: MUSCULAR DEVELOPMENT TRAINING

Phase 3, muscular development training, increases the focus on volume and intensity.

The Phase 3 Olympic lifting program will not look like a typical bodybuilding program because the different lifts used are not typically thought of or used in hypertrophy-based training.

However, there is no reason why these lifts, especially the derivatives, cannot or should not be used. The derivatives can continue to get more advanced but should progress only to the level of the athlete.

There should be continued practice of some technical elements of Olympic lifting, such as catching and pulling from the floor. As seen in traditional hypertrophy training, the idea is to increase total-body volume versus specific body-part volume.

It is strongly suggested that the Sports Performance Coach allow the athlete to have a week of deloading or recovery following Phase 3. Full recovery will be beneficial before Phase 4, maximal strength training, given the high volume and stress placed on the athlete in that phase.

© Tyler Olson/Shutterstock

PHASE 4: MAXIMAL STRENGTH TRAINING

Phase 4, maximal strength training, is the phase in which technique and the additional muscle mass can be transferred into high levels of strength. The loads in this phase will be higher intensity, and the intention to move at a higher velocity should be emphasized. Although the movements in this phase fall on the high-force, low-velocity end of the force–velocity curve, the intention to move fast helps promote maximal recruitment of motor units, rate of force production, and motor unit synchronization. This will translate into increased power output for the athlete and further prepares them for Phases 5 and 6, where power will be maximized.

In Phase 4, squats, pulls, hang power snatches and cleans, and jerks can be emphasized with heavier loads. Again, the term "heavier" must always be relative to the performance client's ability and strength levels. The Sports Performance Coach is encouraged not to sacrifice technique for load. The ability to perform the lifts correctly is essential to how the strength and power output will transfer into the athlete's performance. For example, if the athlete does not achieve an excellent triple extension in the pulls, the transfer to the vertical jump may not be as significant (Suchomel et al., 2015). **Table 15.13** provides an example of appropriate Phase 4 Olympic lifts along with a rationale for their use.

TABLE 15.13 Example Phase 4 Olympic Lifts

OPT Model Phase	Olympic Lifts	Rationale
Maximal strength	1. Push jerk 2. Clean and snatch shrug pulls 3. Split jerk drop-downs 4. Front and overhead squats	1. Total-body strength/power; DB 2. Triple extension with shoulder work; BB 3. Foot speed and agility; KB 4. Leg, core, shoulder, and overhead strength; BB

PHASE 5: POWER TRAINING

Phase 5, power training, is a unique phase of training and can be highly beneficial to performance clients (Cormier et al., 2020; Freitas et al., 2017). It combines high intensity with high-velocity training; thus, it works on both ends of the force–velocity curve. The emphasis in this phase is to increase power by utilizing the stretch–shortening cycle (SSC). Therefore, each exercise tandem in the resistance training section of the program will include a low-intensity, high-velocity plyometric-based movement that follows the high-intensity, low-moderate velocity strength exercise. The high-intensity movement that precedes the high-velocity movement produces an increased post-activation potentiation (PAP). Skill development can be included in the program and will involve more advanced Olympic lift derivatives that include a countermovement. It is imperative that the countermovement (dip to the knees and back up) be a hip hinge and not a squatting motion. **Table 15.14** provides an example of appropriate Phase 5 Olympic lifts along with a rationale for their use.

TABLE 15.14 Example Phase 5 Olympic Lifts

OPT Model Phase	Olympic Lifts	Rationale
Power	1. Split jerk 2. Hang power snatch and clean 3. Front and overhead squats	1. Total-body strength-speed; DB 2. Triple extension with shoulder work; BB 3. Leg, core, shoulder, and overhead strength; BB

PHASE 6: MAXIMAL POWER TRAINING

Phase 6, maximal power training, focuses on optimizing power outputs with high velocity or speed strength. In this training phase, the key is finding the load that allows the greatest speed of loaded movement. For the Olympic lift derivatives, this load is approximately 40% of the 1RM load, with some lifts being slightly higher and others slightly lower (Suchomel et al., 2017). The lifts selected in the Phase 6 program have been shown to result in high velocities, high acceleration, and power. The loads used in this phase should be approximately 30% to 45% of the performance client's 1RM for a power clean.

The athlete should have performed all of the lifts at this point. Thus, the emphasis for the lifts in this phase is speed. Nevertheless, as was discussed for Phase 4 with load, technique should never be sacrificed for speed. The athlete should perform the lifts as fast as they can control. **Table 15.15** provides an example of appropriate Phase 6 Olympic lifts along with a rationale for their use.

TABLE 15.15 Example Phase 6 Olympic Lifts

OPT Model Phase	Olympic Lifts	Rationale
Maximal power	1. Split jerk 2. Hang power snatch and clean	1. Total-body speed-strength; BB 2. Total speed-strength; BB

SUMMARY

Olympic weightlifting is a competitive sport that began in the mid-1800s but whose popularity did not truly grow until the early 1900s. This highly technical sport requires great skill, mobility, strength, coordination, and often years of diligent practice to perfect. Additionally, many of the world's most elite weightlifters have specific body types that give them optimal leverage and a mechanical advantage over other athletes. Traditional Olympic weightlifting consists of snatch, clean, and jerk movements. However, many derivatives that emphasize certain aspects of each lift have been developed during training. Although some athletes may not excel at the two standardized lifts, they can and should employ various derivatives within their training regimen to help maximize power and performance gains.

KEY TAKEAWAYS

- Olympic weightlifting is a highly technical competitive sport that requires advanced training, optimal mobility, high levels of strength, and years of practice to perfect. In addition, correctly executing lifts requires skill and good technique; incorrect execution reduces their effectiveness and increases the chances of injury.
- Key components that increase the effectiveness and safety of Olympic lifting are supervision, education, and equipment.
  - Due to the level of skill required to perform the Olympic lifts, coaches of competitive athletes are often well informed and qualified in the instruction and coaching aspects of these lifts.
  - It is strongly suggested that individuals responsible for overseeing, teaching, and coaching the Olympic lifts be credentialed through an appropriate weightlifting coaching program. Organizations with an extended legacy in Olympic weightlifting, such as Eleiko and USA Weightlifting, provide courses specific to the instruction technique.
  - Proper equipment specifically designed for Olympic weightlifting contributes to safe and effective outcomes. The combination of a bar and bumper plates makes up a barbell.
- The Olympic lifts require more complex neural activation strategies and motor skills to enhance performance. Therefore, identifying and addressing the neuromuscular efficiency of a performance client allows for better planning, programming, and progression toward a successful outcome. Key prerequisites for Olympic weightlifting include mobility, stability, posture, and strength.
- There are two primary full Olympic lifts: the snatch and the clean and jerk. Both lifts involve lifting a barbell from its starting position on the floor to a standing position with the barbell overhead, yet they are uniquely different.

- In the snatch, the lifter moves through six primary phases after the initial setup: first pull, transition, second pull, pull-under, catch, and stand.
- The clean and jerk is a compound movement of two separate stages, the clean and the jerk. The clean follows the same phases as for the snatch. The jerk component has its own set of phases that follow the completion of the clean.
- Compensations during Olympic weightlifting can occur for several reasons, such as structural or congenital and functional issues. Functional reasons include flexibility limitations, pain, mindset, and emotion, as well as motor learning. Structural compensations are typically not correctable to any significant degree, but functional compensations are usually amenable to correction.
- Components of Olympic lifting can be integrated into all phases of NASM's OPT Model.

REFERENCES

Aasa, U., Svartholm, I., Andersson, F., & Berglund, L. (2017). Injuries among weightlifters and powerlifters: A systematic review. *British Journal of Sports Medicine, 51*(4), 211–219. https://doi.org/10.1136/bjsports-2016-096037

Agten, A., Stevens, S., Verbrugghe, J., Eijnde, B. O., Timmermans, A., & Vandenabeele, F. (2020). The lumbar multifidus is characterised by larger type I muscle fibres compared to the erector spinae. *Anatomy & Cell Biology, 53*(2), 143–150. https://doi.org/10.5115/acb.20.009

Alburquerque-Sendín, F., Camargo, P., R., Vieira, A., & Salvini, T., F. (2013). Bilateral myofascial trigger points and pressure pain thresholds in the shoulder muscles in patients with unilateral shoulder impingement syndrome: A blinded, controlled study. *Clinical Journal of Pain, 29*(6), 478–486.

Arabatzi, F., & Kellis, E. (2012). Olympic weightlifting training causes different knee muscle–coactivation adaptations compared with traditional weight training. *Journal of Strength and Conditioning Research, 26*(8), 2192–2201. https://doi.org/10.1519/JSC.0b013e31823b087a

Aspe, R. R., & Swinton, P. A. (2014). Electromyographic and kinetic comparison of the back squat and overhead squat. *Journal of Strength and Conditioning Research, 28*(10), 2827–2836. https://doi.org/10.1519/jsc.0000000000000462

Ayers, J., DeBeliso, M., Sevene, T., & Adams, K. (2016). Hang cleans and hang snatches produce similar improvements in female collegiate athletes. *Biology of Sport, 33*(3), 251–256. https://www.ncbi.nlm.nih.gov/pmc/articles/PMC4993140

Barrett, E., O'Keeffe, M., O'Sullivan, K., McCreesh, K., & Lewis, J. (2016). Is thoracic spine posture associated with shoulder pain, range of motion and function? A systematic review. *Manual Therapy, 25*, e98. https://doi.org/10.1016/j.math.2016.05.171

Bautista, D., Durke, D., Cotter, J. A., Escobar, K. A., & Schick, E. E. (2020). A comparison of muscle activation among the front squat, overhead squat, back extension and plank. *International Journal of Exercise Science, 13*(1), 714–722.

Berton, R., Lixandrão, M. E., Pinto E Silva, C. M., & Tricoli, V. (2018). Effects of weightlifting exercise, traditional resistance and plyometric training on countermovement jump performance: A meta-analysis. *Journal of Sports Sciences, 36*(18), 2038–2044. https://doi.org/10.1080/02640414.2018.1434746

Bousquet, B. A., & Olson, T. (2018). Starting at the ground up. *Strength and Conditioning Journal, 40*(6), 56–67. https://doi.org/10.1519/ssc.0000000000000399

Buckthorpe, M., Stride, M., & Villa, F. D. (2019). Assessing and treating gluteus maximus weakness—A clinical commentary. *International Journal of Sports Physical Therapy, 14*(4), 655–669.

Campbell, A., Kemp-Smith, K., O'Sullivan, P., & Straker, L. (2016). Abdominal bracing increases ground reaction forces and reduces knee and hip flexion during landing. *Journal of Orthopaedic & Sports Physical Therapy, 46*(4), 286–292. https://doi.org/10.2519/jospt.2016.5774

Carlock, J. M., Smith, S. L., Hartman, M. J., Morris, R. T., Ciroslan, D. A., Pierce, K. C., Newton, R. U., Harman, E. A., Sands, W. A., & Stone, M. H. (2004). The relationship between vertical jump power estimates and weightlifting ability: A field-test approach. *Journal of Strength and Conditioning Research, 18*(3), 534–539. https://pubmed.ncbi.nlm.nih.gov/15320676

Case, M. J., Knudson, D. V., & Downey, D. L. (2020). Barbell squat relative strength as an identifier for lower extremity injury in collegiate athletes. *Journal of Strength and Conditioning Research, 34*(5), 1249–1253. https://doi.org/10.1519/jsc.0000000000003554

Chaouachi, A., Hammami, R., Kaabi, S., Chamari, K., Drinkwater, E. J., & Behm, D. G. (2014). Olympic weightlifting and plyometric training with children provides similar or greater performance improvements than traditional resistance training. *Journal of Strength and Conditioning Research, 28*(6), 1483–1496. https://doi.org/10.1519/JSC.0000000000000305

Clarsen, B., Bahr, R., Andersson, S. H., Munk, R., & Myklebust, G. (2014). Reduced glenohumeral rotation, external rotation weakness and scapular dyskinesis are risk factors for shoulder injuries among elite male handball players: A prospective cohort study. *British Journal of Sports Medicine, 48*(17), 1327–1333. https://doi.org/10.1136/bjsports-2014-093702

Cools, A. M., Johansson, F. R., Borms, D., & Maenhout, A. (2015). Prevention of shoulder injuries in overhead athletes: A science-based approach. *Brazilian Journal of Physical Therapy, 19*(5), 331–339. https://doi.org/10.1590/bjpt-rbf.2014.0109

Cormier, P., Freitas, T. T., Rubio-Arias, J. Á., & Alcaraz, P. E. (2020). Complex and contrast training: Does strength and power training sequence affect performance-based adaptations in team sports? A systematic review and meta-analysis. *The Journal of Strength and Conditioning Research, 34*(5), 1461. https://doi.org/10.1519/JSC.0000000000003493

Crosbie, J., Kilbreath, S. L., Hollmann, L., & York, S. (2008). Scapulohumeral rhythm and associated spinal motion. *Clinical Biomechanics, 23*(2), 184–192. https://doi.org/10.1016/j.clinbiomech.2007.09.012

de Oliveira, V. M. A., Pitangui, A. C. R., & de Araújo, R. C. (2019). Factors associated with shoulder deficit in total rotational motion (DTRM) in adolescent athletes. *Journal of Human Sport and Exercise, 15*(1). https://doi.org/10.14198/jhse.2020.151.05

DeWeese, B. H., Suchomel, T. J., Serrano, A. J., Burton, J. D., Scruggs, S. K., & Taber, C. B. (2016). Pull from the knee. *Strength and Conditioning Journal, 38*(1), 79–85. https://doi.org/10.1519/ssc.0000000000000194

Duehring, M. D., Feldmann, C. R., & Ebben, W. P. (2009). Strength and conditioning practices of United States high school strength and conditioning coaches. *Journal of Strength and Conditioning Research, 23*(8), 2188–2203. https://doi.org/10.1519/JSC.0b013e3181bac62d

Durell, D. L., Pujol, T. J., & Barnes, J. T. (2003). A survey of the scientific data and training methods utilized by collegiate strength and conditioning coaches. *Journal of Strength and Conditioning Research, 17*(2), 368–373. https://doi.org/10.1519/00124278-200305000-00026

Ebben, W. P., & Blackard, D. O. (2001). Strength and conditioning practices of National Football League strength and conditioning coaches. *Journal of Strength and Conditioning Research, 15*(1), 48–58.

Ebben, W. P., Carroll, R. M., & Simenz, C. J. (2004). Strength and conditioning practices of National Hockey League strength and conditioning coaches. *Journal of Strength and Conditioning Research, 18*(4), 889–897. https://pubmed.ncbi.nlm.nih.gov/15574099

Ebben, W. P., Hintz, M. J., & Simenz, C. J. (2005). Strength and conditioning practices of Major League Baseball strength and conditioning coaches. *Journal of Strength and Conditioning Research, 19*(3), 538–546. https://pubmed.ncbi.nlm.nih.gov/16095401

Endo, K., Suzuki, H., Sawaji, Y., Nishimura, H., Yorifuji, M., Murata, K., Tanaka, H., Shishido, T., & Yamamoto, K. (2016). Relationship among cervical, thoracic, and lumbopelvic sagittal alignment in healthy adults. *Journal of Orthopaedic Surgery, 24*(1), 92–96. https://doi.org/10.1177/230949901602400121

Faigenbaum, A. D., Kraemer, W. J., Blimkie, C. J., Jeffreys, I., Micheli, L. J., Nitka, M., & Rowland, T. W. (2009). Youth resistance training: Updated position statement paper from the National Strength and Conditioning Association. *Journal of Strength and Conditioning Research, 23*(5 suppl), S60–S79. https://doi.org/10.1519/JSC.0b013e31819df407

Fernández-Pérez, A., M., Villaverde-Gutiérrez, C., Mora-Sánchez, A., Alonso-Blanco, C., Sterling, M., & Fernández-de-Las-Peñas, C. (2012). Muscle trigger points, pressure pain threshold, and cervical range of motion in patients with high level of disability related to acute whiplash injury. *Journal of Orthopedic and Sports Physical Therapy, 42*(7), 634–41.

Fischman, M. G. (2007). Motor learning and control foundations of kinesiology: Defining the academic core. *Quest, 59*(1), 67–76. https://doi.org/10.1080/00336297.2007.10483537

Freitas, T. T., Martinez-Rodriguez, A., Calleja-González, J., & Alcaraz, P. E. (2017). Short-term adaptations following Complex Training in team-sports: A meta-analysis. *PLOS ONE, 12*(6), e0180223. https://doi.org/10.1371/journal.pone.0180223

Gee, T. I., Olsen, P. D., Berger, N. J., Golby, J., & Thompson, K. G. (2011). Strength and conditioning practices in rowing. *Journal of Strength and Conditioning Research, 25*(3), 668–682. https://doi.org/10.1519/JSC.0b013e3181e2e10e

Gullett, J. C., Tillman, M. D., Gutierrez, G. M., & Chow, J. W. (2009). A biomechanical comparison of back and front squats in healthy trained individuals. *Journal of Strength and Conditioning Research, 23*(1), 284–292. https://doi.org/10.1519/jsc.0b013e31818546bb

Hackett, D., Davies, T., Soomro, N., & Halaki, M. (2016). Olympic weightlifting training improves vertical jump height in sportspeople: A systematic review with meta-analysis. *British Journal of Sports Medicine, 50*(14), 865–872. https://doi.org/10.1136/bjsports-2015-094951

Hadi, G., Akkuş, H., & Harbili, E. (2012). Three-dimensional kinematic analysis of the snatch technique for lifting different barbell weights. *Journal of Strength and Conditioning Research, 26*(6), 1568–1576. https://doi.org/10.1519/jsc.0b013e318231abe9

Haff, G. G., & Nimphius, S. (2012). Training principles for power. *Strength and Conditioning Journal, 34*(6), 2–12. https://doi.org/10.1519/ssc.0b013e31826db467

Haugen, T., Seiler, S., Sandbakk, Ø., & Tønnessen, E. (2019). The training and development of elite sprint performance: An integration of scientific and best practice literature. *Sports Medicine: Open, 5*(1). https://doi.org/10.1186/s40798-019-0221-0

Heneghan, N. R., Lokhaug, S. M., Tyros, I., Longvastøl, S., & Rushton, A. (2020). Clinical reasoning framework for thoracic spine exercise prescription in sport: A systematic review and narrative synthesis. *BMJ Open Sport & Exercise Medicine, 6*(1), e000713. https://doi.org/10.1136/bmjsem-2019-000713

Heneghan, N. R., Webb, K., Mahoney, T., & Rushton, A. (2019). Thoracic spine mobility, an essential link in upper limb kinetic chains in athletes: A systematic review. *Translational Sports Medicine, 2*(6), 301–315. https://doi.org/10.1002/tsm2.109

Hermassi, S., Chelly, M. S., Bragazzi, N. L., Shephard, R. J., & Schwesig, R. (2019). In-season weightlifting training exercise in healthy male handball players: Effects on body composition, muscle volume, maximal strength, and ball-throwing velocity. *International Journal of Environmental Research and Public Health, 16*(22), 4520. https://doi.org/10.3390/ijerph16224520

Hodges, P. W., & Tucker, K. (2011). Moving differently in pain: A new theory to explain the adaptation to pain. *Pain, 152*, S90–S98.

Hoffman, J. R., Cooper, J., Wendell, M., & Kang, J. (2004). Comparison of Olympic vs. traditional power lifting training programs in football players. *Journal of Strength and Conditioning Research, 18*(1), 129–135. https://pubmed.ncbi.nlm.nih.gov/14971971

Hoffman, J., & Gabel, P. (2013). Expanding Panjabi's stability model to express movement: A theoretical model. *Medical Hypotheses, 80*(6), 692–697. https://doi.org/10.1016/j.mehy.2013.02.006

Hori, N., Newton, R. U., Nosaka, K., & Stone, M. H. (2005). Weightlifting exercises enhance athletic performance that requires high-load speed strength. *Strength and Conditioning Journal, 27*(4), 50–55. https://journals.lww.com/nsca-scj/Abstract/2005/08000/Weightlifting_Exercises_Enhance_Athletic.8.aspx

Howe, L. P., & Blagrove, R. C. (2015). Shoulder function during overhead lifting tasks. *Strength and Conditioning Journal, 37*(5), 84–96. https://doi.org/10.1519/ssc.0000000000000163

Ibrahim, A., Murrell, G., & Knapman, P. (2007). Adductor strain and hip range of movement in male professional soccer players. *Journal of Orthopaedic Surgery, 15*(1), 46–49. https://doi.org/10.1177/230949900701500111

James, L. P., Comfort, P., Suchomel, T. J., Kelly, V. G., Beckman, E. M., & Haff, G. G. (2019). Influence of power clean ability and training age on adaptations to weightlifting-style training. *Journal of Strength and Conditioning Research, 33*(11), 2936–2944. https://doi.org/10.1519/JSC.0000000000002534

James, L. P., Gregory Haff, G., Kelly, V. G., Connick, M. J., Hoffman, B. W., & Beckman, E. M. (2018). The impact of strength level on adaptations to combined weightlifting, plyometric, and ballistic training. *Scandinavian Journal of Medicine & Science in Sports, 28*(5), 1494–1505. https://doi.org/10.1111/sms.13045

Jones, T. W., Smith, A., Macnaughton, L. S., & French, D. N. (2016). Strength and conditioning and concurrent training practices in elite rugby union. *Journal of Strength and Conditioning Research, 30*(12), 3354–3366. https://doi.org/10.1519/jsc.0000000000001445

Keogh, J. W., & Winwood, P. W. (2017). The epidemiology of injuries across the weight-training sports. *Sports Medicine (Auckland, NZ), 47*(3), 479–501. https://doi.org/10.1007/s40279-016-0575-0

Kim, D. W., & Kim, T. H. (2018). Effects of abdominal hollowing and abdominal bracing during side-lying hip abduction on the lateral rotation and muscle activity of the pelvis. *Journal of Exercise Rehabilitation, 14*(2), 226–230. https://doi.org/10.12965/jer.1836102.051

Kim, S.-H., Kwon, O.-Y., Park, K.-N., Jeon, I.-C., & Weon, J.-H. (2015). Lower extremity strength and the range of motion in relation to squat depth. *Journal of Human Kinetics, 45*(1), 59–69. https://www.ncbi.nlm.nih.gov/pmc/articles/PMC4415844/

Kim, T., & Hwang, B. (2019). Change of head position and muscle activities of neck during overhead arm lift test in subjects with forward head posture. *Physical Therapy Korea, 26*(2), 61–68. https://doi.org/10.12674/ptk.2019.26.2.061

Kipp, K. (2020). Relative importance of lower extremity net joint moments in relation to bar velocity and acceleration in weightlifting. *Sports Biomechanics*, 1–13. https://doi.org/10.1080/14763141.2020.1718196

Kroell, J., & Mike, J. (2017). Exploring the standing barbell overhead press. *Strength and Conditioning Journal*, *39*(6), 70–75. https://doi.org/10.1519/ssc.0000000000000324

Kusuma, M., Rilastio, D., Syafei, M., Nugroho, R., & Budiharjo, B. (2018). Biomechanical analysis of snatch technique in conjunction to kinematic motion of Olympic weightlifters. *Advances in Health Science Research, 12*. https://doi.org/10.2991/isphe-18.2018.30

LaPlaca, D. A., & McCullick, B. A. (2020). National Football League scouting combine tests correlated to National Football League player performance. *Journal of Strength and Conditioning Research, 34*(5), 1317–1329. https://doi.org/10.1519/JSC.0000000000003479

Linde, L. D., Archibald, J., Lampert, E. C., & Srbely, J. Z. (2018). The effect of abdominal muscle activation techniques on trunk and lower limb mechanics during the single-leg squat task in females. *Journal of Sport Rehabilitation, 27*(5), 438–444. https://doi.org/10.1123/jsr.2016-0038

Liu, G., Fekete, G., Yang, H., Ma, J., Sun, D., Mei, Q., & Gu, Y. (2018). Comparative 3-dimensional kinematic analysis of snatch technique between top-elite and sub-elite male weightlifters in 69-kg category. *Heliyon, 4*(7), e00658. https://doi.org/10.1016/j.heliyon.2018.e00658

Lloyd, R. S., Faigenbaum, A. D., Stone, M. H., Oliver, J. L., Jeffreys, I., Moody, J. A., Brewer, C., Pierce, K. C., McCambridge, T. M., Howard, R., Herrington, L., Hainline, B., Micheli, L. J., Jaques, R., Kraemer, W. J., McBride, M. G., Best, T. M., Chu, D. A., Alvar, B. A., & Myer, G. D. (2014). Position statement on youth resistance training: The 2014 International Consensus. *British Journal of Sports Medicine, 48*(7), 498–505. https://doi.org/10.1136/bjsports-2013-092952

MacKenzie, S. J., Lavers, R. J., & Wallace, B. B. (2014). A biomechanical comparison of the vertical jump, power clean, and jump squat. *Journal of Sports Sciences, 32*(16), 1576–1585. https://doi.org/10.1080/02640414.2014.908320

Markström, J. L., & Olsson, C. J. (2013). Countermovement jump peak force relative to body weight and jump height as predictors for sprint running performances: (In)homogeneity of track and field athletes? *Journal of Strength and Conditioning Research, 27*(4), 944–953. https://doi.org/10.1519/JSC.0b013e318260edad

Martins, P. C., Teixeira, A. S., Guglielmo, L., Francisco, J. S., Silva, D., Nakamura, F. Y., & Lima, L. (2021). Phase angle is related to 10 m and 30 m sprint time and repeated-sprint ability in young male soccer players. *International Journal of Environmental Research and Public Health, 18*(9), 4405. https://doi.org/10.3390/ijerph18094405

McKean, M. R., & Burkett, B. J. (2015). Overhead shoulder press: In-front of the head or behind the head? *Journal of Sport and Health Science, 4*(3), 250–257. https://doi.org/10.1016/j.jshs.2013.11.007

McMaster, D. T., Gill, N., Cronin, J., & McGuigan, M. (2014). A brief review of strength and ballistic assessment methodologies in sport. *Sports Medicine (Auckland, NZ), 44*(5), 603–623. https://doi.org/10.1007/s40279-014-0145-2

McQuilliam, S. J., Clark, D. R., Erskine, R. M., & Brownlee, T. E. (2020). Free-weight resistance training in youth athletes: A narrative review. *Sports Medicine (Auckland, NZ), 50*(9), 1567–1580. https://doi.org/10.1007/s40279-020-01307-7

Michalak, J., Troje, N., F., Fischer, J., Vollmar, P., Heidenreich, T., & Schulte, D. (2009). Embodiment of sadness and depression: Gait patterns associated with dysphoric mood. *Psychosomatic Medicine, 71*(5), 580–587.

Moon, J.-H., Jung, J.-H., Hahm, S.-C., Oh, H.-K., Jung, K.-S., & Cho, H.-Y. (2018). Effects of lumbar lordosis assistive support on craniovertebral angle and mechanical properties of the upper trapezius muscle in subjects with forward head posture. *Journal of Physical Therapy Science, 30*(3), 457–460. https://doi.org/10.1589/jpts.30.457

Mujika, I., Santisteban, J., Impellizzeri, F. M., & Castagna, C. (2009). Fitness determinants of success in men's and women's football. *Journal of Sports Sciences, 27*(2), 107–114. https://doi.org/10.1080/02640410802428071

Munger, C. N., Archer, D. C., Leyva, W. D., Wong, M. A., Coburn, J. W., Costa, P. B., & Brown, L. E. (2017). Acute effects of eccentric overload on concentric front squat performance. *The Journal of Strength and Conditioning Research, 31*(5), 1192. https://doi.org/10.1519/JSC.0000000000001825

Muramoto, Y., & Kuruma, H. (2020). Comparison between bracing and hollowing trunk exercise with a focus on the change in T2 values obtained by magnetic resonance imaging. *PLoS One, 15*(10), e0240213. https://doi.org/10.1371/journal.pone.0240213

Nicholson, B., Dinsdale, A., Jones, B., & Till, K. (2021). The training of short distance sprint performance in football code athletes: A systematic review and meta-analysis. *Sports Medicine (Auckland, NZ), 51*(6), 1179–1207. https://doi.org/10.1007/s40279-020-01372-y

Norrie, J. P., & Brown, S. H. M. (2020). Brace yourself: How abdominal bracing affects intersegmental lumbar spine kinematics in response to sudden loading. *Journal of Electromyography and Kinesiology, 54*, 102451. https://doi.org/10.1016/j.jelekin.2020.102451

Oosterwijk, S., Rottevell, M., Fischer, A., H., & Hess, U. (2009). Embodied emotion concepts: How generating words about pride and disappointment influences posture. *European Journal of Social Psychology 39*, 457–466.

Richardson, C. (2004). *Therapeutic exercise for lumbo-pelvic stabilisation.* Churchill Livingstone.

Ruiz, J., Feigenbaum, L., & Best, T. M. (2020). The thoracic spine in the overhead athlete. *Current Sports Medicine Reports, 19*(1), 11–16. https://doi.org/10.1249/JSR.0000000000000671

Sadeghisani, M., Manshadi, F. D., Kalantari, K. K., Rahimi, A., Namnik, N., Karimi, M. T., & Oskouei, A. E. (2015). Correlation between hip rotation range-of-motion impairment and low back pain: A literature review. *Ortopedia, Traumatologia, Rehabilitacja, 17*(5), 455–462. https://pubmed.ncbi.nlm.nih.gov/26751745

Sato, K., & Mokha, M. (2009). Does core strength training influence running kinetics, lower-extremity stability, and 5000-m performance in runners? *Journal of Strength and Conditioning Research, 23*(1), 133–140. https://doi.org/10.1519/jsc.0b013e31818eb0c5

Schoenfeld, B. J. (2010). Squatting kinematics and kinetics and their application to exercise performance. *Journal of Strength and Conditioning Research, 24*(12), 3497–3506. https://doi.org/10.1519/jsc.0b013e3181bac2d7

Shinkle, J., Nesser, T. W., Demchak, T. J., & McMannus, D. M. (2012). Effect of core strength on the measure of power in the extremities. *Journal of Strength and Conditioning Research, 26*(2), 373–380. https://doi.org/10.1519/jsc.0b013e31822600e5

Simenz, C. J., Dugan, C. A., & Ebben, W. P. (2005). Strength and conditioning practices of National Basketball Association strength and conditioning coaches. *Journal of Strength and Conditioning Research, 19*(3), 495–504. https://doi.org/10.1519/00124278-200508000-00003

Soriano, M. A., Suchomel, T. J., & Comfort, P. (2019). Weightlifting overhead pressing derivatives: A review of the literature. *Sports Medicine, 49*(6), 867–885. https://doi.org/10.1007/s40279-019-01096-8

Stojiljkovic, N., Ignjatovic, A., Savic, Z., Markovic, Z., & Milanovic, S. (2013). History of resistance training. *Activities in Physical Education and Sport, 3*(1), 135–138.

Stone, M. H., Pierce, K. C., Sands, W. A., & Stone, M. E. (2006). Weightlifting: A brief overview. *Strength and Conditioning Journal, 28*(1), 50. https://journals.lww.com/nsca-scj/Abstract/2006/02000/Weightlifting__A_Brief_Overview.10.aspx

Storey, A., & Smith, H. K. (2012). Unique aspects of competitive weightlifting: Performance, training and physiology. *Sports Medicine (Auckland, NZ), 42*(9), 769–790. https://doi.org/10.1007/BF03262294

Suchomel, T. J., Comfort, P., & Lake, J. P. (2017). Enhancing the force–velocity profile of athletes using weightlifting derivatives. *Strength and Conditioning Journal, 39*(1), 10–20. https://doi.org/10.1519/ssc.0000000000000275

Suchomel, T. J., & Sole, C. J. (2017). Force-time–curve comparison between weight-lifting derivatives. *International Journal of Sports Physiology and Performance, 12*(4), 431–439. https://doi.org/10.1123/ijspp.2016-0147

Teo, S. Y., Newton, M. J., Newton, R. U., Dempsey, A. R., & Fairchild, T. J. (2016). Comparing the effectiveness of a short-term vertical jump vs. weightlifting program on athletic power development. *Journal of Strength and Conditioning Research, 30*(10), 2741–2748. https://doi.org/10.1519/JSC.0000000000001379

Thigpen, C. A., Padua, D. A., Michener, L. A., Guskiewicz, K., Giuliani, C., Keener, J. D., & Stergiou, N. (2010). Head and shoulder posture affect scapular mechanics and muscle activity in overhead tasks. *Journal of Electromyography and Kinesiology, 20*(4), 701–709. https://doi.org/10.1016/j.jelekin.2009.12.003

Todoroff, M. (2017). Dynamic deep squat: Lower-body kinematics and considerations regarding squat technique, load position, and heel height. *Strength and Conditioning Journal, 39*(1), 71–80. https://doi.org/10.1519/ssc.0000000000000278

Tricoli, V., Lamas, L., Carnevale, R., & Ugrinowitsch, C. (2005). Short-term effects on lower-body functional power development: weightlifting vs. vertical jump training programs. *Journal of Strength and Conditioning Research, 19*(2), 433–437. https://pubmed.ncbi.nlm.nih.gov/15903387

Vaičienė, G., Berškienė, K., Slapsinskaite, A., Mauricienė, V., & Razon, S. (2018). Not only static: Stabilization manoeuvres in dynamic exercises: A pilot study. *PLoS One, 13*(8), e0201017. https://doi.org/10.1371/journal.pone.0201017

Vincent, L. M., Blissmer, B. J., & Hatfield, D. L. (2019). National scouting combine scores as performance predictors in the National Football League. *Journal of Strength and Conditioning Research, 33*(1), 104–111. https://doi.org/10.1519/jsc.0000000000002937

Waller, M., Piper, T., & Miller, J. (2009). Overhead pressing power/strength movements. *Strength and Conditioning Journal, 31*(5), 39–49. https://doi.org/10.1519/ssc.0b013e3181b95a49

Waller, M., & Townsend, R. (2007). The front squat and its variations. *Strength and Conditioning Journal, 29*(6), 14. https://journals.lww.com/nsca-scj/abstract/2007/12000/the_front_squat_and_its_variations.2.aspx

Webb, K., Heneghan, N., & Mahoney, T. (2017). The contribution of the thoracic spine to functional shoulder mobility in athletes: A systematic review. *Physiotherapy, 103*, e42–e43. https://doi.org/10.1016/j.physio.2017.11.207

Weldon, A., Duncan, M. J., Turner, A., LaPlaca, D., Sampaio, J., & Christie, C. J. (2022). Practices of strength and conditioning coaches: A snapshot from different sports, countries, and expertise levels. *Journal of Strength and Conditioning Research, 36*(5), 1335–1344. https://doi.org/10.1519/jsc.0000000000003773

Werner, I., Szelenczy, N., Wachholz, F., & Federolf, P. (2021). How do movement patterns in weightlifting (clean) change when using lighter or heavier barbell loads? A comparison of two principal component analysis-based approaches to studying technique. *Frontiers in Psychology, 11.* https://doi.org/10.3389/fpsyg.2020.606070

Wilczyński, B., Wąż, P., & Zorena, K. (2021). Impact of three strengthening exercises on dynamic knee valgus and balance with poor knee control among young football players: A randomized controlled trial. *Healthcare, 9*(5), 558. https://doi.org/10.3390/healthcare9050558

Winwood, P. W., Cronin, J. B., Brown, S. R., & Keogh, J. W. L. (2015). A biomechanical analysis of the strongman log lift and comparison with weightlifting's clean and jerk. *International Journal of Sports Science & Coaching, 10*(5), 869–886. https://doi.org/10.1260/1747-9541.10.5.869

Wirth, K., Hartmann, H., Mickel, C., Szilvas, E., Keiner, M., & Sander, A. (2017). Core stability in athletes: A critical analysis of current guidelines. *Sports Medicine, 47*(3), 401–414. https://doi.org/10.1007/s40279-016-0597-7

Yavuz, H. U., Erdağ, D., Amca, A. M., & Aritan, S. (2015). Kinematic and EMG activities during front and back squat variations in maximum loads. *Journal of Sports Sciences, 33*(10), 1058–1066. https://doi.org/10.1080/02640414.2014.984240

Ziv, G., & Lidor, R. (2010). Vertical jump in female and male volleyball players: A review of observational and experimental studies. *Scandinavian Journal of Medicine & Science in Sports, 20*(4), 556–567. https://doi.org/10.1111/j.1600-0838.2009.01083.x

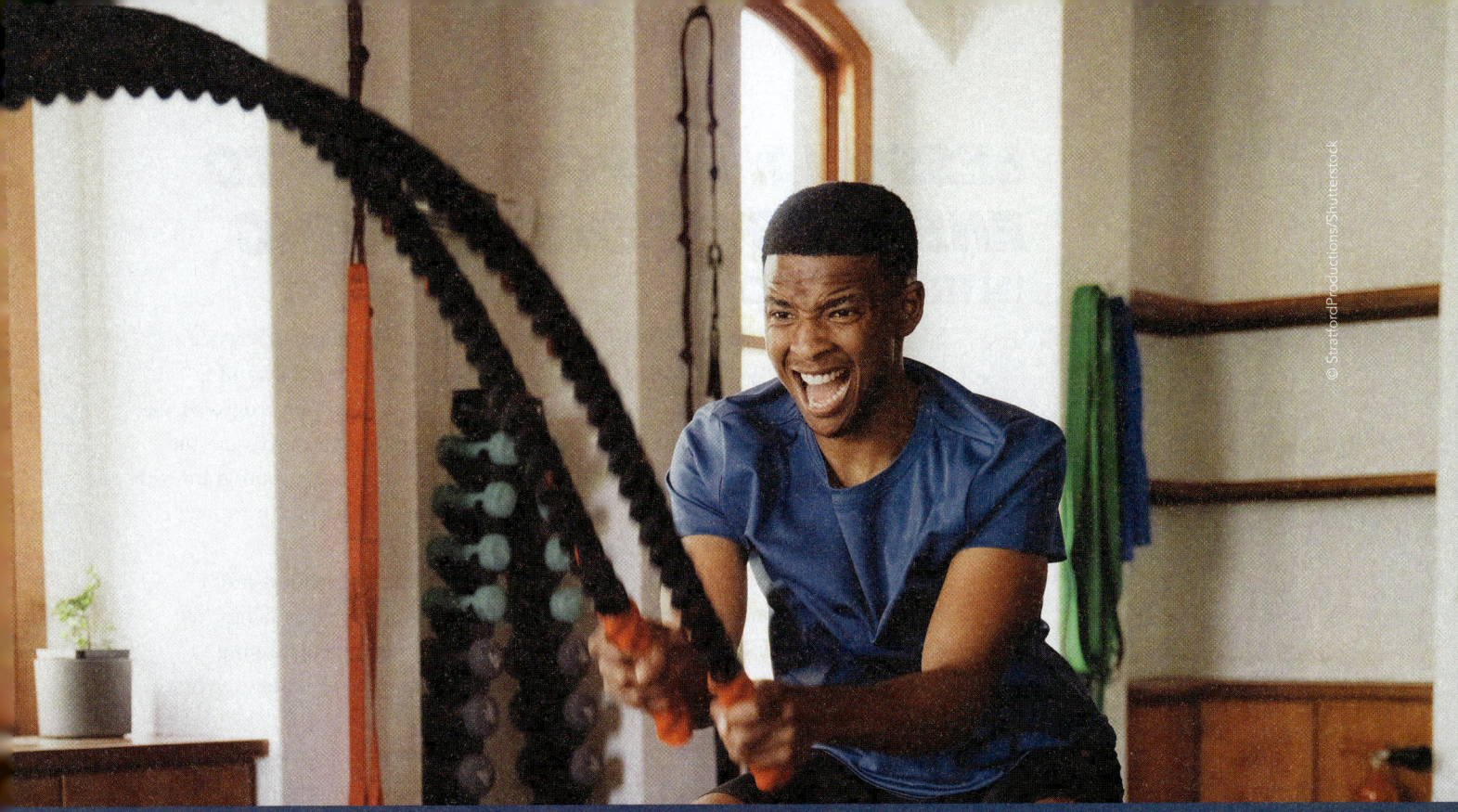

ENERGY SYSTEMS TRAINING FOR SPORTS PERFORMANCE

CHAPTER SIXTEEN

LEARNING OBJECTIVES

Upon completion of this chapter, the Sports Performance Coach will be able to:

- **Summarize** the importance of energy systems training for athletes with differing performance-related goals.
- **Describe** various modalities for energy systems training.
- **Identify** appropriate acute training variables using FITTE-VP to target specific energy systems.
- **Select** the appropriate energy systems training programs or techniques based on athlete needs or sports requirements.

LESSON 1: INTRODUCTION TO ENERGY SYSTEMS TRAINING

INTRODUCTION

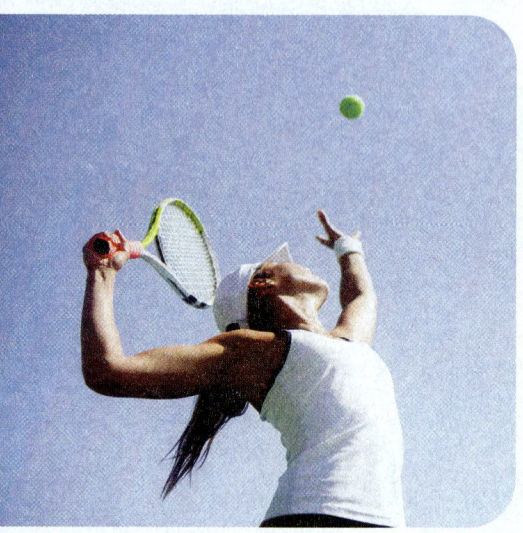

© NDAB Creativity/Shutterstock

Sports Performance Coaches must be creative in developing new cardiovascular (metabolic) training experiences. All athletes need goals and proper training guidelines to ensure continued growth, and personalized metabolic programs will go a long way toward achieving specific goals. To have a complete program, the Sports Performance Coach must first assess the athlete, then create a program with specific goals while applying a measurement tool (such as heart rate or rating of perceived exertion) to measure the athlete's progress.

Cardiorespiratory endurance is probably the most misunderstood and underrated component of a physical fitness program. Athletes often fail to understand why building an aerobic base is integral to a complete training program. However, without a proper base, performance may decrease over time, leading to underperformance and possible injury.

Many people incorrectly assume that metabolic energy system training is synonymous with aerobic exercise. This misunderstanding can delay or prevent athletes from realizing success from a program designed to meet goals specific to their sport. Metabolic energy system training is more than just training the aerobic energy system. To meet performance goals, both the anaerobic and aerobic energy systems must be trained. This is especially true for athletes who require top-end anaerobic energy system utilization while maximizing performance and minimizing fatigue (such as tennis players late in a match). This would be impossible if only the aerobic energy system were trained.

ENERGY PATHWAYS OVERVIEW

Without energy, the body cannot survive, much less perform physical work. This energy is provided in the form of adenosine triphosphate (ATP). The body produces ATP from the foods it consumes. ATP is a complex molecule consisting of a nitrogenous base (adenine), a sugar molecule (ribose), and three phosphate groups. The energy that the body gets from ATP is stored in the chemical bonds that hold the three phosphate groups together. When these chemical bonds are broken, energy from one of the phosphates is released for mechanical work (such as performing muscle contraction), leaving behind another molecule called **adenosine diphosphate (ADP)** and an extra phosphate group (**Figure 16.1**). ATP can be produced both aerobically (with oxygen) and anaerobically (without oxygen). The aerobic system is the most efficient and complex of these two methods (Kenney et al., 2020).

The chemical reactions that transform energy in the body's cells are collectively known as metabolism. It has been estimated that if a person could put all of the ATP in their body into a glass, its size might be between a shot glass and a small juice glass. As such a small amount of ATP is present at any given time, the body must continually produce ATP. For the purposes here, metabolism is understood to supply the energy needed to carry out the mechanical work of muscular contraction across the intensity spectrum (Kenney et al., 2020; Powers et al., 2021). At no time is only one system functioning; instead, all three systems supply energy constantly. The most prominent system depends on the duration, as seen in **Table 16.1**.

> **ADENOSINE DIPHOSPHATE (ADP)** →
>
> A high-energy compound occurring in all cells from which adenosine triphosphate is formed.

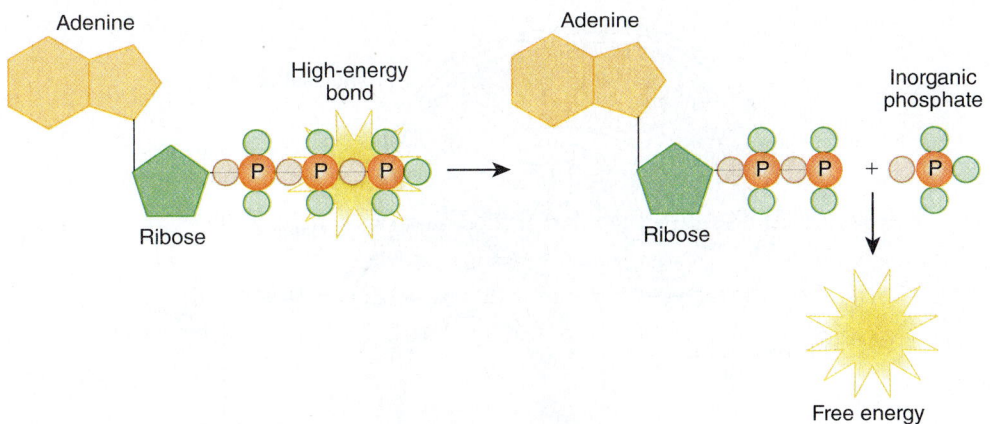

FIGURE 16.1 Conversion of ATP to ADP

TABLE 16.1 Exercise Duration for the Body's Energy Systems and Supplies Used

Estimate Time (s)	Energy System Used	Energy Supply Used
1–4	Anaerobic	ATP in muscle
4–20	Anaerobic	ATP + CP
20–45	Anaerobic	ATP + CP + muscle glycogen
45–120	Anaerobic and lactic	Muscle glycogen
120–240	Aerobic and anaerobic	Muscle glycogen + lactic acid
More than 240	Aerobic	Muscle glycogen + fatty acids

Abbreviations: ATP, adenosine triphosphate; CP, creatine phosphate.

Aerobic training stimulates the heart to adapt by becoming larger and stronger through exercise to supply the body's ever-increasing demand for oxygen. Aerobic energy production requires a constant and adequate supply of oxygen. At rest, the average heart beats approximately 70 beats per minute (bpm) (Kenney et al., 2020). However, the heart rate of a well-trained aerobic athlete can be as low as 40 bpm. The heart adapts to aerobic stress to become a more efficient pump by pumping more blood per beat, meaning it does not need to beat as often to supply the same amount of oxygen.

The respiratory system (**Figure 16.2**) begins with the lungs, which bring oxygen from the air across the alveolar membrane, and into the blood to be carried by hemoglobin. This process is called **pulmonary ventilation**. The movement of oxygen and carbon dioxide into and out of the circulatory system occurs through diffusion (Kenney et al., 2020).

The heart pumps blood out of the left ventricle and into the aorta with each contraction, distending it and creating pressure (systolic) on the vascular wall. During the relaxation phase of the cardiac cycle (between beats), the arterial system's blood pressure (diastolic) declines.

The amount of blood the heart pumps per minute is the **cardiac output**. This volume is determined by multiplying the heart rate by the **stroke volume**, which is the amount of blood pumped with each contraction of the ventricles (Powers et al., 2021). Cardiac

PULMONARY VENTILATION →

Breathing; transfer of oxygen from the air through the lungs into the bloodstream.

CARDIAC OUTPUT →

How much blood the heart pumps each minute; a product of heart rate × stroke volume.

STROKE VOLUME →

How much blood the heart pumps each beat.

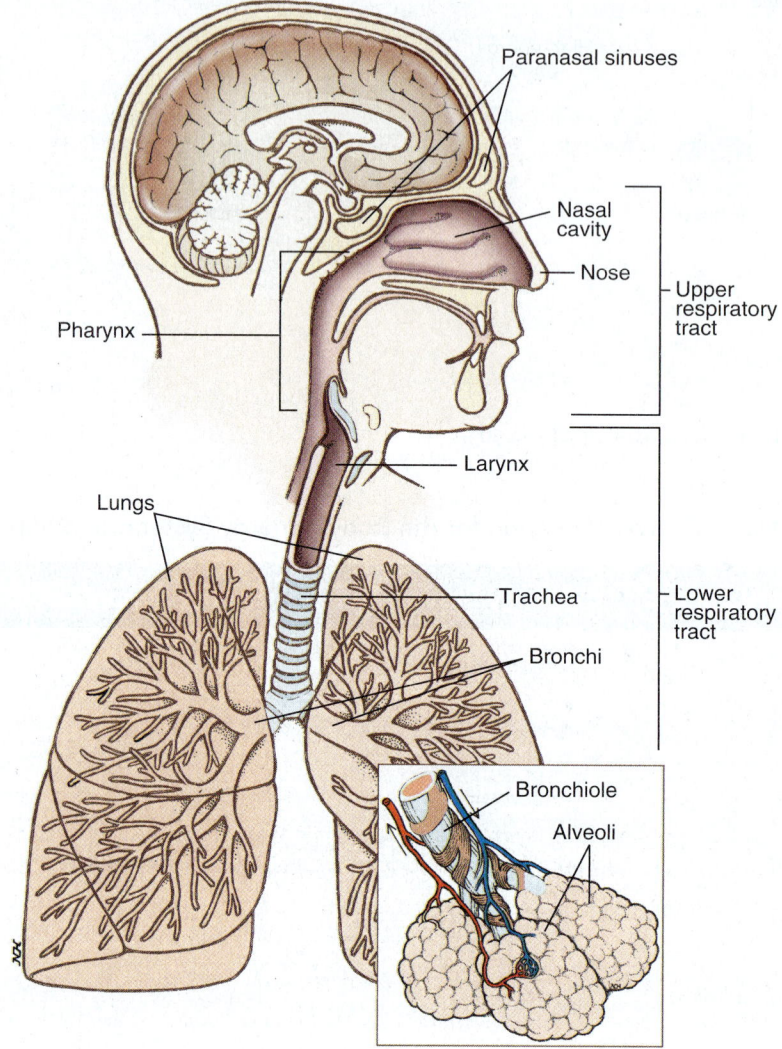

FIGURE 16.2 Respiratory Passages

Reproduced from Clark MA, Lucett SC, Sutton BG. NASM essentials of personal fitness training, 4th ed. Baltimore: Lippincott Williams & Wilkins, 2012. (not printing on page)

output and oxygen consumption are linearly related: As cardiac output increases, oxygen consumption will increase as well.

The body's oxygen requirement at rest (or **steady state**) is constant. A greater stroke volume means the heart beats more slowly. During exercise, the stroke volume generally increases in proportion to the exercise intensity up to approximately 40% of capacity. At that point, the stroke volume starts to plateau. With some elite endurance athletes, the stroke volume may continue to increase as exercise intensity increases above 40% of capacity. However, most athletes' increases in cardiac output that result in more than 40% intensity are due to the increased heart rate. With training, the response of the stroke volume to increasing intensity is the same, but it happens at a higher level due to the heart's increased pumping power. The heart rate response to increasing intensity is linear, and after prolonged training, the maximal heart rate is unchanged or slightly lower. The main reason that maximal cardiac output (and thus oxygen consumption) is improved with training is due to the increase in stroke volume. This change in stroke volume is one of the main central cardiovascular adaptations to training (Kenney et al., 2020; Powers et al., 2021).

STEADY STATE →

An exercise intensity at which the oxygen consumption is constant.

Heart rate can change from rest to its maximum level by approximately a factor of 3 (i.e., from 60 to 180 bpm), whereas stroke volume changes by only a factor of 1.7 (from 70 to 120 mL). Although increasing heart rate is the main factor in increasing cardiac output, if training increases the stroke volume by even a small amount, any increase in heart rate will translate into substantial changes in cardiac output. Resting cardiac output is typically approximately 6 L/min (i.e., 6 liters of blood per minute) at rest and 20 to 25 L/min during maximum exercise, but for aerobic elite athletes (e.g., cross-country skiers, rowers, cyclists), it may be exceed 40 L/min.

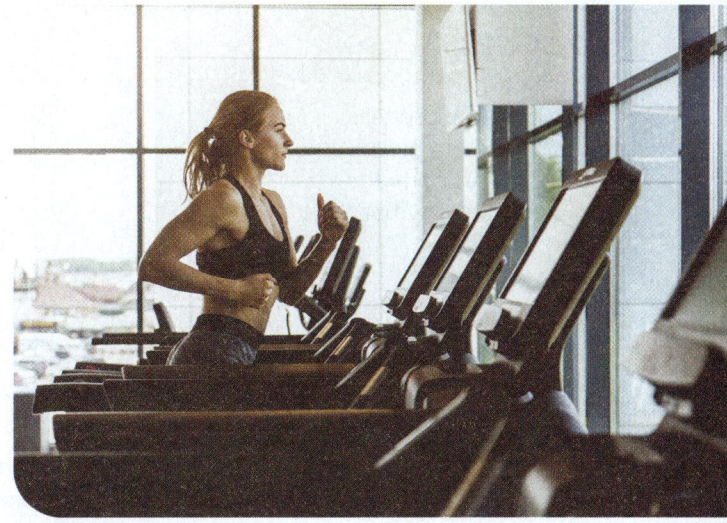

© XArtProduction/Shutterstock

No sport depends on a single energy system, so athletes in each sport need to focus on all of their energy systems during training. An example might be an athlete starting to jog on a treadmill going 7 mph (1.6 km/h). After the first step, the muscles have to increase the rate of ATP utilization to produce the required energy for the new physical demands of the 7-mph pace.

In the transition from rest to moderate exercise, oxygen consumption (or VO_2) increases rapidly and reaches a steady state within 1 to 4 minutes, depending on age and the athlete's level of fitness. The fact that the VO_2 does not increase instantaneously to a steady-state value means an anaerobic energy source has to contribute to the overall production of ATP at the beginning of exercise; at 7 mph, the energy demand of the first steps (well before steady state is reached) is the same as the last steps (well after attaining steady state), so the body must get the needed energy from somewhere. At the same time, the aerobic system "catches up" with its production of energy.

At the onset of exercise, the ATP-creatine phosphate (CP) system is the first active bioenergetic pathway that gives way first to glycolysis and then to aerobic energy production (Brooks, 1986). After a steady state is reached, the body's ATP requirement is met via the balanced delivery and use of oxygen through aerobic metabolism. The energy needed for exercise and sports is not provided by any single bioenergetic pathway, but rather comes from a mixture of several metabolic energy systems that overlap based on the intensity and duration of work.

ATP-CP SYSTEM

The most rapid source of ATP production uses CP to produce ATP anaerobically. This **ATP-CP system** is also referred to as the ATP-PC (phosphocreatine) system or the phosphagen system. The main advantage of the ATP-CP system is the speed at which energy can be supplied (its power). The main drawback is that not as much ATP can be produced as when using the aerobic system (i.e., limited capacity). ATP is produced rapidly via the ATP-CP system, but total production is limited. This system is heavily utilized to produce ATP in very high-power activities but has a low capacity for production (**Figure 16.3**).

The CP molecule is a high-energy compound. Once an ATP molecule has been split and its energy released to fuel mechanical work by the muscle, the energy in the CP molecule can be quickly transferred to the "used" ADP. A free phosphate molecule is attached, making a new ATP molecule. As with the muscle's store of ATP, there is a minimal supply of CP. If this was the sole energy source, exercise might be sustained for approximately 10 to 15 seconds (Kenney et al., 2020; Powers et al., 2021).

> **ATP-CP SYSTEM →**
>
> A rapid-acting energy system that utilizes creatine phosphate to create ATP; also referred to as the ATP-PC or phosphagen system.

GLYCOLYSIS →

A metabolic process that occurs in a cell's cytosol and converts glucose into pyruvate and adenosine triphosphate.

ANAEROBIC THRESHOLD →

The exercise intensity level at which energy demand is greater than the ability of aerobic metabolism to meet those demands.

LACTATE THRESHOLD →

The amount of lactate in the venous blood, which is typically set at 4 mmol/L of blood and at an exercise intensity below the anaerobic threshold.

GLUCOSE →

The simplest form of carbohydrate used by the body for energy.

GLYCOGEN →

Glucose that is deposited and stored in bodily tissues, such as the liver and muscle cells; the storage form of carbohydrates.

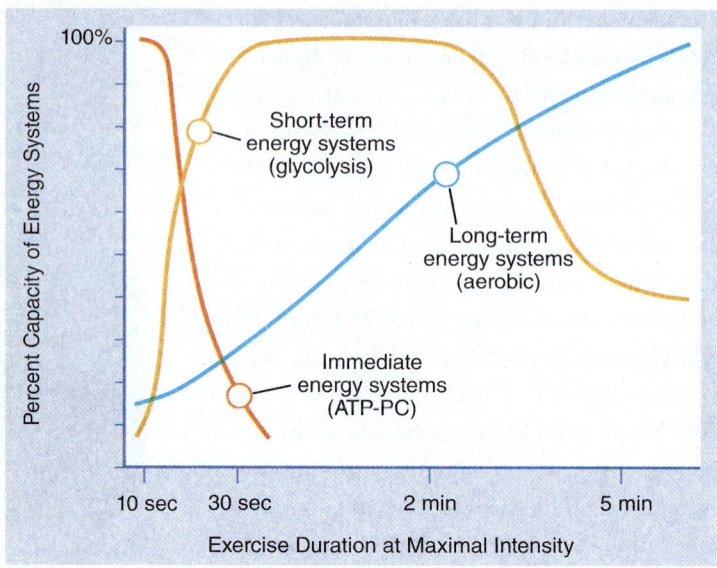

FIGURE 16.3 Energy Systems

Clark MA, Lucett SC, Sutton BG. NASM essentials of personal fitness training, 4th ed. Baltimore: Lippincott Williams & Wilkins, 2012. (not printing on page)

GLYCOLYSIS

Glycolysis, sometimes called the lactic acid (LA) system, is an anaerobic process. This system produces energy by metabolizing carbohydrates in the absence of oxygen. With increasing exercise intensity, the cardiorespiratory system makes every attempt to increase its delivery of oxygen to the mitochondria of the exercising muscle fibers to produce enough ATP aerobically.

At some point during training of increasing intensity, the cardiorespiratory system cannot supply enough oxygen to the exercising muscles, and energy production fails to meet energy needs. In turn, the body increases its reliance on the anaerobic systems to produce ATP rapidly enough to meet those needs. The intensity level at which oxygen supply cannot match the energy demand is referred to as the **anaerobic threshold**, and sometimes (erroneously) called the lactic threshold. Though these terms are often used interchangeably, the actual lactic threshold is reached before the anaerobic threshold.

The **lactate threshold** is determined by serial blood analysis at increasing exercise intensities, whereas the anaerobic threshold can be determined through submaximal VO_2 testing. Although the measurement of oxygen consumption requires some technical expertise and equipment, it is still practical to do in an exercise science setting due to its ease of testing versus the understandable reluctance of athletes to have repeated blood samples taken (Kenney et al., 2020; Powers et al., 2021).

The anaerobic system has high power (can achieve energy quickly) and a limited capacity. This energy pathway is often called the glycolytic (or lactic acid) system. The primary fuel for anaerobic ATP production is **glucose**, which is produced from the conversion of ingested carbohydrates and **glycogen** stored in muscles and the liver. Glycogen, a large molecule made up of chains of glucose, is the carbohydrate storage form. During muscle contraction, glucose is broken down into lactic acid. A small number of high-energy ATP molecules are produced during this breakdown of glucose. If glycolysis were the sole source of fuel for exercise, a person could continue for only a minute or so—hence the need for other energy pathways.

In skeletal muscle, this cycle occurs constantly at the myosin cross-bridges and must be continuously resupplied by ATP from glycolytic and aerobic energy sources. If glycolysis is the prominent source of ATP, an increased lactate level can slow the production of ATP. Lactate can be a precursor for ATP production via aerobic metabolism, but this process occurs more slowly than ATP production via the glycolytic pathway.

Lactic acid is continuously being produced and utilized, even when the body is at rest. When lactic acid is produced faster than it is used, it spills into the blood, and symptoms of fatigue become evident. A primary goal of training should be to minimize lactic acid production while enhancing lactic acid removal during exercise (Powers et al., 2021). One way to accomplish this is by combining high-intensity intervals and prolonged submaximal training.

Interval training helps maximize cardiorespiratory adaptation and increases VO_2 max (Helgerud et al., 2007). The more oxygen that is consumed, the lower the reliance on carbohydrates' anaerobic (especially glycolytic) breakdown will be. Prolonged submaximal training can help to induce an increase in mitochondrial structure and function. These adaptations will help reduce lactic acid formation by increasing the fractional utilization of fatty acids as a mitochondrial fuel source while facilitating lactic acid removal (Brooks, 1986; Donovan & Brooks, 1983).

🤖 GETTING TECHNICAL

What Is Lactic Acid?

During high-intensity exercise, ATP is needed faster than the cardiorespiratory system can deliver oxygen. Therefore, the body relies mainly on the ATP-CP system and glycolysis for energy when intensities push toward maximal levels. As pyruvate accumulates in an anaerobic environment, it is quickly converted to lactate, releasing a free hydrogen ion in the process.

As they are released, these hydrogen ions contribute to decreased muscle pH, a condition known as acidosis. Acidosis can lead to some of the feelings of pain and fatigue associated with intense exercise because the hydrogen ions that lower pH can interfere with muscle contraction. As a result, tissue pH shifts toward becoming acidic; the lactate and hydrogen ions produced during anaerobic glycolysis are often collectively termed lactic acid.

Lactate is not an actual "waste product" in the same way the CO_2 is. Once it has been removed from soft-tissue cells and enters the bloodstream, instead of being removed from the body, lactate is processed by the liver in a separate metabolic process called the Cori cycle. During the Cori cycle, ATP converts lactate in the opposite direction back to pyruvate and subsequently glucose (Cori & Cori, 1929). This glucose is then released back into the bloodstream to be used again. In this way, the Cori cycle plays an essential role in helping keep the body's pH balanced.

OXIDATIVE SYSTEM

Aerobic exercise requires the body to take oxygen from the atmosphere, deliver it to the lungs, transfer it into the blood, and pump it to the working muscles, where it is used to oxidize carbohydrates, fats, and, to a small degree, protein to produce ATP. This energy pathway, which is often termed the **oxidative system**, involves several body systems, including the respiratory, cardiovascular, muscular, and endocrine systems. The oxidative system consists of two energy pathways: the Krebs cycle and the electron transport chain.

Through a complex series of chemical reactions, glycogen and fats are broken down in the presence of oxygen to provide energy to be transferred to ATP. During rest and light, low-intensity activity, the energy required for muscle contraction comes almost entirely from the aerobic production of ATP.

Most cells (including muscle fibers) contain mitochondria, which are the site of aerobic ATP production (**Figure 16.4**). The greater the number and volume of mitochondria, the greater the cell's aerobic energy production capabilities will be. Aerobic reactions generate more than 99% of the energy required during prolonged exercise. These aerobic pathways provide the principal energy supply to all body cells through the metabolism of circulating glucose, stored fats, and stored carbohydrates. Because the amount of stored carbohydrates is limited, one of the most important adaptations to training is the shift by the body from using carbohydrates to using stored fat as a primary fuel for energy (Kenney et al., 2020; Powers et al., 2021).

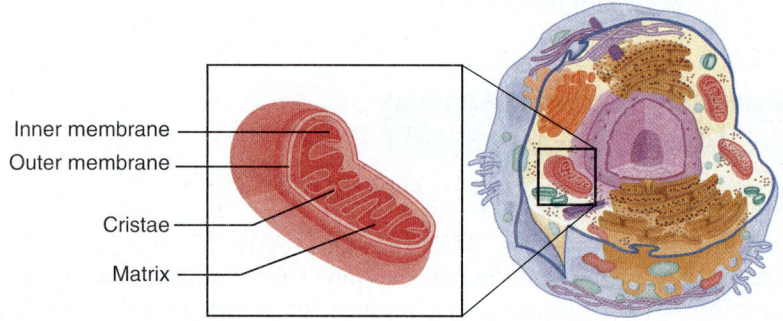

FIGURE 16.4 Mitochondria

When the muscles are used aerobically, they use fat and glucose to produce ATP. The aerobic system makes much more ATP than the anaerobic system does and yields far more ATP when using fat as fuel. This performance primarily reflects the ability to convert fat, which yields 9 calories of energy per gram, whereas glucose produces only about half that amount (4 calories per gram). Additionally, the waste products of aerobic ATP production are water and CO_2, both of which are quickly processed by the body. As a result, aerobic energy production is a more efficient method of generating energy and averting muscle fatigue (Kenney et al., 2020; Powers et al., 2021).

LESSON 2: MECHANISMS OF ENERGY UTILIZATION
ENERGY DURING EXERCISE

During exercise, the body metabolizes ATP as fuel. ATP production comes from all three energy systems, and whatever the duration or intensity of the exercise session, all three energy systems work to provide ATP. The duration and intensity of a session determine the energy contributions from each of the three energy systems. **Table 16.2** shows the energy contributions from each energy system for various activities. As can

TABLE 16.2 Percentage of Each Energy System Used During Sports Activities

Sport	ATP/CP (%)	Glycolysis (%)	Oxidative (%)
Basketball	60	20	20
Fencing	90	10	0
Field events	90	10	0
Golf (swing)	95	5	0
Gymnastics	80	15	5
Hockey	50	20	30
Running (distance)	10	20	70
Rowing	20	30	50
Skiing	33	33	33
Soccer	50	20	30
Sprints	90	10	0
Swimming (1,500 m)	10	20	70
Tennis	20	70	10
Volleyball	80	5	15

be seen in the table, the longer the duration of the activity, the greater the reliance on oxidative metabolism will be. Longer-duration work is typically a steady state or training at a constant intensity for a specific period. The longer the duration and the lower the intensity, the greater the reliance on oxidative metabolism for ATP production will be. Intermittent work typically relies more heavily on the glycolytic and ATP-CP systems for ATP production. Shorter intervals will more strongly tax the ATP-CP system than longer intervals, placing more significant stress on the glycolytic system. Proper metabolic programming includes steady-state and intermittent training sessions, with the programming individualized to each athlete's sports goals.

METABOLISM DURING STEADY-STATE WORK

Steady-state training can be divided into three categories, which differ primarily on the intensity at which the athlete will exercise. These categories are **moderate-intensity continuous training (MICT)**, **race pace (RP)**, and **percentage of maximum heart rate (% HR$_{max}$)**.

The predominant energy system utilized during steady-state work is aerobic metabolism. MICT is almost always at a lower intensity than the other categories of steady-state work. The lower the intensity of steady-state work, the greater the utilization of stored glycogen and fat as a fuel source for the oxidative metabolic system will be.

MODERATE-INTENSITY CONTINUOUS TRAINING (MICT) →

Continuous training at a medium intensity with the goal of completing a set amount of time.

RACE PACE (RP) →

Training at a pace that would be maintained during a competitive event.

PERCENTAGE OF MAXIMUM HEART RATE (% HR$_{MAX}$) →

Training at an intended percentage of maximum heart rate for a continuous amount of time.

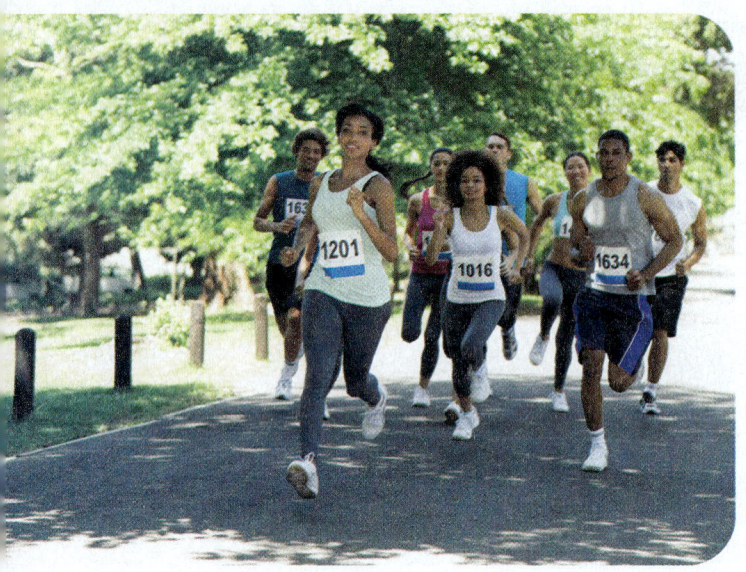
© Wavebreakmedia/Shutterstock

At higher steady-state intensities, such as during RP training, ATP production still occurs primarily from oxidative metabolism, but glucose will be used more significantly as a fuel. This is because there is a greater and faster need for ATP when exercising at higher intensities, and glucose provides a rapid fuel source.

MICT is typically performed for a longer duration and at a low to moderate training intensity. The goal is to complete the amount of time programmed rather than integrating various exercise intensities. This method of training improves maximal aerobic capacity. However, as research has shown, MICT is not the only way to improve aerobic capacity; in some instances, interval training may have similar effects (Nicolò et al., 2014). RP involves training at the same pace maintained during a competitive event.

For those athletes who consistently participate in endurance events, identifying this pace requires calculating the rate from the most recent event. For athletes who compete at various distances, multiple RPs are used. For example, a triathlete might have a 10-kilometer run RP and a half-marathon run RP if they participated in Olympic distance and half Ironman distance events. A time trial can be administered occasionally to identify an RP for those athletes who do not compete in endurance events. Then, this pace is programmed for a specific time to sustain that pace for the entire workout.

Like measuring a one-repetition maximum (1RM) in weight training and using that as a baseline for loading during each workout, calculating a percentage of the RP enables the programming of workouts that alter stress based on maximal effort. This stress can vary between 75% and 110% of RP for various times. Higher intensities are sustained for less time than lower intensities, with each workout contributing to the overall development of metabolic energy system fitness. For example, if an athlete sustained an 8-minute mile pace during a recent half-marathon, this RP could be used to create percentages of pace for training. At 75% of that pace, the athlete would sustain a pace of about 10 minutes per mile; faster paces of 110% could be performed (approximately 7:12 minutes per mile pace) but for shorter distances.

✔ CHECK IT OUT

Race pace will not be performed at 100% of the athlete's maximal effort. Thus, the athlete can train at 110% of their heart rate at RP, as they will not be reaching their HR_{max} effort.

METABOLISM DURING INTERMITTENT WORK

Interval training has drawn significant research attention (Helgerud et al., 2007; Milanović et al., 2015; Weston et al., 2014). This training concept enables higher-intensity effort by providing bouts of recovery between each repetition of exertion. Work-to-rest ratios can be calculated and altered to change the stress applied during each workout. Generally, ratios ranging from 1:1 to 1:5 are utilized to provide adequate recovery within each interval. Higher-intensity efforts and shorter recovery periods increase the training demand and add to the overall stress. Sports Performance Coaches can alter the intensity and work-to-rest ratios to vary training stress throughout the program.

High-intensity intervals challenge the metabolic energy systems by pushing the athlete to near-maximal effort during each repetition. Intervals rely heavily on the ATP-CP and glycolytic energy systems. Shorter-duration and higher-intensity intervals will place more emphasis on the ATP-CP system. The recovery periods are essential to allow the resynthesis of ATP. As the interval length increases, albeit still at intensities well above steady state, there will be increased reliance on the glycolytic energy system for ATP. This switch to glycolysis results in the production of lactic acid. Although lactic acid has been considered a waste product, it is now understood that lactate can be utilized as fuel. Lactate may be used as fuel in the working muscles or transported to other muscle cells for use as fuel. The recovery period also allows buffering of the hydrogen ions from lactic acid, which is essential to execute the next interval at a suitable intensity.

More extended recovery periods are often needed during highly intense intervals to promote recovery in preparation for another bout of intense effort. These intervals are best suited for highly trained athletes or occasional challenges to beginning exercisers. Adequate training and preparation time should enable athletes to prepare for the exertion required in these workouts.

Repeated sprints are a style of interval training shown to be just as effective for improving metabolic energy system fitness as continuous endurance training—only at a reduced total volume—and involve maximal effort in repeated periods of work lasting up to 10 seconds, followed by periods of complete recovery (Gist et al., 2014; Sloth et al., 2013). This type of training is designed to enhance power and power endurance while allowing the metabolic systems ample time to recover between each repetition.

Repeated sprint workouts are highly demanding; athletes must be adequately prepared by completing a considerable amount of time in moderate- and high-intensity interval training, along with sufficient steady-state exercise to build a good foundation of fitness. Once athletes have participated in at least 2 months of consistent interval and steady-state training, they may be prepared for repeated sprint sessions. The Sports Performance Coach should start with short distance sprints (20 to 30 yards) with more extended rest periods between sprints (60 to 90 seconds) to gauge tolerance. If the athlete tolerates this approach, sprint distances may be extended, and rest periods shortened as tolerated by the athlete.

MEASURING INTENSITY

Several methods may be used to measure exercise intensity. Typically, training programs are designed around different levels or percentages of intensity. The decision to utilize a specific strategy will depend on various factors, including, but not limited to, equipment availability, number of athletes, level of athletic performance, and athlete goals. The key point to remember is that whatever intensity measure is chosen should provide valid and reliable data.

The predominant energy system(s) for a sport and equipment availability also help determine the methods used to measure exercise intensity. For example, athletes participating in sports with a heavy reliance on oxidative energy metabolism,

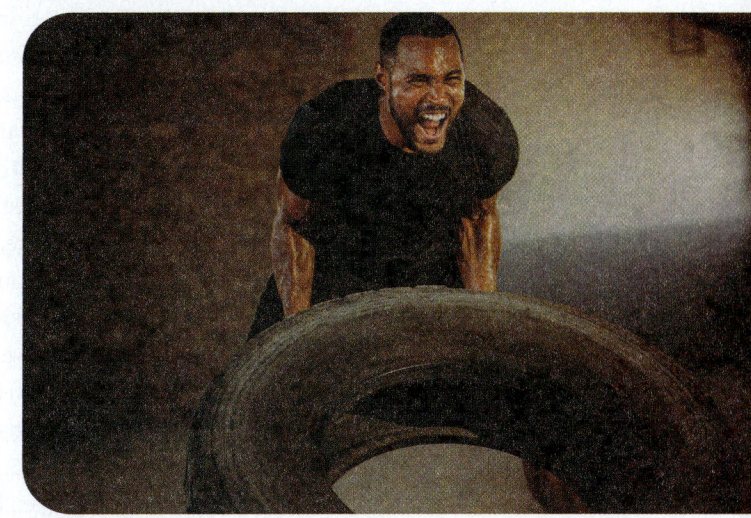

© Jacob Lund/Shutterstock

such as cross-country events, may benefit from measuring the VO_2 max of athletes. However, for athletes participating in sports that are more anaerobic, such as football or sprint events in track, the Sports Performance Coach might want to consider other methods of measuring intensity more applicable to the shorter anaerobic nature of the sport. The talk test or rating of perceived exertion (RPE) can be beneficial, especially when conducting team training sessions with large numbers of athletes.

> ### ⚠ CRITICAL
>
> **Identifying Overtraining**
> Be sure to monitor athletes for signs and symptoms of overtraining, including the following:
>
> - Inability to reach training zones that previously were attainable
> - Disrupted sleep patterns
> - Workouts described by the athlete as "draining"
> - Lack of feeling "refreshed" in the morning or following sufficient recovery time
>
> The importance of recovery days to an athlete's health and progress should be evident. As stress accumulates during a training cycle, monitoring sleep, nutrition, and wellness is essential to ensure sufficient recovery and regeneration between workouts.

VO_2 MAX

VO_2 max (maximum oxygen consumption) is a standard measurement of aerobic capacity that measures the maximal amount of oxygen an individual can consume in a minute. Measurement of VO_2 max usually takes place in a sports science laboratory; however, portable gas analyzers can provide valid and reliable VO_2 max measurements (Guidetti et al., 2018). Once a VO_2 max value is obtained, a training program can be developed based on exercise intensities expressed as a percentage of VO_2 max.

VO_2 max is commonly measured while running, although VO_2 max testing protocols also exist for exercises other than running, including cycling, rowing, and kayaking/canoeing. Most athletes will have the highest VO_2 max levels when tested via a protocol that utilizes the most commonly used exercise type. When an athlete engages in multiple types of exercise (for example, a triathlete), the highest oxygen uptake value obtained is the VO_2 max. Values obtained while testing with other types of exercise are defined as VO_2 peak. For example, a triathlete might have a VO_2 max measured during running, with the highest oxygen uptake seen during cycling being called the cycling VO_2 peak.

Measuring VO_2 max requires the use of a respiratory gas analysis system, which is expensive. It also takes more than 20 minutes to conduct a test, which may mean that it is not a realistic option when working with large groups of athletes. However, if access to the equipment is available, a seasonal or yearly VO_2 max test for athletes who rely heavily on aerobic metabolism may help with long-term program design and metabolic system development.

Sports such as running, rowing, and cycling rely heavily on maintaining or increasing an exercise intensity for 3 minutes or longer and will be highly dependent on maintaining and improving VO_2 max. For athletes participating in these sports, improving VO_2 max and developing glycolytic energy systems will significantly benefit performance. For sports with a smaller reliance on oxidative metabolism, knowing the athlete's maximal oxygen uptake is probably not beneficial. For example, improving aerobic metabolic conditioning for a football player, gymnast, or Olympic weightlifter can enhance training by increasing the recovery rate from high-intensity work. However, because the performance relies heavily on non-oxidative energy sources, knowing the VO_2 max of athletes in these types of sports would not likely influence training program design.

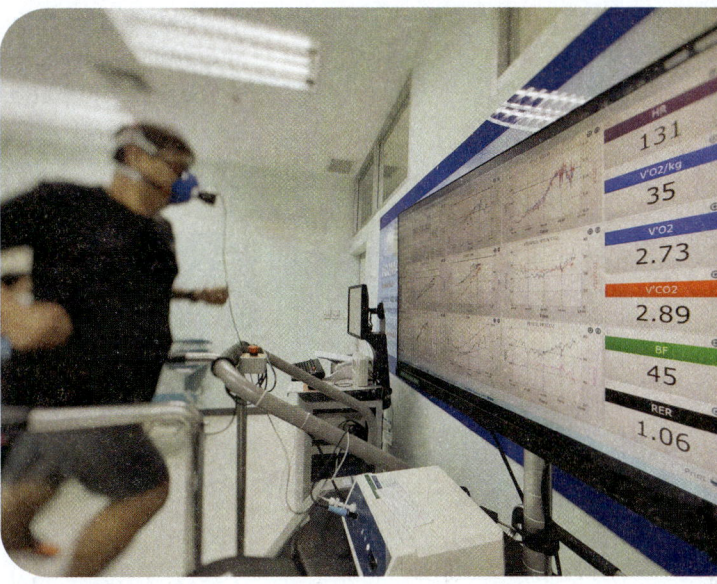

© Sasapin Kanka/Shutterstock

MAXIMUM HEART RATE

Maximum heart rate (HR_{max}) formulas are equations used to estimate HR_{max} for the purpose of developing exercise training intensity zones. The formula 220 – age is probably the most well-known calculation; however, it is not as accurate as the **Tanaka formula** (Nikolaidis et al., 2018; Roy & McCrory, 2015):

$$HR_{max} = 208 - (0.7 \times age)$$

Both the HR_{max}, or estimated HR_{max}, and the resting heart rate (HR_{rest}) are needed to develop training intensities using the Karvonen formula (discussed next). The best time to measure HR_{rest} is immediately after waking in the morning but before getting out of bed. An easy method is to measure the radial pulse on the wrist for 15 seconds and multiply it by 4 to obtain HR_{rest}. If the athlete uses a wearable device that measures heart rate, they can use that to get HR_{rest}.

HEART RATE RESERVE

Heart rate reserve (HRR) is the difference between HR_{max} or estimated HR_{max} and HR_{rest}. The **Karvonen formula** uses the concept of the HRR to determine exercise training zones (Karvonen et al., 1957). There are three standard heart rate training zones ranging from 65% to 95% of HR_{max}, as shown in **Table 16.3**.

TABLE 16.3 Heart Rate Reserve Training Zones Based on % HR_{max} or HRR

HRR Training Zone	% HR_{max}	Purpose
Zone 1	65%–75%	Warm up, cool down, recovery, building an aerobic base
Zone 2	76%–85%	Increase aerobic and anaerobic capacity by "straddling" the energy systems; moderate-intensity interval training and moderate-intensity continuous training
Zone 3	86%–95%	High-intensity interval training

The Karvonen formula is:

$$Target\ heart\ rate = [(HR_{max} - HR_{rest}) \times exercise\ intensity] + HR_{rest}$$

The Karvonen formula gives a reasonable guideline for training heart rate. More precise statements can be made from metabolic measurements such as ventilatory

TANAKA FORMULA →

A formula used to calculate an estimated maximum heart rate: $HR_{max} = 208 - (0.7 \times age)$.

HEART RATE RESERVE (HRR) →

Difference between HR_{max} or estimated HR_{max} and HR_{rest}: $HRR = HR_{max} - HR_{rest}$.

KARVONEN FORMULA →

A formula using the heart rate reserve to calculate exercise intensities: Target heart rate = $[(HR_{max} - HR_{rest}) \times exercise\ intensity] + HR_{rest}$.

thresholds, lactic acid accumulation, or others requiring technical expertise and equipment not available to most Sports Performance Coaches.

These formulas also can have some limitations when applied across the age spectrum. **Table 16.4** provides an example using a 25-year-old athlete.

TABLE 16.4   Estimated Heart Rate Maximum Example

25-Year-Old Athlete with a Resting Heart Rate of 40 bpm	25-Year-Old Athlete with a Resting Heart Rate of 70 bpm
$208 - (0.7 \times 25) = 191$ bpm	$208 - (0.7 \times 25) = 191$ bpm
$191 - 40\ (HR_{rest}) = 151$ bpm	$191 - 70\ (HR_{rest}) = 121$ bpm
$151 \times 85\% = 128$ bpm	$121 \times 85\% = 103$ bpm
$128 + 40 = 168$ bpm	$103 + 70 = 173$ bpm

> **TALK TEST** →
>
> A test used to determine athletes' ability to talk at different exercise intensities.

Many factors could affect heart rate zones, so using a set formula will not always yield a precise result. The Karvonen method, however, provides a usable and widely accepted guideline. For more experienced athletes who train and compete with heart rate monitors, it may be possible to obtain actual HR_{max} values instead of relying on formulas that estimate HR_{max}. Heart rate monitors store heart rates, and the Sports Performance Coach can download these data to determine the highest heart rate achieved by the athlete.

However, using the talk test and the heart rates derived from VT1 and VT2 testing may be a better intensity-monitoring method because they fit better with the stage training model (discussed in the next section).

> **VENTILATORY** →
> **THRESHOLD 1**
> **(VT1)**
>
> The exercise intensity at which talking becomes challenging; at this point, there is a switch from reliance on mostly aerobic metabolism to a greater reliance on anaerobic metabolism.

> ⚠ **CRITICAL**
>
> When using equations that utilize estimates of HR_{max}, remember that the results are estimates. If these equations are used to suggest training intensity, caution is warranted to avoid over- or under-programming of training intensity.

TALK TEST

The **talk test** method can also be used to monitor exercise intensity. As exercise intensity increases, at some point, it will become difficult for the athlete to speak for more than approximately 15 seconds—a point called **ventilatory threshold 1 (VT1)**. As the intensity continues to increase, there will be an intensity level where it is not possible for the athlete to talk, which is termed **ventilatory threshold 2 (VT2)**. Research has found a relationship between the talk test, oxygen uptake, heart rate, and ventilatory threshold during cycling and running (Jeanes et al., 2011; Reed & Pipe, 2016).

> **VENTILATORY** →
> **THRESHOLD 2**
> **(VT2)**
>
> The exercise intensity at which only single-word speech is possible; the highest exercise intensity at which an athlete can work for a few minutes.

One main benefit of using the talk test is that it is easy to administer and does not require extensive equipment. Due to the ease of administration, it is possible to regularly perform the talk test to identify changes in VT1 and VT2 as metabolic conditioning improves. These changes will also allow the Sports Performance Coach to recognize that as VT1 and VT2 change, there are also concomitant changes in the heart rates for the training zones identified from VT1 and VT2.

VT1 testing is aerobic testing described in Chapter 8: Sports Performance Testing and Evaluation. The goal of a VT1 test is to determine the highest level of exercise intensity at which an athlete can speak clearly and consistently for 20 seconds. **Table 16.5** provides an example using a 20-year-old athlete.

TABLE 16.5 Example of VT1 Testing with a 20-Year-Old Female Soccer Athlete

Time (min)	Speed	Talk Test	Heart Rate (bpm)	RPE (0–10)
0–4 (warm-up)	5		120	
5	5.5	Easy	124	3
6	6	Easy	131	3.5
7	6.5	Somewhat easy	135	4
8	7	Somewhat easy	138	4
9	7.5	Challenging	142	5.5
10	8	Difficult	150	6
11–14 (cool-down)				

VT2 testing is a higher-workload aerobic test that is also described in detail in Chapter 8: Sports Performance Testing and Evaluation. VT2 is considered a critical measurement of athletic performance because the intensity immediately below this level represents the exercise pace that an endurance athlete can sustain throughout their race or training to attain their best performance. VT2 testing is recommended only for athletes with endurance performance goals, given the purpose, nature, and intensity required for measuring this physiological marker. **Table 16.6** provides an example using a 20-year-old athlete.

TABLE 16.6 Example of VT2 Testing Running: 20-Year-Old Female Soccer Athlete

Time (Minutes 16–20) of the 20-Minute Test	Heart Rate (bpm)
Minute 16	184
Minute 17	186
Minute 18	186
Minute 19	185
Minute 20	185

Average heart rate = 185.2 × 0.95 = 175.8 rounded up to 176 bpm

VT2 = 176 bpm

RATING OF PERCEIVED EXERTION

Rating of perceived exertion (RPE) is a subjective measure of exercise intensity. The original RPE had values from 6–20 (**Table 16.7**), but a more recently developed scale runs from 0–10 (**Table 16.8**). Individuals rate their exercise intensity subjectively based on physiological factors, including increases in heart rate, breathing rate, sweating, and feelings of fatigue (Williams, 2017). For adults, accurate subjective rating using the 6–20 scale can correspond with heart rate. However, this scale often confuses individuals because it does not start at 1. If the Sports Performance Coach uses RPE for monitoring intensity, then using the 0–10 scale is recommended unless the athlete is already familiar with the original 6–20 scale.

Using RPE to measure exertion has several benefits or advantages for the Sports Performance Coach. It is easy to administer and does not require special equipment other than an RPE chart. It is also easy to administer during a training session, even if the session involves a large number of athletes. Finally, because it is a perceived exertion scale, the RPE scale can potentially identify the need for training session modification. For example, if an athlete enters a training session already fatigued or dehydrated, or the training session is conducted during an unusually hot time, then the RPE rating by the

TABLE 16.7 Original RPE 6–20 Scale

Rating	Perceived Exertion Scale
6	
7	Very, very light
8	
9	Very light
10	
11	Fairly light
12	
13	Somewhat hard
14	
15	Hard
16	
17	Very hard
18	
19	Very, very hard
20	

TABLE 16.8   RPE 1–10 Scale

Rating	Perceived Exertion Scale
0	No exertion, at rest
1	Very light
2–3	Light
4–5	Moderate, somewhat hard
6–7	High, vigorous
8–9	Very hard
10	Maximum effort, highest possible

athlete will take this factor into consideration. This benefits Sports Performance Coaches because they can make immediate adaptations to exercise programming strategies. **Table 16.9** provides a summary of methods for programming cardiorespiratory exercise intensity.

TABLE 16.9   Summary of Cardiorespiratory Exercise Intensity

Method	Description
VO_2 max	Target VO_2 max = VO_2 max $\times$ % intensity desired
Maximal heart rate (HR_{max}) formula	Tanaka HR_{max} formula: 208 – (0.7 $\times$ age) Target heart rate = HR_{max} $\times$ % intensity desired
Heart rate reserve (HRR) formula	Target heart rate = [(HR_{max} – HR_{rest}) $\times$ % intensity desired] + HR_{rest}
Talk test	The ability to speak during activity can identify exercise intensity and ventilatory thresholds (VT1, VT2)
Rating of perceived exertion (RPE)	0–10 scale or 6–20 scale

LESSON 3: ENERGY SYSTEMS TRAINING MODES

TRAINING MODES

As with selection of the exercise type, or modality, various methods can be employed to help athletes reach training goals. Each method differs based on the total stress applied to the metabolic processes by using a unique challenge. For instance, interval training stresses the body's ability to recover from an intense bout of exertion. By comparison, long-distance running presents a more significant challenge to aerobic energy production over time.

By stimulating the body's energy systems in different ways, exercise can promote various physiological adaptations that facilitate overall endurance performance. Training methods can be divided into two main categories: steady-state and interval training. The difference between these categories is the use of consistent, prolonged intensity versus repeating work periods punctuated by recovery segments. Each is highly effective at producing specific performance adaptations, and each has value in strategically improving metabolic energy system fitness within an athlete's training plan.

HIGH-INTENSITY INTERVAL TRAINING

High-intensity interval training (HIIT) is often defined as training at or above 90% of VO_2 peak for bouts lasting seconds to minutes (Gibala & McGee, 2008). HIIT usually involves many repetitions of these short bouts per exercise session interspersed with rest that can be either complete (passive) or active, low-intensity recovery for 2–3 minutes between bouts (Gibala et al., 2012; Gibala & McGee, 2008).

Another example of HIIT frequently used in research studies to elicit the HIIT-induced effects is a session of 4 to 6 back-to-back Wingate tests with about 4 minutes of recovery between each test (Burgomaster et al., 2008; Gibala et al., 2012; Little et al., 2011). Despite the short duration and very high intensity, HIIT specifically targets the cellular pathways involved in aerobic respiration and energy (ATP) generation, rather than the metabolic pathways related to muscle protein synthesis (i.e., mTOR) (Baar, 2006; Bartlett et al., 2012).

HIIT is as good as, but not necessarily superior to, traditional endurance training (i.e., long-slow distance) for increasing mitochondrial content and activity. The advantage of HIIT is the much smaller time investment needed to elicit these adaptations. HIIT is not necessarily a substitute for long-slow distance because longer-duration exercises improve cardiovascular function (stroke volume, cardiac output, vasodilation) and improve running economy (Goodman et al., 2005; Joyner & Coyle, 2008).

However, it is vital to understand the mechanism of HIIT-induced adaptations at the cellular level, so training can be designed to target those adaptations as needed. Specifically, HIIT induces the following adaptations in very time-efficient ways (i.e., 30 total minutes of activity per week [not counting rest] for 2 to 6 weeks):

- Increased synthesis of new mitochondria allows for improved fat oxidation and ATP production.
- Increased mitochondrial biogenesis leads to better energy production (defense of the cellular energy state) and improved fatigue resistance.
- Mitochondria are better able to oxidize fatty acids.
- Sparing muscle glycogen prolongs time to exhaustion, resulting in less lactate production and delayed fatigue.

As a result of these factors, there is a better defense of the cellular energy state, less lactate production, glycogen sparing, increased fatty acid oxidation, and improved fatigue resistance, especially in type II muscle fibers, which have less fatigue resistance in the absence of HIIT training. Understanding the metabolic demands of a specific sport allows for programming that maximizes metabolic system development specific to a sport.

Some sports, such as soccer and basketball, require almost continuous movement during competition, with varying intensities. HIIT programming for sports like these may benefit from active rest to best mimic the intermittent nature of the sport. Other sports, such as golf, field events, and sprints (track and field), require a single high-intensity activity, followed by a significant period before the next exercise. Programming HIIT for these sports should be designed to mimic the lower load and higher intensity

HIGH-INTENSITY INTERVAL TRAINING (HIIT) →

Training intensities that range from seconds to minutes; usually multiple repetitions, with rest between each repetition.

demands. HIIT programming, as with all aspects of metabolic programming, considers the sport-specific needs, training status, and goals of each athlete.

TABATA TRAINING

Tabata training is a HIIT protocol designed by Japanese researcher Izumi Tabata (Tabata et al., 1996). The Tabata protocol is a cycle ergometer protocol of seven or eight 20-second intervals with 10 seconds of rest between each interval (Tabata, 2019). The goal is exhaustion after the seventh or eighth interval. The benefits of Tabata training match those described for HIIT. A strict Tabata training session is not commonly done because the interval intensities are well above VO_2 max, and the protocol lasts for only 4 minutes. However, the principles of Tabata training may be used when designing HIIT sessions.

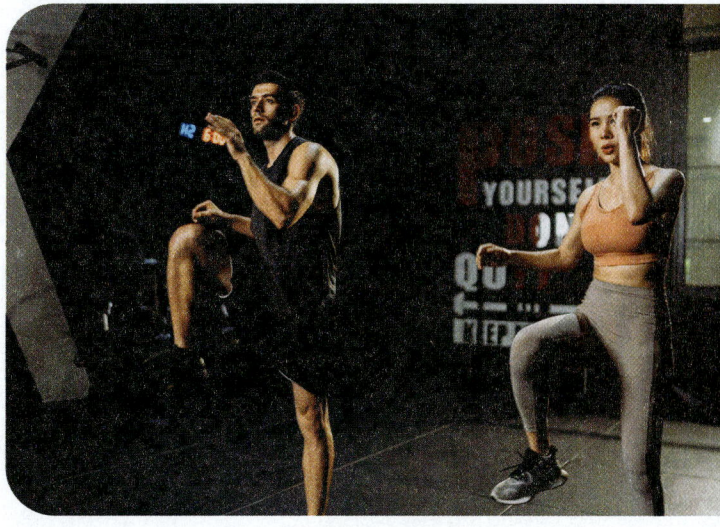

© MMD Creative/Shutterstock

Tabata training should be incorporated judiciously into an athlete's overall training regimen. Coaches and athletes should always consider individual fitness levels, sport-specific demands, and recovery needs when devising any training program. Athletes engaged in sports that require intermittent bursts of high-intensity effort, such as soccer, basketball, hockey, or rugby, stand to gain significantly from this training method. The intense bursts of exercise in Tabata training mirror the high-intensity sprints and efforts seen in these sports, helping athletes improve their ability to recover quickly and perform at their best during critical game moments.

FARTLEK TRAINING

Fartlek training, also known "speed play," is a Swedish term. This type of interval training is unstructured: There are no set work or recovery periods, and the exercise intensity is typically unstructured. The idea is to combine some of the benefits of aerobic and anaerobic training into a single workout. Traditionally, fartlek workouts were running activities, but many athletes may find this training beneficial when combined with other types of exercise such as cycling. Team sports such as soccer, field hockey, and lacrosse can also benefit from integrating fartlek training. Train runs (caboose runs) can be used as a form of interval training. In sports with athletes of various fitness levels, dividing the team into several fitness levels, with separate fartleks for each fitness level, can help with metabolic conditioning. Fartlek training does not require a set or measured interval distance. It can reduce the boredom of moderate-intensity interval training and low-intensity continuous interval training for athletes with heavy training loads; moreover, fartlek training may improve muscular endurance (Palanisamy, 2020; Shingala & Shukla, 2019).

MODERATE-INTENSITY INTERVAL TRAINING

Moderate-intensity interval training (MIIT) involves exercise at a medium intensity, with the athlete aiming to complete a set number of programmed intervals rather than reach maximal- or near-maximal effort during each interval. Moderate intensities are best for beginning exercisers and for periodic reductions in overall training stress to avoid overtraining, making these workouts an excellent tool for day-after recovery following highly intense training days or competitive events.

TABATA TRAINING →

A type of HIIT with seven or eight 20-second intervals with 10 seconds of rest between each interval.

FARTLEK TRAINING →

Speed play; a style of endurance training that uses unstructured intervals to include higher-intensity periods of work within the context of a long-slow distance training stimulus.

MODERATE-INTENSITY INTERVAL TRAINING (MIIT) →

Interval training at a medium intensity with the goal to complete a set number of intervals.

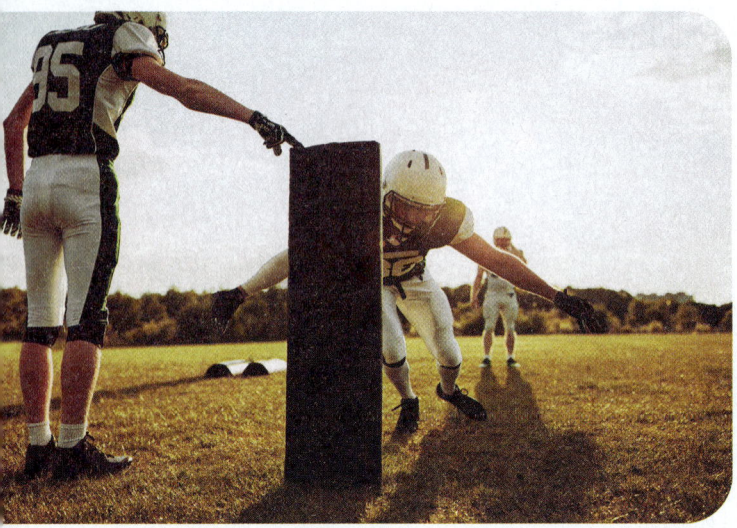

© Ground Picture/Shutterstock

MIIT can also be beneficial for athletes returning from injury or in the off-season phase of their training cycle. Following an injury, it is crucial to gradually rebuild fitness levels to avoid reinjury. MIIT offers a controlled way to reintroduce training and progressively increase intensity as the athlete's recovery progresses. It can also be advantageous for athletes who participate in endurance sports, as it helps to build a solid aerobic base without placing undue stress on the body. MIIT can help enhance aerobic capacity and endurance without the high risk of injury or overtraining that can come with consistent high-intensity workouts.

CONTINUOUS TRAINING

Continuous training occurs at the same intensity for a set period. Moderate-intensity continuous training (MICT; sometimes termed long-slow distance [LSD]), RP, and % HR_{max} are all types of continuous training. MICT is typically conducted around VT1 intensity, and the duration of MICT training sessions generally is more extended than RD or % HR_{max} training. MICT is primarily used to develop aerobic endurance; training at a higher % HR_{max} will also stress the lactic acid energy system. Similarly, RP training supports the development of the lactic acid and aerobic systems. The MICT intensity can also be helpful for warm-up, cool-down, and days when the goal is to keep training intensities low. The higher-intensity continuous training seen with RP and % HR_{max} is used in conjunction with the lower-intensity training in such a case.

The Sports Performance Coach should keep in mind the physiologic demands of the sport. Solo sports such as running and field sports such as soccer and field hockey require athletes to run for significant amounts of time during competition. Regular, continuous run training will help prepare the athlete's musculoskeletal system for this activity and improve their oxidative metabolic system. Sports with less continuous activity requirements, such as track and field events, football, and golf, may be better trained using a variety of interval training sessions.

STAGE TRAINING

NASM uses a five-stage programming system with four intensity zones for training (**Table 16.10**). The intensity zones can be based on the talk test, RPE, or heart rate based on VT1 and VT2 testing values. Whatever the stage, a complete warm-up and cool-down should be performed before and after the activity, respectively. The training progresses systematically to ensure the athlete is adequately prepared for the training load. Attempting to progress training too rapidly or without systematic progression increases the risk of injury and decreases the effectiveness of the programming.

> **CONTINUOUS → TRAINING**
>
> Training at a constant intensity for a specific period of time.

👍 **HELPFUL HINT**

Stage training is individualized and progressive. Training should always be based on the metabolic and training demands of the sport. The overall goal is to enhance performance in the sport, not make metabolic training the priority.

TABLE 16.10 Summary of Cardiorespiratory Programming Methods

Stage Training Zone	Talk Test	RPE 1–10	RPE 6–20	Example Heart Rate**	Description
Zone 1	Below VT1	3–4	12–13	<142 bpm	• Light to moderate • Sweating begins • Conversation is easy
Zone 2	VT1 to midpoint*	5–7	14–15	142–159 bpm	• Challenging to hard • Sweating • Noticeable breathing • Continual conversation becomes challenging
Zone 3	Midpoint to VT2	7–8	16–17	160–175 bpm	• Vigorous to very hard • Heavy sweating • Hard breathing • Ability to talk is limited to short phrases
Zone 4	Above VT2	9–10	18–20	>175	• Very hard to maximal effort • Breathing as hard as possible • Speaking limited to single words or not possible

*Midpoint: The intensity level halfway between VT1 and VT2.

**Example heart rate as a percentage of VT1 and VT2 uses the VT1 and VT2 test of a 20-year-old female soccer player.

Stage training is systematically developed. Training is adapted as an athlete's fitness increases, with a systematic addition of work in higher stages. For example, a new runner with the goal to run a 5-kilometer race might have a small percentage of training in Stage 4 compared to a high-level 5-kilometer runner, who will have a higher total volume of training with more time spent in all the stages compared to the less experienced athlete.

STAGE 1

The first stage of this process is designed to develop a foundation of aerobic endurance. It primarily utilizes long, slow, steady-state training and moderately intense intervals (Zones 1 and 2) for 4 to 6 days per week. Long-slow training sessions should start at 20 to 30 minutes and gradually increase to 40 to 60 minutes per session (**Table 16.11**). The goal is to complete the amount of time set at a pace that can be sustained throughout the session and to increase the rate over time.

Moderately intense interval workouts would last 15 to 30 minutes, and the interval length would be 1 to 3 minutes with a 1-minute recovery between intervals (**Table 16.12**). A mixture of steady-state and interval workouts should be included in Stage 1, with two or three workouts in the week.

Stage 1 training will be a significant part of training for sports that rely heavily on aerobic metabolism. The longer the duration of the sport, the more time that will be spent with Stage 1 training. Stage 1 training can also be used for all athletes to enhance

TABLE 16.11   Example Stage 1 Workout Steady-State Training

	Zone 1 (Light to Moderate)	Zone 2 (Challenging, Hard)	Zone 3 (Vigorous, Very Hard)	Zone 4 (Very Hard, Maximum Effort)
Warm-up	5–10 minutes			
Workout	40 minutes of Zone 1 staying below VT1			
Cool-down	5–10 minutes			

TABLE 16.12   Example Stage 1 Workout with Moderate-Intensity Intervals

	Zone 1 (Light to Moderate)	Zone 2 (Challenging, Hard)	Zone 3 (Vigorous, Very Hard)	Zone 4 (Very Hard, Maximum Effort)
Warm-up	5–10 minutes			
Workout	Interval: 2 minutes in Zone 1, staying below VT1 Recovery: 1 minute in Zone 1 Repetitions: 7			
Cool-down	5–10 minutes			

metabolic conditioning and for more anaerobic sports athletes as an active recovery session. For athletes in sports that place a lower emphasis on oxidative metabolism, Stage 1 intervals are preferred to steady-state training.

👍 **HELPFUL HINT**

Identifying training zones—for example, setting Zone 1 based on the talk test and RPE results—can ensure training is appropriate and considers other influencing factors such as environmental conditions or an athlete who has just completed a stressful school day.

STAGE 2

The second stage of metabolic energy system training keeps athletes at intensity levels of Zones 1 and 2. It may include a combination of continuous training and intervals that go just above VT1 (**Table 16.13**). A total of 4 to 6 workouts should be included in the week, with a mixture of steady-state and interval workouts. Intervals should start with

TABLE 16.13 Example Stage 2 Workout Intervals

	Zone 1 (Light to Moderate)	Zone 2 (Challenging, Hard)	Zone 3 (Vigorous, Very Hard)	Zone 4 (Very Hard, Maximum Effort)
Warm-up	5–10 minutes			
Workout	Interval: 1 minute in Zone 2, just above VT1 Recovery: 3 minutes in Zone 1, below VT1 Repetitions: 4			
Cool-down	5–10 minutes			

30- to 60-second durations and progress to as long as 3 minutes, with the work–rest ratio gradually decreasing from 1:3 to 1:1.

Athletes who participate in sports that emphasize the body's anaerobic energy systems will rely more heavily on Stage 2 intervals than athletes who rely heavily on oxidative energy metabolism. Athletes engaged in extremely long events such as Ironman triathlon training may use predominantly Stage 1 and 2 training. This is because sports performance occurs almost exclusively in Zones 1 and 2, and the high training volumes often preclude higher-intensity work. Stage 2 is a valuable part of the training program for more explosive sports; however, the interval intensities are lower than those in higher stages. The training in Stage 2 can also help improve aerobic capacity, which is beneficial for recovery.

STAGE 3

The third stage progresses to higher percentages of RP or competition intensity with the continued use of high-intensity interval workouts, continuous heart rate training sessions in Zone 3, and gradual inclusion of repeated sprint training (**Table 16.14**). This stage is completed after adequate training time in Stages 1 and 2 have been completed. This programming ensures that each athlete is adequately prepared for the stress of

TABLE 16.14 Example Stage 3 Workout Repeated Sprint Training

	Zone 1 (Light to Moderate)	Zone 2 (Challenging, Hard)	Zone 3 (Vigorous, Very Hard)	Zone 4 (Very Hard, Maximum Effort)
Warm-up	5–10 minutes			
Workout	Interval: Gradually increase intensity over 2 minutes, reaching Zone 3 for the last 40–45 seconds, staying below VT2 for each interval Recovery: 1 minute in Zone 2 Repetitions: 6			
Cool-down	5–10 minutes			

high-intensity exercise. Repeated sprint workouts and RP or competition intensities of 95% to 110% will promote improved anaerobic power and power endurance and continued improvements in aerobic endurance. Fewer workouts are performed each week to allow for more significant recovery between sessions, with 3 to 4 sessions per week being sufficient for improved fitness.

Repeated sprint workouts consisting of 5 to 20 sprints of 5 to 10 seconds are effective during Stage 3. When using supra-maximal race pacing (more than 100% of maximal RP), the Sports Performance Coach must ensure athletes can perform those intensities safely. For instance, a workout of 110% of RP would be performed for only 70% to 90% of the total distance that maximal effort could be sustained. Once again, in Stage 3, monitoring of soreness and fatigue are necessary, with reduced training loads occurring when more recovery is needed.

Activities of shorter duration that rely heavily on oxidative metabolism often use Stage 3 training to enhance glycolytic and high-level oxidative metabolism. The shorter-duration intervals or sprints can help improve velocity, and the higher intensity, which produces high levels of lactic acid, can help develop the aerobic system in a shorter period than is seen with steady-state exercise. For sports such as soccer, lacrosse, and field hockey, work in this stage can mimic some of the intensities seen during athletic competitions. For sports that require extremely high intensities, Stage 3 programs can help prepare the athlete to perform Stage 4 training without injury or excessive fatigue.

STAGE 4

Stage 4 training is a crucial part of metabolic development; it focuses on stressing the anaerobic energy systems, which are critical for anaerobic capacity and power development. Athletes training in Stage 4 spend time in all four training stages, with most of the time being spent in the initial three stages and the shortest amount of time in Stage 4. The goal is to overload the anaerobic systems without overly fatiguing the athlete (**Table 16.15**).

TABLE 16.15 Example Stage 4 Workout

	Zone 1 (Light to Moderate)	Zone 2 (Challenging, Hard)	Zone 3 (Vigorous, Very Hard)	Zone 4 (Very Hard, Maximum Effort)
Warm-up	5–10 minutes			
Workout	Interval: Gradually increase the intensity from Zone 1 to Zone 4 with 45–60 seconds spent in Zones 1–3 and 10–15 seconds above VT2 in Zone 4 Recovery: 2 minutes in Zone 1 Repetitions: 5			
Cool-down	5–10 minutes			

When adding Stage 4 work to an athlete's training program, the Sports Performance Coach should understand the metabolic demands of the athlete's sport. Each athlete's response to the training should be monitored to minimize the potential for overtraining or injury. It is a good idea to communicate with the athlete about their recovery, sleep quality, and mood. Even if programming is designed around other intensity measures, monitoring

RPE is useful. If the athlete does not appear to recover successfully, the intensity and duration of Stage 4 training should be reduced.

Stage 4 is performed at a very high intensity, progressing into Zone 4 for heart rate. The volume is lower than in any other stage, given the high intensity. Monitoring each athlete in each session is essential to minimize the risk of overload. Team sport athletes can benefit from Stage 4 training, which offers the potential to manipulate the intervals and recovery to match the specific demands of the sport. Similarly, track athletes and other athletes, such as skiers, golfers, and fencers, can use Stage 4 training to help enhance their work capacity during their sports activity.

STAGE 5

Stage 5 training is used with all athletes and utilizes sports-specific drills and skill work done at levels to mimic competition intensity. It is helpful to collaborate with all coaches to ensure skill work and drills are appropriate for the specific athletes and the specific time in the competition season. For team sports athletes, Stage 5 training can be vital for developing the aerobic energy system, which is essential to support high-level performance and optimal recovery (Harrison et al., 2015; Stone & Kilding, 2009).

LESSON 4: ENERGY SYSTEMS TRAINING CONSIDERATIONS
TECHNOLOGY USED TO MONITOR AND MANAGE METABOLIC SYSTEMS TRAINING

Technology allows the Sports Performance Coach to obtain physiological data quite rapidly. However, these data will be useful only if they are correctly interpreted and applied to design or modify training programs. An excellent initial technology adaptation is the regular measurement of heart rate. Heart rate monitors are reasonably priced, and the data obtained can provide valuable information, especially when athletes are monitored throughout the entire season.

HEART RATE MONITORS

Heart rate monitors are relatively inexpensive, and the data they collect are often available to download for analysis. Given their ready availability and ease of use, these devices are excellent tools to monitor training intensity and recovery. Heart rate monitors can help athletes understand the relationship between heart rate and exercise intensity. The ability to identify the heart rate at a specific time is beneficial for showing the athlete the importance of warming up before a training session and taking advantage of the rest periods during interval training. Once a coach/athlete regularly uses a heart rate monitor, it is also possible to use these data during a training session to determine if the session needs to be modified or stopped. For example, if heart rate stays elevated during a rest

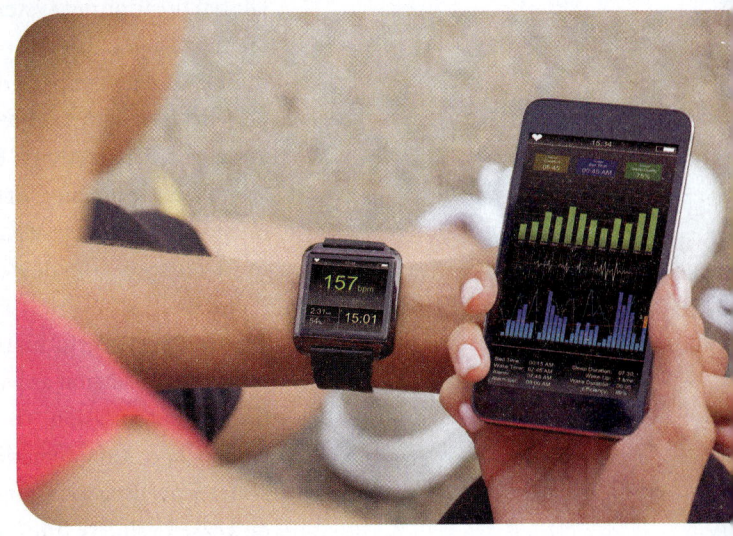

© Andrey_Popov/Shutterstock

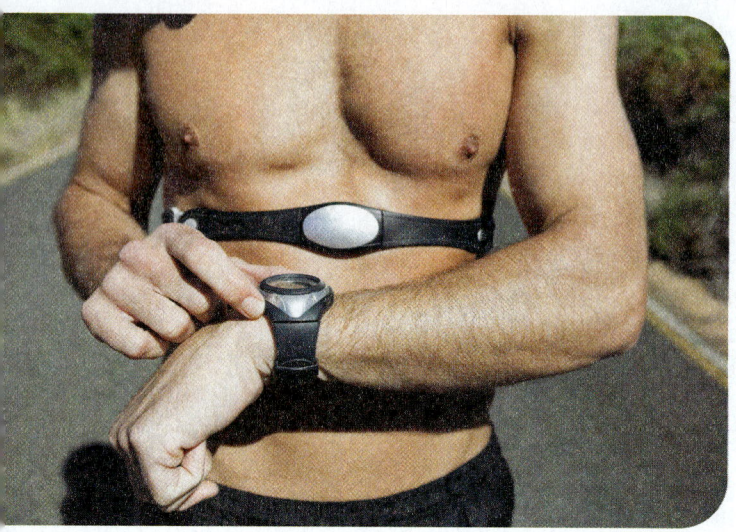
© Wavebreakmedia/Shutterstock

period of an interval training session, it is a potential indication that the athlete might need a longer rest interval or might not be adequately recovered from a previous training session. Heart rate values can help the Sports Performance Coach develop a successful metabolic training program for each athlete.

CHEST STRAP VERSUS OPTICAL SENSORS

The first heart rate monitors used a chest strap with electrodes that sent a signal to a wrist receiver. Today, heart rate monitors can also detect heart rate via a wrist device. In this case, heart rate is measured optically using infrared light-emitting diodes (LEDs) to measure blood flow. Research has consistently shown that a properly positioned chest strap provides heart rate values consistent with an electrocardiogram (EKG). Conversely, some research reports an inconsistency in the accuracy of heart rates among various brands of wrist monitors (Chow & Yang, 2020; Etiwy et al., 2019).

A variety of other devices are marketed to measure heart rate optically; they rely on placement on different parts of the body, such as the forearm/biceps, ear, and finger. A recent field study examined the accuracy of a number of these devices, including a chest strap, during a trail run. The results showed that only the chest strap provided consistent and accurate heart rate measurements (Navalta et al., 2020). Thus, a good recommendation is not to rely solely on devices that are not chest straps to ensure that exercise intensities are not providing inconsistent or erroneous measurements (Chow & Yang, 2020; Navalta et al., 2020).

An optical monitor may be easier to use than a chest strap. However, the Sports Performance Coach needs to recognize the limits of optical heart rate sensors. Any optical monitor must maintain contact with the body without excessive movement so the infrared LEDs can measure blood flow. Suppose the decision is made to use a specific sensor. In that case, the device should be field-tested to ensure that the heart rate values measured by the device are consistent with the values measured by a chest strap.

GLOBAL POSITIONING SYSTEM

Global positioning system (GPS) devices are readily available as individual units and as team packages. The individual units, often worn on the wrist, allow athletes to measure their distance and pace during a training session. In addition, packages of multiple GPS devices with telemetry allow a Sports Performance Coach to monitor team sport athletes during activity. Research reviews have found that GPS devices are useful and reliable tools for measuring distance and velocity when properly calibrated, with errors most likely to occur at higher velocities (Johnston et al., 2012; Scott et al., 2016). The most accurate GPS devices capture data at 10 times per second, often measured as hertz (Scott et al., 2016).

The Sports Performance Coach can use GPS systems to measure the distance traveled in a training session as well as individual athletes' average velocity and velocity trends throughout a session. These values can help identify each athlete's fitness level and personal position demands in a specific sport, and may potentially be used to identify athletes needing a training program modification. For example, if an athlete shows decreased velocity from one training session to another, perhaps the training is too intense or additional recovery measures need to be adapted to allow successful metabolic development.

BIOMETRICS FOR OPTIMAL PROGRAMMING

Sports Performance Coaches can use biometric data to help assess the effects that training has on athletes. Heart rate variability (HRV) is a valuable piece of biometric data that provides insights into an individual's autonomic nervous system. It measures the variation in time between each heartbeat. Contrary to what one might expect, a higher HRV is typically a sign of healthy, responsive physiological systems. Regular monitoring of HRV can offer deep insights into an individual's stress levels, recovery status, and overall well-being.

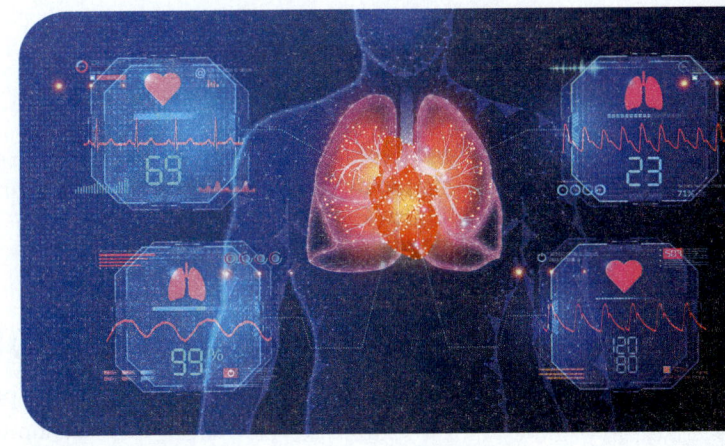

© ArtemisDiana/Shutterstock

A variety of devices are available that can measure HRV. Some measure only HRV, especially those associated with a smartphone app. Others are part of a wearable device. In addition, some smartphone apps measure HRV by measuring blood flow through the finger using the camera as an optical device.

Because training is a stressor, monitoring HRV can allow potential identification of athletes who are not recovering or who might be able to tolerate a higher training load. Recent studies have used HRV tracking to help identify the effect of training load on HRV (Plews et al., 2012) and have shown a relationship between a decreasing HRV and an increased risk of injury (Williams et al., 2017).

Daily HRV measurements can be tracked, and the Sports Performance Coach can use the changes to help determine the effectiveness or ineffectiveness of a training program. Changes in HRV reflect changes in an athlete's sympathetic and parasympathetic nervous system activity. These changes are influenced by training and other factors, such as personal relationships, school/work responsibilities, sleep quality, and alcohol consumption.

HRV is a valuable tool for the Sports Performance Coach. Understanding that the changes in HRV directly result from various good and bad stressors can allow for rapid intervention. For example, a lowered HRV, indicative of increased sympathetic nervous system activity, does not necessarily mean a training session should be canceled. Communication with the athlete can help identify the cause of the change. The introduction of activities that increase parasympathetic nervous system activation, such as a float tank therapy session, deep breathing exercises, or meditation, can all be beneficial to help increase HRV values. Over time, the Sports Performance Coach can help each athlete understand which factors result in lowered HRV values and identify tools to help maintain consistent HRV values. Rarely should a coach solely rely on an HRV value to determine specific programming. Instead, this information simply allows the coach to better understand when they should maintain the current training status and when a change might be necessary.

When athletes are educated about HRV and how various life factors can influence, they can appreciate the helpful nature of changes in HRV values. For example, suppose an athlete's HRV score consistently decreases over many days (indicating an increase in sympathetic nervous system activity). In that case, the Sports Performance Coach and the athlete can work together to understand whether this change relates to training load, life factors, or a combination of the two.

CLIMATE CONSIDERATIONS

The environment places physiologic stress on an individual. When designing a training program, cold, heat, humidity, altitude (high), and air quality are essential factors to consider. Knowing where the athlete trains and competes is necessary because specific environmental conditions may influence program design.

HEAT AND HUMIDITY

Heat and humidity are interrelated environmental factors, and both influence the ability of an athlete to dissipate heat. The Sports Performance Coach should collaborate with the sports medicine team to ensure a safe athletic training and competition environment. Training in hot and humid conditions may require program modifications, and these conditions may reduce exercise capacity because the athlete must cope with the additional stressors of heat and humidity (No & Kwak, 2016).

Measuring **wet bulb global temperature (WBGT)** will help determine whether training or competition should be modified or delayed. WBGT measures heat stress and accounts for the actual temperature (T_{dry}), the temperature based on the effect of humidity (T_{wet}), and the temperature based on the radiant heat or sunlight ($T_{black globe}$). It is calculated using the following formula:

$$WBGT = (0.7 \times T_{wet}) + (0.2 \times T_{black globe}) + (0.1 \times T_{dry})$$

As the equation shows, humidity and, to a lesser extent, radiant heat have a more significant influence on WBGT than temperature does. The higher the humidity, the more difficult it is for sweat to evaporate so that the athlete can dissipate the heat produced by the working muscles. **Table 16.16** shows the training modifications suggested by several governing bodies based on WBGT.

Sports Performance Coaches should also be aware of the importance of acclimatization to heat and humidity when beginning athlete training sessions or when athletes compete in a warmer environment than the training environment. Generally, acclimatization takes up to 10 to 14 days. The physiologic adaptations include increased sweating, earlier onset of sweating, and more dilute sweat. All of these adaptations help to improve the athlete's exercise capacity. **Table 16.17** shows several training methods to help athletes acclimate.

Sweat only cools the body when it evaporates. The more humid the environment, the harder it is for sweat to evaporate because the atmosphere contains a high level of water vapor. Higher humidity levels are more physiologically stressful for the athlete at a given temperature.

COLD

Training and competing in cold environments can have a negative influence on performance. The main concern when exercising in cold temperatures is avoiding hypothermia and cold-related skin injuries, such as frostbite.

WET BULB GLOBAL TEMPERATURE (WBGT) →

A measurement of heat stress based on temperature, humidity, and radiant temperature: WBGT = $(0.7 \times T_{wet})$ + $(0.2 \times T_{black globe})$ + $(0.1 \times T_{dry})$.

TABLE 16.16 Recommendations for Practice Modifications Based on WBGT

WGBT	Organization	Athlete Concerned	Recommendation
32.3°C 90.1°F	American College of Sports Medicine (ACSM)	Acclimatized, fit, and low-risk individuals	Participation cut off
32.2°C 90.0°F	International Tennis Federation (ITF)	Junior and wheelchair tennis players	Immediate suspension of play
32.2°C 90.0°F	Women's Tennis Association (WTA)	Female tennis players	Immediate suspension of play
32.0°C 89.6°F	Federation Internationale de Football Association (FIFA)	Football players	Additional cooling break at 30 and 75 minutes
30.1°C 86.2°F	ACSM	Non-acclimatized, unfit, and high-risk individuals	Participation cut off
30.1°C 86.2°F	ITF-WTA	Junior and female tennis players	10-minute break between second and third sets
28.0°C 82.4°F	Australian Open	Tennis players	10-minute break between second and third sets
21.0°C 69.8°F	Marathon in northern latitudes	Runners in mass-participation events	Cancel marathon

Data from Racinais, S., Alonso, J. M., Coutts, A. J., Flouris, A. D., Girard, O., González-Alonso, J., Hausswirth, C., Jay, O., Lee, J. K. W., Mitchell, N., Nassis, G. P., Nybo, L., Pluim, B. M., Roelands, B., Sawka, M. N., Wingo, J., & Périard, J. D. (2015). *Consensus recommendations on training and competing in the heat. British Journal of Sports Medicine, 49*(18), 1164. https://doi .org/10.1136/bjsports-2015-094915

TABLE 16.17 Methods of Heat Acclimatization

	Objective	Duration	Period	Content	Environment
Pre-season/ in-season training camp	Enhance/boost the training stimulus	1–2 weeks	Pre-season or in-season	Regular or additional training (75–90 min/day) to increase body temperature and induce profuse sweating	Natural or artificial heat stress
Target competition preparatory camp	Optimize future reacclimatization and evaluate individual responses in the heat	2 weeks	1 month before competing in the heat	Regular or additional training, simulated competition and heat response test	Equivalent to or more stressful than target competition
Target competition final camp	Optimize performance in the heat	1–2 weeks, depending on results of preparatory camp	Just before the competition	Precompetition training	Same as competition

Data from Racinais, S., Alonso, J. M., Coutts, A. J., Flouris, A. D., Girard, O., González-Alonso, J., Hausswirth, C., Jay, O., Lee, J. K. W., Mitchell, N., Nassis, G. P., Nybo, L., Pluim, B. M., Roelands, B., Sawka, M. N., Wingo, J., & Périard, J. D. (2015). *Consensus recommendations on training and competing in the heat. British Journal of Sports Medicine, 49*(18), 1164. https:// doi.org/10.1136/bjsports-2015-094915

Hypothermia is a condition in which the body temperature drops below 95°F (35°C). When hypothermia occurs, the body loses heat faster than it can produce heat. Frostbite is a condition in which the skin or the tissues below the skin become frozen. Proper clothing choices and awareness of the temperature and the windchill are effective strategies for minimizing these risks when exercising in the cold. Windchill considers wind's effect on body cooling (Fudge, 2016). The Wind Chill Temperature Index Chart (**Figure 16.5**) shows the effects of temperature and wind speed on the time it takes for frostbite to occur.

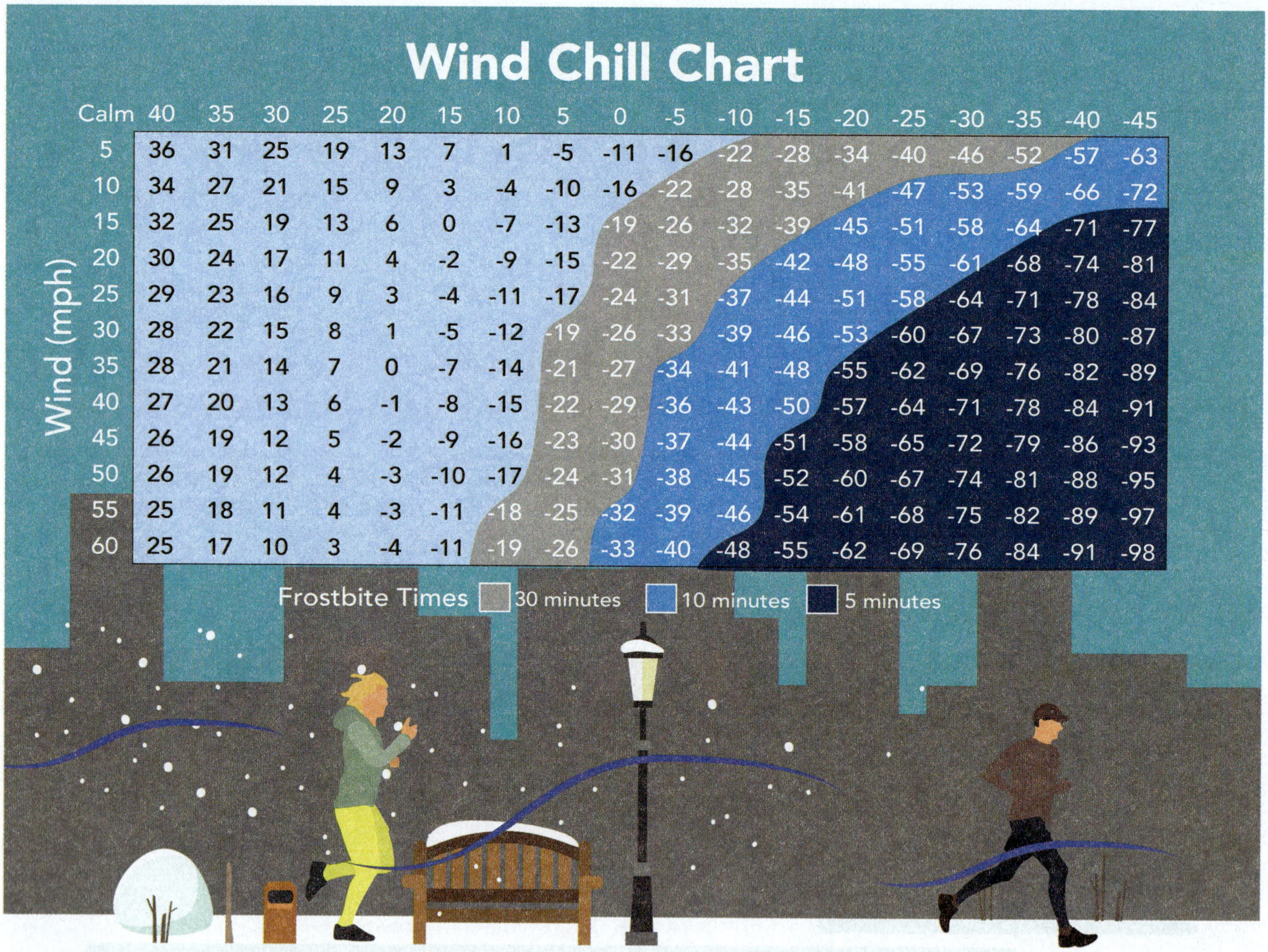

Wind Chill Chart

Wind (mph) \ Calm	40	35	30	25	20	15	10	5	0	-5	-10	-15	-20	-25	-30	-35	-40	-45
5	36	31	25	19	13	7	1	-5	-11	-16	-22	-28	-34	-40	-46	-52	-57	-63
10	34	27	21	15	9	3	-4	-10	-16	-22	-28	-35	-41	-47	-53	-59	-66	-72
15	32	25	19	13	6	0	-7	-13	-19	-26	-32	-39	-45	-51	-58	-64	-71	-77
20	30	24	17	11	4	-2	-9	-15	-22	-29	-35	-42	-48	-55	-61	-68	-74	-81
25	29	23	16	9	3	-4	-11	-17	-24	-31	-37	-44	-51	-58	-64	-71	-78	-84
30	28	22	15	8	1	-5	-12	-19	-26	-33	-39	-46	-53	-60	-67	-73	-80	-87
35	28	21	14	7	0	-7	-14	-21	-27	-34	-41	-48	-55	-62	-69	-76	-82	-89
40	27	20	13	6	-1	-8	-15	-22	-29	-36	-43	-50	-57	-64	-71	-78	-84	-91
45	26	19	12	5	-2	-9	-16	-23	-30	-37	-44	-51	-58	-65	-72	-79	-86	-93
50	26	19	12	4	-3	-10	-17	-24	-31	-38	-45	-52	-60	-67	-74	-81	-88	-95
55	25	18	11	4	-3	-11	-18	-25	-32	-39	-46	-54	-61	-68	-75	-82	-89	-97
60	25	17	10	3	-4	-11	-19	-26	-33	-40	-48	-55	-62	-69	-76	-84	-91	-98

Frostbite Times: 30 minutes | 10 minutes | 5 minutes

FIGURE 16.5 Wind Chill Temperature Index Chart

Data from National Oceanic and Atmospheric Administration. (n.d.). Wind Chill Chart. National Weather Service. https://www.weather.gov/safety/cold-wind-chill-chart

The most significant risk for hypothermia or frostbite arises when cool or cold temperatures are combined with wind. Risk factors such as wet clothing, exposure to the wind, and stop-and-start activities are more likely to cause cold injury in this condition. Knowing the temperature and wind speed allows the Sports Performance Coach to utilize the Wind Chill Temperature Index Chart to gauge the risk of cold injury. Understanding the risks can facilitate training modifications, such as shorter practice sessions and training that provides warming periods. Clothing adaptations such as sweat wicking and wind blocking, but also the ability to "breathe" to allow sweat dissipation, are potential ways to minimize problems when training in the cold (Fudge, 2016).

HIGH ALTITUDE

Training and competing at altitude will influence performance. Generally, 8,000 feet and higher elevations are considered high altitudes (Khodaee et al., 2016). However, elevations can affect performance starting at approximately 5,000 feet above sea level.

It is beneficial for athletes who live at altitude to do some of their higher-intensity training at lower elevations (Brocherie et al., 2015). This is especially true if the competition will occur at sea level. Training at a lower elevation allows for higher intensities than is possible when training at higher elevations.

Acclimatization is important for athletes who live at sea level but will be competing at a higher elevation to allow maximum performance and decrease the potential for illness and injury.

For many athletes, traveling to a competition locale weeks before an event is not feasible. However, arriving at least 48 hours before the event is suggested rather than coming on the day of the competition (Burtscher et al., 2018).

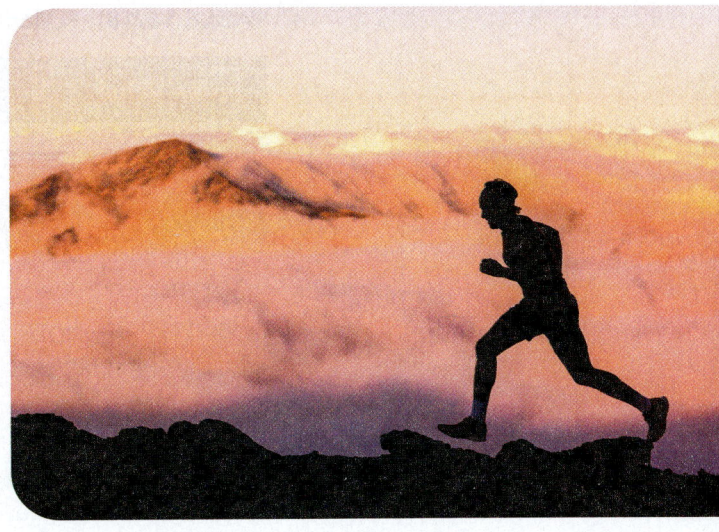

© Maridav/Shutterstock

AIR QUALITY

Air quality can be influenced by air pollution. The effects of air pollution can be acute or chronic, and can significantly affect people with preexisting conditions such as asthma or other lung diseases. However, all athletes can have adverse effects because the pollutants can act as respiratory tract irritants and potentially decrease oxygen uptake, even at rest (Tsegaw & Alemayehu, 2019).

If possible, athletes should avoid training near known pollution sites or areas with heavy automobile traffic. If this is impossible, attempts should be made to train when air quality is highest. For example, a triathlete would avoid training on or near roads during rush-hour traffic.

Sports Performance Coaches can monitor air quality through weather websites. The weather site will show the Pollution Standard Index (PSI), which measures the pollution in the air. **Table 16.18** shows the PSI.

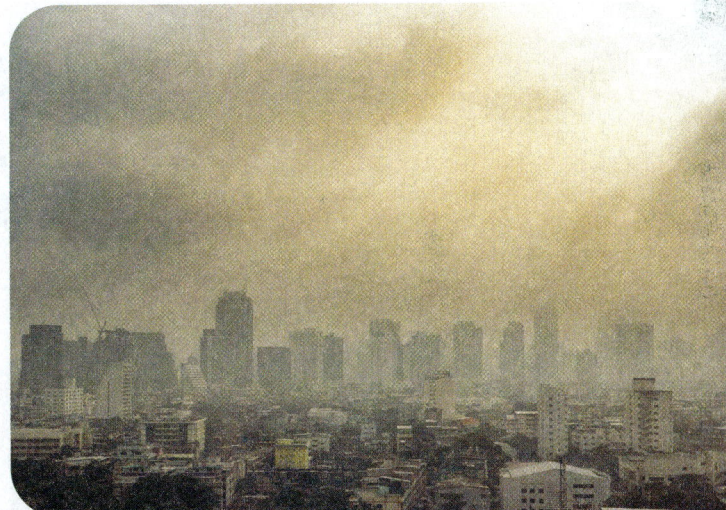

© NEwyyy/Shutterstock

> **⚠ CRITICAL**
>
> It is important to be aware of athletes' medical history. Athletes with respiratory conditions such as asthma may be more sensitive to air pollution than athletes without respiratory conditions.

TABLE 16.18 Pollution Standard Index

Index Value	Air Quality Index (AQI)	Color
< 50	Good	Green
51–100	Moderate	Yellow
101–150	Unhealthy for sensitive groups*	Orange
151–200	Unhealthy	Red
201–300	Very unhealthy	Purple
>301	Hazardous	Maroon

*People with asthma, people with allergies, and active people.

Reproduced from Tsegaw, G., & Alemayehu, Y. (2019). Principal air pollutants and their effects on athletes' health and performance: A critical review. *Scientific Research and Essays*, 14, 44-52. https://doi.org/10.5897/SRE2019.6603

LESSON 5: PRINCIPLES OF ENERGY SYSTEMS TRAINING
ENERGY SYSTEM TRAINING GUIDELINES

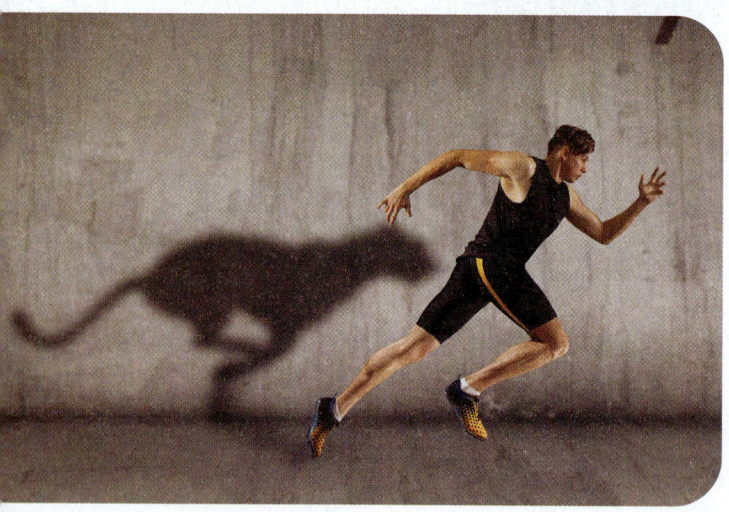

© Andrey Burmakin/Shutterstock

Metabolic energy system training should be planned, organized, and progressive, similar to the design of the OPT Model. Various stages are followed to ensure the correct progression of training stressors in preparation for higher-intensity and more-demanding challenges. This progressive training process ensures safety and effectiveness with the least risk of overtraining.

Much like the dynamic considerations required during each phase of the OPT Model, the Sports Performance Coach must make decisions regarding training stress, rest and recovery, and acute variable manipulation through each metabolic energy system training stage. Acute metabolic energy system training variables include modality or exercise type, intensity, duration, and frequency. Each acute variable influences the others, making this an integrated process. For instance, higher intensities generally require reduced workout duration; several high-effort workouts in a single week will require longer recovery between sessions and, thus, a reduction in training frequency. The key is applying the right amount of stress with proper recovery between training sessions. When repeated over time, this process improves metabolic energy system fitness and performance.

USING NEEDS ANALYSIS AND ASSESSMENT INFORMATION

If access is available, metabolic testing can help identify strengths and weaknesses, providing a benchmark for monitoring improvements over time. Lab-based testing can give a very detailed evaluation of fitness; however, it requires expensive equipment and advanced training to interpret the results. Field tests have been developed to assess individuals' fitness without the need for lab equipment.

Although monitoring changes in fitness over time is of primary importance, the athlete's VO_2 max can be compared to percentile ranks to interpret and evaluate their current fitness level (Kaminsky et al., 2015). Those with higher levels of beginning fitness will then be able to start training at a higher stage.

A heart rate monitor worn during the assessment and training may provide helpful information to track progress and identify changes over time. Monitoring heart rates offers valuable information regarding training effects; as an athlete's fitness continues to improve, the heart rate during maximal and submaximal efforts will change over time, signifying greater efficiency during exercise.

When incorporating heart rate zone training, comparing heart rate patterns during VO_2 max testing can help validate the training zones. Heart rate may decrease at the same test pace over time, signaling an improved metabolic function and the ability of the athlete to push even harder. Conversely, if the exercise heart rate increases along with the pace, that might reflect improved muscular endurance and signal the need for additional training in metabolic efficiency (e.g., high-intensity intervals). This information is essential to monitor during training to verify effectiveness.

When a Sports Performance Coach begins to work with any athlete, the training program design should consider the results of the needs analysis and movement assessment. The assessment results and understanding of the athlete's specific goals are critical to proper metabolic programming. The movement assessment testing provides the Sports Performance Coach with information about any movement impairments. Metabolic programming should ensure that the training does not increase such impairments.

Metabolic programming is adaptable and can be used to maximize metabolic training without increasing movement impairment. Athletes who exhibit specific movement impairment syndromes may require modification of their metabolic program. For example, an athlete diagnosed with pes planus distortion syndrome may not be able to perform running activities at the same volume as an athlete without this syndrome. However, the Sports Performance Coach can design a program incorporating running and other activities such as cycling or swimming to develop the metabolic energy systems without causing injury.

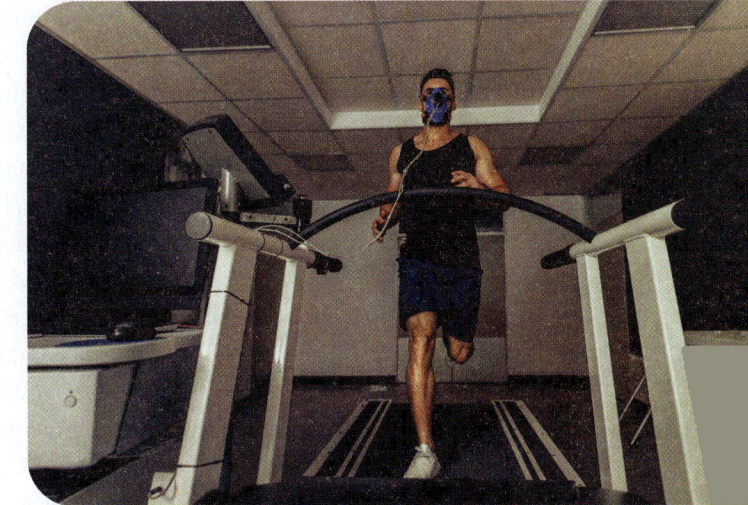

© Jacob Lund/Shutterstock

PROGRESSING ENERGY SYSTEMS TRAINING

One of the most consistent ways to design and progress a program is using FITTE-VP. This standard model for general fitness can be adapted for competitive sports. To successfully adapt it to a specific athlete and sport, the Sports Performance Coach needs to understand the sport's metabolic demands and the competitive level. Communication with specific sports coaches is beneficial for gaining knowledge and understanding. The demands of a competitive sport typically require a higher fitness level than what is necessary for general fitness. The FITTE-VP method can facilitate an excellent and adaptable program design for optimal energy system development.

FITTE-VP PRINCIPLES

Training programs should be individualized to allow maximum training benefits. The **FITTE-VP** method allows for this individualization (Garber et al., 2011). This method defines a training program's frequency, intensity, time, type, enjoyment, volume, and progression.

Frequency refers to the number of times an activity is performed in a time period, typically one week. The Sports Performance Coach recognizes that the frequency may need to be more than most athletes' general fitness recommendations. Competitive swimmers may swim 10 or more sessions each week, in addition to dry-land training. Similarly, an athlete training for an Ironman distance triathlon could have 10 to 12 training sessions divided between the sports. As a final example, a high school football player could have five to six practices weekly and a game once a week. A properly designed program is essential to ensure that the athlete has adequate time to recover from each training session.

Intensity is the level of effort at which the athlete works. Intensity can be measured in several ways, including VO_2 max, % HR_{max}, talk test, or RPE. Generally, for adaptions to occur, intensity needs to be at least 65% of HR_{max}, corresponding to an RPE of at least 3 out of 10 or 12 out of 20, depending on which RPE scale is used. Moreover, intensity must be progressive and systematic as athletes continue improving their cardiorespiratory fitness.

Time refers to the duration of time spent on each activity. The recommendation for general fitness is 20 to 60 minutes for each session, and this time does not include warm-up or cool-down time. General fitness is a concern when working with injured athletes and programming during early off-season periods. Each sport has specific requirements, which are often dependent on competition level. For example, high school cross-country athletes run a 5-kilometer race distance, whereas collegiate men run 10-kilometer races. Women's basketball is another example, with 32-minute games being made up of 8-minute quarters for high school athletes, but 40-minute games, with 10-minute quarters, being played at the collegiate level. The Sports Performance Coach should consider the sport and the competition level when designing metabolic programming for a specific sport.

Type refers to the exercise activity selected. If the athlete is involved in a sport that focuses on a specific mode, performing most metabolic training with that mode is beneficial. For example, a triathlete would do most metabolic training with running, biking, and swimming modes. Other methods might be utilized outside of competition for a mental break and to reduce the risk of repetitive movement injuries. Team sport athletes often benefit physically and psychologically by performing sessions in the pool. Depending on ability, swimming is beneficial for reducing joint stress. A variety of deep-water activities provide training diversification and the benefits of moving differently from what is typical in a sport. Many athletes can also benefit by incorporating mind–body training sessions, such as yoga, into their training programs. This type of activity can be part of the recovery or introduced to integrate alternative movements in a training plan.

Enjoyment refers to the pleasure of participating in the activity. At high levels of athletic training, not all training sessions will be enjoyable. However, the Sports Performance Coach can often utilize an individualized program design to minimize the potential adverse effects of attempting to complete activities that the athlete dislikes. Understanding an athlete's short-term and long-term goals can help inform programs that maximize performance enhancement and enjoyment. Regular communication with the athlete about the purpose of a training session in relation to the long-term goals will also help maximize enjoyment. Including alternative activities such as rest or recovery can enhance training enjoyment. Communicating with the athlete and other sports coaches about alternative workouts can help the Sports Performance Coach determine potentially beneficial activities. Activities such as yoga can work on flexibility and balance and enhance parasympathetic nervous system activity, which is essential for recovery. Pool running sessions—easy runs, intervals, or drills—conducted once a week for athletes who compete in running events can provide a metabolic benefit and enhance the enjoyment lost when training volumes are high.

Volume refers to the time spent each week training. Volume will be sport and sport-level specific. The volume will be greater at higher performance levels. As with time, the Sports Performance Coach should recognize that different competition levels will require other training volumes. The volume needed to improve fitness and successfully compete in a 10-kilometer run in college will be lower than the volume needed for participation in a marathon by the post-collegiate runner. Similarly, the volume required to have the fitness to compete at a high level in college basketball will need to be higher than it is for high school because collegiate games are of longer duration. The Sports Performance Coach should identify athletes moving up in competition and recognize the potential to increase volume too rapidly. Monitoring and communicating with the athlete and the sport-specific coaches can help minimize the development of injury or overtraining.

Progression means that exercise volume is systematically increased, albeit typically no more than 10% each week. For base fitness, the goal is usually 150 minutes or more of moderate-intensity activity spread out over 5 days or 75 minutes or more of vigorous-intensity activity over 3 days (Garber et al., 2011). The Sports Performance Coach should use this recommendation as a starting point and carefully consider factors such as the metabolic requirements of the athlete's sport, individual goals, and age. When an athlete is moving up in competition—for example, from high school to college—the coach should recognize that the increased duration of competition and practice may be significant. Careful and systematic planning usually makes it possible to keep progression increases at 10% or less each week.

DESIGNING AN ATHLETE'S PROGRAM

The first consideration in the programming for metabolic energy system fitness is selecting the proper training mode. Research has shown little difference in general metabolic energy system improvements when comparing training using running, cycling, swimming, and elliptical machines (Mastroianni et al., 2000; Morio et al., 2016; Scott et al., 2006).

However, performance improvements appear to be specific to the mode of training. For example, if progress in cycling performance is desired, cycling should be the primary training mode. Cross-training (i.e., the use of modes other than those involved in competition) can be beneficial to present a unique variation in stress while avoiding repetitive stress injuries. However, the specificity of training should be considered when specialized adaptations are necessary.

For athletes competing in a specific activity, the most significant correlation of fitness training to performance will be seen when the sport of choice is the primary mode of exercise.

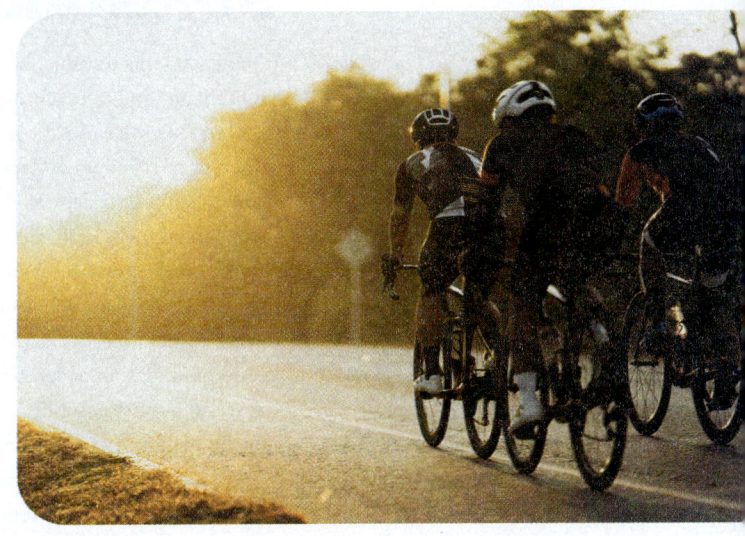
© TORWAISUDIO/Shutterstock

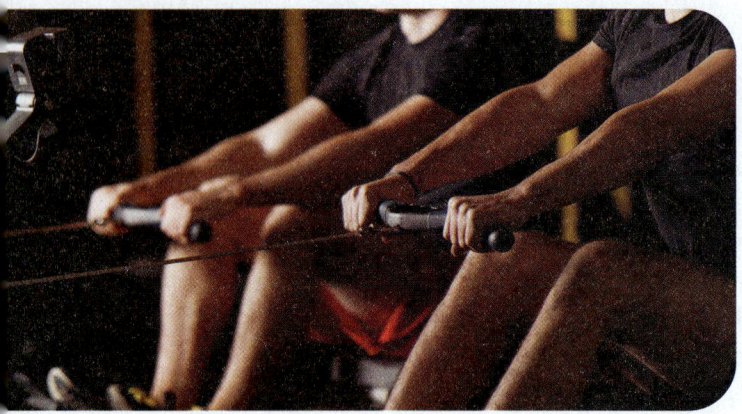
© Berkomaster/Shutterstock

For example, although swimming and cycling may be effective in developing general fitness, running will have a greater influence on performance during run-based sports. Thus, athletes whose sport involves running (e.g., football, basketball, soccer) should perform the bulk of their metabolic energy system training while running.

Each training modality applies a specific type of stress to the body, making each unique regarding the amount of muscle tissue activated and the specific muscle groups recruited during the activity. However, the metabolic stress of each modality is related more to the volume and intensity of training rather than the specific activity. A heart rate of 150 bpm while road cycling represents the same level of metabolic stress as 150 bpm while running. However, the amount of muscle tissue activated during running is more significant than that activated during cycling due to the increased involvement of the upper-body and additional lower-body impact forces. Therefore, heart rate is often higher during running than in cycling, representing a greater overall metabolic demand. Similarly, activities that require both upper- and lower-body muscle activation (i.e., swimming, rowing) can further increase the metabolic demand due to higher rates of muscle tissue recruitment that force the body to meet greater energy demands. These lower-impact forms of exercise may be good options during rehabilitation or to add more metabolic energy system training to an athlete's regimen while preventing overuse injuries.

Recreational sports are often utilized for metabolic energy system training and may represent an enjoyable form of exercise. However, it is difficult to control and monitor acute variables such as volume and intensity during these activities. Recreational activities should be encouraged as a form of daily physical activity that contributes to overall caloric expenditure and promotes overall cardiovascular health, even though more control over the training environment is necessary to achieve the greatest results with metabolic exercise. Modalities such as walking or running, cycling, swimming, rowing, and elliptical machines represent the most effective modalities and should be relied on more than recreational games in the performance enhancement arena.

SUMMARY

Energy systems training for maximal performance is tailored to the specific sport and the athlete. This chapter provides a broad overview of the energy systems and the different training methods used to maximize metabolic development. Each of the training systems discussed stimulates slightly different physiological adaptations. In turn, the Sports Performance Coach should connect the fitness training strategy to the demands of the specific sport. A well-rounded, long-term training plan should include all metabolic energy system training methods, though a greater focus on sport-specific practices is important for peak performance.

The training year should involve a periodized plan, including changing the training focus over time. For interval sports, the off-season should include a mixture of training methods to develop a good foundation of aerobic fitness. Thus, greater reliance on steady-state training is appropriate. However, as the season draws closer, more reliance on interval training will help prepare the athlete for the specific metabolic demands of an interval sport.

In-season metabolic energy system training will depend on the individual athlete. This training should be sufficient to maintain fitness gains, but should not have detrimental effects on performance. Athletes who play a great deal in games may not require a specific metabolic training program. However, those who do not get as much playing time will not benefit from the cardiovascular impact of regular playing. A solid metabolic energy system training program will be vital for them to maintain the gains they made throughout the off-season and pre-season training program.

KEY TAKEAWAYS

- All athletes need goals and proper training guidelines to ensure continued growth, and personalized metabolic programs will go a long way toward achieving specific goals. To have a complete program, the Sports Performance Coach must first assess the athlete, then create a program with specific goals while applying a measurement tool (such as heart rate or rating of perceived exertion) to measure the athlete's progress.
- Longer-duration work is training at a constant intensity for a specific period. The longer the duration and the lower the intensity, the greater the reliance on oxidative metabolism for ATP production will be.
- Intermittent work typically relies more heavily on the glycolytic and ATP-CP systems for ATP production. Shorter intervals will stress the ATP-CP system more than longer intervals, placing more significant stress on the glycolytic system.
- Proper metabolic programming includes steady-state and intermittent training sessions, with the programming individualized to each athlete's sports goals.
- Training programs are designed around different levels or percentages of intensity. The specific strategy used depends on equipment availability, number of athletes, level of athletic performance, and athlete goals.
- The predominant energy systems for a sport and equipment availability help determine the methods used to measure exercise intensity.
- Stage training is a five-stage programming system that uses four intensity zones to systematically progress the athlete while ensuring adequate training load. Training is adapted as an athlete's fitness increases, with a systematic addition of work in higher stages.
- The Sports Performance Coach should know where an athlete trains and factor in specific environmental considerations when designing energy systems development programs.

REFERENCES

Baar, K. (2006). Training for endurance and strength: Lessons from cell signaling. *Medicine & Science in Sports & Exercise, 38*(11), 1939–1944. https://doi.org/10.1249/01.mss.0000233799.62153.19

Bartlett, J. D., Hwa Joo, C., Jeong, T.-S., Louhelainen, J., Cochran, A. J., Gibala, M. J., Gregson, W., Close, G. L., Drust, B., & Morton, J. P. (2012). Matched work high-intensity interval and continuous running induce similar increases in PGC-1α mRNA, AMPK, p38, and p53 phosphorylation in human skeletal muscle. *Journal of Applied Physiology (1985), 112*(7), 1135–1143. https://doi.org/10.1152/japplphysiol.01040.2011

Brocherie, F., Millet, G. P., Hauser, A., Steiner, T., Rysman, J., Wehrlin, J. P., & Girard, O. (2015). "Live high–train low and high" hypoxic training improves team-sport performance. *Medicine & Science in Sports & Exercise, 47*(10). https://doi.org/10.1249/MSS.0000000000000630

Brooks, G. A. (1986). The lactate shuttle during exercise and recovery. *Medicine & Science in Sports & Exercise, 18*(3), 360–368. https://doi.org/10.1249/00005768-198606000-00019

Burgomaster, K. A., Howarth, K. R., Phillips, S. M., Rakobowchuk, M., Macdonald, M. J., McGee, S. L., & Gibala, M. J. (2008). Similar metabolic adaptations during exercise after low volume sprint interval and traditional endurance training in humans. *Journal of Physiology, 586*(1), 151–160. https://doi.org/10.1113/jphysiol.2007.142109

Burtscher, M., Niedermeier, M., Burtscher, J., Pesta, D., Suchy, J., & Strasser, B. (2018). Preparation for endurance competitions at altitude: Physiological, psychological, dietary and coaching aspects: A narrative review. *Frontiers in Physiology, 9*, 1504. https://doi.org/10.3389/fphys.2018.01504

Chow, H.-W., & Yang, C.-C. (2020). Accuracy of optical heart rate sensing technology in wearable fitness trackers for young and older adults: Validation and comparison study. *JMIR mHealth and uHealth*, *8*(4), e14707. https://doi.org/10.2196/14707

Cori, C. F., & Cori G. T. (1929). Glycogen formation in the liver from D- and L-lactic acid. *Journal of Biological Chemistry*, 81, 389–403.

Donovan, C. M., & Brooks, G. A. (1983). Endurance training affects lactate clearance, not lactate production. *American Journal of Physiology*, *244*(1), E83–E92. https://doi.org/10.1152/ajpendo.1983.244.1.E83

Etiwy, M., Akhrass, Z., Gillinov, L., Alashi, A., Wang, R., Blackburn, G., Gillinov, S. M., Phelan, D., Gillinov, A. M., Houghtaling, P. L., Javadikasgari, H., & Desai, M. Y. (2019). Accuracy of wearable heart rate monitors in cardiac rehabilitation. *Cardiovascular Diagnosis and Therapy*, *9*(3), 262–271. https://doi.org/10.21037/cdt.2019.04.08

Fudge, J. (2016). Preventing and managing hypothermia and frostbite injury. *Sports Health: A Multidisciplinary Approach*, *8*(2), 133–139. https://doi.org/10.1177/1941738116630542

Garber, C. E., Blissmer B., Deschenes, M. R., Franklin, BA, Lamonte, M. J., Lee, I. M., Nieman, D. C., & Swain, D. P. (2011). American College of Sports Medicine position stand: Quantity and quality of exercise for developing and maintaining cardiorespiratory, musculoskeletal, and neuromotor fitness in apparently healthy adults: Guidance for prescribing exercise. *Medicine & Science in Sports & Exercise.*, *43*(7), 1334–1359. https://doi.org/10.1249/MSS.0b013e318213fefb

Gibala, M. J., Little, J. P., Macdonald, M. J., & Hawley, J. A. (2012). Physiological adaptations to low-volume, high-intensity interval training in health and disease. *Journal of Physiology*, *590*(5), 1077–1084. https://doi.org/10.1113/jphysiol.2011.224725

Gibala, M. J., & McGee, S. L. (2008). Metabolic adaptations to short-term high-intensity interval training: A little pain for a lot of gain? *Exercise and Sport Sciences Reviews*, *36*(2), 58–63. https://doi.org/10.1097/JES.0b013e318168ec1f

Gist, N., Fedewa, M., Dishman, R., & Cureton, K. (2014). Sprint interval training effects on aerobic capacity: A systematic review and meta-analysis. *Sports Medicine*, *44*(2), 269–279. https://doi.org/10.1007/s40279-013-0115-0

Goodman, J. M., Liu, P. P., & Green, H. J. (2005). Left ventricular adaptations following short-term endurance training. *Journal of Applied Physiology*, *98*(2), 454–460. https://doi.org/10.1152/japplphysiol.00258.2004

Guidetti, L., Meucci, M., Bolletta, F., Emerenziani, G. P., Gallotta, M. C., & Baldari, C. (2018). Validity, reliability and minimum detectable change of COSMED K5 portable gas exchange system in breath-by-breath mode. *PloS One*, *13*(12), e0209925. https://doi.org/10.1371/journal.pone.0209925

Harrison, C. B., Gill, N. D., Kinugasa, T., & Kilding, A. E. (2015). Development of aerobic fitness in young team sport athletes. *Sports Medicine*, *45*(7), 969–983. https://doi.org/10.1007/s40279-015-0330-y

Helgerud, J., Hoydal, K., Wang, E., Karlsen, T., Berg, P., Bjerkaas, M., Simonsen, T., Helgesen, C., Hjorth, N., Bach, R., & Hoff, J. (2007). Aerobic high-intensity intervals improve VO_2max more than moderate training. *Medicine & Science in Sports & Exercise*, *39*(4), 665–671. https://doi.org/10.1249/mss.0b013e3180304570

Jeanes, E. M., Foster, C., Porcari, J. P., Gibson, M., & Doberstein, S. (2011). Translation of exercise testing to exercise prescription using the talk test. *Journal of Strength and Conditioning Research*, *25*(3), 590–596. https://doi.org/10.1519/JSC.0b013e318207ed53

Johnston, R. J., Watsford, M. L., Pine, M. J., Spurrs, R. W., Murphy, A. J., & Pruyn, E. C. (2012). The validity and reliability of 5-hZ global positioning system units to measure team sport movement demands. *Journal of Strength and Conditioning Research*, *26*(3), 758–765. https://doi.org/10.1519/JSC.0b013e318225f161

Joyner, M. J., & Coyle, E. F. (2008). Endurance exercise performance: The physiology of champions. *Journal of Physiology*, *586*(1), 35–44. https://doi.org/10.1113/jphysiol.2007.143834

Kaminsky, L. A., Arena, R., & Myers, J. (2015). Reference standards for cardiorespiratory fitness measured with cardiopulmonary exercise testing: Data from the Fitness Registry and the Importance of Exercise National Database. *Mayo Clinic Proceedings*, *90*(11), 1515–1523. https://doi.org/10.1016/j.mayocp.2015.07.026

Karvonen, M. J., Kentala, E., & Mustala, O. (1957). The effects of training on heart rate: A longitudinal study. *Annales Medicinae Experimentalis et Biologiae Fenniae*, *35*(3), 307–315.

Kenney, W. L., Wilmore, J. H., & Costil, D. L. (2020). *Physiology of sport and exercise* (7th ed.). Human Kinetics.

Khodaee, M., Grothe, H. L., Seyfert, J. H., & VanBaak, K. (2016). Athletes at high altitude. *Sports Health*, *8*(2), 126–132. https://doi.org/10.1177/1941738116630948

Little, J. P., Safdar, A., Bishop, D., Tarnopolsky, M. A., & Gibala, M. J. (2011). An acute bout of high-intensity interval training increases the nuclear abundance of PGC-1α and activates mitochondrial biogenesis in human skeletal muscle. *American Journal of Physiology: Regulatory, Integrative and Comparative Physiology*, *300*(6), R1303–R1310. https://doi.org/10.1152/ajpregu.00538.2010

Mastroianni, G. R., Zupan, M. F., Chuba, D. M., Berger, R. C., & Wile, A. L. (2000). Voluntary pacing and energy cost of off-road cycling and running. *Applied Ergonomics, 31*(5), 479–485. https://doi.org/10.1016/s0003-6870(00)00017-x

Milanović, Z., Sporiš, G., & Weston, M. (2015). Effectiveness of high-intensity interval training (HIT) and continuous endurance training for VO₂max improvements: A systematic review and meta-analysis of controlled trials. *Sports Medicine, 45*(10), 1469–1481. https://doi.org/10.1007/s40279-015-0365-0

Morio, C., Haddoum, M., Fournet, D., & Gueguen, N. (2016). Influence of exercise type on metabolic cost and gross efficiency: Elliptical trainer versus cycling trainer. *Journal of Sports Medicine & Physical Fitness, 56*(5), 520–526. https://pubmed.ncbi.nlm.nih.gov/25665747

Navalta, J. W., Montes, J., Bodell, N. G., Salatto, R. W., Manning, J. W., & DeBeliso, M. (2020). Concurrent heart rate validity of wearable technology devices during trail running. *PloS One, 15*(8), e0238569. https://doi.org/10.1371/journal.pone.0238569

Nicolò, A., Bazzucchi, I., Haxhi, J., Felici, F., & Sacchetti, M. (2014). Comparing continuous and intermittent exercise: An "isoeffort" and "isotime" approach. *PloS One, 9*(4), e94990. https://doi.org/10.1371/journal.pone.0094990

Nikolaidis, P. T., Rosemann, T., & Knechtle, B. (2018). Age-predicted maximal heart rate in recreational marathon runners: A cross-sectional study on Fox's and Tanaka's equations. *Frontiers in Physiology, 9*(226). https://doi.org/10.3389/fphys.2018.00226

No, M., & Kwak, H.-B. (2016). Effects of environmental temperature on physiological responses during submaximal and maximal exercises in soccer players. *Integrative Medicine Research, 5*(3), 216–222. https://doi.org/10.1016/j.imr.2016.06.002

Palanisamy, D. (2020). Effect of fartlek training on muscular endurance among cross country runners. *Think India Journal, 22*(4), 1750–1753.

Plews, D. J., Laursen, P. B., Kilding, A. E., & Buchheit, M. (2012). Heart rate variability in elite triathletes: Is variation in variability the key to effective training? A case comparison. *European Journal of Applied Physiology, 112*(11), 3729–3741. https://doi.org/10.1007/s00421-012-2354-4

Powers, S. K., Howley, E. T., & Quindry, J. (2021). *Exercise physiology: Theory and application to fitness and performance* (11th ed.). McGraw-Hill.

Racinais, S., Alonso, J. M., Coutts, A. J., Flouris, A. D., Girard, O., González-Alonso, J., Hausswirth, C., Jay, O., Lee, J. K. W., Mitchell, N., Nassis, G. P., Nybo, L., Pluim, B. M., Roelands, B., Sawka, M. N., Wingo, J., & Périard, J. D. (2015). Consensus recommendations on training and competing in the heat. *British Journal of Sports Medicine, 49*(18), 1164. https://doi.org/10.1136/bjsports-2015-094915

Reed, J. L., & Pipe, A. L. (2016). Practical approaches to prescribing physical activity and monitoring exercise intensity. *Canadian Journal of Cardiology, 32*(4), 514–522. https://doi.org/10.1016/j.cjca.2015.12.024

Roy, S., & McCrory, J. (2015). Validation of maximal heart rate prediction equations based on sex and physical activity status. *International Journal of Exercise Science, 8*(4), 318–330.

Scott, C. B., Littlefield, N. D., Chason, J. D., Bunker, M. P., & Asselin, E. M. (2006). Differences in oxygen uptake but equivalent energy expenditure between a brief bout of cycling and running. *Nutrition & Metabolism, 3*, 1. https://doi.org/10.1186/1743-7075-3-1

Scott, M. T. U., Scott, T. J., & Kelly, V. G. (2016). The validity and reliability of global positioning systems in team sport: A brief review. *Journal of Strength and Conditioning Research, 30*(5), 1470–1490. https://doi.org/10.1519/jsc.0000000000001221

Shingala, M., & Shukla, Y. (2019). Effectiveness of fartlek training on cardiorespiratory fitness and muscular endurance in young adults: A randomized control trial. *Indian Journal of Physiotherapy and Occupational Therapy, 13*(2), 86–89. https://doi.org/10.5958/0973-5674.2019.00051.0

Sloth, M., Sloth, D., Overgaard, K., & Dalgas, U. (2013). Effects of sprint interval training on VO₂max and aerobic exercise performance: A systematic review and meta-analysis. *Scandinavian Journal of Medicine & Science in Sports, 23*(6). https://doi.org/10.1111/sms.12092

Stone, N. M., & Kilding, A. E. (2009). Aerobic conditioning for team sport athletes. *Sports Medicine, 39*(8), 615–642. https://doi.org/10.2165/00007256-200939080-00002

Tabata, I. (2019). Tabata training: One of the most energetically effective high-intensity intermittent training methods. *Journal of Physiological Sciences, 69*(4), 559–572. https://doi.org/10.1007/s12576-019-00676-7

Tabata, I., Nishimura, K., Kouzaki, M., Hirai, Y., Ogita, F., Miyachi, M., & Yamamoto, K. (1996). Effects of moderate-intensity endurance and high-intensity intermittent training on anaerobic capacity and VO₂max. *Medicine & Science in Sports & Exercise, 28*(10), 1327–1330. https://doi.org/10.1097/00005768-199610000-00018

Tsegaw, G., & Alemayehu, Y. (2019). Principal air pollutants and their effects on athletes' health and performance: A critical review. *Scientific Research and Essays*, *14*(7), 44–52. https://doi.org/10.5897/SRE2019.6603

Weston, M., Taylor, K., Batterham, A., & Hopkins, W. (2014). Effects of low-volume high-intensity interval training (HIT) on fitness in adults: A meta-analysis of controlled and non-controlled trials. *Sports Medicine*, *44*(7), 1005–1017. https://doi.org/10.1007/s40279-014-0180-z

Williams, N. (2017). The Borg Rating of Perceived Exertion (RPE) scale. *Occupational Medicine*, *67*(5), 404–405. https://doi.org/10.1093/occmed/kqx063

Williams, S., Booton, T., Watson, M., Rowland, D., & Altini, M. (2017). Heart rate variability is a moderating factor in the workload-injury relationship of competitive CrossFit™ athletes. *Journal of Sports Science & Medicine, 16*(4), 443–449.

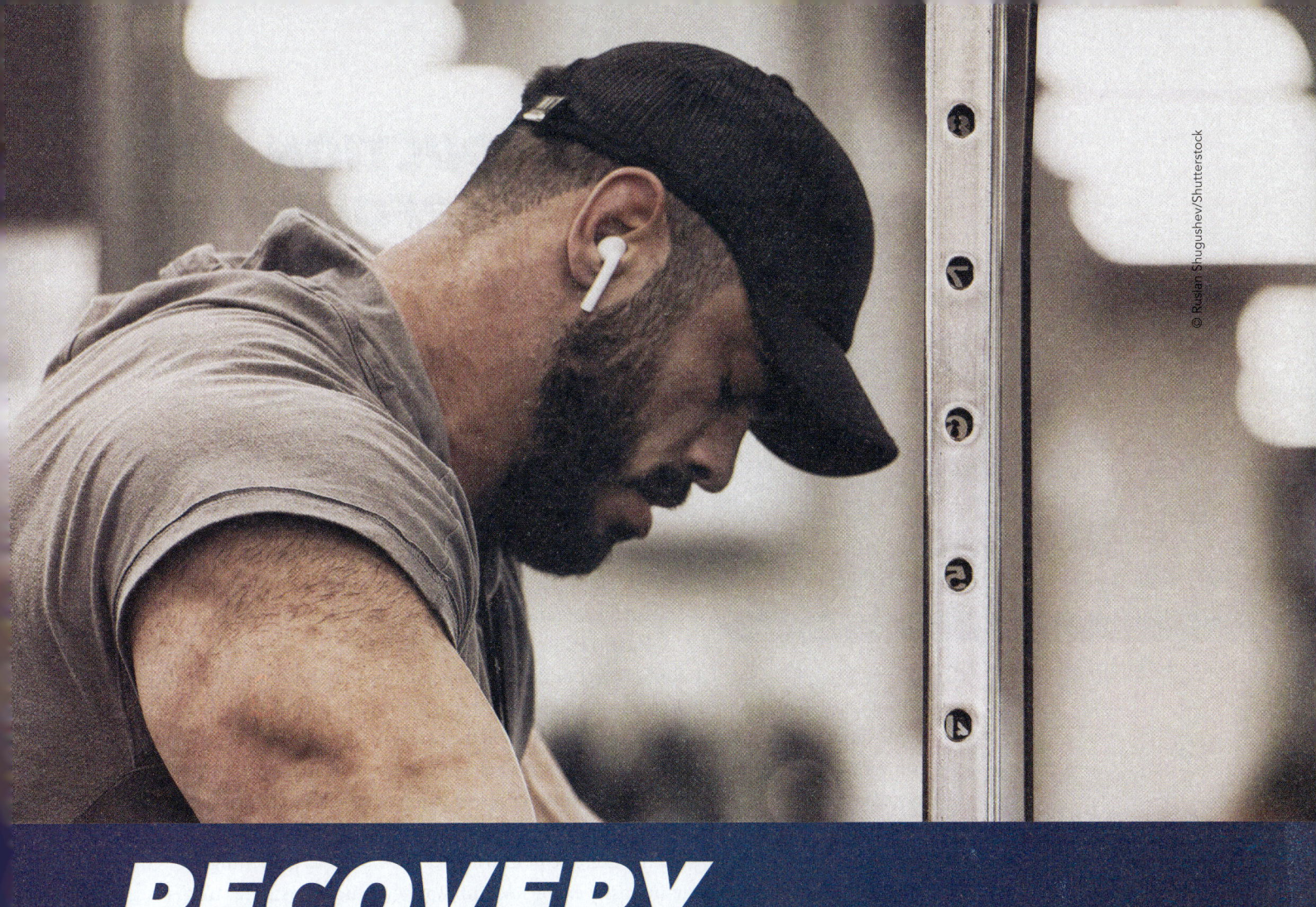

RECOVERY FOR SPORTS PERFORMANCE

CHAPTER SEVENTEEN

LEARNING OBJECTIVES

Upon completion of this chapter, the Sports Performance Coach will be able to:

- **Summarize** the importance of recovery for athletes with differing performance-related goals.
- **Explain** the scientific rationale for integrating rest and recovery into sports performance training.
- **Identify** methods to optimize an athlete's rest and recovery to maximize training adaptations.
- **Evaluate** rest and recovery methods for reliability and credibility.
- **Describe** rest and recovery through the levels of the OPT™ Model.

LESSON 1: INTRODUCTION TO RECOVERY FOR PERFORMANCE
INTRODUCTION

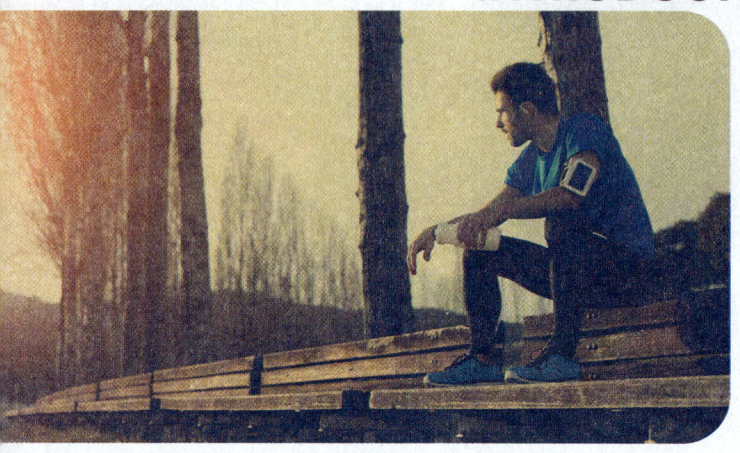

© Alex from the Rock/Shutterstock

Over the past few decades, the idea that rest and recovery allow for performance gains has gained momentum, but it remains less discussed or planned between athletes and their coaching teams. Including a rest and recovery strategy helps ensure a well-designed training plan has the best chance of success. Unfortunately, far too many athletes have not seen planned performance gains due to a lack of rest and recovery.

This chapter outlines which physiological considerations should be taken into account in a recovery strategy, how to implement rest and recovery into training, and how to monitor and adapt rest and recovery.

Rest is the removal of a training stimulus, activity, or stress. Rest can occur during an activity bout (time between intervals or sets) or between activity bouts. Although no concrete definition of rest exists in the context of exercise, an essential component of it is the removal of work. This consideration is important because activity outside of traditional exercise can still apply stress to organ systems. For example, a runner might consider rest starting at the end of a running session; however, the activities following the exercise bout affect whether the individual is actually "resting." Following the exercise bout with activities such as gardening, walking the dog, chores, low-intensity exercises, and more does not constitute "true" rest. Management of these activities can alter how an individual will recover in relation to a training plan.

Recovery is the concept of adaptive processes to repair, restore, and return the athlete to a normal or supercompensatory state. Outside of this chapter, "recovery" may be used in some contexts to describe intrasession components of exercise, such as the time between intervals or sets. In this chapter, we will discuss recovery in the sense of interventions between training sessions. The concept of recovery can be more encompassing than exercise and rest, but a properly designed training program should discuss recovery as a piece of the performance plan. These recovery factors can be related to sleep, nutrition, and tools, using biometrics and subjective data to quantify recovery and even rest.

> ### REST →
> The removal of a training stimulus, activity, or stress.

> ### RECOVERY →
> The adaptive processes to repair, restore, and return the athlete to a normal or supercompensatory state.

THE CONSEQUENCES OF A LACK OF REST AND RECOVERY

Training and recovery cannot exist without each other. Training induces stress that is required to stimulate adaptations and decreases physical function temporarily. Without recovery, exercise would be bad for an athlete; with recovery, it leads to increases in performance. Without training, there would be no performance deficit from which to recover. Therefore, the balance of training stress, recovery, and supercompensation (as part of the recovery response from training) determines the athlete's progression.

Many coaches, athletes, and scientists refer to overtraining as "under-recovering." Although this is not a scientific term, its usage illustrates the importance of balancing training and recovery. Overtraining is marked by a decrease in performance despite steady or increased exercise. Affected athletes commonly demonstrate signs of exhaustion, burnout, and fatigue, although they are not requisite for overtraining syndrome. Many athletes may not know that they are in an overtrained state, which may lead to them wanting to push harder to combat the decline in performance.

It is essential to discuss with the athlete the signs of overtraining and how recovery and rest can be implemented to either avoid or rectify overtraining. Although it is usually too late for many athletes by the time they undergo rest, early identification can lead to a quicker return to "normal" than waiting too long. Additionally, implementing proper rest and recovery may help athletes avoid the injuries that are a typical result of overtraining.

Unfortunately, overtraining can be difficult to quantify objectively. From a practical standpoint, some bad performances may not be overtraining—but how can the athlete, coach, or trainer know for sure? Although there is no objective way to find out, screening for psychological factors

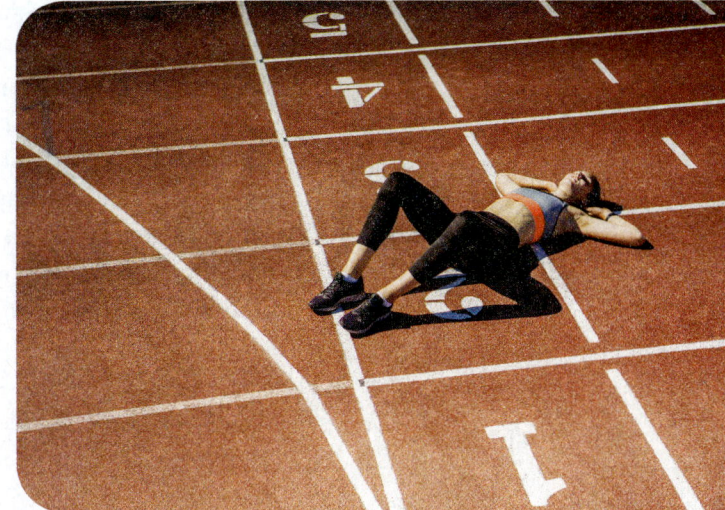

© Comeback Images/Shutterstock

(especially mood) and examining sleep patterns and biometrics will allow tracking of an athlete over time. Many of these will change together and noticeably when an athlete is exhibiting overtraining. Due to the uncertain nature of identifying overtraining, athlete success teams must be diligent in monitoring a wide array of high-frequency measures to understand the individual athlete's profile. Members of the athlete's success team (e.g., coaches, trainers, parents) must be in constant communication to catch deviations early and rectify them as soon as possible.

OVERTRAINING SYNDROME

Overtraining syndrome (OTS) is a complex condition marked by an athlete's performance decrement and increased fatigue in response to training (Cadegiani & Kater, 2019). Although this condition has been known to exist for many decades, its notoriety has grown over more recent history with growth of the scientific literature, public discussion, and advances in training optimizations. OTS can be easily identifiable in some situations, but a wide variety of presentations are possible, making it difficult in some cases to diagnose and manage appropriately.

The two phases of OTS help clarify the progression and recognition of OTS—namely, overreaching and overtraining. An overview of overtraining was provided earlier in this chapter. Overreaching can best be described as exceeding the capabilities of an individual based on their current fitness level and activity type. This can include individual components of exercise, including duration of activity bouts, frequency of exercise sessions, intensity of each session, or anything that contributes to the total volume of physical activity over some time.

FUNCTIONAL OVERREACHING

Functional overreaching is a commonly used approach to push the limits and capabilities of an athlete. This phase is typically brought about as part of the training design, and focuses on increasing training demands to lead to adaptation. However, rest and recovery are essential factors to consider between training sessions.

Mismanagement of rest and recovery is typically thought of as a critical contributor to nonfunctional overreaching. An improper balance of training, rest, and recovery does not allow organ systems in the body a chance to adapt to the demands of training, significantly increasing the risk of overtraining or injury. Should an athlete begin to show signs of

**OVERTRAINING →
SYNDROME
(OTS)**

A complex condition marked by an athlete's decrement in performance and increase in fatigue in response to training.

**FUNCTIONAL →
OVERREACHING**

Intentionally increasing training volume or intensity beyond an athlete's recovery capacity for a short period of time.

nonfunctional overreaching, such as fatigue, decreased performance, mood disturbances, or poor sleep, rest should be the primary focus to allow the body to adapt, enabling proper recovery to occur. Recovery without rest is tough to obtain during nonfunctional overreaching.

This phase is highly athlete-dependent. Some athletes can manage a high training load and use recovery modalities and typical amounts of rest to make it through this phase. Other athletes may need to be more attentive to proper rest to allow for appropriate restorative recovery. Due to the delicate nature of functional overtraining, mismanagement of rest and recovery can easily lead to *nonfunctional* overreaching. In contrast, adequate rest and recovery help an individual absorb the training, maximizing their benefit.

ATHLETE-INDUCED STRESS/DEPRESSION

Athlete-induced stress/depression is a highly complex condition involving both physiological and psychological responses. Its early stages tend to promote anxiety and restlessness (Goldstein-Piekarski et al., 2018). When left unchecked, a positive-feedback loop can occur in which stress and anxiety hamper the body's ability to recover, leading to disrupted sleep patterns, such as insomnia, which in turn further increases stress. This cycle, which frequently overlaps with overtraining, creates a heavy burden of mental stress and could progress into feelings of depression. Although some athletes may be more prone to athlete-induced stress/depression, evaluating mood and other psychological factors is crucial when determining how an athlete responds and recovers during a training cycle.

As a Sports Performance Coach, the signs and symptoms of stress and depression are often more visible to you than to the athlete. Focusing on recovery (through reduced training load and stress, nutrition interventions, and psychological counseling) should lead to restorative function and reduced stress brought about by training.

The Sports Performance Coach must recognize that stress is cumulative. Athletes experience many stressors during training on top of their "normal" life. This leads to many expectations, highs and lows, and other factors influencing an athlete's mental health. It is crucial to monitor and consider these factors and their effects. Training stress, which alters endocrine profiles, has been noted to lead to athlete stress, anxiety, and depression (Anderson et al., 2021; Elliott-Sale et al., 2018; Kamimura et al., 2020). It is a common occurrence for most athletes, despite being seldom talked about, affecting about one-third of all athletes (Hammond et al., 2013).

On top of daily psychological stress, specific events can mentally and physically tax a person. Travel, environmental changes, and competitions are all examples of these scenarios. Traveling is stressful for athletes (Huyghe et al., 2018) and can include long hours of inactivity, unpredictable nutrition, and unexpected, stressful changes. Acute changes in the environment, such as abrupt seasonal changes, going to altitude, traveling to a new climate, or similar events, can all impact a person physiologically, influencing their mood. Lastly, competitions can be a huge source of exhaustion for athletes.

Athletes, coaches, trainers, and other professionals involved in athlete success should monitor mood, behavior, communication, and performance to determine whether an athlete is demonstrating signs of overreaching/overtraining-induced anxiety and depression. Several questionnaires can be used to assess for these outcomes and may provide reliable ways for the athlete's success team to quantify an athlete's progression.

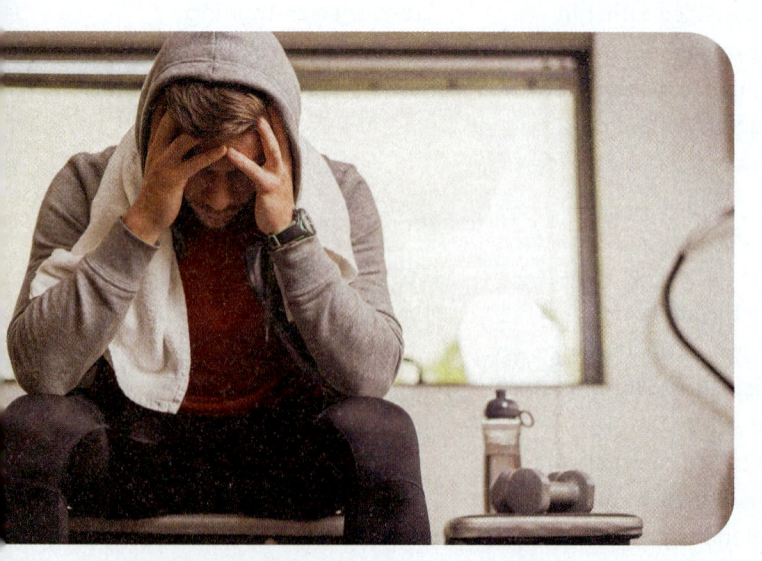

© Starstuff/Shutterstock

COACH'S CORNER

It's crucial for the Sports Performance Coach to detect early signs of stress in athletes, such as fatigue, increased perceived exertion, irritability, depression, and more, as athletes might not recognize these symptoms themselves. Engaging with athletes and tracking these signs using systems such as journaling or digital platforms can be helpful in monitoring gradual changes. These platforms can use daily questionnaires and data analytics to record psychological states. Although some might be costly, custom solutions, including free online forms, can also provide valuable insights. However, if an athlete shows signs of stress or depression, a Sports Performance Coach's role is to notice and track these changes and then refer the athlete to the appropriate professional.

FEMALE ATHLETE TRIAD →

A medical condition in highly athletic women characterized by low energy availability, menstrual dysfunction, and low bone mineral density.

LOW ENERGY AVAILABILITY (LEA) →

A mismatch between energy in and energy out that leaves an inadequate supply of energy for the body to maintain processes that ensure health and wellness. It can occur even if the subject is weight stable.

FEMALE ATHLETE TRIAD

The **female athlete triad** (**Figure 17.1**) describes the interrelationship of **low energy availability (LEA)**, menstrual function, and low bone mineral density (Nazem & Ackerman, 2012). This condition has been discussed for several decades but is drawing new attention today due to increased awareness and greater acceptance of training/recovery balance. An energy imbalance primarily brings about the triad (kilocalories expended versus consumed) (Mountjoy et al., 2018). It is most common in female athletes participating in endurance sports, where caloric expenditure is high and there is an increased desire to have a lighter weight. When large caloric deficits are paired with high training loads, endocrine dysfunction can cause women to become amenorrhoeic (loss of menstruation) (Dipla et al., 2021). Amenorrhea in women often leads to loss of minerals from the bones and disruptions in bone maintenance, which decreases bone mineral density. If allowed to progress, this condition leads to osteopenia and osteoporosis.

The female athlete triad can occur in any premenopausal woman. However, during high school and college, there are many societal and athletic pressures to reduce weight, either for physical performance or for appearance. This may occur with or without the presence of an eating disorder, which could accelerate this process.

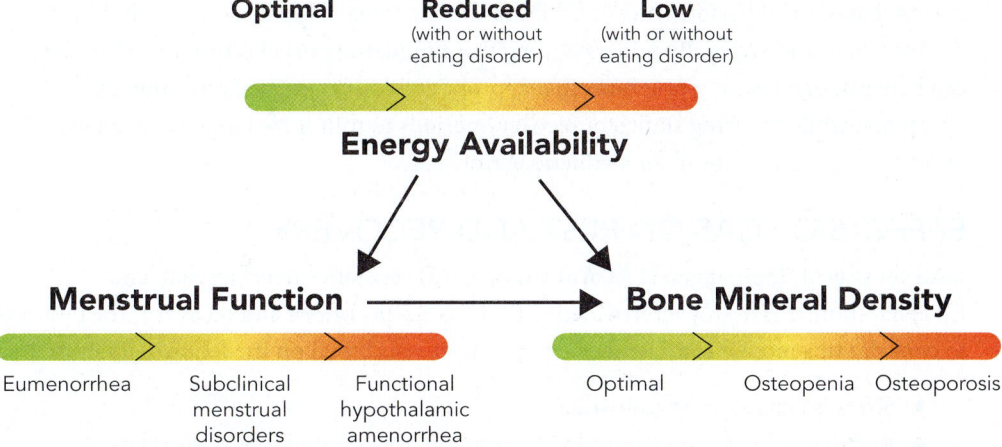

FIGURE 17.1 The Female Athlete Triad

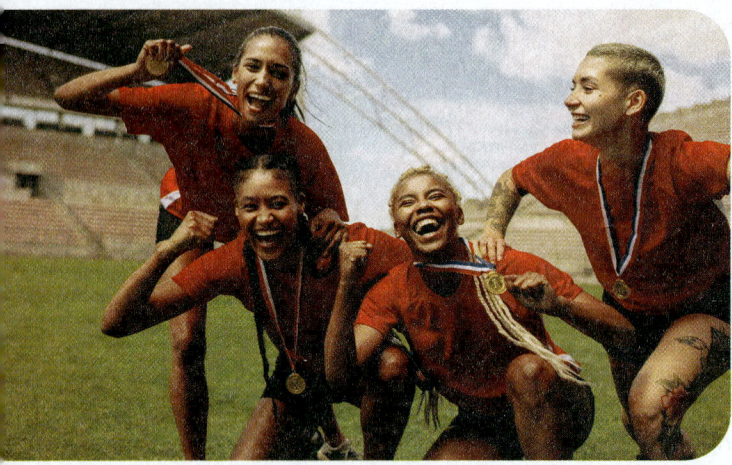

© Jacob Lund/Shutterstock

Additionally, females tend to build bone mineral density from birth to the mid-twenties, after which a decline occurs in each decade of life (Riggs et al., 2008). When bone mineral density is decreased during the early years, the mid-twenties peak will be much lower than in athletes who have not succumbed to the female athlete triad (Birch, 2005). Ultimately, this leads to stress fractures in young women and osteoporosis at an earlier age—sometimes as early as age 30 (Beals & Meyer, 2007).

Many physicians and coaches recommend dietary interventions to combat the female athlete triad, but rest is also an essential strategy in balancing training/recovery loads. Reducing lesser-functional training aspects (e.g., "junk miles"), prescribing fewer intense reps/sessions, and implementing rest days can help reduce the overall stress that female athletes' systems face.

📋 COACH'S CORNER

Recognizing the female athlete triad—a condition involving disordered eating, menstrual irregularities, and low bone density—requires sensitivity due to the personal nature of the symptoms. Training staff should emphasize the importance of healthy body composition and proper nutrition while fostering a supportive community. If monitoring bone mineral density and menstrual irregularities is impractical or inappropriate, tracking nutrition and energy balance could be more feasible, though care must be taken with athletes prone to disordered eating. As tracking these indicators can be challenging, the key lies in communication and education. It is essential to encourage athletes to consult with physicians, engage with nutritionists, and promote a culture that values healthy eating and training habits.

GENERAL ADAPTATION SYNDROME AND FITNESS–FATIGUE MODEL

General adaptation syndrome (GAS) and the fitness–fatigue model are crucial frameworks for optimizing athlete recovery because they offer insights into how the body responds to stress and exercise. GAS outlines how the body initially reacts to stress, adapts over time, and potentially experiences exhaustion without adequate recovery. The fitness–fatigue model, in contrast, suggests that training both improves fitness and induces fatigue, and asserts that optimal performance is achieved when fatigue dissipates faster than fitness declines during recovery. By understanding these models, Sports Performance Coaches can better design training programs that appropriately stress the body to stimulate adaptation while ensuring sufficient recovery periods to minimize fatigue and avoid overtraining, thereby optimizing athletic performance.

EFFECTS OF GAS ON REST AND RECOVERY

GAS consists of three stages: (1) alarm reaction, (2) resistance development, and (3) exhaustion. It is highly intertwined with the concepts of rest and recovery. The best way to consider this model from the recovery perspective is based on the following points:

- Stress is applied to an individual.
- Rest and recovery alter an individual's ability to cope with the acute stress.
- The adaptation response is dictated by the remainder of the stress and recovery.

The alarm phase is a normal response to any stressor, including exercise. This phase may differ among individuals, partly due to their stress responses. Training effectiveness depends on rest and recovery to help an individual move through the alarm phase. Adding in recovery and rest will not eliminate the alarm phase, as it is a requisite part of adaptation; instead, the goal is to balance stress and recovery to make this phase sustainable.

During the resistance development phase, stress hormones and autonomic system activation will still be higher than in the pre-alarm phase. However, the repair and fortification of beneficial pathways are activated simultaneously. The balance of these two pathways can determine the magnitude of benefit to an athlete: Too little recovery and maintenance of stressors may lead to an overall decline in net benefit; adequate recovery and stress reduction will lead to a net benefit in adaptation after the alarm phase.

The exhaustion phase, which is brought about by reduced adaptive (beneficial) responses, leads to a high imbalance of stress and physiological responses. Ideally, exhaustion will not be reached in a properly designed training cycle, although some cycles may bring individuals close to this point. If an individual has reached this stage, a reduction of total systemic stress must occur because the applied stress has brought them to the exhaustion phase. Sustaining this stress will lead to prolonged exhaustion, whereas removing stress will allow adaptive pathways to recover and lead to adaptation.

Upon early signs of exhaustion, recovery modalities may not be enough to manage stress—that is, rest is essential for reducing the training stressors. Simply put, post-exercise attempts to acutely recover from hard training once the point of exhaustion has been reached likely will not be enough; instead, overall training volume and intensity must be reduced until a normal adaptation has recovered. In addition to the reduction in training, involving an athlete's health team may be beneficial for the athlete's return; including doctors, nutritionists, and therapists in the athlete's recovery plan is likely to yield better results than a reduction in training alone, as there may be a recovery deficit in more than one area of life.

📋 COACH'S CORNER

Monitoring for signs of exhaustion in athletes is crucial, as they may overlook these symptoms, attributing them to their regular training. Indicators to watch for include heightened fatigue, diminished motivation, anxiety, and depression. Less commonly, some athletes may experience gastrointestinal issues and sleep disturbances as signs of exhaustion (Adamsson & Bernhardsson, 2018). Recognizing these symptoms early can prevent overtraining and promote optimal performance and overall well-being.

FITNESS–FATIGUE MODEL OF REST AND RECOVERY

The fitness–fatigue model is used to discuss the cumulative effects of beneficial adaptations of training as well as the degradative results (**Figure 17.2**). The fundamental approach is an extension of the GAS, in the sense that the model includes the assumption that stress can be both bad and good when applied to an individual. Exercise-induced stress is known to lead to fatigue, damage, and degradation.

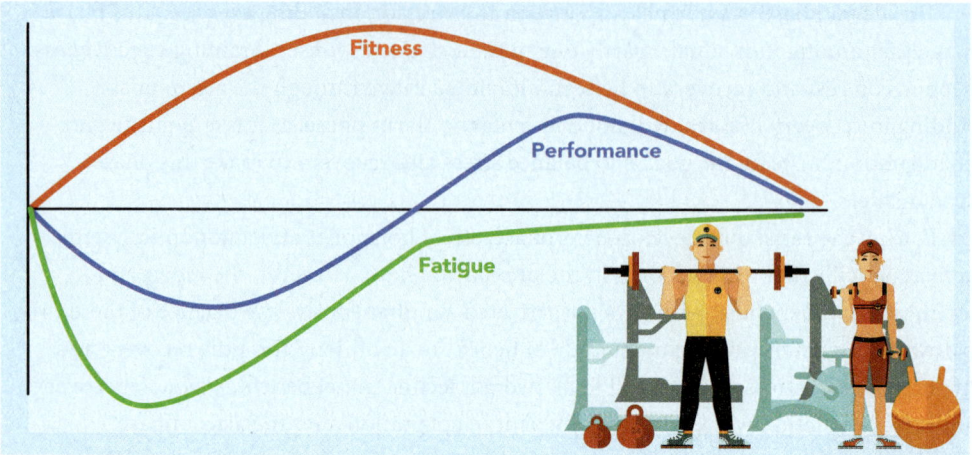

FIGURE 17.2 The Fitness–Fatigue Curves and Cumulative Performance Curve

For example, extensive eccentric contractions may lead to muscle damage in the form of myofibril damage, which will take time to repair so that the athlete can regain function. In most cases, when adequate recovery of function is ensured, physiological pathways are built back with better function than in the previous state. In the case of muscle damage, that means more myofibrils and supporting structures, allowing for greater capacity to handle the mechanical load (Laumonier & Menetrey, 2016).

As the fitness–fatigue model's name implies, the overall curve has two main components: fitness and fatigue. The fitness curve conceptualizes the beneficial responses to exercise. Exercise training can and should lead to increased performance, which demonstrates fitness. Similarly, fitness follows the principle of reversibility, meaning the benefit is transient; lack of exercise-induced stress leads to decreased performance and, therefore, to reduced fitness.

In contrast, fatigue can be described as a transient decrement in overall performance related to prior stress within or after an exercise session. Simply put, a strenuous exercise session leads to muscular damage, metabolic distress, hormonal adaptations, "central governor" or central nervous system limitations, and many other physiological responses that induce a relatively short-lived decrement in performance. These adverse effects are transient and signal the body to build back and fortify its physiological pathways; this increases the individual's ability to manage similar stress in the future, thereby improving performance. In general, the higher the "dose" of exercise (greater intensity or longer duration), the greater the performance decrement will be.

THE CUMULATIVE CURVE

The cumulative fitness–fatigue curve, which is the sum of the positive (fitness) and negative (fatigue) effects, has an oscillatory shape with two distinct parts (**Figure 17.3**). Those parts depict the reality that beneficial adaptations to exercise often take time to occur due to biological signaling/repair mechanisms. For example, muscle damage happens rapidly, whereas muscle repair occurs over days. Thus, after a moderate- to high-intensity exercise session, it is common to see a diminished performance in the short term. The return toward the baseline represents faster-acting restoration in physiological function as beneficial adaptations begin to be seen.

The curve does cross a theoretical zero point at the end of the negative side of the curve, reflecting a net zero change in performance. This does not mean an individual is fully ready for the next session, as there is still residual fatigue. However, performance

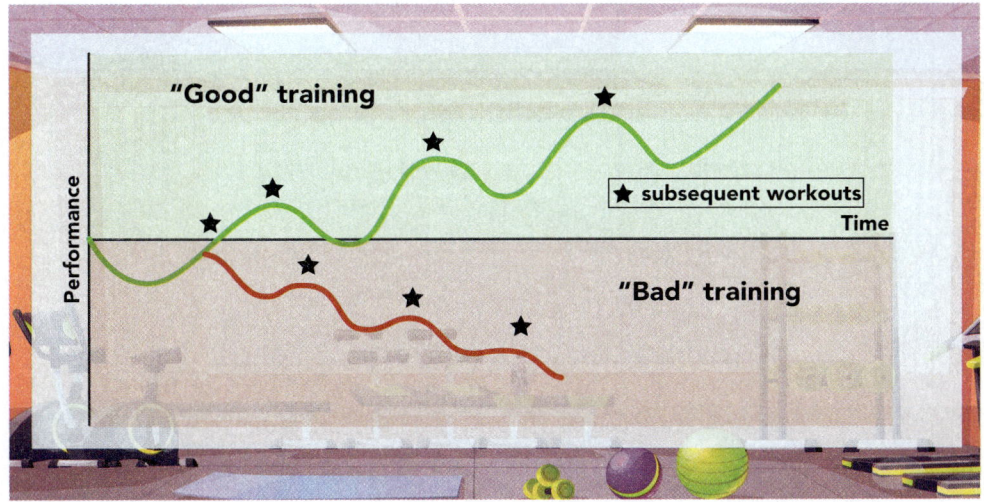

FIGURE 17.3 Subsequent Session Timing and Its Effect on the Fitness–Fatigue Curve

gains can theoretically occur after this stage. Thus, many coaches suggest timing sessions during the second positive part of the curve, which is the area of supercompensation, as fitness is elevated past the initial point before exercise. Repeatedly timing exercise sessions during the supercompensation phase should lead to additive supercompensation—that is, an upward trend in fitness over time.

The second part of the cumulative curve is largely positive compared to the baseline and represents fitness gains exceeding the remaining (if any) fatigue. Recall that some beneficial physiological pathways and responses to stress take hours or days to yield results (e.g., structural or enzymatic protein restoration, glycogen supercompensation, adrenal balance, and neural adaptations, among others). By the time these benefits have been maximized, fatigue, under this model, has subsided enough to yield a *net* beneficial response. This does not necessarily mean that fatigue is absent, but rather that the performance benefits of added fitness outweigh the remaining fatigue.

The last part of the cumulative fitness–fatigue curve is a return to baseline, which suggests that fatigue has returned to baseline and fitness gains have now attenuated, resulting in a net zero change. Note that this curve represents a response to a single exercise bout, meaning the changes over time depend on the timing of the following exercise session (net downward, no change, or net upward trends) (Zatsiorsky et al., 2020).

EFFECT OF EXERCISE DOSING ON THE FITNESS–FATIGUE CURVE

Exercise dose, a function of exercise intensity and duration, affects each curve component (**Figure 17.4**). Typically, intensity and duration will make the curve larger in both the negative and positive directions, reflecting more fatigue from the workout and more net benefit. Additionally, the curve will be stretched rightward due to the time it takes to recover and manifest positive adaptive changes (Kreider et al., 1998).

EFFECTS OF REST AND RECOVERY

Rest and recovery, in theory, can affect this curve as well. Typically, improving rest and recovery affects the speed at which the negative effects are overcome and the rate at which benefits come. Therefore, the curve (**Figure 17.5**) can be "stretched" horizontally (rightward if recovery is suboptimal, leftward if recovery is optimal).

EXERCISE DOSE →

A theoretical quantification of an exercise session, which is a function of both its intensity and its duration.

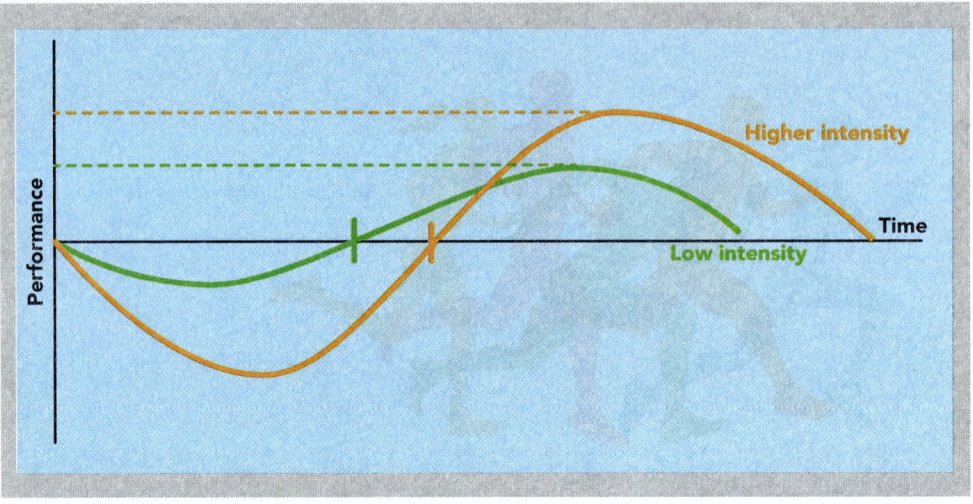

FIGURE 17.4 Effects of Intensity on the Performance Curve

Data from Kreider, R. B. 1962-, Fry, A. C. 1956-, O'Toole, M. Louise., Kreider, R. B. 1962-, Fry, A. C. 1956-, & O'Toole, M. Louise. (1998). Overtraining in Sport. Human Kinetics; WorldCat.org.

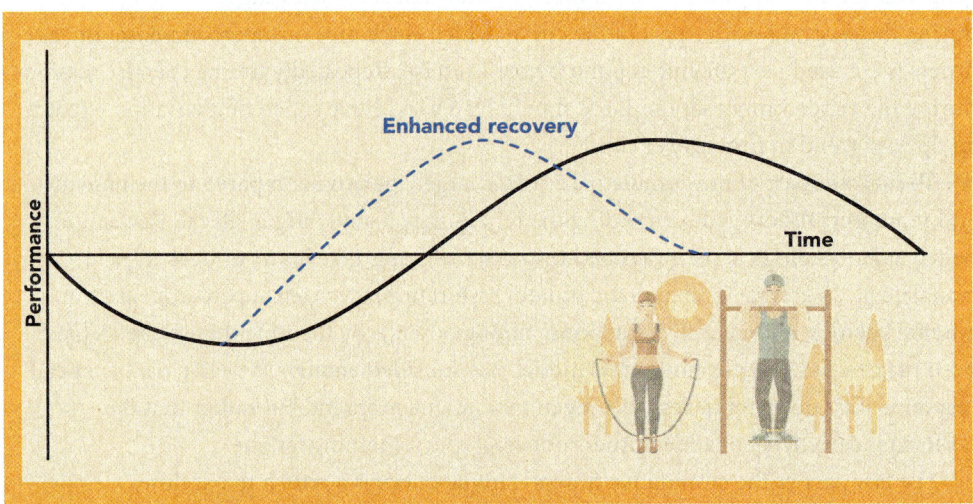

FIGURE 17.5 Conceptual Effects of Enhanced Recovery

LESSON 2: RECOVERY PROGRAMMING METHODS
EVIDENCE-BASED REST AND RECOVERY METHODS

In athletic development, the implementation of validated rest and recovery methods has been shown to optimize performance and promote overall athlete well-being. These multidimensional methods encompass elements such as quality sleep, proper nutrition and hydration, manual recovery techniques, and mindfulness practices. Sleep is considered a crucial pillar, given its role in physiological repair and cognitive function; achieving sufficient and quality sleep is thus an area of key focus. Nutrition and hydration, meanwhile, provide the vital macronutrients, micronutrients, and fluids that replenish energy stores and aid in tissue repair and rehydration. Manual recovery techniques, including myofascial rolling, massage, and compression, alleviate muscle tension and promote soft-tissue health. Lastly, meditation and breath work provide psychological rest, helping athletes manage stress and improve mental resilience. Based on the scientific evidence, each method appears to contribute uniquely to the comprehensive rest and recovery program, emphasizing the interconnectedness of physical, nutritional, and mental recovery in athletic performance.

SLEEP METHODS

Sleep is vital for normal physiological functioning. Perhaps unsurprisingly, it can be a pivotal contributor to recovery and athletic success. Sleep helps athletes recover and restores their systems from previous stressors. Although a single night of sleep cannot fully recover or restore function from an exhaustive day, special sleep considerations can accelerate recovery, and poor sleep quality can hinder recovery.

Four major stages of sleep are distinguished based on whether they include **rapid eye movement (REM) sleep** or **non-rapid eye movement (NREM) sleep** (Rodenbeck et al., 2006) (**Table 17.1**). REM sleep is a sleep state in which the brain's electrical activity is dyssynchronous; this activity reflects brain cells that are very active, firing rapidly at different times. NREM sleep is a sleep state in which the brain's electrical activity is synchronous; this activity reflects neurons that are firing slowly and together.

TABLE 17.1 Major Stages of Sleep

NREM1	The lightest stage of sleep; often represents the transition to NREM2 sleep from an awake state and is brief (5–15 minutes). Not many benefits of sleep are observed during this stage.
NREM2	A stage of light sleep, where arousal can easily occur; typically makes up most of the sleep in the total number of minutes. During light sleep, the body benefits mildly from sleep, and most of the night of sleep is spent in this stage. Waking and movement during this stage are common.
NREM3	Also known as slow-wave sleep (SWS) or delta-wave sleep; often considered "deep sleep." This stage is the most restorative, where most of the therapeutic process has the most significant impact (e.g., secretion of growth hormone, which aids in tissue growth and repair). Deep sleep makes up roughly 20% of sleep each night and occurs primarily in the first half of the night; the second half is composed more of REM sleep.
REM	Characterized by the rapid movement of the eyes; considered "paradoxical sleep" because it is a state in which an individual is hardest to wake up from, yet physiological signals, including heart rate, respiratory rate, and brain waves, are closer to the signals during awake periods. It is thought that most memory formation, cognitive processing, and other psychological effects occur during this stage, leading to a slightly heightened sense of physiological state. However, neurotransmitters paralyze muscles during this stage, so individuals do not act out dreams that might occur.

Data from Rodenbeck, A., Binder, R., Geisler, P., Danker-Hopfe, H., Lund, R., Raschke, F., Weeß, H.-G., & Schulz, H. (2006). A Review of Sleep EEG Patterns. Part I: A Compilation of Amended Rules for Their Visual Recognition according to Rechtschaffen and Kales. *Somnologie, 10*(4), 159–175. https://onlinelibrary.wiley.com/doi/abs/10.1111/j.1439-054x.2006.00101.x

RAPID EYE MOVEMENT (REM) SLEEP →

A sleep state in which the brain's electrical activity is dyssynchronous; an electroencephalo-graph (EEG) shows this as low-voltage, high-frequency activity. This activity reflects brain cells that are very active, firing rapidly at different times.

NON-RAPID EYE MOVEMENT (NREM) SLEEP →

A sleep state in which the brain's electrical activity is synchronous; it is measured by an elec-troencephalograph (EEG) as high-voltage, low-frequency brain activity. This activity reflects neurons that are firing slowly and together.

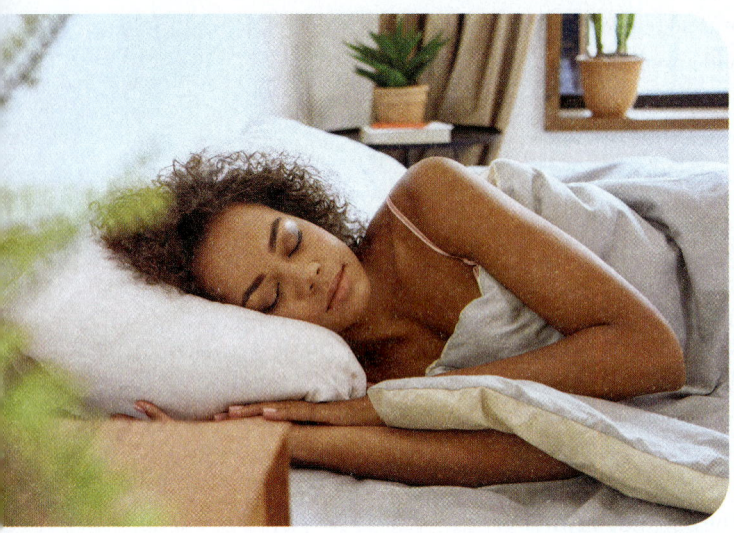
© Ground Picture/Shutterstock

Not all sleep is considered equally beneficial. Larger total and relative amounts of deep sleep correlate with better physical and cognitive function (Nofsinger & Shank, 2019). As such, counting hours of sleep may not be enough to track sleep and its effects on performance and recovery. In general, more sleep may lead to better performance, but if sleep is restless or predominantly light, sleep's effectiveness may not reach its full potential.

Any factors that increase sleep quality can be seen as performance and recovery enhancing (Bird, 2013). Some of these factors include sleeping in colder environments, reducing exposure to blue light in the evening, being consistent with regular sleep and wake times, minimizing consumption of foods before sleep, reducing stressful activities (work and exercise) closer to bedtime, and improving mattress and pillow quality.

Certain supplements, such as tryptophan, B-vitamins (B_3, B_6, and B_{12}), zinc, magnesium, and melatonin, are widely available and are claimed to improve sleep quality (Ordóñez et al., 2017). Other recovery strategies (e.g., massage, light therapy, meditation) have been shown to have some efficacy in improving sleep quality, particularly in reducing **sleep latency**, but more research is required to understand the full nature of dosing and quality control.

Because of the many small changes that can be made to improve sleep consistency, quality, and duration, many sleep experts recommend finding a pre-bedtime routine that enhances sleep and sticking to this routine as best as possible. Many of these behaviors send signals to the central nervous system to encourage hormonal cycles, such as melatonin production (Prayag et al., 2019).

SLEEP LATENCY →

The time taken between lying down and falling asleep.

📋 COACH'S CORNER

Despite prevailing cultural beliefs suggesting an inverse relationship between sleep and productivity, embodied in mantras like "rise and grind" and "training while others are sleeping," research consistently affirms the opposite is true. Rather than detracting from productivity, increased sleep has been shown to enhance cognitive performance, physical function, and overall productivity, thereby bolstering athletic performance. This underscores the principle of "sharpening the axe," where time invested in sleep heightens efficiency. Consequently, Sports Performance Coaches should prioritize getting optimal sleep for athletes—typically 7 to 9 hours per night—over extending training sessions, recognizing its pivotal role in athletic development and performance.

NUTRITION AND HYDRATION METHODS

The role of nutrition and hydration as significant performance enhancers in sports and athletic endeavors is well established. Numerous studies have explored their direct impacts on enhancing athletic performance, fueling physical exertion, and improving endurance. However, the intricate connection between these elements and recovery—an equally essential component of an athlete's regimen—is an area that is increasingly drawing research interest. Though sometimes overshadowed by performance-centric perspectives, the nexus of nutrition, hydration, and recovery is central to creating a comprehensive athlete development strategy. This involves understanding an athlete's specific nutritional and hydration needs post-exercise, and meeting them in ways that contribute to immediate recovery, overall resilience, and long-term performance enhancement.

For purposes ranging from replenishing glycogen stores to facilitating muscle repair, consuming the proper nutrients and sufficient fluids is crucial. Consequently, nutrition strategies must extend beyond performance fueling to encompass these crucial recovery aspects, fostering a more balanced and sustainable athletic development approach.

PRE-EXERCISE

The effects of pre-exercise nutrition are well documented in relation to performance improvements for the exercise session, especially regarding carbohydrate and fluid consumption. By comparison, only minimal evidence supports the notion that pre-exercise nutrition aids recovery. This is not due to a lack of findings; rather, only a limited number of studies have been performed in this area. Given the benefits of recovery from nutrition taken during and after exercise (outlined in the following subsections), pre-exercise nutrition may be an excellent way to set up good practices earlier. After all, heading into a workout when ill prepared is likely to increase metabolic stress, increasing recovery demand.

PERI-EXERCISE

The concept of nutrition and hydration during exercise is familiar to many athletes and coaches as a way to maintain performance during an exercise session or competition, so much so that an entire industry has developed around it. In addition, some studies illustrate that peri-exercise nutrition and hydration can improve recovery from that individual session. This consideration is important because many training programs comprise a series of exercise training sessions, including times when sessions may be separated by less than 24 hours.

In most of the studies performed, carbohydrates and water were provided as peri-exercise nutrition. Properly fueling the body with carbohydrates and water appears to reduce cortisol and improve heart rate variability–based stress markers of stress post-exercise (McAnulty et al., 2003; Peçanha et al., 2014). Therefore, post-exercise stress may be slightly lower when proper nutrition is considered during exercise.

Although no specific guidelines exist for *recovery* purposes, it appears that intake of approximately 30 to 60 grams of carbohydrates per hour of prolonged exercise is best for performance (Rosenbloom et al., 2012) and approximately 6 to 12 fluid ounces of water every 15 to 30 minutes of the exercise session (Manore, 2005).

POST-EXERCISE

Many athletes understand the value of post-exercise nutrition, which is why the sports nutrition industry offers a seemingly endless array of recovery drinks, mixes, and supplements. Numerous studies have been performed to illustrate the benefits of such nutrition. This section will not present a comprehensive review of these options, but rather reminds coaches that starting recovery as soon as possible has known benefits.

Many researchers agree that taking a mixture of water, carbohydrates, and protein after exercise yields the best absorption and utilization of nutrients, which provides the

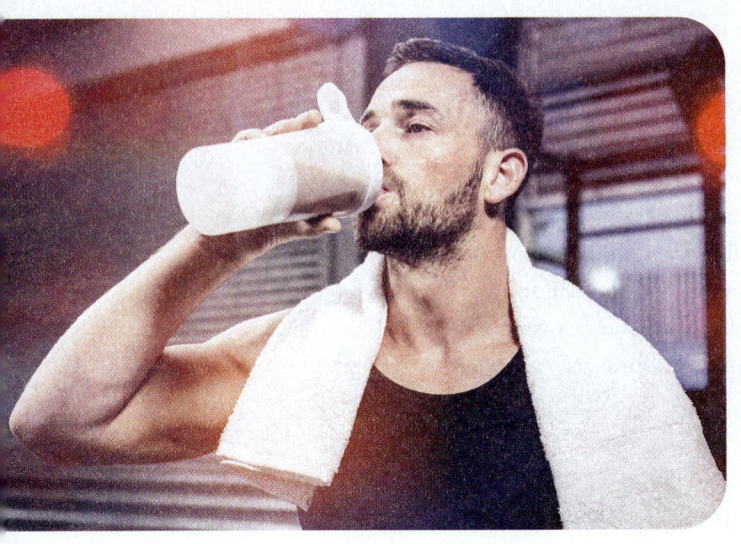

© Vectorfusionart/Shutterstock

necessary nutrients quickly and effectively. Note that missing the timing window or not consuming the correct ratios of macronutrients does not ruin recovery; many individuals will still recover as long as their dietary needs are met over the following 12 to 24 hours (Parkin et al., 1997).

However, optimal timing and composition of diet post-exercise are most important when recovery must be quick, as in subsequent workouts or competitions—for example, later in the day or first thing the following morning after a late session. Optimizing nutrient intake for recovery means taking in 30 to 60 grams of carbohydrates within 30 minutes of the end of an activity due to the upregulation of enzymes and glucose transporters (Derave et al., 1999).

Additionally, a larger composition of carbohydrates mixed with protein within 2 hours of exercise yields higher glucose absorption due to increased insulin responses, but may not produce increased glycogen synthesis and remains a point of debate (Alghannam et al., 2018). During this 2-hour window, intake of approximately 20 to 25 grams of protein appears to benefit protein synthesis as well (Beelen et al., 2010). Beyond this window, eating well-balanced, nutritional meals as part of a "typical" diet is acceptable to facilitate proper recovery.

MANUAL RECOVERY METHODS

Manual techniques have long been a staple in the recovery of high-performing athletes. More recently, attention and marketing of these methods have focused on nonprofessional athletes. After all, anyone who engages in exercise training is likely to deal with muscle and joint pain that would benefit from manual techniques. Traditionally, professional athletes can utilize athletic trainers, manual and physical therapists, chiropractors, and other clinicians who can apply massage, dry needling, acupuncture, or other modalities. However, self-massage has been shown to bring similar results, with far less cost and time.

When used as a recovery modality, self-myofascial techniques aim to address areas of tension or tightness and to encourage fluid movement through muscle tissue. Although this has implications for performance, the movement of fluids can also benefit lymphatic uptake (Mortimer et al., 1990) by facilitating proper cell function and waste removal. Typically, blood flow handles most of these tasks; however, if blood flow is reduced (as in sedentary states), nutrient delivery and waste removal can be blunted. Massaging or otherwise applying pressure to a tight muscle may increase local blood flow to the area, bringing more fluids to the local tissues and helping to "turn" the extracellular space fluid, which is absorbed by the lymphatic system. This movement of fluids is helpful for the maintenance and return to a proper physiological state.

This modality can be beneficial to many athletes regardless of activity level or competitiveness. A recreationally active person who has a sedentary desk job may have muscle tightness from sitting all day; an elite amateur may not have the time or money for a physical or manual therapist to aid in recovery after hard training; a person overcoming a surgery who may not exercise but wants to regain function in their joints may benefit from these modalities as well. Thankfully, many of these techniques are now available to the average consumer.

When managing recent injuries, it is important to be cautious about applying manual therapies requiring physical contact, pressure, or vibration. Pressure and manual techniques can aggravate inflammation and interrupt healing. Any individual with a fresh injury should consult with a sports medicine practitioner. Individuals with neuropathies, osteoporosis, or joint disorders (including arthritis) may require extra consideration when introducing foam rolling and percussive or compression devices.

MYOFASCIAL ROLLING

Myofascial rollers are one of the most widely used and adopted technologies by athletes at every level. They can be used for most of the lower legs, back, and selected regions around the neck and chest. These rollers are often most effective when muscles are tight, as the pressure from body weight can be used broadly or pinpoint to a region to release myofascial tension. Even so, 20 minutes of myofascial rolling at the end of a session appears to positively affect recovery and subsequent performance (Rey et al., 2019). This may be partly due to observed improvements in arterial function (Okamoto et al., 2014).

Similar techniques include the use of hard or soft balls (e.g., softballs, tennis balls, lacrosse balls) to increase pressure in certain regions, such as the calf, gluteal muscles, shoulder, or other hard-to-reach areas. In addition, massage sticks may be used to apply pressure with the hands instead of gravity; and other specialty-shaped tools to apply pressure in certain regions in specific ways. While caution should always be used when rolling, extra care should be given when using a roller that is not intended for soft-tissue work (e.g., lacrosse balls) to avoid injury because the ergonomics are not explicitly designed for the pressure distribution of rolling.

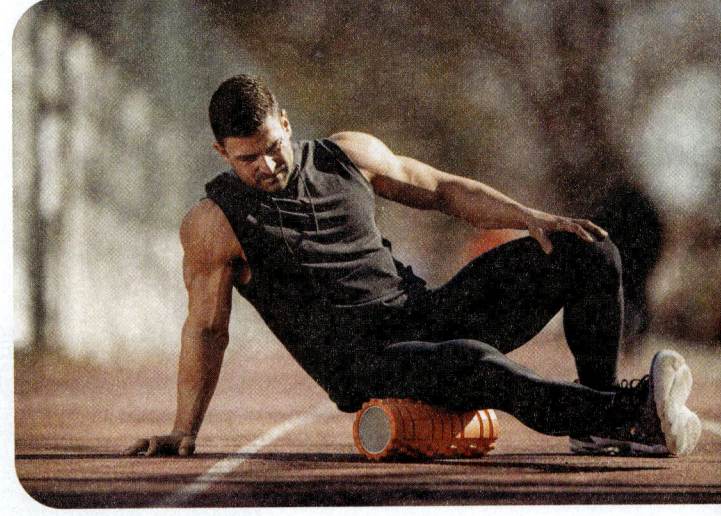

© Just Life/Shutterstock

As a form of recovery, athletes are encouraged to use myofascial rolling on areas identified as short and overactive via movement assessments. In addition, the prime movers utilized during physical training can be targeted post-exercise to help mitigate delayed-onset muscle soreness (DOMS). For example, suppose an athlete has a training day that includes heavy squats. In that case, they will want to perform myofascial rolling on the gluteal, quadriceps, and calf complex during their post-exercise session. Spending 30 seconds to 2 minutes per muscle group can provide benefits in ROM and soreness, although additional application time does not appear to be detrimental (Behm et al., 2020).

MUSCLE VIBRATION

Muscle vibration is another way of eliciting similar responses without the direct, localized application of pressure. In theory, the vibration of a muscle body causes back-and-forth movement on a small but fast scale, leading to the mechanical release of actin–myosin binding sites and relieving tension in fascial tissues. Popular examples of muscle vibration tools include the Hyperice Vyper and Therabody Core Roller, which add multiple levels of muscle vibration into the common massage ball and foam roller tools.

An important distinction to make is between muscle vibration and whole-body vibration *training*. Although more research needs to be done to elucidate the characteristics and benefits of each of these categories, whole-body vibration training tends to utilize contractile elements of muscle sarcomeres to dampen vibration (Wakeling et al., 2002) and may have effects on neural activation. Lower doses may provide performance benefits (Cardinale & Bosco, 2003), but higher doses, especially load-bearing vibration, may lead to peripheral fatigue (Adamo et al., 2002).

Local muscle vibration, which does not rely on concomitant contraction, has been noted to improve blood perfusion (Fuller et al., 2013), which aids in muscle fiber recovery, allowing for both nutrient uptake and waste removal. In addition, this modality facilitates the movement of fluids in a way similar to myofascial rolling, which increases lymphatic uptake. Vibration therapy can improve performance in activities requiring high neural capacity (Osawa et al., 2013) but requires more research. In support of the purported neural adaptations, one study found an increase in pressure pain tolerance after vibrating foam rolling compared to regular foam rolling (Cheatham et al., 2019).

Although more research needs to be done to examine its neural effects, local vibration appears to have some transient effects. For example, one study noted that older adults who received local vibration therapy performed better on strength and functional measures (Lau et al., 2011). While many studies of this recovery method have been conducted, a wide variety of protocols are used, and recommendations cannot be made. However, many studies used 30 to 60 Hz, 3 to 6 mm of displacement, and 8 to 15 minutes of cumulative duration (some protocols were noncontinuous) (Germann et al., 2018).

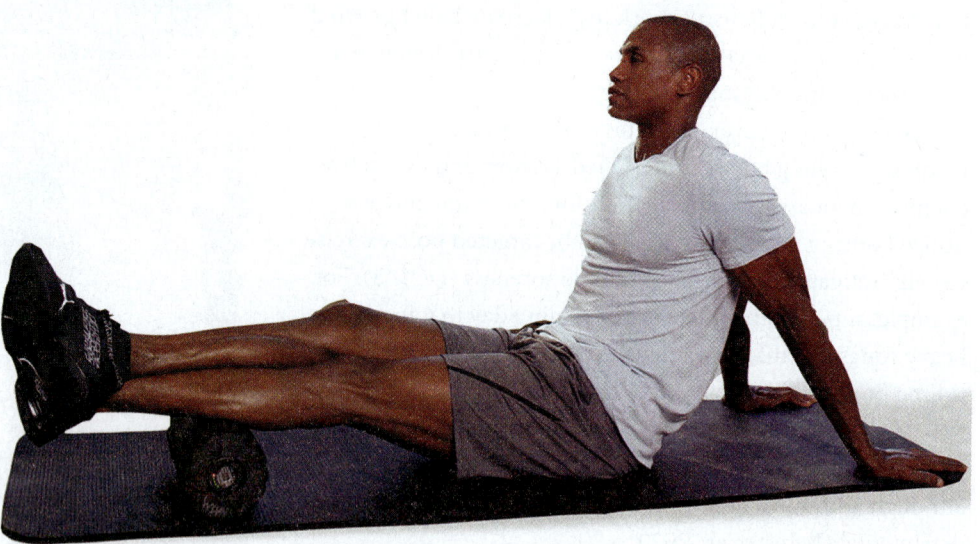

Self-Myofascial Release with Vibrating Roller

PERCUSSION DEVICES

Percussion devices have become a popular way to obtain results more quickly and easily than is possible with foam rolling and vibration techniques. Many percussion devices are handheld electronic devices that oscillate back and forth, with soft heads that impact the muscle. These devices usually have variable oscillation frequencies that can be tuned for specific athlete preferences. With different heads and an overall more focused location than a foam roller, targeting individual spots, particularly ones deep in the muscle, is more easily achievable with percussion massagers.

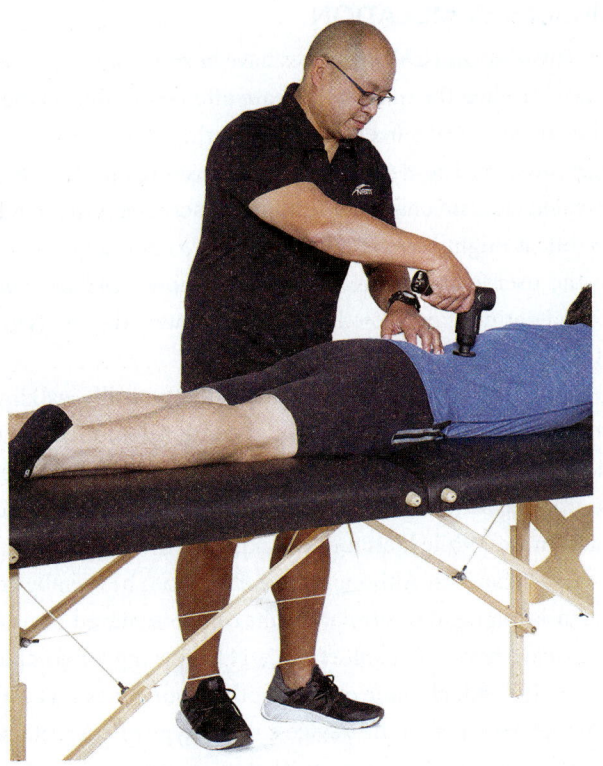

STRETCHING

Stretching of any type may aid recovery when performed as part of a post-workout session. It allows for tension release in muscles and reset of the muscle sensors (spindles and Golgi tendon organs), which may lead to less tightness later. However, stretching may have only minimal effects on soreness related to muscle damage (Herbert et al., 2011).

Additionally, it is suggested that this recovery method may increase parasympathetic activity acutely after stretching, but more studies are needed to confirm these findings (Eda et al., 2020; Farinatti et al., 2011). When practicing stretching, caution is advised for individuals with current musculoskeletal injuries or superficial wounds, as stretching may disrupt local healing or aggravate injured areas.

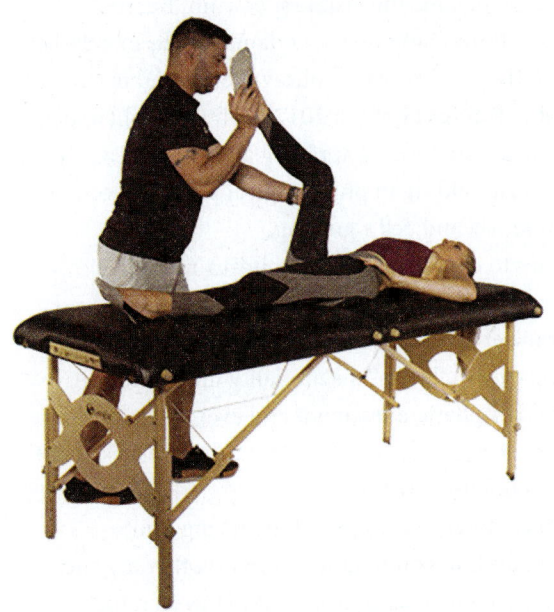 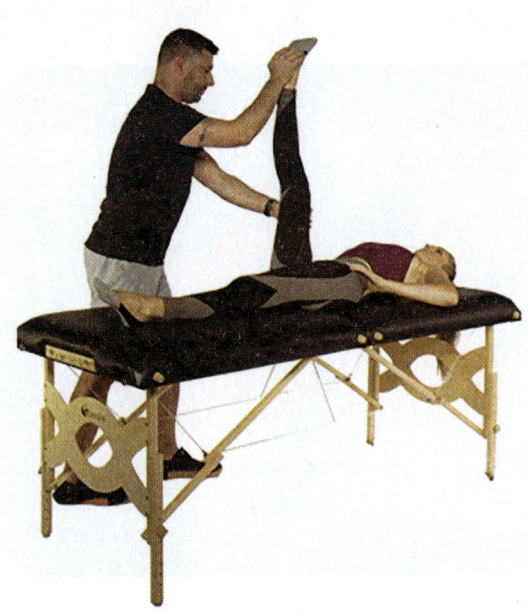

ELECTRONIC MUSCLE STIMULATION

Electronic muscle stimulation (EMS) devices have become ubiquitous as more affordable options have reached the market; they are often employed as therapy for injury recovery. EMS applies an electrical current on the skin through electrodes, which can be placed over the target muscles. The electrical current causes the muscle to contract by stimulating voltage-gated calcium channels, leading to increased intracellular calcium and troponin binding. While it might seem counterintuitive to contract muscles for recovery, EMS is a passive-to-the-user form of active recovery. Notably, EMS also appears to benefit injury recovery by accelerating axon growth and bone mineral density (Dudley-Javoroski & Shields, 2008; Fu et al., 2020).

It is plausible that muscle contractions at low intensity (typically walking, easy swimming, some yoga/Pilates, and so on) can lead to better subsequent performance because of increased blood flow (Varatharajan et al., 2015), lymphatic movement (Burgess et al., 2019), glucose uptake (Sanchez et al., 2020), neural tuning (Vanderthommen & Duchateau, 2007), and more. While literature is lacking on this topic, many top-level coaches encourage these behaviors. Although these effects can be seen by going for a walk at the end of a hard training day, similar results can be achieved for isolated muscles and without having to leave home (Babault et al., 2011), allowing for completion of other activities that require an individual's time or use of other modalities that can aid in recovery.

Recommended usage depends on the device and the type of current used, but many portable devices have preprogrammed sessions that may serve as a good starting point. Beginning with 10- to 15-minute sessions at a tolerable intensity, with contraction-to-rest ratios of approximately 1:3, may yield the best benefits when starting out (Nussbaum et al., 2017). As familiarity with the device increases, the intensity and duration can be increased to comfort, primarily when EMS is used as a recovery method (not pre-exercise). EMS should be limited or avoided when an individual has a pacemaker (use on the chest region), over sensitive areas (e.g., transcranial, eyes, carotid arch, genitalia), or on the torso during pregnancy.

INFRARED AND RED-LIGHT THERAPY

Infrared and red-light therapy is a form of photo-biomodulation that remains lesser known in the athletic and scientific communities but shows promise as a recovery method. Infrared light is a lower-energy light outside the visible spectrum. Because of its low energy, infrared light does not damage cells or cellular components in the same way that ultraviolet or higher-energy wavelengths do (Tsai & Hamblin, 2017). Infrared light appears to primarily act as a method of applying an external energy source (felt as heat), aiding in physiological pathways centered on the mitochondria and cell signaling.

Most studies to date demonstrate mild-to-moderate improvements in exercise performance with use of infrared light (Dellagrana et al., 2018), though little research has been done on the recovery effects. This modality may improve blood flow and lymphatic movement and even have calming effects on the central nervous system (Mitchell & Mack, 2013; Vatansever & Hamblin, 2012).

De Marchi et al. (2017) suggested that using photo-biomodulation, both in combination with cryotherapy and on its own, may attenuate oxidative stress. However, the

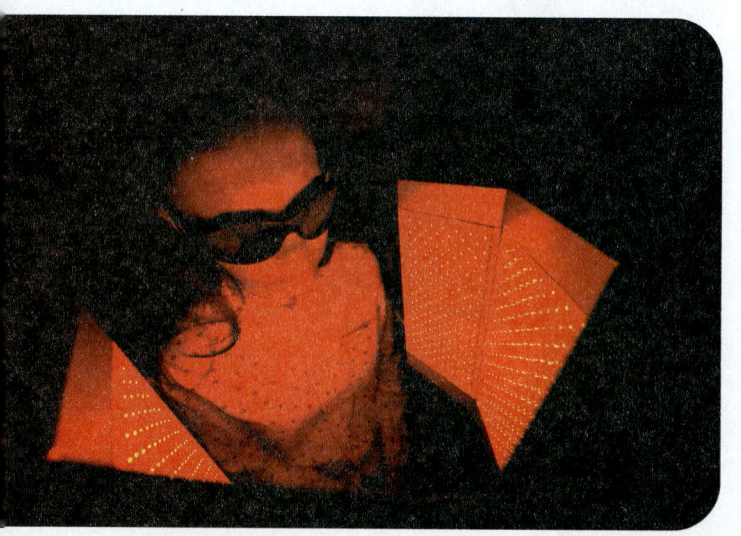

© Evgeniy Kalinovskiy/Shutterstock

mechanism is unknown (De Marchi et al., 2017). While more research needs to be done to understand the physiological effects, infrared light is a popular solution for in-home saunas, which may provide similar benefits.

Currently, due to device differences, it is challenging to make dosing recommendations. Concentrated delivery appears to be best, at a level of 30 to 60 joules per muscle (Dellagrana et al., 2018; De Marchi et al., 2017). The dosing guidelines for whole-body exposure (e.g., infrared saunas, LED panels) are less clear due to variations in proximity to the light, number of LEDs, and wavelengths used. It is best to follow the manufacturer's recommended guidelines as a starting point.

> ⚠ **CRITICAL**
>
> When applying light therapy, contraindications include photosensitivity, epilepsy, alcohol use, and pregnancy (although individuals may consult with their doctor to determine the validity of this contraindication). Because light therapy has similar effects to a sauna, proper hydration is recommended.

COMPRESSION THERAPY

Compression therapy is similar to massage and myofascial rolling in that it applies an external force to a limb, joint, or muscle to facilitate blood flow, improve tissue oxygen saturation and lymphatic movement, and ease muscle tension (Keith et al., 1992; Ménétrier et al., 2011). Two types of compression are generally used in commercial products—inflatable compression and compression fabric garments. Inflatable compression consists of sleeves made for different parts of the body, which inflate bladders much like a blood pressure cuff. Many devices utilize computer interfaces to control the pumps and, therefore, can offer different pressures, patterns, and compression modalities. Because these devices are powered, they do not require physical input from the user to obtain the intended benefit.

By comparison, compression garments have been used longer and more widely due to the relatively simple technology and low-cost approach. These garments are designed to be worn over targeted tissues and apply a constant mild pressure (lower than that of inflatable devices). Compression can differ among garments based on the garment's size, fabric, and cut, and can also be "tuned" to add more compression in some areas and less in others. These garments are more popular for individuals with circulation issues, often encouraging lymphatic return, reducing swelling and edema in limbs, and reducing embolism risk during inactivity (Eppsteiner et al., 2010).

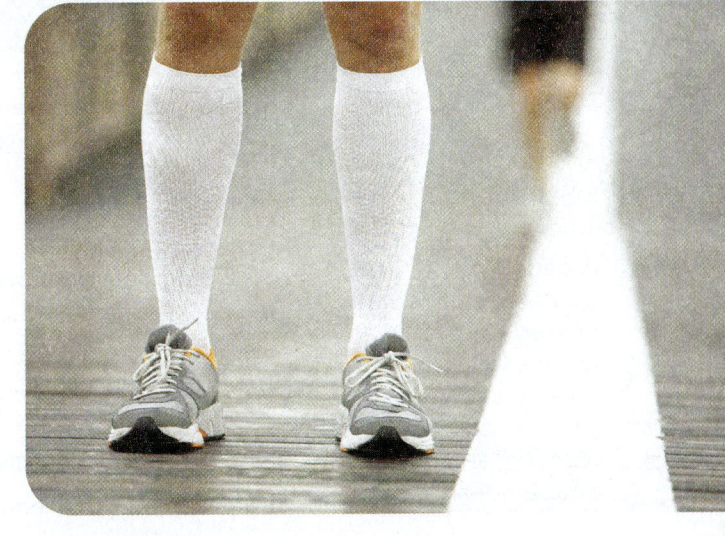

© Maridav/Shutterstock

Compression garments offer a wide variety of constant or variable pressures in different wearable forms, making dosing challenging to understand. Commercially available products that rely on pneumatic pressure have their own protocols; for best results, starting with 15 minutes at lower pressure settings may be an excellent choice for recovery protocols, with the duration and pressures being adjusted over time to the individual's preferences. As when considering the use of manual techniques, individuals who have muscle pain, fresh injuries, joint disorders, or neuropathies should seek advice from their medical practitioner before undertaking such therapy.

CRYOTHERAPY

Cryotherapy utilizes cold air or water to stimulate physiological responses that are intended to improve recovery. Many kinds of cryotherapies are available, including both whole-body and localized options. Whole-body modalities tend to have more global effects for widespread change, whereas local therapies may be targeted to get a specific response from an individual muscle (Rose et al., 2017). Cryotherapy produces the following global changes (Loap & Lathe, 2018; Nasi et al., 2020):

- Metabolic shifts, which activate thermogenesis and can lead to "browning" of adipose tissue (converting it to a more "energy-burning" form of adipose tissue)
- Increased levels of anabolic hormones such as growth hormone and testosterone
- Global vasoconstriction, which may transiently encourage lymphatic uptake, followed by an influx of blood flow upon cessation of cryotherapy

Leveraging changes in blood flow to cold (vasoconstriction) and subsequently warm (vasodilation) is a common strategy to facilitate the "pumping" of blood and may enhance certain outcomes such as lymphatic movement compared to cryotherapy alone (Kim et al., 2020).

Two critical considerations of cryotherapy are the temperature and the cooling modality; convection and conduction are elemental in heat transfer. Water transfers heat at a rate 25 times faster than air. In consequence, it takes less time to reach critical hypothermia if temperatures are too low, and the water temperature should be seen as not comparable to the air temperature. Additionally, the presence of a convection source may increase cooling. For water cryotherapy, temperatures ranging from 10°C to 15°C (50°F to 59°F) for 10 to 15 minutes are sufficient.

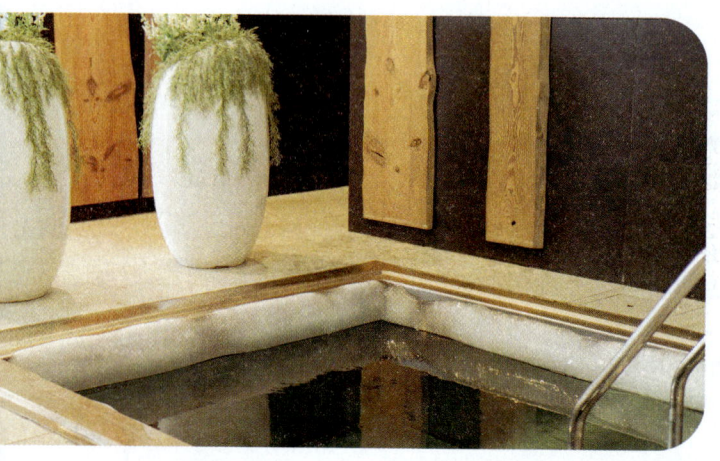

© Nieriss/Shutterstock

TRY THIS

If you take an ice bath, after a few minutes, stir the water around and notice how much colder it gets. This is why convection makes a considerable difference.

If completing a contrast protocol, timing should consist of a 1:1 to 1:4 ratio of cold to warm, where "warm" is 38°C to 40°C (100°F to 104°F). Contraindications include hypersensitivity to cold, open wounds (for water immersion), impaired circulation, and severe cardiovascular conditions.

DELOAD PROGRAMMING

Deload training is a commonly used strategy in periodized programming, in which volume and intensity are significantly reduced, allowing for recovery and adaptation. This programming is highly recommended for all athletes because application of a consistent stimulus and pushing harder may not allow enough time for the athlete to adapt to training fully. While maintaining movements at low intensities, neural recruitment and underlying fitness can be maintained, whereas taking a week off from training may cause more issues than it solves. Most exercises that are prescribed movements or activities can be included during deloading if the intensity is able to be greatly reduced.

The primary goals are to use the same muscle groupings with less mechanical stress, support blood flow, retain some neural and physiological pathways, and prevent deconditioning compared to sedentary rest. In theory, deloading is like a taper. However, because peak performance is not the end goal, high-intensity sessions need not be leveraged. In fact, they are discouraged in most cases due to the increased risk of adverse effects, such as injuries, overexertion, or creating too much stress during a deloading period.

It may be hard to convince some athletes of the value of the deloading approach, but the top athletes in most sports do, in fact, utilize some form of deloading. This allows for mesocycles that build toward functional overreaching and then back off to allow the body to recover. After a deloading week, the goal is to deliver the athlete to the following cycle with full readiness to handle the next mesocycle.

MEDITATION AND BREATH WORK METHODS

Meditation has been shown to aid in recovery by activating the parasympathetic pathways. Many meditation practices aim to remove outside stressors and focus inwardly on the body, particularly on breathing. By eliminating external stimuli and thoughts and paying attention to the body, many athletes notice a reduction in perceived stress, improved physiological indicators of parasympathetic activity, and better overall mood and mindset.

Mindfulness may offer similar results, although mindfulness and meditation are practiced in different ways. Mindfulness is typically more focused on intention, whereas meditation emphasizes the removal or direction of thoughts (Van Dam et al., 2018). Due to constraints in mindfulness practices, many research studies show mixed results for this modality, albeit similar directionality to meditation (Christodoulou et al., 2020).

Many top athletes use meditation or variants of it (such as mindfulness or sensory deprivation) to "train" the parasympathetic response to calm their mind and body (Zhang et al., 2019). These effects can be seen when the athlete practices for as little as a few minutes a day (Chang et al., 2020). Indeed, meditation can show effects in as little as 1 minute (Nair et al., 2017), but more can be better, to an extent. Meditating 15 minutes once or twice daily seems to be an effective and practical way to achieve most of the effects with minimal time commitment (Prasad et al., 2011). In summary, meditation can be a straightforward approach that has real, tangible effects on reducing stress and improving recovery.

Similarly, sensory reduction has become more common in recent years, particularly in the form of "float tanks." These isolated pods contain a high-specific-gravity saline solution, which allows an individual to float and be removed from environmental stimuli when the pod is closed. Although novel, this method appears to improve subsequent performance parameters compared to passive recovery (Broderick et al., 2019) as well as to improve mood states (Driller & Argus, 2016).

Breath training is, in essence, an isolated form of meditation; that is, breathing awareness contributes to many of the benefits of meditation. Despite the focus on breathing, the goal for recovery is not to improve the physiological function of the pulmonary system. Instead, the athlete seeks to focus attention on the breathing rate and depth to calm their parasympathetic pathway. Studies have noted that respiratory sensors

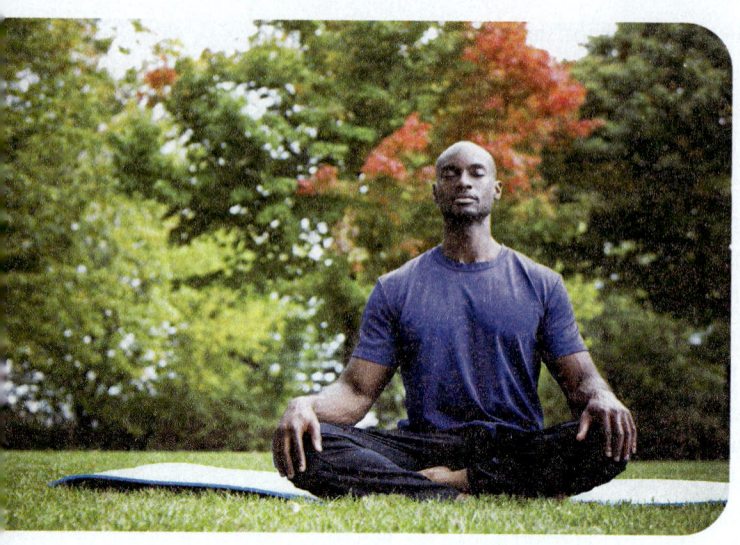

© Zdenka Darula/Shutterstock

(chemoreceptors, mechanoreceptors, and baroreceptors) send information to the brain's respiratory centers (Brinkman et al., 2021), which are located in the medulla oblongata. This center is also responsible for controlling cardiovascular responses, so it is no surprise that pulmonary input prompts the medulla oblongata to send signals to the heart to modulate contractile processes.

One notable phenomenon is respiratory sinus arrhythmia, which is the observation that heart rate tends to speed up with inspiration and slow down with expiration. This is merely a demonstration of the interconnection of the two systems. Nevertheless, studies have shown that breathing work enormously influences cardiovascular parameters, specifically heart rate and heart rate variability (Kromenacker et al., 2018), as well as decision making (De Couck et al., 2019).

⚙ TRY THIS

Find your pulse, close your eyes, and begin to take deeper and slower breaths. You will notice your pulse speed up and slow down with each breath, and likely slowing down overall the longer you go.

LESSON 3: CLIENT-CENTRIC RECOVERY PROGRAMMING
COMMUNICATING ABOUT REST AND RECOVERY

As a Sports Performance Coach, it is important not only to understand the material around rest and recovery, but also to be able to communicate these ideas. For many athletes, other parties may influence their actions, such as their parents, family, coaches, and friends. While rest and recovery are gaining recognition as critical aspects of athletic performance, many people still insist on outdated approaches, such as going hard every workout, not taking rest days, and physically and mentally demanding too much.

Because coaches, trainers, physicians, family, and friends are all invested in an athlete's success, it is crucial to recognize that everyone involved is on the same team and that working together and agreeing on a methodology may translate into better success. Specifically, by communicating and practicing the importance of rest and recovery, the likelihood of the athlete meeting their goals in a training cycle increases significantly (Li et al., 2019; Roos et al., 2015).

The integral role of rest and recovery in an athlete's success is often underestimated by the people involved in their development journey. Therefore, clearly conveying this importance to the athlete and their support team, including coaches, family, and friends, is crucial. Although some may perceive a dichotomy between training and recovery, a deeper understanding of their synergy can reshape these perceptions, highlighting that effective training is intertwined with adequate rest and recovery. Facilitating this shared understanding encourages a cohesive approach to athletic development, with specific recommendations including scheduled rest days, adequate sleep, proper nutrition and hydration, and incorporation of mindfulness practices.

COMMUNICATING ABOUT RECOVERY TO ATHLETES

Despite the prevalence of the attitude that "doing more is better" among athletes, this belief results from not knowing how to get better and not trusting that rest and recovery are key to success. Most athletes love to perform better and are highly invested in their bodies, so they are usually receptive to hearing messages about rest and recovery. That said, implementation can be challenging due to prior habits and the perception of "falling behind" in their training on easier days.

To combat this misinformation, the Sports Performance Coach can highlight that for the athlete to get better initially, the hard days must be hard—and for that to happen, the easy days must be easy. Reminding the athlete that change and progress come from high-intensity training rather than moderate-intensity workouts may yield some results, but ultimately the athlete may feel as if they can go hard all the time. Remind the athlete that going into the workout fresher means a few extra percent more, which adds up over time, and those last few percent gains come when the body is allowed to recover.

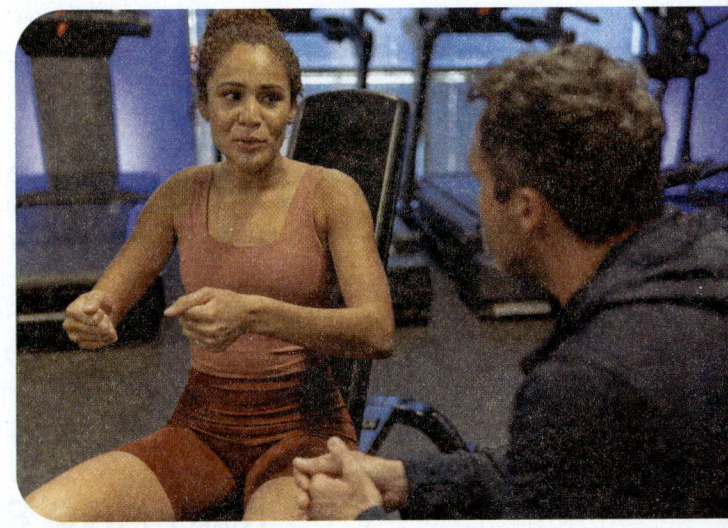

This encouragement is not necessarily needed on the hard days, but rather on the easy days, when many athletes report feeling guilt or feeling that they are falling behind. This is an excellent opportunity to remind them how beneficial rest and recovery are and how it will give them an advantage.

COMMUNICATING ABOUT RECOVERY TO COACHES

Ideally, coaches will already understand the benefits of recovery and rest for their athletes. However, if coaches do not appreciate the value of these concepts, then mismanagement of athletes is likely. A common perception among coaches is that the time in front of their athletes must be high quality (generally true), but many misinterpret high quality as a lot of work. This myth is generally more commonly encountered in youth and team sports, where discussing individual performance and recovery strategies may be challenging. Additionally, coaches may assume that rest and recovery fall outside the time athletes spend with them and take less of a role in this area.

Making assumptions about what a coach does or does not know is not recommended. Instead, it is vital to approach a coach or coaching staff by discussing strategies they recommend to their athletes for rest and recovery and asking how they have structured it into their plan to yield better performance. Focusing the discussion on implementation makes it more athlete-focused, and often will reflect what coaches do or do not know without addressing any misperceptions directly. For team sports, in particular, discussing strategies to screen for exhaustion, fatigue, or burnout is essential to the success of the athlete and team.

COMMUNICATING ABOUT RECOVERY TO PARENTS

Working with youth athletes has a unique set of challenges. It is a time when youth are physically developing, focusing on education, and immersed in social life—and yet, at the end of the day, parents have control over what they do. Generally speaking, parents are very receptive to professionals who coach and train their kids; after all, most parents want their kids to be healthy and well. In some cases, however, parents may be difficult to communicate with because they are emotionally invested in their kid's performance. These cases have become fewer in number as education around rest and recovery has improved, but parents who were former athletes and were used to pushing hard themselves may still have some unhelpful habits to break.

In all likelihood, even the parents who may be hard to communicate with regarding rest and recovery still want their child to be healthy and succeed. Therefore, the communication should be similar to talking to the athlete, with the discussion focusing on how allowing easy days and being attentive to exhaustion and fatigue can balance out stress and yield better results in the long term. This may require a two-way conversation about what parents think rest and recovery looks like and when to implement it. Often, having them explain their interpretation may allow them to see why a properly designed strategy can work better.

One last consideration: Imagine a child on an athletic team who comes home frustrated about not performing well. Some parents interpret bad performance as lousy coaching, and respond by saying their kid needs to be pushed harder to "whip them into shape." This is a complex situation in which the parent thinks they know best, but the root problem may be that the athlete needs some rest and recovery to perform better. This parent may not like hearing the message that their child needs to take it easy, and the cumulative stress at home may push the athlete even further into exhaustion. This scenario is brought up because communication with the parents may prevent a lot of undue stress on the athlete and build trust with the rest of the training staff responsible for the athlete's success. Additionally, a specific recovery strategy, when outlined, communicated, and agreed upon in advance, may help hold all parties accountable.

REST AND RECOVERY PROGRAMMING

A properly designed sports performance program should include both rest and recovery. After all, rest and recovery are periods when training is absorbed and the body can prepare for more stress. As with training, failure to have a well-thought-out plan will lead to failure to optimize the outcomes, and not all athletes can use the same program—specificity and individual responses still apply.

IN-SEASON

In-season recovery is highly sought after but can be the most challenging to implement, depending on the sport. As competitions are highly demanding both mentally and physically, it is no surprise that athletes can be fatigued longer after a competition than after a typical training session. Combined with frequent events, cumulative fatigue can build up over the course of a season if rest and recovery are not properly managed.

A wide variety of nutritional, mechanical, and sleep-oriented recovery tactics are recommended to be implemented as soon as possible after a competition. Many athletes report being less willing to put in efforts toward recovery after demanding competition, which can ultimately slow the recovery time, taking away valuable time during in-season training. When competitions occur every 3 to 5 days, as is the case with many competitive team sports, quickly recovered athletes can engage in higher-quality skill-based sessions between competitions, allowing for preparations for the next match.

Recovery when athletes compete more frequently, such as every other day or multiple times a day, requires more rigorous attention. While applying recovery tactics can aid recovery, vigorous exercise/competition will lead to fatigue that necessitates rest and/or during-play management, if possible. When competitions occur every other day or every day, the focus should be on sleep and practice at a low intensity to facilitate familiarity with the sport and movements without accumulating additional stress.

When athletes compete multiple times per day, rest and recovery should primarily focus on proper nutrition and hydration to restore glycogen and body water and alleviate inter-competition stress. Inter-play stressors may include planning meals, media obligations, prepping equipment, and keeping track of competitors and standings, among other things. Minimizing these stressors is highly individualized, but adds up between competition. An athlete with a plan to reduce stress or perhaps to have a friend, family member, or staff take care of some of these activities may demonstrate better recovery and performance.

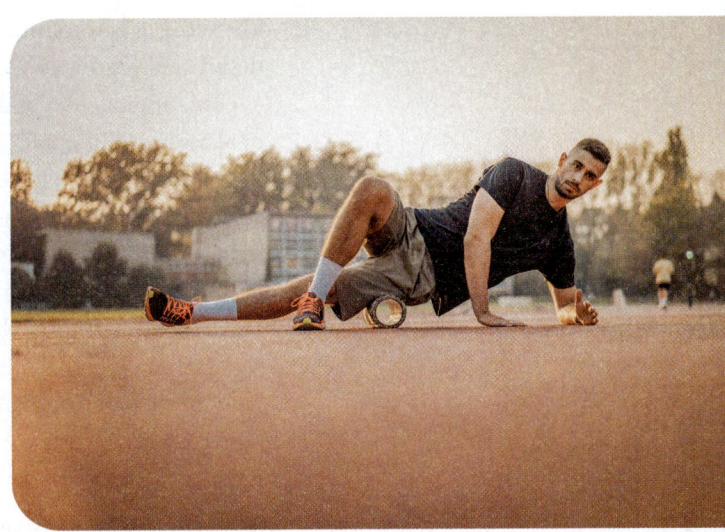
© Vladimir Borovic/Shutterstock

Many athletes use an arsenal of recovery tactics between frequent events to recover between sessions. To date, relatively few studies have examined the use of recovery modalities in between short succession. It is well known that hydration and nutrition between events can affect subsequent performance, particularly when replenishment needs are not met. Myofascial rolling appears to be a viable strategy to mitigate the performance decline due to acute fatigue, especially in activities involving high neural recruitment, such as power production, sprinting, and jumping (Jo et al., 2018; Kaya et al., 2021; Pearcey et al., 2015). Studies of wearing compression garments over prime movers in between repeated competitions have yielded mixed results, but some demonstrate improvements in high-intensity aerobic sports such as running and cycling time trials (Brophy-Williams et al., 2019; de Glanville & Hamlin, 2012; Williams et al., 2020). Other novel recovery methods, including photo-biomodulation and cryotherapy, have been studied less often, though a few studies support each of these methods (Aleixo-Junior et al., 2021; da Costa Santos et al., 2014).

Given the limited research on back-to-back exercise/competition, it is clear that more research is needed to validate these findings. However, these strategies should be experimented with before the athlete enters these settings to understand their willingness and response to each modality. What works best for an individual athlete is likely the best option for between-competition strategies, as long as it is not detrimental or taxing.

OFF-SEASON

The off-season is an important time in athlete development. Too little work and the athlete may be ill prepared for the preseason; too much work and the athlete may reach exhaustion before the season begins. Many athletes and coaches take different approaches to the off-season, but it is important to recognize the importance of rest and recovery to all of them. Resting immediately after a season is a common practice among elite athletes.

Taking time for the mind and body to reset, repair, and prepare for off-season training is highly recommended. Successful athletes also report higher instances of rest days during the off-season, as it may be essential to balance external life factors. Recovery is often overlooked when rest levels are high, with many individuals assuming they are the same. However, as previously mentioned, not all rest is created equally. Rest does allow deloading, but sitting on the couch may not facilitate proper musculoskeletal care.

Therefore, it is recommended to normalize recovery modalities during the off-season, despite many athletes feeling less of a "need."

This approach to bodily maintenance allows for consistency, which is often a hallmark of success. Additionally, many athletes struggle to consider the effects of nutrition and its impact on recovery. As the stakes are not as high during the off-season, many athletes report inconsistent diets, which can affect their recovery and sleep, making a quiet but sizable impact on their in-season performance.

For some athletes, small recovery deficits throughout this period may be easy to ignore. However, according to the GAS model, correcting these deficits by enhancing recovery may prevent an unwanted downward trend in performance by returning an athlete to baseline or supercompensation prior to the next training session.

PRE-SEASON

Pre-season training is often when training truly ramps up for many athletes, preparing them for the next season's demands. This time is vital for proper bodily function, which can be partially managed by rest and recovery. When training increases in volume or intensity, athletes may report more soreness, aches, pains, and potential injuries. It is vital for the entire athlete success team (trainers, coaches, family, and athlete) to maintain open communication with one another. This allows the athlete to regularly discuss how they are adapting to increases in training demand, which then aids in screening for injuries and overtraining.

Proper communication and monitoring of an athlete's response to training are vital to the athlete's success. Additionally, by being attentive to nutrition, body care, and strategic rest periods, athletes can build more volume and intensity safely than if they ignored rest and recovery considerations. Athletes should be guided and encouraged during the pre-season to diligently follow the recovery plan. Off-season compliance may vary among athletes, however, and the new demands of pre-season training may compete for their time and focus.

DAILY, WEEKLY, AND MONTHLY RECOVERY PROGRAMS

To incorporate a strategy for recovery and rest, it is important to consider the daily, weekly, and monthly patterns and how to manage them. Daily rest and recovery should be a large portion of the initial design and discussion of the training program with an athlete, as it allows for insight into their everyday life and their schedule and abilities. An athlete who trains late in the evening should have a different recovery strategy than an athlete who engages in early morning sessions, especially when athletes are doing multiple sessions a day. Topics of discussion should include timing of nutrition, what availability is like post-session to initiate recovery, what the rest of the day's demands are, and how to improve nighttime and sleep strategies.

Weekly discussions should revolve around allocating recovery efforts to address the most challenging points during the week, so individuals can maximize their recovery between sessions and absorb training properly. Although weekly discussions may be a good starting point, be aware that some athletes may be more open than others. These differences may require more frequent outreach to some athletes who need it, or open availability for discussion to those who are more proactive—after all, stress, performance, and recovery can change quickly and require rapid action.

Additionally, workouts should be planned in an appropriate sequence, but it is still crucial to think about any complications that an individual may have in their weekly schedule. It may be necessary to move hard, easy, and rest days around the other life demands of the week, as cumulative stress can unwind a plan that is good only on paper.

Just as periodization can dictate the workouts in a cycle, a recovery pattern can and should be considered when planning the program, especially during recovery weeks. The primary consideration for recovery weeks is that many athletes ease up on nutrition and recovery practices because they are not "doing as much." This pattern can inhibit the absorption and adaptations occurring during a recovery week; emphasis on maintaining nutrition, recovery modalities, sleep, and other factors should all be communicated to the athlete. The goal of a rest week is to maximize recovery so that the athlete can approach the next block in a fitter condition and can optimally prepare to handle more work.

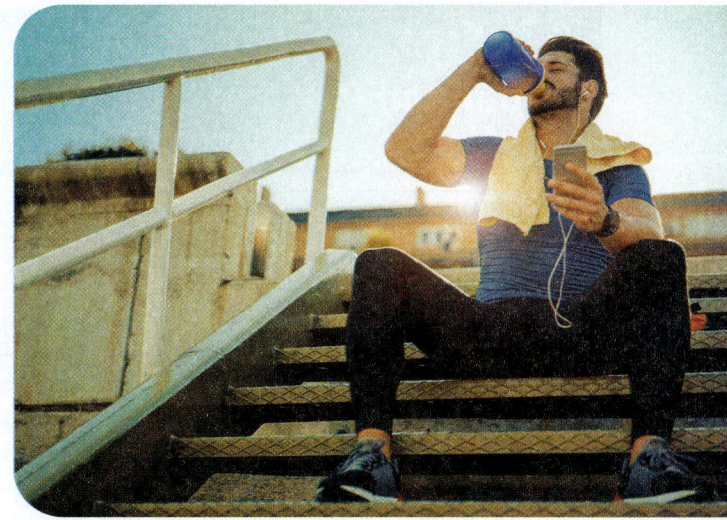
© Ivanko80/Shutterstock

REST AND RECOVERY USING NASM'S OPT MODEL

NASM's Optimum Performance Training (OPT) Model periodizes exercise training to maximize the benefits of training; it should comes as no surprise that offering periodized recovery may offer a similar strategy. Different phases of the OPT Model may warrant different recovery modalities and techniques, and periodization can occur on micro-, meso-, and macro-cycle levels.

STABILIZATION

In the stabilization level of the OPT Model, rest and recovery may be overlooked as a performance improvement method. Although the demands on the athlete's muscles and other organ systems may be relatively low, the neural system must be at the forefront of consideration. This is a great time to implement and train an athlete to have consistency in recovery and rest, as it is easier to focus on the details during this phase. Similarly, an athlete may be encouraged to try different recovery modalities, strategies, and timing, as the consequences of adjusting a recovery plan in this phase are minimized. Allowing for basic maintenance and emphasis on sleep will allow neural adaptations necessary for development. **Figure 17.6** provides a basic example of manual recovery methods that can be integrated into a training session.

STRENGTH

In the strength level, recovery modalities such as nutrition, myofascial maintenance, and sleep will yield superior results, as these are critical components of muscle adaptations. As training demands increase, especially with the specific purpose of overload and functional overreaching, recovery will reduce stressors, helping to avoid overtraining. Ideally, coming from the stabilization phase, where messages about consistency in rest and recovery were solidified, athletes will better understand how to take an active role in recovery. **Figure 17.7** provides an example of how to incorporate stabilization days, with an emphasis on recovery, into a strength training cycle.

POWER

Rest and recovery are essential in the power level but may look different than in the strength phase. Whereas the strength phase relies on fundamental physiology and managing the stress that comes with high-volume training, the power phase stresses

Optimum Performance Training®

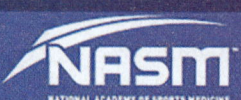

EXERCISE	SETS	REPS	TEMPO	REST	NOTES
CLIENT'S NAME:					
GOAL:					
PHASE:					
DATE:					
WARM-UP					
Myofascial Rolling	1-3	1	30s	NA	
Static Stretching	1	1	30s	NA	
Dynamic Stretching	1-3	10-15	Mod+	NA	
Cardio (Optional)	1	1	NA	NA	
ACTIVATION (core & balance)					
SKILL DEVELOPMENT (plyometric & SAQ)					
RESISTANCE TRAINING					
CLIENT'S CHOICE					
E-Stim (optional)	1	1	30-120	NA	Large muscle groups & pained areas
COOL-DOWN					
Myofascial Rolling	1-3	1	30s	NA	Remaining tight areas
Static Stretching	1-3	1-2	30s	NA	Prime movers
Cryotherapy	1	1	NA	NA	Targeted or global, 2-3 min

Coaching Tips: Be sure to practice extra recovery habits during the remainder of the day. Mindfulnes/meditation, hydration, healthy and nutritious foods. Prior to bed, use myofascial techniques if tightness occurs, IR therapy, if desired, and get good quality sleep.

FIGURE 17.6 Using Stabilization Endurance to Focus on Recovery

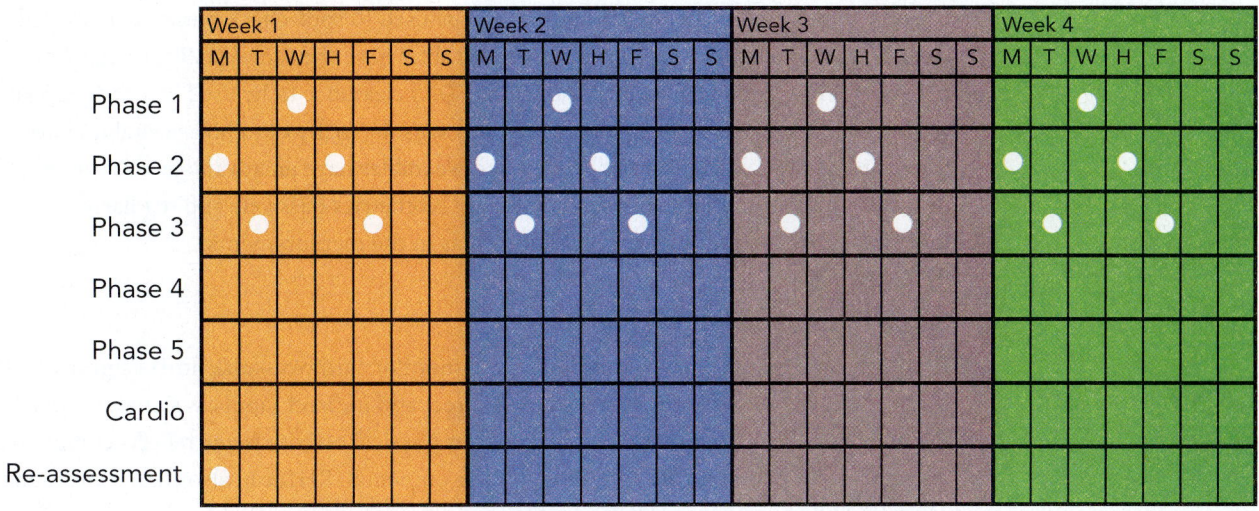

FIGURE 17.7 Mesocycle Incorporating Stabilization Days for Recovery During a Strength Phase

the sympathetic responses more heavily. Sleep, psychological recovery, and nutrient timing will be more heavily weighted in this phase. **Figure 17.8** provides an example of incorporating multiple stabilization days, with an emphasis on recovery, into a higher-intensity strength and power training cycle.

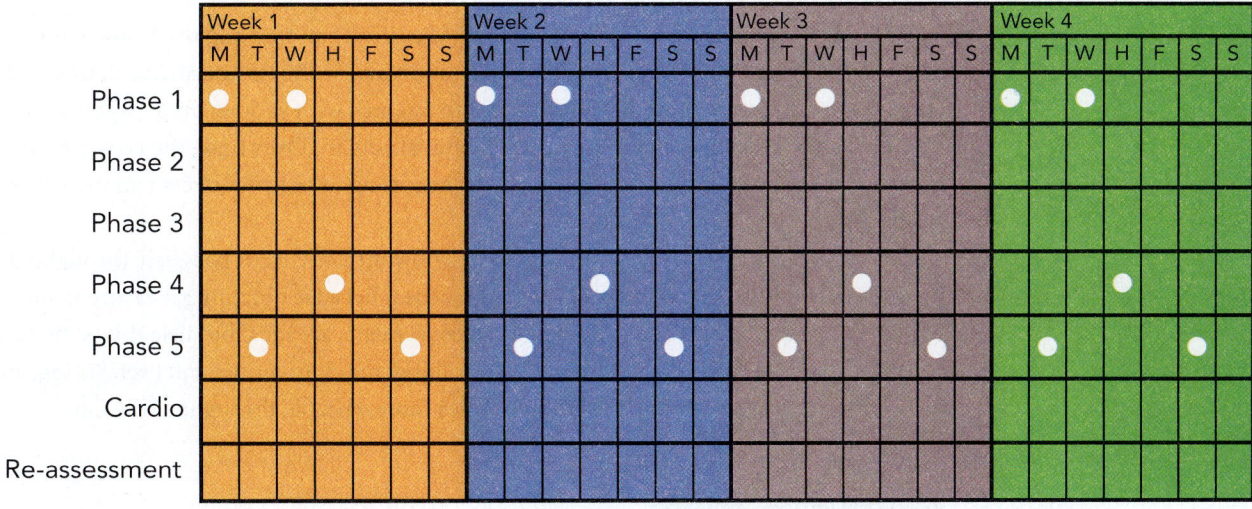

FIGURE 17.8 Mesocycle Incorporating Stabilization Days for Recovery During a Power Phase

LESSON 4: INCORPORATING BIOMETRICS
INCORPORATING BIOMETRICS FOR RECOVERY

In the past, tracking biometrics were reserved for use with medical equipment and research and typically required expensive machinery. With technological advances, many biometrics can now be measured using more affordable, noninvasive technology. Many individuals are already familiar with the biosensors integrated into "smart" wearable products, particularly watches and bands.

Additionally, home health equipment can be used to spot-check measurements and sometimes offers better reliability. Not all wearables have the same quality, as many do not require Food and Drug Administration (FDA) clearance to be used in a commercial setting. With advancements in algorithms and sensors, many of today's wearables have improved reliability and accuracy. Integrated wearables have an advantage over home health equipment in that they usually measure biometrics passively and regularly throughout the day and night, which limits bias in the measurements.

RESTING HEART RATE

Resting heart rate (RHR) is a common way to monitor cardiovascular fitness and stress. The sympathetic nervous system perceives both direct and indirect inputs as signals to speed up the heart rate. Hence, an increase in RHR when physical activity is low reflects cumulative stress, whether psychological, physical, or environmental. RHR can also change over longer periods of time in response to changes in cardiovascular fitness. Cardiovascular training increases the left ventricle's size and the amount of blood pumped with each beat, with fewer beats being required to deliver the same amount of blood. Conversely, cardiovascular deconditioning can lead to the heart becoming less efficient and increase the RHR.

Normal RHR ranges are 60 to 100 beats per minute (bpm). An RHR greater than 100 bpm (tachycardia) indicates increased cardiovascular dysfunction, and less than 60 bpm (bradycardia) is commonly associated with athletes. However, reduced metabolism can lower heart rate.

Although ranges are helpful for health risk classification, tracking over days, weeks, or months can provide deeper insights into an individual's fitness and stress. RHR should change only minimally from day to day ($\pm$ 3 to 5 bpm), with sudden, more significant increases often reflecting elevated stress (Quer et al., 2020). Over time, the goal should be to decrease RHR with training, as this trend demonstrates lower stress and increased cardiac efficiency.

Many fitness wearables and clinical devices now measure RHR passively throughout the day and night. This passive measurement is ideal because obtaining measurements requires no extra effort. Passive overnight measurements are ideal because this is the time when the external stress is the lowest. Upon waking, moving, eating, and even sitting, an individual's heart rate increases, and it becomes more variable throughout the day.

> ### ⚙ TRY THIS
>
> Take your RHR first thing upon waking. Then take it sporadically throughout the day and notice the difference. Stressors of the day will increase RHR a good bit. First thing in the morning tends to be the most stable time to measure RHR.

HEART RATE VARIABILITY

Although RHR is a valuable tool for understanding stress, it changes only a small amount compared to heart rate variability (HRV), which provides another dimension of stress quantification. Typically, hearts beat at irregular intervals, but are not perfectly timed. The HRV quantifies how irregular the beat-to-beat intervals are. Notably, sympathetic activity makes heartbeats more regular (decreased variability), whereas parasympathetic activity makes heartbeats more irregular (higher variability). Therefore, HRV is considered an indicator of central nervous system balance. At similar heart rates, stress may appear equal, but HRV may indicate differences in stress levels.

As with RHR, the best time to measure HRV is overnight, when external stressors are minimized. HRV is usually lower at the beginning of sleep and peaks around waking time. After waking, HRV decreases moderately and then varies throughout the day based on cumulative stressors. Lower levels of HRV throughout sleep and upon waking appear to be correlated with poorer recovery; thus, they may serve as an index of recovery and readiness. It is typically considered beneficial to have a high HRV relative to the typical values, indicating better parasympathetic activation, decreased stress, and better recovery.

Of course, this metric, like most others, is not a perfect indicator for any particular condition. HRV is highly individualized and is not easily compared between individuals. Understanding what is "typical" for an athlete and tracking substantial changes, both high and low, will provide the most helpful insights. Because of the highly individualized nature of HRV, there are currently no recommended or standard ranges for this metric. Instead, HRV should be used over time and with other metrics, including subjective metrics, to determine recovery and readiness.

🤖 GETTING TECHNICAL

There are many types of measurements for HRV, including root mean square of successive differences (RMSSD), standard deviation of RR intervals (SDRR), number of pairs of successive NN intervals that differ by more than 50 ms (NN50), entropy, and frequency analysis. RMSSD is the most popular in the literature and commercial wearables. Be sure to identify which method is used, as they are not comparable.

SLEEP TRACKING

Sleep is one of the most important and underutilized training and recovery tools. This is when the body undergoes recovery, repair, and restoration, allowing for proper adaptations to training. Many are familiar with the idea of sleep quantity, as recommendations have been made for it. For example, the National Sleep Foundation recommends 8 to 10 hours of sleep per night for teenagers, 7 to 9 hours for young adults, and 7 to 8 hours for older adults (Hirshkowitz et al., 2015).

However, sleep duration is intended to be the number of hours of sleep, not time in bed. Many wearables can detect sleep onset and wake time by tracking heart rate, HRV, movement, skin temperature, and more. Many individuals do not spend 100% of their time in bed sleeping, especially individuals with sleep disorders. Time spent attempting to fall asleep and awakenings through the night count toward total awake time. Using a wearable or other health device can allow for better tracking and logging, which can serve as an area to track improvement or explain training behavior patterns.

It is not uncommon to see high-level athletes utilizing naps as an addition to their sleep strategy. Studies demonstrate that napping improves cognitive and physical performance,

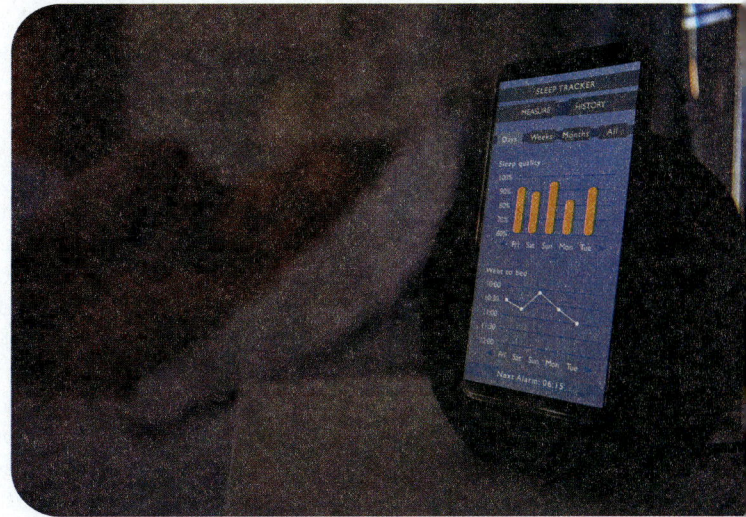

© Monkey Business Images/Shutterstock

especially in response to sleep deprivation (Ajjimaporn et al., 2020; Gillberg et al., 1996; Lovato & Lack, 2010). Although it is difficult to determine the equivalence of napping and sleeping, it appears that total sleep that includes napping—not just sleep *or* napping—may be a better indicator of some health conditions (Cohen-Mansfield & Perach, 2012; Li et al., 2021), suggesting a somewhat additive effect.

Sleep efficiency is a metric that expresses the time spent asleep to the time in bed as a proportion. For example, an individual who spends 9 hours in bed but a total of 8 hours asleep has a sleep efficiency of 89%. While more is better, 100% sleep efficiency is not necessarily attainable or healthy. Sleep latency influences sleep efficiency and reflects the time it takes from attempting to fall asleep to the time it takes to actually fall asleep. Typically, 10 to 30 minutes is considered normal, with less than 5 minutes reflecting severe exhaustion (Ohayon et al., 2004). Other factors influencing sleep latency are alcohol, medications, exercise, diet, blue light exposure, and other pre-bedtime activities (Kräuchi & Wirz-Justice, 2001).

Sleep stages can be approximated by many wearables and health devices, allowing users to understand sleep quality as more than just duration. Deep sleep, or slow wave sleep, is the most important stage of sleep for physical recovery and can be tracked in this manner. Deep sleep typically accounts for 13% to 23% of nightly sleep (Colten & Altevogt, 2006) and, like other metrics, should be tracked over time. A significant decrease in the number of deep sleep minutes can provide insight into poor recovery and performance, even if the total sleep duration remains unchanged.

A lesser-known variable is sleep consistency, which reflects regularity in bed and wake times. Many devices may or may not present this information as a specific metric, but it is something that anyone can keep track of and aim to act upon. Because the endocrine system has a significant influence over 24-hour rhythms and sleep affects this process, keeping a consistent sleep–wake schedule leads to less overall endocrine disturbance and sleep disturbance and reduces stress (Abbott et al., 2019; Huang & Redline, 2019).

⚙ TRY THIS

Many successful athletes wake up at the same time each day, even on rest days. Although it may be tempting to sleep in, having inconsistent bed and wake times often leads to poorer overall sleep quality and can lead to suboptimal recovery. Try a nap in the afternoon rather than sleeping later in the morning.

📋 COACH'S CORNER

When interacting with athletes, you should be attentive to all aspects of performance, including signs of fatigue, performance, mental health, and overall mood. Given the importance of sleep, screening for abnormal sleep patterns or changes in sleep habits is recommended for almost any scenario involving these symptoms. Because many of the signs and symptoms of poor sleep overlap with many other conditions, it may be hard to spot sleep issues if you do not ask about them.

Asking simple questions such as "How many hours are you sleeping?", "Are you having difficulties falling asleep?", "Are you having difficulties staying asleep?", and "Are you feeling refreshed after sleep?" may be adequate to screen for sleep abnormalities, but without tangible data, it may be hard to spot changes or abnormalities. For example, if someone is used to waking up frequently throughout the night, they may not see that as "abnormal," but it may indicate sleep disorders.

SUMMARY

Rest and recovery warrant a great deal of consideration from fitness professionals training athletes. Just as exercise training requires a well-thought-out, individualized plan, so does rest and recovery. Recovery methods may aid in athlete success during training or competition, and rest is an invaluable tool to promote recovery. Balancing rest, recovery, and training is challenging, but proper rest and recovery complement training in a way that maximizes the possible benefits.

This chapter underscored the vital importance of integrating rest and recovery into athletic development based on the fundamental biological processes of human physical performance. Key components of evidence-based rest and recovery methods include quality sleep, proper nutrition and hydration, manual recovery techniques, and mindfulness practices. The chapter debunked common misconceptions about sleep and productivity, emphasizing the role of quality sleep—around 7 to 9 hours per night—as an essential performance enhancer. Nutrition and hydration also serve as performance drivers and integral elements of the recovery process. The need for a comprehensive approach, balancing training with adequate recovery, requires a shared understanding between the athlete and their support team. The chapter concluded with recommendations for integrating rest and recovery into athletic development, emphasizing a holistic approach to achieving optimal athletic performance.

KEY TAKEAWAYS

- Rest and recovery should be discussed with each athlete, making a plan tailored to them and their training plan, allowing flexibility and adaptability as training and stress change.
- Stress, including life stressors, is cumulative and can impact recovery and performance.
- Recovery modalities can have many benefits and can help an athlete cope with hard training cycles.
- Sleep, nutrition, myofascial and physiological techniques, and psychological interventions all affect the quality of recovery.
- Sleep does not include just the number of hours of sleep. Sleep stages, number of awakenings, and biometrics during sleep describe how effective the sleep session was. Sleep quality and consistency are some of the most important factors for recovery.
- Rest should be used regularly and should be included in contingency plans when an athlete demonstrates signs of exhaustion or overtraining.
- Monitoring health via biometrics can provide insights into the quality of recovery and the need to implement extra recovery or rest.

REFERENCES

Abbott, S. M., Weng, J., Reid, K. J., Daviglus, M. L., Gallo, L. C., Loredo, J. S., Nyenhuis, S. M., Ramos, A. R., Shah, N. A., Sotres-Alvarez, D., Patel, S. R., & Zee, P. C. (2019). Sleep timing, stability, and BP in the Sueño Ancillary Study of the Hispanic Community Health Study/Study of Latinos. *Chest*, *155*(1), 60–68. https://doi.org/10.1016/j.chest.2018.09.018

Adamo, D. E., Martin, B. J., & Johnson, P. W. (2002). Vibration-induced muscle fatigue, a possible contribution to musculoskeletal injury. *European Journal of Applied Physiology*, *88*(1–2), 134–140. https://doi.org/10.1007/s00421-002-0660-y

Adamsson, A., & Bernhardsson, S. (2018). Symptoms that may be stress-related and lead to exhaustion disorder: A retrospective medical chart review in Swedish primary care. *BMC Family Practice*, *19*, 172. https://doi.org/10.1186/s12875-018-0858-7

Ajjimaporn, A., Ramyarangsi, P., & Siripornpanich, V. (2020). Effects of a 20-min nap after sleep deprivation on brain activity and soccer performance. *International Journal of Sports Medicine*, *41*(14), 1009–1016. https://doi.org/10.1055/a-1192-6187

Aleixo-Junior, I. de O., Leal-Junior, E. C. P., Leal-Junior, E. C. P., Leal-Junior, E. C. P., Casalechi, H. L., Vanin, A. A., de Paiva, P. R. V., Machado, C. dos S. M., Dias, L. B., Lino, M. M. A., Teixeira, A. M., Johnson, D. S., &

Tomazoni, S. S. (2021). Immediate effects of photobiomodulation therapy combined with a static magnetic field on the subsequent performance: A preliminary randomized crossover triple-blinded placebo-controlled trial. *Biomedical Optics Express, 12*(11), 6940–6953. https://doi.org/10.1364/BOE.442075

Alghannam, A. F., Gonzalez, J. T., & Betts, J. A. (2018). Restoration of muscle glycogen and functional capacity: Role of post-exercise carbohydrate and protein co-ingestion. *Nutrients, 10*(2), 253. https://doi.org/10.3390/nu10020253

Anderson, T., Wideman, L., Cadegiani, F. A., & Kater, C. E. (2021). Effects of overtraining status on the cortisol awakening response—endocrine and metabolic responses on overtraining syndrome (EROS-CAR). *International Journal of Sports Physiology and Performance, 16*(7), 965–973. https://doi.org/10.1123/ijspp.2020-0205

Babault, N., Cometti, C., Maffiuletti, N. A., & Deley, G. (2011). Does electrical stimulation enhance post-exercise performance recovery? *European Journal of Applied Physiology, 111*(10), 2501–2507. https://doi.org/10.1007/s00421-011-2117-7

Beals, K. A., & Meyer, N. L. (2007). Female athlete triad update. *Clinics in Sports Medicine, 26*(1), 69–89. https://doi.org/10.1016/j.csm.2006.11.002

Beelen, M., Burke, L. M., Gibala, M. J., & van Loon L, J. C. (2010). Nutritional strategies to promote postexercise recovery. *International Journal of Sport Nutrition and Exercise Metabolism, 20*(6), 515–532. https://doi.org/10.1123/ijsnem.20.6.515

Behm, D. G., Alizadeh, S., Hadjizadeh Anvar, S., Mahmoud, M. M. I., Ramsay, E., Hanlon, C., & Cheatham, S. (2020). Foam rolling prescription: A clinical commentary. *Journal of Strength & Conditioning Research, 34*(11), 3301–3308. https://doi.org/10.1519/JSC.0000000000003765

Birch, K. (2005). Female athlete triad. *BMJ, 330*(7485), 244–246. https://doi.org/10.1136/bmj.330.7485.244

Bird, S. P. (2013). Sleep, recovery, and athletic performance: A brief review and recommendations. *Strength and Conditioning Journal, 35*(5), 43–47. https://doi.org/10.1519/SSC.0b013e3182a62e2f

Brinkman, J. E., Toro, F., & Sharma, S. (2021). Physiology, respiratory drive. In *StatPearls*. StatPearls Publishing. http://www.ncbi.nlm.nih.gov/books/NBK482414/

Broderick, V., Uiga, L., & Driller, M. (2019). Flotation-restricted environmental stimulation therapy improves sleep and performance recovery in athletes. *Performance Enhancement & Health, 7*(1), 100149. https://doi.org/10.1016/j.peh.2019.100149

Brophy-Williams, N., Driller, M. W., Kitic, C. M., Fell, J. W., & Halson, S. L. (2019). Wearing compression socks during exercise aids subsequent performance. *Journal of Science and Medicine in Sport, 22*(1), 123–127. https://doi.org/10.1016/j.jsams.2018.06.010

Burgess, L., Immins, T., Swain, I. D., & Wainwright, T. (2019). Effectiveness of neuromuscular electrical stimulation for reducing oedema: A systematic review. *Journal of Rehabilitation Medicine, 51*(4), 237–243.

Cadegiani, F. A., & Kater, C. E. (2019). Novel insights of overtraining syndrome discovered from the EROS study. *BMJ Open Sport & Exercise Medicine, 5*(1), e000542. https://doi.org/10.1136/bmjsem-2019-000542

Cardinale, M., & Bosco, C. (2003). The use of vibration as an exercise intervention. *Exercise and Sport Sciences Reviews, 31*(1), 3–7. https://doi.org/10.1097/00003677-200301000-00002

Chang, K.-M., Wu Chueh, M.-T., & Lai, Y.-J. (2020). Meditation practice improves short-term changes in heart rate variability. *International Journal of Environmental Research and Public Health, 17*(6), 2128. https://doi.org/10.3390/ijerph17062128

Cheatham, S. W., Stull, K. R., & Kolber, M. J. (2019). Comparison of a vibration roller and a nonvibration roller intervention on knee range of motion and pressure pain threshold: A randomized controlled trial. *Journal of Sport Rehabilitation, 28*(1), 39–45. https://doi.org/10.1123/jsr.2017-0164

Christodoulou, G., Salami, N., & Black, D. S. (2020). The utility of heart rate variability in mindfulness research. *Mindfulness, 11*(3), 554–570. https://doi.org/10.1007/s12671-019-01296-3

Cohen-Mansfield, J., & Perach, R. (2012). Sleep duration, nap habits, and mortality in older persons. *Sleep, 35*(7), 1003–1009. https://doi.org/10.5665/sleep.1970

Colten, H. R., & Altevogt, B. M. (Eds.). (2006). Sleep physiology. In *Sleep disorders and sleep deprivation: An unmet public health problem*. National Academies Press. https://www.ncbi.nlm.nih.gov/books/NBK19956/

da Costa Santos, V. B., de Paula Ramos, S., Milanez, V. F., Corrêa, J. C. M., de Andrade Alves, R. I., Dias, I. F. L., & Nakamura, F. Y. (2014). LED therapy or cryotherapy between exercise intervals in Wistar rats: Anti-inflammatory and ergogenic effects. *Lasers in Medical Science, 29*(2), 599–605. https://doi.org/10.1007/s10103-013-1371-9

De Couck, M., Caers, R., Musch, L., Fliegauf, J., Giangreco, A., & Gidron, Y. (2019). How breathing can help you make better decisions: Two studies on the effects of breathing patterns on heart rate variability and decision-making in business cases. *International Journal of Psychophysiology, 139*, 1–9. https://doi.org/10.1016/j.ijpsycho.2019.02.011

de Glanville, K. M., & Hamlin, M. J. (2012). Positive effect of lower body compression garments on subsequent 40-km cycling time trial performance. *Journal of Strength and Conditioning Research, 26*(2), 480–486. https://doi.org/10.1519/JSC.0b013e318225ff61

Dellagrana, R. A., Rossato, M., Sakugawa, R. L., Baroni, B. M., & Diefenthaeler, F. (2018). Photobiomodulation therapy on physiological and performance parameters during running tests: Dose–response effects. *Journal of Strength and Conditioning Research, 32*(10), 2807–2815. https://doi.org/10.1519/JSC.0000000000002488

De Marchi, T., Schmitt, V. M., Machado, G. P., de Sene, J. S., de Col, C. D., Tairova, O., Salvador, M., & Leal-Junior, E. C. P. (2017). Does photobiomodulation therapy is better than cryotherapy in muscle recovery after a high-intensity exercise? A randomized, double-blind, placebo-controlled clinical trial. *Lasers in Medical Science, 32*(2), 429–437. https://doi.org/10.1007/s10103-016-2139-9

Derave, W., Lund, S., Holman, G. D., Wojtaszewski, J., Pedersen, O., & Richter, E. A. (1999). Contraction-stimulated muscle glucose transport and GLUT-4 surface content are dependent on glycogen content. *American Journal of Physiology, 277*(6), E1103-1110. https://doi.org/10.1152/ajpendo.1999.277.6.E1103

Dipla, K., Kraemer, R. R., Constantini, N. W., & Hackney, A. C. (2021). Relative energy deficiency in sports (RED-S): Elucidation of endocrine changes affecting the health of males and females. *Hormones, 20*(1), 35–47. https://doi.org/10.1007/s42000-020-00214-w

Driller, M. W., & Argus, C. K. (2016). Flotation restricted environmental stimulation therapy and napping on mood state and muscle soreness in elite athletes: A novel recovery strategy? *Performance Enhancement & Health, 5*(2), 60–65. https://doi.org/10.1016/j.peh.2016.08.002

Dudley-Javoroski, S., & Shields, R. K. (2008). Muscle and bone plasticity after spinal cord injury: Review of adaptations to disuse and to electrical muscle stimulation. *Journal of Rehabilitation Research and Development, 45*(2), 283–296.

Eda, N., Ito, H., & Akama, T. (2020). Beneficial effects of yoga stretching on salivary stress hormones and parasympathetic nerve activity. *Journal of Sports Science & Medicine, 19*(4), 695–702.

Elliott-Sale, K. J., Tenforde, A. S., Parziale, A. L., Holtzman, B., & Ackerman, K. E. (2018). Endocrine effects of relative energy deficiency in sport. *International Journal of Sport Nutrition and Exercise Metabolism, 28*(4), 335–349. https://doi.org/10.1123/ijsnem.2018-0127

Eppsteiner, R. W., Shin, J. J., Johnson, J., & van Dam, R. M. (2010). Mechanical compression versus subcutaneous heparin therapy in postoperative and posttrauma patients: A systematic review and meta-analysis. *World Journal of Surgery, 34*(1), 10–19. https://doi.org/10.1007/s00268-009-0284-z

Farinatti, P. T. V., Brandão, C., Soares, P. P. S., & Duarte, A. F. A. (2011). Acute effects of stretching exercise on the heart rate variability in subjects with low flexibility levels. *Journal of Strength and Conditioning Research, 25*(6), 1579–1585. https://doi.org/10.1519/JSC.0b013e3181e06ce1

Fu, T., Jiang, L., Peng, Y., Li, Z., Liu, S., Lu, J., Zhang, F., & Zhang, J. (2020). Electrical muscle stimulation accelerates functional recovery after nerve injury. *Neuroscience, 426*, 179–188. https://doi.org/10.1016/j.neuroscience.2019.10.052

Fuller, J. T., Thomson, R. L., Howe, P. R. C., & Buckley, J. D. (2013). Effect of vibration on muscle perfusion: A systematic review. *Clinical Physiology and Functional Imaging, 33*(1), 1–10. https://doi.org/10.1111/j.1475-097X.2012.01161.x

Germann, D., El Bouse, A., Shnier, J., Abdelkader, N., & Kazemi, M. (2018). Effects of local vibration therapy on various performance parameters: A narrative literature review. *Journal of the Canadian Chiropractic Association, 62*(3), 170–181.

Gillberg, M., Kecklund, G., Axelsson, J., & Åkerstedt, T. (1996). The effects of a short daytime nap after restricted night sleep. *Sleep, 19*(7), 570–575. https://doi.org/10.1093/sleep/19.7.570

Goldstein-Piekarski, A. N., Greer, S. M., Saletin, J. M., Harvey, A. G., Williams, L. M., & Walker, M. P. (2018). Sex, sleep deprivation, and the anxious brain. *Journal of Cognitive Neuroscience, 30*(4), 565–578. https://doi.org/10.1162/jocn_a_01225

Hammond, T., Gialloreto, C., Kubas, H., & Hap Davis, H. (2013). The prevalence of failure-based depression among elite athletes. *Clinical Journal of Sport Medicine: Official Journal of the Canadian Academy of Sport Medicine, 23*(4), 273–277. https://doi.org/10.1097/JSM.0b013e318287b870

Herbert, R. D., Noronha, M. de, & Kamper, S. J. (2011). Stretching to prevent or reduce muscle soreness after exercise. *Cochrane Database of Systematic Reviews, 7*. https://doi.org/10.1002/14651858.CD004577.pub3

Hirshkowitz, M., Whiton, K., Albert, S. M., Alessi, C., Bruni, O., DonCarlos, L., Hazen, N., Herman, J., Katz, E. S., Kheirandish-Gozal, L., Neubauer, D. N., O'Donnell, A. E., Ohayon, M., Peever, J., Rawding, R., Sachdeva, R. C., Setters, B., Vitiello, M. V., Ware, J. C., & Adams Hillard, P. J. (2015). National Sleep Foundation's sleep time duration recommendations: Methodology and results summary. *Sleep Health, 1*(1), 40–43. https://doi.org/10.1016/j.sleh.2014.12.010

Huang, T., & Redline, S. (2019). Cross-sectional and prospective associations of actigraphy-assessed sleep regularity with metabolic abnormalities: The multi-ethnic study of atherosclerosis. *Diabetes Care*, *42*(8), 1422–1429. https://doi.org/10.2337/dc19-0596

Huyghe, T., Scanlan, A. T., Dalbo, V. J., & Calleja-González, J. (2018). The negative influence of air travel on health and performance in the National Basketball Association: A narrative review. *Sports*, *6*(3), 89. https://doi.org/10.3390/sports6030089

Jo, E., Juache, G. A., Saralegui, D. E., Weng, D., & Falatoonzadeh, S. (2018). The acute effects of foam rolling on fatigue-related impairments of muscular performance. *Sports*, *6*(4), 112. https://doi.org/10.3390/sports6040112

Kamimura, A., Kawata, Y., Raedeke, T. D., & Hirosawa, M. (2020). Association of athlete burnout with depression among Japanese university athletes. *Juntendo Medical Journal, 66*(3), 221–232. https://doi.org/10.14789/jmj.2020.66.JMJ19-OA24

Kaya, S., Cug, M., & Behm, D. G. (2021). Foam rolling during a simulated half-time attenuates subsequent soccer-specific performance decrements. *Journal of Bodywork and Movement Therapies*, *26*, 193–200. https://doi.org/10.1016/j.jbmt.2020.12.009

Keith, S. L., McLaughlin, D. J., Anderson, F. A., Jr., Cardullo, P. A., Jones, C. E., Rohrer, M. J., & Cutler, B. S. (1992). Do graduated compression stockings and pneumatic boots have an additive effect on the peak velocity of venous blood flow? *Archives of Surgery*, *127*(6), 727–730. https://doi.org/10.1001/archsurg.1992.01420060107016

Kim, J., Jung, H., & Yim, J. (2020). Effects of contrast therapy using infrared and cryotherapy as compared with contrast bath therapy on blood flow, muscle tone, and pain threshold in young healthy adults. *Medical Science Monitor: International Medical Journal of Experimental and Clinical Research*, *26*, e922544-1-e922544-8. https://doi.org/10.12659/MSM.922544

Kräuchi, K., & Wirz-Justice, A. (2001). Circadian clues to sleep onset mechanisms. *Neuropsychopharmacology*, *25*(1), S92–S96. https://doi.org/10.1016/S0893-133X(01)00315-3

Kreider, R. B., Fry, A. C., & O'Toole, M. L (1998). *Overtraining in sport*. Human Kinetics.

Kromenacker, B. W., Sanova, A. A., Marcus, F. I., Allen, J. J. B., & Lane, R. D. (2018). Vagal mediation of low-frequency heart rate variability during slow yogic breathing. *Psychosomatic Medicine*, *80*(6), 581–587. https://doi.org/10.1097/PSY.0000000000000603

Lau, R. W., Liao, L.-R., Yu, F., Teo, T., Chung, R. C., & Pang, M. Y. (2011). The effects of whole body vibration therapy on bone mineral density and leg muscle strength in older adults: A systematic review and meta-analysis. *Clinical Rehabilitation*, *25*(11), 975–988. https://doi.org/10.1177/0269215511405078

Laumonier, T., & Menetrey, J. (2016). Muscle injuries and strategies for improving their repair. *Journal of Experimental Orthopaedics*, *3*(1), 15. https://doi.org/10.1186/s40634-016-0051-7

Li, C., Zhu, Y., Zhang, M., Gustafsson, H., & Chen, T. (2019). Mindfulness and athlete burnout: A systematic review and meta-analysis. *International Journal of Environmental Research and Public Health*, *16*(3), 449. https://doi.org/10.3390/ijerph16030449

Li, W., Taskin, T., Gautam, P., Gamber, M., & Sun, W. (2021). Is there an association among sleep duration, nap, and stroke? Findings from the China Health and Retirement Longitudinal Study. *Sleep and Breathing*, *25*(1), 315–323. https://doi.org/10.1007/s11325-020-02118-w

Loap, S., & Lathe, R. (2018). Mechanism underlying tissue cryotherapy to combat obesity/overweight: Triggering thermogenesis. *Journal of Obesity*, *2018*, e5789647. https://doi.org/10.1155/2018/5789647

Lovato, N., & Lack, L. (2010). The effects of napping on cognitive functioning. In G. A. Kerkhof & H. P. A. van Dongen (Eds.), *Progress in brain research* (Vol. 185, pp. 155–166). Elsevier. https://doi.org/10.1016/B978-0-444-53702-7.00009-9

Manore, M. M. (2005). Exercise and the Institute of Medicine recommendations for nutrition. *Current Sports Medicine Reports*, *4*(4), 193–198. https://doi.org/10.1097/01.CSMR.0000306206.72186.00

McAnulty, S. R., McAnulty, L. S., Nieman, D. C., Morrow, J. D., Utter, A. C., Henson, D. A., Dumke, C. L., & Vinci, D. M. (2003). Influence of carbohydrate ingestion on oxidative stress and plasma antioxidant potential following a 3 h run. *Free Radical Research*, *37*(8), 835–840. https://doi.org/10.1080/1071576031000136559

Ménétrier, A., Mourot, L., Bouhaddi, M., Regnard, J., & Tordi, N. (2011). Compression sleeves increase tissue oxygen saturation but not running performance. *International Journal of Sports Medicine*, *32*(11), 864–868. https://doi.org/10.1055/s-0031-1283181

Mitchell, U. H., & Mack, G. L. (2013). Low-level laser treatment with near-infrared light increases venous nitric oxide levels acutely: A single-blind, randomized clinical trial of efficacy. *American Journal of Physical Medicine & Rehabilitation*, *92*(2), 151–156. https://doi.org/10.1097/PHM.0b013e318269d70a

Mortimer, P. S., Simmonds, R., Rezvani, M., Robbins, M., Hopewell, J. W., & Ryan, T. J. (1990). The measurement of skin lymph flow by isotope clearance: Reliability, reproducibility, injection dynamics, and the effect of massage. *Journal of Investigative Dermatology*, *95*(6), 677–682. https://www.jidonline.org/article /0022-202X(90)90038-8/abstract

Mountjoy, M., Sundgot-Borgen, J. K., Burke, L. M., Ackerman, K. E., Blauwet, C., Constantini, N., Lebrun, C., Lundy, B., Melin, A. K., Meyer, N. L., Sherman, R. T., Tenforde, A. S., Klungland Torstveit, M., & Budgett, R. (2018). IOC consensus statement on relative energy deficiency in sport (RED-S): 2018 update. *British Journal of Sports Medicine*, *52*(11), 687–697. https://doi.org/10.1136/bjsports-2018-099193

Nair, A. K., Sasidharan, A., John, J. P., Mehrotra, S., & Kutty, B. M. (2017). Just a minute meditation: Rapid voluntary conscious state shifts in long term meditators. *Consciousness and Cognition*, *53*, 176–184. https://doi.org/10.1016/j.concog.2017.06.002

Nasi, M., Bianchini, E., Lo Tartaro, D., De Biasi, S., Mattioli, M., Paolini, A., Gibellini, L., Pinti, M., De Gaetano, A., D'Alisera, R., Roli, L., Chester, J., Mattioli, A. V., Polverari, T., Maietta, P., Tripi, F., Stefani, O., Guerra, E., Savino, G., … Cossarizza, A. (2020). Effects of whole-body cryotherapy on the innate and adaptive immune response in cyclists and runners. *Immunologic Research*, *68*(6), 422–435. https://doi .org/10.1007/s12026-020-09165-1

Nazem, T. G., & Ackerman, K. E. (2012). The female athlete triad. *Sports Health*, *4*(4), 302–311. https://doi .org/10.1177/1941738112439685

Nofsinger, J. R., & Shank, C. A. (2019). DEEP sleep: The impact of sleep on financial risk taking. *Review of Financial Economics*, *37*(1), 92–105. https://doi.org/10.1002/rfe.1034

Nussbaum, E. L., Houghton, P., Anthony, J., Rennie, S., Shay, B. L., & Hoens, A. M. (2017). Neuromuscular electrical stimulation for treatment of muscle impairment: Critical review and recommendations for clinical practice. *Physiotherapy Canada*, *69*(5), 1–76. https://doi.org/10.3138/ptc.2015-88

Ohayon, M. M., Carskadon, M. A., Guilleminault, C., & Vitiello, M. V. (2004). Meta-analysis of quantitative sleep parameters from childhood to old age in healthy individuals: Developing normative sleep values across the human lifespan. *Sleep*, *27*(7), 1255–1273. https://doi.org/10.1093/sleep/27.7.1255

Okamoto, T., Masuhara, M., & Ikuta, K. (2014). Acute effects of self-myofascial release using a foam roller on arterial function. *Journal of Strength and Conditioning Research*, *28*(1), 69–73. https://doi.org/10.1519 /JSC.0b013e31829480f5

Ordóñez, F. M., Oliver, A. J. S., Bastos, P. C., Guillén, L. S., & Domínguez, R. (2017). Sleep improvement in athletes: Use of nutritional supplements. *Archivos de Medicinadel Deporte*, *34*(2), 93–99.

Osawa, Y., Oguma, Y., & Ishii, N. (2013). The effects of whole-body vibration on muscle strength and power: A meta-analysis. *Journal of Musculoskeletal Neuronal Interactions*, *13*(3), 380–390.

Parkin, J. A., Carey, M. F., Martin, I. K., Stojanovska, L., & Febbraio, M. A. (1997). Muscle glycogen storage following prolonged exercise: Effect of timing of ingestion of high glycemic index food. *Medicine & Science in Sports & Exercise*, *29*(2), 220–224. https://doi.org/10.1097/00005768-199702000-00009

Pearcey, G. E. P., Bradbury-Squires, D. J., Kawamoto, J.-E., Drinkwater, E. J., Behm, D. G., & Button, D. C. (2015). Foam rolling for delayed-onset muscle soreness and recovery of dynamic performance measures. *Journal of Athletic Training*, *50*(1), 5–13. https://doi.org/10.4085/1062-6050-50.1.01

Peçanha, T., Paula-Ribeiro, M., Campana-Rezende, E., Bartels, R., Marins, J. C. B., & de Lima, J. R. P. (2014). Water intake accelerates parasympathetic reactivation after high-intensity exercise. *International Journal of Sport Nutrition and Exercise Metabolism*, *24*(5), 489–496. https://doi.org/10.1123/ijsnem.2013-0122

Prasad, K., Wahner-Roedler, D. L., Cha, S. S., & Sood, A. (2011). Effect of a single-session meditation training to reduce stress and improve quality of life among health care professionals: A "dose-ranging" feasibility study. *Alternative Therapies in Health and Medicine*, *17*(3), 46–49.

Prayag, A. S., Najjar, R. P., & Gronfier, C. (2019). Melatonin suppression is exquisitely sensitive to light and primarily driven by melanopsin in humans. *Journal of Pineal Research*, *66*(4), e12562. https://doi .org/10.1111/jpi.12562

Quer, G., Gouda, P., Galarnyk, M., Topol, E. J., & Steinhubl, S. R. (2020). Inter- and intraindividual variability in daily resting heart rate and its associations with age, sex, sleep, BMI, and time of year: Retrospective, longitudinal cohort study of 92,457 adults. *PLoS One*, *15*(2), e0227709. https://doi.org/10.1371/journal.pone.0227709

Rey, E., Padrón-Cabo, A., Costa, P. B., & Barcala-Furelos, R. (2019). Effects of foam rolling as a recovery tool in professional soccer players. *Journal of Strength and Conditioning Research*, *33*(8), 2194–2201. https://doi .org/10.1519/JSC.0000000000002277

Riggs, B. L., Melton, L. J., Robb, R. A., Camp, J. J., Atkinson, E. J., McDaniel, L., Amin, S., Rouleau, P. A., & Khosla, S. (2008). A population-based assessment of rates of bone loss at multiple skeletal sites: Evidence for substantial trabecular bone loss in young adult women and men. *Journal of Bone and Mineral Research*, *23*(2), 205–214. https://doi.org/10.1359/jbmr.071020

Rodenbeck, A., Binder, R., Geisler, P., Danker-Hopfe, H., Lund, R., Raschke, F., Weeß, H.-G., & Schulz, H. (2006). A review of sleep EEG patterns. Part I: A compilation of amended rules for their visual recognition according to Rechtschaffen and Kales. *Somnologie*, *10*(4), 159–175. https://onlinelibrary.wiley.com/doi/abs/10.1111/j.1439-054x.2006.00101.x

Roos, L., Boesch, M., Sefidan, S., Frey, F., Mäder, U., Annen, H., & Wyss, T. (2015). Adapted marching distances and physical training decrease recruits' injuries and attrition. *Military Medicine*, *180*(3), 329–336. https://doi.org/10.7205/MILMED-D-14-00184

Rose, C., Edwards, K. M., Siegler, J., Graham, K., & Caillaud, C. (2017). Whole-body cryotherapy as a recovery technique after exercise: A review of the literature. *International Journal of Sports Medicine*, *38*(14), 1049–1060. https://doi.org/10.1055/s-0043-114861

Rosenbloom, C., Coleman, E., & Academy of Nutrition and Dietetics. (2012). *Sports nutrition: A practice manual for professionals* (5th ed.). Academy of Nutrition and Dietetics.

Sanchez, M., Galvan, M., Nacim, D., & Bajpeyi, S. (2020). Improved glucose tolerance and glucose utilization with neuromuscular electrical stimulation. *International Journal of Exercise Science: Conference Proceedings*, *2*(12). https://digitalcommons.wku.edu/ijesab/vol2/iss12/85

Tsai, S.-R., & Hamblin, M. R. (2017). Biological effects and medical applications of infrared radiation. *Journal of Photochemistry and Photobiology B: Biology*, *170*, 197–207. https://doi.org/10.1016/j.jphotobiol.2017.04.014

Van Dam, N. T., van Vugt, M. K., Vago, D. R., Schmalzl, L., Saron, C. D., Olendzki, A., Meissner, T., Lazar, S. W., Kerr, C. E., Gorchov, J., Fox, K. C. R., Field, B. A., Britton, W. B., Brefczynski-Lewis, J. A., & Meyer, D. E. (2018). Mind the hype: A critical evaluation and prescriptive agenda for research on mindfulness and meditation. *Perspectives on Psychological Science*, *13*(1), 36–61. https://doi.org/10.1177/1745691617709589

Vanderthommen, M., & Duchateau, J. (2007). Electrical stimulation as a modality to improve performance of the neuromuscular system. *Exercise and Sport Sciences Reviews*, *35*(4), 180–185. https://doi.org/10.1097/jes.0b013e318156e785

Varatharajan, L., Williams, K., Moore, H., & Davies, A. H. (2015). The effect of footplate neuromuscular electrical stimulation on venous and arterial haemodynamics. *Phlebology*, *30*(9), 648–650. https://doi.org/10.1177/0268355514542682

Vatansever, F., & Hamblin, M. R. (2012). Far infrared radiation (FIR): Its biological effects and medical applications. *Photonics & Lasers in Medicine*, *4*, 255–266. https://doi.org/10.1515/plm-2012-0034

Wakeling, J. M., Nigg, B. M., & Rozitis, A. I. (2002). Muscle activity damps the soft tissue resonance that occurs in response to pulsed and continuous vibrations. *Journal of Applied Physiology*, *93*(3), 1093–1103. https://doi.org/10.1152/japplphysiol.00142.2002

Williams, E. R., McKendry, J., Morgan, P. T., & Breen, L. (2020). Enhanced cycling time-trial performance during multiday exercise with higher-pressure compression garment wear. *International Journal of Sports Physiology and Performance*, *16*(2), 287–295. https://doi.org/10.1123/ijspp.2019-0716

Zatsiorsky, V. M., Kraemer, W. J., & Fry, A. C. (2020). *Science and practice of strength training*. Human Kinetics. https://books.google.com/books?id=3v3FDwAAQBAJ

Zhang, Q., Wang, Z., Wang, X., Liu, L., Zhang, J., & Zhou, R. (2019). The effects of different stages of mindfulness meditation training on emotion regulation. *Frontiers in Human Neuroscience*, *13*, 208. https://doi.org/10.3389/fnhum.2019.00208

SECTION 5

PERIODIZATION AND PROGRAMMING

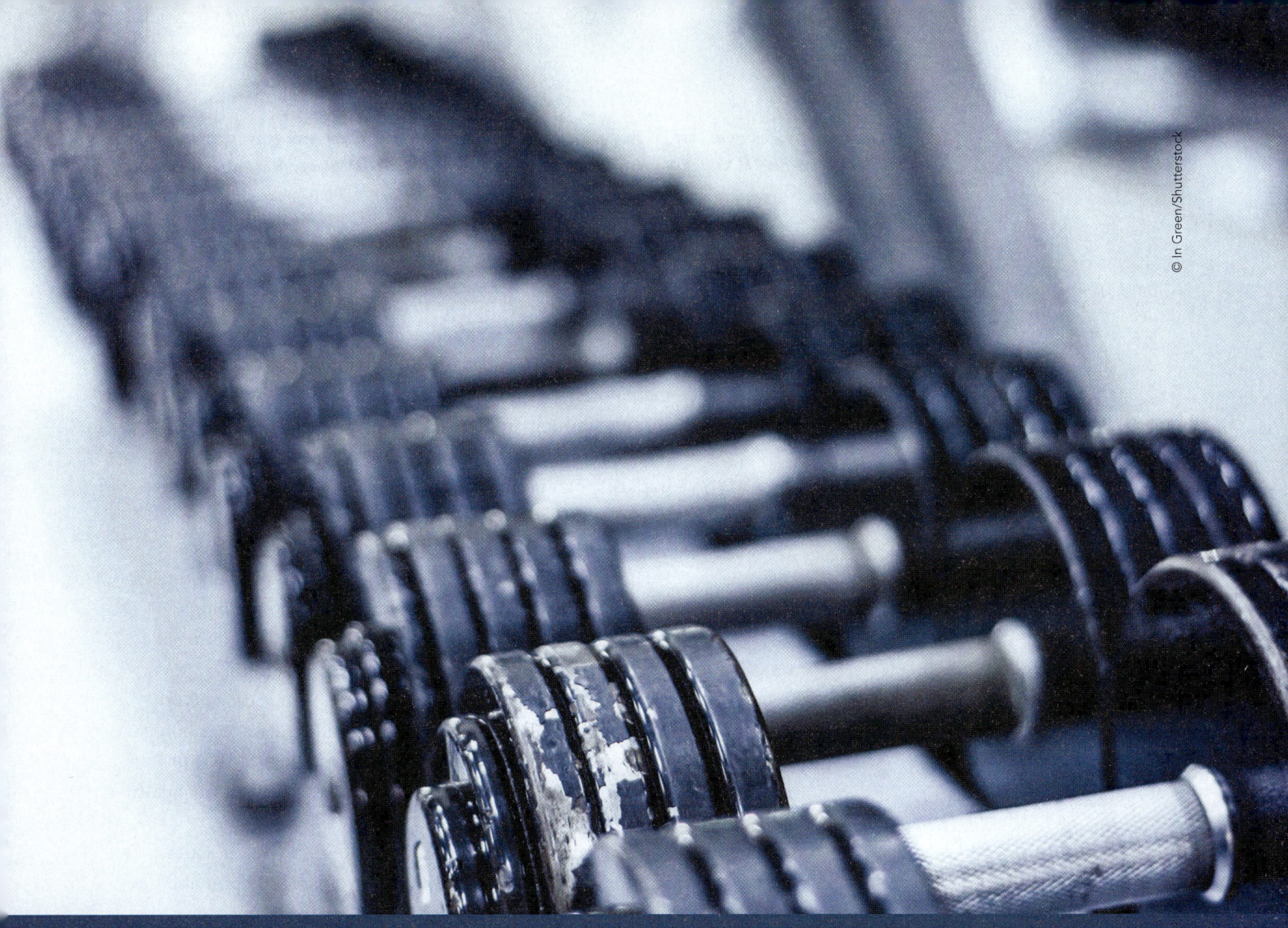
© In Green/Shutterstock

THE SCIENCE OF PERIODIZATION

CHAPTER EIGHTEEN

LEARNING OBJECTIVES

Upon completion of this chapter, the Sports Performance Coach will be able to:

- **Identify** biomotor abilities related to sports performance.
- **Define** periodization.
- **Differentiate** between models of periodization.
- **Explain** periodization as it relates to biomotor abilities.
- **Differentiate** between periodized programs for endurance and strength and power athletes.

LESSON 1: BIOMOTOR ABILITIES AND PERIODIZATION
INTRODUCTION

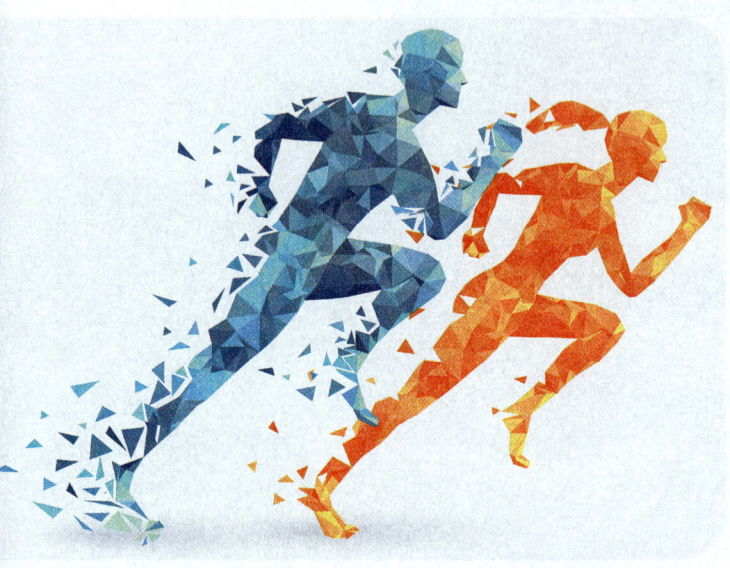

© Dina Winter/Shutterstock

Improving physical performance is dependent on the enhancement of strength, power, speed, and endurance. These attributes of performance are the dominant biomotor abilities that Sports Performance Coaches seek to build through specific training programs. The Sports Performance Coach must have in-depth knowledge of how these biomotor abilities impact sports performance and how physical training aims to maximize their development. Gaining detailed insight into these biomotor abilities also requires that the Sports Performance Coach understand the foundational components of each one. Once an understanding of biomotor ability development is established, the Sports Performance Coach must then explore proven methods of programming. Sports Performance Coaches aim to improve, in some capacity, all the dominant biomotor abilities through structured training programs designed to elicit certain adaptations at specific points in an athlete's training regimen. This is most frequently done using well-validated periodized models.

Many proven methods of periodization have been established in the past decades, along with a variety of programming tools. This chapter aims to define biomotor abilities and outline fundamental principles for their development. Further, this chapter provides detailed insights into the importance of periodization, how to structure an **annual plan**, and a summary of the most common periodized models.

> **ANNUAL PLAN →**
>
> The entire training year, which is broken into three distinct phases of periodization: preparation, competition, and transition.

BIOMOTOR ABILITIES

A diverse skill set of sport-specific movements allows athletes to effectively participate in their selected sports. The expression of these movements can be impressive and is useful for success in athletics.

All of these skills are supported by biomotor abilities, which are fundamental elements of skill-related fitness that create a foundation, extending the ceiling for skill acquisition and implementation. The general development of supporting abilities lets athletes train harder and perform better than if they were to neglect training for attributes such as power, speed, and endurance.

The sequential introduction of biomotor abilities is often used in sports performance to optimize training outcomes at specific times. Properly peaking key biomotor abilities at the right time in relation to competitions is predicated on a structured approach to performance training, where technical and tactical skills are built on a foundation of vital biomotor abilities. The amount of positive transfer, or the expression of these biomotor abilities in a sport-specific context, should be the ultimate goal for any athletic performance program.

Many methods are available to the coach to implement for athletes. Each method has merit, but many of them require advanced knowledge to know when, why, and how implementation can directly influence positive transfer to athletic performance.

An important feature of advanced programming is ensuring the direct application to athletic performance is built on the fundamental biomotor abilities that are not neglected during a training program in favor of flashier, advanced techniques. Just because a training tactic is available, that does not mean it should be implemented haphazardly at any point in the program. Any program should include a plan for developing foundational attributes progressively over time to maximize the influence that these attributes—such as strength, power, speed, and endurance—have on athletic performance.

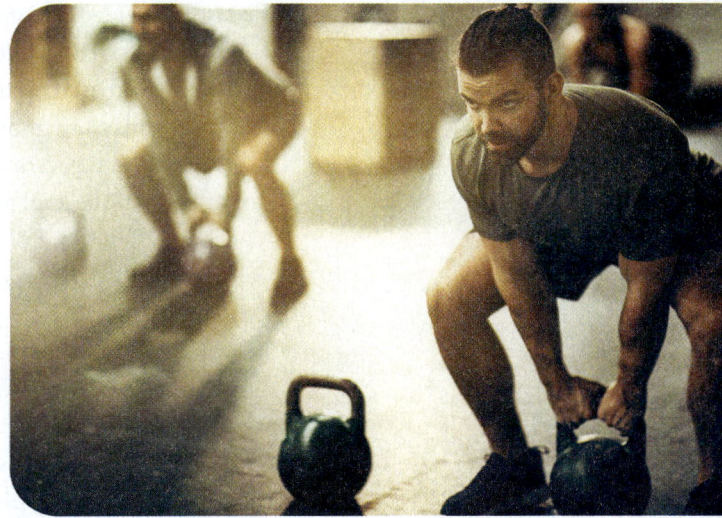

© Ground Picture/Shutterstock

STRENGTH DEVELOPMENT

Traditionally, three specific types of strength are considered the key to athletic development: strength endurance/muscular development (hypertrophy), maximal strength/absolute strength, and explosive strength/power. Within strength training, there are also avenues for muscular development and maximal power associated with strength development. An effective manner to organize the three forms of strength development is outlined in **Table 18.1**.

TABLE 18.1 Strength Development Strategies

Method	Description of Method
Repeated effort	An athlete uses any exercise and lifts a nonmaximal load to failure.
Maximal effort	An athlete lifts a maximal load or exercises against a maximal resistance.
Dynamic effort	An athlete uses maximal speed to lift or throw a nonmaximal load.

These specific strategies enable athletes to develop not only strength but also an improved rate of force development and explosive strength. Rate of force development, defined as the development of maximal force in minimal time, is typically used as an index of explosive strength (McLellan et al., 2011). The aim of rate of force development is to increase speed for high-force output.

✔ CHECK IT OUT

Consider the following scenario. Two football players are attempting a deadlift at 405 pounds. If the first player has a high rate of force development, then the deadlift will be completed in 1.5 seconds. The second player, who has a lower rate of force development, may complete the deadlift in 2.25 seconds. Although this difference might seem insignificant, the first player will have tremendous carryover to the playing field because they can quickly produce force and perhaps outjump a defensive player who is attempting to get the same ball.

Utilizing the three methods of strength as a key for developing training cycles, adjustments can be made to formulate the best plans for the athlete. Developing subcategories based on these methods can help the Sports Performance Coach create effective plans throughout the entire annual plan.

Table 18.2 suggests how the coach could prioritize training to increase the stimulus for athletes at the appropriate time of their training phase. For example, suppose the coach is trying to get players to gain muscle mass during the preparatory phase. They will want to use the repeated effort method because of the number of repetitions that will be completed during that time, but with a potential adjustment of the repetition tempo to provide the muscles more time under tension. If the athlete were to complete 12 repetitions at 70% of their one-repetition maximum (1RM), they might complete this exercise with a slower eccentric phase, a short pause, and then a slightly faster concentric phase. This is a positive stimulus for increasing hypertrophy of specific muscle groups that could be lacking in a specific athlete.

TABLE 18.2 Methods of Strength Development Examples

Strength Endurance Muscular Development with Repeated Effort	Maximal Strength Absolute Strength with Maximal Effort	Explosive Strength Power with Dynamic Effort
• Train to failure: Loads between 5% and 85% • Modified repeated effort: A taxing repetition range but within limits, leaving one to two reps in the tank • Repetition tempo: Manipulating eccentric, concentric, and amortization states for increased time under tension	• Maximum effort training: Training at or above 90% of the 1RM • Submaximal effort training: Training between 75% and 88% of 1RM • True maximum effort training: Establishing daily training maximums of specified movements	• 30% to 55% of 1RM for deadlifts, squatting, and pressing with implantation of accommodating resistance • 40% to 70% of 1RM for deadlift, squatting, and pressing with barbell load • 70% to 76% of 1RM for Olympic weightlifting lifts (snatch and clean and jerk)

Data from Kenn, J. (2003). The coach's strength training playbook. Monterey, CA: Coaches Choice.

POWER, SPEED, AND ENDURANCE DEVELOPMENT

Foundational attributes, such as power, speed, and endurance, can be overlooked or underemphasized in an athletic performance program in favor of more strength training. Each of these factors interrelates not only with the others but also with sport-specific skills (Allen & Hopkins, 2015). Depending on the skill's complexity and the athlete's age, power, speed, and endurance may have more or less of a dominant effect on sport-specific performance. A highly complex skill, such as a golf swing, may have less direct benefit for an athlete with great power ability because of the relatively higher level of importance of motor learning for this particular skill. Similarly, a younger athlete with less technical ability may gain more benefit from neuromuscular training and motor learning for a complex skill than from raw power training. These facts notwithstanding, if neuromotor ability is held constant and power is improved, it is likely to have a positive transfer to either athlete's golf swing. The ability to express power is positively associated with speed, and both metrics are higher for athletes competing at an elite level compared to lower-level competitors (Hansen et al., 2011).

Reilly et al. (2000) reported the differences in power, speed, and endurance for elite versus sub-elite young male soccer athletes. The elite athletes had higher vertical jumps (an expression of power), were significantly faster over 5-, 15-, 25-, and 30-m sprints, and had higher VO_2 max values and better fatigue tolerance. Although research entailed a cross-sectional comparison instead of an intervention, precluding a causative conclusion, it is still interesting to note the profound differences in fundamental skills for elite athletes compared to age-matched, non-elite peers. Logically, these fitness skills provide a better foundation for athletes to express soccer-specific skills and reach higher levels of competition.

The importance of power, speed, and endurance is further supported by the emphasis on these attributes in long-term athlete development (LTAD) models (Balyi & Hamilton, 2004; Lloyd & Oliver, 2012). Beginning with fundamental training in an unstructured and play-oriented environment, youth athletes begin training power, speed, and endurance to create a foundation that can reach its peak around the time very highly structured and targeted approaches to training are applicable—generally, from late high school into the collegiate years. A long-term approach to training these athletes is important because of how the components of speed and power can positively influence sports performance. Training the right biomotor ability at the right time in an athlete's training helps promote optimized adaptations. As opposed to strength improvements, power, speed, and endurance development must be completed in different manners and generally with different equipment.

COMPONENTS OF SPEED AND POWER

Any conversation about the applicability of speed and power for sports performance should be supported by specific characteristics of these relatively broad terms. The expression of speed and power can be different for different athletes. Additionally, both terms are not unidimensional and have subcomponents that are important to understand.

Speed

From a simplistic point of view, speed is a measure of how rapidly an athlete can progress from one point to the next. Linear speed can be differentiated from lateral speed based on the forward–backward orientation versus side-to-side movement, respectively. Acceleration is a component of speed that measures the rate of change. Athletes completing short sprints will generally be more reliant on their accelerative abilities, whereas an athlete sprinting over longer distances will require top speed, which is where additional acceleration is not possible (Cronin & Hansen, 2005) (**Figure 18.1**).

Track and field sprinters will reach top speeds after 50 to 60 m (Brown & Vescovi, 2012). Theoretically, if team sports more commonly cover distances of 20 to 30 m per sprint effort, it might be concluded that top speed should be excluded

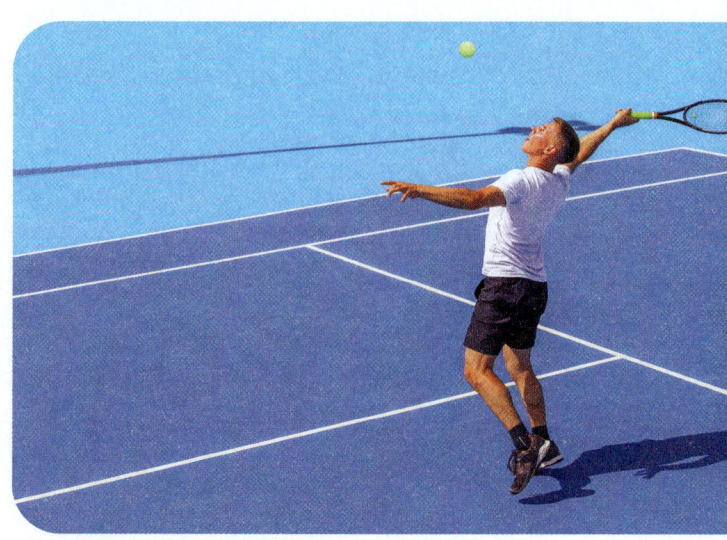

© PalSand/Shutterstock

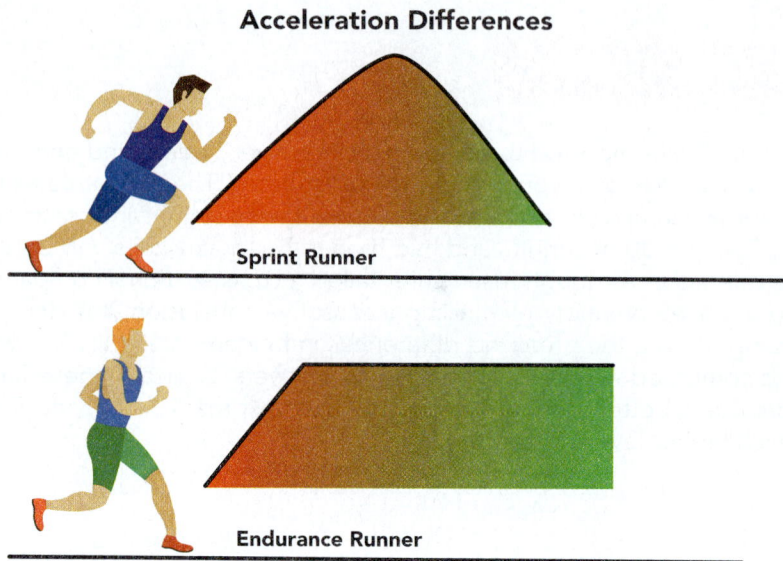

Acceleration Differences

Sprint Runner

Endurance Runner

FIGURE 18.1 Acceleration Differences

from training in favor of acceleration training (Rumpf et al., 2016). However, caution is warranted when trying to make these distinctions absolute (Brown & Vescovi, 2012). In reality, speed and acceleration are complementary and both should be addressed in training in the context of the sport.

In tennis, an athlete will rarely reach top speed, so training for a tennis athlete might focus on acceleration. Alternatively, a 100-m sprinter will reach their top speed; thus, their training focus should emphasize both acceleration and top speed.

Located in between the tennis athlete and the sprinter is the American football player, who frequently needs short distance acceleration and top speed capabilities. Open-field sprinting is a part of the positional requirements for American football, but a significant amount of change of direction is also involved. Thus, top speed is relevant, especially with specific routes that could be 15 to 20 yards and longer. For shorter routes, the emphasis shifts toward acceleration. While the context of speed and acceleration are important, coaches should avoid eliminating either form of training from a comprehensive training program.

Moreover, longer time to top speed might be a sport-specific tactic rather than a training rule (Cronin & Hansen, 2005). In fact, elite sprinters have been documented as completing 50- to 60-m races faster than the 50- to 60-m splits in a world record 100-m race (Brown & Vescovi, 2012). In combine testing for the National Football League, athletes accelerated through the first 20 yards and maintained peak speed over the remaining 20 yards of a 40-yard dash (Clark et al., 2019). Based on the training goals, the acceleration profile and distance to top speed were different in these two testing scenarios. Furthermore, track and field sprinting begins from a static start, whereas team sports such as soccer or rugby are more likely to feature some degree of walking or jogging before a sprint effort occurs, such that these athletes require a shorter distance to reach top speed (Duthie et al., 2006). Therefore, both top speed and acceleration appear to be relevant metrics for team sports (Rumpf et al., 2016).

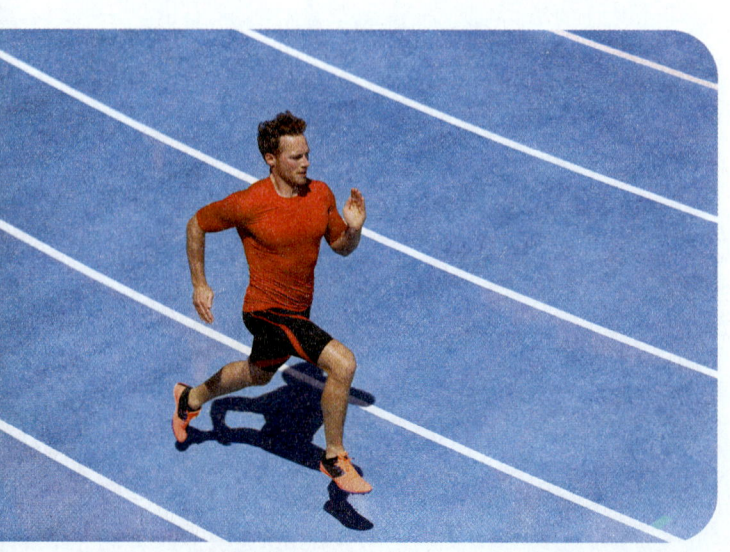

© Maridav/Shutterstock

Top speeds are possible in games but their relevance may depend on both the sport and the context of play. For example, elite field hockey athletes had average peak speeds during a four-game tournament that were slightly less than 85% of the peak speeds measured during fitness testing (Lythe & Kilding, 2011). Some things to consider when interpreting the need for speed versus acceleration include the sprint mechanics of the sport, patterns of play, and field dimensions. For example, the bent-over nature of field hockey may limit the overall expression of speed compared to fitness testing, which means the application of speed and acceleration are different, but not irrelevant. In another example from elite field hockey, 5% to 8% of the total distance covered during games was in the highest speed zone, with an average of 34 unique sprint efforts throughout the game (McGuinness et al., 2019). Clearly, speed is a relevant skill for field hockey.

Power

Power can be understood as the neurophysiological adaptation that underpins speed development. Certain mechanical aspects of sprinting are important to efficiently express power, but the root of speed can be traced back to the body's ability to produce force rapidly (**Figure 18.2**).

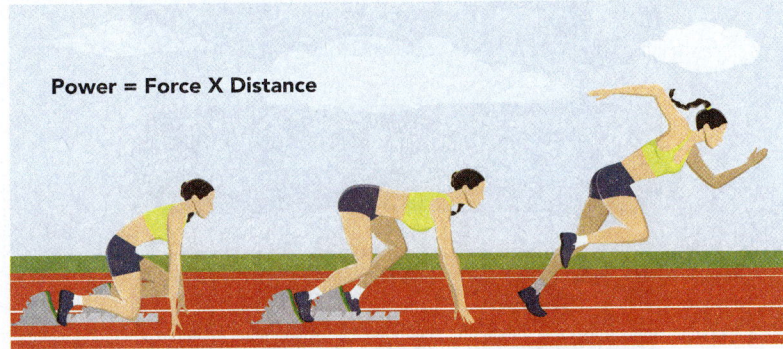

Power = Force X Distance

FIGURE 18.2 Power Defined

When applied to performance, the concept of power is the ability to produce as much force as possible over the distance required for the skill in the least amount of time possible. This positive influence on performance holds true for endurance, power, and team sport athletes, with all categories of athletes testing significantly higher on power metrics compared to non-athletes (Degens et al., 2019). All else equal, an athlete who can generate more force over a fixed amount of time will be more powerful. Such a sprinter demonstrates higher forces and can achieve faster sprint times (Weyand et al., 2000). Faster sprinters also have shorter ground contact time compared to slower sprinters (Paradisis et al., 2019), with reduced ground contact times being significantly related to maximal sprint speed (Nummela et al., 2007). As the equation for power suggests, if more work (higher forces) can be done in a shorter time (less ground contact), both of these mechanisms will lead to a more powerful athlete.

Application of the power equation can be further understood by referring to the force–velocity curve. The goal of training is to shift this curve up and to the right such that an increased amount of force can be produced at a given speed, thereby increasing power. Research shows there is more of a difference between elite sprinters and nonspecialists on the velocity part of the curve than on the force part, implicating the rate of force development as a key performance indicator in sprinting (Bissas & Havenetidis, 2008; Morin et al., 2012). This notion is also supported in team sports such as hockey, where Division I players have shown significantly higher top speeds (flying start—blue line to blue line) and peak power (vertical jumps and Wingate anaerobic tests) compared to Division III players (Peterson et al., 2004). With only a limited amount of ground contact time, an athlete who can generate more force faster will likely be the faster sprinter and more powerful in general (Turner et al., 2021).

COMPONENTS OF ENDURANCE

Whereas speed and power are explosive skills, endurance is the physiological backing that allows an athlete to repeat efforts without experiencing avoidable fatigue. Due to the deleterious effects of fatigue on the rate of force development, it is important to have the endurance foundation to withstand as many sport-specific expressions of speed and power as possible (D'Emanuele, 2021). As a generic construct, endurance can be defined as submaximal repeated efforts completed relatively continuously. Endurance can be broken down into three primary categories: anaerobic, aerobic, and muscular (**Figure 18.3**).

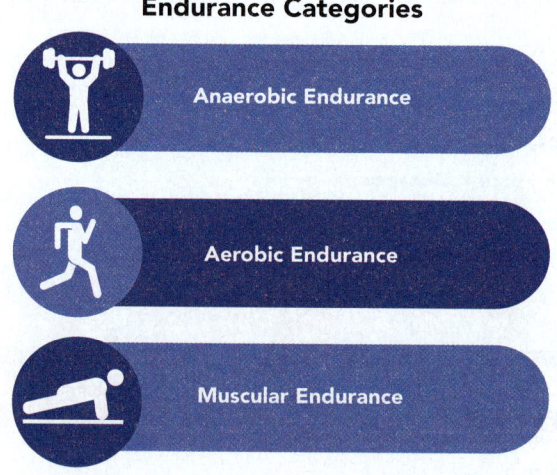

Endurance Categories

Anaerobic Endurance

Aerobic Endurance

Muscular Endurance

FIGURE 18.3 Endurance Categories

Anaerobic Endurance

Anaerobic endurance relies on adenosine triphosphate (ATP) replenishment through anaerobic mechanisms (i.e., without oxygen) (Green & Dawson, 1993). With continuous, high-intensity effort, the anaerobic endurance of an individual will quickly be exhausted, leading to a decline in work output. Some sports directly challenge anaerobic endurance with steady-state activities; examples include a 400-m sprint, a 500-m row, and a 100-m swim.

In team sports, the pattern of play is often far more intermittent—hence, the coining of the term "repeated sprint ability." Repeated sprint ability is generally characterized by sprints lasting less than 10 seconds followed by incomplete recovery of less than 60 seconds (Girard et al., 2011). The better an athlete can maintain speed over each subsequent sprint, the higher that athlete's anaerobic endurance is. Depending on the total number of repeated sprints, substantial support may also be provided by the aerobic energy system.

Aerobic Endurance

Aerobic endurance is often associated with steady-state performance in endurance sports. This is an accurate representation of the term, but the importance of aerobic endurance on recovery during the rest periods between intermittent sprint efforts is often underemphasized.

Sports such as basketball are characterized by sprints interspersed with lower-intensity periods of recovery. Generally, the anaerobic system is credited with providing energy during sprints; yet, as the number of sprints increases, there is a higher amount of support from aerobic endurance. In a group of college male basketball athletes, Gantois et al. (2017) found an increasingly strong association between VO_2 max and speed during 30-m sprints in a set of six sprints separated by 20 seconds of recovery. Longer protocols requiring higher volume—such as three sets of five 40-m sprints with 1 minute of recovery between reps and 1.5 minutes of recovery between sets—are associated with greater aerobic demand, with aerobic fitness being a "precious asset" for sustained performance (Thébault et al., 2011). Sports such as soccer and handball are other examples in which sustained speed is related to decreased performance when recovery is suboptimal (Gharbi et al., 2015).

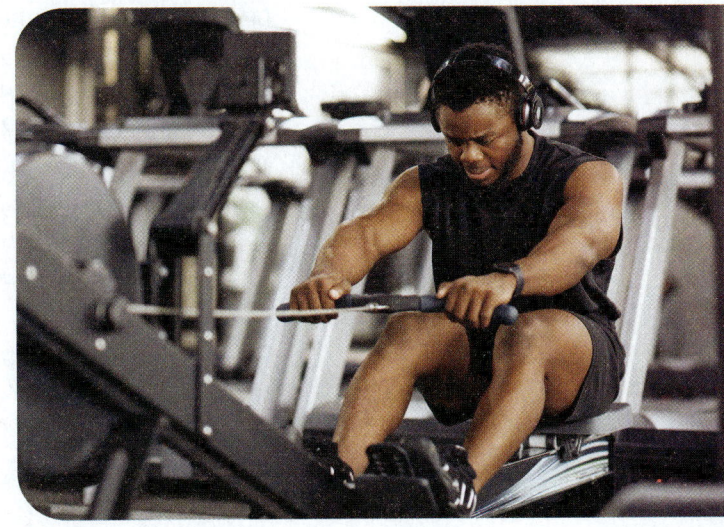
© Prostock-studio/Shutterstock

Muscular Endurance

Muscular endurance is the ability of a muscle to repeatedly contract at a submaximal intensity (Azeem & Al Ameer, 2013). Another way to think about muscular endurance is as the muscle's ability to resist fatigue under repeated exposure and continuous repetitions. For example, Hayes et al. (2011) demonstrated that running economy is strongly correlated with muscular endurance, implicating a regulatory role for muscular endurance in running performance.

Muscular endurance also must be considered in the context of absolute strength. Theoretically, if absolute strength increases, it is sensible to consider that submaximal strength would demonstrate a concomitant increase. With higher levels of maximal strength, sport-specific expressions of submaximal strength are further from peak ability, which could stave off fatigue. Semiprofessional rugby league players, for example, had better tackling ability under conditions of fatigue when they tested high on maximal strength using a 4RM squat protocol (Gabbett, 2016). This highlights that muscular endurance is a submaximal expression of strength; in turn, improving maximal strength is likely to benefit muscular endurance performance.

LESSON 2: INTRODUCTION TO PERIODIZATION
PERIODIZATION

Performance coaches aim to improve, in some capacity, all of the dominant biomotor abilities through structured training programs designed to elicit certain adaptations at specific points in an athlete's training regimen. This is most frequently done using well-validated, periodized models. **Periodization** is most easily defined by breaking up annual training plans into smaller, more distinct phases so as to segment training more

PERIODIZATION →

A systematic, planned, and sequential approach to strength and conditioning programming that divides training programs into smaller, progressive stages with the aim of driving physical and metabolic adaptations to improve performance.

manageably and better prepare for competition at all levels (Hoover et al., 2016). Periodization aims to divide periods of training into cycles or segments, enabling the coach to target specific adaptations during each cycle for higher focus on improving overall performance (**Figure 18.4**). Benefits of periodization include devoting the appropriate amounts of time to various aspects of training; developing an arsenal of sport skills by refining and perfecting each skill component technically, tactically, and psychologically; preventing fatigue and burnout by increasing work capacity; and acclimating athletes to competition demands through matched training (Lidor et al., 2016).

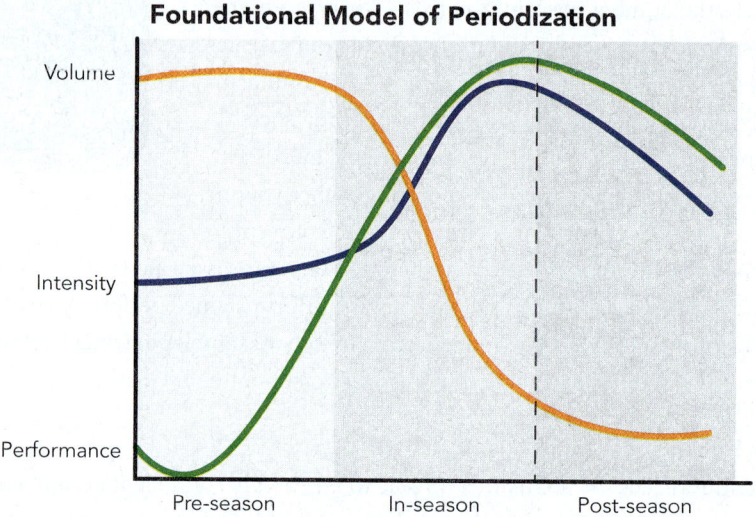

FIGURE 18.4 Foundational Model of Periodization

The foundations for periodization lie in the general adaptation syndrome (GAS), a concept introduced by Hans Selye that focuses on the relationship between a stressor and the time course of adaptation (Cunanan et al., 2018) (**Figure 18.5**). GAS, when applied to training, is characterized by an alarm phase in which performance is temporarily reduced based on the introduction of a training stressor. In this phase, recovery strategies should be emphasized over new training stimuli.

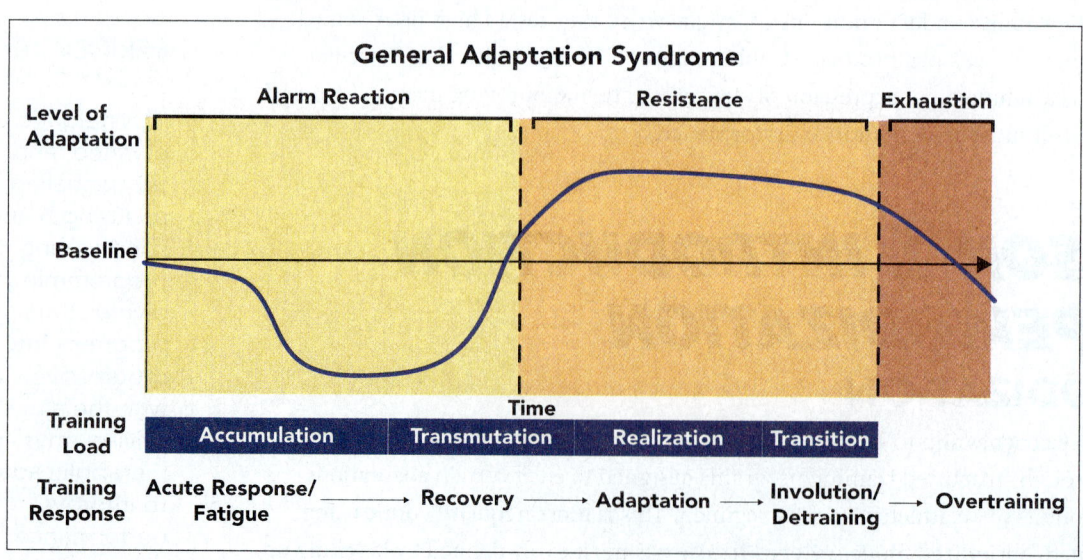

FIGURE 18.5 General Adaptation Syndrome

In response to the training stimulus, the body begins to adapt in the resistance phase, as recovery takes place and the body overcompensates to create a new and higher baseline for performance. This is the optimal time to introduce a new training stressor. If too much time passes between the previous training stressor and the introduction of the new one, detraining will occur. If not enough time is allocated for recovery, the athlete will enter into the exhaustion phase, which is characterized by reduced performance due to accumulated fatigue. Periodization provides a structure through which the timing of each training stressor can be optimized to manage fatigue and maximize the training effects.

✔ CHECK IT OUT

The concept of periodization originated in ancient writings from Greek and Spanish philosophers and was used by Romans, Greeks, and Chinese to train their armies. USSR physiologist Lenoid Matveyev, the "Father of Periodization," later advanced this concept, applying it to training of Olympic track and field teams. Hans Selye further contributed with his GAS model, highlighting the relationship between stress and adaptation. Thus, as scholars and practitioners alike have recognized the impact of stress on the body and the necessity of proper recovery, periodization has been applied in settings ranging from ancient soldier training to modern performance coaching, emphasizing the critical role of timing in achieving optimal results. Whether on a battlefield or a sports field, effective periodization is key to high-level performance.

Whereas programming focuses on immediate adaptations, periodization addresses the long-term adaptations of the athlete. Periodization follows a pathway in which general training yields to specific training, and lower intensity and higher volume yield to higher intensity and lower volume (Mujika et al., 2018; Stone et al., 2021).

✔ CHECK IT OUT

Periodization and programming, while interconnected, serve distinct roles in athletic training. Periodization is akin to a roadmap, outlining the broad approach, current state, and desired goal. It defines the macro-level objectives and sequence of training priorities. By comparison, programming is the chosen route to the end goal, dictating the micro-level, day-to-day decisions, such as specific sets and reps or exercise choices. Therefore, while two coaches may follow the same periodization model, their specific programming may differ based on individual methods and decisions.

PREPARATORY PHASE →

The pre-season; the periodization phase that emphasizes the development of the foundational biomotor abilities required for the specific sport to the highest level possible.

COMPETITIVE PHASE →

The in-season period; the periodization phase in which peak performance is planned to be reached. This phase is generally characterized by decreases in training volume and increases in training intensity.

TRANSITION PHASE →

The off-season; the periodization phase that serves as a rest period for physical and psychological recovery. This phase is generally characterized by the athlete not engaging in formal competitions.

Table 18.3 presents a model of periodization that divides an athlete's annual plan or macro-cycle into three or four sequential training phases or mesocycles: (1) the **preparatory phase** or pre-season; (2) the **competitive phase** or in-season; and (3) the **transition phase** or off-season (Plisk & Stone, 2003). The sequence of training goals ought to follow the fundamental progression of biomotor abilities, with each subsequent

TABLE 18.3 Periodization Phases

	Annual Plan/Macro-Cycle			
	General Preparatory Off-season	**Specific Preparatory** Pre-season	**Competition** In-season	**Active Recovery** Post-season
Goals	Strength and endurance	Basic strength	Strength and power	Variable
	Metabolic endurance	Repeated sprint ability	Speed	Variable

Data from Plisk, S. S., & Stone, M. H. (2003). Periodization strategies. *Strength & Conditioning Journal, 25*(6), 19-37.

GENERAL PREPARATORY PHASE →

The early weeks of the preparatory phase, which include more general training and an emphasis on aerobic conditioning.

SPECIFIC PREPARATORY PHASE →

The portion of the preparatory phase in which programming shifts toward developing biomotor abilities in a more specific manner required for the athlete's sport—traditionally, shifting to a more anaerobic capacity emphasis using tactics that target repeated sprint ability.

attribute building on the adaptations of the preceding ability (Turner, 2011). In most cases, training programs progress from less task specificity to greater task specificity, and from higher volume and lower intensity to lower volume and higher intensity (Stone et al., 2021).

THE PREPARATORY PHASE

The preparatory phase, also referred to as the pre-season, emphasizes the development of the foundational biomotor abilities required for the specific sport to the highest level possible to improve performance in each subsequent year (Bompa, 2004). If a Sports Performance Coach does not spend adequate time in this phase, it may impede the achievement of higher-level performance adaptations. During the preparatory phase, athletes generally do not have formal competitions and have fewer structured practice sessions. Therefore, more time can be spent on enhancing their basic physical abilities.

In many cases, the preparatory phase is divided into the **general preparatory phase** and the **specific preparatory phase**. That is, the early weeks of the preparatory phase include more general training that emphasizes aerobic conditioning through either steady-state distance runs or aerobic intervals of greater than 3 minutes with about equal time working and resting. Resistance training follows, with volume accumulating to create strength and endurance and improve overall work capacity. Sets will generally be higher (3 to 6) with repetitions on the higher end as well (6 to 12) and lighter loads. Exercise selection will also be higher, with more volume dedicated to accessory lifts.

As the training moves into the specific preparatory phase, programming should shift toward developing biomotor abilities in a more specific manner required for the athlete's sport. Traditionally, shifting to a more anaerobic capacity emphasis uses tactics that target repeated sprint ability. Shorter intervals of around 30 seconds can be used with 2 to 4 minutes of recovery, or shorter distances (10 to 40 yards) can be used with incomplete recovery time of less than 60 seconds. Resistance training begins to progress through muscular development to a more maximum strength focus, which requires less volume and higher intensity (more than 85% 1RM).

Progression within a training block can add volume with increased repetitions, add training density by reducing rest periods, or increase intensity with faster speeds over a fixed distance. This training foundation prepares an athlete for the higher-intensity speed work performed during in-season training.

THE COMPETITIVE PHASE

The competitive phase, or in-season period, is when peak performance is planned to be reached (Bompa, 2004). This phase is generally characterized by decreases in training volume and increases in training intensity. Additionally, practice time generally increases, with more time being devoted to skill technique and game strategy, leaving less time available for other aspects of physical conditioning. The primary goal of the competitive phase is to get the athlete into peak condition for the competitive season (Bompa & Haff, 2009). Competition periods vary among sports, with some lasting as little as 3 weeks and others spanning many months.

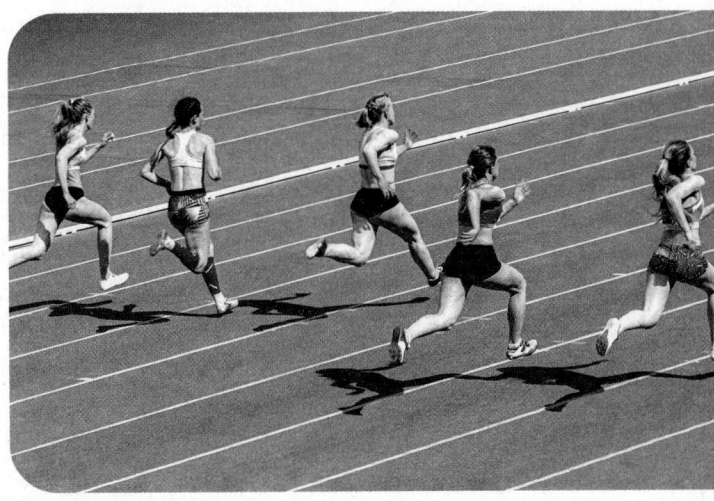

© Real Sports Photos/Shutterstock

One notable concern with traditional periodization is that peak performance cannot be maintained for long periods due to accumulated fatigue. Therefore, the competitive phase must be planned accordingly. If the athlete faces a long competitive season, the coach must manipulate the training variables by varying intensity, duration, and total volume to avoid overtraining and burnout (Bompa & Haff, 2009). In these cases, the goals are to preserve performance levels through moderation rather than trying to improve performance (Bompa & Haff, 2009). Utilizing various periodization models, such as block periodization, can be one way to mitigate accumulated fatigue and maintain performance over longer periods (Stone et al., 2021).

TRANSITION PHASE

The transition phase, or off-season, is used as a rest period for physical and psychological recovery. This phase is generally characterized by the athlete not engaging in formal competitions. However, they should still seek to maintain general physical conditioning; thus, the transition phase is an active rest period. The transition phase can last from one to several weeks in length. Longer periods in this phase make it ideal for injury rehabilitation.

Some coaches and researchers have encouraged the use of two transition periods (Bompa & Haff, 2009). The first transition period occurs between the preparatory and competitive phases, before the athlete begins more high-volume, high-intensity training (Bompa, 2004). This transition can serve as an active rest week with the athlete revisiting corrective exercise and recovery strategies to prepare for the next phase. The second transition falls between the competitive preparatory phases and is generally longer in duration.

Despite the sequential nature of the overarching goals, the conceptualization of periodization as a linear model is somewhat misleading (Stone et al., 2021). Although sequential changes do occur from one phase to the next, the actual loading strategies used in programming will be far more cyclical. Often, a 3:1 loading strategy is used in which 3 weeks of accumulated training stress precede 1 week of a reduction in stress, called a deload (Turner, 2011). To avoid detraining, the reduction in stress can be accomplished by reducing overall volume while maintaining the training intensity that matches the goals for the training phase. This kind of planned recovery with cyclical loading strategies is especially important for advanced athletes, who need higher-volume loads to facilitate further adaptations. The importance of fatigue management for optimal training and adaptation cannot be emphasized enough. Refer to the Sample Training Week in Appendix E for an example of weekly training for each phase of periodization for a competitive athlete.

To properly design a comprehensive and effective program, the Sports Performance Coach must consider the timing of a stimulus and the resultant adaptation that occurs. As an analogy, consider the process of baking bread. When baking bread, a cook must have the right ingredients (reps, sets, exercises, etc.) and must follow the instructions (frequency, intensity, length, type of exercise). However, without proper timing, the result will be either a soggy lump of dough in a pan or a hard-as-a-rock loaf of bread. Similarly, when the right ingredients and instructions are not accompanied by the proper timing, the athlete will likely not be ready to start the season and compete at the highest level.

The Sports Performance Coach should operate as a structured practitioner, serving many roles in the athletic development process. One objective for the Sports Performance Coach is to have a solid grasp of the principles of periodization. Proper implementation of these principles will establish the necessary baselines needed to maximize athletic performance, thereby increasing team and individual potentials. It is imperative to understand how periodization is a blueprint, permitting coaches to predict and then assign periods of time for achieving and demonstrating specific fitness characteristics (Cunanan et al., 2018). As with any program, however, adaptability is critical to athlete and team sport development; therefore, the periodization model must be updated on an as-needed basis dependent on evaluations of the team dynamics.

For the Sports Performance Coach, programming aimed at maximizing performance must be purposeful, integrated, and timely to ensure constant improvement. It is imperative that periodization goes beyond proper placement of acute variables for training in appropriate time frames surrounding a sport's season. There must be additional ways to provide the athlete with a complete training package that includes the use of diet and psychological skills during the appropriate training phases (Mujika et al., 2018). If athletes can optimize their training, diet, and mindset, their contributions to the team or individual sport will be the highest and most fulfilling.

LESSON 3: STRUCTURING THE YEARLY TRAINING SCHEDULE
PERIODIZATION OF THE ANNUAL PLAN

Periodization is about properly timing or scheduling training routines that lead to the athletic season. Annual plans must be implemented using specific training parameters so that an athlete can recover in the post-season, enhance their physical attributes and improve their skills during off-season training, and peak at the right time right before the in-season to perform optimally without undue fatigue. The annual plan spans the entire training year and is specifically broken into the three distinct phases of periodization: preparation, competition, and transition.

Using the annual plan, the coach can determine when the next season starts and plan out the athlete's macro-, meso- and micro-cycles that will dictate training and recovery parameters. The athlete or team will benefit from an annual plan because they can execute the necessary steps of the daily program and know what to expect as the plan moves into the subsequent phases. When athletes understand their training routines, they can adjust their schedules to get the most out of their training plans. They also know how to prepare mentally and physically for not only the next workout, but also what comes in the next cycle. Mental preparedness is just as important as physical preparedness with training, so it is optimal for the athlete to know what to expect moving forward—it should not comes as a surprise.

Athletes and coaches in all sports need to have a coordinated approach regarding how to move in and out of their season. Using proper transition periods, preparation, and competition phases will align players and coaches on how to progress through each time frame of the annual plan. The coach will optimize performance through the correct acute training variables and the necessary recovery, so players are fresh moving into their next training session and into the season. Players and coaches need to understand the need for being at a peak level of performance at the correct time so that the need for rest and recovery does not affect the playing season. No matter the sport or player position, it is imperative that all athletes are trained according to the annual plan so that they are prepared for the demands of both the pre-season and the post-season. When using an annual plan, the coach will coordinate training with the athlete's competitive season. If working with middle school, high school, and collegiate-level athletes, the Sports Performance Coach will most likely follow the academic calendar when setting up this plan (**Table 18.4**).

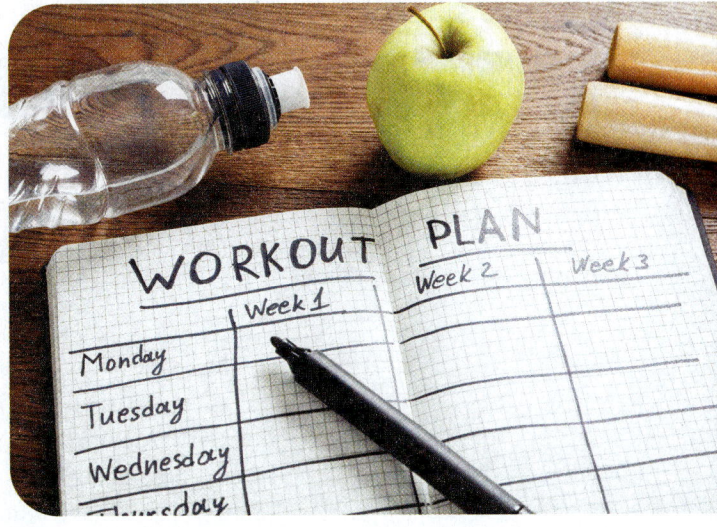

© Andrey_Popov/Shutterstock

TABLE 18.4 Example Template for Annual Plan

Training Phases	Preparatory Phase			Competitive Phase			Transition
Macro-cycles							
Micro-cycles							

STARTING AND ENDING DATES

The Sports Performance Coach must understand that the annual plan starting and ending dates are dependent on the athlete's specific sport. In regard to the calendar, the annual plan will begin at the end of the current season and span until the last day before the start of the future season. For example, in the National Football League (NFL), the current season ends with the Super Bowl, which is usually played in February. Thus, the annual plan for the next season starts on the day after the Super Bowl and ends with the Super Bowl in the next year.

All sports have different starting and ending dates for their respective seasons, and the dates will also differ depending on how well a player/team performs. As the starting time for the annual plan begins the day after the previous season ends, the initial weeks of the annual plan will begin with recovery. Therefore, the first day of the off-season truly marks the initiation of the annual plan, as the coach starts implementing the proper protocols for the athletes at this point. **Table 18.5** provides an example annual plan where the competitive season ends November 30.

TABLE 18.5 Example Annual Plan

Month	1	2	3	4	5	6	7	8	9	10	11	12
Periodization (phases)	Preparatory						Competition					Transition
	General preparatory			Specific preparatory			Competitive/maintenance					Recovery

Once the season gets under way, the annual plan equates to 52 weeks out of the year (a full calendar), though it can be extended if necessary. If teams make the playoffs or, even better, the championship game, additional weeks of training may be needed that push the players beyond the limits of the 52-week annual plan. Player load and volume of training must be taken into consideration so as to not increase risk of injury to these players who have been competing for extended periods of time. These factors must be taken into account at the start of every season, and alterations must be put in place to accommodate them.

After the yearly calendar has been established, but before the coach begins the process of developing the upcoming plans for a specific sport, key factors—more specifically, dates—need to be accounted for. These distractions to the training process can be considered uncontrollable factors. Uncontrollable factors are those factors that the coach cannot manipulate when designing the annual plan for a sport. They can lead to adjustments of the programs and cycles because they were not taken into account when the annual plan was developed. To save time, before beginning to build out the annual plan, it is recommended that the Sports Performance Coach creates a table or list of specific concerns that may affect program design and then acquire the necessary calendars and dates needed to plot those dates (**Table 18.6**).

TABLE 18.6 Factors That May Affect the Annual Plan

Uncontrollable Factors of the Annual Plan	Important Dates of the Annual Plan
Holidays	In-season schedule
Semester breaks	Playoff schedule
Exam schedule	Tournament schedule
On-site training versus off-site training time	Spring or fall out-of-season practice
College/university semester/quarter system	Training camp

Once the corresponding dates have been established, the next step is to input the competition schedule into the annual plan. This includes such information as the spring/fall practice schedule, off-season training activities, the in-season schedule, and the playoff schedule (if needed).

ANNUAL CYCLE TRAINING PLANNING

Annual cycle training planning is a structured approach to training designed to optimize performance by systematically varying training intensity, volume, and specificity throughout the year. This method aims to prepare an athlete to peak at the most crucial times of the season. Among the various types of periodization, the three main options are mono-cycle, bi-cycle, and tri-cycle plans.

The type of cycle chosen may vary depending on the number of competitive seasons that fall within a calendar year. Whereas some athletes have only one competitive season that lasts for a relatively short period, other athletes may need a training schedule that preps for peaking multiple times per year.

MONO-CYCLE

According to Bompa and Buzzichelli (2019), a **mono-cycle** is a plan that provides a long preparatory phase, allowing the athlete to develop a stronger foundation for skill development without the higher stress of competitions. A mono-cycle is often used in seasonal sports and sports that emphasize endurance (Bompa & Buzzichelli, 2019). In such a case, the annual plan is developed so that the athlete can peak prior to their competitive season. For younger athletes, seasonal sports include football, hockey, soccer, and baseball. **Figure 18.6** provides a mono-cycle example, showing a 5-month competitive season.

MONO-CYCLE →

Annual plan with only one peak or competitive season.

Month	1	2	3	4	5	6	7	8	9	10	11	12
Periodization (Phase)	Preparatory						Competition					Transition

FIGURE 18.6 Mono-Cycle Example

BI-CYCLE

As the name implies, a **bi-cycle** features two peaks in the athlete's annual plan. This approach is more suitable for advanced athletes but should still include a long preparatory phase for the development of foundational skills (Bompa & Buzzichelli, 2019). **Figure 18.7** provides a bi-cycle example, showing a sport with two competitive seasons in the same calendar year.

BI-CYCLE →

Annual plan with two peaks or competitive seasons.

Month	1	2	3	4	5	6	7	8	9	10	11	12
Periodization (Phase)	Preparatory 1			Competitive 1			T1	Preparatory 2		Competitive 1		T2

FIGURE 18.7 Bi-Cycle Example

TRI-CYCLE

Elite athletes, or those with significant training experience and physiological maturity who can handle multiple training peaks per year, can follow a **tri-cycle** or multiple-peak cycle (Bompa & Buzzichelli, 2019). It is important for the coach to recognize that the preparatory phase is significantly reduced when planning for multiple peaks per year. As Hoover et al. (2016) note, a tri-cycle is typically used with Olympic-style sports such as boxing, wrestling, and gymnastics, which require athletes to peak for national championships, international qualifiers, and international championships all within the same year. In other words, this cycle style is appropriate for those athletes who need to peak multiple times throughout the year. Sports such as football, basketball, and baseball would not use this type of cycle format because they have distinct peaking schedules. **Figure 18.8** provides a tri-cycle example, showing a sport with three competitive seasons in the same calendar year.

TRI-CYCLE →

Annual plan with three peaks or competitive seasons.

Month	1	2	3	4	5	6	7	8	9	10	11	12
Periodization (Phase)	Prep. 1	Competitive 1	T1		Prep 2	Competitive 2	T2		Prep. 3		Comp. 3	T3

FIGURE 18.8 Tri-Cycle Example

CYCLE TRAINING

The coach must now take the three main phases of the annual plan and put together the details that will lead to improved athletic performance on the playing field. Timing can be dictated by specific cycles that ensure an athlete does not spend too much time in one distinct area of training, thereby potentially hurting performance. **Cycle training** is critical to the success of the overall training plan, and comprises the content in each cycle that provides the stimulus to improve performance. These cycles (which are traditionally described as micro-, meso-, and macro-cycles) have been used extensively to help enhance performance and facilitate proper recovery (Cross et al., 2019).

MICRO-CYCLES

An individual training week, which traditionally consists of 7 consecutive days, is classified as a micro-cycle (Chena et al., 2021). The micro-cycle usually contains daily programming details such as sets, reps, intensity, and rest periods. Depending on these variables, micro-cycles may actually last between 7 to 14 days, as the coach may have specific variables planned due to a need or goal that must be achieved within that block of time.

Micro-cycles are traditionally positioned to serve a single goal or work toward the development of a small subset of biomotor abilities. In this context, the coach can utilize active rest, base, load, and deload micro-cycles to prioritize specific adaptations.

ACTIVE REST MICRO-CYCLE

The **active rest micro-cycle** is the primary micro-cycle used during the initial weeks of the preparatory phase. Its implementation within the developmental stage usually means a transition from one cycle to another, a program change, or a stage change. This cycle can be utilized as an aid in recovery, reconditioning, or rehabilitation, or as a time of complete rest.

If a period of complete rest is chosen, the athlete is not required to participate in any formal training. Sometimes it is necessary to give the athlete complete rest to assure both physical and mental recovery. Generally, 5 to 7 days of rest will not affect the athlete's fitness levels. After 7 days, however, the athlete may begin to detrain and their progress may begin to diminish. For a high school or collegiate athlete, this micro-cycle can be implemented during classroom examinations or during holidays. It may also be used after an extended period of uninterrupted training in which the athlete has completed a full week of performance testing. During complete rest periods, it is still in the athlete's best interest to engage in some extremely light activity (walking), and this message should be communicated by the Sports Performance Coach.

BASE MICRO-CYCLE

When developing a new training plan or phase, the first week of formal training is referred to as a **base micro-cycle**. This introductory cycle sets the precedent for the progressive micro-cycles that follow. During this week, new training parameters are implemented and new exercises may be introduced. In most cases, this cycle will include a lower training intensity and higher volume compared to the load and performance. The base micro-cycle

---

CYCLE TRAINING →

Use of the three main phases of the annual plan to develop the annual training program.

ACTIVE REST MICRO-CYCLE →

The primary micro-cycle used during the initial weeks of the preparatory phase.

BASE MICRO-CYCLE →

The first week of formal training.

---

typically focuses on developing stabilization and muscular endurance to establish a solid foundation for higher load training.

LOAD MICRO-CYCLE

A **load micro-cycle** will generally follow the base micro-cycle and build on the volume and intensity scale in a step-loaded pattern. In a step-loaded plan, training intensity usually increases from the previous week's work. Training intensity is higher in this micro-cycle, and volume is manipulated as well. The exercise choice and order remain in place.

✔ **CHECK IT OUT**

A step-loading pattern is another way of explaining the classical periodization approach. The aim is to increase intensity, or training weight, while simultaneously decreasing the volume to offset the heavier loads (Kell, 2011). This approach is not new and should continue to be used because of the ability to increase strength in a progressively overloaded manner.

For linking micro-cycles, an additional load week is usually implemented. In a standard plan where there is a specific increase in training intensity and possibly volume, with no other adjustments, this micro-cycle acts as a second load micro-cycle and the athlete completes the prescribed workload.

DELOAD MICRO-CYCLE

The deload micro-cycle is implemented to give the athlete the ability to physically and mentally recharge before higher levels of training are required. Deloading provides for a reduction of training volume load, similar to tapering, through a reduction in training volume and training intensity (Vann et al., 2021). The exercise order and the selection of exercises remain the same. In general, this period of deloading marks the end of a specific period of development. It is implemented to break up the continuous increase in training intensity that could lead to an overtraining state and possible injury.

Unlike the active rest micro-cycle, which can act as a stand-alone cycle, the deload micro-cycle is similar in structure to the progressive cycles. With a reduction in training intensity and the loads being decreased, this micro-cycle can be used to refocus on the technical efficiency of the main movements. A deload workout can use corrective or stabilization training to ensure training intensity and volume are not excessive and do not put undue strain on the athlete.

MESOCYCLES

A typical **mesocycle** is created by linking micro-cycles together; it makes up a traditional monthly or multi-month plan. This middle-length cycle (DeWeese et al., 2015; Issurin, 2008) may consist of any phase within the traditional periodization arrangement. Within the phases, the coach will make sure to provide specific variations in training, and different goals may need to be achieved throughout. According to DeWeese et al. (2015), a mesocycle can potentially consist of one distinct phase of training as well. For example, an athlete might stay in one mesocycle that revolves around the preparatory phase of training. Both aspects are common and should be used correctly by the coach to enhance performance throughout each mesocycle.

A standard mesocycle, as typically used in strength training planning, consists of three progressive micro-cycles: two load cycles and one base cycle, followed by a deload micro-cycle for recovery. This structure is commonly seen in plans where training intensity increases progressively over 3 weeks, often by 5% per week in a step-loaded pattern (**Figure 18.9**). Accompanying this intensity increase, training volume is adjusted accordingly. Generally, the deload micro-cycle reduces the training intensity by about 5%, returning to levels comparable to the base micro-cycle.

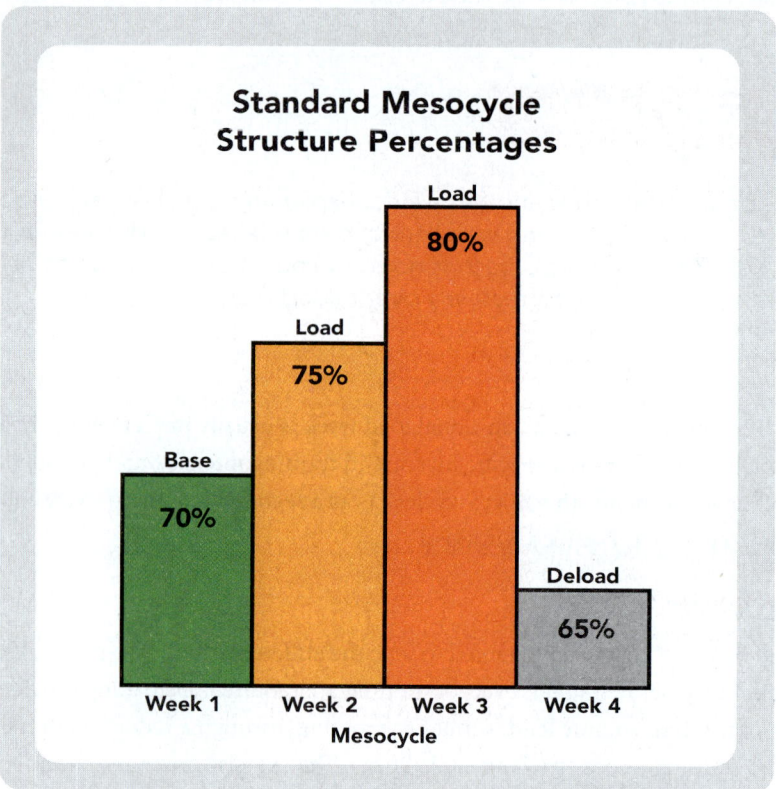

FIGURE 18.9 Standard Mesocycle Structure Percentages

👍 HELPFUL HINT

Weekly training intensity will usually increase in increments of 2.5%, 3%, 5%, 6%, and possibly as high as 7.5% per week. This is usually determined based on how many mesocycles are linked together and the specific goals of each cycle.

🤖 GETTING TECHNICAL

In an ideal training world, the Sports Performance Coach would be able to develop 4-week mesocycles that cover the entire year. This is rarely possible, however, because of the uncontrollable factors associated with the annual plan. When 4 weeks is not an option, there are a couple of recommendations. In the case of a 3-week block of time, remove the deload micro-cycle and utilize the three progressive micro-cycles (base, load, and load) as the mesocycle. In the case of a 2-week block of time, utilize the base micro-cycle and one load micro-cycle (**Figure 18.10**).

Mesocycle Comparison

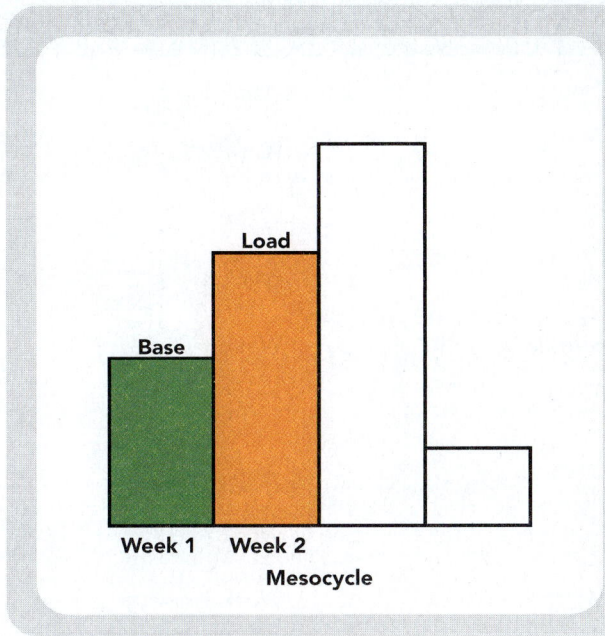
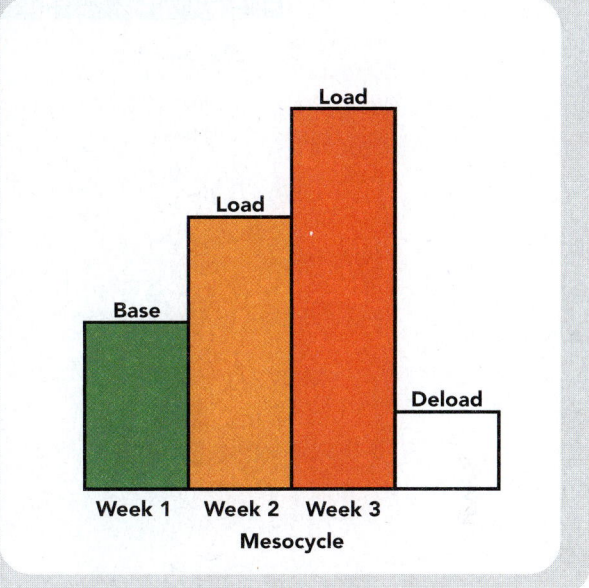

FIGURE 18.10 Mesocycle Comparison

MACRO-CYCLES

A **macro-cycle** is a complete season that an athlete will endure, including both the training component and the competition component (Naclerio et al., 2013). The macro-cycle varies according to the sport played, the amount of time the competition season takes up out of the whole year, the position that an athlete plays, and how many different phases the athlete must complete for performance enhancement. The coach must be aware of all these aspects so that they can create the best plan for the individual or team. Moreover, the coach must pay attention to the details of the specific sport because multiple seasons sometimes occurs within the same macro-cycle (Naclerio et al., 2013). This is especially important for swimming, track and field, and potentially soccer and baseball, as some geographic locations may offer these sports on a year-round basis.

A macro-cycle is frequently described as a generalized training program that spans one year. However, this term can also describe the linking of two more mesocycles in succession to form a defined time period. Macro-cycles are usually established when there is long period of training time, and programs and mesocycles are linked together to create desired training outcomes during that specific stage of training. In team sports, the longest uninterrupted training period is usually the competitive stage. In this stage, the pre-season, in-season, and possibly post-season programs may encompass as many as six or more mesocycles. Macro-cycle development combined with multiple complete mesocycles to improve training outcomes is ideal for most athletes. However, these cycles are particularly important in the long-term athletic development of youth athletes, whose training age is low and in whom most biomotor abilities are underdeveloped. **Table 18.7** provides an example annual macro-cycle with corresponding mesocycles and micro-cycles. Only 3 months are shown in the table, but this pattern would repeat for the entire calendar year.

> **MACRO-CYCLE →**
>
> An annual or seasonal training plan that demonstrates how a training program will progress for the long term, from month to month, to meet the desired goal.

TABLE 18.7   Example Macro-Cycle

Macro-Cycle	Mesocycle	Micro-Cycle
Calendar year	January	Week 1
		Week 2
		Week 3
		Week 4
	February	Week 1
		Week 2
		Week 3
		Week 4
	March	Week 1
		Week 2
		Week 3
		Week 4

LESSON 4: PLANNING STRENGTH TRAINING PHASES
PERIODIZATION OF STRENGTH CYCLES

In practice, periodization can take many forms. However, some popular and evidence-based models are available that should be the primary sources for informing coaching practice. The traditional or classic model of periodization has been emphasized so far in this chapter. The following advanced models can also be applied depending on the context and the athlete's needs (other models exist as well). These periodization models include linear, block, undulating, and conjugate sequencing (coupled successive). Each of these specific models can be integrated into the traditional model in a way that fits the athlete's training needs, the time of year, and the number of training goals.

LINEAR PERIODIZATION

Linear periodization is characterized by an initial high-volume, low-intensity form of training, with decreases in volume and increases in intensity then occurring gradually, usually over a period of months (Harries et al., 2015; Mann et al., 2010). The term "linear" typically implies that something flows in a straight line, making it easier to implement and execute. With performance training, linear periodization progresses from cycle to cycle in a manner in which the athlete overloads the system with weight versus volume to elicit the necessary changes according to the training program. This linear progression of the training load is the premise for progressive overload training.

Using linear periodization, the athlete would progressively increase the intensity of training over the training period (e.g., 50% to 60% to 70%). Conversely, the volume of training would systematically decrease, also in a linear fashion. This may require up to 6 months of uninterrupted training, as each phase traditionally lasts at least 4 weeks. Athletes who have a short competition season or compete only a few times per year may be ideal candidates for linear periodization models.

Although linear periodization can be a great approach to training, sometimes certain factors may prevent an athlete from training in this manner. Therefore, it is up to the Sports Performance Coach to determine if linear periodization is the best option, especially if the athlete has a demanding schedule or other factors that could prevent them from getting the most out of this option. **Figure 18.11** shows basic weekly progressions that can be utilized for linear periodization.

ACCUMULATION →

Similar to traditional periodization; aims to provide general preparation.

Basic Linear Periodization/Progression Overload Example

	Week 1	Week 2	Week 3	Week 4	Week 5	Week 6	Week 7	Week 8	Week 9	Week 10	Week 11	Week 12	Week 13	Week 14	Week 15	Week 16	Week 17	Week 18	Week 19	Week 20
%	50	52.5	55	57.5	60	62.5	65	67.5	70	72.5	75	77.5	80	82.5	85	87.5	90	92.5	95	100
SxR	1x20	1x20	1x20	1x20	1x15	1x15	1x15	1x12	1x12	1x10	1x10	1x9	1x8	1x7	1x6	1x5	1x4	1x3	1x2	1x1

FIGURE 18.11 Basic Linear Periodization/Progressive Overload Example

BLOCK PERIODIZATION

Block periodization is a progression of the traditional model that employs a more targeted and sequential approach compared to the broader, more simultaneous development that occurs with the traditional model. Block periodization is characterized by a focus on one training adaptation for a given time, usually blocks of 1 month (mesocycle), followed by a large change in acute variables to focus on a different goal (Ranisavljevic & Ilic, 2010). Because of the extreme focus on specific acute variables, the coach must be aware of the highly concentrated training workloads and how those workloads cannot be managed simultaneously. Therefore, the number of variables being developed at the same time should be drastically reduced (Issurin, 2008). Also, the Sports Performance Coach must ensure that the acute variables addressed in that particular block do not completely negate the need to maintain the other variables within the training program (Rønnestad et al., 2014).

The biomotor abilities of strength, power, and speed garner the most attention with this approach, with the primary adaptations being hypertrophy/strength endurance, maximum/absolute strength, and explosive strength/power. Block periodization specifies which specific trait will be emphasized and trained for in that specific mesocycle before changing the goals and moving forward. Commonly, block periodization is subdivided into three parts: **accumulation**, **transmutation**, and **realization** (Marques et al., 2017; Wetmore et al., 2020). As in traditional periodization, accumulation aims to provide general preparation, transmutation is for special preparation (specific to the sport), and realization is the competition and tapering. As the training program progresses, each biomotor ability will be given different levels of priority according to the overarching goals of the training phase (Kirby et al., 2010). **Figure 18.12** shows how when one biomotor ability receives emphasis, the other two must receive less emphasis for optimal adaptation.

TRANSMUTATION →

Sport-specific and skill training that takes advantage of the progress experienced in the accumulation phase.

REALIZATION →

The competition and tapering phase/stage of training.

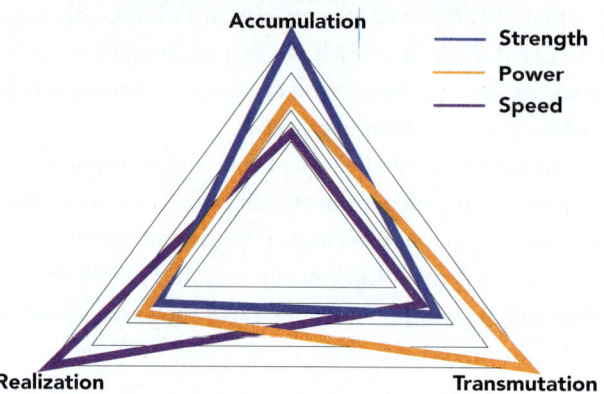

Relative Training Emphasis of Biomotor Abilities with Block Periodization

— Strength
— Power
— Speed

FIGURE 18.12 Relative Training Emphasis of Biomotor Abilities with Block Periodization

As an example, a baseball player who has just completed the regular season and no playoffs would use their general preparation to reestablish symmetry in the body (corrective) and begin to transition from stabilization and strength endurance to hypertrophy, through strength and maximal strength, and then power. During the pre-season, the transition would be to specific sports training (transmutation), which would then move to tapering directly before the competition and competition training. **Table 18.8** shows the transitions, moving from left to right, from accumulation through realization.

TABLE 18.8 Baseball Player Example of Block Periodization Transitions

Accumulation			Transmutation	Realization
Corrective exercise Stabilization endurance Strength endurance	Muscular development Maximal strength	Power Maximal power	Sport-specific training Maintain accumulation tasks	Taper Competition Competition training

This type of training traditionally utilizes a linear approach, as training intensity and volume will be varied in a linear fashion. The programming may not always follow a perfect path from high volume and low intensity to low volume and high intensity, but the blocks provide a more definite structure around the adaptation focus (**Figure 18.13**).

✔ CHECK IT OUT

Vladimir Issurin (2008) developed the concept of block periodization, which emphasizes the sequential development of biomotor abilities to avoid use of conflicting training methods. This approach focuses on a single training aspect at a time while de-prioritizing others, thereby reducing the total training load. It is especially beneficial for elite athletes who need a potent stimulus for continuous adaptations and has been applied effectively in Olympic sports such as swimming and canoeing/kayaking.

Accumulation Block Periodization Example

	Week 1	Week 2	Week 3	Week 4	Week 5	Week 6	Week 7	Week 8	Week 9	Week 10	Week 11	Week 12
	Hypertrophy/Strength Endurance				Maximum/Absolute Strength				Explosive Strength/Power			
%	60-75%				80-95%				50-60%			
SxR	3-5x8-12				3-5x2-6				6-8x1-3			

FIGURE 18.13 Accumulation Block Periodization Example

UNDULATING PERIODIZATION

Undulating periodization has been described as more frequent changes in volume and intensity, often on a daily or weekly basis (Harries et al., 2015). Daily undulating periodization is the manipulation of volume and intensities with the training sessions of the week. In the example shown in Figure 18.14, each individual training session of the week has a specific trait that is being emphasized, along with appropriate intensities and volume for that adaptation. The daily undulating model also fits well with the concept of microdosing, where shorter, more frequent training sessions are spread throughout the week to accommodate in-season requirements (Cuthbert et al., 2021). Many coaches will allocate one to two training sessions per week in-season to avoid unnecessary fatigue while also preventing the detraining of relevant biomotor abilities. Weekly undulating periodization is similar, but the volume and intensity changes occur weekly rather than daily.

In the example shown in Figure 18.15, all training sessions of the week emphasize the same traits. This results in specific goal changes for each training session in the daily undulating scheme; however, in weekly undulating plans, the goals remain the same for the entire week and change per micro-cycle. As opposed to prolonged linear periodization, undulating periodization does not allow for potential neural fatigue that could lead to a lack of strength development (Kok et al., 2009). If the Sports Performance Coach believes the athlete would benefit from undulating periodization by not incurring excessive fatigue across mesocycles, it is their responsibility to program each micro-cycle appropriately so

UNDULATING PERIODIZATION →

The manipulation of volume and intensities with the training sessions of the week.

MICRODOSING →

The programming tactic of introducing shorter, more frequent exercise stimuli to spread out the weekly training load and manage fatigue.

Daily Undulating Periodization Example

	Monday	Wednesday	Friday
	Hypertrophy/Strength Endurance	Maximum/Absolute Strength	Explosive Strength/Power
%	60-75%	80-95%	50-60%
SxR	3-5x8-12	3-5x2-6	6-8x1-3

FIGURE 18.14 Daily Undulating Periodization Example

Weekly Undulating Periodization Example

	Week 1	Week 2	Week 3
	Hypertrophy/Strength Endurance	Maximum/Absolute Strength	Explosive Strength/Power
%	60-75%	80-95%	50-60%
SxR	3-5x8-12	3-5x2-6	6-8x1-3

FIGURE 18.15 Weekly Undulating Periodization Example

as to not overextend the athletes. The Sports Performance Coach must be detailed and organized with undulating plans to ensure progressions are applied correctly.

CONJUGATE PERIODIZATION

The **conjugate periodization** model, also known as conjugate sequences or the coupled successive system, is considered advanced and should be reserved for athletes with a strong training foundation and a high training age (Plisk & Stone, 2003). The rationale for not implementing this model with beginners is that it uses blocks of concentrated loading to intentionally overreach and promote fatigue in an accumulation block of training, which are not appropriate for the training tolerances of novice athletes (Turner, 2011). During the fatiguing accumulation blocks of 2 to 8 weeks, advanced athletes will temporarily experience reductions in certain biomotor abilities, which will then be restored during subsequent restitution blocks characterized by reduced training volume and a shift in priority (Stone et al., 2021).

As an example, **Figure 18.16** depicts the conjugate sequence for an athlete whose first accumulation block is characterized by concentrated loading for explosive strength, which leans toward the force side of the force–velocity curve, with a strength-speed goal. To saturate this ability, a coach might program 6 to 10 exercises on a 4-day-a-week split during an accumulation block, then reduce the volume by focusing on 3 to 5 exercises twice a week during a restitution block where 2 to 3 days of speed training become the emphasis. With this periodization plan, fatigue accumulates for approximately 4 weeks, but then the target goal is switched to a speed emphasis for 4 weeks and considerably less volume is dedicated to explosive strength.

Conjugate Sequence to Develop Speed

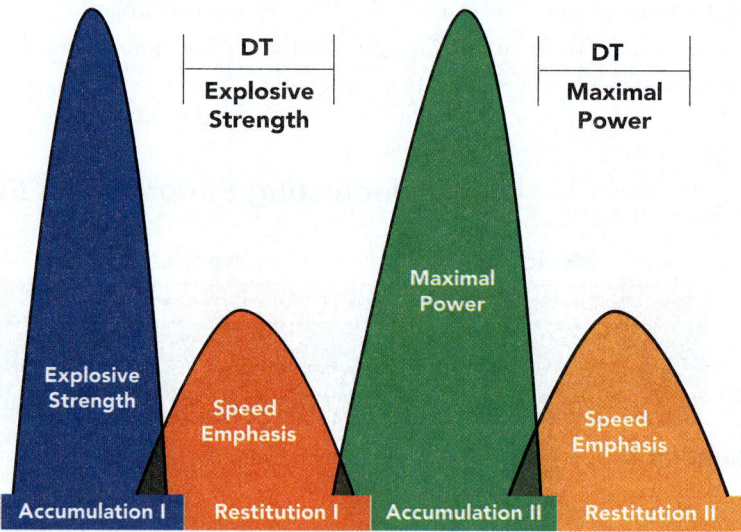

FIGURE 18.16 Conjugate Sequence to Develop Speed

A temporary reduction in power and speed is expected during the accumulation block. However, due to the delayed training effect, the restitution phase will demonstrate enhanced performance when recovery is optimized, despite the removal of a considerable volume of explosive strength training. This sequence is repeated with an accumulation block focused on maximum power, followed by another restitution block focused on speed.

The key aim of this model is to push the boundaries of fatigue, then rely on intentional recovery to apply the adaptations from the previous training block. The balance between fatigue and recovery is more tenuous in this model, as it is designed to push the upper limits of an athlete's ability with the intention of promoting continued adaptations.

Conjugate periodization is often preferred for athletes who must demonstrate maximal strength and explosiveness. The goal in such cases is to continually and progressively develop hypertrophy/strength endurance, maximum/absolute strength, and explosive strength/power within the same mesocycle (**Figure 18.17**).

Conjugate Periodization Example

	Monday	Wednesday	Friday	Saturday
	Lower Body	Upper Body	Lower Body	Upper Body
1	Maximum/Absolute Strength	Maximum/Absolute Strength	Explosive Strength/Power	Explosive Strength/Power
2	Hypertrophy/Strength Endurance	Hypertrophy/Strength Endurance	Hypertrophy/Strength Endurance	Hypertrophy/Strength Endurance

FIGURE 18.17 Conjugate Periodization Example

SELECTIVE PERIODIZATION

Selective periodization is a method that tailors the periodization model and annual training plan to the individual athlete, taking into consideration their performance schedule and experience level. Much of the existing research on periodization models focuses on elite athletes with extensive training experience, making some models potentially unsuitable for younger or less experienced athletes. As such, the athlete's experience should align with the complexity of the training cycles employed. For instance, an athlete who is relatively new to a sport or physiologically immature may start with a simpler plan, such as a mono-cycle, and progressively advance to more complex plans like a bi-cycle as their experience grows. Key to the success of this approach is the thoughtful variation of the training plan, which requires a deep understanding of the athlete's sport, its schedule, and the individual athlete.

✔ CHECK IT OUT

In the periodized plan, the goals and development of the running/field plan (aerobic endurance, speed, and agility) should coincide with the goals of the strength program. Higher volumes in the strength program should coincide with longer bouts of conditioning. As volumes change and the goals of strength and power are manipulated, the programming of linear and lateral speed, change of direction, plyometric training, and position-specific conditioning should match with the goals of each program written by the Sports Performance Coach.

SUMMARY

Periodization models and annual training plans should be tailored to the athlete's performance schedule, experience level, and physiological maturity. Not all models will suit younger or novice athletes, as most research has been conducted on elite athletes. Novice athletes may start with more straightforward plans such as a mono-cycle and gradually progress to bi-cycle and tri-cycle plans.

Variation in training, carefully planned around the sport's schedule, is crucial. Different periodization models, such as the linear, block, conjugate, or undulated options, could be utilized depending on the off-season duration or time between events. For example, athletes recovering from injuries or long gaps between bouts might benefit from a full linear schedule, while in-season training might require an undulated approach.

Periodization also involves managing training stress in relation to competition stress. Coaches should adjust the training volume and intensity during periods of high competitive stress to avoid overtraining and ensure sufficient recovery. Athlete playing time, position, acute stress levels, training status, and season schedule should all be considered when developing a training program.

Enhancing foundational biomotor abilities such as strength, power, speed, and endurance is essential for peak performance. Advanced training programs and appropriate periodization models, including cycle training, can help develop these abilities effectively. Coaches should understand the fundamentals of fitness, explore various training options, and implement the most suitable program to elicit high levels of adaptation and performance in athletes.

KEY TAKEAWAYS

- Biomotor abilities such as strength, power, speed, and agility are the foundational skills on which performance programs are built.
- Vital targets to enhance performance are maximal strength and rate of force development; these interrelated concepts can be best understood through applications of the force–velocity curve.
- The benefits of periodization include devoting the appropriate amounts of time to various aspects of training; developing an arsenal of sport skills by refining and perfecting each skill component technically, tactically, and psychologically; preventing fatigue and burnout by increasing work capacity; and acclimating athletes to competition demands through matched training.
- Periodization is based on the general adaptation syndrome (GAS), which focuses on the relationship between a stressor and the time course of adaptation. When applied to training, GAS is defined by the alarm, resistance, and exhaustion phases.
- Cycle training is used for overall programming schedules and essentially lays out the necessary performance-improving stimuli. These cycles, which are traditionally described as micro-, meso-, and macro-cycles, have been used extensively to enhance performance and facilitate proper recovery.
- Day-to-day programming decisions for training methods should be determined by the overarching structure of the goals for a long-term program, which can be defined through periodized models such as block periodization, conjugated sequencing, and daily undulating periodization.

REFERENCES

Allen, S. V., & Hopkins, W. G. (2015). Age of peak competitive performance of elite athletes: A systematic review. *Sports Medicine, 45*(10): 1431–1441. https://doi.org/10.1007/s40279-015-0354-3

Azeem, K., & Al Ameer, A. (2013). Effect of weight training programme on body composition, muscular endurance, and muscular strength of males. *Annals of Biological Research, 4*(2), 154–156.

Balyi, I., & Hamilton, A. (2004). Long-term athlete development: Trainability in childhood and adolescence. *Olympic Coach, 16*(1), 4–9.

Bissas, A., & Havenetidis, K. (2008). The use of various strength-power tests as predictors of sprint running performance. *Journal of Sports Medicine and Physical Fitness, 48*(1), 49–54.

Bompa, T. O. (2004). Primer on periodization. *Olympic Coach, 18*(2): 4–7.

Bompa, T. O., & Buzzichelli, C. A. (2019). *Periodization: Theory and methodology of training* (6th ed.). Human Kinetics.

Bompa, T. O., & Haff, G. G. (2009). *Periodization: Theory and methodology of training* (5th ed.). Human Kinetics.

Brown, T. D., & Vescovi, J. (2012). Maximum speed: Misconceptions of sprinting. *Strength and Conditioning Journal, 34*(2), 37–41. http://doi.org/10.1519/SSC.0b013e31824ea156

Chena, M., Morcillo, J. A., Rodríguez-Hernández, M. L., Zapardiel, J. C., Owen, A., & Lozano, D. (2021). The effect of weekly training load across a competitive microcycle on contextual variables in professional soccer. *International Journal of Environmental Research and Public Health, 18*(10), 5091. https://doi.org/10.3390/ijerph18105091

Clark, K. P., Rieger, R. H., Bruno, R. F., & Stearne, D. J. (2019). The National Football League combine 40-yd dash: How important is maximum velocity? *Journal of Strength and Conditioning Research, 33*(6), 1542–1550. https://doi.org/10.1519/jsc.0000000000002081

Cronin, J. B., & Hansen, K. T. (2005). Strength and power predictors of sports speed. *Journal of Strength and Conditioning Research, 19*(2), 349–357. https://pubmed.ncbi.nlm.nih.gov/15903374

Cross, R., Siegler, J., Marshall, P., & Lovell, R. (2019). Scheduling of training and recovery during the in-season weekly micro-cycle: Insights from team sport practitioners. *European Journal of Sport Science, 19*(10), 1287–1296. https://doi.org/10.1080/17461391.2019.1595740

Cunanan, A. J., DeWeese, B. H., Wagle, J. P., Carroll, K. M., Sausaman, R., Hornsby, W. G., 3rd, Haff, G. G., Triplett, T., Pierce, K. C., & Stone, M. H. (2018). The general adaptation syndrome: A foundation for the concept of periodization. *Sports Medicine, 48*(4), 787–797. https://doi.org/10.1007/s40279-017-0855-3

Cuthbert, M., Haff, G. G., Arent, S. M., Ripley, N., McMahon, J. J., Evans, M., & Comfort, P. (2021). Effects of variations in resistance training frequency on strength development in well-trained populations and implications for in-season athlete training: A systematic review and meta-analysis. *Sports Medicine, 51*(9), 1967–1982. https://doi.org/10.1007/s40279-021-01460-7

Degens, H., Stasiulis, A., Skurvydas, A., Statkeviciene, B., & Venckunas, T. (2019). Physiological comparison between non-athletes, endurance, power and team athletes. *European Journal of Applied Physiology, 119*(6), 1377–1386. https://doi.org/10.1007/s00421-019-04128-3

D'Emanuele, S., Maffiuletti, N. A., Tarperi, C., Rainoldi, A., Schena, F., & Boccia, G. (2021). Rate of force development as an indicator of neuromuscular fatigue: A scoping review. *Frontiers in Human Neuroscience, 15*, 701916. https://doi.org/10.3389/fnhum.2021.701916

DeWeese, B. H., Hornsby, G., Stone, M., & Stone, M. H. (2015). The training process: Planning for strength-power training in track and field. Part 2: Practical and applied aspects. *Journal of Sport and Health Science, 4*(4), 318–324. https://doi.org/10.1016/j.jshs.2015.07.002

Duthie, G. M., Pyne, D. B., Marsh, D. J., & Hooper, S. L. (2006). Sprint patterns in rugby union players during competition. *Journal of Strength and Conditioning Research, 20*(1), 208–214. https://pubmed.ncbi.nlm.nih.gov/16506864

Gabbett, T. J. (2016). Influence of fatigue on tackling ability in rugby league players: Role of muscular strength, endurance, and aerobic qualities. *PLOS One, 11*(10), e0163161.

Gantois, P., Aidar, F. J., De Matos, D. G., De Souza, R. F., Da Silva, L. M., De Castro, K. R., Medeiros, R.C., & Cabral, B. G. (2017). Repeated sprints and the relationship with anaerobic and aerobic fitness of basketball athletes. *Journal of Physical Education and Sport, 17*(2), 910.

Gharbi, Z., Dardouri, W., Haj-Sassi, R., Chamari, K., & Souissi, N. (2015). Aerobic and anaerobic determinants of repeated sprint ability in team sports athletes. *Biology of Sport, 32*(3), 207–212. https://www.ncbi.nlm.nih.gov/pmc/articles/PMC4577558

Girard, O., Mendez-Villanueva, A., & Bishop, D. (2011). Repeated-sprint ability: Part I. *Sports Medicine, 41*(8), 673–694.

Green, S., & Dawson, B. (1993). Measurement of anaerobic capacities in humans: Definitions, limitations and unsolved problems. *Sports Medicine, 15*(5), 312–327. https://doi.org/10.2165/00007256-199315050-00003

Hansen, K. T., Cronin, J. B., Pickering, S. L., & Douglas, L. (2011). Do force–time and power–time measures in a loaded jump squat differentiate between speed performance and playing level in elite and elite junior rugby union players? *Journal of Strength and Conditioning Research, 25*(9), 2382–2391. https://doi.org/10.1519/JSC.0b013e318201bf48

Harries, S. K., Lubans, D. R., & Callister, R. (2015). Systematic review and meta-analysis of linear and undulating periodized resistance training programs on muscular strength. *Journal of Strength and Conditioning Research, 29*(4), 1113–1125. https://doi.org/10.1519/jsc.0000000000000712

Hayes, P. R., French, D. N., & Thomas, K. (2011). The effect of muscular endurance on running economy. *Journal of Strength and Conditioning Research, 25*(9), 2464–2469.

Hoover, D. L., VanWye, W. R., & Judge, L. W. (2016). Periodization and physical therapy: Bridging the gap between training and rehabilitation. *Physical Therapy in Sport, 18,* 1–20. http://doi.org/10.1016/j.ptsp .2015.08.003

Issurin, V. (2008). Block periodization versus traditional training theory: A review. *Journal of Sports Medicine and Physical Fitness, 48*(1), 65–75.

Kell, R. T. (2011). The influence of periodized resistance training on strength changes in men and women. *Journal of Strength and Conditioning Research, 25*(3), 735–744. https://doi.org/10.1519/jsc.0b013e3181c69f22

Kenn, J. (2003). *The coach's strength training playbook.* Coaches Choice.

Kirby, T. J., Erickson, T., & McBride, J. M. (2010). Model for progression of strength, power, and speed training. *Strength & Conditioning Journal, 32*(5), 86–90.

Kok, L.-Y., Hamer, P. W., & Bishop, D. J. (2009). Enhancing muscular qualities in untrained women. *Medicine & Science in Sports & Exercise, 41,* 1797–1807.

Lidor, R., Tenenbaum, G., Ziv, G., & Issurin, V. (2016). Achieving expertise in sport: Deliberate practice, adaptation, and periodization of training. *Kinesiology Review, 5*(1), 129–141. https://doi.org/10.1123/kr.2015-0004

Lloyd, R. S., & Oliver, J. L. (2012). The youth physical development model: A new approach to long-term athletic development. *Strength & Conditioning Journal, 34*(3), 61–72.

Lythe, J., & Kilding, A. E. (2011). Physical demands and physiological responses during elite field hockey. *International Journal of Sports Medicine, 32*(07), 523–528. https://doi.org/10.1055/s-0031-1273710

Mann, J. B., Thyfault, J. P., Ivey, P. A., & Sayers, S. P. (2010). The effect of autoregulatory progressive resistance exercise vs. linear periodization on strength improvement in college athletes. *Journal of Strength and Conditioning Research, 24*(7), 1718–1723. https://doi.org/10.1519/jsc.0b013e3181def4a6

Marques, L., Franchini, E., Drago, G., Aoki, M. S., & Moreira, A. (2017). Physiological and performance changes in national and international judo athletes during block periodization training. *Biology of Sport, 34*(4), 371–378. https://doi.org/10.5114%2Fbiolsport.2017.69825

McGuinness, A., Malone, S., Petrakos, G., & Collins, K. (2019). Physical and physiological demands of elite international female field hockey players during competitive match play. *Journal of Strength and Conditioning Research, 33*(11), 3105–3113. https://doi.org/10.1519/jsc.0000000000002158

McLellan, C. P., Lovel, D. I., & Gass, G. C. (2011). The role of rate of force development on vertical jump performance. *Journal of Strength and Conditioning Research, 25*(2), 379–385. https://doi.org/10.1519 /jsc.0b013e3181be305c

Morin, J.-B., Bourdin, M., Edouard, P., Peyrot, N., Samozino, P., & Lacour, J.- R. (2012). Mechanical determinants of 100-m sprint running performance. *European Journal of Applied Physiology, 112*(11), 3921–3930.

Mujika, I., Halson, S., Burke, L. M., Balagué, G., & Farrow, D. (2018). An integrated, multifactorial approach to periodization for optimal performance in individual and team sports. *International Journal of Sports Physiology and Performance, 13*(5), 538–561. https://doi.org/10.1123/ijspp.2018-0093

Naclerio, F., Moody, J., & Chapman, M. (2013). Applied periodization: A methodological approach. *Journal of Human Sport & Exercise, 8*(2), 350–366. http://doi.org/10.4100/jhse.2012.82.04

Nummela, A., Keränen, T., & Mikkelsson, L. O. (2007). Factors related to top running speed and economy. *International Journal of Sports Medicine, 28*(8), 655–661. https://doi.org/10.1055/s-2007-964896

Paradisis, G. P., Bissas, A., Pappas, P., Zacharogiannis, E., Theodorou, A., & Girard, O. (2019). Sprint mechanical differences at maximal running speed: Effects of performance level. *Journal of Sports Sciences, 37*(17), 2026–2036. https://doi.org/10.1080/02640414.2019.1616958

Peterson, M. D., Rhea, M. R., & Alvar, B. A. (2004). Maximizing strength development in athletes: A meta-analysis to determine the dose–response relationship. *Journal of Strength and Conditioning Research, 18*(2), 377–382. https://doi.org/10.1519/r-12842.1

Plisk, S. S., & Stone, M. H. (2003). Periodization strategies. *Strength & Conditioning Journal, 25*(6), 19–37.

Ranisavljevic, I., & Ilic, V. (2010). Periodization variants in strength training throughout microcycles and mesocycles. *Proceedings of the Faculty of Physical Education, 2010*(2), 304–311.

Reilly, T., Williams, A. M., Nevill, A., & Franks, A. (2000). A multidisciplinary approach to talent identification in soccer. *Journal of Sports Sciences, 18*(9), 695–702. https://doi.org/10.1080/02640410050120078

Rønnestad, B. R., Ellefsen, S., Nygaard, H., Zacharoff, E. E., Vikmoen, O., Hansen, J., & Hallén, J. (2014). Effects of 12 weeks of block periodization on performance and performance indices in well-trained cyclists. *Scandinavian Journal of Medicine & Science in Sports, 24*(2), 327–335. https://doi.org/10.1111/sms.12016

Rumpf, M. C., Lockie, R. G., Cronin, J. B., & Jalilvand, F. (2016). Effect of different sprint training methods on sprint performance over various distances: A brief review. *Journal of Strength and Conditioning Research, 30*(6), 1767–1785. https://doi.org/10.1519/jsc.0000000000001245

Stone, M. H., Hornsby, W. G., Haff, G. G., Fry, A. C., Suarez, D. G., Liu, J., Gonzalez-Rave, J. M., Pierce, K. C. (2021). Periodization and block periodization in sports: Emphasis on strength-power training: A provocative and challenging narrative. *Journal of Strength and Conditioning Research, 35*(8), 2351–2371. https://doi.org /10.1519/JSC.0000000000004050

Thébault, N., Léger, L. A., & Passelergue, P. (2011). Repeated-sprint ability and aerobic fitness. *Journal of Strength and Conditioning Research, 25(10)*, 2857–2865.

Turner, A. N. (2011). The science and practice of periodization: A brief review. *Strength and Conditioning Journal, 33*(1), 34–46. http://doi.org/10.1519/SSC.0b013e3182079cdf

Turner, A. N., Comfort, P., McMahon, J., Bishop, C., Chavda, S., Read, P., Mundy, P., & Lake, J. (2021). Developing powerful athletes: Part 2: Practical applications. *Strength and Conditioning Journal, 43*(1), 23–31. https://doi .org/10.1519/SSC.0000000000000544

Vann, C. G., Haun, C. T., Osburn, S. C., Romero, M. A., Roberson, P. A., Mumford, P. W., Mobley, C. B., Holmes, H. M., Fox, C. D., Young, K. C., & Roberts, M. D. (2021). Molecular differences in skeletal muscle after 1 week of active vs. passive recovery from high-volume resistance training. *Journal of Strength and Conditioning Research, 35*(8), 2102–2113. https://doi.org/10.1519/jsc.0000000000004071

Wetmore, A. B., Moquin, P. A., Carroll, K. M., Fry, A. C., Hornsby, W. G., & Stone, M. H. (2020). The effect of training status on adaptations to 11 weeks of block periodization training. *Sports, 8*(11), 145. https:// doi.org/10.3390/sports8110145

Weyand, P. G., Sternlight, D. B., Bellizzi, M. J., & Wright, S. (2000). Faster top running speeds are achieved with greater ground forces not more rapid leg movements. *Journal of Applied Physiology, 89*(5), 1991–1999.

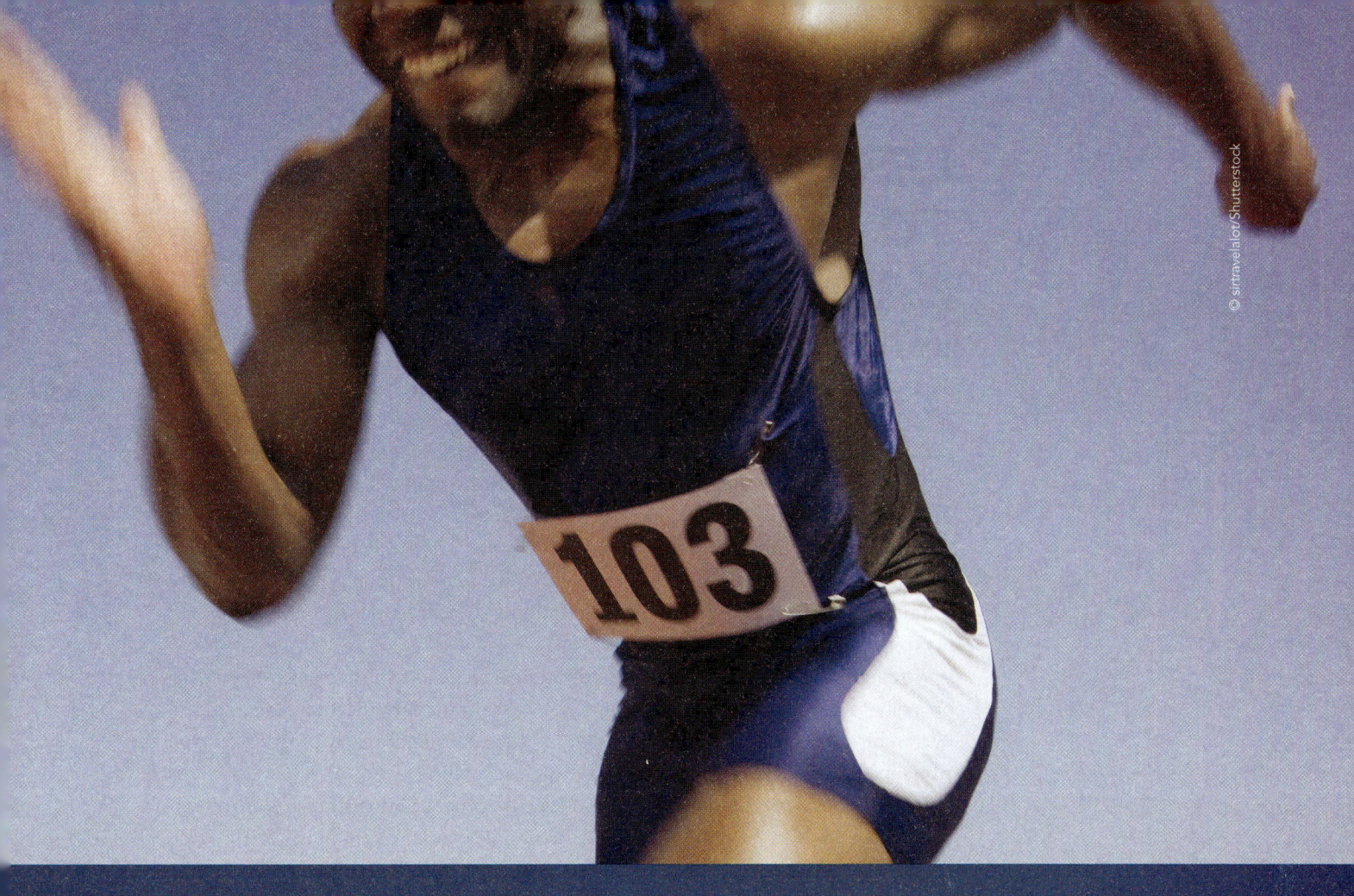

PROGRAMMING FOR SPORTS PERFORMANCE

CHAPTER NINETEEN

LEARNING OBJECTIVES

Upon completion of this chapter, the Sports Performance Coach will be able to:

- **Identify** common acute training variables.

- **Describe** the relationship between training variables and desired adaptations.

- **Determine** appropriate exercise selection for specified training phases.

- **Select** training phases that align with desired outcomes for program design.

- **Describe** the programming process.

LESSON 1: INTRODUCTION TO PROGRAMMING USING NASM'S OPT™ MODEL

INTRODUCTION

Successful athletic performance reaches its culmination when the foundational principles of human movement science are combined with the scientific strategies of periodization. Periodization is a term that is widely applied, yet inconsistent in its definition and application. In this chapter, periodization describes a structured approach to training designed to elicit specific adaptations at specific points in an athlete's training program. The details of periodization were provided in Chapter 18: The Science of Periodization. The Sports Performance Coach must recognize that periodization is the key to structured training that optimizes the timing of each training stressor to manage fatigue and maximize the training effects.

Programming is a vital part of periodization because it defines the microlevel decisions on a day-to-day and session-to-session basis. By contrast, periodization defines the overarching objectives and adaptations, but it is the daily and weekly program to apply the stressors to help the athletes safely achieve each adaptation.

The various periodization models and effective programming strategies are often confusing and overwhelming. NASM's Optimum Performance Training™ (OPT™) Model creates a foundation to advance an athlete's performance. When the Sports Performance Coach uses the OPT Model correctly, they can align periodization models and simplify the programming process. The OPT Model does not inform the Sports Performance Coach exactly how to write each program for all athletes, but instead provides specific parameters and programming guidelines for each day, week, and month (**Figure 19.1**).

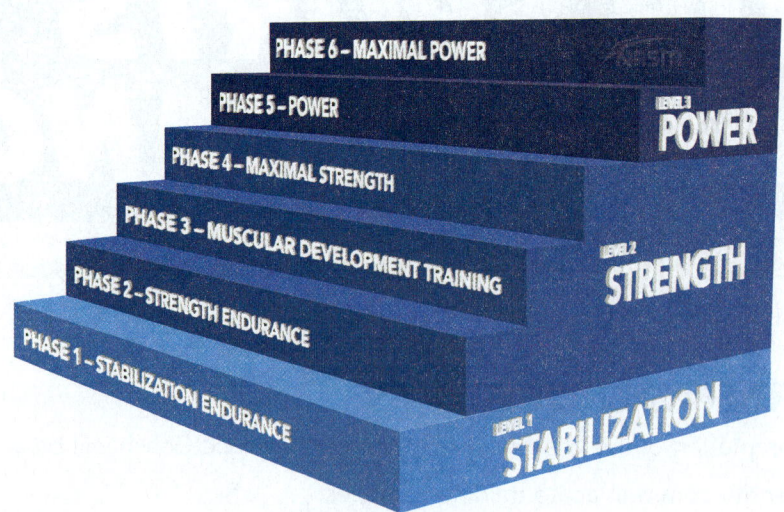

FIGURE 19.1 NASM'S OPT™ Model

NASM'S OPT MODEL

NASM's OPT Model was one of the first models of training to integrate multidisciplinary research from across the globe and to blend performance-enhancement outcomes with an injury-prevention focus. This model aims to improve all components of human movement through a progressive and systematic approach. It has withstood rigorous testing both in the laboratory and with real-life athletes and is an effective evidence-based model (DiStefano et al., 2013). The OPT Model is integrated and includes guidance for flexibility; core; balance; plyometrics; speed, agility, and quickness (SAQ); metabolic; and strength training. Further, the model was predicated on the sequential progressions of standard acute training variables.

PROGRAM DESIGN CONTINUUM

NASM's OPT Model takes the guesswork out of program design and allows for a planned, systematic progression by preassigning specific acute variables for each training phase to elicit the desired adaptation (dos Santos et al., 2017). The acute training variables are the foundation of program design and fall within the **Program Design Continuum** (**Table 19.1**). Program design is a process of decision making based on needs and goals, with each acute training variable being altered individually. To create a workout program, depending on the training phase, the Sports Performance Coach progresses through a series of decisions based on the unique needs of the individual athlete. These decisions include identifying the appropriate volume and intensity of training, selecting the appropriate tempo, setting optimal rest intervals, determining exercise frequency, selecting the best training duration, and identifying the most appropriate exercises.

PROGRAM DESIGN CONTINUUM →

A comprehensive approach to designing a training program, considering various acute training variables that can be adjusted to meet desired training adaptations.

TABLE 19.1 Program Design Continuum

Adaptation	Reps	Sets	Intensity	Rest Period
Power	1–10	3–6	30%–45% of one rep max or ≤ 10% of body weight	3–5 minutes
Strength	1–12	3–6	70%–100%	45 seconds to 5 minutes
Stabilization	12–25	2–3	50%–70%	0 seconds to 1.5 minutes

REPETITIONS + INTENSITY AND THE OPT MODEL

All acute training variables have an interdependent relationship with each other. Repetitions are inversely related to intensity. Training intensity for optimal stress is essential to ensure adaptations occur and to minimize the risk of injury. The Sports Performance Coach will use the inverse relationship when designing strength programs. For example, maximal strength is best achieved with lower repetitions (1 to 5) and higher loads (80% to 100% of a one-repetition maximum [1RM]). In contrast, muscular endurance is achieved with a higher repetition range and lighter loads lifted (Fleck & Kraemer, 2014; Hatfield et al., 2006; Tan, 1999).

Research demonstrates that training in an exact range of repetitions with the recommended intensity yields specific adaptations. The athlete's goals and the precise time of season will help determine the training phase, dictating the precise repetition ranges and intensities (**Table 19.2**) (Baz-Valle et al., 2018).

TABLE 19.2   Repetition and Intensity Continuum

Phase	Repetition Range	Training Intensity
Stabilization/strength endurance	12–25	50%–70%
Muscular development	6–12	75%–85%
Maximal strength	1–5	85%–100%
Power	1–10	30%–45% or ≤ 10% of body weight

✔ **CHECK IT OUT**

Using percentages of 1RM is not the only method of identifying optimal training loads. However, it is commonly used in practice and often the most recommended method. This method requires periodic testing of 1RM to allow for adjustments in relative intensity. The more fit an athlete is, the greater the intensity that will be needed to promote optimal gains in muscular fitness (Peterson et al., 2004; Rhea et al., 2003).

The OPT Model systematically utilizes the repetition and intensity continuum to provide the stimulus for the desired adaptations. The beginning phases involve higher repetition schemes with lower intensities that help build stability, endurance, and connective tissue strength, which is especially important for the beginning athlete. However, a mistake made by many advanced athletes is failing to follow a planned training program that alternates periods of low-repetition training with periods of high-repetition training. Higher training intensities (with fewer repetitions) can be sustained for only a short time without running the risk of overtraining (Häkkinen, 1994; Peterson et al., 2004). The OPT Model guides the Sports Performance Coach and the athlete through a systematic training approach that minimizes the risk of overtraining and maximizes specific results using planned training intervals.

Training in an unstable environment increases the training intensity because it requires more motor unit recruitment (Anderson & Behm, 2005; Behm, 1995; Behm & Anderson, 2006; Kornecki et al., 2001) and more energy expenditure per exercise (Cressey et al., 2007; Ogita et al., 2000; Williford et al., 1998), leading to the development of neuromuscular efficiency. Changing other acute training variables, such as rest periods and tempo, also changes the relative training intensity at a given load and the intensity of the entire workout. Thus, intensity is a function of more than just external resistance. An integrated training program will focus on a holistic approach, leading to continued adaptations.

In the practical setting, the Sports Performance Coach should consider training intensity as a training load based on a percentage of the athlete's specific maximum effort for movement. This requires that an athlete's maximum be tested.

Example of training intensity:

- Athlete training max = 400
- Prescribed workload = 70%
- Actual training load = 400 × 70% = 280
- Prescribed repetitions = 12
- Athlete's training session = 12 reps at 280 lb

VOLUME AND THE OPT MODEL

There is also an inverse relationship between sets, repetitions (training volume), and intensity. The athlete performs fewer sets when executing higher repetitions at a lower intensity (endurance and muscular development adaptations) and more sets when using lower repetitions at a higher intensity (Chandler & Brown, 2019; Ratamess et al., 2009). Essentially, these are strength and power adaptations (Campos et al., 2002; Kraemer et al., 2000; Tan, 1999).

Training volume, generally represented by the number of sets per exercise performed, must be appropriately managed to stimulate specific adaptations and avoid overtraining (**Table 19.3**). The total volume is determined by the combination of the weight lifted, repetitions, and sets. As an athlete becomes more highly trained, more significant amounts of stress are needed to continue to prompt adaptations (Peterson et al., 2004; Rhea et al., 2003). Therefore, long-term athlete development may require gradual progression in daily, weekly, and monthly training volume.

TABLE 19.3 Volume Continuum

Phase	Sets	Repetitions	Training Volume
Stabilization/strength endurance	1–3	12–25	36–75 (repetitions/exercise)
Muscular development	3–4	6–12	27–36 (repetitions/exercise)
Maximal strength	3–6	1–5	18–24 (repetitions/exercise)
Power	3–6	1–10	12–20 (repetitions/exercise)

The Sports Performance Coach must consider total training volume and intensity over a specific period of time (periodization) when designing advanced training programs. However, initially focusing on sets per exercise is an effective approach. Note that the stress accumulated through the training volume is muscle group specific, with those muscles acting as primary movers and synergists encountering the stress applied. Therefore, sets per muscle group is a more appropriate volume designation, as multiple exercises targeting the same muscle groups may be used in a single training session.

The inverse relationship between volume and intensity is one of the most important concepts to remember. When working with loads exceeding 90% of an athlete's maximum, a workout may involve a total volume of 20 repetitions (4 sets of 3 to 5 repetitions) per exercise. However, when working with loads of 60% of maximum, a workout may involve a volume of 36 to 60 repetitions per exercise (3 sets of 12 to 20 repetitions). The exception is the beginner athlete, who may perform only 12 to 25 repetitions per exercise (1 set of each exercise). The readiness of the athlete, training phase, and training goal dictate the optimal number of repetitions, while the number of sets, intensity, rest, tempo, and the combination of these dictate the volume (Campos et al., 2002; Chandler & Brown, 2019; Kraemer et al., 2000; Tan, 1999).

📋 COACH'S CORNER

The Sports Performance Coach should use volume to help monitor the load on an athlete to avoid overtraining, decreased performance, and potential increases in injury. Volume has distinct measurements, repetition volume, and weight volume.

- Repetition volume (total reps): 5 sets of 10 repetitions: $5 \times 10 = 50$ total reps
- Weight volume (total weight): 5 sets of 10 repetitions at 150 pounds per rep: $5 \times 10 \times 150 = 7,500$ lb

The Sports Performance Coach should look at these numbers regularly and determine how to manage one or both of these amounts to help athletes maintain progress with their performance.

REPETITION TEMPO AND THE OPT MODEL

REPETITION TEMPO →

The speed at which each repetition is performed.

Repetition tempo is important for achieving specific training objectives such as endurance, hypertrophy, strength, and power (Chandler & Brown, 2019; Fleck & Kraemer, 2014; Ratamess et al., 2009; Tan, 1999). Repetition tempo, like other acute training variables, is interrelated with intensity. For adaptations of stabilization and endurance (using lower intensities and higher rep ranges), the total tempo can be slower. However, for adaptations of muscular development, strength, and power (using progressively higher training intensities), the repetition tempo must increase (**Table 19.4**).

TABLE 19.4 Tempo Continuum (Eccentric/Isometric/Concentric/Isometric)

Phase	Tempo
Stabilization/strength endurance	Slow (4/2/1/1)
Muscular development	Moderate (2/0/2/0)
Maximal strength	Moderate (2/0/2/0)
Power	Fast/explosive

The tempo also determines the time under tension, referring to the duration for which a muscle is under load during a set. A longer time under tension, often resulting from slower tempos, stimulates muscle growth and endurance, whereas a shorter time using faster tempos can enhance power and speed. Additionally, slower tempos can improve neuromuscular coordination and proprioception, aiding the development of better movement mechanics and stability.

REST INTERVALS AND THE OPT MODEL

Rest intervals are vital because they allow the body to replenish its primary energy reserves. The primary energy used during training depends on the training phase, exercise intensity, and goal. Therefore, the ability to replenish adenosine triphosphate (ATP) and creatine phosphate (CP) rapidly is crucial. The length of the rest periods is contingent on the current training phase, the exercise intensity, and the overarching training objectives. Factors such as the speed of ATP/CP recovery, the intensity and volume of the training, and the specific athletic goals dictate the duration of these intervals. For instance, shorter rest periods may limit the athlete's ability to maintain a high intensity throughout multiple sets due to incomplete recovery. Conversely, longer rest intervals promote a more thorough recovery, facilitating sustained high-intensity performance, which is critical for strength and power development.

Furthermore, rest interval length should align with specific training goals: shorter intervals for enhancing muscular endurance or aerobic capacity, and longer intervals for strength, power, or hypertrophy objectives (**Table 19.5**). Longer intervals also aid in more effective lactate clearance, facilitating recovery and reducing muscle fatigue. Therefore, strategically adjusting rest intervals in a training program, while carefully considering the training phase, exercise intensity, and overall goals, is crucial for maximizing sports performance.

> **REST INTERVAL →**
>
> The time taken to recuperate between sets, exercises, or both.

TABLE 19.5 Rest Interval Continuum

Phase	Rest Interval
Stabilization/strength endurance	0–90 seconds
Muscular development	0–180 seconds
Maximal strength	3–5 minutes
Power	3–5 minutes

TRAINING FREQUENCY AND THE OPT MODEL

The optimal number of training sessions per week or month is determined by many factors, such as goals, health, work capacity, nutrition, overall recoverability, and other factors. In addition, the Sports Performance Coach must consider outside factors such as additional practice, skill development, and other activities when designing a training program. For example, a Sports Performance Coach could program five to seven training sessions per week if the sessions alter the stress placed on the body to avoid targeting the same muscle groups more than two to three times per week. **Table 19.6** lists the

TABLE 19.6 Training Frequency Recommendations

Phase	Recommended Sessions per Week
Overall performance improvement	5–7 variable sessions, including additional practice and skill development
Strength/power development	2–4 sessions
Maintenance	1–2 sessions

recommended sessions per week based on intended outcomes. This schedule should include other activities. Training status appears to influence tolerance of higher-frequency training (Peterson et al., 2004; Rhea et al., 2003) but is highly affected by training volume and intensity. More advanced athletes may perform higher-volume and more-intense efforts in each workout than less advanced athletes. However, they will require more extended recovery periods between workouts, resulting in lower frequency.

TRAINING DURATION AND THE OPT MODEL

Training duration has two essential connotations: One refers to the span of a single workout, from its commencement to completion; the other relates to the period, typically measured in weeks, spent in a specific training phase or period. The length of a training phase hinges on an athlete's physical ability level, targeted goal, and adherence to the program. Such a phase commonly lasts approximately 4 weeks, reflecting the average time required for the body to adapt to a new training stimulus. However, some training phases could be shorter or longer depending on various factors. It is generally understood that most adaptations to a new stimulus occur within 4 weeks. The training stimulus then needs to be increased to stimulate further adaptations after this period (Bompa & Calcina, 1993). The importance of training duration is accentuated in team settings and within the framework of sports governing bodies' rules and regulations, underlining the need to account for uncontrollable factors, such as imposed daily and weekly time limitations on athletes.

EXERCISE SELECTION AND THE OPT MODEL

For several reasons, exercise selection is crucial in designing a training program for athletic development. First, specificity is paramount; the selected exercises should closely mirror the unique demands and movements intrinsic to the athlete's sport, enabling the training to enhance performance and decrease injury risk. Second, individual needs and attributes must be considered, as every athlete presents distinct physical abilities and constraints. Consequently, the exercises in the program should be challenging, yet enable the athlete to perform them effectively and safely. Third, exercise selection must facilitate advances through progressive overload, which involves gradually increasing exercise intensity over time, which is crucial for sustained improvement and physiological adaptation. Lastly, a well-rounded selection of exercises is essential for balanced muscular development. This prevents potential muscle imbalances that can contribute to injuries. For example, equal emphasis should be placed on exercises that work for both the anterior and posterior muscle groups.

The OPT Model is a comprehensive framework that categorizes exercises directed at all components of athletic training: flexibility, core, balance, plyometrics, SAQ, and resistance training. These exercises are segmented based on the training phase and the primary adaptation they aim to achieve.

For instance, exercises utilized in Phase 1 of the OPT Model, which targets stabilization endurance, are termed "stabilization-focused exercises." They aim to progress muscular endurance and stability. Exercises used in Phases 2 to 4, which aim to enhance strength, are referred to as "strength-focused exercises." Those employed in Phases 5 and 6, which concentrate on power, are called "power-focused exercises." Through a comprehensive assessment and a review of specific training goals, the OPT Model equips the Sports Performance Coach to select suitable exercises for each athlete, integrating them into a well-planned training program (**Table 19.7**).

TABLE 19.7 Exercise Selection Examples

Goal	Total Body	Multiple-Joint	Single Joint
Stabilization-focused	Step-up balance to overhead press	Single-leg tubing chest press Single-leg cable row Single-leg dumbbell shoulder press	Single-leg dumbbell curl
Strength-focused	Squat curl to overhead press	Bench press Seated row machine Shoulder press machine squat	Standing barbell curl
Power-focused	Power clean	Two-arm medicine ball chest pass Medicine ball pullover throw Medicine ball oblique throw	Not applicable

Traditional exercises are adapted to less stable environments, such as standing positions (two-leg, staggered-stance, single-leg) or unstable surfaces (e.g., Airex pad, stability ball, BOSU ball) to optimize stability. Research supports that exercises in unstable environments yield superior results for stabilizing and training the core muscles (Clark et al., 2018; Olivia-Lozano & Muyor, 2020). Examples include the kneeling kettlebell bottoms-up press, single-leg kettlebell deadlift, and supine ball dumbbell triceps extensions.

Strength can be developed through any resistance exercise, provided the load is adequate to improve force development. Total-body and multiple-joint exercises are particularly effective for developing strength and muscle coordination (Azegami et al., 2007), as they increase neural demands by requiring several muscle groups to coordinate in timing and force of contraction. Given the complexity of most athletic skills, total-body exercises such as the barbell deadlift; shrug to calf raise; and squat, curl to two-arm press can enhance the transference of training from exercise to sport.

For optimal power development, plyometrics and explosive medicine ball exercises can be performed during functional movement patterns (Yanghattee & Srihirun, 2021). Examples of power exercises include the squat jump, medicine ball pullover throw, and barbell push press.

LESSON 2: PRINCIPLES AND APPLICATIONS OF NASM'S OPT™ MODEL
PROGRAMMING WITH NASM'S OPT MODEL

The OPT Model simplifies the development of biomotor abilities into three distinct yet interdependent levels (stabilization, strength, and power) and six phases (stabilization endurance, strength endurance, muscular development, maximal strength, power, and maximal power) (**Figure 19.2**). A sequential approach to training helps the Sports Performance Coach focus on specific adaptations needed for sports performance enhancement while ensuring the athlete stays within recommended intensities and training volumes to avoid overtraining and injury. The model has been designed to accommodate many periodization methods and follows established principles of human movement science. Beginning with developing joint stabilization and muscular endurance, it progresses to strength development and power production, and ultimately to promoting the skills necessary for the athlete to express this strength and power during sports. The OPT Model encourages all athletes to develop a solid foundation on which higher performance levels can be built. The model is progressive and flexible enough to accommodate any athlete at any level of performance. The OPT Model does not precisely tell the Sports Performance coach what to do, but rather provides specific parameters and guidelines to help simplify the programming process.

✔ CHECK IT OUT

In many cases, movement impairments and muscle imbalances are expected when athletes train and compete at high levels. Therefore, it is vital to discuss corrective exercise (CEx). CEx can be considered an "active recovery phase" using traditional periodization; it is used to improve faulty movement patterns by addressing muscle imbalances, joint dysfunction, neuromuscular deficits, and postural malalignment. In many cases, athletes may benefit from a few or even several weeks in a CEx training phase before beginning Phase 1 of the OPT Model. If this is unfeasible due to time constraints, CEx programming may be done concurrently or integrated within other training phases.

CEx uses a four-step process:

1. Inhibit overactive muscles using self-myofascial techniques or manual therapy.
2. Lengthen short muscles using static, neuromuscular, or assisted-stretching techniques.
3. Activate underactive muscles using isolated strengthening.
4. Integrate the neuromuscular system with specific, total-body movement patterns.

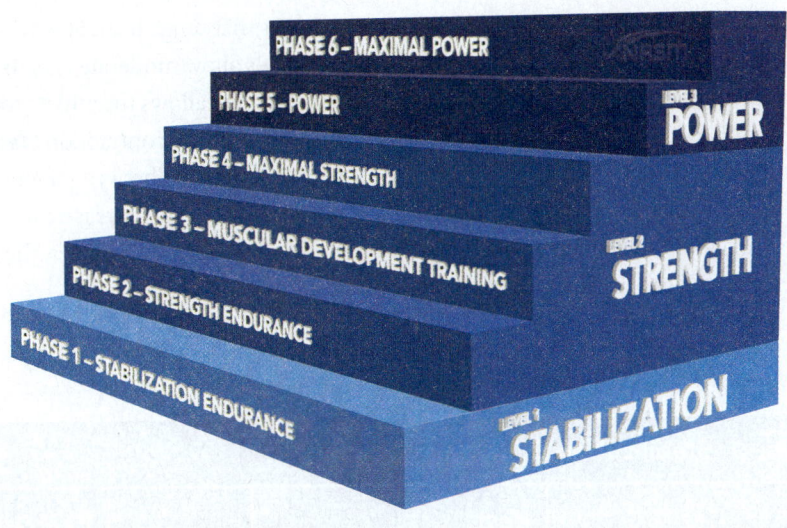

FIGURE 19.2 NASM's OPT™ Model

STABILIZATION (ACTIVE RECOVERY PHASE/GENERAL PREPARATORY PHASE)

The stabilization level consists of one phase, stabilization endurance training, and is the first phase in the OPT Model. Phase 1 lays the foundation by improving muscular endurance, joint stabilization, and neuromuscular coordination, which are required to further develop strength, power, and speed in later training phases.

PHASE 1: STABILIZATION ENDURANCE

Stabilization endurance training creates foundational levels of stabilization strength, postural control, and muscular endurance to prepare the body for the more demanding phases. This focus develops the biomotor abilities of muscle and aerobic endurance. Stabilization endurance training can also be used between periods of higher-intensity training, as seen in Phases 2 through 6, to allow for proper recovery and to maintain optimal levels of stabilization, control, and endurance throughout the training period.

The primary focus when progressing in Phase 1 is on increasing the proprioceptive demand of the exercises rather than just load or volume. Thus, Phase 1 focuses on the following aspects of performance:

- Increasing stability
- Improving muscular endurance
- Increasing neuromuscular efficiency
- Improving intermuscular and intramuscular coordination

When considering general periodization principles, the stabilization level of the OPT Model is closely aligned with active recovery (post-season) and leading up to the general preparatory phase (off-season). In active recovery, Phase 1 integrates flexibility methods focused on improving muscle imbalances and reestablishing optimal movement patterns. These include, but are not limited to, self-myofascial rolling and static and assisted stretching. Furthermore, given the lower relative intensity of exercises, Phase 1 is suited for post-season recovery training and can be progressed into the general preparatory phase. Further, Phase 1 can be utilized throughout the competition phase to maintain specific performance attributes.

The resistance training section of Phase 1 uses intensities that range from 50% to 70% of the athlete's estimated 1RM. The lower to moderate intensities allow moderate (12) to high (20) repetitions to be performed. Further, the intensity of Phase 1 allows the athlete to perform the exercise with a slower tempo (4/2/1/1), emphasizing the eccentric contraction (**Table 19.8**). The Sports Performance Coach must consider the inverse relationship between intensity and repetitions when progressing the athlete during this phase. As intensity increases, sets should decrease. While these are presented as a linear progression in the following tables, the Sports Performance Coach can utilize undulating periodization as desired.

TABLE 19.8 Stabilization Endurance Acute Training Variables

Phase 1: Stabilization Endurance Training								
	Reps	Sets	Tempo	% Intensity	Rest Interval	Frequency	Duration	Exercise Selection
Flexibility	1	1–3	30–seconds hold	N/A	N/A	3–7 times/ week	4–6 weeks	SMT and static
Core	12–20	1–4	Slow 4/2/1	N/A	0–90 seconds	2–4 times/ week	4–6 weeks	1–4 stabilization level
Balance	12–20 6–10(SL)*	1–3	Slow 4/2/1	N/A	0–90 seconds	2–4 times/ week	4–6 weeks	1–4 stabilization level
Plyometric*	5–8	1–3	3–5 seconds hold on landing	N/A	0–90 seconds	2–4 times/ week	4–6 weeks	0–2 stabilization level
SAQ	15–20 yards	3–4 2–4	Controlled	N/A	1:3** 1:5**	2–4 times/ week	4–6 weeks	3–4 technique drills 3–5 speed of movement drills (linear/ multidirectional speed)
Resistance training	12–20	1–3	4/2/1	50–70%	0–90 seconds	2–4 times/ week	4–6 weeks	1–2 stabilization progressions per body part

Abbreviations: N/A = not applicable; SL = single-leg (6–10) on each leg; SMT = self-myofascial technique.

*If an athlete does not have ample amounts of core stability and balance, plyometric exercises may not be included in the phase of training until these components are developed.

**1:3 = 3 minutes of rest for 1 minute of work, 1:5 = 5 minutes of rest for 1 minute of work.

Beginning or deconditioned athletes with no significant muscle imbalances can begin Phase 1 by performing a single set with fewer repetitions. Weekly progressions can include increasing both sets and repetitions. The intensity (% of 1RM) will remain low to allow the athlete to focus on stability, coordination, and control. A primary goal for such an athlete is to learn to execute the fundamental movements correctly and successfully progress to the other training phases. The Sports Performance Coach should design the program to continually challenge proprioception for optimal neuromuscular efficiency. A well-designed program will have an athlete in this training phase until the appropriate adaptations are met in preparation for the demands of Phase 2, strength endurance training. This phase or cycle of training usually lasts between 3 and 6 weeks.

Experienced or conditioned athletes with no significant muscle imbalances can begin Phase 1 by performing a single set with more repetitions. Their higher level of conditioning should allow the athlete to perform more repetitions while maintaining optimal form and control. Weekly progressions can follow a more traditional approach of increasing sets and intensity while decreasing repetitions (**Table 19.9**) to establish the necessary levels of muscular endurance and strength in the stabilizing muscles.

TABLE 19.9 Stabilization Endurance Example Progressions

		Weekly Progression			
		Week 1	Week 2	Week 3	Week 4
Core	Sets	1	2	3	3
	Reps	20	20	15	15
Balance	Sets	1	2	3	3
	Reps	20	20	15	15
Plyometric	Sets	1	2	3	3
	Reps	6	6	6	8
SAQ	Sets	3/3	3/3	4/3	4/4
	Reps	15 yards	20 yards	20 yards	20 yards
Resistance training	Sets	1–2	2	3	3
	Reps	20	15	15	12
	Intensity	60%	65%	65%	70%

⚠ **CRITICAL**

One of the most common errors in programming for Phase 1 is not utilizing the correct intensity for a given number of repetitions. For example, if an athlete is performing 3 sets at 70% estimated 1RM for 12 reps, they should hit a state of fatigue or near-failure at 12 repetitions. Often, an athlete stops at the prescribed number of reps but still has a few left "in the tank." In this case, what was thought to be the optimal intensity for the given exercise was too low, and the desired adaptation will not be achieved.

STRENGTH (GENERAL PREPARATORY PHASE/SPECIFIC PREPARATORY PHASE)

The second level of training in the OPT Model focuses on the primary adaptation of strength, which includes strength endurance, muscular development, and maximal strength. It is designed to maintain stability while increasing the stress placed on the body so as to increase muscle size and strength.

This training period is necessary to develop muscle size, strength, and overall general performance. Enhancing muscular strength is a vital attribute for all athletes because of its underlying influence on performance skills such as jumping, sprinting, and change of direction (Suchomel et al., 2016). It has been proposed that additional performance benefits are apparent for athletes back-squatting up to twice their body weight. Conversely, a strength deficit would be defined by a relative back squat strength of less than 0.5 times body weight and emphasizes motor learning and initial skill acquisition. Translation into performance improvements comes with the association phase of 0.5 to 2.0 times body weight, with additional yet diminishing benefits occurring in the strength reserve phase. It is important to note this theoretical model was developed specific to the back squat and may be adjusted based on sport-specific requirements (**Figure 19.3**).

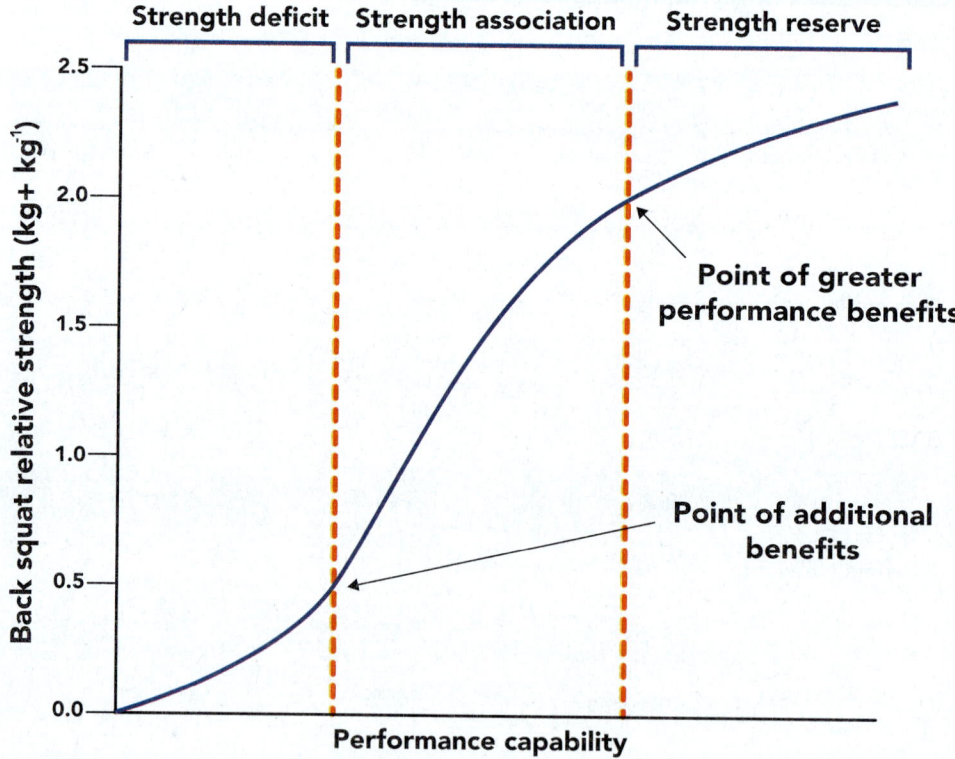

FIGURE 19.3 Back Squat Relative Strength Versus Performance Capability

Data from Suchomel, T. J., Nimphius, S., & Stone, M. H. (2016). The importance of muscular strength in athletic performance. *Sports Medicine, 46*(10), 1419-1449.

Strength training increases the following attributes of the athlete:

- The ability of the core musculature to stabilize the pelvis and spine under heavier loads through more complete ranges of motion
- The load-bearing capabilities of muscles, tendons, ligaments, and joints
- The volume of training with more reps, sets, and intensity

- Metabolic demand by taxing the ATP/CP and glycolytic energy systems to induce cellular changes in muscle (weight loss, hypertrophy, or both)
- Motor unit recruitment, frequency of motor unit recruitment, and motor unit synchronization (maximal strength)

The strength level of the OPT Model focuses on progressive strength development and consists of three phases: strength endurance (Phase 2), muscular development (Phase 3), and maximal strength (Phase 4). When compared to traditional principles of periodization, the strength level of the OPT Model most closely aligns with the general preparatory phase and progresses into the specific preparatory phase. Phases 3 and 4 are generally suited for the specific preparatory phase in an annual plan (pre-season) to enhance an athlete's strength before moving into a competition phase. As athletes transition from stabilization into strength, flexibility techniques can become more active than static. However, if an athlete is still dealing with muscle imbalances, some static techniques can continue to be included. The Sports Performance Coach should plan to include whatever static stretching is needed directly after self-myofascial rolling and then have the athlete perform a few active or even dynamic stretches before engaging in the higher-intensity lifts.

PHASE 2: STRENGTH ENDURANCE

Strength endurance training further enhances the biomotor ability of muscular endurance by using the complex training methodology of supersets performed with contrasting loads and repetitions during resistance training programming. In this phase, the athlete performs a traditional strength exercise, such as a bench press (**Figure 19.4**), at a moderate intensity, followed by an exercise that utilizes the same prime mover(s) and has similar joint dynamics but requires greater stabilization to execute, such as a stability ball push-up (**Figure 19.5**). The biomechanically similar exercises, when performed back-to-back, stimulate the adaptations of strength and muscular endurance. However, hypertrophy can also be experienced due to the higher training volumes.

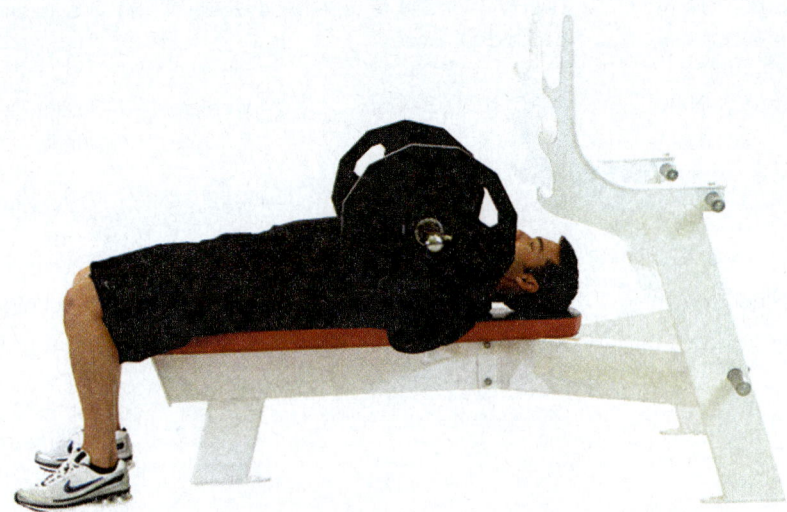

FIGURE 19.4 Bench Press

The two exercises in the superset have different acute training variables that align with the different intensities. The first exercise, performed at 70% to 80%, will utilize repetitions that align with strength development (8 to 12 reps) and a faster tempo

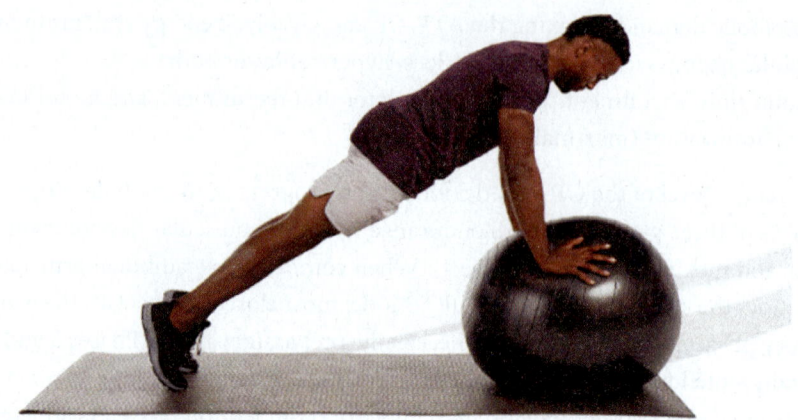

FIGURE 19.5 Stability Ball Push-up

(2/0/2/0). The Sports Performance Coach can vary the tempo if desired, but it is important to recognize that as the load increases, the tempo generally increases. The second exercise in the superset closely follows the acute training variables of Phase 1, including the lower intensity (50% to 70%) and slower tempo (4/2/1/1) (**Table 19.10**).

TABLE 19.10   Strength Endurance Acute Training Variables

Phase 2: Strength Endurance Training								
	Reps	Sets	Tempo	% Intensity	Rest Interval	Frequency	Duration	Exercise Selection
Flexibility	5–10	1–2	1–2 seconds hold	N/A	N/A	3–7 times/ week	4 weeks	SMT and dynamic (optional)
Core	8–12	2–3	Moderate	N/A	0–90 seconds	2–4 times/ week	4 weeks	1–3 core strength
Balance	8–12	2–3	Moderate	N/A	0–90 seconds	2–4 times/ week	4 weeks	1–3 balance strength
Plyometric	8–10	2–3	Repeating	N/A	0–60 seconds	2–4 times/ week	4 weeks	1–3 plyometric strength
SAQ	15–20 yards	3–4 2–4	Controlled	N/A	1:3 1:5	2–4 times/ week	4 weeks	2–3 technique drills 5–7 speed of movement drills (linear/ multidirectional speed)
Resistance training	8–12	2–4	2/0/2/0	70–80%	0–60 seconds	2–4 times/ week	4 weeks	1 strength
	8–12		4/2/1/1	50–70%				1 stabilization

Abbreviations: N/A = not applicable; SMT = self-myofascial technique.

However, repetitions differ because the total between the two exercises should equal approximately 20. Therefore, if an athlete performs a strength exercise for 12 reps at 70%, the stabilization exercise should be performed at the higher end of the stabilization intensity range (approximately 70%) for 8 reps, thus totaling 20 repetitions. At the other end of the spectrum, if the strength exercise is performed for 8 reps at 80%, then the stabilization should be performed at the lower end of the stabilization range (approximately 50%) for 12 reps. Again, there is a total of 20 repetitions to achieve the adaptation of muscular endurance. The combined number of reps will be essential to remember as the phase progresses over the desired weeks.

Beginning athletes will progress to Phase 2 after completing Phase 1 of the OPT Model. While muscular development could be obtained in Phase 2, this is not a primary goal. For this reason, sets, repetition, and intensity ranges will remain moderate. Weekly progressions can follow a traditional approach of increasing sets and intensity while decreasing repetitions (**Table 19.11**). An athlete can stay in Phase 2 for 3 to 6 weeks, depending on their goals and the time available for training.

TABLE 19.11   Strength Endurance Example Progressions

Weekly Progression					
		Week 1	**Week 2**	**Week 3**	**Week 4**
Core	Sets	2	2	3	3
	Reps	12	12	10	8
Balance	Sets	2	2	3	3
	Reps	12	12	10	8
Plyometric	Sets	2	3	3	3
	Reps	8	8	10	10
SAQ	Sets	3/3	3/3	4/3	4/4
	Reps	15 yards	20 yards	20 yards	20 yards
Resistance training	Sets	2	3	3	4
	Reps	12 strength 8 stabilization	10 strength 10 stabilization	8 strength 12 stabilization	8 strength 12 stabilization
	Intensity	70% strength 70% stabilization	75% strength 65% stabilization	80% strength 60% stabilization	80% strength 55% stabilization

More advanced and well-conditioned athletes with no significant muscle imbalances can potentially bypass Phase 1 and begin in Phase 2. The goals of joint stabilization and muscular endurance overlap between the two phases. Thus, an athlete will still obtain increased stabilization and endurance in Phase 2. However, Phase 1 should be used for the advanced athlete as a form of active recovery between more intense training sessions. Further, the Sports Performance Coach can adjust supersets for the advanced athlete. Given the wide variety of demands included in sports, programming a stabilization exercise prior to a strength exercise could lead to a desirable transfer effect in some cases.

✔ CHECK IT OUT

Supersets are crucial to Phase 2 of the OPT Model, bridging the gap between the stabilization and strength levels for a smooth transition. They involve pairing a traditional strength exercise with a stabilization exercise, balancing the increase in prime mover strength with a challenge to the stabilization system. This approach aligns with the "drop set" principle, where a high-intensity exercise, recruiting more type II motor units, is followed by a lower-intensity one, engaging type I motor units. This pattern ensures that the athlete maintains joint stabilization and muscular endurance even when prime movers are fatigued. Once foundational levels of joint stabilization and muscular endurance are achieved, the sequence can be altered with a stabilization exercise preceding a strength one. This way, the stabilization system is "primed" before the load increases, facilitating the efficient recruitment of motor units. Coaches can start with traditional Phase 1, then transition into Phase 1, followed by a Phase 2 superset for 2 weeks, and finally move to Phase 2, followed by a Phase 1 superset for the remaining time in Phase 2.

Week 1	Week 2	Week 3	Week 4	Week 5	Week 6	Week 7	Week 8
Stabilization	Stabilization	Stabilization	Strength + stabilization	Strength + stabilization	Strength + stabilization	Strength + stabilization	Strength + stabilization

---

PHASE 3: MUSCULAR DEVELOPMENT

Muscular development training focuses on the adaptation of maximal muscle growth (i.e., hypertrophy). Phase 3 introduces higher levels of volume with minimal rest periods to force cellular changes that result in an overall increase in muscle size. However, flexibility, core, balance, plyometric, and SAQ training remain relatively consistent with Phase 2.

Phase 3 is appropriate for those athletes seeking to improve body composition or requiring increased muscle mass. In terms of biomotor ability development, increasing the cross-sectional area of a muscle (hypertrophy) enhances its ability to produce higher levels of force. Therefore, Phase 3 is advantageous to developing fundamental strength and further establishes the foundation for optimal power production. However, this phase is considered optional for the athlete restricted by a weight class who does not desire an increase in muscle mass. As mentioned, hypertrophy can be experienced in Phase 2; thus, some athletes can progress from Phase 2 to Phase 4 or 5.

Although its content varies, Phase 3 generally includes traditional strength exercises, such as bench presses, squats, deadlifts, and barbell rows. Muscular development requires moderate to higher intensities (75% to 85%), performed for a moderate repetition range (6 to 12), and at a consistent tempo (2/0/2/0) (**Table 19.12**). The Sports Performance

TABLE 19.12 Muscular Development Acute Training Variables

	Reps	Sets	Tempo	% Intensity	Rest Interval	Frequency	Duration	Exercise Selection
Flexibility	5–10	1–2	1–2 seconds hold	N/A	N/A	3–7 times/ week	4 weeks	SMT and dynamic* (optional)
Core*	8–12	2–3	Moderate	N/A	0–60 seconds	3–6 times/ week	4 weeks	0–4 core strength
Balance*	8–12	2–3	Moderate	N/A	0–60 seconds	3–6 times/ week	4 weeks	0–4 balance strength
Plyometric*	8–10	2–3	Repeating	N/A	0–60 seconds	3–6 times/ week	4 weeks	0–4 plyometric strength
SAQ*	15–20 yards	3–4 2–4	Controlled	N/A	1:3 1:5	2–4 times/ week	4 weeks	2–3 technique drills 5–7 speed of movement drills (linear/ multidirectional speed)
Resistance training	6–12	3–5	2/0/2/0	75–85%	0–180 seconds	3–6 times/ week	4 weeks	2–4 strength level exercises per body part
Comments:	Total of 24–36 sets per workout Light day = 20–24 total sets Moderate day = 24–30 total sets Heavy day = 30–36 total sets							

Abbreviations: N/A = not applicable; SMT = self-myofascial technique.

*Because of the goal, core, balance, plyometric, and SAQ training may be optional in this phase of training (although recommended). Such training can also be performed on nonresistance training days.

Coach should know that muscular development is directly related to training volume. In a meta-analysis that included both untrained and trained participants, higher weekly training volumes resulted in more significant muscle hypertrophy, with each additional set equating to a 0.36% increase in hypertrophy (Schoenfeld et al., 2017). Trained athletes generally need higher volumes to induce muscular development than untrained athletes. Rest intervals for muscular development remain a point of controversy (see the Getting Technical feature). However, the Sports Performance Coach can alternate rest intervals (between 1 and 3 minutes) with intensities to obtain the best results.

Progressions generally follow a linear periodization model with increasing intensity and decreasing repetitions (**Table 19.13**).

TABLE 19.13 Muscular Development Example Progressions

Weekly Progression					
		Week 1	Week 2	Week 3	Week 4
Core	Sets	2	2	3	3
	Reps	12	12	10	8
Balance	Sets	2	2	3	3
	Reps	12	12	10	8
Plyometric	Sets	2	3	3	3
	Reps	8	8	10	10
SAQ	Sets	3/3	3/3	4/3	4/4
	Reps	15 yards	20 yards	20 yards	20 yards
Resistance training	Sets	3	3	4	5
	Reps	12	10	8	6
	Intensity	75%	80%	80%	85%
	Rest interval	1 minute	1.5 minutes	2 minutes	2.5–3 minutes

🤖 GETTING TECHNICAL

Some controversy exists regarding the optimal rest interval for muscular development training. Rahimi et al. (2010) found that shorter rest periods during traditional strength exercises (bench press and squat, performed at 85%) resulted in greater anabolic hormone concentration. This supports the findings of de Salles et al. (2009), who pointed out that shorter rest periods (less than 60 seconds) might be preferred when using moderate intensities during hypertrophy training because of the increase in growth hormone associated with this type of training. Increases in such anabolic hormones support enhanced muscular development post-training.

However, total training volume decreases at moderate to higher intensities (75% to 85%) as rest periods decrease (Hernandez et al., 2021; Ratamess et al., 2009). In support of these findings, Longo et al. (2022) and Schoenfeld et al. (2016) found moderate- to higher-intensity resistance training exercises produced greater hypertrophy in some muscle groups when utilizing a 3-minute rest interval compared to a 1-minute rest interval.

PHASE 4: MAXIMAL STRENGTH

Maximal strength training focuses on increasing the load placed on the tissues for the adaptation of strength. Phase 4 is the last phase in the strength level and uses near-maximal strength to enhance the biomotor ability of strength through improvements in the following attributes:

- Motor unit recruitment
- Motor unit synchronization
- Rate of force production

Strength is the amount of force a muscle or muscle group can produce. Force equals mass multiplied by acceleration, so force production can be increased by increasing the mass (i.e., load/intensity) and the acceleration (i.e., speed of the contraction). However, the demonstration of strength by an athlete can vary depending on the speed of the contraction. Improving recruitment and synchronization of motor units work synergistically to improve the rate of force production, which is optimized in the power level of training.

Phase 4 uses traditional, more compound/multiple-joint strength training movements. However, the specific needs of certain athletes may dictate the use of less-traditional variations. These exercises are performed at near maximal intensities (85% to 100%), for fewer repetitions (1 to 5), and with more sets (4 to 6) (**Table 19.14**). Given the higher training intensity, a longer rest interval (3 to 5 minutes) is required for the optimal regeneration of ATP between sets. Rest interval is a vital component of this phase and is often overlooked. Due to the low repetitions, a Sports Performance Coach may believe an athlete is fully prepared for a subsequent set before the rest interval expires. However, shortening the rest interval can lead to early fatigue, such that the athletes do not reach the desired total training volume for strength adaptations (Hernandez et al., 2021; Ratamess et al., 2009).

Further, the repetition tempo must be examined. The athlete must try to move the load quickly and safely. However, given the relative weight of the load (i.e., 100% of 1RM), the athlete generally does not move the load very fast. Thus, the athlete attempts to move explosively, but the weight itself moves slowly. For example, consider a defensive lineman who is attempting a bench press at two different percentages, 65% and 90% of 500 pounds. At 65%, the player can lift 325 pounds, and at 90%, he can lift 450 pounds. The force–velocity curve indicates that the heavier the weight, the more slowly that weight moves in an upward direction (Harris et al., 2000). Therefore, if this football player lifts closer to his 1RM (450 pounds), the weight will move more slowly. Also, more type II motor units

TABLE 19.14 Maximal Strength Acute Training Variables

	Reps	Sets	Tempo	% Intensity	Rest Interval	Frequency	Duration	Exercise Selection
Flexibility	5–10	1–2	1–2 seconds hold	N/A	N/A	3–7 times/ week	4 weeks	SMT and dynamic* (optional)
Core*	8–12	2–3	Moderate	N/A	0–60 seconds	2–4 times/ week	4 weeks	0–3 core strength
Balance*	8–12	2–3	Moderate	N/A	0–60 seconds	2–4 times/ week	4 weeks	0–3 balance strength
Plyometric*	8–10	2–3	Repeating	N/A	0–60 seconds	2–4 times/ week	4 weeks	0–3 plyometric strength
SAQ*	15–20 yards	3–4 2–4	Fast	N/A	1:3 1:5	2–4 times/ week	4 weeks	2–3 technique drills 5–7 speed of movement drills (linear/ multidirectional speed)
Resistance training	1–5	4–6	As fast as can be controlled	85%–100%	3–5 minutes	2–4 times/ week	4 weeks	1–3 strength-level exercises per body part

Abbreviations: N/A = not applicable; SMT = self-myofascial technique.

*Because of the goal, core, balance, plyometric, and SAQ training may be optional in this phase of training (although recommended). This training can also be performed on nonresistance training days.

will be called upon during the lift to help overcome the load (Grgic & Schoenfeld, 2018; Morton et al., 2019).

As in Phase 3, flexibility, core, balance, plyometric, and SAQ training do not change in Phase 4. Further, due to the types of lifts used in Phase 4 (e.g., squats, deadlifts, bench press), core, balance, plyometric, and SAQ training are optional, though recommended for certain athletes. A Sports Performance Coach should also recognize that training with maximal intensity is demanding for all muscle groups. Thus, an athlete should not fatigue any specific region, specifically the core musculature, before performing maximal-intensity lifts. In these cases, the Sports Performance Coach may program core and balance training at the end of the program rather than at the beginning or include these other training components on nonresistance training days.

Phase 4 is required for most athletes because an improvement in maximal strength is usually beneficial in sports. Weekly progressions can follow a traditional approach of increasing training intensity and minimal increases in overall volume (**Table 19.15**). The length of time spent in Phase 4 will vary between athletes, with the average time being 4 to 6 weeks. Once Phase 4 is completed, the athlete can cycle back through Phases 1, 2, and 3 if needed and time permits, or move on to the power level.

TABLE 19.15 Maximal Strength Example Progressions

		Weekly Progression			
		Week 1	Week 2	Week 3	Week 4
Core	Sets	2	2	3	3
	Reps	12	12	10	8
Balance	Sets	2	2	3	3
	Reps	12	12	10	8
Plyometric	Sets	3	2	3	3
	Reps	8	8	10	10
SAQ	Sets	3/3	3/3	4/3	4/4
	Reps	15 yards	20 yards	20 yards	20 yards
Resistance training	Sets	4	5	5	6
	Reps	5	5	4	3
	Intensity	85%	85%	89%	93%
	Rest interval	3 minutes	3 minutes	3.5 minutes	4 minutes

POWER (SPECIFIC PREPARATORY PHASE/COMPETITION PHASE)

The power level is designed to increase the rate of force production (or speed of muscle contraction). This form of training uses the strength and stabilization adaptations acquired in the previous training phases, but applies them with more realistic speeds and forces that the body will encounter in sports.

Power is calculated as force multiplied by velocity ($P = F \times V$). Therefore, any increase in either force, velocity, or both will produce an increase in power. In training, this is accomplished by increasing the load (i.e., force) or speed (i.e., velocity). The combined effect is a better rate of force production during athletic activities.

Athletes must train with heavy loads (85% to 100%) at low speeds and light loads (30% to 45%) at high speeds to maximize power development. The focus of power training is to enhance the following attributes:

- Motor unit recruitment
- Motor unit synchronization
- Speed of motor unit activation (Matavuli et al., 2001; Saunders et al., 2006)

The power level of training in the OPT Model consists of two phases of training: power training (Phase 5) and maximal power training (Phase 6). Phase 5 generally aligns with the end of the specific preparatory phase, whereas Phase 6 is best aligned with the competition phase.

PHASE 5: POWER

Phase 5, like Phase 2, uses the complex training methodology of supersets performed with contrasting loads in resistance training programming. This phase serves as a bridge for the transition of basic strength to power and speed. Here, the athlete performs an exercise that requires maximal strength to complete (85% to 100%), followed by an exercise that utilizes the same prime movers and is biomechanically similar but performed with a lower intensity (30% to 45%, or up to 10% body weight when using a medicine ball) at higher speeds. A simple example of this type of superset is a heavy barbell bench press (**Figure 19.6**), followed by a medicine ball chest pass (**Figure 19.7**).

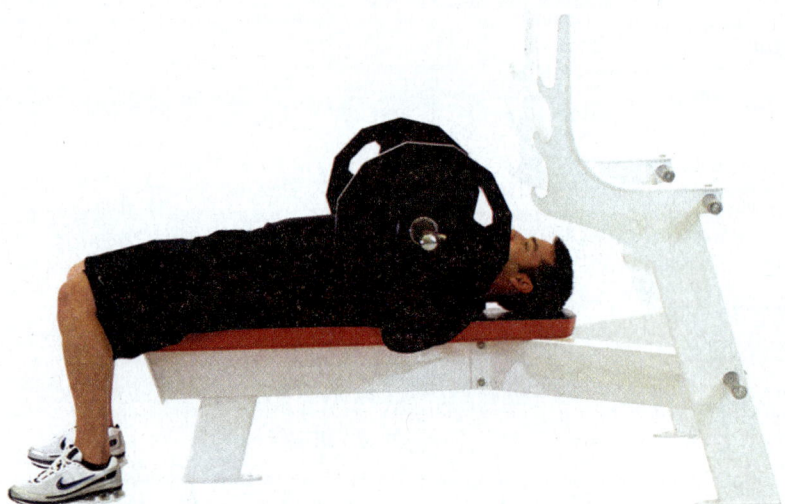

FIGURE 19.6 Bench Press

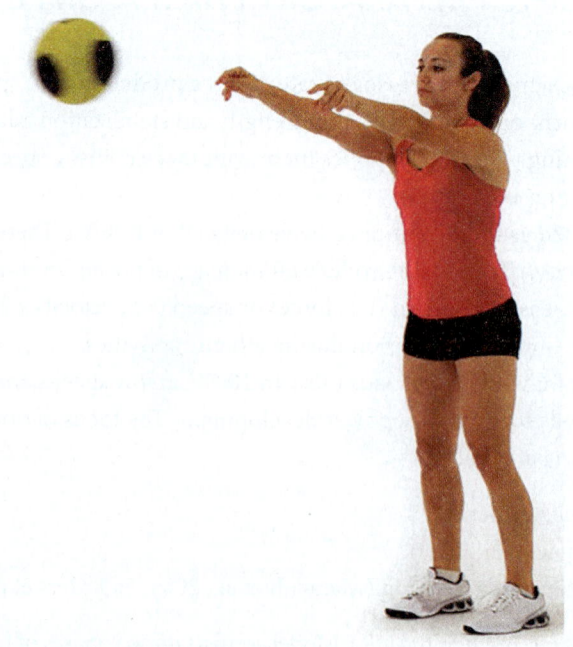

FIGURE 19.7 Medicine Ball Chest Pass

An athlete can produce high power outputs by using a high resistance with explosive movement (although the actual velocity may be slow because of the resistance) and low resistance with a high velocity (Ebben & Blackard, 1997; Newton et al., 2002). This training method elicits a post-activation potentiation (PAP) effect whereby the high-force exercise temporarily spikes performance via motor unit activation. Recall that the power equation is $P = F \times V$. The first exercise in this superset format focuses on the force side of the power equation, as it utilizes near-maximum or maximum loads. The second exercise focuses on the velocity side of the equation, as it utilizes lighter loads performed quickly. For example, the 30% to 45% intensity could be used for jump squats or plyometric push-ups, where the exercise is performed explosively and quickly with a low load. When using medicine ball training, the athlete will choose a ball up to 10% of their body weight. The lower intensity of the medicine ball allows the athlete to focus on quick, powerful, and repetitive movements. To this end, all exercises used to address the velocity side of the equation should include quick, powerful, and repetitive movements. Thus, the exercises must have a powerful release (e.g., throwing, jumping) and minimal transition time between repetitions.

📋 COACH'S CORNER

Phase 5, power training, includes a superset with one maximal strength training exercise followed by a power exercise. If an athlete's training calendar does not allow 4 to 6 weeks of specific maximal-strength training, the Sports Performance Coach can progress them from Phase 2 or 3 directly into Phase 5 to achieve maximal strength adaptations. However, some modifications to intensity may need to be made to ensure a safe transition when skipping Phase 4.

Considering the nature of the strength and power superset, athletes will develop core, balance, and plyometric strength during the resistance training portion of the program design. Further, it is imperative that the Sports Performance Coach not prematurely induce fatigue by including too many core or plyometric exercises before resistance training. Therefore, these are optional in the power level. Due to the higher neuromuscular demands of power training, SAQ exercises should ideally be performed on nonresistance training days.

The repetitions align with the relative intensity of the exercise. Thus, the first exercise in the superset (strength) will use 1 to 5 repetitions, while the second exercise (power) uses 8 to 10 repetitions. Both exercises should be performed at higher intensities (the athlete should be attempting to generate power as rapidly as possible during the power exercise), and a rest interval of up to 2 minutes can be allowed between sets or different exercises. However, the rest interval between the two exercises in the superset should be minimal. For example, if performing a bench press followed by a medicine ball chest throw, the athlete should move directly from the bench press to the medicine ball exercise without rest. However, once the medicine ball chest throw has been completed, the athlete is allowed a 1- to 2-minute break.

Because the goal of this phase of training is primarily power, the program design will focus on progressing intensity and velocity (**Table 19.16**). In Phase 5, the athlete can also begin to integrate sport-specific skills and drills that will be applied in the competition phase. Phase 5 is considered mandatory for most athletes, as increased power production directly relates to an increase in overall performance.

TABLE 19.16 Power Acute Training Variables

Phase 5: Power Training								
	Reps	Sets	Tempo	% Intensity	Rest Interval	Frequency	Duration	Exercise Selection
Flexibility	10–15	1–2	Controlled	N/A	N/A	3–7 times/week	4 weeks	SMT and dynamic; 3–5 exercises
Core*	8–12	2–3	As fast as can be controlled	N/A	0–60 seconds	2–4 times/week	4 weeks	0–2 core-power level
Balance*	8–12	2–3	Controlled	N/A	0–60 seconds	2–4 times/week	4 weeks	0–2 balance-power level
Plyometric*	8–12	2–3	As fast as possible	N/A	0–60 seconds	2–4 times/week	4 weeks	0–2 plyometric-power level
SAQ**	15–20 yards	3–4 2–4	Fast	N/A	1:3 1:5	2–4 times/week	4 weeks	1–2 technique drills 7–10 speed of movement drills (linear/multidirectional speed)
Resistance training	1–5 strength	3–5	As fast as can be controlled	85–100%	No rest between supersets	2–4 times/week	4 weeks	1–2 strength with 1–2 power per body part
	8–10 power		Explosive	30–45 at <10% body weight	1–2 minutes			

Abbreviations: N/A = not applicable; SMT = self-myofascial technique.

*Because of the goal, core, balance, plyometric, and SAQ training may be optional in this phase of training (although recommended). This training can also be performed on nonresistance training days.

**SAQ drills should be done on separate days.

An athlete in Phase 5 will generally stay in this phase of training for 4 to 6 weeks before cycling back through Phases 1 or 2 or progressing to Phase 6, maximal power training (**Table 19.17**).

TABLE 19.17 Power Example Progressions

		Weekly Progression			
		Week 1	Week 2	Week 3	Week 4
Core	Sets	2	2	3	3
	Reps	12	12	10	8
Balance	Sets	2	2	3	3
	Reps	12	12	10	8
Plyometric	Sets	2	3	3	3
	Reps	8	8	10	10
SAQ	Sets	3/3	3/3	4/3	4/4
	Reps	15 yards	20 yards	20 yards	20 yards
Resistance training	Sets	3	4	4	5
	Reps	5 strength 8 power	4 strength 9 power	4 strength 9 power	2–3 strength 10 power
	Intensity	85% strength as necessary per exercise	90% strength as necessary per exercise	90% strength as necessary per exercise	95% strength as necessary per exercise

---

✔ CHECK IT OUT

In Phase 5 of the OPT Model, supersets are key to transitioning between the strength and power levels. These pairs consist of a traditional strength exercise followed by a power exercise, allowing the athlete to work on adaptations of the prior level. The strength exercise potentiates the system, leading to more explosive power movements. Utilizing heavy loads may activate the recruitment of type II motor units, which enhances maximal muscle recruitment necessary for power development. Despite the general size principle, research has shown that preferential recruitment of large type II motor units can occur in ballistic muscle actions, enhancing muscular force (Dideriksen et al., 2020). Therefore, the sequence could start with a ballistic (power) movement to potentiate the system to enhance muscular force for the strength exercise. When an athlete is in Phase 4, the Sports Performance Coach can continue with the traditional progressions of Phase 5, flip the superset for 2 weeks, and finally move into Phase 6 for the remainder of the phase.

Week 1	Week 2	Week 3	Week 4	Week 5	Week 6	Week 7	Week 8	Week 9	Week 10	Week 11
Maximum strength	Maximum strength	Maximum strength	Maximum strength	Maximum strength + power	Maximum strength + power	Power + maximum strength	Power + maximum strength	Power	Power	Power

PHASE 6: MAXIMAL POWER

Maximal power training focuses on high-velocity training to further develop the biomotor abilities of power and speed. Traditional training techniques often emphasize concentric strength and do not allow maximum acceleration throughout the range of motion. Research demonstrates that approximately 25% to 40% of a traditional explosive power lift requires deceleration (Kraemer et al., 2000). Therefore, athletes who follow traditional training techniques may not be able to express their speed strength throughout the necessary range of motion when required in sport, so they cannot achieve optimal performance.

Phase 6 focuses solely on increasing the velocity side of the power equation by training with 30% to 45% of an athlete's maximum strength and accelerating through the entire range of motion. This physically and mentally demanding phase most closely aligns with actual performance in sports, with sport-specific drills being performed at real-time playing speeds. To enhance the transfer of exercise to sport, the Sports Performance Coach should carefully review the sport-specific demands for each athlete and ensure that the program design coincides with the sport. Phase 6 is considered a specialized form of training and should be implemented only by those athletes who have successfully demonstrated adequate coordination, control, and foundational levels of strength. It is best implemented before a short recovery period (approximately 1 week), with the athlete then entering the competitive season.

Phase 6 generally includes total-body explosive lifts, which are often similar or directly related to movements used during sports. Such exercises include jump squats, lunge jumps, plyometric push-ups, medicine ball slams/rotational throws, and Olympic-style lifts. Given the training style, core, balance, and plyometric exercises would not be necessary to ensure the athlete does not overtrain. Further, core and balance exercises can be integrated into the athlete's dynamic warm-up. SAQ training should be included on separate days to help mitigate neuromuscular fatigue. The athlete should use the power acute training variables from Phase 5. Intensity is reduced to 30% to 45% (or up to 10% of body weight for medicine ball training) with 8 to 10 repetitions during resistance training exercises (**Table 19.18**). The athlete must approach each exercise with the same demeanor and intensity as they would use in the actual sport and focus on accelerating through the entire range of motion of a movement or exercise.

TABLE 19.18 Maximal Power Acute Training Variables

Phase 6: Maximal Power Training								
	Reps	Sets	Tempo	% Intensity	Rest Interval	Frequency	Duration	Exercise Selection
Flexibility	10–15	1–2	Controlled	N/A	N/A	3–7 times/ week	4 weeks	SMT and dynamic; 3–5 exercises
Core*	N/A	N/A	N/A	N/A	N/A	N/A	N/A	N/A
Balance*	N/A	N/A	N/A	N/A	N/A	N/A	N/A	N/A
Plyometric*	N/A	N/A	N/A	N/A	N/A	N/A	N/A	N/A

Phase 6: Maximal Power Training								
	Reps	Sets	Tempo	% Intensity	Rest Interval	Frequency	Duration	Exercise Selection
SAQ**	15–20 yards	3–4 2–4	Fast	N/A	1:3 1:5	2–4 times/ week	4 weeks	1–2 technique drills 7–10 speed of movement drills (linear/ multidirectional speed)
Resistance training	10	4–6	As fast as can be controlled	30–45% Maximum: 10% body weight	3–5 minutes	1–2 times/ week	4 weeks	2–3 per body part
Comments:	4–6 total exercises							

Abbreviations: N/A = not applicable; SMT = self-myofascial technique.

*Because of the use of core-power, balance-power and plyometric-power exercises in the resistance training portion of this program, it is not necessary to perform these exercises prior to the resistance training portion of the program. These components can be included in the dynamic flexibility warm-up portion of this program.

**SAQ drills should be done on separate days.

Because the goal of this phase is power development, the progressions will focus on increasing velocity and volume, with minimal relative progressions in intensity. Athletes will generally stay in this training phase for 3 to 4 weeks before cycling through Phase 1 or 2. (**Table 19.19**).

TABLE 19.19 Maximal Power Example Progressions

Weekly Progression						
		Week 1	Week 2	Week 3	Week 4
Core	Sets	N/A	N/A	N/A	N/A
	Reps	N/A	N/A	N/A	N/A
Balance	Sets	N/A	N/A	N/A	N/A
	Reps	12	N/A	N/A	N/A
Plyometric	Sets	N/A	N/A	N/A	N/A
	Reps	N/A	N/A	N/A	N/A

(*continues*)

TABLE 19.19 Maximal Power Example Progressions (*continued*)

		Weekly Progression			
		Week 1	Week 2	Week 3	Week 4
SAQ	Sets	3/3	3/3	4/3	4/4
	Reps	15 yards	20 yards	20 yards	20 yards
Resistance training	Sets	3	4	4	5
	Reps	10 power	10 power	8 power	8 power
	Intensity	Power 5% body weight	Power 5% body weight	Power 8% body weight	Power 10% body weight

> ⚠ **CRITICAL**
>
> Phase 6 is the most physically and mentally demanding phase in the OPT Model. Therefore, the Sports Performance Coach must monitor fatigue and pay attention to signs of overtraining. In addition, the Sports Performance Coach should integrate Phase 1 as an active recovery phase within the cycle of Phase 6 training. Similarly, the Coach should plan for an athlete to return to Phase 1 after Phase 6.

LESSON 3: FOUNDATIONS OF INTEGRATED SPORTS PERFORMANCE TRAINING
INTEGRATED TRAINING COMPONENTS AND THE OPT MODEL

Comprehensive sports training programs should utilize all practical methods available to enhance athletic performance without compromising the athlete's safety, ethics, or integrity. As mentioned, NASM's OPT Model is a truly integrated model that draws on the collective research on performance enhancement and injury prevention. Integrated training is a concept that combines all forms of physical training into one system: flexibility, core, balance, plyometric, SAQ, resistance, and cardio endurance/respiratory training. This all-inclusive approach to sports performance training can improve overall performance, health, and wellness.

Using the principles of integrated training, a Sports Performance Coach can discover many effective programming strategies, methods, and techniques to include in an athlete's comprehensive program that provide several benefits:

- Psychological: improved mood, improved sleep, and stress relief
- Physiological: improved cardiovascular, respiratory, musculoskeletal, and endocrine functionality

- Performance: improved strength, flexibility, endurance, and power
- Safety: reduced risk of overtraining or undertraining

The Sports Performance Coach should also recognize that integrated training encourages the use of multiple training modalities, emphasizing the entire muscle action spectrum and all planes of motion. Incorporating different types of training in all planes can improve movement quality, speed and agility, strength, endurance, flexibility, and power better than isolated resistance training programs (DiStefano et al., 2013). NASM strongly encourages the use of integrated training programs to improve athletes' performance.

FLEXIBILITY TRAINING

Flexibility training involves techniques to improve tissue extensibility, with the aim of increasing range of motion. NASM recommends that Sports Performance Coaches use a variety of options systematically and progressively to achieve optimal results. These stretching techniques include self-myofascial techniques, such as foam rolling, and static, active, and dynamic stretching. The Sports Performance Coach can also include percussion and assisted-stretching techniques when appropriate and if properly trained. Flexibility training offers the following benefits:

- Decreased chance of injury
- Prevention of muscle imbalances
- Correction of existing muscle imbalances
- Improved posture
- Enhanced joint range of motion

DESIGNING A STABILIZATION-LEVEL FLEXIBILITY TRAINING PROGRAM

The flexibility techniques used within the stabilization level include self-myofascial techniques (SMT), static stretching, and dynamic stretching. Dynamic stretching in this level is optional based on the athlete's assessment results and goals. The flexibility program should be based on the results of a comprehensive assessment, including transitional, mobility, and dynamic assessments. NASM recommends that flexibility training be performed as part of a comprehensive warm-up. The athlete must perform flexibility exercises before cardio warm-up to avoid exacerbating existing compensations.

When performing SMT, the recommendation is to target muscles identified as short/overactive in the assessment process (refer to Chapter 7 for transitional, mobility, and dynamic movement assessment compensation charts). In general, the Sports Performance Coach should choose one to three muscle groups and have the athlete slowly roll each muscle, holding pressure on tender areas for a minimum of 30 seconds. Refer to Chapter 9 for more information on how to perform SMT.

After completing SMT, the athlete should then perform static stretching. In most cases, it is best to statically stretch the same muscles targeted during SMT because both techniques elicit a better overall response and increase in range of motion (Fairall et al., 2017; Mohr et al., 2014; Škarabot et al., 2015). The Sports Performance Coach should have the athlete hold each static stretch for a minimum of 30 seconds for the best increase in range of motion (Behm et al., 2016). Refer to Chapter 9 for more information on static stretching.

Dynamic stretching is optional in this level of training, depending on the severity of movement compensations and the athlete's goals. Due to the complexity of dynamic stretches, the Sports Performance Coach must ensure that the athlete does not make compensations worse or move poorly when performing dynamic stretching. However, including dynamic stretching within a flexibility routine may increase joint range of motion while increasing the potential expression of strength and power output (Behm et al., 2016; Opplert & Babault, 2018). If dynamic stretching is part of the routine, choose one set of 3 to 10 stretches using a repetition range of 10 to 15. Refer to Chapter 9 for more information on dynamic stretching. **Tables 19.20**, **19.21**, and **19.22** provide examples of flexibility programs for common movement impairments.

TABLE 19.20 Stabilization-Level Flexibility Training Exercises for Foot Turn-Out Impairment

Exercise Selection	Sets	Reps	Tempo	Frequency	Duration
Self-myofascial techniques: • Calves • Biceps femoris • Tenor fascia latae	1–3	1	Slow; hold pressure on tender spots for 30–60 seconds	5–7 days per week	Per-session times vary; 4–6 weeks total depending on goals
Static stretching: • Standing calf stretch • Standing lateral hamstrings stretch • Kneeling hip flexor stretch	1–3	1	Slow; hold end range for approximately 60 seconds	5–7 days per week	
Dynamic stretching (optional): • Lunge with rotation	1	10–15	Moderate/controlled	5–7 days per week	

TABLE 19.21 Stabilization-Level Flexibility Training Exercises for Knee Valgus Impairment

Exercise Selection	Sets	Reps	Tempo	Frequency	Duration
Self-myofascial techniques: • Calves • Adductor complex	1–3	1	Slow; hold pressure on tender spots for 30–60 seconds	5–7 days per week	Per-session times vary; 4–6 weeks total depending on goals
Static stretching: • Standing calf stretch • Standing adductor stretch	1–3	1	Slow; hold end range for approximately 60 seconds	5–7 days per week	
Dynamic stretching (optional): • Multiplanar lunge	1	10–15	Moderate/controlled	5–7 days per week	

TABLE 19.22 Stabilization-Level Flexibility Training Exercises for Arms Fall Forward Impairment

Exercise Selection	Sets	Reps	Tempo	Frequency	Duration
Self-myofascial techniques: • Pectorals • Latissimus • Thoracic spine	1–3	1	Slow; hold pressure on tender spots for 30–60 seconds	5–7 days per week	Per-session times vary; 4–6 weeks total depending on goals
Static stretching: • Standing pectoral stretch • Stability ball latissimus stretch • Seated thoracic spine rotation stretch	1–3	1	Slow; hold end range for approximately 60 seconds	5–7 days per week	
Dynamic stretching (optional): • Reverse lunge to overhead reach	1	10–15	Moderate/controlled	5–7 days per week	

DESIGNING A STRENGTH-LEVEL FLEXIBILITY TRAINING PROGRAM

The flexibility techniques used within the strength level include SMT, active stretching, and dynamic stretching. Dynamic stretching in this level is optional based on the athlete's assessment results and goals. The flexibility program in the strength level is generally similar to that in the stabilization program, with the focus on the same muscles in most cases. The target muscles include those identified as short/overactive in the assessment process or muscles that may have a propensity to become overactive due to the athlete's sport. In general, choose one to three muscle groups and have the athlete slowly roll each muscle, holding pressure on tender areas for a minimum of 30 seconds. Active stretches require 5 to 10 repetitions in which the stretched position is held for 1 to 2 seconds. If dynamic stretching is part of the routine, choose one set of 3 to 10 stretches using a repetition range of 10 to 15. **Tables 19.23**, **19.24**, and **19.25** provide example flexibility programs for common movement impairments.

TABLE 19.23 Strength-Level Flexibility Training Exercises for Foot Turn-Out Impairment

Exercise Selection	Sets	Reps	Tempo	Frequency	Duration
Self-myofascial techniques: • Calves • Biceps femoris • Tenor fascia latae	1–3	1	Slow; hold pressure on tender spots for 30–60 seconds	5–7 days per week	Per-session times vary; 4–6 weeks total depending on goals

(continues)

TABLE 19.23 Strength-Level Flexibility Training Exercises for Foot Turn-Out Impairment (*continued*)

Exercise Selection	Sets	Reps	Tempo	Frequency	Duration
Active stretching: • Standing calf stretch • Standing lateral hamstrings stretch • Kneeling hip flexor stretch	1–3	1	Hold each stretch for 1–2 seconds	5–7 days per week	
Dynamic stretching (optional): • Lunge with rotation	1	10–15	Moderate/controlled	5–7 days per week	

TABLE 19.24 Strength-Level Flexibility Training Exercises for Knee Valgus Impairment

Exercise Selection	Sets	Reps	Tempo	Frequency	Duration
Self-myofascial techniques: • Calves • Adductor complex	1–3	1	Slow; hold pressure on tender spots for 30–60 seconds	5–7 days per week	Per-session times vary; 4–6 weeks total depending on goals
Active stretching: • Standing calf stretch • Standing adductor stretch	1–3	1	Hold each stretch for 1–2 seconds	5–7 days per week	
Dynamic stretching (optional): • Multiplanar lunge	1	10–15	Moderate/controlled	5–7 days per week	

TABLE 19.25 Strength-Level Flexibility Training Exercises for Arms Fall Forward Impairment

Exercise Selection	Sets	Reps	Tempo	Frequency	Duration
Self-myofascial techniques: • Pectorals • Latissimus • Thoracic spine	1–3	1	Slow; hold pressure on tender spots for 30–60 seconds	5–7 days per week	Per-session times vary; 4–6 weeks total depending on goals

Exercise Selection	Sets	Reps	Tempo	Frequency	Duration
Active stretching: • Standing pectoral stretch • Stability ball latissimus stretch • Seated thoracic spine rotation stretch	1–3	1	Hold each stretch for 1–2 seconds	5–7 days per week	
Dynamic stretching (optional): • Reverse lunge to overhead reach	1	10–15	Moderate/controlled	5–7 days per week	

DESIGNING A POWER-LEVEL FLEXIBILITY TRAINING PROGRAM

The flexibility techniques used in the power level include SMT and dynamic stretching. A similar progression can continue by including muscles that were identified as short/overactive in the assessment process or muscles that may have a propensity to become overactive due to the athlete's sport for SMT. However, the athlete should have shown some reduction in movement compensations before beginning in the power level. Dynamic flexibility exercises can also include these muscles but should focus more on movement patterns similar to the planned activities. In general, choose one to three muscle groups and have the athlete slowly roll each muscle, holding pressure on tender areas for a minimum of 30 seconds. After completing SMT, move directly into dynamic stretching and choose one set of 3 to 10 stretches using a repetition range of 10 to 15. **Tables 19.26**, **19.27**, and **19.28** provide flexibility programs for common movement impairments.

TABLE 19.26 Power-Level Flexibility Training Exercises for Foot Turn-Out Impairment

Exercise Selection	Sets	Reps	Tempo	Frequency	Duration
Self-myofascial techniques: • Calves • Biceps femoris • Tenor fascia latae	1–3	1	Slow; hold pressure on tender spots for 30–60 seconds	5–7 days per week	Per-session times vary; 4–6 weeks total depending on goals
Dynamic stretching (optional): • Bodyweight squat • Reverse lunge • Medicine ball woodchop	1	10–15	Moderately fast to fast	5–7 days per week	

TABLE 19.27 Power-Level Flexibility Training Exercises for Knee Valgus Impairment

Exercise Selection	Sets	Reps	Tempo	Frequency	Duration
Self-myofascial techniques: • Calves • Adductor complex	1–3	1	Slow; hold pressure on tender spots for 30–60 seconds	5–7 days per week	Per-session times vary; 4–6 weeks total depending on goals
Dynamic stretching (optional): • Multiplanar lunge with reach • Frontal plane leg swings	1	10–15	Moderately fast to fast	5–7 days per week	

TABLE 19.28 Power-Level Flexibility Training Exercises for Arms Fall Forward Impairment

Exercise Selection	Sets	Reps	Tempo	Frequency	Duration
Self-myofascial techniques: • Pectorals • Latissimus • Thoracic spine	1–3	1	Slow; hold pressure on tender spots for 30–60 seconds	5–7 days per week	Per-session times vary; 4–6 weeks total depending on goals
Dynamic stretching (optional): • Reverse lunge to overhead reach • Squat to overhead press • Push-up to rotation	1	10–15	Moderately fast to fast	5–7 days per week	

👍 **HELPFUL HINT**

Flexibility training in the power level does not typically include static or active stretching. However, if an athlete still demonstrates minor compensations or can otherwise benefit from either technique, the Sports Performance Coach is encouraged to include it before the dynamic stretches.

CORE TRAINING

Athletes in any sport require optimal function for enhanced performance. Core stability is the ability to control the position and motion of the trunk over the pelvis and legs for optimal production, transfer, and control of force and motion (Manchado et al., 2017). Exercises that integrate all planes of motion and include the entire core as a unit should be used (i.e., spinal stabilizers, abdominal complex, lower back, obliques, and gluteal complex) rather than focusing on only the anterior core muscles in the sagittal plane. Core training offers the following benefits:

- Enhanced posture and spinal health
- Improved balance, stabilization, and coordination of the kinetic chain
- Improved low-back pain symptoms
- Improved vertical jump
- Improved core activation patterns for enhanced strength, power, and skill-related movements

DESIGNING A STABILIZATION-LEVEL CORE TRAINING PROGRAM

Stabilization-level core exercises should emphasize core stabilization and intervertebral stability. These exercises primarily target the local core muscles, such as the rotators, multifidus, transverse abdominis, and diaphragm. To accomplish this, core exercises in this level of training should focus on isometric contractions utilizing the drawing-in maneuver and little to no motion at the spine. These exercises focus on motor control of the core (**Table 19.29**). If the movement of limbs is included, it should occur with a slow repetition tempo. An example of slow repetition is 4-2-1-1 (4-second eccentric, 2-second isometric, 1-second concentric, and 1-second isometric). The volume and intensity of core exercises in this level should be relatively low because the goal is to activate—rather than exhaust—the local core musculature before more intense exercise begins. Choose between 1 and 4 core exercises with a repetition range of 12 to 20 and 1 to 3 sets. Progressions within this level of core training involve altering body positions (e.g., from supine to side-lying to standing), adding movement of the limbs (e.g., supine drawing-in to dead bug), and decreasing external stability (e.g., floor bridge to floor bridge with a foam roller).

TABLE 19.29 Stabilization-Level Core Training Example

Exercise Selection	Sets	Reps	Tempo	Frequency	Duration
Motor control core training: • Crook-lying drawing in maneuver • Side-lying drawing in maneuver • Dead bugs	1–10	10-second isometric holds 12–20 reps	N/A Slow	2–4 times per week	Per-session times vary; 4–6 weeks total depending on goals
Advanced motor control core training: • Clamshells • Bench bridge with chains	2–3	60- to 90-second holds or 12–20 reps	N/A Slow	2–4 times per week	

Core training within the stabilization level can continue to progress to advanced motor control core training. These exercises focus on keeping the lumbo-pelvic-hip complex (LPHC) in a neutral position while improving isometric strength. Demonstrating isometric strength from functional positions is imperative for athletes. Therefore, advanced motor control core training is essential before progressing to the strength level. Refer to Chapter 10 for more information on core training.

DESIGNING A STRENGTH-LEVEL CORE TRAINING PROGRAM

Core training should be progressed from the stabilization level to the strength level by becoming more strength-biased and involving more dynamic eccentric and concentric movements of the spine. In other words, the strength-level core exercises involve flexion, extension, and rotation with slightly faster tempos (**Table 19.30**). Choose between 1 and 4 exercises, using a moderate tempo of 2-0-2-0 (2-second eccentric, 0-second isometric, 2-second concentric, and 0-second isometric). The athlete should demonstrate control in the sagittal and frontal planes before including transverse plane exercises. Choose between 1 and 4 core exercises with a repetition range of 8 to 12 and 2 to 4 sets. Although it is recommended to progress exercises to include movement in the spine, the Sports Performance Coach can still include stabilization-level exercises when appropriate. Refer to Chapter 10 for more information on core training.

TABLE 19.30   Strength-Level Core Training Example

Exercise Selection	Sets	Reps	Tempo	Frequency	Duration
Strength-biased core training: • Pike-up to reverse crunch • Back extensions • Cable chops	2–4	8–12 reps	Slow to moderate	2–4 times per week	Per-session times vary; 4–6 weeks total depending on goals

DESIGNING A POWER-LEVEL CORE TRAINING PROGRAM

Due to the increased demands of power-level training programs, core training is optional in this level. The Sports Performance Coach can include core training but should use caution to avoid fatiguing the core musculature before other components of the training program are initiated. If core exercises are programmed, they should involve exercises that focus on applying the concepts of motor control and strength-biased core training to sport-specific actions. This integration-biased core training prepares athletes to perform at real-time speeds.

Many of these exercises involve explosive movements designed to increase the rate of force production of the core musculature (**Table 19.31**). Progressions of integration-biased core training within the power level can include the addition of jumping–landing, acceleration, and deceleration in all planes of motion and using resistance bands to facilitate proximal-to-distal movement production. Choose between 1 and 2 core

TABLE 19.31   Power-Level Core Training Example

Exercise Selection	Sets	Reps	Tempo	Frequency	Duration
Integration-biased core training: • Medicine ball overhead throw • Drop step to sprint stand with medicine ball rotation	1–3	8–12 reps	Fast/explosive	2–4 times per week	Per-session times vary; 4–6 weeks total depending on goals

exercises using a repetition range of 8 to 12 with an explosive tempo and 1 to 3 sets. However, the Sports Performance Coach is encouraged to incorporate core exercises from the stabilization and strength levels when appropriate. Refer to Chapter 10 for more information on core training.

📋 **COACH'S CORNER**

Medicine ball exercises are commonly recommended because the athlete needs to generate maximal power to throw the ball as explosively as possible. Although other tools, such as resistance tubing, can be utilized, they do not provoke the full expression of power because the athlete never actually releases the resistance tubing.

BALANCE TRAINING

Balance is the ability to maintain, achieve, or restore a specific state of balance without falling (Callesen et al., 2018). Optimal balance is essential for athletes to control their center of mass while performing complex movements at various speeds in all planes of motion. In addition, balance training is used to improve postural control by challenging the alignment of the body's center of gravity with the base of support (Lesinski et al., 2015). Further, balance training may reduce the occurrence of ankle sprains in athletes (Bellows & Wong, 2018). Balance training offers the following benefits:

- Reduced risk of ankle sprains
- Improved landing mechanics
- Improved proprioception and lower-extremity awareness
- Enhanced execution of agility-based outcomes
- Stronger hip musculature

DESIGNING A STABILIZATION-LEVEL BALANCE TRAINING PROGRAM

Like all components of an integrated training program, balance training must be systematic and progressive. The main goal of this training is to continually increase the athlete's awareness of their stability limits by creating controlled instability. Not following progressions can lead to movement compensations and improper execution of exercises, which decreases the effectiveness and increases the risk for injury. The initial exercises focus on static balance and are designed to improve reflexive joint stabilization contractions so as to increase joint stability (**Table 19.32**). Progressions within this level can include the introduction of perturbations to induce a heightened reflexive stabilization

TABLE 19.32 Stabilization-Level Balance Training Example

Exercise Selection	Sets	Reps	Tempo	Frequency	Duration
Static-balance training: • Single-leg balance reach • Single-leg stance with upper-extremity perturbations	1–3	12–20 (6–10 on each leg)	Slow or isometric	2–4 times per week	Per-session times vary; 4–6 weeks total depending on goals

response. Choose between 1 and 4 balance exercises with a repetition range of 12 to 20 (6 to 10 repetitions on each leg) using a controlled movement if appropriate and 1 to 3 sets. Refer to Chapter 11 for more information on balance training.

> ### 📋 COACH'S CORNER
>
> Balance tools, such as balance discs and foam pads, can be included in the program, but the Sports Performance Coach should ensure that the athlete maintains the proper form and kinetic chain alignment.

DESIGNING A STRENGTH-LEVEL BALANCE TRAINING PROGRAM

As in core training, the progression of balance exercises includes introducing dynamic eccentric and concentric movements in the balance leg. Movements in sports require dynamic control through the midrange of motion and isometric stabilization at the end ranges of movement. Therefore, dynamic balance training can introduce changes to body positions that further challenge neuromuscular control (**Table 19.33**). The speed and neural demand of these exercises are also progressed. Choose between 1 and 4 balance exercises using a repetition range of 8 to 12 with a moderate tempo and 2 to 4 sets. The Sports Performance Coach has the discretion to continue to include stabilization-level exercises if appropriate. Refer to Chapter 11 for more information on balance training.

TABLE 19.33   Strength-Level Balance Training Example

Exercise Selection	Sets	Reps	Tempo	Frequency	Duration
Dynamic balance training: • Single-leg squat • Single-leg Romanian deadlift • Hip airplanes	2–4	8–12	Moderate/ controlled	2–4 times per week	Per-session times vary; 4–6 weeks total depending on goals

DESIGNING A POWER-LEVEL BALANCE TRAINING PROGRAM

The balance exercises used in the power level are a progression from previous phases. They are designed to emphasize eccentric deceleration ability to move the body from a dynamic state to a controlled position (**Table 19.34**). Beginning athletes can begin with assisted controlled eccentric balance training and progress to hopping motions. In contrast, advanced athletes may begin with hopping. Assisted eccentric training differs from dynamic balance training in that the time spent in the eccentric phase of the contraction is accentuated by an increased time or range of motion. The athlete will hold the landing position for 3 to 5 seconds when using single-leg hops. Like core training in the power level, balance training may be optional depending on the level of athlete, specific training program, and goals. Refer to Chapter 11 for more information on balance training.

TABLE 19.34 Power-Level Balance Training Example

Exercise Selection	Sets	Reps	Tempo	Frequency	Duration
Eccentric control and deceleration balance training: • Single-leg lowering • Multiplanar hop with stabilization	2–4	8–12	Moderate/controlled	2–4 times per week	Per-session times vary; 4–6 weeks total depending on goals

---

📋 COACH'S CORNER

The 3- to 5-second hold is meant to reinforce optimal alignment of the landing position. Therefore, if the athlete lands with less than desirable form, the Sports Performance Coach should correct their alignment and then have the athlete hold for 3 to 5 seconds. Also, this hold should be in the landing position (i.e., athletic stance) rather than with the athlete standing upright.

PLYOMETRIC/REACTIVE STRENGTH TRAINING

Plyometric training has also been described as reactive strength training. In essence, plyometric training is used to enhance reactive strength. It is a safe and effective mode of exercise for many populations, but is especially important for athletes because it is characterized by the expression of muscular power (Mansur et al., 2018). Plyometric exercises improve the stretch–shortening cycle, which enhances an athlete's ability to react and move explosively (Ramirez-Campillo et al., 2015). Plyometric training offers the following benefits:

- Improved soft-tissue strength and decreased risk of injury
- Improved lower-body strength and power
- Improved motor synchronization
- Improved performance in speed- and agility-based outcomes

DESIGNING A STABILIZATION-LEVEL PLYOMETRIC TRAINING PROGRAM

Even for skilled athletes, plyometric training in the stabilization level should emphasize optimal deceleration, stability, and kinetic chain alignment. These exercises initially involve small jumps (lower amplitude), while focusing on an ideal landing (**Table 19.35**).

TABLE 19.35 Stabilization-Level Plyometric Training Example

Exercise Selection	Sets	Reps	Tempo	Frequency	Duration
Plyometric stabilization: • Squat jump with stabilization • Box jump with stabilization	1–3	5–8	Hold landing position for 3–5 seconds	2–4 times per week	Per-session times vary; 4–6 weeks total depending on goals

When the athlete lands, they should correct any faulty postures and hold the position for 3 to 5 seconds. Although this level involves small jumps, the athlete should still achieve the optimal range of motion during the movement. For example, the athlete should reach full triple extension during a jump. Choose between 1 and 3 plyometric exercises with a repetition range of 5 to 8 and perform 1 to 3 sets. Refer to Chapter 12 for more information on plyometric training.

📋 COACH'S CORNER

The Sports Performance Coach should constantly consider progressions and regressions. A training program should challenge an athlete but always remain within their boundaries of ability. As part of planning, the coach should question whether progressing within a session is necessary. In theory, if an exercise such as the squat jump with stabilization presents a challenge to the athlete, then a box jump with stabilization may be too difficult for the athlete to perform well. Conversely, if an athlete can perform a box jump with stabilization with optimal form, then a regular squat jump with stabilization may be too easy to stimulate additional adaptions.

DESIGNING A STRENGTH-LEVEL PLYOMETRIC TRAINING PROGRAM

Plyometric exercises for the strength level should involve a jump with more amplitude and reduced time spent on the ground (i.e., decreased amortization phase). These exercises, similar to those performed for the stabilization level, are performed repetitively, with the athlete no longer holding the landing for 3 to 5 seconds (**Table 19.36**). In theory, the athlete should have learned optimal posture in the stabilization level, so now they can speed up the movement while demonstrating control and coordination of the kinetic chain checkpoints. Select between 1 and 4 plyometric exercises with a repetition range of 8 to 12 and perform for 2 to 4 sets. Refer to Chapter 12 for more information on plyometric training.

TABLE 19.36 Strength-Level Plyometric Training Example

Exercise Selection	Sets	Reps	Tempo	Frequency	Duration
Plyometric strength: • Squat jump • Power step-ups	2–4	8–12	Moderate/ no hold upon landing	2–4 times per week	Per-session times vary; 4–6 weeks total depending on goals

DESIGNING A POWER-LEVEL PLYOMETRIC TRAINING PROGRAM

Plyometric training in the power level progresses from the previous level by introducing quicker, more explosive, and more powerful movements mimicking real-time playing speed. These exercises are designed to further improve the rate of force production and the eccentric strength of the entire kinetic chain (**Table 19.37**). As with the progression between the stabilization and strength levels, exercises in the power level will further reduce the time spent in contact with the ground. Thus, some exercise options for this phase may involve low-amplitude movements but are performed as rapidly as possible, such as proprioceptive hops. Choose between 1 and 4 exercises with a repetition range of 8 to 12 and 3 to 5 sets. Given the increased demands created in this level of training, plyometric exercise may be optional to prevent fatigue. The Sports Performance Coach

TABLE 19.37 Power-Level Plyometric Training Example

Exercise Selection	Sets	Reps	Tempo	Frequency	Duration
Plyometric power: • Ice skaters • Single-leg power step-ups • Proprioceptive hops	3–5	8–12	Fast/controlled	2–4 times per week	Per-session times vary; 4–6 weeks total depending on goals

should use their discretion when deciding whether to include plyometric exercises from prior levels. Refer to Chapter 12 for more information on plyometric training.

SPEED, AGILITY, AND QUICKNESS TRAINING

SAQ training is a system of progressive exercises and instruction aimed at developing fundamental motor abilities to enhance the capability of athletes to be more skillful at real-time speeds and with greater precision (Chandrakumar & Ramesh, 2015). SAQ training can improve reaction time, sprinting velocity, and lower-body power. SAQ training offers the following benefits:

- Improved acceleration/deceleration and change of direction at top-speed performance
- Improved reaction time
- Improved sprinting and change of direction mechanics

DESIGNING A STABILIZATION-LEVEL SAQ TRAINING PROGRAM

SAQ programs may vary within the OPT Model. However, most athletes will begin by seeking to improve their technique and linear speed. These exercises are generally simpler and allow the athlete to focus on the optimal technique and front-side and back-side sprinting mechanics (**Table 19.38**). Choose between 3 and 4 technique-focused exercises

TABLE 19.38 Stabilization-Level SAQ Training Example

Exercise Selection	Sets	Reps (yards)	Work:Rest Ratio	Tempo	Frequency	Duration
Technique drills: • Ladder drills: 1–2 inches • A-skips • Cycling B-skips	3–4	15–20	1:3	Moderate/controlled	2–4 times per week	Per-session times vary; 4–6 weeks total depending on goals
Speed of movement/linear speed/MDS: • 1/3/5 wall drill • Arm swings • 5-yard dash	2–4	15–20	1:5			

with a repetition range of 15 to 20 yards using a moderate yet controlled movement and 3 to 4 sets. Additionally, choose between 3 and 5 speeds of movement, linear speed, or multidirectional speed (MDS)-focused exercises with a repetition range of 15 to 20 yards using a moderate yet controlled movement and 2 to 4 sets. Refer to Chapter 13 for more information on SAQ training.

DESIGNING A STRENGTH-LEVEL SAQ TRAINING PROGRAM

Progressions within SAQ training focus on reducing the emphasis on technique, as the athlete should have learned this in the prior level. The strength level begins to emphasize the speed of movement (**Table 19.39**). Also, these drills progressively become more complex, including overspeed or resisted speed training. Refer to Chapter 13 for more information on SAQ training.

TABLE 19.39 Strength-Level SAQ Training Example

Exercise Selection	Sets	Reps (yards)	Work:Rest Ratio	Tempo	Frequency	Duration
Technique drills: • Ladder drills • Jumping jacks, side shuffle • Lateral A-skips	3–4	15–20	1:3	Moderate/ controlled	2–4 times per week	Per-session times vary; 4–6 weeks total depending on goals
Speed of movement/ linear speed/MDS: • 20-yard dash • Line-stop deceleration drill • Resisted sprints • Assisted sprints • 5-10-5 drill	2–4	15–20	1:5			

🤖 GETTING TECHNICAL

Assisted sprint training, such as downhill running, high-speed towing, or treadmill sprinting, effectively enhances stride frequency and influences sprinting acceleration (Clark et al., 2021). Resisted sprint training boosts force production at high speeds; it includes uphill running, sled towing, parachute running, and weighted-vest sprints (Cahill et al., 2020). Both methods provide a specific additional stimulus, particularly for initial acceleration (Rumpf et al., 2016). Coaches often use these forms of training to help athletes meet the high neuromuscular demands of sprinting. However, if a satisfactory sprint training program already exists, these methods might not be necessary.

DESIGNING A POWER-LEVEL SAQ TRAINING PROGRAM

The last SAQ progressions within the OPT Model focus more on the speed of movement, linear speed, and MDS, with less emphasis placed on technique. This last level also includes increased complexity with more MDS and the introduction of a lack of predictability (**Table 19.40**). In other words, instead of the athlete running a predetermined drill (e.g., box drill), they will begin to respond to visual or auditory cues (e.g., partner-mirror drill). Refer to Chapter 13 for more information on SAQ training.

TABLE 19.40 Power-Level SAQ Training Example

Exercise Selection	Sets	Reps (yards)	Work:Rest Ratio	Tempo	Frequency	Duration
Technique drills: • Ladder drills • Out-out-in-in • Lateral 1/3/5 wall drill	3–4	15–20	1:3	Fast/ controlled	2–4 times per week	Per session times vary; 4–6 weeks total depending on goals
Speed of movement/ linear speed/MDS: • Push-up sprints • Parachute resisted sprints • T-drill • Modified box drill • Partner-mirror drill • Turn and grab card drill • T-drill with audible/visual cues	2–4	15–20	1:5			

📋 COACH'S CORNER

SAQ exercises in the power level of the OPT Model progress by simply replacing a typical pattern with a visual or auditory cue. For example, when performing the T-drill, the Sports Performance Coach can have the athlete respond to the direction the coach is pointing or calling out rather than the traditional pattern.

⚠ CRITICAL

Progressions for SAQ training are not as straightforward as for other training components. Exercise selection should depend on the athlete's skills, abilities, and goals. SAQ training might be considered optional, but at least some such training is highly recommended within all levels of the model to ensure the athlete is continually working on agility and reactive ability.

RESISTANCE TRAINING

Resistance training is well known to promote significant increases in muscle strength and hypertrophy in athletes from a wide range of demographics (Schoenfeld et al., 2016). In addition, resistance training is vital in improving various performance measures and rehabilitation from musculoskeletal injury (Kristensen & Franklyn-Miller, 2011; Vesci et al., 2017). Thus, the overall impact of resistance training on athletic performance and overall health cannot be overemphasized, and the Sports Performance Coach should have a strong understanding of its benefits and different programming strategies. Resistance training offers the following benefits:

- Increased endurance, strength, and power
- Improved resting heart rate and blood pressure regulation
- Improved overall athletic performance
- Decreased risk of injury due to enhanced strength of all soft tissues

📋 COACH'S CORNER

Ideally, resistance training exercises in the stabilization level will include movements that integrate the total-body musculature. However, an athlete can perform some isolated movements if needed or desired using the acute training variables recommended to achieve muscular endurance.

DESIGNING A STABILIZATION-LEVEL RESISTANCE TRAINING PROGRAM

Resistance training exercises in the stabilization level are designed to improve neuromuscular efficiency and stability by having the athlete perform the exercise in an unstable yet controllable environment. These exercises generally help to teach fundamental movement patterns (e.g., squat, hip hinge) and rely on the athlete to produce internal stability rather than external stability (**Table 19.41**). The Sports Performance Coach must consider the athlete's training goals and the results of the transitional, mobility, and dynamic assessments when designing the resistance training program in the stabilization phase. NASM discourages using exercises that may exacerbate the athlete's movement compensations. For example, if an athlete demonstrates feet turning out, the

TABLE 19.41 Stabilization-Level Resistance Training Example

Exercise Selection	Sets	Reps	Intensity	Tempo	Frequency	Duration
• Squat to row • Standing cable chest press • Step-up to scaption raise • Reverse lunge to balance	1–3	12–20	50–70% 1RM	Slow: 4/2/1/1	2–4 times per week	Per-session times vary; 4–6 weeks total depending on goals

Sports Performance Coach should not include an exercise such as calf raises. Similarly, if an athlete demonstrates the arms fall forward impairment, then the latissimus pull-down could be replaced with a wide-grip row to emphasize the mid- and upper-back musculature. Refer to Chapter 7 for transitional, mobility, and dynamic movement assessment compensation charts. Choose between 1 and 2 resistance training exercises per body part, performed with a repetition range of 12 to 20 and at low to moderate intensity (50% to 70% 1RM), and perform 1 to 3 sets. Refer to Chapter 14 for more information on resistance training.

DESIGNING A STRENGTH-LEVEL RESISTANCE TRAINING PROGRAM

Resistance training exercises within the strength level of the OPT Model are designed to enhance prime-mover strength by having the athlete perform these exercises in more stable environments. Recall that the strength level includes three phases. These exercises progress from the stabilization level by transitioning to more traditional exercises performed at progressively higher intensities. Depending on the adaption desired, repetitions will range from 6 to 12 and intensities from 75% to 100% 1RM. Phase 2 uses supersets at varying intensities and reps (**Table 19.42**), Phase 3 includes traditional exercises aimed at muscular development (**Table 19.43**), and Phase 4 uses traditional exercises aimed at strength development (**Table 19.44**). Refer to Chapter 14 for more information on resistance training.

TABLE 19.42 Strength-Level Resistance Training Example (Strength Endurance)

Exercise Selection	Sets	Reps	Intensity	Tempo	Frequency	Duration
• Bench press	2–4	8–12	70%–80%	2/0/2/0	2–4 times per week	Per-session times vary; 4–6 weeks total depending on goals
• Stability ball push-up		8–12	50%–70%	4/2/1/1		
• Squat		8–12	70%–80%	2/0/2/0		
• Reverse lunge to balance		8–12	50%–70%	4/2/1/1		
• Bent-over barbell row		8–12	70%–80%	2/0/2/0		
• Single-arm standing cable row		8–12	50%–70%	4/2/1/1		

TABLE 19.43 Strength-Level Resistance Training Example (Muscular Development)

Exercise Selection	Sets	Reps	Intensity	Tempo	Frequency	Duration
• Bench press	3–5	6–12	75%–85%	2/0/2/0	2–4 times per week	Per-session times vary; 4–6 weeks total depending on goals
• Squat						
• Bent-over barbell row						

TABLE 19.44 Strength-Level Resistance Training Example (Maximal Strength)

Exercise Selection	Sets	Reps	Intensity	Tempo	Frequency	Duration
• Bench press • Squat • Bent-over barbell row	4–6	1–5	85%–100%	As fast as can be controlled	2–4 times per week	Per-session times vary; 4–6 weeks total depending on goals

DESIGNING A POWER-LEVEL RESISTANCE TRAINING PROGRAM

Resistance training exercises within the power level of the OPT Model are designed to improve the rate of force production and overall muscular power by having the athlete perform them as fast and explosively as possible. Recall that the power level includes two phases. These exercises progress from the strength level by emphasizing the rate of force production through explosive movements. Repetitions will range from 1 to 10, with intensities varying between 30% and 100%. Phase 5 includes varying intensities, reps, and speeds (**Table 19.45**), whereas Phase 6 utilizes traditional exercises aimed at power development (**Table 19.46**). Refer to Chapter 14 for more information on resistance training.

TABLE 19.45 Power-Level Resistance Training Example (Power)

Exercise Selection	Sets	Reps	Intensity	Tempo	Frequency	Duration
• Bench press • Medicine ball chest pass • Squat • Ice skater • Bent-over barbell row • Medicine ball slam	3–5	1–5 8–10 1–5 8–10 1–5 8–10	85%–100% <10% body weight for medicine ball 85%–100% body weight 85%–100% <10% body weight for medicine ball	As fast as can be controlled; as explosively as possible	2–4 times per week	Per-session times vary; 4–6 weeks total depending on goals

TABLE 19.46 Power-Level Resistance Training Example (Maximal Power)

Exercise Selection	Sets	Reps	Intensity	Tempo	Frequency	Duration
• Medicine ball chest pass • Ice skater • Medicine ball slam	3–5	8–10	<10% body weight 30%–45% body weight <10% body weight	As explosively as possible	2–4 times per week	Per-session times vary; 4–6 weeks total depending on goals

ENERGY SYSTEMS DEVELOPMENT

Proper development of energy systems serves as the metabolic foundation for all other athletic efforts, providing the physiological backing for the repeated efforts needed during sports training and competition. Therefore, Sports Performance Coaches must systematically develop cardiovascular (metabolic) training programs to optimize the energy systems. For athletes participating in endurance sports, aerobic endurance is the key to success. For athletes participating in team sports, there tends to be a minimum threshold for aerobic capacity required to support the anaerobic side of metabolism, which is often termed "repeated sprint ability." Most athletes in team sports will need to express high-intensity efforts repeatedly throughout a competition, necessitating some endurance training in their training program.

Sports Performance Coaches must understand that optimal energy system development results in increased performance in all sports. Energy systems development offers the following benefits:

- Increased stroke volume and cardiac output
- Improved gas exchange, decreased airway resistance, and improved oxygen uptake
- Decreased blood flow resistance and increased blood volume
- Enhanced overall athletic performance and recovery
- Decreased risk of acute fatigue, overtraining, and associated injuries (Anderson et al., 2016; Garber et al., 2011).

STAGE TRAINING

As discussed in Chapter 16, NASM recommends using a five-stage programming system with four intensity zones for training. Stage training organizes training strategies into a progressive sequence of training tactics. The Sports Performance Coach can utilize the talk test, rating of perceived exertion (RPE), or heart rate based on VT1 and VT2 testing values to monitor training intensity. Energy systems development should always be individualized and based on the metabolic demands of the specific sport. When developing a metabolic conditioning program, the athlete's aerobic capacity should determine where they begin. For example, a well-conditioned athlete (i.e., performed well on aerobic tests) can begin at higher stages. In contrast, a less well-conditioned athlete will begin at lower stages.

From a general perspective, the goals of stage training align with the primary objectives of traditional periodization and the OPT Model (**Table 19.47**). For example, when beginning in the general preparatory phase, the athlete will focus on improving muscular endurance and joint stabilization (i.e., Phase 1 of the OPT Model). At the same time, they begin in Stage 1 to develop or improve aerobic endurance. When considering the specifics of energy systems, Phase 1 training includes low-intensity, high-repetition work that primarily utilizes the oxidative pathway. Similarly, Stage 1 includes lower- to moderate-intensity work primarily utilizing the oxidative pathway. These similarities continue throughout the OPT Model. Nevertheless, this is not a hard-fast rule; the results of the testing should determine where an athlete begins.

TABLE 19.47 Periodization and Stage Training

Periodization Phase	Stage Training
Preparatory phase (general and specific preparatory phase)	Stage 1: aerobic endurance
	Stage 2: increased work capacity/workload
	Stage 3: progresses to a higher percentage of competition intensity, increased anaerobic power, and power endurance
Competition phase	Stage 4: additional increases in intensity to maximize anaerobic power and power endurance
	Stage 5: sports-specific drills and skill work done at competition intensity
Transition phase	Stage 1: recovery/active rest periods

DESIGNING A STABILIZATION-LEVEL METABOLIC CONDITIONING PROGRAM

Recall that the stabilization level of the OPT Model has the primary goals of improving foundational levels of stabilization strength, postural control, and muscular and aerobic endurance. This level most closely aligns with the active recovery and general preparatory phase. Therefore, metabolic conditioning focused on the development or improvement of aerobic endurance could benefit athletes at this training level. If utilizing Stage 1, the Sports Performance Coach could program a basic training schedule designed to improve aerobic endurance and facilitate recovery (**Table 19.48**).

TABLE 19.48 Stage 1 Metabolic Training Example

Steady-State Training	Modality	Zone 1 (Light to Moderate)
Warm-up	Walk on treadmill	5–10 minutes
Workout	Light jog on treadmill	40 minutes of Zone 1 staying below VT1
Cool-down	Walk on treadmill	5–10 minutes

The Sports Performance Coach should also recognize that appropriate aerobic adaptations can be achieved within a resistance training session when utilizing the OPT Model correctly. For example, if using vertical loading (i.e., circuit training), the athlete can stay within the recommended VT1 (**Table 19.49**). When using resistance training in this manner, the Sports Performance Coach must use the intensity of the load (i.e., level of resistance) to control the training zone.

TABLE 19.49 Stage 1 Circuit Training Example

Steady-State Training	Modality	Sets × Reps	Tempo	Rest	Zone 1 (Light to Moderate)
Warm-up	Core, balance, and plyometric circuit	2 × 12	Slow, controlled	No rest between exercises; 30–60 seconds between sets	5–10 minutes
Workout	Squat to row Step-up to scaption raise Stability ball dumbbell press Lateral lunge to overhead press Single-leg curl Prone stability ball triceps extension	3 × 15	4/2/1/1		40 minutes of Zone 1 staying below VT1
Cool-down	Walk on treadmill				5–10 minutes

The Sports Performance Coach may also integrate Stage 2 training with the stabilization level. Stage 2 progresses with more interval training and increased volume (**Table 19.50**).

DESIGNING A STRENGTH-LEVEL METABOLIC CONDITIONING PROGRAM

Recall that the strength level's primary focuses include endurance, muscular development, and maximal strength. This level most closely aligns with the ending weeks of the general preparatory phase and progressing into the specific preparatory phase. Therefore, metabolic conditioning can improve work capacity and workload (Stage 2), progress to

TABLE 19.50 Stage 2 Metabolic Training Example

Steady-State Training	Modality	Zone 1 (Light to Moderate)	Zone 2 (Challenging, Hard)
Warm-up	Walk on treadmill	5–10 minutes	
Workout	Interval: light jog on treadmill Recovery: walk on treadmill Repeat 4 times	1 minute at Zone 2, just above VT1 3 minutes at Zone 1, below VT1	
Cool-down	Walk on treadmill	5–10 minutes	

a higher percentage of competition intensity, and increase anaerobic power and power endurance (Stage 3). In addition, the Sports Performance Coach should recognize that the development of anaerobic power and power endurance provide an advantage to the athlete who is focused on muscular development and maximal strength. Therefore, the Sports Performance Coach could design a training program emphasizing these aspects (**Table 19.51**).

TABLE 19.51 Stage 3 Metabolic Training Example

Steady-State Training	Modality	Zone 1 (Light to Moderate)	Zone 2 (Challenging, Hard)	Zone 3 (Vigorous, Very Hard)
Warm-up	Walk on treadmill	5–10 minutes		
Workout	Interval: jog/run on treadmill Recovery: light jog on treadmill Repeat 3–4 times	Gradually increase intensity over 2 minutes, reaching Zone 3 for the last 40–45 seconds, staying below VT2 for each interval 1-minute recovery in Zone 2		
Cool-down	Walk on treadmill	5–10 minutes		

Within the strength level—specifically, Phase 2 of the OPT Model—the Sports Performance Coach can take advantage of the supersets used during resistance training to achieve similar metabolic adaptations as Stage 2 cardiorespiratory training (**Table 19.52**). Note, however, that the second exercise in the superset is performed at a lower (i.e., recovery) intensity.

Using a resistance training circuit to match Stage 3 training presents some challenges. However, the Sports Performance Coach may include it if the athlete has limited time or other hurdles prevent them from undertaking specific metabolic conditioning. The example in **Table 19.53** uses a Phase 3 resistance training program.

DESIGNING A POWER-LEVEL METABOLIC CONDITIONING PROGRAM

The OPT Model's power level primarily aims to improve the force production rate, thereby enhancing power output. Increasing power results from increasing the velocity of a

TABLE 19.52 Stage 2 Circuit Training Example

Steady-State Training	Modality	Sets × Reps	Tempo	Rest	Zone 1 (Light to Moderate)	Zone 2 (Challenging, Hard)
Warm-up	Core, balance, and plyometric circuit	2 × 10	Medium, controlled	No rest between exercises; 30–60 seconds between sets	5–10 minutes	
Workout	• Seated military press	3 × 10	2/0/2/0			First exercise in steady state: 1 minute at Zone 2, just above VT1
	• Single-leg scaption raise	3 × 10	4/2/1/1			Second exercise in steady state: 2 minutes at Zone 1, below VT1
	• Barbell squat	3 × 10	2/0/2/0			
	• Lateral lunge	3 × 10	4/2/1/1			
	• Seated cable row	3 × 10	2/0/2/0			
	• Bent-over single-arm dumbbell row	3 × 10	4/2/1/1			
Cool-down	Walk on treadmill				5–10 minutes	

TABLE 19.53 Stage 3 Circuit Training Example

Steady-State Training	Modality	Sets × Reps	Tempo	Rest	Zone 1 (Light to Moderate)	Zone 2 (Challenging, Hard)	Zone 3 (Vigorous, Very Hard)
Warm-up	Core, balance, and plyometric circuit	2 × 10	Medium, controlled	No rest between exercises; 30–60 seconds between sets	5–10 minutes		
Workout	Seated military press Barbell squat Bent-over barbell row Barbell bench press	4 × 8	2/0/2/0	60 seconds between exercises and sets	At higher training intensities, the athlete should reach Zone 3 for the last 10 seconds of each set, staying below VT2 1-minute recovery in Zone 2		
Cool-down	Walk on treadmill				5–10 minutes		

contraction or increasing force. Optimizing power development requires athletes to train with heavy loads or at high speeds. Both require the rapid production of ATP, which is enhanced through Stage 4 and 5 training. Therefore, the Sports Performance Coach could design a training program focused on these aspects (**Table 19.54**).

TABLE 19.54 Stage 4 Metabolic Training Example

Steady-State Training	Modality	Zone 1 (Light to Moderate)	Zone 2 (Challenging, Hard)	Zone 3 (Vigorous, Very Hard)	Zone 4 (Very Hard, Maximum Effort)
Warm-up	Walk on treadmill	5–10 minutes			
Workout	Interval: run/maximum sprint on treadmill Recovery: light jog/walk on treadmill Repeat 5 times	Interval: gradually increase the intensity from Zone 1 to Zone 4, with 45–60 seconds spent in Zones 1–3 and 10–15 seconds above VT2 in Zone 4 2-minute recovery in Zone 1			
Cool-down	Walk on treadmill	5–10 minutes			

As in Stage 3, using a resistance training circuit to match Stage 4 training recommendations presents some challenges. However, the Sports Performance Coach may include it if the athlete has limited time or other hurdles prevent them from undertaking specific metabolic conditioning. The example in **Table 19.55** uses a Phase 5 resistance training program.

TABLE 19.55 Stage 4 Circuit Training Example

Steady-State Training	Modality	Sets × Reps	Tempo	Rest	Zone 1 (Light to Moderate)	Zone 2 (Challenging, Hard)	Zone 3 (Vigorous, Very Hard)	Zone 4 (Very Hard, Maximum Effort)
Warm-up	Core, balance, and plyometric circuit	2 × 10	Medium/controlled	No rest between exercises; 30–60 seconds between sets	5–10 minutes			
Workout	• Barbell squat • Squat jump • Bent-over barbell row • Medicine ball slam • Barbell bench press • Plyometric push-up	4 × 10 4 × 10 4 × 10 4 × 10 4 × 10 4 × 10	As fast as can be controlled	No rest between supersets 1–2 minutes between exercise or 3 minutes between sets	The combination of maximum load and maximum velocity of the supersets should reach Zone 4 for the last 10 seconds of each set; above VT2 2-minute recovery in Zone 2			
Cool-down	Walk on treadmill				5–10 minutes			

Small-Sided Games

The Sports Performance Coach can integrate Stage 5 metabolic conditioning into the power level. Recall that Stage 5 focuses on sport-specific drills and skill work at actual competition levels. Therefore, the inclusion of well-designed small-sided games would be appropriate.

🤖 GETTING TECHNICAL

The play pattern in small-sided games influences the physiological stimuli and adaptations. Hauer et al. (2018) compared heart rate responses and aerobic capacity improvements in lacrosse players during intermittent and continuous small-sided games. One group participated in 4-minute games with 3-minute active recovery periods, while another group played for 25 continuous minutes. The intermittent group spent more time in lower heart rate zones (less than 85% HR_{max}), while the continuous group spent more time in the highest zone (more than 90% HR_{max}). Both groups showed similar performance improvements on the yo-yo intermittent shuttle test. Thus, both intermittent and continuous small-sided game formats appear to effectively improve aerobic capacity.

LESSON 4: DEVELOPING A TRAINING PROGRAM
THE PROGRAMMING PROCESS

Athletes at all levels have different desires and needs based on various factors. The Sports Performance Coach must thoroughly understand the integrated training components discussed in this chapter to ensure that programming for the individual athlete is tailored appropriately. In addition, the coach must incorporate the information provided in the needs analysis and performance testing into the daily, weekly, and monthly program design.

NEEDS ANALYSIS

Every athlete will have specific needs based on their unique abilities as an athlete combined with their specific sport. For example, a younger athlete may need more foundational training to increase maximal strength compared to an athlete with a higher training age who has already developed above-average base levels of strength. The difference between an athlete who has participated in ballistic strength training (e.g., Olympic lifting, plyometrics) and an athlete who has participated only in their sport is profound. Even athletes with an advanced training age may have skipped over certain aspects of training. For example, an athlete who is fast because of their dedication to sprint training may not have completed strength and power training, possibly leaving performance improvements yet to be realized. Chapter 7 reviews the needs analysis in detail.

Each sport has unique requirements for the exact expression of performance attributes. For example, the curvilinear speed required by a baseball runner rounding second base is quite different than the accelerative speed necessary for a soccer goalie moving across

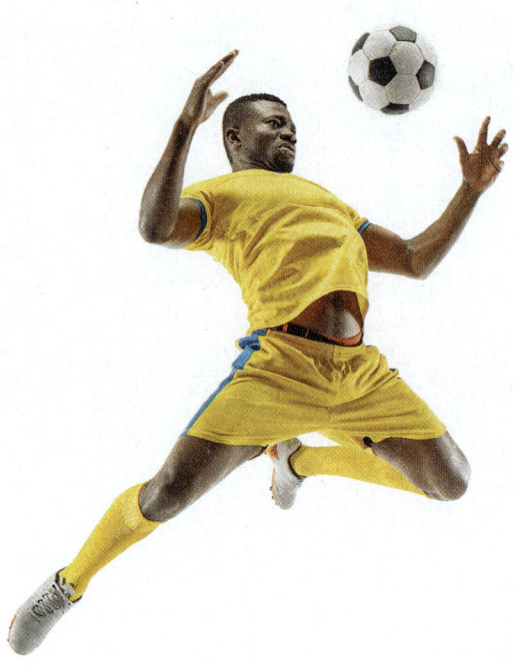

© Master1305/Shutterstock

the goal face to make a play on a shot. In the former case, the sagittal plane is dominant, whereas the latter is likely to require a greater inclusion of movement in the frontal plane. Similarly, the vertical power required for a basketball or volleyball athlete to jump for a shot or spike differs from the horizontal and lateral power a lacrosse goalie needs to step into a save.

Even if movements are similar, a sport's relative work-to-rest ratios may differ from those in other sports. For example, the intermittent nature of tennis or volleyball is different than the more continuous nature of a sport like field hockey, which is far different than the concentrated loads of ice hockey, despite the recovery time between shifts. When analyzing a sport, key aspects of movement should be considered, such as the planes of motion, the direction of movement, the biomechanical attributes, and the pattern of play.

PERFORMANCE TESTING

Many methods exist to assess an athlete's ability to produce power and speed. To ensure the needs analysis reveals truly valuable information, the Sports Performance Coach should select an assessment that mimics the needs of the sport as closely as possible during testing. For example, basketball and volleyball players can often benefit from increased jump height. Thus, the Sports Performance Coach needs to include tests that measure lower-extremity power production for these athletes. Further, athletes in almost all sports, including soccer, tennis, and football, can benefit from improved cutting and acceleration ability, so the coach should include tests that measure agility, quickness, and acceleration. Refer to Chapter 8 for more information on performance testing.

Sports Performance Coaches should familiarize themselves with the characteristics of each sport to have a more thorough understanding of the performance tests needed. For example, sports that include sprinting, running, jumping, cutting, or any lower-body power production require significant gluteus maximus strength. Therefore, testing the gluteus maximus is important for athletes in such sports. Various assessments and tests can be used for the gluteus maximus, such as the overhead squat, single-leg squat, 3 to 5 reps maximum squat, or the vertical jump.

Acceleration to top speed is also vital to success as an athlete. Most athletes will be able to reach top speed within 40 yards, making this distance a popular test in sports such as football (Clark et al., 2019). However, the greatest acceleration comes from the first half of efforts over the longer distance, so split times are also often employed. For example, a coach could measure the times at 5, 10, 20, and 40 yards to determine if an athlete has appropriate acceleration ability compared to their overall time and top speed. As most athletes in team sports accelerate within a span of 20 meters or so (Rumpf et al., 2016), most speed-based performance testing does not require use of long distances. However, coaches in some sports may consider looking at an athlete's ability to sustain top speed over a longer duration. For example, it is possible (though rare) for a football or a soccer athlete to sprint for 100 yards, so a 100-yard sprint test may be useful.

Other sports may select less conventional distances that focus more intently on acceleration, such as a baseball team selecting the 30 yards between bases as a sport-specific testing protocol. Similarly, hockey athletes often use the distance from blue line to blue line (approximately 17 yards) as a sport-specific sprint distance (Peterson et al., 2015). It is sensible for coaches to select testing protocols with distances that match the characteristics of athlete requirements during competition.

The ability to accelerate or hit top speed is important for many sports, but other sports require more consistent efforts; thus, repeated sprint ability may be tested in the latter sports. Many different iterations have been used to test repeated sprint ability. For example, a testing design of 12 × 20 meters, with 20 seconds of recovery, has been applied to young basketball and rugby athletes, among others (Johnston & Gabbett, 2011; Meckel et al., 2009). A fatigue index can be used to determine the drop-off in speed from the first sprint to the last. Ideally, the athlete will maintain their speed through the last rep. However, accumulating fatigue generally does not allow this to happen, as the test is designed to push the boundaries of glycolysis and will require increased contributions from aerobic metabolism with subsequent sprints (Girard et al., 2011). Sport performance coaches can use assessments of repeated sprint ability to distinguish between speed and endurance. In summary, each test selected should cover a vital biomotor ability such that the combination of all test results gives a comprehensive performance profile for each athlete.

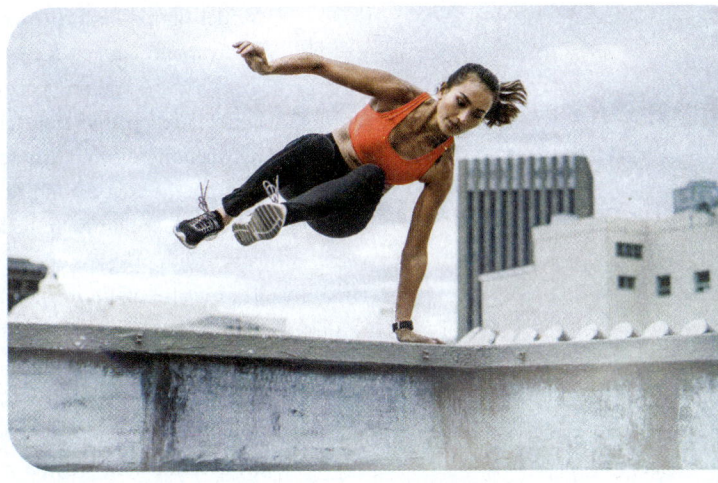
© Jacob Lund/Shutterstock

PROGRAM DESIGN

First and foremost, the Sports Performance Coach must understand that program design is guided by the needs analysis, assessments, and performance testing. The Sports Performance Coach must use the needs analysis to explore the demands of the sport as well as additional tests required for participation. For example, the National Football League uses the bench press test to measure strength and endurance. Therefore, the coach must integrate this skill into programming at some point in the athlete's training. As explained in Chapter 8, performance tests can serve two purposes: (1) to identify an athlete's strengths and weaknesses, and (2) to serve as an objective measure of improvement.

Movement assessments must also be considered. In many cases, the results of the movement assessments take priority over performance testing. An athlete who demonstrates movement compensations cannot be expected to perform at their best due to postural malalignments. Therefore, the Sports Performance Coach must program for the movement pattern before focusing on improvements in any specific performance test. However, performance on tests is likely to improve along with improvement in movement patterns due to increased movement efficiency.

The Sports Performance Coach should use the OPT Model as a framework for programming that guides the selection of acute training variables, progressions and regressions, and exercise choice. The OPT Model should be viewed as a comprehensive system that takes the guesswork out of the programming process. The Sports Performance Coach is encouraged to view this model holistically, understanding that it is adaptable to each athlete and each situation. While the OPT Model fits nicely into traditional linear periodization, it is flexible enough to be used for almost any periodization model.

SUMMARY

Coaches and athletes must dedicate themselves to improving foundational biomotor abilities such as strength, power, speed, and endurance to maximize performance. Without a fitness foundation, sport-specific requirements may be limited. To develop targeted biomotor abilities, athletes can participate in advanced training programs that progressively enhance the training stimuli. By following periodization principles and utilizing an integrated training model, such as NASM's OPT

Model, Sports Performance Coaches can structure training programs to enhance athletes' sports performance and efficacy.

With any training program, the Sports Performance Coach must be consistently aware of the anticipated positive transfer of biomotor development to sport-specific skills. The direct connection between these two attributes can be determined by the needs analysis and monitored regularly using a comprehensive testing battery. The performance tests selected should provide a complete picture of the athlete's abilities in the areas most relevant to their sport. In addition, regular testing provides the coach with progress checks to ensure that the method of programming and periodization is effective. Testing also offers an effective way to individualize training programs based on the specific needs and weaknesses of every athlete.

The information presented in this chapter provides the Sports Performance Coach with the tools necessary to understand why the fundamental biomotor abilities create the foundation of athletic ability and how these abilities can be targeted through intentional training. Many methods are available that provide various options to fit the unique demands of any athlete for any sport. Although certain principles are relatively universal, their specific applications will vary. Ultimately, coaches are responsible for understanding the fundamental aspects of fitness, weighing their training options to target these aspects, and implementing the best program possible to elicit the highest levels of adaptation and performance for athletes.

KEY TAKEAWAYS

- Biomotor abilities such as strength, power, speed, and agility are the foundational skills on which performance programs are built.
- Acute training variables are vital for the Sports Performance Coach to understand because they determine the stresses applied to the athlete and direct the training outcomes.
- The Sports Performance Coach must understand each acute training variable's direct or inverse relationship with the other variables. For example, intensity is inversely related to reps, but is directly related to the rest period. In other words, as intensity increases, reps decrease and rest periods increase.
- Athletic performance relies on human movement science and periodization, a structured training approach designed to elicit specific adaptations at precise points in an athlete's training program.
- The OPT Model provides an easy-to-follow framework for program design that can align with various periodization models.
- The OPT Model combines all forms of physical training into one integrated system to improve overall performance, health, and wellness without compromising the athlete's safety, ethics, or integrity.
- Benefits of integrated training programs include psychological improvements such as better mood and sleep, physiological benefits such as enhanced cardiovascular and endocrine functionality, performance enhancements such as improved strength and endurance, and safety aspects such as reducing the risk of overtraining or undertraining.
- Day-to-day programming decisions for training methods should be determined by the overarching structure of the goals for a long-term program, which can be defined through periodized models.
- Programming is integral to periodization; it involves micro-level decisions that apply stressors to help athletes achieve adaptations safely on a daily or weekly basis.
- Athletes' specific training needs will depend on their unique abilities and their specific sport. Recognizing this allows for more personalized and effective training programs that address gaps in athletes' existing training or skills.

REFERENCES

Anderson, K. & Behm, D.G. (2005). The impact of instability resistance training on balance and stability. *Sports Medicine, 35*(1), 43–53.

Anderson, L., Thompson, D. R., Oldridge, N., Zwisler, A.-D., Rees, K., Martin, N., & Taylor, R. S. (2016). Exercise-based cardiac rehabilitation for coronary heart disease. *Cochrane Database of Systematic Reviews, 1,* CD001800. https://doi.org/10.1002/14651858.cd001800.pub3

Azegami, M., Ohira, M., Miyoshi, K., Kobayashi, C, Hongo, M., Yanagihashi, R., Sadoyama, T. (2007). Effect of single and multi-joint lower extremity muscle strength on the functional capacity and ADL/IADL status in Japanese community-dwelling older adults. *Nursing & Health Sciences, 9*(3), 168–176.

Baz-Valle, E., Fontes-Villalba, M., & Santos-Concejero, J. (2018). Total number of sets as a training volume quantification method for muscle hypertrophy: A systematic review. *Journal of Strength and Conditioning Research, 35*(3), 870–878.

Behm, D. G. (1995). Neuromuscular implications and applications of resistance training. *Journal of Strength and Conditioning Research, 9*(4), 264–274.

Behm, D. G., & Anderson, K. G. (2006). The role of instability with resistance training. *Journal of Strength and Conditioning Research, 20*(3), 716–722.

Behm, D. G., Anderson, K., & Curnew, R. S. (2002). Muscle force and activation under stable and unstable conditions. *Journal of Strength and Conditioning Research, 16*(3), 416–422. https://doi.org /10.1519 /1533-4287(2002)0162.0.co;2

Behm, D. G., Blazevich, A. J., Kay, A. D., & McHugh, M. (2016). Acute effects of muscle stretching on physical performance, range of motion, and injury incidence in healthy active individuals: A systematic review. *Applied Physiology, Nutrition, and Metabolism, 41*(1), 1–11. https://doi.org/10.1139/apnm-2015-0235

Bellows, R., & Wong, C. K. (2018). The effect of bracing and balance training on ankle sprain incidence among athletes: A systematic review with meta-analysis. *International Journal of Sports Physical Therapy, 13*(3), 379–388. https://doi.org/10.26603/ijspt20180379

Bompa, T. O., & Calcina, O. (1993). *Periodization of strength: The new wave in strength training.* Veritas.

Cahill, M. J., Oliver, J. L., Cronin, J. B., Clark, K., Cross, M. R., Lloyd, R. S., & Lee, J. E. (2020). Influence of resisted sled-pull training on the sprint force-velocity profile of male high-school athletes. *Journal of Strength and Conditioning Research, 34*(10), 2751–2759. https://doi.org/10.1519/JSC.0000000000003770

Callesen, J. L., Brincks, J., Cattaneo, D., & Dalgas, U. (2018). How does strength training and balance training affect gait and fatigue in patients with multiple sclerosis? A study protocol of a randomized controlled trial. *NeuroRehabilitation, 42*(2), 131–142. https://doi.org/10.3233/NRE-172238

Campos, G. E. R., Luecke, T. J., Wendeln, H. K., Toma, K., Hagerman, F. C., Murray, T. F., Ragg, K. E., Ratamess, N. A., Kraemer, W. J., & Staron, R. S. (2002). Muscular adaptations in response to three different resistance-training regimens: Specificity of repetition maximum training zones. *European Journal of Applied Physiology, 88*(1), 50–60.

Chen, Y.-T., Hsieh, Y.-Y., Ho, J.-Y., Lin, T.-Y., & Lin, J.-C. (2022). Two weeks of detraining reduces cardiopulmonary function and muscular fitness in endurance athletes. *European Journal of Sport Science, 22*(3), 399–406. https://doi.org/10.1080/17461391.2021.1880647

Chandler, T. J., & Brown, L. E. (2019). *Conditioning for strength and human performance* (3rd ed.).

Chandrakumar, N., & Ramesh, C. (2015). Effect of ladder drill and SAQ training on speed and agility among sports club badminton players. *International Journal of Applied Research, 1*(12), 527–529. https://www .allresearchjournal.com/archives/?year=2015&vol=1&issue=12&part=H&ArticleId=1129

Clark, D. R., Lambert, M. I., & Hunter, A. M. (2018). Contemporary perspectives of core stability training for dynamic athletic performance: A survey of athletes, coaches, sports science and sports medicine practitioners. *Sports Medicine - Open, 4*(1), 32. https://doi.org/10.1186/s40798-018-0150-3

Clark, K., Cahill, M., Korfist, C., & Whitacre, T. (2021). Acute kinematic effects of sprinting with motorized assistance. *Journal of Strength and Conditioning Research, 35*(7), 1856–1864. https://doi.org/10.1519 /JSC.0000000000003051

Clark, K. P., Rieger, R. H., Bruno, R. F., & Stearne, D. J. (2019). The National Football League combine 40-yd dash: How important is maximum velocity? *Journal of Strength and Conditioning Research, 33*(6), 1542–1550.

Cressey, E. M., West, C. A., Tiberio, D. P., Kraemer, W. J., & Maresh, C. M. (2007). Unstable surface training on markers of athletic performance. *Journal of Strength and Conditioning Research, 21*(2), 561–567.

De Salles, B. F., Simão, R., Miranda, F., Da Silva Novaes, J., Lemos, A., & Willardson, J. M. (2009). Rest interval between sets in strength training: *Sports Medicine, 39*(9), 765–777. https://doi.org/10.2165 /11315230-000000000-00000

Dideriksen, J. L., Del Vecchio, A., & Farina, D. (2020). Neural and muscular determinants of maximal rate of force development. *Journal of Neurophysiology, 123*(1), 149–157. https://doi.org/10.1152/jn.00330.2019

DiStefano, L. J., Clark, M. A., & Padua, D. A. (2009). Evidence supporting balance training in healthy individuals: A systemic review. *Journal of Strength and Conditioning Research, 23*(9), 2718–2731. https://doi.org/10.1519 /jsc.0b013e3181c1f7c5

DiStefano, L. J., DiStefano, M. J., Frank, B. S., Clark, M. A., & Padua, D. A. (2013). Comparison of integrated and isolated training on performance measures and neuromuscular control. *Journal of Strength and Conditioning Research, 27*(4), 1083–1090. https://doi.org/10.1519/jsc.0b013e318280d40b

dos Santos, W. D. N., Gentil, P., de Moraes, R. F., Junior, J. B. F., Campos, M. H., de Lira, C. A. B., Junior, R. F., Bottaro, M., & Vieira, C. A. (2017). Chronic effects of resistance training in breast cancer survivors. *BioMed Research International, 2017*, 1–18.

Ebben, W. P., & Blackard, D. O. (1997). Complex training with combined explosive weight and plyometric exercises. *Olympic Coach, 7*(4), 11–12.

Fairall, R. R., Cabell, L., Boergers, R .J., & Battaglia, F. (2017). Acute effects of self-myofascial release and stretching in overhead athletes with GIRD. *Journal of Bodywork and Movement Therapies, 21*(3), 648–652. https://doi.org/10.1016/j.jbmt.2017.04.001

Fitts, R. H. (1994). Cellular mechanism of muscle fatigue. *Physiology Reviews, 74*(1), 49–94.

Fleck, S. J., & Kraemer, W. J. (2014). *Designing resistance training programs* (4th ed.). Human Kinetics.

Garber, C. E., Blissmer, B., Deschenes, M. R., Franklin, B. A., Lamonte, M. J., Lee, I.-M., Neiman, D. C., & Swain, D. P. (2011). Quantity and quality of exercise for developing and maintaining cardiorespiratory, musculoskeletal, and neuromotor fitness in apparently healthy adults: Guidance for prescribing exercise. *Medicine & Science in Sports & Exercise, 43*(7), 1334–1359. https://doi.org/10.1249/MSS.0b013e318213fefb

Girard, O., Mendez-Villanueva, A., & Bishop, D. (2011). Repeated-sprint ability: Part I. *Sports Medicine, 41*(8), 673–694.

Grgic, J., & Schoenfeld, B. J. (2018). Are the hypertrophic adaptations to high and low-load resistance training muscle fiber type specific? *Frontier Physiology, 9*(402), 1–6.

Häkkinen, K. (1994). Neuromuscular adaptation during strength training, ageing, detraining, and immobilization. *Critical Reviews in Physical and Rehabilitation Medicine, 14*(1994), 161–198.

Harris, G. R., Stone, M. H., O'Bryant, H. S., Proulx, C. M., & Johnson, R. L. (2000). Short-term performance effects of high power, high force, or combined weight-training methods. *Journal of Strength and Conditioning Research, 14*(1), 14–20.

Hatfield, D. L., Kraemer, W. J., Spiering, B. A., Häkkinen, K., Volek, J. S., Shimano, T., Spreuwenberg, L. P. B., Silvestre, R., Vingren, J. L., Fragala, M. S., Gómez, A. L., Fleck, S. J., Newton, R. U., & Maresh, C. M. (2006). The impact of velocity of movement on performance factors in resistance exercise. *Journal of Strength and Conditioning Research, 20*(4), 760–766.

Hauer, R., Tessitore, A., Binder, N., & Tschan, H. (2018). Physiological, perceptual, and technical responses to continuous and intermittent small-sided games in lacrosse players. *PloS One, 13*(10), e0203832.

Hernandez, D. J., Healy, S., Giacomini, M. L., & Kwon, Y. S. (2021). Effect of rest interval duration on the volume completed during a high-intensity bench press exercise. *Journal of Strength and Conditioning Research, 35*(11), 2981–2987. https://doi.org/10.1519/JSC.0000000000003477

Johnston, R. D., & Gabbett, T. J. (2011). Repeated-sprint and effort ability in rugby league players. *Journal of Strength and Conditioning Research, 25*(10), 2789–2795.

Kornecki, S., Kebel, A., & Siemieński, A. (2001). Muscular co-operation during joint stabilization, as reflected by EMG. *European Journal of Applied Physiology, 84*(5), 453–461.

Kraemer, W. J., Ratamess, N., & Fry, A. C. (2000). Influence of resistance training volume and periodization on physiological and performance adaptations in collegiate women tennis players. *American Journal of Sports Medicine, 28*(5), 626–633.

Kristensen, J., & Franklyn-Miller, A. (2011). Resistance training in musculoskeletal rehabilitation: A systematic review. *British Journal of Sports Medicine, 46*(10), 719–726. https://doi.org/10.1136/bjsm.2010.079376

Lesinski, M., Hortobagyi, T., Muehlbauer, T., Gollhofer, A., & Granacher, U. (2015). Effects of balance training on balance performance in healthy older adults: A systematic review and meta-analysis. *Sports Medicine, 45*(12), 1721–1738. https://doi.org/10.1007/s40279-015-0375-y

Longo, A. R., Silva-Batista, C., Pedroso, K., de Salles Painelli, V., Lasevicius, T., Schoenfeld, B. J., Aihara, A. Y., de Almeida Peres, B., Tricoli, V., & Teixeira, E. L. (2022). Volume load rather than resting interval influences muscle hypertrophy during high-intensity resistance training. *Journal of Strength and Conditioning Research, 36*(6), 1554–1559. https://doi.org/10.1519/JSC.0000000000003668

Manchado, C., Garcia-Ruiz, J., Cortell-Tormo, J. M., & TortosaMartinez, J. (2017). Effect of core training on male handball players' throwing velocity. *Journal of Human Kinetics, 56*(1), 177–185. https://www.ncbi.nlm.nih.gov/pmc/articles/PMC5384065

Mansur, M., Irianto, S., & Kurniawan, F. (2018). The effect of plyometric training to speed of volleyball athletes. *Advances in Social Science, Education and Humanities Research, 278*, 357–358. https://doi.org/10.2991/yishpess-cois-18.2018.88

Matavulj, D., Kukolj, M., Ugarkovic, D., Tihanyi, J., & Jaric, S. (2001). Effects of plyometric training on jumping performance in junior basketball players. *Journal of Sports Medicine and Physical Fitness, 41*(2), 159–164.

Meckel, Y., Gottlieb, R., & Eliakim, A. (2009). Repeated sprint tests in young basketball players at different game stages. *European Journal of Applied Physiology, 107*(3), 273–279.

Mohr, A. R., Long, B. C., & Goad, C. L. (2014). Effect of foam rolling and static stretching on passive hip-flexion range of motion. *Journal of Sport Rehabilitation, 23*(4), 296–299. https://doi.org/10.1123/jsr.2013-0025

Newton, R. U., Häkkinen, K., Hakkinen, A., McCormick, M., Volek, J., & Kraemer, W. J. (2002). Mixed-methods resistance training increases power and strength of young and older men. *Medicine and Science in Sports and Exercise, 34*(8), 1367–1375.

Ogita, F., Stam, R. P., Tazawa, H. O., Toussaint, H. M., & Hollander, A. P. (2000). Oxygen uptake in one-legged and two-legged exercise. *Medicine and Science in Sports and Exercise, 32*(10), 1737–1742.

Oliva-Lozano, J. M., & Muyor, J. M. (2020). Core muscle activity during physical fitness exercises: A systematic review. *International Journal of Environmental Research and Public Health, 17*(12), 4306. https://doi.org/10.3390/ijerph17124306

Opplert, J., & Babault, N. (2018). Flexibility and performance: An analysis of the current literature. *Sports Medicine, 48*, 299–325.

Peterson, B. J., Fitzgerald, J. S., Dietz, C. C., Ziegler, K. S., Ingraham, S. J., Baker, S. E., & Snyder, E. M. (2015). Division I hockey players generate more power than Division III players during on-and off-ice performance tests. *Journal of Strength and Conditioning Research, 29*(5), 1191–1196.

Peterson, M. D., Rhea, M. R., & Alvar, B. A. (2004). Maximizing strength development in athletes: A meta-analysis to determine the dose–response relationship. *Journal of Strength and Conditioning Research, 18*(2), 377–382.

Rahimi, R., Qaderi, M., Faraji, H., & Boroujerdi, S. S. (2010). Effects of very short rest periods on hormonal responses to resistance exercise in men. *Journal of Strength and Conditioning Research, 24*(7), 1851–1859. https://doi.org/10.1519/JSC.0b013e3181ddb265

Ramirez-Campillo, R., Henriquez-Olguin, C., Burgos, C., Andrade, D. C., Martinez, C., Alvarez, C., Baez, E. I., Castro-Sepúlveda, M., Peñailillo, L., & Izquierdo, M. (2015). Effect of progressive volume-based overload during plyometric training on explosive and endurance performance in young soccer players. *Journal of Strength and Conditioning Research, 29*(7), 1884–1893. https://doi.org/10.1519/JSC.0000000000000836

Ratamess, N. A., Alvar, B. A., Evetoch, T. K., Housh, T. J., Kibler, W. B., Kraemer, W. J., & Triplett, N. T. (2009). American College of Sports Medicine position stand: Progressive models in resistance training for healthy adults. *Medicine and Science in Sports and Exercise, 41*(3), 687–708.

Rhea, M. R., Alvar, B. A., Burkett, L. N., & Ball, S. D. (2003). A meta-analysis to determine the dose response for strength development. *Medicine and Science in Sports and Exercise, 35*(3), 456–464.

Rumpf, M. C., Lockie, R. G., Cronin, J. B., & Jalilvand, F. (2016). Effect of different sprint training methods on sprint performance over various distances: A brief review. *Journal of Strength and Conditioning Research, 30*(6), 1767–1785.

Saunders, P. U., Telford, R. D., Pyne, D. B., Peltola, E. M., Cunningham, R. B., Gore, C. J., & Hawley, J. A. (2006). Short-term plyometric training improves running economy in highly trained middle and long distance runners. *Journal of Strength and Conditioning Research, 20*(4), 947–954.

Schoenfeld, B. J., Ogborn, D., & Krieger, J. W. (2017). Dose–response relationship between weekly resistance training volume and increases in muscle mass: A systematic review and meta-analysis. *Journal of Sports Science, 35*(11), 1073–1082.

Schoenfeld, B. J., Wilson, J. M., Lowery, R. P., & Krieger, J. W. (2016). Muscular adaptations in low- versus high-load resistance training: A meta-analysis. *European Journal of Sport Science, 16*(1), 1–10. https://doi.org/10.1080/17461391.2014.989922

Škarabot, J., Beardsley, C., & Štirn, I. (2015). Comparing the effects of self-myofascial release with static stretching on ankle range-of-motion in adolescent athletes. *International Journal of Sports Physical Therapy, 10*(2), 203–212.

Suchomel, T. J., Nimphius, S., & Stone, M. H. (2016). The importance of muscular strength in athletic performance. *Sports Medicine, 46*(10), 1419–1449.

Tan, B. (1999). Manipulating resistance training program variables to optimize maximum strength in men: A review. *Journal of Strength and Conditioning Research, 13*(3), 289–304.

Vesci, A. S., Webster, K. A., Sich, M., & Marinko, L. N. (2017). Resistance training in youth improves athletic performance: A systematic review. *Athletic Training & Sports Health Care, 9*(4), 184–192. https://doi.org/10.3928/19425864-20170504-01

Williford, H. N., Olson, M. S., Gauger, S., Duey, W. J., & Blessing, D. L. (1998). Cardiovascular and metabolic costs of forward, backward, and lateral motion. *Medicine and Science in Sports and Exercise, 30*(9), 1419–1423.

Yanghattee, J., & Srihirun, K. (2021). The effect of complex training with barbell thruster and medicine ball wood chop on Ippon-Seoinage throwing performance in male judo players. *JEPonline, 24*(5), 1–9.

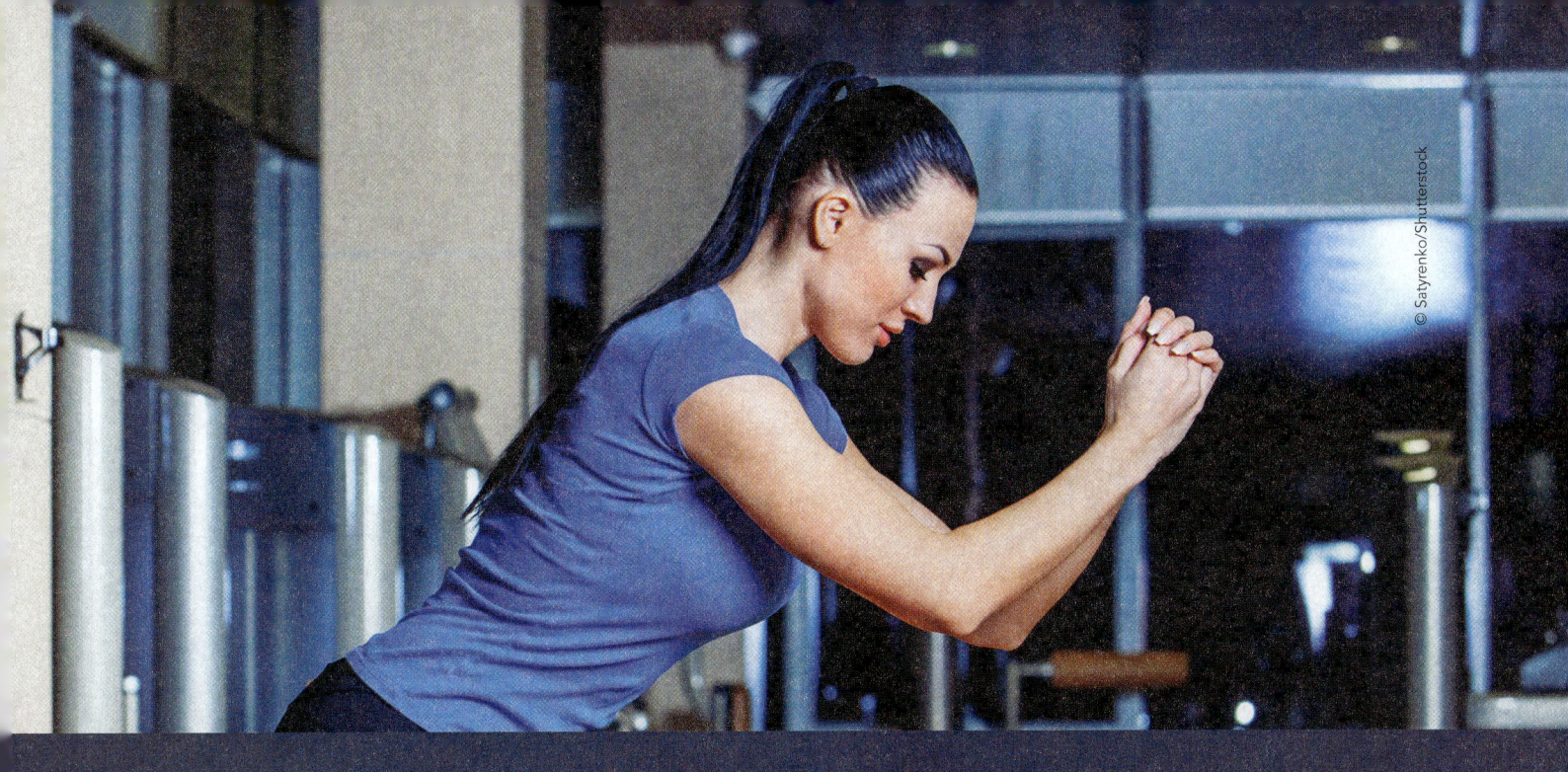

INJURY RESISTANCE AND RETURN TO PERFORMANCE AFTER INJURY

CHAPTER TWENTY

LEARNING OBJECTIVES

Upon completion of this chapter, the Sports Performance Coach will be able to:

- **Explain** the relationship between training and sports injury.
- **Identify** common overuse and noncontact sports injury mechanisms.
- **Explain** the role of training and acute variables in building injury resilience.
- **Identify** the scope of practice for the Sports Performance Coach after injury.
- **Differentiate** appropriate training strategies for return to performance after injury.

LESSON 1: INTRODUCTION TO TRAINING FOR INJURY RESISTANCE

INTRODUCTION

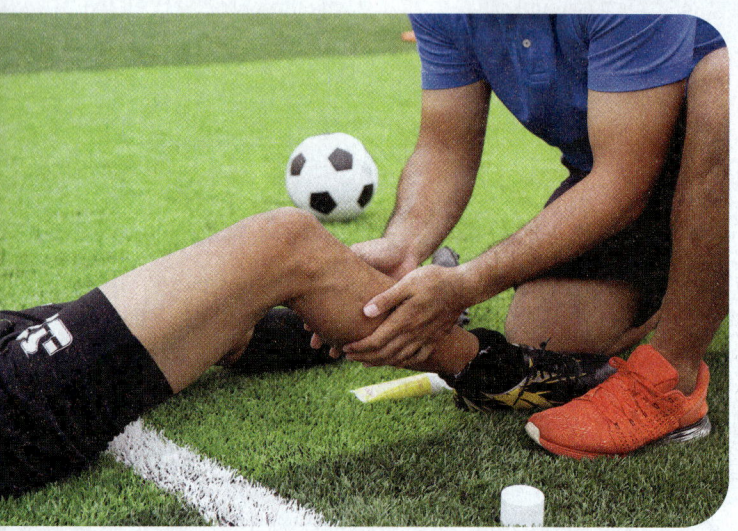

© Nirat.pix/Shutterstock

Injury is an unfortunate but almost inevitable part of sports participation that poses a significant challenge to athletes. Of greater concern, however, is the specter of reinjury, a menace that has been haunting athletes and sports professionals for decades. A study by Hootman et al. (2007) revealed that a previous injury is the strongest predictor of future injury, emphasizing the critical importance of effective recovery strategies and preventive training.

In the world of sports, injuries can jeopardize not only an athlete's current performance but also their long-term career. Various factors influence return-to-play outcomes, including the severity of the injury, the intricacy of the medical or surgical care required, the quality of the rehabilitation process, the restoration of sport-specific conditioning and energy systems, and the psychological readiness of the athlete. Each of these factors underlines the complex and multifaceted nature of injury prevention and post-injury recovery.

In sports where cutting and jumping are fundamental, such as basketball and football, athletes often encounter injuries stemming from overtraining, poor neuromuscular control, arthrokinetic dysfunction, or improper biomechanics. The frequency and intensity of injuries to key areas—the foot, ankle, knees, hips, low back, shoulders, head, and neck—are truly alarming, necessitating a comprehensive approach to injury prevention.

This chapter delves into the role of Sports Performance Coaches in facilitating recovery and preventing injuries. It seeks to elucidate the nature of common sports injuries and the challenges they present. Further, we explore various operational models that guide critical thought processes and inform strategies for ensuring a safe and effective return to play. The goal of this chapter is to underscore the importance of a comprehensive programming strategy, designed to return athletes to their pre-injury status and bolster their resilience against future injuries. This is pivotal in securing the health and longevity of athletes' careers.

THE MULTIDISCIPLINARY TEAM

In the sphere of sports and athlete development, a multidisciplinary team approach is paramount. It involves professionals from different backgrounds, including physicians, physiotherapists, nutritionists, psychologists, and Sports Performance Coaches, all working collaboratively toward the common goal of optimizing the athlete's performance and well-being. The Sports Performance Coach plays a key role in the multidisciplinary team that provides the entire continuum of care—that is, the care from the time of injury through the athlete's rehabilitation and complete return to participation (Lafave et al., 2015) (**Figure 20.1**). This care model is inherently complicated, as all multidisciplinary team members come with their own knowledge, skills, training, and experiences. Team members will inevitably adopt differing approaches while seeking to attain the same goal:

Process	Provider	Role
Medical treatment	• Physicians	Examine, re-evaluate, diagnose, surgical correction
	• Physical Therapists • Athletic Trainers Physicians	Manage pain, limit swelling, protect injured tissues
Rehabilitation	• Athletic Trainers • Physical Therapists	Restore motion, neuromuscular control of individual muscle/muscle groups
End-stage rehabilitation	• Athletic Trainers • Physical Therapists • Sports Performance Coaches	Restore balance, reflex control, strength, endurance
Generic-specific development	• Sports Performance Coaches	Restore most basic physical performance functions
Sports-specific development	• Sports Coaches • Sports Performance Coaches	Restore competitive performance functions

FIGURE 20.1 Roles and Responsibilities

to safely return the injured athlete to full participation and apply prevention measures that reduce the risk of recurrence. Therefore, strong communication skills are a critical success factor in the multidisciplinary team including physicians, physical therapists, athletic trainers, and coaching administration, especially considering that these roles are increasingly overlapping. To communicate effectively, team members should clarify their specific roles and responsibilities and openly discuss theories, methods, philosophies, and protocols to address each component of the full care continuum. An incomplete and ineffective communication approach slows or prevents athletes from returning to peak performance and could increase the risks for recurrence and even more debilitating injuries (Kraemer et al., 2009).

SCOPE OF PRACTICE FOR THE SPORTS PERFORMANCE COACH AND STANDARDS OF CARE

Determining the scope of practice has traditionally been a procedure reserved for medical experts, who describe the services that a qualified specialist is competent to perform and permitted to undertake, in keeping with the terms of their professional license (Wilhite, 2012). In the case of the Sports Performance Coach, a state (or national) regulatory body does not issue a professional license; instead, individual agencies provide regulations via certifications. In many applied-skills professions, widely recognized certifications allow professionals to operate by meeting entry-level requirements and continuing education mandates. The concept of the scope of practice can apply to the Sports Performance Coach, as it clarifies roles and responsibilities to protect athlete health and safety. State and local laws, education, training, experience, credentials, and employer policies determine the scope of practice.

Sports Performance Coaches work with populations for which the development and maintenance of performance-based qualities are critical for success in athletics and similar occupations. Key responsibility areas for them include physical assessment, exercise program development, exercise technique, technical coaching, monitoring the physiologic and psychologic effects of fatigue, program evaluation, and facility maintenance (**Figure 20.2**). To further clarify the way services are delivered by the Sports Performance Coach, additional standards of practice are necessary.

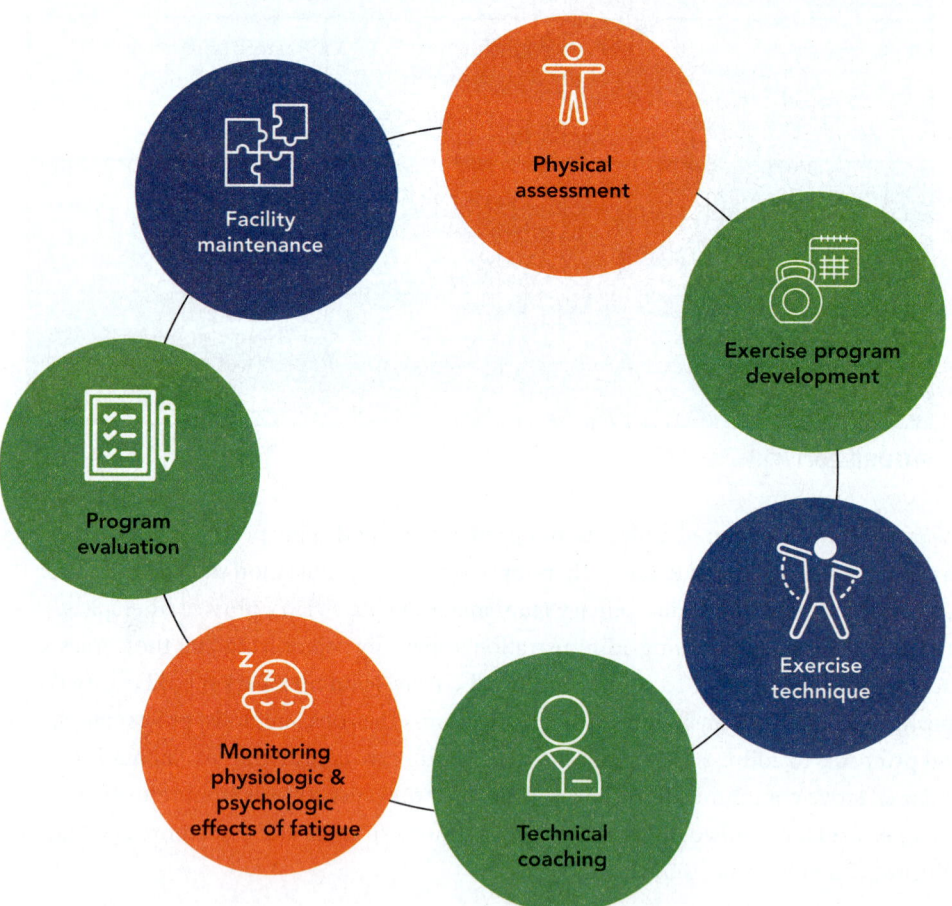

Key Responsibilities of a Sports Performance Coach

FIGURE 20.2 Key Responsibilities of a Sports Performance Coach

STANDARDS OF PRACTICE RECOMMENDATIONS

In addition to the NASM Code of Professional Conduct, additional **standards of practice** have been developed to promote athlete safety and mitigate catastrophic injuries and death in sports. Epidemiologic studies have identified two primary mechanisms by which these events occur: traumatic and nontraumatic (Casa, 2012; Parsons et al., 2020).

Traumatic injuries are bodily injuries caused by direct participation in a sports activity, such as a spinal cord injury caused by a tackle in football. Nontraumatic injuries result from exertion while participating or preparing for the sport, such as a hamstring strain or sudden cardiac arrest during basketball practice (**Figure 20.3**). Hamstring strains and other musculoskeletal injuries are common in sports participation and related training and conditioning sessions. Although described as nontraumatic injuries, they often lead to more severe conditions.

Since 1970, fatalities due to nontraumatic injuries have outnumbered traumatic fatalities in both high school and collegiate football (Parsons et al., 2020). These events rarely occur during game competitions, but are more prevalent in off-season or pre-season conditioning sessions (Casa, 2012; Parsons et al., 2020). To address these trends, an inter-association task force produced best-practice recommendations that have been adopted by 13 prominent organizations, including the National Academy of Sports Medicine. Some of these best practices are highlighted here (Casa, 2012; Parsons et al., 2020):

- All strength and conditioning sessions should be evidence-based, sport-specific, intentionally administered, appropriately monitored, and nonpunitive in nature.
- All training and conditioning activities should be introduced intentionally, gradually, and progressively to encourage proper exercise acclimatization.
- All conditioning programs should begin with the work-to-rest ratio intervals for the training session's goals, allowing for proper recovery.
- All training sessions should be documented, including the exercises, training volume, intensity, duration, and environmental conditions (indoor/outdoor, temperature, humidity) where applicable.

Traumatic vs. Nontraumatic Injuries

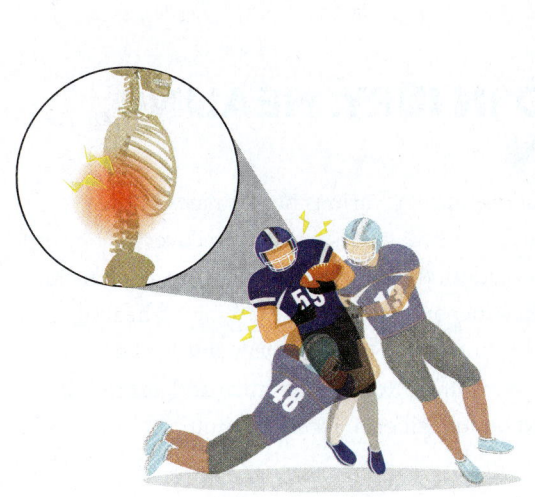

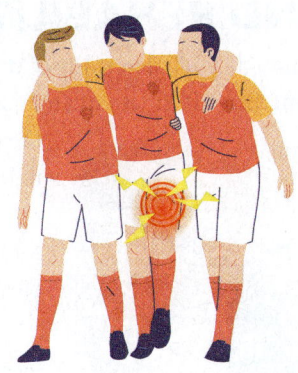

Traumatic injuries

Bodily injuries caused by direct participation in a sport activity.

Nontraumatic

Result of exertion while participating in a sport or in preparation for the sport activities.

FIGURE 20.3 Traumatic Versus Nontraumatic Injuries

- All comprehensive Emergency Action Plans should be developed and rehearsed to care for common catastrophic events (head and neck injury, cardiac arrest, heat illnesses, exertional rhabdomyolysis, exertional or nonexertional collapse, asthma, diabetic emergency, and mental health emergency).

EXERTIONAL RHABDO-MYOLYSIS →

A potentially life-threatening metabolic condition caused by extreme physical exertion that causes the cellular breakdown of muscle cell components, resulting in kidney failure.

🤖 GETTING TECHNICAL

Exertional rhabdomyolysis results from extreme fatigue, producing rapid muscle tissue breakdown that releases a protein (myoglobin) into the blood. Excessive muscular activity results in a state in which ATP production cannot meet the demand, which eventually exhausts the cellular energy supplies and leads to the failure of muscle cell membranes. Insufficient ATP levels produce cellular death of the muscle cells, allowing large volumes of intracellular electrolytes to rush into circulation, which increases the blood's acidity (lowering pH) and produces a flood of myoglobin. The large molecular size of myoglobin impairs the circulation and immediately impacts kidney function, leading to systemic failure (Khan, 2009; Rathi, 2014; Torres et al., 2015). Approximately 33% (Khan, 2009) to 50% (Huerta-Alardín et al., 2005) of patients diagnosed with rhabdomyolysis develop rapid-onset kidney failure, and up to 8% (Khan, 2009) of all cases are fatal. Recovery requires immediate supervised medical care.

Symptoms of rhabdomyolysis include dark, reddish urine, a decreased amount of urine, weakness, and severe muscle aches and stiffness. Early symptom intervention with aggressive fluid replacement and emergent medical care can reduce the risk of kidney damage (Casa, 2012; Connes, 2015; Khan, 2009). A phased return to play/performance should be implemented to safely return the athlete to physical activity (Schleich et al., 2016).

TISSUE RESPONSE TO INJURY, HEALING, AND REHABILITATION

Although a detailed study of the histological response of various body tissues in the immediate aftermath of an injury and the different milestones of injury recovery is beyond the scope of this section, the Sports Performance Coach needs to be aware of the independent responses to injury, healing, and rehabilitation. This knowledge provides valuable background for creating programming intended to return athletes to full participation and build resilience for future injury.

TISSUE RESPONSE TO INJURY

Injuries occur when mechanical loads exceed the tolerance of specific tissues to distribute that load safely. These injuries are often painful and require rest, modification of training practices, and sometimes surgical intervention. Injuries rarely are limited to affecting a single tissue or structure. Each tissue responds to stress in unique ways, so it is vital to know the type of tissue(s) involved to estimate the time required for complete healing and return to sport.

© Wachiwit/Shutterstock

MUSCLE

Anatomic muscle attachments are slightly off-axis, which allows for the production of a variety of multiplanar functions. Each muscle has individuality and different force–length, force–velocity, and torque–velocity characteristics, which depend on the joint's position.

In turn, injuries to muscle tissue have broad impacts on its functional capabilities. Muscle injuries generally are categorized as either compression (contusion) or strain (stretch) injuries. A **contusion** (bruise) is a compression injury in which the blood discharges into the muscle tissue, creating discoloration. A strain is trauma to the muscle or the musculotendinous junction (Starkey & Johnson, 2006). Typically, strain injuries occur during forceful contraction or an extreme stretch. Muscle strains are graded according to the severity of the damage (**Figure 20.4**).

Grades of Muscle Strains

Grade Type	Severity of Damage
Grade I	An overstretching of the muscle fibers, producing no palpable defect, resulting in tearing of less than 10% of the muscle fibers.
Grade II	Moderate strains with 10%-50% muscle fibers tearing and producing a palpable deficit at the injury site.
Grade III	Muscle strains are more extensive resulting in tearing of 50% (or more) of the muscle fibers.

FIGURE 20.4 Grades of Muscles Strains

TENDON

Tendons are semi-fibrous connective tissues that join muscle to bone (**Figure 20.5**). They differ considerably in their overall shape and how they attach to bone. Overall, tendons are very effective at resisting mechanical loads. In some instances, the tendon aspect may constitute 75% of the entire muscle–tendon–bone length, as in the plantaris (wrist flexors). The osteotendinous junction (enthesis) is the point at which the muscle–tendon bundle inserts into bone (Kannus, 2000). It is a central point of stress concentration and is prone to overuse inflammatory responses called tendonitis (Benjamin et al., 2006; Starkey & Johnson, 2006).

LIGAMENT

Ligaments are strong connective tissues that join bone to bone. These structures primarily provide joint stability and act as a guide for dynamic joint motion. Ligamentous injuries, referred to as sprains, are among the most common causes of joint pain and disability (Hauser et al., 2013). Ligament sprains are commonly graded according to the severity of the damage. A Grade I sprain involves a mild tear, Grade II involves a moderate tear, and

Tendons

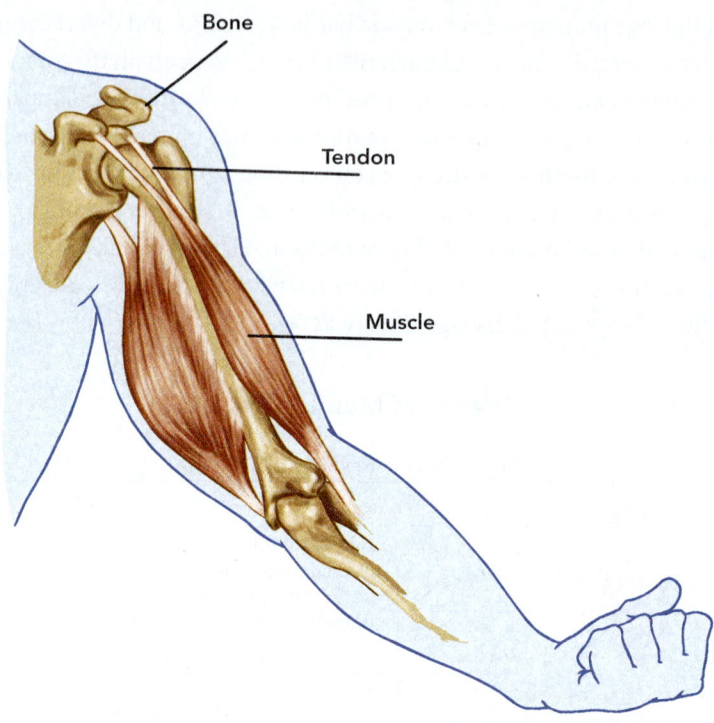

FIGURE 20.5 Tendons

WOLFF'S LAW →

States that bone tissue will adapt to the loads placed upon it along the lines of stress.

RELATIVE ENERGY DEFICIENCY IN SPORT (RED-S) SYNDROME →

A condition characterized by the interrelationship of low energy availability and menstrual dysfunction, which impair bone structure health. Formerly known as female athlete triad.

Grade III is a complete tear or rupture. Healing time is often complicated and determined by any accessory joint or tissue damage, the need for surgical intervention, and the overall load tolerance expectations of the sport or position (**Figure 20.6**).

Multiple ligaments at joints with many degrees of freedom usually contribute to stability in various directions. For example, the knee has four ligaments: anterior cruciate, posterior cruciate, lateral collateral, and medial collateral. The lateral and medial collateral ligaments provide side-to-side stability, whereas the anterior and posterior cruciate ligaments provide front-to-back stability.

BONE

Bone injuries generally fall into two categories: acute (fractures) and chronic (stress reactions) (Neumann, 2017; Starkey & Johnson, 2006). Bone is active and continually changing to balance new bone formation and reabsorption. According to **Wolff's law**, bones adapt to the loads placed upon them; stress is the primary stimulus for these changes (Prendergast & Huiskes, 1995). Acute bone fractures are typically immobilized initially; they generally heal in 6 weeks and continue to mature for many months. Chronic (stress fractures) reactions are more complicated and generally improve over time with a reduction in training loads and, in some cases, immobilization.

Specific considerations should be made for athletes assigned female at birth who report bone pain due to **relative energy deficiency in sport (RED-S) syndrome** (Mountjoy et al., 2018; Nazem & Ackerman, 2012). This condition (sometimes known as female athlete triad) is defined as the interrelationship of low energy availability (with or without disordered eating patterns) and menstrual dysfunction. These factors impair bone structural health, further undermining the ability to handle high repetitive training loads (Barrack et al., 2014).

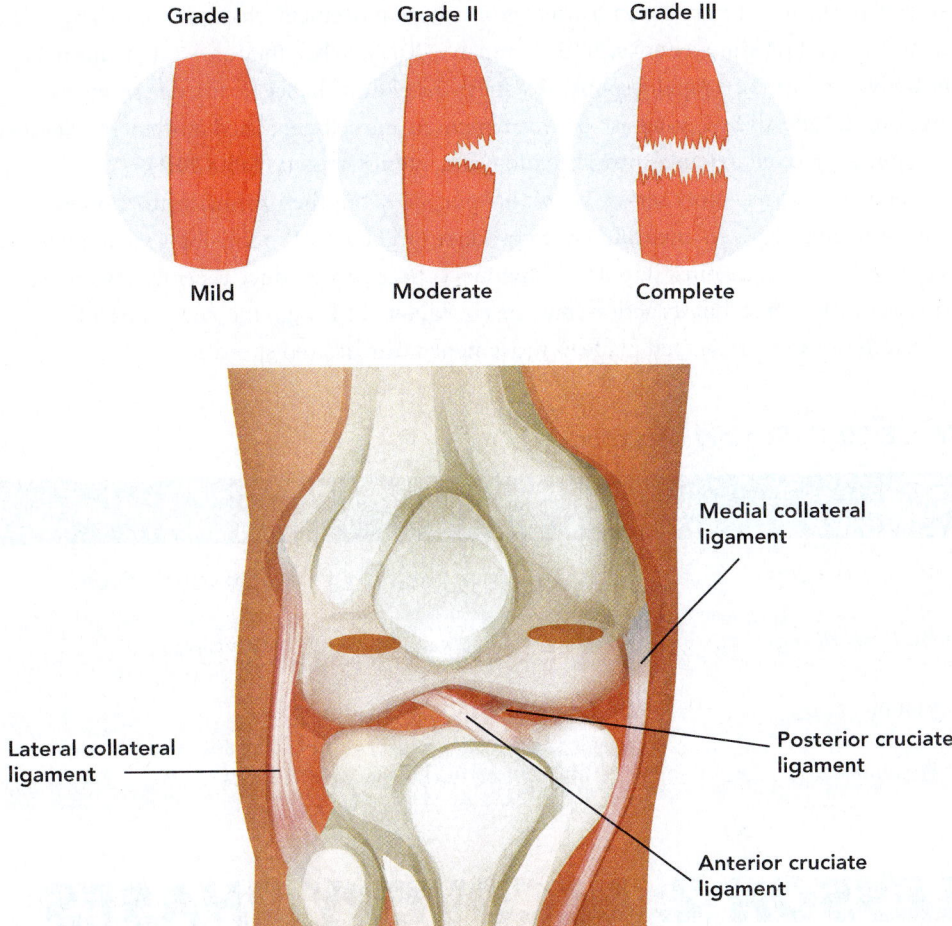

Grade I   Grade II   Grade III

Mild   Moderate   Complete

Medial collateral ligament

Lateral collateral ligament

Posterior cruciate ligament

Anterior cruciate ligament

FIGURE 20.6 Grades of Ligament Tears

CARTILAGE

Cartilage is a highly specialized tissue located within articular (joint) spaces. Its primary function is to transfer compressive loads across joint surfaces and provide a smooth, lubricated surface for efficient joint movement (Little et al., 2011; Starkey & Johnson, 2006). Cartilage tissue is avascular, meaning that it has no direct blood supply. This lack of internal circulation impedes the delivery of nutrition and removal of waste by-products, thus making healing of cartilage a prolonged process. Nutrition to the cartilage is provided by gentle compression/decompression of the joint spaces.

Cartilage is also an aneural tissue, meaning it has no nerve supply. Therefore, the lack of nerve endings impairs the sensation of joint pain. Pain generally does not manifest until the cartilage tissue has degraded significantly and begun to impair surrounding areas, such as bony surfaces or ligaments. Chronic damage to cartilage is the leading cause of osteoarthritis—a condition that is highly prevalent in the United States and a leading cause of disability. An estimated 14 million people in the United States have knee osteoarthritis; most notably, more than half of these individuals are older than 65 years of age (Vina & Kwoh, 2018).

NEUROMUSCULAR CONSIDERATIONS

Soft-tissue and joint injuries interfere with the normal function of sensory receptors. Sensory receptors (also called mechanoreceptors) are pathways used by the central nervous system to provide information regarding limb orientation, rate of movement, changes in joint angles, and changes in joint pressures (Enoka, 2002; Neumann, 2017). When they are working normally, the body can organize a rapid response to a mechanical disturbance (load), determine its position, and effectively distinguish between imposed and self-generated movements. Sensory receptors are located in joints' muscle, tendon, and interior aspects (**Table 20.1**).

Each of these receptors serves individual purposes, but their primary function is to work in an integrated environment to produce (and control) multi-joint movement patterns. Each muscle must have the individual capacity to produce eccentric, isometric, and concentric force, but its action must be coordinated through the neuromuscular system to work in the desired plane of movement at the desired speed.

TABLE 20.1 Sensory Receptors

Type	Location
Muscle spindles	Within muscles, parallel to muscle fibers
Golgi tendon organs (GTO)	Located in the musculotendinous junction
Ruffini endings	Found within joint spaces
Pacinian corpuscles	Located in the joint space

LESSON 2: RECOVERY PHASES
STAGES OF HEALING

Following an injury, a predictable cascade of events occurs in the involved tissues that is generally referred to as the healing process. These stages of healing do not exist in isolation; rather, much overlap occurs between each stage. Injuries vary in severity, and an athlete's response is highly individualized; however, an understanding of the three stages of healing (*inflammatory, proliferative, remodeling*) is essential to estimate the athlete's potential downtime, identify possible limitations, and determine reconditioning requirements (Hauser et al., 2013; Starkey & Johnson, 2006) (**Figure 20.7**). It is important to note that Sports Performance Coaches should not take the lead in the early phases of injury rehabilitation.

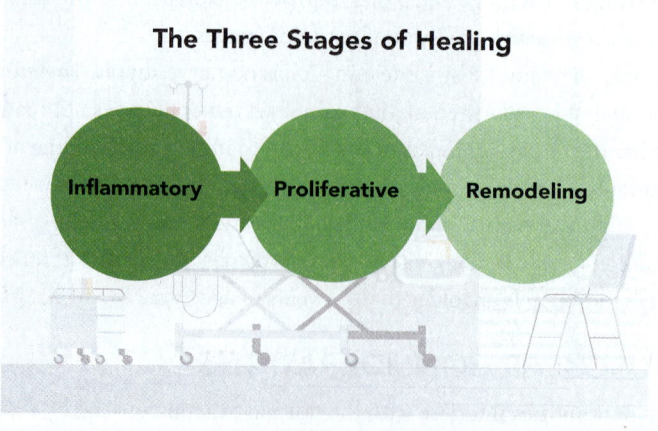

The Three Stages of Healing

Inflammatory → Proliferative → Remodeling

FIGURE 20.7 The Three Stages of Healing

STAGE 1: INFLAMMATION

The **inflammatory stage** begins with the onset of the injury. Inflammation is a nonspecific response to physical injury that represents the body's attempt to limit the extent of the injury and initiate the tissue repair process (Hauser et al., 2013; Pauyo et al., 2017; Starkey & Johnson, 2006). It is a necessary and critical element of the injury response process, yet has both positive and negative effects. Beneficial aspects include producing antibodies, mitigating the effects of toxins, and providing necessary nutrition to the injury site. However, inflammation also produces pain, swelling, and limited function. During this stage, a brief period of immobilization (usually 3 to 7 days) may be beneficial to reduce pain and optimize the cellular response to injury.

STAGE 2: PROLIFERATION

During the **proliferative stage**, macrophages are introduced to the injury site (Hauser et al., 2013; Pauyo et al., 2017; Starkey & Johnson, 2006). These specialized cells remove dead tissue, dried blood, and other residual factors. This stage typically lasts 2 to 4 weeks, but is longer in the case of bone fracture (roughly 6 weeks). Bony tissue heals only through the formation of new bone.

Muscles, tendons, and ligaments heal by forming semi-rigid scar tissue. Additional specialty cells (fibroblasts) produce a collagen matrix in which fibers are aligned in a cross-hatch matrix to optimize the initial stability of the injured area. These early formations of scar tissue are resistant to stretch and serve the purpose of holding the damaged tissue together.

STAGE 3: REMODELING

During the **remodeling stage**, the injured tissue begins to respond to stress and continues to mature (Hauser et al., 2013; Pauyo et al., 2017; Starkey & Johnson, 2006). This continual and gradual process typically allows tissue to reach its full tensile strength by the 12th week (**Figure 20.8**). Appropriate training stress allows for the cross-hatched collagen fiber matrix to realign along those approved lines of stress. This mechanism underpins the importance of ideal exercise technique and of never training through obvious movement compensations. Such habitual, compensatory, and modifiable patterns increase abnormal

Tendon Healing Stages

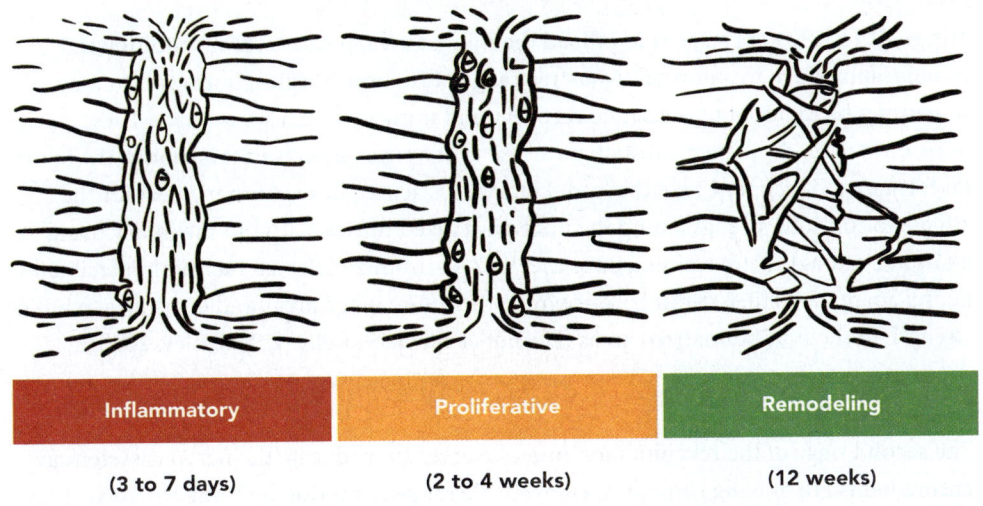

Inflammatory	Proliferative	Remodeling
(3 to 7 days)	**(2 to 4 weeks)**	**(12 weeks)**

Adapted from Strickland, 2000.

FIGURE 20.8 Stages of Tendon Healing

tissue and joint stress, impair recovery and regeneration, and decrease the likelihood of a successful return to participation.

INJURY REHABILITATION

A rehabilitation program aims to return the athlete to competition safely. The focus of the Sports Performance Coach should be on developing strength programs that will complement the protocols put in place by licensed medical and allied healthcare professionals (e.g., athletic trainers, physical therapists, team physicians). All team members need to effectively communicate to facilitate the development of a holistic rehabilitation program that will return the athlete safely to play. To mitigate future injury, it is essential for the Sports Performance Coach not to lose focus on maintaining the uninjured areas of the athlete. Therapeutic rehabilitation can be mnemonically represented by the **4-R system** (*Restore, Reeducate, Recondition, Return to Play*) defined by the athlete's symptomology and recovery trajectory (**Figure 20.9**).

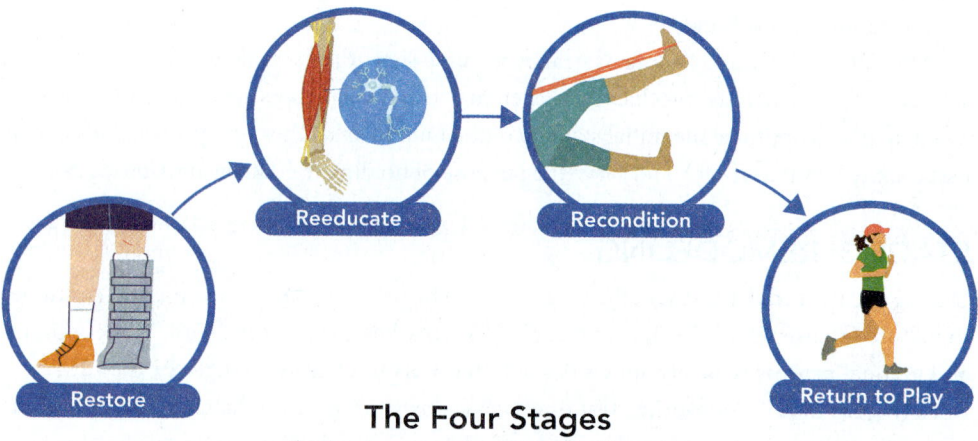

The Four Stages of Therapeutic Rehabilitation

FIGURE 20.9 The Four Stages of Therapeutic Rehabilitation

RESTORE

The goal of the restore stage is to offload the injured area, protect it from additional trauma, and return to a normal, pain-free range of motion. Surgical intervention may sometimes be required to accelerate recovery and mitigate injury recurrence. These decisions are made by medical staff; however, in the latter aspects of this model, the Sports Performance Coach may take the lead. During this acute phase, it is beneficial for the athlete to continue strengthening the nontraumatized muscles around the injury using isolateral or single-limb training once the pain is minimized. Isolateral training facilitates neural adaptations that minimize atrophy in the traumatized areas and continues to build strength in the nontraumatized areas (Harput et al., 2019; Kelly & Beardsley, 2016).

REEDUCATE

The second stage of the rehabilitation process serves to reeducate the nervous system to ensure joints are moving through their available range of motion by firing the correct sequence of muscle fibers. Long periods of recovery can increase the complexity of this step. An effective method to restore ideal neuromuscular firing patterns is through controlled, isolated, single-muscle or single-joint exercises. These movements are not intended to produce strength per se, but rather to improve the isolated coordination of the muscular contraction and single-joint movement. This stage will introduce progressive resistance training exercises to gradually improve tissue tolerance to load (Ratamess et al., 2009; Schoenfeld et al., 2017).

RECONDITION

Once isolated muscle function has been restored, the reconditioning stage begins to coordinate isolated muscle functions with other muscle groups and joint complexes. Various types of reconditioning exercises can support the athlete's full return to play. Resistance training activities are both therapeutic and progressive. Strength training facilitates increased blood circulation to the traumatized area to promote healing while returning the traumatized area to functional capacity. In this stage, the focus is on optimizing performance in exercises that stress the primary functional subsystems and follow the **neuromuscular training continuum** (Appendix E).

RETURN TO PLAY

The return to play stage focuses on returning the traumatized area to baseline or greater than pre-injury performance levels. In addition to gaining strength, emphasis is directed at increasing the athlete's specific metabolic conditioning needs.

Additional sport-specific attention to other performance attributes is required for safe participation. **Figure 20.10** identifies activities in which too much exposure too early should be avoided.

> **NEURO-MUSCULAR TRAINING CONTINUUM** →
>
> Model of exercise progression to optimally develop neuromuscular coordination.

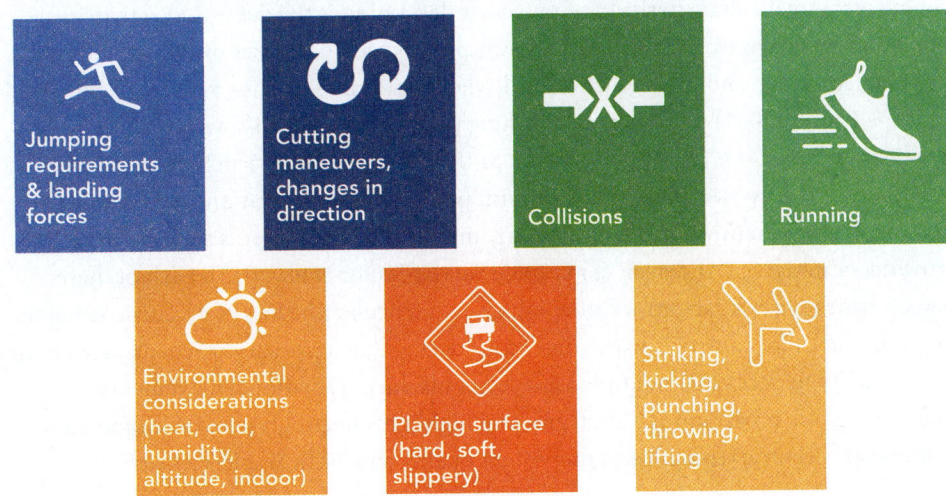

Return to Play: Safe Participation
Watch out for these sport-specific movements.

Jumping requirements & landing forces

Cutting maneuvers, changes in direction

Collisions

Running

Environmental considerations (heat, cold, humidity, altitude, indoor)

Playing surface (hard, soft, slippery)

Striking, kicking, punching, throwing, lifting

FIGURE 20.10 Return to Play: Safe Participation

In this stage, the Sports Performance Coach adopts an injury prevention mindset. At its core, this process aims to continually identify and manage modifiable risk factors—for example, movement quality, range of motion, energy system efficiency, capacity to decelerate in multiple planes of motion, speed, and agility, balance, as well as muscular endurance, strength, and power. More details, considerations, and models to guide reentry to sports are provided later in the chapter.

DETRAINING AND IMMOBILIZATION CHARACTERISTICS

DAVIS'S LAW →

States that soft tissues (muscle and connective) will remodel along the lines of stress.

Muscles, tendons, ligaments, and bony structures respond to the stresses imposed on them. According to Wolff's law, bone tissue will adapt based on the demands placed upon it (Pendergast, 1995). Additionally, **Davis's law** states that soft tissues (muscle and connective) will remodel along the lines of stress (Cyron & Humphrey, 2017; Fahmy, 2022). During the initial treatment of some injuries, immobilization is a standard of care. Although immobilization may provide the ideal environment to optimize healing and repair, the lack of movement, absence of exposure to compression/decompression, and lack of stretch–shortening cycles will cause predictable physiological changes, all of which negatively affect athletic performance. Structured training regimens allow for muscular improvements, enabling increased exercise tolerance. These muscular improvements include improved strength, endurance, cross-sectional area, power, tissue vascularity, and metabolic efficiency to maintain force production. In contrast, and inherent to the principle of reversibility, when training is discontinued, these training-induced adaptations are compromised, negatively affecting athletic performance (Santos-Júnior et al., 2013).

One of the main characteristics of muscular detraining is the decreased activity of mitochondrial enzymes; their capacity to transport oxygen decreases by 30% in the first 3 weeks of detraining, and by as much as 40% when detraining reaches 6 weeks (Coyle, 1990; Mujika & Padilla, 2001). Long-term detraining periods have been shown to shift muscle fiber distribution (from fast-twitch type IIa to IIb), decrease slow-twitch fibers, reduce muscle size and cross-sectional area, diminish or alter neural activation, and lead to a loss of eccentric strength production, particularly in unloaded movements such as running, throwing, or jumping (Andersen et al., 2005; Santos-Júnior et al., 2013). Each of these characteristics is a risk factor for future injury. In particular, the loss of eccentric strength and neuromuscular control is worrisome, considering that a primary mechanism for injury is the inability to decelerate multiple joint segments during rotational movements (Clark, 2000). Therefore, programming strategies that highlight the progressive development of multiplanar eccentric strength and movement quality should be implemented.

LESSON 3: SPORTS INJURIES
COMMON SPORTS INJURIES

The Sports Performance Coach plays an essential role in transitioning from a controlled, supervised rehabilitation program to the return-to-participation process because they have the specific knowledge and appropriate exercise techniques to develop and supervise effective reconditioning and injury prevention programs. To best utilize this process, knowledge, awareness, and familiarity with common sports injuries and known risk factors are essential. This chapter highlights some common sports injuries and ailments, specific exercise considerations, and return-to-play criteria from an injury resilience perspective. However, a detailed, individualized return-to-play program for each ailment is beyond the scope of this chapter.

INJURY RISK FACTORS

Sports-related injuries are complex, and many factors must be considered. Some of these elements can be modified through physical rehabilitation, planned training programs, and improved recovery habits.

The various risk factors can generally be categorized as either intrinsic or extrinsic. **Intrinsic risk factors** are internal to the athlete, including age, gender, previous injury history, and physical fitness (Pizzari et al., 2020). Conversely, **extrinsic risk factors** are external to the athlete. They include such variables as the type of sport, the amount of lifetime sports experience (including early sport specialization), and the competition or practice environment (i.e., heat, cold, humidity, altitude, indoor, outdoor). **Table 20.2** provides a more detailed list of these risk factors.

INTRINSIC → RISK FACTORS

Individual characteristics or conditions that increase a person's susceptibility to physical harm or injury. These can be physiological, psychological, or related to personal habits and behaviors.

EXTRINSIC → RISK FACTORS

Environmental, situational, or circumstantial elements that increase an individual's likelihood of sustaining injury.

TABLE 20.2   Intrinsic and Extrinsic Injury Risk Factors

Intrinsic Risk Factors	Extrinsic Risk Factors
• Previous injury	• Overall lifestyle*
• Bone mass*, structure*	• Amount of intentional recovery*
• Decreased joint motion*	• Footwear, uniform limitations
• Muscle imbalances*	• Physical activity (too much or too little)*
• Biomechanical*, movement quality*	• Playing experience
• Body weight*, composition*	• Early sport/skill specialization
• Age	• Practice/competition environment
• Gender	• Type of sport
• Ethnicity	• Training focus or intensity
• Dietary and hydration habits*	• Physical demands of practice and competition
• Psychological readiness and motivation*	• Movement repetition
• Muscular strength*, endurance*, power*	• Unilateral versus symmetrical
	• Number of contact/collisions
	• Training technique efficiency

*This risk factor can be changed or controlled.

Some of these factors are modifiable with planned training and individualized support, whereas others are not (Pizzari et al., 2020). Physical fitness is somewhat unique and has been described as having a U-shaped effect on injury risk (Wilson et al., 2020). Regular physical training has been shown to reduce the risks of injury, whereas high levels of exercise increase the chances of injury (Wilson et al., 2020).

In general terms, these risk factors apply to most athletes, but their specific impact is highly individualized. Thus, it is important to disassociate known risk factors from the probability of injury. The simple presence of these risk factors does not predict future injury. However, from a programming perspective, the Sports Performance Coach must manage these considerations to effectively develop return-to-play protocols and athletic performance training sessions.

COMMON FOOT AND ANKLE INJURIES

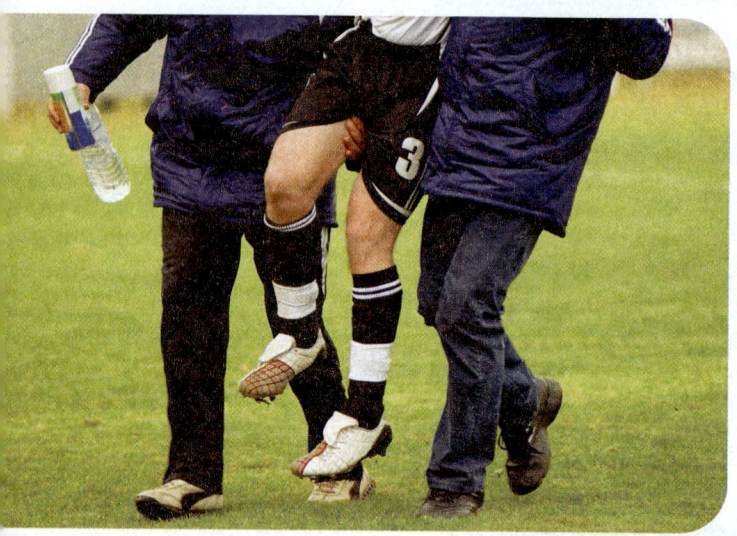

© Synto/Shutterstock

Many foot and ankle injuries can result from acute trauma or overuse. Specific populations have been reported to be at greater risk for these injuries, including runners, athletes assigned female at birth, and individuals with high body mass index (BMI) (Caldemeyer et al., 2020). Ankle sprains are reported to be the most common sports-related injury and the number one injury in terms of time lost from sport participation (Caldemeyer et al., 2020). Approximately 47% to 73% of individuals who suffer an initial ankle sprain will reinjure their ankle (Gribble et al., 2014). Ankle trauma and a history of ankle sprains are also associated with the development of osteoarthritis (Bagherian et al., 2018), chronic ankle instability (Doherty et al., 2016), a reduction in activity level (Saltzman et al., 2005; Valderrabano et al., 2006), and impaired quality of life (Koshino et al., 2020).

Common factors contributing to chronic foot and ankle injuries that the Sports Performance Coach can actively address include muscle weakness, restricted joint movement, and altered movement biomechanics. These factors are modifiable and can be improved with individualized, targeted, progressive exercise and flexibility programs.

Specific muscle weaknesses that should be addressed to reduce the risk of foot and ankle injury include the hip abductors (Fredericson et al., 2000), hip external rotators (Leetun et al., 2004), and ankle inverters (McKeon et al., 2008). Strength deficits within these muscles have been identified as a contributing factor to ankle injuries. Muscle weakness allows for the early and excessive medial collapse of the medial longitudinal arch (Khamis & Yizhar, 2007), which initiates a cascade of related movement impairments throughout the kinetic chain (Clark, 2000). A targeted training program that includes progressive resistance exercises of the gluteus maximus, gluteus medius, and anterior tibialis can address the kinetic chain dysfunctions that place an athlete at risk for an ankle injury.

Normal motion of the ankle joints can become limited by muscle tightness of the gastrocnemius and soleus muscles (Caldemeyer et al., 2020; Donovan et al., 2020). Tightness in the calf musculature limits the available range of motion for dorsiflexion and effective eccentric muscle contractions. Deficits in ankle dorsiflexion have been associated with an increased risk of sustaining an ankle injury and the creation of altered biomechanics along the kinetic chain (Tabrizi et al., 2000).

Additionally, restricted dorsiflexion alters dynamic balance (Hoch et al., 2011) and muscular-activation patterns (Bell et al.,, 2012; Bell-Jenje et al., 2016; Macrum et al., 2012), increases medial knee displacement during squatting movements (Bell-Jenje et al., 2016; Macrum et al., 2012; Stanley et al., 2019), and has been implicated in injury patterns up the kinetic chain in the knee (Macrum et al., 2012; Stanley et al., 2019), hip (Fredericson et al., 2000; Neumann, 2010), and lumbar spine (Bell-Jenje et al., 2016; Hootman et al., 2007).

Decreased eccentric force production in the ankle places abnormal stresses on other joints, such as the patellofemoral and hip acetabulum, when the athlete is attempting to complete jumping and running-type activities (Malliaras et al., 2006). A targeted flexibility program should be implemented to address this range of motion deficit.

Increased forefoot pronation and collapse of the medial longitudinal arch produce an increased anterior pelvic tilt (Khamis & Yizhar, 2007). This relationship between foot-to-hip and hip-to-foot is essential when working with athletes with a prior injury history. Considering the biomechanical link between the foot and ankle complex up to the lumbar spine, effective exercise programs must be progressive, individualized, systematic, and multisensory (Caldemeyer et al., 2020).

Exercises rich in multiplanar neuromuscular stimulation are preferred for athletes recovering from foot and ankle injuries and have been shown to improve risk factors associated with reinjury, such as postural and neuromuscular control (DiStefano et al., 2009; McKeon et al., 2008). Exercises are advanced gradually by increasing load (intensity, sets, repetitions, speed) or neurological demand (movement complexity, range of motion, sensorimotor challenge). Though often overlooked, exercises focusing on the foot's intrinsic muscles are a critical part of successful reconditioning programs (McKeon et al., 2015). These muscles support the foot arches and are highly active during dynamic activities such as walking, running, and jumping. **Table 20.3** lists common foot and ankle injuries and conditions.

TABLE 20.3 Common Foot and Ankle Injuries and Conditions

First Metatarsal Joint Sprain ("Turf Toe")	
Injury overview	Capsuloligamentous sprain is typically caused by forced hyperextension of the first metatarsophalangeal (MTP) joint (great toe) and is usually combined with ankle dorsiflexion. Normal foot mechanics place significant stress on the first MTP joint. Activities such as running and jumping increase stress magnitude by 3 to 8 times body weight.
Surgical and rehabilitative management	Surgery is generally not required. Rest, including partial or non-weight bearing, and limiting the amount of toe extension typically decrease symptoms. Using stiff shoe insoles and supportive taping can provide passive stability throughout the healing process.
Return-to-play exercise and conditioning considerations	Use the results from movement quality assessments to guide exercise selection. Implement a progressive neuromuscular approach to strengthen intrinsic and extrinsic muscles in the foot, ankle, knee, and hip. Begin with bilateral exercises, progressing to single-leg functional activities.
Return-to-play criteria	Full range of motion (70 degrees of passive extension of first MTP joint) and single-leg balance efficiency. Athletes should be able to push off forcefully, tolerate changes in direction, and demonstrate good landing techniques during jumping or running activities.
Estimated timeline	2–8 weeks, depending on the initial degree of damage and related mechanical contributing factors.

(continues)

TABLE 20.3 Common Foot and Ankle Injuries and Conditions (*continued*)

Ankle Sprain	
Injury overview	Lateral sprain involving damage to the anterior talofibular ligament, calcaneofibular ligament, and posterior talofibular ligament. Medial sprains involve injury to the broad-oriented deltoid ligament. These ligaments together provide sensory feedback and overall joint stability for the ankle. Damage to these structures impairs the normal function of the ankle.
Surgical and rehabilitative management	In most cases, ankle sprains are managed nonsurgically. In more severe cases, in conjunction with bony fracture and syndesmosis disruption, surgical intervention is recommended. Active range-of-motion exercises usually begin early (2–5 days post-injury). Isolated resistance exercises are introduced as tolerated, and exercise intensity increases once full weight-bearing is restored.
Return-to-play exercise and conditioning considerations	Restore normal gait and movement patterns without compensation. Stress the importance of the neuromuscular exercise continuum for progressions. Assessments include the star balance excursion test, shark skill test, 5–10–5, and T-drill.
Return-to-play criteria	Successful completion of a dynamic skill battery (based on specific sports needs) on back-to-back days without complications.
Estimated timeline	Nonsurgical: 2–6 weeks. Surgical: can exceed 8 weeks, depending on the scale of intervention performed.

Achilles Tendinopathy	
Injury overview	Response to chronic overload to the protective sheath covering the Achilles tendon (most often, the actual tendon is not damaged).
Surgical and rehabilitative management	Rehabilitation efforts focus on eccentric strengthening of the gastrocnemius and soleus in multiplanar positions. Persistence of symptoms lasting 6–8 months could lead to surgical intervention.
Return-to-play exercise and conditioning considerations	Restore normal gait and movement patterns without compensation. Stress the importance of neuromuscular exercise continuum for progressions.
Return-to-play criteria	Assessments include the star balance excursion test, shark skill test, 5-10-5, T-drill, and triple hop for distance.
Estimated timeline	2 weeks to 6 months. Generally dependent on the amount of stress reduction (rest) allowed to optimize healing. Since this is self-limiting, athletes commonly continue to participate in their sport with modifications.

Plantar Fasciitis	
Injury overview	Under normal conditions, the plantar fascia distributes forces in the foot while weight-bearing. Chronic overuse produces microtears that heal inadequately, leaving scar tissue that is resistant to stretching, and leading to stiff plantar fascia.
Surgical and rehabilitative management	Surgical repair is typically not needed but can be helpful for chronic conditions that include the formation of bone spurs (calcitrant) on the heel. The use of a night splint can be an effective support device. It will position the foot in dorsiflexion during the sleeping hours, allowing the tissues to heal under a gentle stretch (as opposed to the typical plantar-flexed foot posture during sleeping).
Return-to-play exercise and conditioning considerations	Towel crunches, single-leg longitudinal balance, balance training exercises, and stretching of gastrocnemius/soleus complex.
Return-to-play criteria	Assessments include the star balance excursion test, shark skill test, 5-10-5, and T-drill.
Estimated timeline	2 weeks to 4 months.

Neuroma	
Injury overview	Referred to as Morton's neuroma or plantar neuroma. This inflammation occurs in the neural tissue between the metatarsals, usually between the second and third metatarsal heads. Repetitive stress (running, jumping, tight-fitting shoes, high-heeled shoes) causes scar tissue formation around the nerve.
Surgical and rehabilitative management	Generally, not needed. Ensure proper footwear and fit.
Return-to-play exercise and conditioning considerations	Balance training continuum and landing mechanics education.
Return-to-play criteria	Assessments include the star balance excursion test, shark skill test, 5-10-5, and T-drill.
Estimated timeline	In most instances, this is a self-limiting ailment. Surgical cases will require 4–8 weeks of recovery.

COMMON KNEE INJURIES

After studying 15 collegiate sports over 16 years, Hootman et al. (2007) concluded that lower-extremity injuries accounted for more than 50% of all sports injuries, with the knee being the predominant joint affected. Two of the more common diagnoses resulting from physical activity are patellofemoral pain (PFP) and anterior cruciate ligament (ACL) sprains.

PFP is a general term used to define knee pain during activities involving motion at the patellofemoral joint and increased pressure of the patella against the femoral condyles (Arnoldi, 1991). The development of PFP can also be devastating due to the recurrence of symptoms. In a retrospective investigation, 91% of individuals diagnosed with PFP reported continued knee pain for 4 to 18 years post-presentation, with 36% of these individuals having restricted physical activity (Stathopulu & Baildam, 2003). Surgical treatment is an option for PFP; however, little evidence exists favoring surgical intervention over conservative management (Sandow & Goodfellow, 1985).

Approximately 150,000 ACL injuries occur annually (Bram et al., 2021); these injuries rank second (to ankle sprains) as the most common injury in collegiate athletics, accounting for more than 50% of the total (Fernandez et al., 2008). The ACL is one of the knee's primary stabilizing ligaments, whose primary function is to prevent the tibia from moving forward on the femur (**Figure 20.11**). Secondary injuries to the medial collateral ligament (MCL), medial meniscus, or lateral meniscus may also occur simultaneously with an ACL injury.

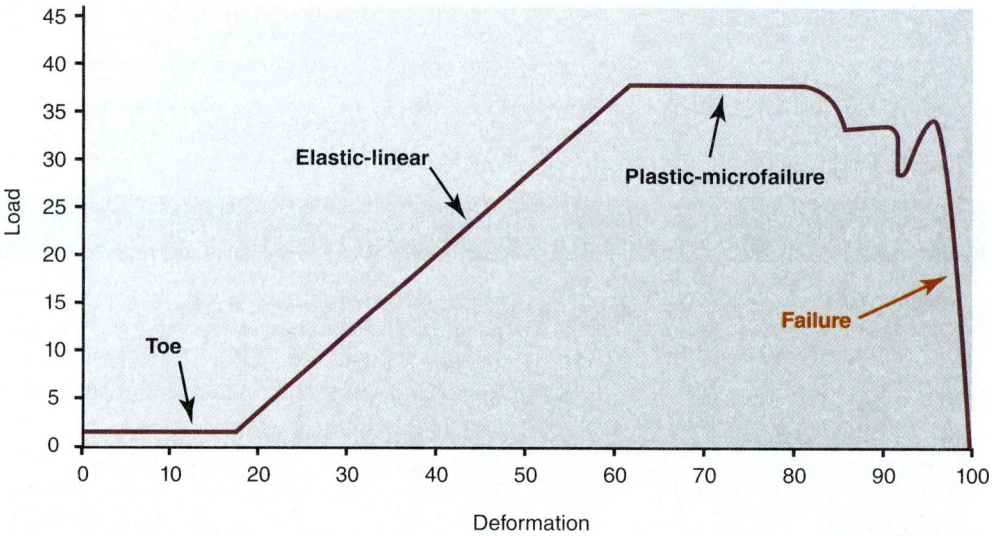

FIGURE 20.11 Mechanism of ACL Injury

Across multiple sports, the overall incidence of ACL injuries is similar between the sexes (Bram et al., 2021). However, in sports where athletes of all genders compete (e.g., soccer, basketball, volleyball), the injury rate is higher for competitors assigned female at birth (Agel et al., 2015; Bram et al., 2021). Those individuals who suffer an ACL injury and undergo surgical intervention face a lengthy rehabilitation process ranging from 6 to 36 months. Only 75% of these individuals return to their previous activity levels (Bram et al., 2021; Huang et al., 2020). Furthermore, individuals who sustain an acute knee injury, such as ACL damage, are seven times more likely to develop knee osteoarthritis approximately 25 years following the initial injury than those with no history of acute knee injury (Wilder et al., 2002).

ACL injuries are overwhelmingly noncontact in nature (70% to 75%) and almost always occur as the body undergoes rapid deceleration (Bram et al., 2021). The three major noncontact events responsible for ACL injury are planting and cutting, straight knee landing, and one-step landing with a hyperextended knee (Hewett et al., 2005; Padua et al., 2015). Specific movement patterns commonly occurring during ACL and lower-extremity injury include knee valgus, excessive leg rotation, and decreased knee flexion (Eckard et al., 2018b; Shultz, 2015). A large amount of stress is placed on the ACL during tibial rotation and knee valgus (Shultz, 2015) (**Figure 20.12**).

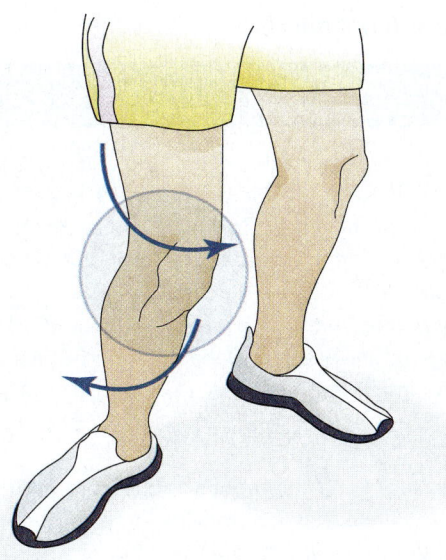

FIGURE 20.12 Tibial Rotation and Knee Valgus

Faulty movement patterns, such as those described earlier, are modifiable through targeted, individualized exercise and flexibility training (Eckard et al., 2018b; Mauntel et al., 2013; Padua et al., 2012). An exercise-based injury prevention program that successfully improves movement patterns by decreasing the visible knee valgus, minimizing tibial rotation, and increasing knee flexion angles can reduce the incidence of a knee injury during sports and recreational activities (Davies et al., 2017; Eckard et al., 2018b; Huang et al., 2020). **Table 20.4** lists common knee injuries and conditions.

TABLE 20.4   Common Knee Injuries and Conditions

Patellofemoral Pain Syndrome	
Injury overview	This is a general term used to describe a broad range of pain in the anterior aspect of the knee.
Surgical and rehabilitative management	Surgical intervention is typically not required. Initial rehabilitation will focus on inflammation management and gentle exercises through pain-free ranges of motion.
Return-to-play exercise and conditioning considerations	Exercises should focus on correcting altered biomechanical factors contributing to poor movement quality of the hip, knee, and foot/ankle, and improving the efficiency of multi-joint, multiplanar movement.
Return-to-play criteria	Hip extension ROM (0 degrees) when combined with knee flexion, hip internal rotation ROM (45 degrees), ankle dorsiflexion ROM (20 degrees). Completion of sport-specific functional test battery without complication.
Estimated timeline	Most cases will resolve to full participation within 1–4 weeks.

(continues)

TABLE 20.4 Common Knee Injuries and Conditions (*continued*)

Patellar Tendinopathy	
Injury overview	Common in sports with an emphasis on jumping and cutting, such as basketball, soccer, and volleyball. Patellar tendonitis ("jumper's knee") is an overuse injury of the patellar tendon, which produces pain at the anterior aspect of the patella and often localized tenderness to the inferior aspect of the patella.
Surgical and rehabilitative management	Immobilization may be recommended when a painful ROM exists. Crutches may alleviate pain during weight-bearing. Rehabilitation begins quickly within pain-free ROMs to control inflammation and restore normal muscle activation patterns. Surgical interventions are rare.
Return-to-play exercise and conditioning considerations	Flexibility to address functional limitations and restore normal range of knee extension (with the hip flexed), ankle dorsiflexion (straight and bent knee), and hip internal rotation. A slow introduction of eccentric training for the quadriceps.
Return-to-play criteria	Pain-free ROM and comparable strength symmetry. Hip internal ROM (45 degrees); hip extension 90/90 (20 degrees); ankle dorsiflexion ROM (20 degrees). Sport-specific functional test battery completed without complications.
Estimated timeline	Conservatively, symptoms usually subside within 1–4 weeks.

Osteoarthritis (OA)	
Injury overview	This chronic condition involves degeneration of the articular cartilage, which will reduce the intra-articular space, affect joint stability and surface integrity, cause pain, and affect the long-term quality of life and disability. OA results from chronic overuse, altered joint mechanics, and poor movement quality.
Surgical and rehabilitative management	Surgical interventions do not eliminate OA but may effectively mitigate current mechanisms contributing to symptoms (i.e., removal of bone spurs, reshaping of bony structures, microfracture procedure to produce postsurgical scarring effect to "regenerate" the smooth articular surface).
Return-to-play exercise and conditioning considerations	Pain-free ROM and comparable strength symmetry. Hip internal ROM (45 degrees); hip extension 90/90 (25 degrees); ankle dorsiflexion ROM (20 degrees). Sport-specific functional test battery completed without complications (including the star balance excursion test, shark skill test, triple hop for distance, 5–10–5 test, and T-drill).
Return-to-play criteria	Continue progressing overall metabolic specificity and conditioning to preserve core strength, balance, upper-body strength, and power, speed, and agility.
Estimated timeline	Return to participation is usually a self-limited scenario. Typically, athletes can return once symptoms are managed.

Anterior Cruciate Ligament (ACL) Sprain

Injury overview	Sprain of this ligament is common with rapid deceleration or change of direction with knee valgus position and planted foot, typically without contact.
Surgical and rehabilitative management	Following an acute injury, there is a period of non-weight-bearing until pain-free ROM and normal muscle activation of the quadriceps are regained. Some injuries can be managed through comprehensive exercise training, sports participation limitations, and protective bracing. Surgical interventions are common and, when performed early, restore dynamic stability of the joint and minimize the risks of OA development (long term). Rehabilitation focuses on inflammation and pain management, progressing to therapeutic exercises to restore normal ROM and joint arthrokinematics. Closed- and open-chain exercises are then introduced to improve the ability to produce and reduce forces dynamically.
Return-to-play exercise and conditioning considerations	Continue progressing overall metabolic specificity and conditioning to preserve core strength, balance, upper-body strength, and power, speed, and agility.
Return-to-play criteria	Sport-specific functional performance battery without complication (including the star balance excursion test, shark skill test, triple hop for distance, 5–10–5 test, and T-drill).
Estimated timeline	Nonsurgical: 2–4 weeks. Surgical: 6–9 months.

Medial Collateral Ligament (MCL)

Injury overview	Injury to the supporting ligament to the inner (medial) side of the knee. Typically, these occur from a direct blow to the outside of the knee, creating pain to the medial joint surface and producing feelings of joint instability.
Surgical and rehabilitative management	Surgical interventions are generally not required if the injury is contained to the MCL. Should the damaged tissues include the ACL and meniscus, it is a likely case for surgical repair. Rehabilitation programs will include an initial focus on inflammation and pain management, restoration of flexibility and balance deficits, and inclusion of progressive resistance exercises. Using a protective (hinged) knee brace is considered a best practice.
Return-to-play exercise and conditioning considerations	Continue progressing overall metabolic specificity and conditioning to preserve core strength, balance, upper-body strength, and power, speed, and agility.
Return-to-play criteria	Sport-specific functional performance battery without complication (including the star balance excursion test, shark skill test, triple hop for distance, 5–10–5 test, and T- drill).
Estimated timeline	1–2 weeks for minor sprain, extending to 3 months for more severe sprains (with or without surgical intervention). If surgical repair includes other structures, this timeline is extended.

(continues)

TABLE 20.4 Common Knee Injuries and Conditions (*continued*)

Posterior–Lateral Complex	
Injury overview	This term encompasses injuries to the lateral collateral ligament (LCL), posterior cruciate ligament (PCL), lateral meniscus, and proximal fibular head fractures. Injuries that involve only the LCL are rare; more structures are usually damaged.
Surgical and rehabilitative management	Surgical interventions are common to rapidly restore joint stability and normal movement biomechanics. Nonsurgical treatments are also an option, though the lack of joint stability increases OA risks (which impacts the long-term quality of life).
Return-to-play exercise and conditioning considerations	Continue progressing overall metabolic specificity and conditioning to preserve core strength, balance, upper-body strength, and power, speed, and agility.
Return-to-play criteria	Sport-specific functional performance battery without complication (including the star balance excursion test, shark skill test, triple hop for distance, 5–10–5 test, and T-drill).
Estimated timeline	1–2 weeks for a minor sprain, extending up to a year depending on the specific structures damaged and the time between the injury date and the surgery date. The best outcomes are achieved when the repair is within 2 weeks of the initial injury date.

Meniscal Tear	
Injury overview	Under normal conditions, the medial and lateral meniscus provides joint cushioning and stability and allows for smooth joint movement. The vascular structure provides some complications, as not all sections of the meniscus have good blood flow. The location of the lesion will determine whether the injury can heal without surgical intervention.
Surgical and rehabilitative management	Surgical repairs include suturing or removing meniscal sections to create a smooth joint surface. Rehabilitative management is initially dependent on the specific surgical procedures performed. Partial meniscectomy generally has the athlete back to controlled weight-bearing activities within 1 week. In contrast, those with meniscal repairs require straight-leg immobilization and non-weight-bearing for 4 weeks.
Return-to-play exercise and conditioning considerations	Continue progressing overall metabolic specificity and conditioning to preserve core strength, balance, upper-body strength, and power, speed, and agility.
Return-to-play criteria	Sport-specific functional performance battery without complication (including the star balance excursion test, shark skill test, triple hop for distance, 5–10–5 test, and T-drill).
Estimated timeline	Conservative approach: 2–6 weeks. Surgical partial meniscectomy: 4–6 weeks. Surgical meniscal repair: 10 weeks, up to 6 months.

COMMON HIP INJURIES

Injuries to the hip complex can limit athletic participation and have a broad impact throughout the entire kinetic chain. The hip joint is a central point of rotation for the whole body. Hip-area injuries include muscular strains, articular cartilage damage, maladaptive bony changes, and chronic lower abdominal and groin pain (Cohen et al., 2016; Freehill & Safran, 2011b; Geisler, 2021; Salas et al., 2020). Cadaveric studies demonstrate that 29 muscles begin or terminate around the hips (Neumann, 2010, 2017). Each muscle can display various functions that extend beyond force control at the hip and have primary roles in movements above and below the region. For example, the gluteus maximus controls the rate of internal (medial) rotation of the tibia during functional tasks under load (Preece et al., 2008). During dynamic activities such as walking, the gluteus maximus works to decelerate hip flexion, hip abduction via the iliotibial band (Stecco et al., 2013), and internal (medial) rotation of the tibia (Neumann, 2010; Preece et al., 2008). This forms the functional sagittal plane longitudinal subsystem (Clark, 2000; Neumann, 2017). **Table 20.5** lists common hip injuries and conditions.

TABLE 20.5 Common Hip Injuries and Conditions

Hamstring Muscle Strain	
Injury overview	These injuries are commonly caused by forceful eccentric contractions of the hamstring muscle. Athletes will have altered gait patterns with acute muscle strains.
Surgical and rehabilitative management	Surgical repairs are required only in severe cases.
Return-to-play exercise and conditioning considerations	Continue progressing overall metabolic specificity and conditioning to preserve core strength, balance, upper-body strength, and power, speed, and agility. Include eccentric hamstring strengthening gradually and as part of an injury prevention program.
Return-to-play criteria	Sport-specific functional performance battery without complication (including the star balance excursion test, shark skill test, triple hop for distance, 5–10–5 test, and T-drill).
Estimated timeline	Time lost is dependent on the degree of tissue damage and the specific demands of this muscle during sports participation, lasting from a couple of days (minor) to 6 (or more) months for a complete rupture.
Adductor Muscle Strain	
Injury overview	Also known as "groin strains," these injuries are commonly caused by rapid passive lengthening combined with a forceful contraction of the hip adductors. Athletes will have altered gait patterns with acute muscle strains.
Surgical and rehabilitative management	Surgical repairs are required only in severe cases.
Return-to-play exercise and conditioning considerations	Continue progressing overall metabolic specificity and conditioning to preserve core strength, balance, upper-body strength, and power, speed, and agility.
Return-to-play criteria	Sport-specific functional performance battery without complication (including the star balance excursion test, shark skill test, triple hop for distance, 5–10–5 test, and T-drill).
Estimated timeline	Time lost is dependent on the degree of tissue damage and the specific demands of this muscle during sports participation, lasting from a couple of days (minor) to 6 (or more) months for a complete rupture.

(continues)

TABLE 20.5 Common Hip Injuries and Conditions (*continued*)

Quadriceps Muscle Strain

Injury overview	Of the four muscles in the quadriceps muscle group, the rectus femoris crosses two joints, predisposing it to injury.
Surgical and rehabilitative management	Surgical repairs are required only in severe cases.
Return-to-play exercise and conditioning considerations	Continue progressing overall metabolic specificity and conditioning to preserve core strength, balance, upper-body strength, and power, speed, and agility.
Return-to-play criteria	Sport-specific functional performance battery without complication (including the star balance excursion test, shark skill test, triple hop for distance, 5–10–5 test, and T-drill).
Estimated timeline	Time lost is dependent on the degree of tissue damage and the specific demands of this muscle during sports participation, lasting from a couple of days (minor) to 6 (or more) months for a complete rupture.

Greater Trochanter Pain Syndrome ("Bursitis")

Injury overview	Although a direct (acute) contusion can cause this condition, it is more commonly seen as a chronic condition caused by friction between the trochanter and the bursa. This friction sometimes produces a "snapping" hip sensation, leading to pain.
Surgical and rehabilitative management	Surgery is typically not required. Rehabilitation will focus on symptom management, progressing to resisted exercise within pain-free ROM.
Return-to-play exercise and conditioning considerations	Continue progressing overall metabolic specificity and conditioning to preserve core strength, balance, upper-body strength, and power, speed, and agility.
Return-to-play criteria	Sport-specific functional performance battery without complication (including the star balance excursion test, shark skill test, triple hop for distance, 5–10–5 test, and T-drill).
Estimated timeline	Time lost is dependent on the degree of tissue damage and the specific demands of this muscle during sports participation, lasting from a couple of days (minor) to 6 (or more) months for a complete rupture.

Chronic Pubalgia ("Sports Hernia," "Athletic Hernia")

Injury overview	Chronic lower abdominal and groin pain without a true hernia. This condition often occurs in conjunction with other hip and pelvic ailments (i.e., acetabular labral tears, femoroacetabular (FA) impingement, trochanteric bursitis) and primarily affects athletes participating in activities that require repetitive turning and twisting, such as ice hockey and soccer.
Surgical and rehabilitative management	Surgical repair of the pubalgia alone has a poor success rate. However, since pubalgia is compounded by the bony formation in the hip (FA impingement), when surgical interventions correct both the pubalgia and the FA impingement, the rate of return to sport outcomes approaches 90%.

Return-to-play exercise and conditioning considerations	Continue progressing overall metabolic specificity and conditioning to preserve core strength, balance, upper-body strength, and power, speed, and agility.
Return-to-play criteria	Sport-specific functional performance battery without complication (including the star balance excursion test, shark skill test, triple hop for distance, 5–10–5 test, and T-drill).
Estimated timeline	Time lost is dependent on the degree of tissue damage and the specific demands of this muscle during sports participation, lasting from a couple of days (minor) to 6 (or more) months for a complete rupture.

Piriformis Syndrome

Injury overview	Common in runners, weightlifters, and baseball/softball catchers, this condition involves muscle tightness of the piriformis muscle compressing on the sciatic nerve.
Surgical and rehabilitative management	Surgery is typically not required. Rehabilitation involves an integrated flexibility program to restore multiplanar mobility of the hip, combined with progressive core stability and a balance training program.
Return-to-play exercise and conditioning considerations	Continue progressing overall metabolic specificity and conditioning to preserve core strength, balance, upper-body strength, and power, speed, and agility.
Return-to-play criteria	Sport-specific functional performance battery without complication (including the star balance excursion test, shark skill test, triple hop for distance, 5–10–5 test, and T- drill).
Estimated timeline	Return to full participation generally occurs quickly. Continued maintenance is required to improve all modifiable factors contributing to faulty movement quality.

COMMON LOW BACK INJURIES

Low back pain is among the most frequent complaints reported among people living both active and sedentary lifestyles (Coulombe et al., 2017; Maselli et al., 2020; Skundric et al., 2021). Approximately 6% to 15% of athletes experience low back pain each year, resulting in decreased training levels, conditioning, and overall performance levels (Fett et al., 2019; Wilson et al., 2020). The generalized low back pain symptoms usually take 4 to 6 weeks to resolve (Trainor & Wiesel, 2002). It is important to remember that athletes who suffer one low back injury are significantly more likely to suffer additional low back injuries, further increasing their training and competition time lost (Wilson et al., 2020). Repeated injuries to the back may predispose the athlete to future OA and long-term disability (Skundric et al., 2021). Prevention of the first injury is the most effective way to promote athletes' health and performance.

Vertebral disc injuries occur when the outer fibrous structure of the disc (annulus fibrosus) fails, allowing the internal contents of the disc (nucleus pulposus) to be pushed out and irritate the nerves that exit the spinal cord at the intervertebral foramen (**Figure 20.13**). The exact mechanism is generally thought to be due to a combination of motion with compressive loading. Increases in disc pressures and stresses are influenced by the movement occurring at the lumbar spine (Drake et al., 2005; Schmidt & Kohlmann, 2005). Disc pressure increases during lumbar flexion and decreases during extension, with a combination of flexion and lateral bending being demonstrated to increase significant strain on the discs (Schmidt & Kohlmann, 2005).

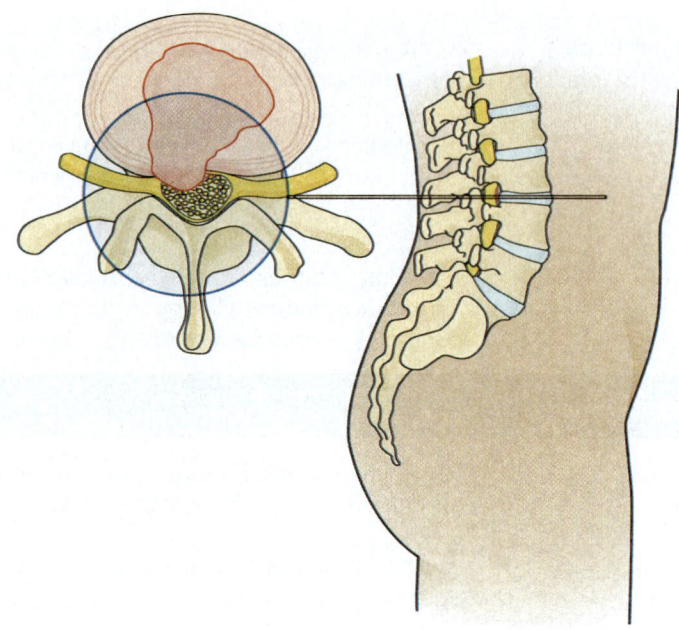

FIGURE 20.13 Disc Injury

Exercise recommendations center on progressive core stability training (Coulombe et al., 2017; Huxel-Bliven & Anderson, 2013; McGill et al., 2009), balance training (Behm & Colado, 2013; DiStefano et al., 2009), and flexibility, focused on hip musculature (Litwin et al., 2011; McGill et al., 2009). Poor core stability endurance is strongly associated with nonspecific low back pain. Training programs to develop injury resistance should follow a systematic programming model, beginning with a focus on increased core endurance (Abdelraouf & Abdel-Aziem, 2016; Huxel-Bliven & Anderson, 2013; McGill et al., 2009; Overley et al., 2016). The inclusion of balance training is vital to address the postural and neuromuscular disorders commonly associated with lower back pain.

Individuals with chronic lower back pain have been found to have altered postural control. A flexibility program that targets hip extension ROM deficits may also alleviate the athlete's low back pain. **Table 20.6** lists common low back injuries and conditions.

TABLE 20.6 Common Low Back Injuries and Conditions

Nonspecific Low Back Pain	
Injury overview	This general term describes the collection of soft-tissue musculoskeletal injuries in sports, which typically involve the paraspinal muscles. Poor posture, inefficient movement patterns, and faulty training techniques elevate the risk of soft-tissue injuries to the lower back.
Surgical and rehabilitative management	Surgery is rarely required. Rehabilitation begins to control pain, inflammation, and loss of daily function. Then rehabilitation progresses to address flexibility deficits and improve posture/core stability, balance control, and functional strength.
Return-to-play exercise and conditioning considerations	Pain-free ROM of spinal flexion, extension, lateral flexion (to each side), and lumbar rotation (to each side). Establish comprehensive baseline ROM data to guide continued training and serve as a comparator in the event of reinjury.

Return-to-play criteria	Multiplanar and multi-segmental stability are primary focus areas.
Estimated timeline	Variable. One day to several weeks, depending on the degree of damage and reliance on low back area function during sport-specific tasks.

Disc Herniation

Injury overview	Intervertebral discs are positioned between vertebral segments and function to maintain consistent joint spacing and provide cushioning. Disc herniations (bulging) predominantly occur in the posterior aspect of the lumbar spine at L4–L5 and L5–S1. These segments have the greatest stress on the lumbar spine during forward bending and rotation activities. During the herniation, disc particulates enter the spinal column, creating mechanical pain and chemical irritation, elevating the pain and discomfort levels an athlete encounters.
Surgical and rehabilitative management	Conservative rehabilitation is typically initiated first, focusing on inflammation and pain control, then gradually increasing therapeutic exercises. Should this approach fail, surgical repair is recommended.
Return-to-play exercise and conditioning considerations	Base training programs on the core stability and neuromuscular training continuum to account for the athlete's ability to dynamically stabilize multiple joint segments at the right time, with the right amount of force.
Return-to-play criteria	Pain-free ROM (flexion, extension, lateral flexion, and rotation). Completion of a sport-specific performance test battery to include the upper-extremity closed kinetic chain stability test. Goniometric values should be within 80% of normal for all hip measures and ankle dorsiflexion.
Estimated timeline	2 weeks to 2 months.

Spondylosis and Spondylolisthesis

Injury overview	Commonly appearing in the lumbar spine (L5–S1), spondylolysis is a fracture defect in the vertebral arch. When the vertebral body below the defect slips anteriorly, the condition is known as spondylolisthesis. Either condition can contribute to low back pain and related movement dysfunction.
Surgical and rehabilitative management	Surgical repair is necessary for persistent symptoms or spine instability. Following surgery, the use of back braces is common to immobilize the area and allow the best opportunity for the fusion to heal.
Return-to-play exercise and conditioning considerations	Develop a comprehensive spinal stability program; however, avoid hyperextension-type exercises.
Return-to-play criteria	Normal, pain-free ROM and completion of a sport-specific performance test battery without complications.
Estimated timeline	2 weeks to 2 months (if a surgical repair was completed, this would extend an additional 6 months).

COMMON SHOULDER INJURIES

Shoulder pain is common in athletes and the general population. Approximately 21% of the population experiences shoulder pain (Bongers, 2001), with 40% having pain that persists for at least 1 year (Van der Heijden, 1999). Pain in the shoulder region is common in athletes who perform overhead motions (Fares et al., 2020; Laudner et al., 2020). Shoulder impingement is the most prevalent diagnosis, accounting for 40% to 65% of reported shoulder pain (Berget et al., 2006), while traumatic shoulder dislocations account for an additional 15% to 25% of shoulder pain reports (Borsa et al., 2008).

The persistent nature of shoulder pain may result from degenerative changes to the shoulder's capsuloligamentous structures, articular cartilage, and tendons (Bergert et al., 2006). Degenerative changes may also affect the rotator cuff by weakening the tendons over time through various risk factors (Carpenter et al., 1998; Yamaguchi et al., 2006). These risk factors include repetitive overhead use, increased loads raised above shoulder height (National Institute for Occupational Safety and Health, 1997), head-forward and rounded shoulder posture (Diab, 2012; Szeto et al., 2002), and altered scapular kinematics and muscle activity (Borsa et al., 2008). These factors are theorized to overload the shoulder muscles, which can lead to shoulder pain and dysfunction.

Shoulder injuries can be broadly categorized into those that affect the rotator cuff muscles and those that affect the capsuloligamentous structures of the shoulder (**Figure 20.14**). Rotator cuff strains occur when a muscle group is overexerted, causing micro-damage within the muscle belly and tendon, and resulting in immediate inflammation and decreased muscle function (Bergert et al., 2006). In contrast, injuries to the capsuloligamentous structures lead to deficits in the passive stabilizing structures of the shoulder, such as the anterior, posterior, or inferior glenohumeral ligaments and the glenoid labrum (Michener et al., 2018). Rotator cuff and capsuloligamentous injuries are devastating to the shoulder's ability to reach forward or perform overhead tasks.

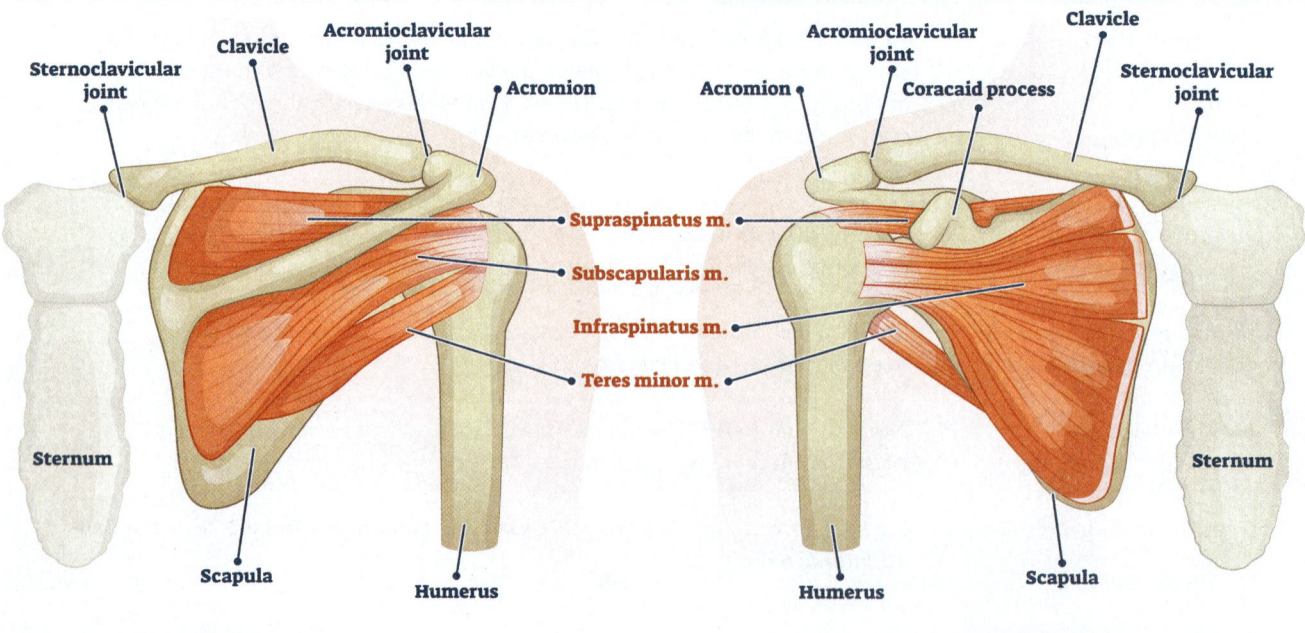

SHOULDER ANATOMY

FIGURE 20.14 Rotator Cuff
© VectorMine/Shutterstock

Another commonly diagnosed source of shoulder pain is **subacromial impingement syndrome**, broadly defined as compression of the structures that run beneath the coracoacromial arch (Bergert et al., 2006) (**Figure 20.15**). The impinged structures include the supraspinatus and infraspinatus tendons, the subacromial bursa, and the long head of the biceps tendon (**Figure 20.16**). Repetitive compression of these structures with the overhead motions required in many sports can lead to irritation and inflammation

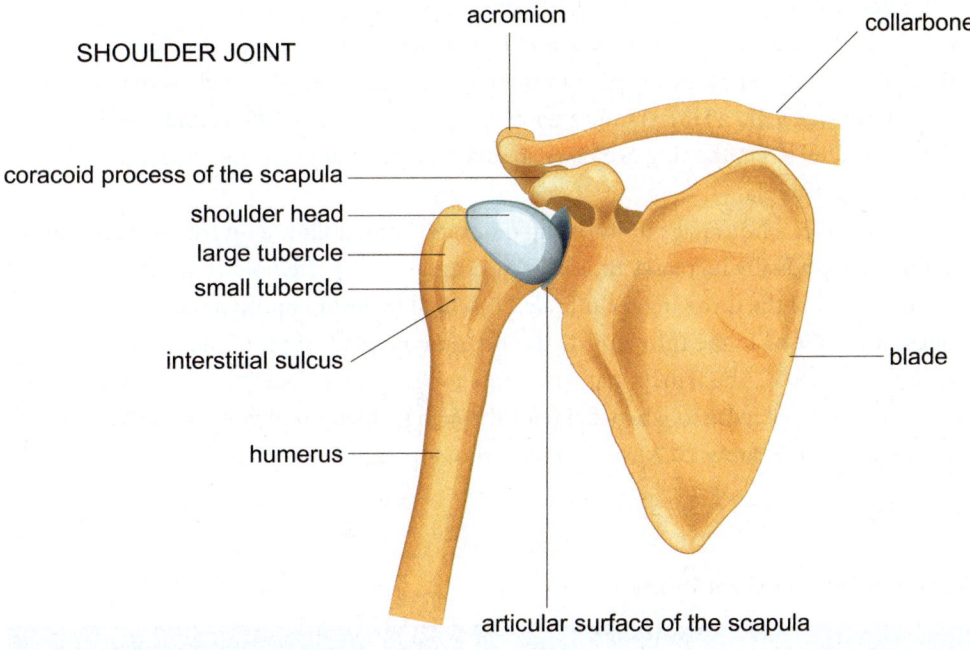

FIGURE 20.15 Coracoacromial Arch
© Artemida-psy/Shutterstock

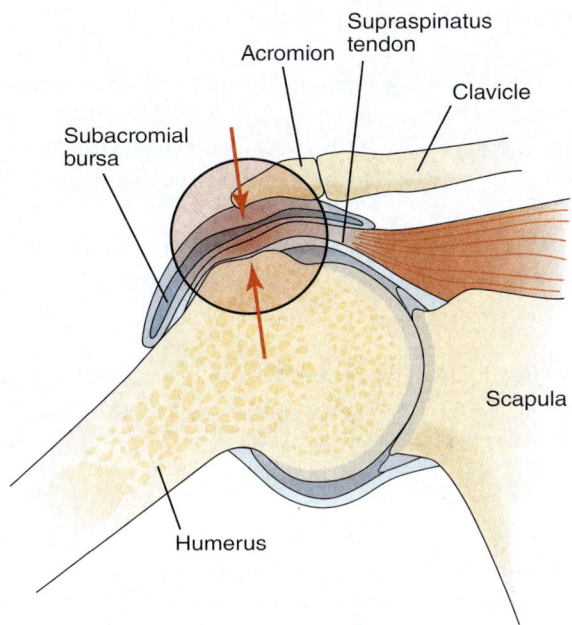

FIGURE 20.16 Subacromial Impingement

(Bergert et al., 2006). In turn, prolonged inflammation can cause muscular inefficiency affecting the rotator cuff muscles. Subacromial impingement syndrome may result from bony deformity of the acromion, underlying rotator cuff weakness, shoulder instability, or scapular dyskinesis (Thigpen et al., 2005).

Shoulder instability most often manifests itself as anterior or multidirectional. The most common cause is an acute injury from an abducted and externally rotated arm. This damages the anterior or inferior glenohumeral ligament and often the glenoid labrum. It usually leads to the athlete having a significant disability with overhead activities and often requires surgical repair (Buss et al., 2004).

Shoulder injury prevention strategies include soft-tissue mobilization and self-myofascial release techniques that increase the overactive muscles' extensibility (Michener et al., 2018). Static or neuromuscular stretching exercises, such as the sleeper stretch (Chepeha et al., 2018), should then be performed for 30 to 45 seconds on these muscles. Isolated strengthening exercises should be used to activate the underactive muscles of the scapula.

Those athletes who engage in throwing motions should follow a return-to-throwing program that gradually increases time, distance, and velocity (Reinold et al., 2002).

Supervision of the throwing technique is essential to ensure optimal movement patterns are exposed to the throwing loads and to monitor for signs of tissue failure (Bergert et al., 2006). The Functional Arm Scale for Throwers (FAST) is a valid and reliable patient-reported outcome tool beneficial for throwing athletes returning to participation (Sauers et al., 2017). **Table 20.7** lists common shoulder injuries and conditions.

TABLE 20.7   Common Shoulder Injuries and Conditions

Rotator Cuff Injuries	
Injury overview	Rotator cuff is a single term that describes the combined function of four muscles (teres major, teres minor, subscapularis, and infraspinatus) that provide stability and support for the glenohumeral joint. Common injuries to this collection of muscles include strains, tendinopathies, and impingement.
Surgical and rehabilitative management	Conservative approaches generally improve function and return athletes to full participation within 3–6 months. If symptoms persist beyond that point, surgical repair should be explored. Rehabilitation includes initial inflammation management, followed by a gradual return to resistance exercises within a pain-free ROM.
Return-to-play exercise and conditioning considerations	Avoid early overhead activities and delay throwing (if applicable) until clearance from the medical team.
Return-to-play criteria	Symptom-free, pain-free ROM, normal strength, and endurance. Sport-specific functional performance battery without complication (including the upper-extremity closed kinetic chain stability test). The Functional Arm Scale for Throwers may be a valuable tool.
Estimated timeline	Variable based on the degree of tissue damage and whether the surgical repair was used. Athletes with minor strains can resume full participation in 1–2 weeks, whereas the timeline for those with more complicated cases could extend to 6 months (or more).

Clavicular Joint Sprains

Injury overview	The clavicle has two articulations within the shoulder complex: sternoclavicular (distal end) and acromioclavicular (proximal end). Increased damage to the supportive ligaments that make up each joint allows for accessory motion leading to subluxations (joint slips in/out of normal position) and complete dislocations (joint slips and remains out). These joint injuries can be problematic for athletes in sports that require high-velocity overhead movements (e.g., volleyball spike, baseball throwing, tennis serve) or endure high-load compressive forces (e.g., football tackle, wrestling), considering the end-range strength and stability required for normal joint function.
Surgical and rehabilitative management	Minor sprains can heal relatively quickly when external joint supports are added (bracing, taping) to progressive exercise programs within pain-free ROMs.
Return-to-play exercise and conditioning considerations	Avoid early overhead activities and delay throwing (if applicable) until clearance from the medical team.
Return-to-play criteria	Symptom-free, pain-free ROM, normal strength, and endurance. Sport-specific functional performance battery without complication (including the upper-extremity closed kinetic chain stability test). The Functional Arm Scale for Throwers may be a valuable tool.
Estimated timeline	Return to participation is estimated mainly by the degree of damage, whether the surgical repair was required, the contact nature of the sport, and the location of the injury (e.g., athlete's dominant versus nondominant side). Recovery from less severe sprains may require only 1–2 weeks, but that from more severe surgically repaired injuries can exceed 10 weeks.

Biceps Tendinopathy

Injury overview	In athletics, tendinopathies to the biceps tendon primarily involve the long head of the biceps, which has an intra-articular point of origin. This attachment area is prone to compression (by the acromion) during overhead activities, creating an inflammatory response. During overhead throwing motions, the highest activity of the biceps muscle is during the follow-through stage, when the bicep decelerates dynamic elbow extension.
Surgical and rehabilitative management	Return-to-play outcomes are marginal for surgical repair of the long head of the biceps tendon, particularly for those athletes in roles that require hard throwing.
Return-to-play exercise and conditioning considerations	Emphasis on rotational movements (combined flexion/abduction/external rotation followed by extension/adduction/internal rotation, push-up with rotation) over shoulder abduction exercises (lateral raises, overhead press). Continue to progress isolated rotator cuff performance and integrated multisensory exercises for core stability, endurance, and balance.
Return-to-play criteria	Sport-specific functional performance battery without complication (including the upper-extremity closed kinetic chain stability test).
Estimated timeline	2–6 weeks depending on the degree of damage and the overall requirement to participate in hard-throwing–related activities (e.g., baseball, softball, volleyball, tennis).

(continues)

TABLE 20.7 Common Shoulder Injuries and Conditions (*continued*)

Superior Labrum Anterior–Posterior (SLAP) Lesions	
Injury overview	The labrum is a cartilage tissue that attaches to the glenoid of the humerus. It extends the surface area of the glenoid's small bony surface and passively increases the dynamic joint stability of the glenohumeral joint. A common tear in this tissue is a SLAP lesion. These lesions originate at the superior glenoid (in addition to the long head of the biceps tendon) and run from an anterior-to-posterior direction. Such injuries destabilize the glenohumeral joint and produce pain during high-velocity throwing, requiring rotation ROMs near extreme limits.
Surgical and rehabilitative management	Surgical repair is recommended to restore structural joint stability. Rehabilitation begins following a 3- to 4-week immobilization phase and progresses from that point to improve flexibility, mobility, and stability in a gradual way.
Return-to-play exercise and conditioning considerations	Avoid early overhead activities and delay throwing (if applicable) until clearance from the medical team.
Return-to-play criteria	Normal, pain-free ROM, strength, and endurance. Sport-specific functional performance battery without complication (including the upper-extremity closed kinetic chain stability test).
Estimated timeline	4–6 months, depending on the requirement for the injured area to participate in high-velocity or high-compression activities.

COMMON ELBOW INJURIES

Pain to the elbow is common in athletics requiring high-velocity overhead movements such as baseball, softball, javelin, water polo, tennis, and volleyball (Freehill & Safran, 2011a; Kraan et al., 2019). Common injuries include pain to the medial (inner) and lateral (outer) epicondyles (Miyashita et al., 2008; Neumann, 2017) and ligamentous injury to the medial aspect (Bergert et al., 2006; Freehill & Safran, 2011a) that is often combined with injury to nerve tissues. Mechanisms of injury generally begin from overuse and repetitive stress to the wrist flexor and extensor muscle groups that have their origins in the epicondyles. These muscle groups are nearly exclusively responsible for grip strength and forearm stability (Bergert et al., 2006). From an exercise perspective, it is challenging to list exercises that do not require elements of grip strength to perform. Grip strength is further exposed when the activity requires dynamic control during high-velocity throwing maneuvers.

Hard throwing elevates stress directly to the medial elbow, and stress intensity increases with higher degrees of shoulder external rotation (Freehill & Safran, 2011a; Miyashita et al., 2008). Effective management of elbow injuries requires focusing on the hand/wrists and the shoulder complex. **Table 20.8** lists common elbow injuries and conditions.

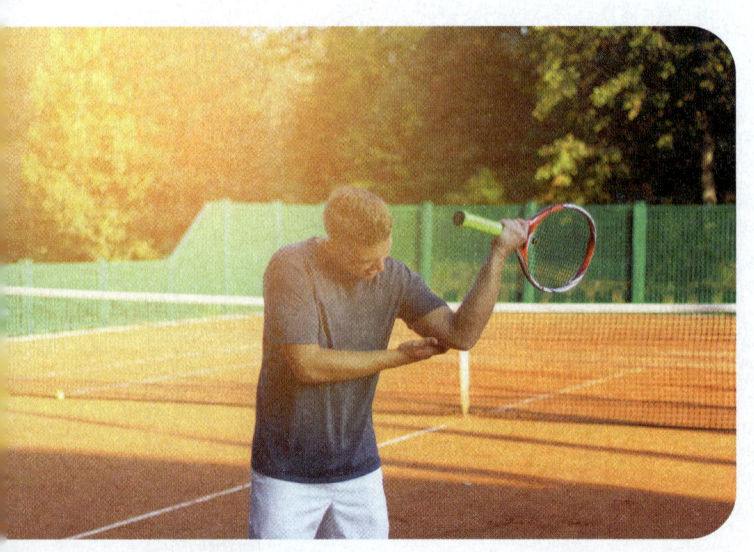
© Nick Bakhur/Shutterstock

TABLE 20.8 Common Elbow Injuries and Conditions

Lateral Epicondylitis ("Tennis Elbow")

Injury overview	Common in tennis players and golfers, this condition develops due to chronic inflammation of the common extensor tendon that originates at the lateral epicondyle. Improper use of the equipment and poor movement techniques can contribute to the onset of lateral epicondylitis.
Surgical and rehabilitative management	Surgical repair is generally not warranted, and the condition improves rapidly with activity modulation and gradual rehabilitation programs.
Return-to-play exercise and conditioning considerations	Include exercises that stress wrist extension in conjunction with varying elbow flexion/extension angles, pronation/supination, and full extension of the fingers.
Return-to-play criteria	Full pain-free ROM, symmetrical grip strength. Sport-specific functional performance battery without complication (including the upper-extremity closed kinetic chain stability test).
Estimated timeline	Acute flare-ups generally resolve within 3 days. Chronic conditions may require significant activity/lifestyle modification to allow the injured tissue to heal and remodel effectively. These more complicated cases can take 4–6 months.

Medial Epicondylitis ("Golfer's Elbow")

Injury overview	This condition involves the common flexor tendon originating on the medial epicondyle. Though its is popularly termed "golfer's elbow," any athlete who participates in activities that produce valgus forces to the medial elbow (e.g., throwing, golf swing) can experience medial epicondylitis.
Surgical and rehabilitative management	Surgical repair is generally not warranted, and the condition improves rapidly with activity modulation and gradual rehabilitation programs.
Return-to-play exercise and conditioning considerations	Avoid (initially) isolated wrist flexion training. Nearly every exercise commonly performed in a sports performance training program involves wrist (and hand) flexion elements. Therefore, additional isolated work in this area is not recommended—including spring-loaded grip trainers and gyroscopic modalities. Supplement existing forearm flexor training with exercises to stress the static crush-grip (i.e., bodyweight hang on pull-up bar) and pinch-grip (i.e., firefighter's carry holding two 10-pound barbell plates together in the same hand).
Return-to-play criteria	Full pain-free ROM, symmetrical grip strength. Sport-specific functional performance battery without complication (including the upper-extremity closed kinetic chain stability test). Standard throwing mechanics (if applicable).
Estimated timeline	Acute flare-ups generally resolve within 3 days. Chronic conditions may require significant activity/lifestyle modification to allow the injured tissue to heal and remodel effectively. These more complicated cases can take 4–6 months.

(continues)

TABLE 20.8 Common Elbow Injuries and Conditions (*continued*)

Ulnar Collateral Ligament Sprain	
Injury overview	The ulnar collateral ligament provides stability to the medial aspect of the elbow and is commonly injured in athletes participating in throwing sports (e.g., baseball, softball, volleyball, javelin). When the stabilizing ligament fails, the medial aspect of the joint is expanded, placing additional stress on the muscular, neural, and vascular tissues.
Surgical and rehabilitative management	The surgical repair, commonly termed the "Tommy John procedure," is named after the first professional baseball player to successfully return to a high level of performance following the surgery. Surgical and rehabilitative outcomes routinely return athletes to their previous level of participation. Valgus stress to the elbow is avoided for the first 4–5 months following surgery.
Return-to-play exercise and conditioning considerations	All athletes recovering from elbow injuries should undertake a comprehensive training program to develop stability and mobility of the shoulder complex, in addition to total integration with the trunk, legs, and back.
Return-to-play criteria	Sport-specific functional performance battery without complication (including the upper-extremity closed kinetic chain stability test).
Estimated timeline	9–12 months is common among athletes with surgical repair. This will fluctuate considering the valgus overload forces required of their sport/position.

VIRAL ILLNESS CONSIDERATIONS

The effects of viral illnesses are widespread and damaging worldwide. Viral illnesses can cause damage to the lungs, heart, and brain, which increases the risk of long-term health problems—not to mention the related negative impacts on athletic performance outcomes (Colombo et al., 2021; Halle et al., 2021; Komici et al., 2021). Viral illness symptoms can sometimes be prolonged, lasting 6 months or more; individuals affected by the prolonged versions are termed "long haulers" (Colombo et al., 2021; Komici et al., 2021).

Common signs and symptoms that can linger over time include the following (Centers for Disease Control and Prevention [CDC], 2019):

- Fatigue
- Headache
- Shortness of breath
- Joint, muscle, or chest pain
- Loss of memory, mental acuity
- Loss of smell or taste
- Worsened symptoms after physical activities

VIRAL ILLNESS RETURN-TO-PLAY GUIDELINES

After they experience a viral infection, athletes should be encouraged to begin gradual, progressive exercise after their recovery from the acute infection (Elliott et al., 2020; Halle et al., 2021). Firm guidelines are not available, as research in this area is lacking. However, it is imperative that all exercise training is individualized to optimize the balance between training load and recoverability. At this time, athletes can generally return to full participation without residual damage to the heart and lungs (Colombo et al., 2021; Halle et al., 2021; Komici et al., 2021; Phelan et al., 2020). Medical professionals should closely monitor the return-to-sport process when extenuating damage to the heart (myocarditis) or lungs (pneumonia, fibrosis) has occurred. Importantly, athletes who have been required to take a long time away from supervised exercise training may have performance deficits in crucial neuromuscular qualities (e.g., coordination, balance, rate of force production, reaction time, multi-segmental stability), which increase their risks of preventable musculoskeletal injuries (Cohen et al., 2021). As a general guideline, return to exercise training should begin following a symptom-free period of (at least) 7 days (**Table 20.9**).

TABLE 20.9 Returning to Exercise Training

	Phase 1	Phase 2	Phase 3	Phase 4	Phase 5	Phase 6
Duration	1–2 days	1+ days	1+ days	1–2 days	1+ days	Gradual return to full participation
Exercise mode	Walking, stationary bike, elliptical (no resistance training)	Light running, stationary bike	Jump rope, sport-specific drills, increased complexity, light resistance training	Normal resistance training, normal conditioning activities	Normal resistance training, normal conditioning activities	
Intensity	Light	Moderate	Moderate	Normal	Normal	
Time	15 minutes	30 minutes	45 minutes	60 minutes	60+ minutes	
Heart rate %	<70%	<80%	<80%	<80%	Normal	

Data from Elliott, N., Martin, R., Heron, N., Elliott, J., Grimstead, D., & Biswas, A. (2020). Infographic. Graduated return to play guidance following COVID-19 infection. *British Journal of Sports Medicine, 54*(19), 1174–1175. https://doi.org/10.1136/bjsports-2020-102637

Cloth face coverings and medical-grade masks are thought to decrease the spread of viral illnesses. As such, use of face coverings has increased in fitness centers and during athletic activities in some sports. During exercise, however, wearing cloth face masks may pose physiological limitations. The use of cloth masks during exercise has been shown to reduce overall exercise time by 14% and to lower VO_2 max by nearly 30%, particularly at higher exercise intensities (Driver et al., 2022). From a practical perspective, the Sports Performance Coach should utilize caution when exercise sessions include wearing cloth face masks and consider modifying the intensity and duration of training sessions.

LESSON 4: BACK TO PERFORMANCE AFTER INJURY
RETURN TO PLAY

Injuries are a common and unfortunate consequence of sports and athletic competition. Previous injury is the most significant influencer of reinjury, leading to a four-fold increase in this outcome (Fuller et al., 2007; Hootman et al., 2007; Shrier, 2015). The long-term goal following an injury is for the athlete to return to full participation at pre-injury performance levels. The decision to return to sport should be based on objective physical and psychological data and consensus among the multidisciplinary care team and the athlete. The data should demonstrate the injured body part has healed, baseline comparisons are within appropriate ranges, and functional and sport-specific performance tasks can be completed without pain or limitation (Clover & Wall, 2010; Creighton et al., 2010). Traditionally, physical testing has been the standard to determine whether an athlete is ready to return. However, this factor alone is no longer considered sufficient. The Sports Performance Coach must also address the athlete's psychological readiness to identify tendencies of apprehension; fear of reinjury; perceived stress from family, friends, and the team; and overall motivation levels.

Returning an athlete to competition is a complex, highly individualized process, and includes much more than physical rehabilitation. The sports performance professional must consider multiple factors to ensure adequate preparation, allow for successful sport reintroduction, and incorporate beneficial strategies to mitigate future injury risks (Clover & Wall, 2010; Michener et al., 2018). To develop injury resistance and account for the abundance of confounding variables, return-to-play (RTP) decisions are critical and often highly scrutinized. Decision-making models provide a systematic approach to RTP and account for the many variables related to the athlete's injury, recovery, sports environment, and overall psychological readiness.

SYSTEMATIC APPROACH TO GUIDE RETURN TO PLAY

Traditionally, RTP decisions were based on limited input from care providers, primarily due to the lack of standardization and models to guide decision making through the entire process. This lack of communication often confused athletes, coaches, physicians, athletic trainers, physical therapists, and Sports Performance Coaches. Only recently has the body of research begun to look at these complexities. Creighton et al. (2010) proposed a three-step model focused on health status, participation risk, and decision modifiers. This model was criticized by clinicians for the inability to manage serious injuries (i.e., concussions, cardiac events) and simultaneous risks (e.g., the short-term risk of reinjury, long-term risk of osteoarthritis). In response, the model was evolved to create the **Strategic Assessment of Risk and Risk Tolerance (StARRT)** framework in 2015 (**Figure 20.17**).

STRATEGIC → ASSESSMENT OF RISK AND RISK TOLERANCE (STARRT)

A three-step framework that describes when an athlete should be deemed ready to return to participation.

StARRT Framework

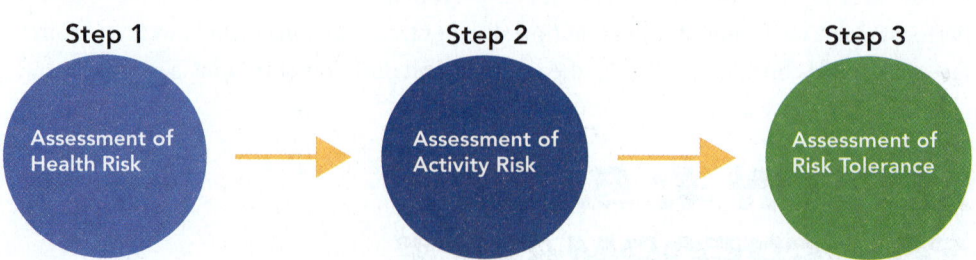

FIGURE 20.17 StARRT Framework

The StARRT framework describes how athletes should be deemed ready to return to play only when the risk assessment (health risk and participation risk) is below the athlete's risk tolerance. If the risk assessment is greater than the risk tolerance, the decision should be made *not* to return to play (Shrier, 2015)—or at least to not return to a level that exceeds the athlete's risk tolerance.

STEP 1: ASSESSMENT OF HEALTH RISK

The first step is to determine the overall ability of the injured tissue(s) to handle loading stress. Determining factors might include current symptoms, injured body parts, surgical intervention (if applicable), personal medical history, medical/physical examination, imaging tests (X-ray, MRI), functional tests, neuromuscular control, and psychological readiness.

Generally accepted RTP best practices are summarized here (Clover & Wall, 2010; Creighton et al., 2010; Miller et al., 2009):

- Strength should be at or near pre-injury levels or symmetrical with the noninvolved side.
- ROM should be pain-free, at or near pre-injury levels, or symmetrical with the noninvolved side.
- No joint instability should be present.
- The injured site should not be painful.
- No tissue inflammation or joint swelling (effusion) should be present.
- Anthropometric measures should be at or near pre-injury levels or symmetrical with the noninvolved side.
- Functional performance (throwing, jumping, running, VO_2 max) should be at or near pre-injury levels or symmetrical with the noninvolved side (where applicable).
- The athlete should be able to reproduce repeated full-participation practices (i.e., back-to-back days) without pain or limitation in the injured body part before full release to sports participation.

STEP 2: ASSESSMENT OF ACTIVITY RISK

The overall dynamic of sporting activities induces various loads (e.g., speed, volume, tension, change of direction) on the body. An injury will occur if these loads exceed the tissue's tolerance level. This step assesses the load (stress) applied to the tissues. Factors considered here include the type of sport (contact versus noncontact), position played, competitive level, repetitive movement dominance, ability to protect the area from future tissue insult, and any environmental concerns (e.g., heat, humidity, cold, altitude).

STEP 3: ASSESSMENT OF RISK TOLERANCE

The final step establishes the threshold for "acceptable risk." This step should include thorough conversations with the entire multidisciplinary care team. Factors to consider include the current timing of the season (pre-season, in-season, post-season), events that occur on a specific date (i.e., marathon, triathlon, Olympic qualifiers), pressure from the athlete to return, the influence of external pressures (e.g., coach, family, friends, teammates, media), and any fears regarding potential litigation.

Operational models, such as the StARRT framework, can help the Sports Performance Coach to categorize related data regarding athlete progress, including functional task performance and overall psychological readiness. This comprehensive framework will promote a standardized approach to guide RTP decisions.

IMPORTANCE OF MOVEMENT QUALITY

Full recovery from injury is never enough to ensure a successful return to participation. Much consideration must be given to tissues and joint structures located both proximal and distal to the injured site. Movement quality is the dynamic representation of the efficient control of the neuromuscular system. From a movement perspective, two primary elements impact capacity for movement: joint stability and joint mobility. These

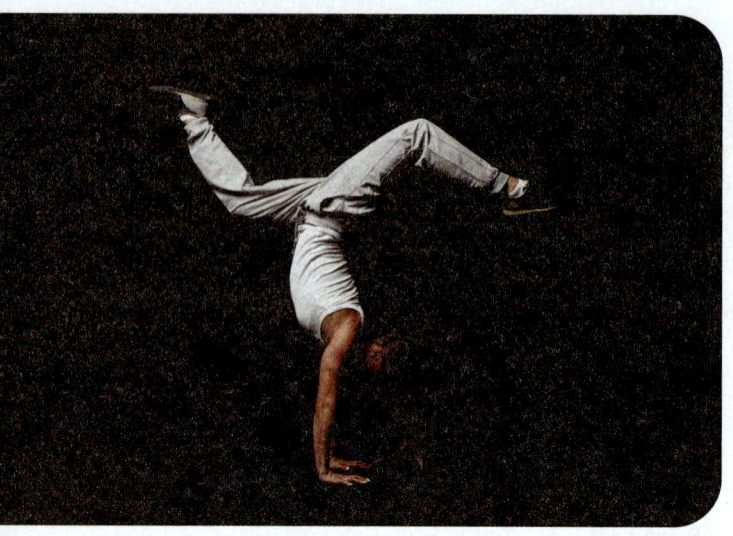

physical attributes work together to allow controlled motion through available joint ranges across multiple joint segments to produce efficient movement. When returning an athlete to participation, it is essential to identify total-body discrepancies in both stability and mobility—as it is likely that each of these contributed to the movement profile leading to the injury.

To illustrate this total-body approach, consider the general relationship between stability and mobility (Cook, 2010), beginning at the foot and working toward the head. The foot, knee, lumbosacral spine, and scapulothoracic joint should be stable, while the ankle, hips, thoracic spine, and glenohumeral joint should be mobile. This is only a generalized process, but assessment of patterns of alternating joint complexes and their ideal goal (stability or mobility) can help improve many movement pattern problems.

Injuries (and recovery from these injuries) alter these general patterns and facilitate motor recruitment strategies that may (unintentionally) elevate injury risk upon the athlete's return to their sport. For example, the natural response to an ankle sprain is restricted mobility in the ankle, which increases mobility demands in the proximal (knee) and distal (foot) joint complexes. The foot, which should ideally be focused on stability, now must demonstrate mobility qualities to allow a greater range of motion in the frontal and transverse plane. These combined motions increase abnormal loading to protective structures and can accelerate the rate of tissue overload. Herein lies both the dilemma and the solution. From a purely movement efficiency perspective, the faster you can restore multiplanar movement that enables the return to the "normal" alternating pattern of stability and mobility, the greater the likelihood of success for the RTP outcome.

To assess lower-extremity movement quality, the double-leg and single-leg squat tests (Hirth, 2007) provide an integrated view of muscle activation patterns (Bagherian et al., 2017; Bell et al., 2008; Bell et al., 2012; Eckard et al., 2018b; Mauntel et al., 2013; Mauntel et al., 2014; Padua et al., 2012) and relationships with ROM of the ankle (Bagherian et al., 2018; Macrum et al., 2012). Additionally, more dynamic activities that identify proficiencies in jump landings, such as the depth jump, may be helpful. It is also essential to look at dynamic scapulothoracic and glenohumeral joint neuromuscular control when combined forces are integrated through the entire kinetic chain. The upper-extremity closed kinetic chain stability test (Davies test) provides an integrated view of upper-extremity function (Goldbeck & Davies 2000; Welch et al., 2020). Electromyography (EMG) and kinematic differences exist between transitional and dynamic movements; therefore, various movement assessments should be used to identify faulty neuromuscular control tendencies to develop comprehensive programs (Mauntel et al., 2018). In combination, these assessments supply abundant information to guide program development and exercise selection.

TRAINING PRINCIPLES FOR RTP

High-quality research is limited in regard to "injured" or "return to sport" athletes, leaving the Sports Performance Coach with little evidence to inform the design and development of resistance training programs for athletes in the advanced stages of injury rehabilitation. The goal is to design comprehensive training programs that facilitate neuromuscular adaptations to build injury resilience and preserve the tissue healing that has already occurred (Bergert et al., 2006; Clover & Wall, 2010; Lorenz & Morrison, 2015).

Movement systems will adapt according to the demands placed upon them. The most common method of increasing the amount of overload is to simply add more resistance. However, additional methods may be just as effective and minimize stress to the healing body part, such as altering rest/recovery periods, changes in velocity, modifying the muscle contraction spectrum (eccentric/isometric/concentric), adjusting the total time under tension, and increasing the number of repetitions and sets (Lorenz et al., 2010; Reiman & Lorenz, 2011). Because all muscles function eccentrically, isometrically, and concentrically in the sagittal, frontal, and transverse planes, an integrated training program should use a multiplanar training approach throughout the entire muscle contraction spectrum (Clark, 2000; Franchi et al., 2017; Reiman & Lorenz, 2011).

Restoration of muscle strength is one of the primary goals of a strength training program (Lorenz & Morrison, 2015). However, force production is just one quality needed for athletic success. A comprehensive program design should equally improve the rate of force production, neuromuscular control, isolated joint and multi-segment stability, energy system efficiency, and (potentially) muscular hypertrophy.

PROGRAM DEVELOPMENT CONSIDERATIONS

The range of physical qualities that can enhance athletic performance is best developed following a systematic and progressive approach. Athletes returning to full participation following the initial rehabilitation stages of injury recovery will also benefit from a comprehensive, multimodal, multiplanar program. However, the specific applications of exercise selection, training frequency, exercise order, rest period, training load, and exercise technique are unique to each athlete, their tissues' tolerance of training loads, and the overall demands of their sport and position.

EXERCISE SELECTION

Exercises encouraging multiplanar, multisensory, and coordinated multi-joint movements should be a primary building block of programming (DiStefano et al., 2013; Hewett & Bates, 2017). Multi-joint movements are typically the most difficult, require the most coordination and skill, and are most taxing to the neuromuscular and metabolic systems (Caldemeyer et al., 2020). Examples include squats, bench presses, pull-ups, and Olympic-style lifts. Eccentric training can help restore normal tissue length in agonist muscles and develop strength throughout improved ROMs through tissue remodeling (Brughelli & Cronin, 2007; Franchi et al., 2017; Reiman & Lorenz, 2011). Training in a controlled, unstable environment often increases motor unit recruitment, significantly reducing the external load (DiStefano et al., 2013; Hewett & Bates, 2017). These movements are instrumental when the goal is optimal muscle activation with submaximal training loads that spare a recovering injury (Reiman & Lorenz, 2011).

TRAINING FREQUENCY

Training frequency depends on the training volume and intensity. Generally, recovery periods of 24 hours between training sessions and 48 hours between sessions that focus on a single body part (Reiman & Lorenz, 2011) are recommended. For example, a split-style routine could be performed daily, where one day would include a "push/pull" model, and the next day's focus would be on the legs. This alternating approach will provide 48 hours of rest between body parts, yet provide sufficient recovery to allow for some training to occur daily (Issurin, 2010). Alternate-day performance scheduling is recommended (initially) to allow an opportunity for recovery and reassessment to evaluate the tissue and structural tolerance of the previous day's level of performance. The injured tissue must be continually monitored for signs of load tolerance failure.

EXERCISE ORDER

The order in which a series of exercises are performed determines the overall outcome. As multi-joint exercises require the highest degree of coordination and metabolic demand, they should be grouped early in the session, followed by exercises focusing on a single joint (Issurin, 2010; Reiman & Lorenz, 2011). Vertical loading offers several advantages, such as enhanced metabolic efficiency, workloads similar to those encountered in an athletic environment, and time efficiency of training. Vertical loading is a circuit-style approach to training in which the athlete performs a series of exercises in succession (Gibala & McGee, 2008; Issurin, 2010). After recovery, they start the next round from the first exercise. Compound training includes biomechanically similar exercises performed in succession (i.e., a superset) with little (or no) rest period between (Issurin, 2010). This style, called strength-endurance training in the OPT™ Model, develops strength, endurance, hypertrophy, and metabolic efficiency. With such training, the strength exercise for that body part is performed first, immediately followed by a (biomechanically similar) stabilization exercise for that same body part. For instance, a bench press immediately followed by push-ups is an example of complex training for the chest/shoulder/triceps muscle groups.

REST PERIOD

The length of the rest period is largely dependent on the exercise training intensity. Higher training intensities will require more extended rest periods.

From a metabolic perspective, the exercise intensity and duration effect (or a combination thereof) depend on the fuel source (Gibala & McGee, 2008; Plews et al., 2013). For example, the phosphagen system provides an instant boost of energy that lasts for only a few seconds. The anaerobic system provides an intermediate energy source for moderate- to high-intensity movements that lasts for a few minutes. The aerobic system relies on sufficient oxygen to produce energy and will provide sustainable energy for long-duration, low-intensity activities. Energy-system development can be a training goal, and rest periods can be manipulated to keep work-to-rest ratios in line with these ranges (Plews et al., 2013; Reiman & Lorenz, 2011) (**Table 20.10**).

TABLE 20.10 Energy System Development

	Phosphagen (Glycolytic)	Anaerobic	Aerobic (Oxidative)
Work-to-rest ratio	1:50 to 1:30	1:10 to 1:30	1:1 to 10+:1

COMBINED TRAINING LOAD

Training loads are typically the product of recommended weekly repetitions, sets, and sessions. Traditionally, these loads have been represented as a percentage of a single-repetition maximum (%1RM) for each exercise. This approach is not practical for the athlete recovering from injury, however, as training with maximal resistance is not recommended in this context (Clover & Wall, 2010; Gabbett et al., 2021). Submaximal training loads within particular volume (sets and repetitions) ranges can provide specific adaptations. These training loads can be combined to deliver specific outcomes, such as strength, stability, endurance, and power. However, each training adaptation may interfere with one another, thereby limiting the optimized development of one specific element (Issurin, 2010). The popularization of sports performance training has stimulated modern research in recovery and regeneration, with recent studies providing evidence on the necessity of maintaining a balance between training, rest, and recovery (Gabbett et al., 2021; Hamlin et al., 2019).

MOVEMENT AND EXERCISE TECHNIQUE

Faulty movement patterns cause abnormal stress to joint surfaces and connective tissues and lead to early fatigue (Eckard et al., 2018a). Exercise-induced fatigue of the lower extremities alters ROM, joint stiffness, and ability to effectively control reactive ground forces and knee valgus moments (Cornell et al., 2021; Hewett & Bates, 2017), thus demonstrating the adverse effects of neuromuscular fatigue on the overall performance decline of a multi-joint system (Cornell et al., 2021; Padua et al., 2012; Zhang et al., 2018). To identify modifiable factors (e.g., strength, mobility, stability, neuromuscular control) contributing to the faulty movement, the Sports Performance Coach can perform a variety of movement-based assessments (Lorenzetti et al., 2018; Sheriff et al., 2021).

CORRECTIVE EXERCISE CONTINUUM

In addition to following a systematic, progressive, comprehensive approach for performance enhancement, an effective model to utilize in the RTP phase is NASM's Corrective Exercise (CEx) Continuum (**Figure 20.18**). Originally described as an individualized warm-up program lasting 10 minutes, its conceptual basis allows for

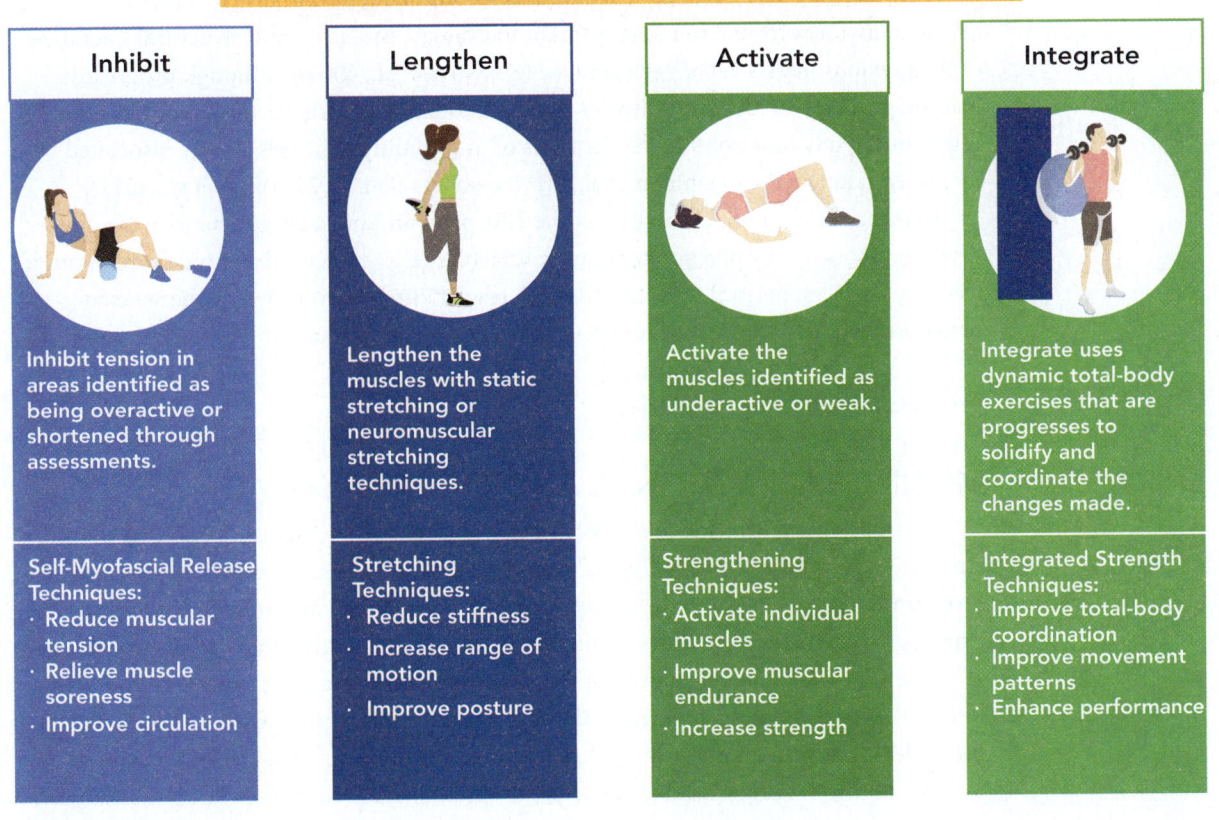

FIGURE 20.18 Corrective Exercise Continuum

an expanded application to accommodate the stimulus (volume, sets, load, number of exercises) required to deliver the intended adaptations. The CEx Continuum, as a programmatic model, aims to mitigate the effects of identified neuromuscular control deficits. Implementing the CEx Continuum involves a four-step process: Inhibit, Lengthen, Activate, and Integrate.

The CEx Continuum is most successful when the specific exercises selected are directly linked to data obtained from movement assessments. **Table 20.11** provides a simplified example for an athlete demonstrating knee valgus. Using this programmatic template, the Sports Performance Coach can add additional exercises, sets, and repetitions while manipulating rest periods to deliver the desired adaptations preserving the injured tissues from potentially damaging stress.

TABLE 20.11 Example of a Corrective Exercise Program for Knee Valgus

Short and overactive	Adductors
Long and underactive	Gluteal complex (gluteus medius)
Step 1: inhibit	SMT adductors, 1 × 30 seconds
Step 2: lengthen	Static stretch adductors, 1 × 30 seconds
Step 3: activate	Side-lying hip abduction (gluteus medius), 1 × 12 reps
Step 4: integrate	Single-leg balance reach, 1 × 12 reps

Alternate-day performance scheduling is recommended (initially) to allow an opportunity for recovery and reassessment to evaluate the tissue and structural tolerance of the previous day's level of performance (Kraemer et al., 2009). Although progressive loading provides an ideal stimulus for tissue remodeling, Sports Performance Coaches must continually monitor athletes for signs of overloading, which is closely associated with increased reinjury risks (Dhillon et al., 2017; Gabbett et al., 2021; Weiss et al., 2017).

To extend the simplified version of the CEx program into a comprehensive training program, modify the appropriate training variables (e.g., exercise selection, exercise order, training load, rest period) to match the athlete's status while considering the specific details of the individual's sport and position. The CEx Continuum model seamlessly aligns with long-term performance training and is appropriate for athletes returning to full participation following an injury.

MONITORING INTERNAL AND EXTERNAL LOAD

The critical challenge for the Sports Performance Coach is to balance intentional training stress with adequate recovery. Throughout the injury rehabilitation and RTP process, programming strategies to improve the load tolerance of the compromised tissues are the primary focus. As training shifts to introduce more sport-specific movements and training at greater intensities, it is helpful to utilize tools to quantify training loads (external and internal) to prevent undertraining and buffer against overtraining. External load refers to the athlete's performance efforts (e.g., repetitions, weight lifted, distance, time running, number of throws, or peak velocity), whereas internal loads comprise the biomechanical, physiologic, and psychologic effects of the external loads (**Table 20.12**). From a

TABLE 20.12 Internal vs. External Load

Internal Load ("What happened to you")	External Load ("What you did")
• Metabolic changes • Muscle hypertrophy • Muscular strength • Improved vertical jump • Changes in resting heart rate • Sleep quality	• Total repetitions • Training intensity • Total pounds lifted • Distance of running • Speed of running

measurement perspective, external loads are simple to document. In contrast, the accurate representation of the internal loads is more complex.

The **session rating of perceived exertion (sRPE)** is the most widely used athlete-reported outcome method to quantify internal response to training loads (Foster et al., 2001). These data can be tracked over time to identify trends and ensure the athlete's perceived effort matches the expected response according to the predetermined training goals for that session (Gabbett et al., 2021). Training responses are highly individualized, and often differences in sRPEs are common among team members completing the same training session under the same conditions (Bowen et al., 2020; Gabbett et al., 2021; Impellizzeri, Menaspà, et al., 2020).

However, it is vital to put each session into a broader context to determine the relationships between how the training loads in a single training session compare to those averaged over the prior 4 weeks (Blanch & Gabbett, 2016). The intention is to look at the athlete's chronic, long-term training habits compared to their more recent habits as a method to monitor modifiable factors that increase injury risk (Eckard et al., 2018a). Athletes with patterns of consistent, progressive training programs tend to be more resilient to changes in workload and generally experience lower injury risk (Nielsen et al., 2017).

The **acute-to-chronic workload ratio (ACWR)** is a clinical tool to compare the effects of fatigue (acute workload) to levels of fitness (chronic workload). When represented as a ratio of acute-to-chronic workload (ACWR), the data can be used to quantify training outcomes (Impellizzeri, McCall, et al., 2020; Morton et al., 1990). To promote the most significant fitness gains and injury resilience, the ACWR should be between 1.0 and 1.5, with a higher risk of injury associated with a higher ratio (Blanch & Gabbett, 2016). Athletes with ACWRs greater than 1.5 are 2 to 4 times more likely to experience an injury (Gabbett, 2020), and those with ACWRs of 2.0 or greater may be at up to 7 times greater risk (Bowen et al., 2020). **Table 20.13** provides an example calculation of the ACWR for a runner at the end of the ideal range and trending toward increased injury risks.

SESSION RATING OF PERCEIVED EXERTION (sRPE) →

A self-reported outcome measure used to monitor the perceived difficulty of a training session.

ACUTE-TO-CHRONIC WORKLOAD RATIO (ACWR) →

A clinical tool used to measure the effects of fatigue (acute workload) on fitness levels (chronic workload).

TABLE 20.13 Example Calculation: ACWR for a Runner

Average Milage	New Milage	ACWR Calculation
50 miles per week for 4 weeks	75 miles	75 ÷ 50 = 1.5 ACWR

ACWR can also be calculated using sRPE (**Table 20.14**). The sRPE method is intended to provide the Sports Performance Coach with a simple, valid, and reliable tool to measure the athlete-reported response to training loads.

TABLE 20.14 Example Calculation: ACWR for sRPE

Past Daily Average sRPE	New Daily Average sRPE	ACWR Calculation
6.5 for 4 weeks	4 for the past week	4 ÷ 6.5 = 0.62 ACWR

The value obtained in Table 20.14, 0.62, falls below the ideal range (1.0 to 1.5) (**Figure 20.19**), indicating that this athlete is on a detraining trajectory and not maintaining adaptations earned through prior training. This subjective rating tool, which is based on a limited range (1-to-10) scale, certainly has limitations—particularly when fitness levels generally improve over time, which could alter workload perceptions, and the timing of the training calendar may be geared toward a higher acute training load (e.g., pre-season). The ACWR should not be used to modify specific training programs (Impellizzeri et al., 2019; Impellizzeri, McCall, et al., 2020; Impellizzeri, Menaspà, et al., 2020) but can have practical value in guiding decision making (Gabbett et al., 2021).

1	Nothing
2	Very Easy
3	Easy
4	Comfortable
5	Somewhat Difficult
6	Difficult
7	Hard
8	Very Hard
9	Extremely Hard
10	Maximal/Exhaustion

FIGURE 20.19 Session Rating of Perceived Exertion

PSYCHOLOGICAL CONSIDERATIONS

Injury rehabilitation primarily speaks to physiological damage and repair. Equally crucially, the psychological aspects must be addressed to optimize the continued recovery and reintroduction to sports/team activities. Feelings of discouragement and disappointment will inevitably have to be managed. Athletes must be encouraged and motivated through the process. The Sports Performance Coach must recognize negative attitudes and redirect the athlete toward focusing on what must be done to return the athlete to competition. The psychological impact of injuries must be a continual area of focus throughout the RTP process.

Concerns over reinjury, regaining team status, and failing to perform can affect psychological readiness and thus influence the rate of recovery and the successful outcomes of the RTP process (Kraemer et al., 2009). Psychological readiness is primarily influenced by the athlete's emotions and confidence; this term is frequently used to describe the mental factors influencing return to sports after injury (Webster & Feller, 2018). Such factors include realistic expectations, confidence in performance, high levels of self-efficacy, and low levels of fear and anxiety (Faleide et al., 2020). Notably, low fear of reinjury and high psychological readiness have been found to favor a return to pre-injury level of the sport (Ardern et al., 2016) **(Figure 20.20)**.

Psychological Readiness

- Confidence in performance

- High levels of self-efficacy

- Realistic expectations

- Low levels of fear and anxiety

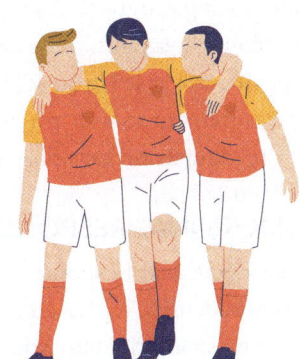

FIGURE 20.20 Factors Associated with Psychological Readiness

Athletes who experience high stress levels (on or off the field) are consistently at the highest risk of injury. In response to stress, athletes may experience a variety of emotional responses, with these reactions following no predictable pattern or sequence (Kraemer et al., 2009). Common signs of stress and emotional responses to stress are listed in **Table 20.15**.

TABLE 20.15 Common Signs and Emotional Responses to Stress

Common Signs of Stress	Common Emotional Responses to Stress
• Behavioral: altered sleep, lack of focus, substance abuse, performance decline in games (versus practice) • Physical: feeling ill, headaches, altered appetite, profuse sweating • Psychological: negativity (thoughts, images, self-talk), inability to focus, self-doubt	• Persistent: altered appetite, disturbed sleep, irritable • Worsening: disordered eating, sadness/depression, disengagement, and alienation • Excessive: anger and rage, substance abuse, emotional outbursts, pain behaviors

The Sports Performance Coach plays a vital role by continuously monitoring the athlete's physical and psychological responses to training. When athletes are in the RTP phase, several factors should be considered that will proactively enable the development of a successful environment that will nurture trust and rapport:

- Identify misinformation about the injury and provide proper education about the injury and recovery process.

- Encourage the use of specific stress coping skills, such as motivation, thought restructuring/replacement, imagery, relaxation skills, and coping simulations (Faleide et al., 2020; Kraemer et al., 2009).
- Use relevant and reliable tools (e.g., ERAIQ, I-PRSS, POMS) as critical resources to monitor psychological readiness following an injury.

RTP RESOURCES

Many resources provide alternative methods of monitoring current status and measuring progress. This section highlights some widely used patient-reported outcome measures. They can serve as objective measures that may be applied to specific use cases in an RTP setting. Although a comprehensive array of outcome measurement tools is provided here, there are undoubtedly other valid resources used by rehabilitation care providers.

EMOTIONAL RESPONSE OF ATHLETES TO INJURY QUESTIONNAIRE

The Emotional Response of Athletes to Injury Questionnaire (ERAIQ) is a comprehensive tool used to assess the athlete's sports preferences, motivation, number of sports participation hours (per week) before and after injury, perceived athleticism, perceived recovery, goals (including those before and after the injury), presence of fears associated with RTP, and perceived support and pressures to return (from family, friends, teammates, coaches, and media) (Smith et al., 1990). The full ERAIQ can be found in Appendix E.

INJURY-PSYCHOLOGICAL READINESS TO RETURN TO SPORT

The Injury-Psychological Readiness to Return to Sport (I-PRRS) is a tool that focuses on the athlete's perceived confidence to return to their sport safely while considering levels of pain, self-appraisal of skill and ability, motivation and desire, and satisfactory injury recovery to handle the demands of the sport/activity (Glazer, 2009). Athletes answer six questions on a scale from 0 to 100, set in 10-point increments. A score of 0 implies the athlete has little or no confidence, whereas a score of 100 implies that they have the highest level of confidence in that item. Upon completion, the scores are summed, then divided by 10. A final score of 60 indicates the highest level of confidence to return to sport; a score of 40 shows only moderate confidence; and a score of 20 indicates low overall confidence. The full I-PRRS can be found in Appendix E.

PROFILE OF MOOD STATES

The Profile of Mood States (POMS) is used to primarily measure the athlete's emotional response to injury and the changes in mood state throughout the recovery period/process. This quick survey provides a critical index of mood alterations after an injury as measured by six mood states—tension, depression, anger, vigor, fatigue, and confusion (Grove & Prapavessis, 1992). The full POMS can found in Appendix E.

ACL-RETURN TO SPORT AFTER INJURY SCALE

The ACL-Return to Sport After Injury (ACL-RSI) scale was developed to measure psychological readiness to return to sport following an ACL injury, surgical intervention, and lengthy physical therapy regimen. This 12-item scale measures an athlete's emotions, confidence in performance, and risk appraisal (Webster & Feller, 2018). The full ACL-RSI can be found in Appendix E.

SINGLE ASSESSMENT NUMERIC EVALUATION

The Single Assessment Numeric Evaluation (SANE) tool, which was established initially as a patient-reported outcome measure after shoulder surgery, can be adapted to suit various needs. The SANE rating (Williams et al., 1999) is based on the athlete's response to a single question: "How would you rate your [shoulder] today as a percentage of normal (0% to 100% scale, with 100% being normal)?" This model can be adapted to objectify the status of any body part and continues to be helpful long after the athlete has successfully returned to full participation. The full SANE tool is found in Appendix E.

FUNCTIONAL ARM SCALE FOR THROWERS

The Functional Arm Scale for Throwers (FAST), a patient-reported outcome scale, is an upper-extremity region-specific tool for throwers that measures status across five domains: pain, throwing, activities of daily living, psychological impact, and advancement (Sauers et al., 2017). This scale is appropriate for any athlete recovering from a shoulder injury, but particularly those in racquet and throwing sports. The full FAST can be found in Appendix E.

INTERVAL THROWING PROGRAM

The Interval Throwing Program is designed to progressively reintroduce throwing-related forces to healing tissues and gradually return the athlete to full participation (Reinold et al., 2002). A critical focus of this program is on proper throwing mechanics. A specialized throwing (pitching) coach or biomechanist may be a helpful resource to guide advancement through the program. The Interval Throwing Program can be found in Appendix E.

The RTP process is a multifaceted approach that involves evaluating an athlete's health risk, activity risk, and risk tolerance. Considerations include the nature and severity of the injury, the athlete's physical and psychological readiness, the demands of the sport or activity, and the athlete's and stakeholders' acceptance of risk. The goal is not just to help the athlete recover from the injury, but also to ensure safe and effective performance while minimizing the risk of reinjury. The RTP decision is often made using standardized models and frameworks, such as the StARRT framework, and should involve a comprehensive, multimodal, and individualized rehabilitation and training program.

LESSON 5: APPLIED LEARNING
CASE STUDIES

Translations from theory to practice can be challenging. A practical method to better visualize implementation is scenario-based learning and population-specific personas. The case studies presented in this section offer a unique opportunity to develop a programmatic strategy that aligns with the athlete's training constraints, performance goals, and injury history. Physical training exercises simply supply elements of overload intended to develop or enhance particular physiologic attributes that deliver a performance advantage. This chapter has focused on planned, intentional training to reduce injury risk and improve overall resilience to preventable musculoskeletal injury. Therefore, commentary specific to these personas will be limited to typical injuries associated with these sports/activities.

The template popularized in NASM's Corrective Exercise Continuum is used to guide program development. Of course, the list of exercises and stretches continues to expand. The ones provided here are intended for demonstration purposes only. Individual athletes may respond to exercises, order, repetitions, and sets in a different fashion than other athletes. The Sports Performance Coach should be prepared to utilize a variety of movement patterns to address complex movement impairment concerns.

Exercise selection should target mechanical drivers of increased foot pronation, knee valgus, and internal femoral rotation. Beginning with the Flexibility section, the focus is on inhibitory and lengthening techniques targeting muscle groups that tend to be overactive. Next, the Activation stage strives to improve isolated motor activity to a functional antagonist (e.g., adductors are inhibited and lengthened; hip abductors are activated). Finally, the Integration stage is more transitional and accounts for more dynamic control of body weight through all three planes of motion.

CASE STUDY 1: JIM

Jim is a young, apparently healthy, fit athlete with an appropriate body weight. He is a competitive triathlete with a goal to improve his performance in the run stage of the event. Occasionally, he gets soreness in his feet and knees. His training goal is to improve his running economy, neuromuscular efficiency, and long-duration stability of the lower extremity. In a basic sense, triathlons require extremes of physical strength, stamina, and mental focus. However extreme, these abundant (and frequent) running, swimming, and cycling training volumes should factor into the volume recommendations for supplemental training in the weight room. Exercises of value promote sustained postural control of the foot, particularly when combined with proper alignment of the hips (level) and knee (aligned over second toe). Jim's program can be found in Appendix E.

CASE STUDY 2: MARIA

Maria is a young, competitive soccer player. Currently, she plays the forward position, which requires her to initiate body contact with opponents and have frequent, short-duration/high-intensity sprinting bouts. Currently, she reports no general health concerns; however, her sport ranks high on the list of activities in which participants sustain ACL injuries. Such injuries (and related recovery) will almost certainly end a competitive season. Therefore, the nature of her sport dictates that Maria's program follows the progressive neuromuscular guidelines to protect the ACL and develop short-burst, sport-specific running speed. A program of this nature will address her current limitations in hip mobility and deficits in core strength, and properly prepare her for the cutting and jumping demands of soccer. Maria's program can be found in Appendix E.

CASE STUDY 3: MIKA

Mika is a 30-year-old software company executive with ambitions to complete a 10K adventure obstacle race. A review of his height and weight suggests he is fit and proportioned with adequate muscle mass. To complete his 10K race, he will need to improve his overall endurance and ability to actively recover from obstacle challenges as he continues the run portion of the event. In the past, Mika has dealt with intermittent foot pain. Exercise selection should address mechanical drivers of foot pronation, knee adduction, and internal femoral rotation, as well as improve his overall balance, power, upper-extremity stability, and grip strength. Mika'a event is a year away, which should allow ample time to progressively and systematically implement goal-specific training phases to address his physical and metabolic needs. Mika's program can be found in Appendix E.

CASE STUDY 4: DAVE

Dave is a middle-aged, former collegiate golfer who wants to compete in a 4-day golf tournament in 6 months. His consistent participation in golf and regular exercise has been limited by injuries to his lower back. Dave has recently been under the care of a physician, who has recommended a return to structured training to develop better flexibility and core strength. Exercise program development should consider the rapid (sometimes violent) acceleration required in an effective golf swing. To enhance club head velocity, focus on exercises that improve hip internal rotation, external rotation, abduction, extension, and rotary stability through the trunk. Dave's program can be found in Appendix E.

SUMMARY

Any return-to-play strategy aims to achieve readiness: a condition where the athlete has no physical performance impairment, mental fatigue, or excessive psychological stress. While sports-related injuries are common, the Sports Performance Coach has the knowledge and ability to develop programming designed to build injury resilience and support desired performance outcomes. This requires a knowledge of the epidemiology of the injury and an understanding of prevention strategies to prepare athletes for the demands of the sport. Prevention strategies are vital to an athlete's health and career longevity. The influence of poor biomechanics, neuromuscular dysfunctions, overtraining, and decreased flexibility contribute to injury. Research has provided evidence supporting preventive strategies that include integrated flexibility, proprioceptive training, strengthening, a focus on proper technique, and implementation of progressive plyometric intervention strategies.

Once the athlete returns to their competitive domain, the work of the performance enhancement specialist continues with a focus on injury risk mitigation and fitness optimization. This is best achieved by following a comprehensive, systematic, and individualized approach to training the human movement system (Clark, 2000), which will deliver optimal development of biomechanical, physiological, and psychological systems.

KEY TAKEAWAYS

- Movement quality is key. An abundance of research demonstrates the adverse effects of poor movement quality (i.e., fatigue, muscle weakness, pain/injury, altered muscle activation patterns, diminished rate of force production, and decreased performance outcomes). Perform movement quality assessments to identify modifiable factors (strength, mobility, stability, neuromuscular control) that can be used to guide exercise selection. Implementing multiple checks to identify faulty movement patterns will yield the best results. Performance on one assessment does not dictate performance in another evaluation.
- Exercise technique matters. Especially with an athlete in the return-to-play stage, movement under load must be in biomechanically appropriate ranges. Feet should be forward during the two-legged squat (weighted or not). Allowing for knees-in, knees-out, toes-in, and toes-out position places unnecessary stress on the tissue and joint surfaces and may contribute to joint pathologies.
- All training programs should be evidence based, intentionally administered, progressive, gradual, appropriately monitored, and nonpunitive in nature.

- Improve proximal stability before distal mobility (local → global). Prime movers can be activated only to the degree to which joints are stabilized. To boost force production in prime movers, first improve neuromuscular control, coordination and stability—and strive to restore the mobility/stability relationship among alternating joint complexes throughout the kinetic chain.
- Return to play is a constantly evolving process. As neuromuscular coordination improves, so does tissue tolerance, which accelerates multi-segmental movement efficiency. These developments collectively contribute to a safe reintroduction to the sport.
- Begin with the end in mind. What will the joints be expected to do? Which forces should the muscles be prepared to distribute safely? Is there time in the current season for the athlete to successfully return to their sport? Consider all these factors when developing return-to-play programs.
- Utilization of tools and resources to monitor external and internal training loads, functional status, and psychological readiness is a best practice.
- Reintroduction to full participation does not end the return-to-play process, but rather is another milestone in the ongoing recovery process. Continue to monitor for aberrant tissue responses to stress—and adjust accordingly.
- Utilize performance and sport-specific tests as opportunities to compare the athlete's level of achievement to baseline values and objectively gauge progress.
- Work as a team, and prioritize 360-degree communication in which you lead with accurate and timely information sharing among members of the care team (athletic trainer, physical therapist, team physician), coaches, sports performance support staff, and the athlete.

REFERENCES

Abdelraouf, O. R., & Abdel-Aziem, A. (2016). The relationship between core endurance and back dysfunction in collegiate male athletes with and without nonspecific low back pain. *International Journal of Sports Physical Therapy, 11*(3), 337–344.

Agel, J., Arendt, E., & Bershadsky, B. (2015). Anterior cruciate ligament injury in National Collegiate Athletic Association basketball and soccer: A 13-year review. *American Journal of Sports Medicine, 33*, 524–530. https://doi.org/10.1177/0363546504269937

Andersen, L. L., Andersen, J. L., Magnusson, S. P., Suetta, C., Madsen, J. L., Christensen, L. R., & Aagaard, P. (2005). Changes in the human muscle force–velocity relationship in response to resistance training and subsequent detraining. *Journal of Applied Physiology (Bethesda, MD: 1985), 99*(1), 87–94. https://doi.org/10.1152/japplphysiol.00091.2005

Ardern, C. L., Kvist, J., & Webster, K. E. (2016). Psychological aspects of anterior cruciate ligament injuries. *Operative Techniques in Sports Medicine, 24,* 77-83.

Arnoldi, C. C. (1991). The patellar pain syndrome. *Actaorthpaedica Scandinavica Supplementum, 244,* 62.

Bagherian, S., Ghasempoor, K., Rahnama, N., & Wikstrom, E. A. (2017). The effect of core stability training on functional movements in college athletes. *Journal of Sport Rehabilitation, 28*(5), 444–449.

Bagherian, S., Rahnama, N., Wikstrom, E. A., Clark, M. A., & Rostami, F. (2018). Characterizing lower extremity movement scores before and after fatigue in collegiate athletes with chronic ankle instability. *International Journal Athletic Therapy and Training, 23,* 27–32.

Barrack, M. T., Gibbs, J. C., De Souza, M. J., Williams, N. I., Nichols, J. F., Rauh, M. J., & Nattiv, A. (2014). Higher incidence of bone stress injuries with increasing female athlete triad-related risk factors: A prospective multisite study of exercising girls and women. *American Journal of Sports Medicine, 42*(4), 949–958. https://doi.org/10.1177/0363546513520295

Behm, D. G., & Colado, J. C. (2013). Instability resistance training across the exercise continuum. *Sports Health, 5*(6), 500–503. https://doi.org/10.1177/1941738113477815

Bell, D. R., Padua, D. A., & Clark, M. A. (2008). Muscle strength and flexibility characteristics of people displaying excessive medial knee displacement. *Archives of Physical Medicine and Rehabilitation, 89*(7), 1323–1328. https://doi.org/10.1016/j.apmr.2007.11.048

Bell, D. R., Vesci, B. J., DiStefano, L. J., Guskiewicz, K. M., Hirth, C. J., & Padua, D. A. (2012). Muscle activity and flexibility in individuals with medial knee displacement during the overhead squat. *Athletic Training and Sports Health Care, 4*(3), 117–125.

Bell-Jenje, T., Olivier, B., Wood, W., Rogers, S., Green, A., & McKinon, W. (2016). The association between loss of ankle dorsiflexion range of movement, and hip adduction and internal rotation during a step down test. *Manual Therapy, 21*, 256–261. https://doi.org/10.1016/j.math.2015.09.010

Benjamin, M., Toumi, H., Ralphs, J. R., Bydder, G., Best, T. M., & Milz, S. (2006). Where tendons and ligaments meet bone: Attachment sites ("entheses") in relation to exercise and/or mechanical load. *Journal of Anatomy, 208*(4), 471–490. https://doi.org/10.1111/j.1469-7580.2006.00540.x

Bergert, N., Harmon, B., & Yocum, L. (2006). Shoulder injuries. In *Athletic training and sports medicine.* (pp. 267–335). Jones & Bartlett Learning.

Blanch, P., & Gabbett, T. J. (2016). Has the athlete trained enough to return to play safely? The acute:chronic workload ratio permits clinicians to quantify a player's risk of subsequent injury. *British Journal of Sports Medicine, 50*(8), 471–475. https://doi.org/10.1136/bjsports-2015-095445

Bongers, P. M. (2001). The cost of shoulder pain at work. *BMJ (Clinical Research ed.), 322*(7278), 64–65. https://doi.org/10.1136/bmj.322.7278.64

Borsa, P. A., Laudner, K. G., & Sauers, E. L. (2008). Mobility and stability adaptations in the shoulder of the overhead athlete: A theoretical and evidence-based perspective. *Sports Medicine (Auckland, NZ), 38*(1), 17–36. https://doi.org/10.2165/00007256-200838010-00003

Bowen, L., Gross, A. S., Gimpel, M., Bruce-Low, S., & Li, F. X. (2020). Spikes in acute:chronic workload ratio (ACWR) associated with a 5–7 times greater injury rate in English Premier League football players: A comprehensive 3-year study. *British Journal of Sports Medicine, 54*, 731–738.

Bram, J. T., Magee, L. C., Mehta, N. N., Patel, N. M., & Ganley, T. J. (2021). Anterior cruciate ligament injury incidence in adolescent athletes: A systematic review and meta-analysis. *The American Journal of Sports Medicine, 49*(7), 1962–1972. https://doi.org/10.1177/0363546520959619

Brughelli, M., & Cronin, J. (2007). Altering the length–tension relationship with eccentric exercise: implications for performance and injury. *Sports Medicine (Auckland, NZ), 37*(9), 807–826. https://doi.org/10.2165/00007256-200737090-00004

Buss, D. D., Lynch, G. P., Meyer, C. P., Huber, S. M., & Freehill, M. Q. (2004). Nonoperative management for in-season athletes with anterior shoulder instability. *American Journal of Sports Medicine, 32*(6), 1430–1433. https://doi.org/10.1177/0363546503262069

Caldemeyer, L. E., Brown, S. M., & Mulcahey, M. K. (2020). Neuromuscular training for the prevention of ankle sprains in female athletes: A systematic review. *Physician and Sportsmedicine, 48*(4), 363–369. https://doi.org/10.1080/00913847.2020.1732246

Carpenter, J. E., Flanagan, C. L., Thomopoulos, S., Yian, E. H., & Soslowsky, L. J. (1998). The effects of overuse combined with intrinsic or extrinsic alterations in an animal model of rotator cuff tendinosis. *American Journal of Sports Medicine, 26*, 801–807.

Casa, D. J. (2012). *Preventing sudden death in sport and physical activity.* Jones & Bartlett Learning.

Centers for Disease Control and Prevention. (2019). *Post-COVID conditions: Information for healthcare providers.* https://archive.cdc.gov/www_cdc_gov/coronavirus/2019-ncov/hcp/clinical-care/post-covid-conditions.html

Chepeha, J. C., Magee, D. J., Bouliane, M., Sheps, D., & Beaupre, L. (2018). Effectiveness of a posterior shoulder stretching program on university-level overhead athletes: Randomized controlled trial. *Clinical Journal of Sport Medicine: Official Journal of the Canadian Academy of Sport Medicine, 28*(2), 146–152. https://doi.org/10.1097/JSM.0000000000000434

Clark, M. A. (2000). *Integrated training for the new millennium.* National Academy of Sports Medicine.

Clover, J., & Wall, J. (2010). Return-to-play criteria following sports injury. *Clinics in Sports Medicine, 29*(1). https://doi.org/10.1016/j.csm.2009.09.008

Cohen, B., Kleinhenz, D., Schiller, J., & Tabaddor, R. (2016). Understanding athletic pubalgia: A review. *Rhode Island Medical Journal (2013), 99*(10), 31–35.

Cohen, D. D., Restrepo, A., Richter, C., Harry, J. R., Franchi, M. V., Restrepo, C., Poletto, R., & Taberner, M. (2021). Detraining of specific neuromuscular qualities in elite footballers during COVID-19 quarantine. *Science and Medicine in Football.* https://doi.org/10.1080/24733938.2020.1834123

Colombo, C. S. S. S., Leitão, M. B., Avanza Junior, A. C., Borges, S. F., Silveira, A. D., Braga, F., Camarozano, A. C., Kopiler, D. A., Lazzoli, J. K., Freitas, O. G. A., Grossman, G. B., Milani, M., Nunes, M. B., Ritt, L. E. F., Sellera, C. A. C., & Ghorayeb, N. (2021). Position statement on post–COVID-19 cardiovascular preparticipation screening: Guidance for returning to physical exercise and sports–2020. *Arquivos Brasileiros de Cardiologia, 116*(6), 1213–1226.

Connes, P. (2015). Sickle cell trait, exertional rhabdomyolysis, and compartment syndrome. *Lancet, 385*(9981), 1948. https://doi.org/10.1016/s0140-6736(15)60961-8

Cook, G. (2010). *Functional movement systems: Screening, assessment, and corrective strategies.* On Target Publications.

Cornell, D. J., Ebersole, K. T., Azen, R., Zalewski, K. R., Earl-Boehm, J. E., & Alt, C. A. (2021). Measures of functional movement quality among firefighters. *Athletic Training & Sports Health Care, 13*(5), e262–e270. https://doi.org/10.3928/19425864-20201117-01

Coulombe, B. J., Games, K. E., Neil, E. R., & Eberman, L. E. (2017). Core stability exercise versus general exercise for chronic low back pain. *Journal of Athletic Training, 52*(1), 71–72. https://doi.org/10.4085/1062-6050-51.11.16

Coyle, E. F. (1990). Detraining and retention of training-induced adaptations. *Sports Science Exchange, 2,* 1–5.

Creighton, D. W., Shrier, I., Shultz, R., Meeuwisse, W. H., & Matheson, G. O. (2010). Return-to-play in sport: A decision-based model. *Clinical Journal of Sport Medicine: Official Journal of the Canadian Academy of Sport Medicine, 20*(5), 379–385. https://doi.org/10.1097/JSM.0b013e3181f3c0fe

Cyron, C. J., & Humphrey, J. D. (2017). Growth and remodeling of load-bearing biological soft tissues. *Meccanica, 52*(3), 645–664. https://doi.org/10.1007/s11012-016-0472-5

Davies, G. J., McCarty, E., Provencher, M., & Manske, R. C. (2017). ACL return to sport guidelines and criteria. *Current Reviews in Musculoskeletal Medicine, 10*(3), 307–314. https://doi.org/10.1007/s12178-017-9420-9

Dhillon, H., Dhillon, S., & Dhillon, M. S. (2017). Current concepts in sports injury rehabilitation. *Indian Journal of Orthopaedics, 51*(5), 529–536. https://doi.org/10.4103/ortho.IJOrtho_226_17

Diab, A. A. (2012). The role of forward head correction in management of adolescent idiopathic scoliotic patients: A randomized controlled trial. *Clinical Rehabilitation, 26*(12), 1123–1132. https://doi.org/10.1177/0269215512447085

DiStefano, L. J., Clark, M. A., & Padua, D. A. (2009). Evidence supporting balance training in healthy individuals: A systemic review. *Journal of Strength and Conditioning Research, 23*(9), 2718–2731. https://doi.org/10.1519/JSC.0b013e3181c1f7c5

DiStefano, L. J., DiStefano, M. J., Frank, B. S., Clark, M. A., & Padua, D. A. (2013). Comparison of integrated and isolated training on performance measures and neuromuscular control. *Journal of Strength and Conditioning Research, 27*(4), 1083–1090. https://doi.org/10.1519/JSC.0b013e318280d40b

Doherty, C., Bleakley, C., Hertel, J., Caulfield, B., Ryan, J., & Delahunt, E. (2016). Recovery from a first-time lateral ankle sprain and the predictors of chronic ankle instability: A prospective cohort analysis. *American Journal of Sports Medicine, 44*(4), 995–1003. https://doi.org/10.1177/0363546516628870

Donovan, L., Hetzel, S., Laufenberg, C. R., & McGuine, T. A. (2020). Prevalence and impact of chronic ankle instability in adolescent athletes. *Orthopaedic Journal of Sports Medicine, 8*(2), 2325967119900962. https://doi.org/10.1177/2325967119900962

Drake, J. D., Aultman, C. D., McGill, S. M., & Callaghan, J. P. (2005). The influence of static axial torque in combined loading on intervertebral joint failure mechanics using a porcine model. *Clinical Biomechanics (Bristol, Avon), 20*(10), 1038–1045. https://doi.org/10.1016/j.clinbiomech.2005.06.007

Driver, S., Reynolds, M., Brown, K., Vingren, J. L., Hill, D. W., Bennett, M., Gilliland, T., McShan, E., Callender, L., Reynolds, E., Borunda, N., Mosolf, J., Cates, C., & Jones, A. (2022). Effects of wearing a cloth face mask on performance, physiological and perceptual responses during a graded treadmill running exercise test. *British Journal of Sports Medicine, 56*(2), 107–113. https://doi.org/10.1136/bjsports-2020-103758

Eckard, T. G., Padua, D. A., Hearn, D. W., Pexa, B. S., & Frank, B. S. (2018a). The relationship between training load and injury in athletes: A systematic review. *Sports Medicine (Auckland, NZ), 48*(8), 1929–1961. https://doi.org/10.1007/s40279-018-0951-z

Eckard, T. G., Padua, D. A., Mauntel, T., Frank, B., Pietrosimone, L., Begalle, R., Goto, S., Clark, M., & Kucera, K. (2018b). Association between double-leg squat and single-leg squat performance and injury incidence among incoming NCAA Division I athletes: A prospective cohort study. *Physical Therapy in Sport: Official Journal of the Association of Chartered Physiotherapists in Sports Medicine, 34,* 192–200. https://doi.org/10.1016/j.ptsp.2018.10.009

Elliott, N., Martin, R., Heron, N., Elliott, J., Grimstead, D., & Biswas, A. (2020). Infographic. Graduated return to play guidance following COVID-19 infection. *British Journal of Sports Medicine, 54*(19), 1174–1175. https://doi.org/10.1136/bjsports-2020-102637

Enoka, R. M. (2002). *Neuromechanics of human movement* (3rd ed.). Human Kinetics.

Fahmy, R. (2022). *NASM essentials of corrective exercise training* (2nd ed.). Jones & Bartlett Learning.

Faleide, A., Inderhaug, E., Vervaat, W., Breivik, K., Bogen, B. E., Mo, I. F., Trøan, I., Strand, T., & Magnussen, L. H. (2020). Anterior Cruciate Ligament—Return to Sport After Injury Scale: Validation of the Norwegian language version. *Knee Surgery, Sports Traumatology, Arthroscopy: Official Journal of the ESSKA, 28*(8), 2634–2643. https://doi.org/10.1007/s00167-020-05901-0

Fares, M. Y., Fares, J., Baydoun, H., & Fares, Y. (2020). Prevalence and patterns of shoulder injuries in Major League Baseball. *Physician and Sports Medicine, 48*(1), 63–67. https://doi.org/10.1080/00913847.2019.1629705

Fernandez, W. G., Yard, E. E., & Comstock, R. D. (2008). Epidemiology of lower extremity injuries among U.S. high school athletes. *Academic Emergency Medicine: Official Journal of the Society for Academic Emergency Medicine, 14*(7), 641–645. https://onlinelibrary.wiley.com/doi/10.1111/j.1553-2712.2007.tb01851.x

Fett, D., Trompeter, K., & Platen, P. (2019). Prevalence of back pain in a group of elite athletes exposed to repetitive overhead activity. *PLOS One, 14*(1), e0210429. https://doi.org/10.1371/journal.pone.0210429

Foster, C., Florhaug, J. A., Franklin, J., Gottschall, L., Hrovatin, L. A., Parker, S., Doleshal, P., & Dodge, C. (2001). A new approach to monitoring exercise training. *Journal of Strength and Conditioning Research, 15*(1), 109–115.

Franchi, M. V., Reeves, N. D., & Narici, M. V. (2017). Skeletal muscle remodeling in response to eccentric vs. concentric loading: Morphological, molecular, and metabolic adaptations. *Frontiers in Physiology, 8,* 447.

Fredericson, M., Cookingham, C. L., Chaudhari, A. M., Dowdell, B. C., Oestreicher, N., & Sahrmann, S. A. (2000). Hip abductor weakness in distance runners with iliotibial band syndrome. *Clinical Journal of Sport Medicine: Official Journal of the Canadian Academy of Sport Medicine, 10*(3), 169–175. https://doi.org/10.1097/00042752-200007000-00004

Freehill, M. T., & Safran, M. R. (2011a). Diagnosis and management of ulnar collateral ligament injuries in throwers. *Current Sports Medicine Reports, 10*(5), 271–278. https://doi.org/10.1249/JSR.0b013e31822d4000

Freehill, M. T., & Safran, M. R. (2011b). The labrum of the hip: Diagnosis and rationale for surgical correction. *Clinics in Sports Medicine, 30*(2), 293–315. https://doi.org/10.1016/j.csm.2010.12.002

Fuller, C. W., Bahr, R., Dick, R. W., & Meeuwisse, W. H. (2007). A framework for recording recurrences, reinjuries, and exacerbations in injury surveillance. *Clinical Journal of Sport Medicine, 17*(3), 197–200. https://doi.org/10.1097/JSM.0b013e3180471b89

Gabbett, T .J. (2020). Debunking the myths about training load, injury and performance: empirical evidence, hot topics and recommendations for practitioners. *British Journal of Sports Medicine, 54*(1), 58–66.

Gabbett, T., Sancho, I., Dingenen, B., & Willy, R. W. (2021). When progressing training loads, what are the considerations for healthy and injured athletes? *British Journal of Sports Medicine, 55*(17), 947–948. https://doi.org/10.1136/bjsports-2020-103769

Geisler, P. R. (2021). Current clinical concepts: Synthesizing the available evidence for improved clinical outcomes in iliotibial band impingement syndrome. *Journal of Athletic Training, 56*(8), 805–815. https://doi.org/10.4085/1062-6050-548-19

Gibala, M. J., & McGee, S. L. (2008). Metabolic adaptations to short-term high-intensity interval training: A little pain for a lot of gain? *Exercise and Sport Sciences Reviews, 36*(2), 58–63. https://doi.org/10.1097/JES.0b013e318168ec1f

Glazer, D. D. (2009). Development and preliminary validation of the Injury-Psychological Readiness to Return to Sport (I-PRRS) scale. *Journal of Athletic Training, 44*(2), 185–189. https://doi.org/10.4085/1062-6050-44.2.185

Goldbeck, T. G, & Davies, G. J. (2000). Test–retest reliability of the closed kinetic chain upper extremity stability test: A clinical field test. *Journal of Sport Rehabilitation, 9*(1), 35–45.

Gribble, P. A., Delahunt, E., Bleakley, C. M., Caulfield, B., Docherty, C. L., Fong, D. T., Fourchet, F., Hertel, J., Hiller, C. E., Kaminski, T. W., McKeon, P. O., Refshauge, K. M., van der Wees, P., Vicenzino, W., & Wikstrom, E. A. (2014). Selection criteria for patients with chronic ankle instability in controlled research: A position statement of the International Ankle Consortium. *Journal of Athletic Training, 49*(1), 121–127. https://doi.org/10.4085/1062-6050-49.1.14

Grove, J. R., & Prapavessis, H. (1992). Preliminary evidence for the reliability and validity of an abbreviated Profile of Mood States. *International Journal of Sport Psychology, 23*(2), 93–109.

Halle, M., Bloch, W., Niess, A. M., Predel, H. G., Reinsberger, C., Scharhag, J., Steinacker, J., Wolfarth, B., Scherr, J., & Niebauer, J. (2021). Exercise and sports after COVID-19: Guidance from a clinical perspective. *Translational Sports Medicine, 4*(3), 310–318. https://doi.org/10.1002/tsm2.247

Hamlin, M. J., Wilkes, D., Elliot, C. A., Lizamore, C. A., & Kathiravel, Y. (2019). Monitoring training loads and perceived stress in young elite university athletes. *Frontiers in Physiology, 10,* 34. https://doi.org/10.3389/fphys.2019.00034

Harput, G., Ulusoy, B., Yildiz, T. I., Demirci, S., Eraslan, L., Turhan, E., & Tunay, V. B. (2019). Cross-education improves quadriceps strength recovery after ACL reconstruction: A randomized controlled trial. *Knee Surgery, Sports Traumatology, Arthroscopy: Official Journal of the ESSKA, 27*(1), 68–75. https://doi.org/10.1007/s00167-018-5040-1

Hauser, R. A., Dolan, E. E., Phillips, H. J., Newlin, A. C., Moore, R. E., & Woldin, B. A. (2013). Ligament injury and healing: A review of current clinical diagnostics and therapeutics. *Open Rehabilitation Journal, 6,* 1–20.

Hewett, T. E., & Bates, N. A. (2017). Preventive biomechanics: A paradigm shift with a translational approach to injury prevention. *American Journal of Sports Medicine, 45*(11), 2654–2664. https://doi.org/10.1177/0363546516686080

Hewett, T. E., Myer, G. D., Ford, K. R., Heidt, R. S. Jr, Colosimo, A. J., McLean, S. G., van den Bogert, A. J., Paterno, M. V., & Succop, P. (2005). Biomechanical measures of neuromuscular control and valgus loading of the knee predict anterior cruciate ligament injury risk in female athletes: A prospective study. *American Journal of Sports Medicine, 33*(4), 492–501. https://doi.org/10.1177/0363546504269591

Hirth, C. J. (2007). Clinical movement analysis to identify muscle imbalances and guide exercise. *Athletic Therapy Today, 12*(4), 10–14.

Hoch, M. C., Staton, G. S., & McKeon, P. O. (2011). Dorsiflexion range of motion significantly influences dynamic balance. *Journal of Science and Medicine in Sport, 14*(1), 90–92. https://doi.org/10.1016/j.jsams.2010.08.001

Hootman, J. M., Dick, R., & Agel, J. (2007). Epidemiology of collegiate injuries for 15 sports: Summary and recommendations for injury prevention initiatives. *Journal of Athletic Training, 42*(2), 311–319.

Huang, Y. L., Jung, J., Mulligan, C., Oh, J., & Norcross, M. F. (2020). A majority of anterior cruciate ligament injuries can be prevented by injury prevention programs: A systematic review of randomized controlled trials and cluster-randomized controlled trials with meta-analysis. *American Journal of Sports Medicine, 48*(6), 1505–1515. https://doi.org/10.1177/0363546519870175

Huerta-Alardín, A. L., Varon, J., & Marik, P. E. (2005). Bench-to-bedside review: Rhabdomyolysis: An overview for clinicians. *Critical Care (London, UK), 9*(2), 158–169. https://doi.org/10.1186/cc2978

Huxel-Bliven, K. C., & Anderson, B. E. (2013). Core stability training for injury prevention. *Sports Health, 5*(6), 514–522. https://doi.org/10.1177/1941738113481200

Impellizzeri, F. M., Marcora, S. M., & Coutts, A. J. (2019). Internal and external training load: 15 years on. *International Journal of Sports Physiology and Performance, 14*(2), 270–273. https://doi.org/10.1123/ijspp.2018-0935

Impellizzeri, F. M., McCall, A., Ward, P., Bornn, L., & Coutts, A. J. (2020). Training load and its role in injury prevention, part 2: Conceptual and methodological pitfalls. *Journal of Athletic Training, 55*(9), 893–901.

Impellizzeri, F. M., Menaspà, P., Coutts, A. J., Kalkhoven, J., & Menaspà, M. J. (2020). Training load and its role in injury prevention, part I: Back to the future. *Journal of Athletic Training, 55*(9), 885–892. https://doi.org/10.4085/1062-6050-500-19

Issurin, V. B. (2010). New horizons for the methodology and physiology of training periodization. *Sports Medicine (Auckland, NZ), 40*(3), 189–206. https://doi.org/10.2165/11319770-000000000-00000

Kannus, P. (2000). Structure of the tendon connective tissue. *Scandinavian Journal of Medicine & Science in Sports, 10*(6), 312–320. https://doi.org/10.1034/j.1600-0838.2000.010006312.x

Kelly, S., & Beardsley, C. (2016). Specific and cross-over effects of foam rolling on ankle dorsiflexion range of motion. *International Journal of Sports Physical Therapy, 11*(4), 544–551.

Khamis, S., & Yizhar, Z. (2007). Effect of feet hyperpronation on pelvic alignment in a standing position. *Gait & Posture Journal, 25*, 127–134.

Khan, F. Y. (2009). Rhabdomyolysis: A review of the literature. *Netherlands Journal of Medicine, 67*(9), 272–283.

Komici, K., Bianco, A., Perrotta, F., Dello Iacono, A., Bencivenga, L., D'Agnano, V., Rocca, A., Bianco, A., Rengo, G., & Guerra, G. (2021). Clinical characteristics, exercise capacity and pulmonary function in post-covid-19 competitive athletes. *Journal of Clinical Medicine, 10*(14), 3053. https://doi.org/10.3390/jcm10143053

Koshino, Y., Samukawa, M., Murata, H., Osuka, S., Kasahara, S., Yamanaka, M., & Tohyama, H. (2020). Prevalence and characteristics of chronic ankle instability and copers identified by the criteria for research and clinical practice in collegiate athletes. *Physical Therapy in Sport, 45*, 23–29. https://doi.org/10.1016/j.ptsp.2020.05.014

Kraan, R. B. J., de Nobel, D., Eygendaal, D., Daams, J. G., Kuijer, P. P. F. M., & Maas, M. (2019). Incidence, prevalence, and risk factors for elbow and shoulder overuse in youth athletes: A systematic review. *Translational Sports Medicine, 2*, 186–195.

Kraemer, W. J., Denegar, C., & Flanagan, S. (2009). Recovery from injury in sport: Considerations in the transition from medical care to performance care. *Sports Health, 1*(5), 392–395.

Lafave, M. R., Butterwick, D., & Eubank, B. (2015). Validation of the continuum of care conceptual model for athletic therapy. *Journal of Sports Medicine, 2015*, 391459. https://doi.org/10.1155/2015/391459

Laudner, K., Wong, R., Latal, J., & Meister, K. (2020). Posterior shoulder tightness and subacromial impingement characteristics in baseball pitchers: A blinded, matched control study. *International Journal of Sports Physical Therapy, 15*(2), 188–195.

Leetun, D. T., Ireland, M. L., Willson, J. D., Ballantyne, B. T., & Davis, I. M. (2004). Core stability measures as risk factors for lower-extremity injury in athletes. *Medicine & Science in Sports & Exercise, 36*(6), 926–934.

Little, C. J., Bawolin, N. K., & Chen, X. (2011). Mechanical properties of natural cartilage and tissue-engineered constructs. *Tissue Engineering Part B: Reviews, 17*(4), 213–227.

Litwin, D. E., Sneider, E. B., McEnaney, P. M., & Busconi, B. D. (2011). Athletic pubalgia (sports hernia). *Clinics in Sports Medicine, 30*(2), 417–434. https://doi.org/10.1016/j.csm.2010.12.010

Lorenz, D., & Morrison, S. (2015). Current concepts in periodization of strength and conditioning for the sports physical therapist. *International Journal of Sports Physical Therapy, 10*(6), 734–747.

Lorenz, D. S., Reiman, M. P., & Walker, J. C. (2010). Periodization: Current review and suggested implementation for athletic rehabilitation. *Sports Health, 2*(6), 509–518.

Lorenzetti, S., Ostermann, M., Zeidler, F., Zimmer, P., Jentsch, L., List, R., Tayler, W. R., & Schellenberg, F. (2018). How to squat? Effects of various stance widths, foot placement angles and level of experience on knee, hip and trunk motion and loading. *BMC Sports Science, Medicine and Rehabilitation, 10*(14). https://doi.org /10.1186/s13102-018-0103-7

Macrum, E., Bell, D. R., Boling, M., Lewek, M., & Padua, D. (2012). Effect of limiting ankle-dorsiflexion range of motion on lower extremity kinematics and muscle-activation patterns during a squat. *Journal of Sport Rehabilitation, 21*(2), 144–150. https://doi.org/10.1123/jsr.21.2.144

Malliaras, P., Cook, J. L., & Kent, P. (2006). Reduced ankle dorsiflexion range may increase the risk of patellar tendon injury among volleyball players. *Journal of Science and Medicine in Sport, 9*(4), 304–309.

Maselli, F., Storari, L., Barbari, V., Colombi, A., Turolla, A., Gianola, S., Rossettini, G., & Testa, M. (2020). Prevalence and incidence of low back pain among runners: A systematic review. *BMC Musculoskeletal Disorders, 21*(1), 343. https://doi.org/10.1186/s12891-020-03357-4

Mauntel, T. C., Begalle, R. L., Cram, T. R., Frank, B. S., Hirth, C. J., Blackburn, T., & Padua, D. A. (2013). The effects of lower extremity muscle activation and passive range of motion on single leg squat performance. *Journal of Strength and Conditioning Research, 27*(7), 1813–1823. https://doi.org/10.1519 /JSC.0b013e318276b886

Mauntel, T. C., Cram, T. R., Frank, B. S., Begalle, R. L., Norcross, M. F., Blackburn, J. T., & Padua, D. A. (2018). Kinematic and neuromuscular relationships between lower extremity clinical movement assessments. *Sports Biomechanics, 17*(2), 273–284. https://doi.org/10.1080/14763141.2017.1348536

Mauntel, T. C., Frank, B. S., Begalle, R. L., Blackburn, J. T., & Padua, D. A. (2014). Kinematic differences between those with and without medial knee displacement during a single-leg squat. *Journal of Applied Biomechanics, 30*(6), 707–712. https://doi.org/10.1123/jab.2014-0003

McGill, S. M., Karpowicz, A., Fenwick, C. M., & Brown, S. H. (2009). Exercises for the torso performed in a standing posture: spine and hip motion and motor patterns and spine load. *Journal of Strength and Conditioning Research, 23*(2), 455–464. https://journals.lww.com/nsca-jscr/fulltext/2009/03000/exercises _for_the_torso_performed_in_a_standing.15.aspx

McKeon, P. O., Hertel, J., Bramble, D., & Davis, I. (2015). The foot core system: A new paradigm for understanding intrinsic foot muscle function. *British Journal of Sports Medicine, 49*, 290. https://doi.org /10.1136/bjsports-2013-092690

McKeon, P. O., Ingersoll, C. D., Kerrigan, D. C., Saliba, E., Bennett, B. C., & Hertel, J. (2008). Balance training improves function and postural control in those with chronic ankle instability. *Medicine and Science in Sports and Exercise, 40*(10), 1810–1819. https://doi.org/10.1249/MSS.0b013e31817e0f92

Michener, L. A., Abrams, J. S., Bliven, K., Falsone, S., Laudner, K. G., McFarland, E. G., Tibone, J. E., Thigpen, C. A., & Uhl, T. L. (2018). National Athletic Trainers' Association position statement: Evaluation, management, and outcomes of and return-to-play criteria for overhead athletes with superior labral anterior-posterior injuries. *Journal of Athletic Training, 53*(3), 209–229. https://doi.org/10.4085/1062-6050-59-16

Miller, M. D., Arciero, R. A., Cooper, D. E., Johnson, D. L., & Best, T. M. (2009). Doc, when can he go back in the game? *Instructional Course Lectures, 58*, 437–443.

Miyashita, K., Urabe, Y., Kobayashi, H., Yokoe, K., Koshida, S., Kawamura, M., & Ida, K. (2008). The role of shoulder maximum external rotation during throwing for elbow injury prevention in baseball players. *Journal of Sports Science & Medicine, 7*(2), 223–228.

Morton, R. H., Fitz-Clarke, J. R., & Banister, E. W. (1990). Modeling human performance in running. *Journal of Applied Physiology (Bethesda, MD: 1985), 69*(3), 1171–1177. https://doi.org/10.1152/jappl.1990.69.3.1171

Mountjoy, M., Sundgot-Borgen, J. K., Burke, L. M., Ackerman, K. E., Blauwet, C., Constantini, N., Lebrun, C., Lundy, B., Melin, A. K., Meyer, N. L., Sherman, R. T., Tenforde, A. S., Klungland Torstveit, M., & Budgett, R. (2018). IOC consensus statement on relative energy deficiency in sport (RED-S): 2018 update. *British Journal of Sports Medicine, 52*(11), 687–697. https://doi.org/10.1136/bjsports-2018-099193

Mujika, I., & Padilla, S. (2001). Muscular characteristics of detraining in humans. *Medicine and Science in Sports and Exercise, 33*(8), 1297–1303. https://doi.org/10.1097/00005768-200108000-00009

National Institute for Occupational Safety and Health. (1997). *Musculoskeletal disorders (MSDs) and workplace factors: A critical review of epidemiologic evidence for work-related musculoskeletal disorders of the neck, upper extremity, and low back.* Centers for Disease Control and Prevention.

Nazem, T. G., & Ackerman, K. E. (2012). The female athlete triad. *Sports Health, 4*(4), 302–311.

Neumann, D. A. (2010). Kinesiology of the hip: A focus on muscular actions. *Journal of Orthopaedic & Sports Physical Therapy, 40*(2), 82–94.

Neumann, D. (2017). *Kinesiology of the musculoskeletal system: Foundations for physical rehabilitation* (3rd ed.). Elsevier Mosby.

Nielsen, R. O., Bertelsen, M. L., Moller, M., Hulme, A., Windt, J., Verhagen, E., Mansournia, M. A., Casals, M., & Partner, E. T. (2017). Training load and structure-specific load: Applications for sport injury causality and data analysis. *British Journal of Sports Medicine, 16*(S2), 1–3. https://doi.org/10.1136/bjsports-2017-097838

Overley, S. C., McAnany, S. J., Andelman, S., Patterson, D. C., Cho, S. K., Qureshi, S. A., Hsu, W. K., & Hecht, A. C. (2016). Return to play in elite athletes after lumbar microdiscectomy: A meta-analysis. *Spine, 41*(8), 713–718. https://doi.org/10.1097/BRS.0000000000001325

Padua, D. A., Bell, D. R., & Clark, M. A. (2012). Neuromuscular characteristics of individuals displaying excessive medial knee displacement. *Journal of Athletic Training, 47*(5), 525–536. https://doi.org/10.4085/1062-6050-47.5.10

Padua, D. A., DiStefano, L. J., Beutler, A. I., de la Motte, S. J., DiStefano, M. J., & Marshall, S. W. (2015). The landing error scoring system as a screening tool for an anterior cruciate ligament injury-prevention program in elite-youth soccer athletes. *Journal of Athletic Training, 50*(6), 589–595. https://doi.org/10.4085/1062-6050-50.1.10

Parsons, J. T., Anderson, S. A., Casa, D. J., & Hainline, B. (2020). Preventing catastrophic injury and death in collegiate athletes: Interassociation recommendations endorsed by 13 medical and sports medicine organisations. *British Journal of Sports Medicine, 54,* 208–215.

Pauyo, T., Herbst, E., & Fu, F. H. (2017) Tendon healing. In G. Canata, P. d'Hooghe, & K. Hunt (Eds.), *Muscle and tendon injuries* (pp. 45–50). Springer. https://doi.org/10.1007/978-3-662-54184-5_4

Phelan, D., Kim, J. H., & Chung, E. H. (2020). A game plan for the resumption of sport and exercise after coronavirus disease 2019 (COVID-19) infection. *JAMA Cardiology, 5*(10), 1085–1086. https://doi.org/10.1001/jamacardio.2020.2136

Pizzari, T., Green, B., & van Dyk, N. (2020) Extrinsic and intrinsic risk factors associated with hamstring injury. In K. Thorborg, D. Opar, & A. Shields (Eds.), *Preventing and rehabilitation of hamstring injuries* (pp. 83–115). Springer. https://doi.org/10.1007/978-3-030-31638-9_4

Plews, D. J., Laursen, P. B., Kilding, A. E., & Buchheit, M. (2013). Evaluating training adaptation with heart-rate measures: A methodological comparison. *International Journal of Sports Physiology and Performance, 8*(6), 688–691. https://doi.org/10.1123/ijspp.8.6.688

Preece, S. J., Graham-Smith, P., Nester, C. J., Howard, D., Hermens, H., Herrington, L., & Bowker, P. (2008). The influence of gluteus maximus on transverse plane tibial rotation. *Gait & Posture, 27*(4), 616–621.

Prendergast, P. J., & Huiskes, R. (1995). The Biomechanics of Wolff's law: Recent advances. *Irish Journal of Medical Science, 164*(2), 152–154. https://doi.org/10.1007/BF02973285

Ratamess, N. A., Alvar, B. A., Evetoch, T. K., Housh, T. J., Kibler, W. B., & Kraemer, W. J. (2009). Progression models in resistance training for healthy adults. *Medicine & Science in Sports & Exercise, 41*(3), 687–708. https://doi.org/10.1249/MSS.0b013e3181915670 3

Rathi, M. (2014). Two cases of CrossFit®-induced rhabdomyolysis: A rising concern. *International Journal of Medical Students, 2*(3), 132–134.

Reiman, M. P., & Lorenz, D. S. (2011). Integration of strength and conditioning principles into a rehabilitation program. *International Journal of Sports Physical Therapy, 6*(3), 241–253.

Reinold, M. M., Wilk, K. E., Reed, J., Crenshaw, K., & Andrews, J. R. (2002). Interval sport programs: Guidelines for baseball, tennis, and golf. *Journal of Orthopaedic and Sports Physical Therapy, 32*(6), 293–298. https://doi.org/10.2519/jospt.2002.32.6.293

Salas, C., Sintes, P., Joan, J., Urbano, D., & Sospedra, J. (2020). Conservative management of femoroacetabular impingement (FAI) in professional basketball. *Apunts Sports Medicine, 55*(205), 5–20. https://doi.org/10.1016/j.apunsm.2020.01.001

Saltzman, C. L., Salamon, M. L., Blanchard, G. M., Huff, T., Hayes, A., Buckwalter, J. A., & Amendola, A. (2005). Epidemiology of ankle arthritis: Report of a consecutive series of 639 patients from a tertiary orthopaedic center. *Iowa Orthopaedic Journal, 25,* 44–46.

Sandow, M. J., & Goodfellow, J. W. (1985). The natural history of anterior knee pain in adolescents. *Journal of Bone and Joint Surgery, 67B*, 36–38.

Santos-Júnior, F., Nonato, D. T., Cavalcante, F. S., Soares, P. M., & Ceccatto, V. M. (2013). Consequences of immobilization and disuse: A short review. *International Journal of Basic and Applied Sciences, 2*, 297–302.

Sauers, E. L., Bay, R. C., Snyder Valier, A. R., Ellery, T., & Huxel Bliven, K. C. (2017). The Functional Arm Scale for Throwers (FAST): Part I: The design and development of an upper extremity region-specific and population-specific patient-reported outcome scale for throwing athletes. *Orthopaedic Journal of Sports Medicine, 5*(3), 2325967117698455. https://doi.org/10.1177/2325967117698455

Schleich, K., Slayman, T., West, D., & Smoot, K. (2016). Return to play after exertional rhabdomyolysis. *Journal of Athletic Training, 51*(5), 406–409. https://doi.org/10.4085/1062-6050-51.5.12

Schmidt, C. O., & Kohlmann, T. (2005). Was wissen wir über das Symptom Rückenschmerz? Epidemiologische Ergebnisse zu Prävalenz, Inzidenz, Verlauf, Risikofaktoren [What do we know about the symptoms of back pain? Epidemiological results on prevalence, incidence, progression and risk factors]. *Zeitschrift fur Orthopadie und ihre Grenzgebiete, 143*(3), 292–298. https://doi.org/10.1055/s-2005-836631

Schoenfeld, B. J., Grgic, J., Ogborn, D., & Krieger, J. W. (2017). Strength and hypertrophy adaptations between low- vs. high-load resistance training: A systematic review and meta-analysis. *Journal of Strength and Conditioning Research, 31*(12), 3508–3523. https://doi.org/10.1519/JSC.0000000000002200

Sheriff, T. J., Ebersole, K. T., & Cornell, D. J. (2021). Relationship between gastrocnemius muscle length and overhead squat movement compensations among active-duty firefighters. *International Journal of Athletic Therapy and Training, 26*, 230–235.

Shrier, I. (2015). Strategic Assessment of Risk and Risk Tolerance (StARRT) framework for return-to-play decision-making. *British Journal of Sports Medicine, 49*, 1311–1315.

Shultz, S. J. (2015). ACL injury risk in the physically active: Why are females more susceptible? *Kinesiology Review, 5*, 52–62.

Skundric, G., Vukicevic, V., & Lukic, N. (2021). Effects of core stability exercises, lumbar lordosis and low-back pain: A systematic review. *Journal of Anthropology of Sport and Physical Education, 5*(1), 17–23. https://doi.org/10.26773/jaspe.210104

Smith, A. M., Scott, S. G., O'Fallon, W. M., & Young, M. L. (1990). Emotional responses of athletes to injury. *Mayo Clinic Proceedings, 65*(1), 38–50. https://doi.org/10.1016/s0025-6196(12)62108-9

Stanley, L. E., Harkey, M., Luc-Harkey, B., Frank, B. S., Pietrosimone, B., Blackburn, T. J., & Padua, D. A. (2019). Ankle dorsiflexion displacement is associated with hip and knee kinematics in females following anterior cruciate ligament reconstruction. *Research in Sports Medicine, 27*, 21–33.

Starkey, C. & Johnson, G. (Eds.). (2006). *Athletic training and sports medicine.* Jones & Bartlett Learning.

Stathopulu, E., & Baildam, E. (2003). Anterior knee pain: A long-term follow-up. *Rheumatology, 42*, 380–382.

Stecco, A., Gesi, M., Stecco, C., & Stern, R. (2013). Fascial components of the myofascial pain syndrome. *Current Pain and Headache Reports, 17*(8), 352.

Szeto, G. P., Straker, L., & Raine, S. (2002). A field comparison of neck and shoulder postures in symptomatic and asymptomatic office workers. *Applied Ergonomics, 33*(1), 75–84. https://doi.org/10.1016/s0003-6870(01)00043-6

Tabrizi, P., Mcintyre, W., Quesnel, M., & Howard, A. (2000). Limited dorsiflexion predisposes to injuries of the ankle in children. *Journal of Bone and Joint Surgery—British, 82*(8), 1103–1106. https://doi.org/10.1302/0301-620x.82b8.10134

Thigpen, C. A., Padua, D. A., Xu, N., & Karas, S. G. (2005). Comparison of scapular muscle activity between individuals with and without multidirectional shoulder instability. *Journal of Orthopaedic & Sports Physical Therapy, 35*, A4-PL18.

Torres, P. A., Helmstetter, J. A., Kaye, A. M., & Kaye, A. D. (2015). Rhabdomyolysis: Pathogenesis, diagnosis, and treatment. *Ochsner Journal, 5*(1), 58–69.

Trainor, T. J., & Wiesel, S. W. (2002). Epidemiology of back pain in the athlete. *Clinics in Sports Medicine, 21*(1), 93–103.

Valderrabano, V., Hintermann, B., Horisberger, M., & Fung, T. S. (2006). Ligamentous posttraumatic ankle osteoarthritis. *American Journal of Sports Medicine, 34*(4), 612–620. https://doi.org/10.1177/0363546505281813

Van der Heijden, G. J. (1999). Shoulder disorders: A state-of-the-art review. Bailliere's best practice & research. *Clinical Rheumatology, 13*(2), 287–309. https://doi.org/10.1053/berh.1999.0021

Vina, E. R., & Kwoh, C. K. (2018). Epidemiology of osteoarthritis: Literature update. *Current Opinion in Rheumatology, 30*(2), 160–167. https://doi.org/10.1097/BOR.0000000000000479

Webster, K., & Feller, J. (2018). Development and validation of short version of the Anterior Cruciate Ligament Return to Sport After Injury (ACL-RSI) scale. *Orthopaedic Journal of Sports Medicine, 6*(4), 232596711876376. https://doi.org/10.1177/2325967118763763

Weiss, K. J., Allen, S. V., McGuigan, M. R., & Whatman, C. S. (2017). The relationship between training load and injury in men's professional basketball. *International Journal of Sports Physiology and Performance, 12*(9), 1238–1242. https://doi.org/10.1123/ijspp.2016-0726

Welch, E. S., Watson, M. D., Davies, G. J., & Riemann, B. L. (2020). Biomechanical analysis of the closed kinetic chain upper extremity stability test in healthy young adults. *Physical Therapy in Sport: Official Journal of the Association of Chartered Physiotherapists in Sports Medicine, 45*, 120–125. https://doi.org/10.1016/j.ptsp.2020.06.010

Wilder, F. V., Hall, B. J., Barrett, J. P. Jr., & Lemrow, N. B. (2002). History of acute knee injury and osteoarthritis of the knee: A prospective epidemiological assessment. The Clearwater Osteoarthritis Study. *Osteoarthritis and Cartilage, 10*(8), 611–616. https://doi.org/10.1053/joca.2002.0795

Wilhite, C. L. (2012). Scope of practice . . . Standard of practice . . .Standard of care . . . What is my/your obligation? *Plastic Surgical Nursing Journal, 32*(3), 120–122.

Williams, G. N., Gangel, T. J., Arciero, R. A., Uhorchak, J. M., & Taylor, D. C. (1999). Comparison of the single assessment numeric evaluation method and two shoulder rating scales. Outcomes measures after shoulder surgery. *American Journal of Sports Medicine, 27*(2), 214–221. https://doi.org/10.1177/03635465990270021701

Wilson, F., Ardern, C. L., Hartvigsen, J., Dane, K., Trompeter, K., Trease, L., Vinther, A., Gissane, C., McDonnell, S. J., Caneiro, J. P., Newlands, C., Wilkie, K., Mockler, D., & Thornton, J. S. (2020). Prevalence and risk factors for back pain in sports: A systematic review with meta-analysis. *British Journal of Sports Medicine*, bjsports-2020-102537. https://doi.org/10.1136/bjsports-2020-102537

Yamaguchi, K., Ditsios, K., Middleton, W. D., Hildebolt, C. F., Galatz, L. M., & Teefey, S. A. (2006). The demographic and morphological features of rotator cuff disease: A comparison of asymptomatic and symptomatic shoulders. *Journal of Bone and Joint Surgery, 88*, 1699–1704.

Zhang, X., Xia, R., Dai, B., Sun, X., & Fu, W. (2018). Effects of exercise-induced fatigue on lower extremity joint mechanics, stiffness, and energy absorption during landings. *Journal of Sports Science & Medicine, 17*(4), 640–649.

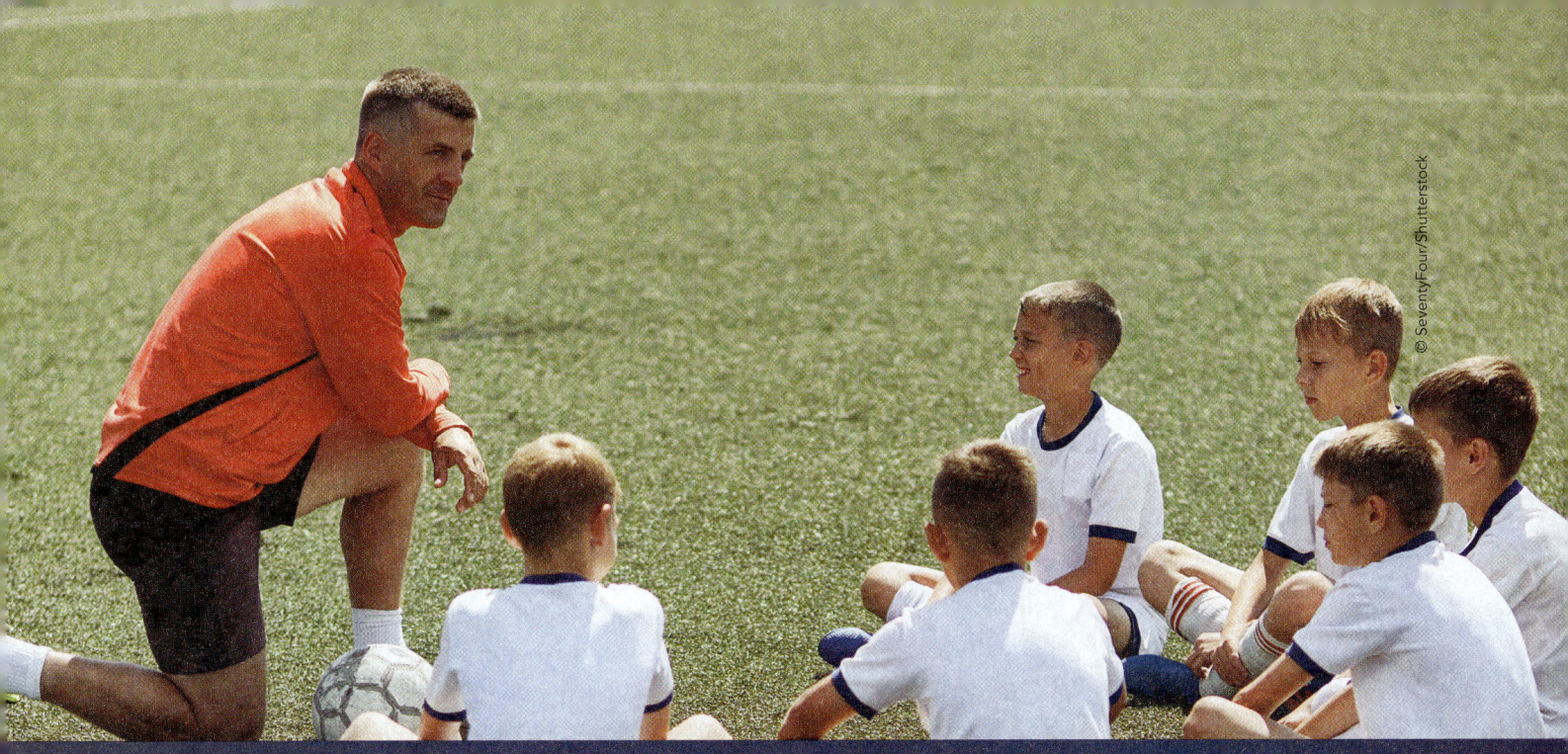

YOUTH TRAINING PRINCIPLES AND LONG-TERM ATHLETE DEVELOPMENT

CHAPTER TWENTY-ONE

LEARNING OBJECTIVES

Upon completion of this chapter, the Sports Performance Coach will be able to:

- **Differentiate** the youth athlete from the adult athlete.
- **Describe** the long-term athlete development (LTAD) model.
- **Identify** growth and development monitoring techniques for the youth athlete to optimize athletic development.
- **Compare** the LTAD model and NASM's OPT Model.
- **Describe** the acute training variables across the stages of long-term athlete development.

LESSON 1: INTRODUCTION TO YOUTH TRAINING AND GENERAL PRINCIPLES OF DEVELOPMENT

INTRODUCTION

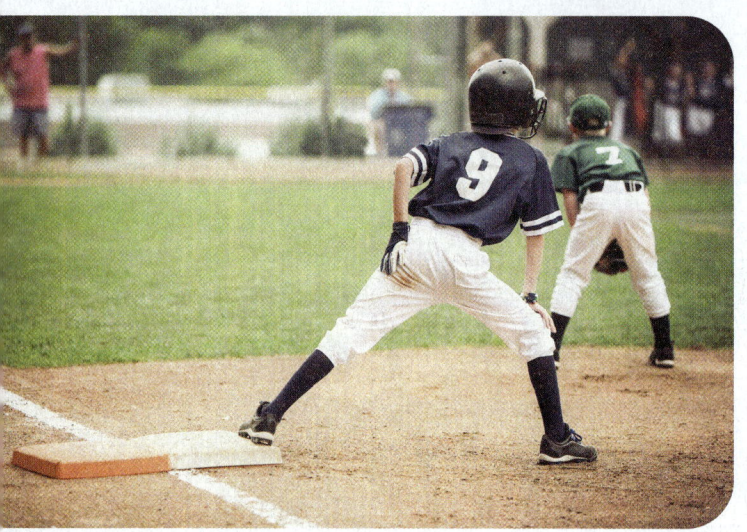

© Suzanne Tucker/Shutterstock

Physical activity, including physical education and youth sports, is assumed to be essential for normal growth, maturation, and development of children and adolescents. Indeed, it is well documented that a positive experience in youth sports and physical activity can enhance the physical, psychological, cognitive, and social health and well-being of young people (Janssen & Leblanc, 2010). However, current estimates suggest that only 24% of children and adolescents meet the physical activity recommendations (**Table 21.1**). Although multiple outlets for physical activity exist, part of this issue may stem from few children attending daily physical education; for example, only 29.9% of high school students participate in such education (Kann et al., 2018). Other aspects (e.g., schools, physical education, active transportation, play, faith-based settings) also collectively impact the overall grade of D-minus on the 2018 United States Report Card on Physical Activity for children and youth (Katzmarzyk et al., 2018).

Regardless of the underlying factors, the lack of physical activity among youth contributes to a major public health issue in the United States and around the world: childhood obesity. Current estimates indicate that approximately one in five children and adolescents are classified as obese, defined as a body mass index (BMI) greater than the

PHYSICAL INACTIVITY TRIAD (PIT) →

A combination of low levels of physical activity, reduced muscular fitness, and poor movement competency.

EXERCISE DEFICIT DISORDER →

Accumulating less than the recommended 60 minutes of moderate- to vigorous-intensity physical activity per day.

TABLE 21.1 Recommendations for Physical Activity in Children and Adolescents Ages 6 to 17

Type of Activity	Description
Aerobic	Most of the 60 minutes or more per day should be either moderate- or vigorous-intensity aerobic physical activity and should include vigorous-intensity physical activity on at least 3 days per week.
Muscle strengthening	As part of their 60 minutes or more of daily physical activity, children and adolescents should include muscle-strengthening physical activity on at least 3 days per week.
Bone strengthening	As part of their 60 minutes or more of daily physical activity, children and adolescents should include bone-strengthening physical activity on at least 3 days per week.

95th percentile of the age- and sex-specific Centers for Disease Control and Prevention (CDC) reference values, and another 18% are classified as overweight, defined as a BMI between the 85th and 95th percentiles (CDC, 2024).

In addition to these epidemics of physical inactivity and obesity, relatively high percentages of youth are physically unfit and possess poor fundamental movement skill competency. Faigenbaum et al. (2018) described this scenario with the youth **physical inactivity triad (PIT)**, which depicts the relationships between **exercise deficit disorder**, pediatric dynapenia, and **physical illiteracy**.

Taken together, the elements of the youth PIT have a myriad of short- and long-term health and psychosocial consequences. In the short term, a young person may be cut from a sports team, be bullied, suffer from mental health issues, or do poorly in school. In the long term, the **hypokinetic**, obese youth is more likely to die prematurely (Faigenbaum et al., 2018).

Youth sports serve a significant role in promoting the health of young people. Youth sports provide a major outlet for physical activity, the development of movement and sport skills, and psychosocial development. Many youths and teens participate in organized sports. Indeed, it is estimated that 72% of 6- to 12-year-olds participate in youth sports and more than 50% (or about 8 million) of high school students participate in scholastic sports (Aspen Institute, 2021; National Federation of State High School Associations, 2019). Despite this widespread participation, several problematic issues are encountered in youth sports, including dropouts, pay-to-play, lack of or inadequate coach education, early specialization, excessive or inappropriate training and competition, burnout, and overuse injury. In fact, the Aspen Institute's (2017) Project Play Report Card on Youth Sports has given the U.S. sports system an overall grade of C.

This chapter covers several aspects of engaging young people in physical activity and training, while focusing on evidence-based principles including the **long-term athlete development (LTAD)** model. First, the general principles of growth, maturation, and development are described to provide an understanding of growing up during the first two decades of life. Next, the chapter addresses gaps in youth training, models, and the LTAD framework. For the Sports Performance Coach, it is important to recognize that the demands of youth sports training are increasing, and specialists should be aware of the physical and mental differences between youth and adult athletes.

GENERAL PRINCIPLES OF GROWTH, MATURATION, AND DEVELOPMENT

"Children are not miniature adults" is a common mantra when it comes to training youth athletes. This statement acknowledges the age- and maturity-related changes that occur during the first two decades of life, including dynamic changes in body size, body composition, physiological function, fitness, cognition, emotions, and behaviors.

To understand the nature of physical activity, training, and sports performance during childhood and adolescence, it is essential that the Sports Performance Coach first understand basic principles of normal growth, maturation, and development. All these factors should be considered when designing, implementing, and evaluating training programs.

AGE: DETERMINING CHRONOLOGICAL AGE

A child's age must be considered due to the varying degrees of physical and cognitive development observed among children. **Chronological age** refers to the exact number of

PHYSICAL ILLITERACY →

Lack of motor competence and confidence to move well and often.

HYPOKINETIC →

A low level of movement throughout the day.

LONG-TERM ATHLETE DEVELOPMENT (LTAD) →

The habitual development of athleticism over time with the goal of improving health, fitness, and physical performance, reducing injury risk, and developing confidence and competence in all youth.

CHRONO-LOGICAL AGE →

The number of years, expressed as a decimal, from the birthdate.

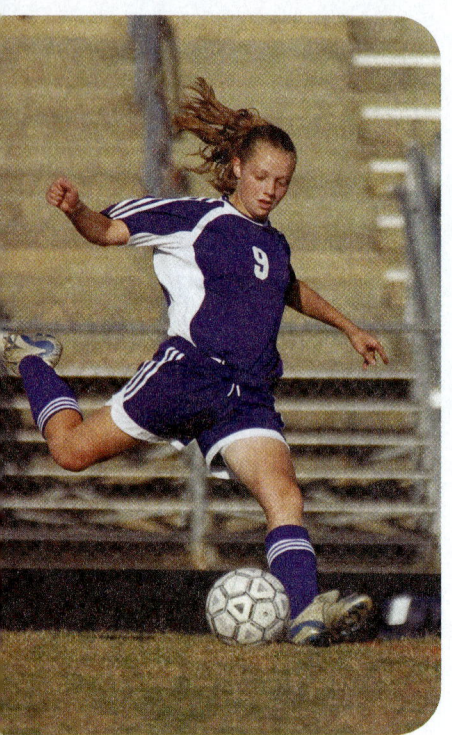

© CLS Digital Arts/Shutterstock

years a person has been alive, whereas **relative age** refers to an individual's age compared to a specific group. For instance, in a youth sports program, the relative age might be significantly different between the youngest and the oldest children in the same group, despite their chronological ages being similar. A child's true chronological age is the decimal age of the time elapsed since the date of birth (**Figure 21.1**).

How to Calculate Chronological Age

Formula	Chronological age = [(Today's Date − Date of Birth) ÷ 365)]
Example	Date of Birth: March 2, 2013 Assessment Date: June 18, 2021 [(6/18/2021 − 3/2/2013) ÷ 365 = 8.3]

FIGURE 21.1 Formula for Calculating Chronological Age

The precise calculation of chronological age is important because two young athletes playing on an 8-year-old soccer team could be nearly a year apart in age, growth, and life experience. This difference also relates to what has been termed the relative age effect. The **relative age effect** was first described based on roster data at a junior hockey game, where it was noticed that several of the players were born in the first quarter of the year (January through March) and relatively few in the last quarter of the year (October through December) (**Figure 21.2**). This phenomenon has been identified in several sports, beginning at a young age, and has implications for talent identification and selection.

RELATIVE AGE →

Birth date relative to age group cut-off dates.

RELATIVE AGE EFFECT →

A phenomenon in which children born in, or close to, a critical age cut-off period may have an advantage in athletic performance.

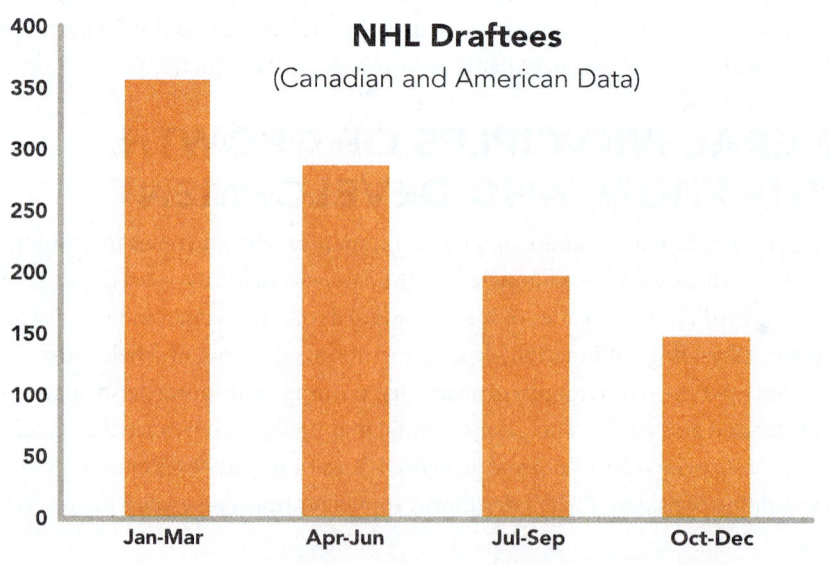

Baker & Logan (2007)

FIGURE 21.2 National Hockey League Draftees by Birth Month

Data from Baker, J., & Logan, A. J. (2007). Developmental contexts and sporting success: birth date and birthplace effects in national hockey league draftees 2000-2005. *British Journal of Sports Medicine, 41*(8), 515–517. https://doi.org/10.1136/bjsm.2006.033977

It is also important to recognize the individual differences in maturation and **biological age**. This is particularly evident during the **adolescent growth spurt**. **Figure 21.3** shows three boys who are 14.75 years of age; however, the early-maturing boy has a biological age of 16.4 years, and the late-maturing boy has a biological age of 12.2 years.

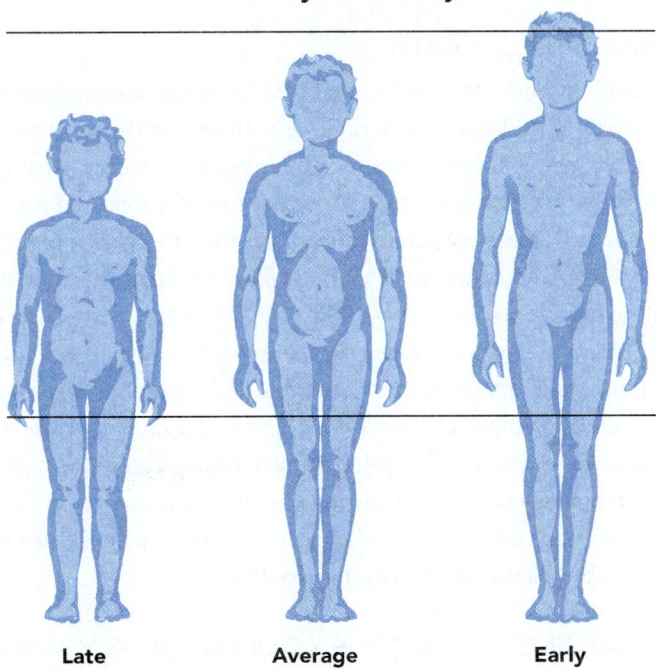

Maturity Variations
14.75-year-old boys

Late   Average   Early

FIGURE 21.3 Maturity Variations

In the context of training and conditioning, the Sports Performance Coach should consider **training age** as well. This factor can also be considered specific to the mode of training (e.g., sport skills, strength training, plyometrics, speed and agility). For example, many 14-year-olds have never been in a weight room, so their strength training age is 0 years. Having these athletes participate in a strength training session designed for experienced athletes may lead to injury, excessive soreness, discouragement, and even embarrassment.

Remember that the training sessions should match the training age of the young athlete. However, coaches often fail to take into account the developmental and **cognitive age** of the young person as they are learning how to behave within their society or culture. This sort of behavioral maturity can have implications for when youth are ready for certain experiences in youth sports. For example, cognitive development of the young athlete affects attention span. Therefore, the complexity of instructions and exercise choice should be taken into consideration.

 COACH'S CORNER

The Sports Performance Coach must consider the combination of all the different ages—chronological, biological, developmental, and training—when designing programs.

BIOLOGICAL AGE →

A measurement of a person's age based on various assessments of biological maturity.

ADOLESCENT GROWTH SPURT →

Period of the lifespan during which a marked increase in growth and puberty occurs.

TRAINING AGE →

The number of years or duration of experience that the athlete has participated in systematic (regular, consistent, organized) training.

COGNITIVE AGE →

Refers to an individual's cognitive abilities or performance relative to their chronological age, focusing specifically on abilities such as memory, problem-solving skills, understanding, and information processing.

PHYSICAL GROWTH AND BIOLOGICAL MATURATION: SEPARATE BUT RELATED CONSTRUCTS

With increasing age during childhood and adolescence come normal physical growth and biological maturation of the body. Although these terms are often used interchangeably, physical growth and biological maturation are separate but interrelated constructs. As children grow, they observably become taller and heavier, and these data are often recorded on a clinical growth chart (CDC, 2017).

THE FOUR PHASES OF GROWTH

The pattern of growth in body size can be organized into four phases: rapid growth in infancy, steady growth in mid-childhood, rapid growth during the adolescent spurt, and deceleration or slowing down of growth until adult height is attained. Changes in body composition also occur, including an overall increase in lean (bone and muscle) and fat tissues. Notably, however, there are gender differences in body composition patterns, with females accruing greater amounts of fat mass than males during adolescence and males gaining more muscle and bone mass. Most organs and organ systems (e.g., heart, lungs) likewise increase in size, following a similar growth pattern to either height or body weight. In turn, functional capacities such as aerobic and anaerobic power and muscle strength increase with age. The nervous system is an exception, as it grows more rapidly during childhood and is near adult size prior to entering adolescence. By comparison, the reproductive system develops slowly during childhood and advances rapidly during puberty. These age-related patterns of development associated with the growth of the body can be characterized by Scammon's curves (**Figure 21.4**).

BIOLOGICAL MATURATION AND THE ADOLESCENT GROWTH SPURT

As the body grows, it is also maturing biologically. **Maturation** refers to progress toward the biologically mature state and varies considerably between individuals in terms of timing (maturity status at a given time) and tempo (maturity progress), especially during

> **MATURATION** →
>
> Progress toward the biologically mature state; varies considerably between individuals in terms of timing (maturity status at a given time) and tempo (maturity progress) especially during adolescence.

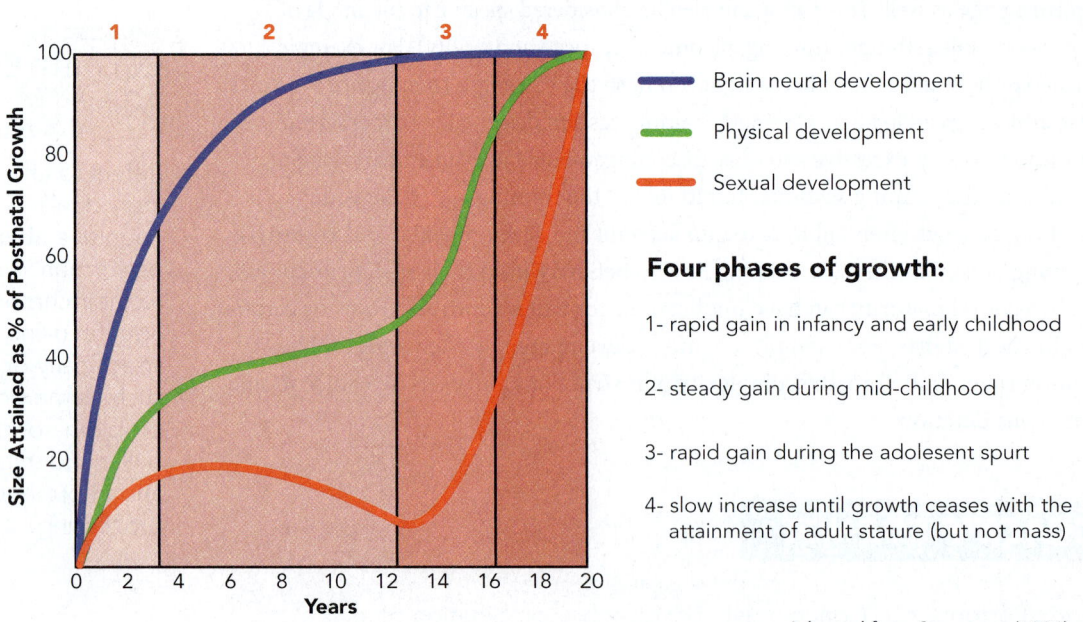

Four phases of growth:

1- rapid gain in infancy and early childhood

2- steady gain during mid-childhood

3- rapid gain during the adolesent spurt

4- slow increase until growth ceases with the attainment of adult stature (but not mass)

Adapted from Scammon (1930)

FIGURE 21.4 Scammon's Curves and the Four Phases of Growth

Copyright 1930 by the University of Minnesota. Reprinted, by permission, from R.E. Scammon, 1930, The Measurement of Man, edited by J.A. Harris et al., Minneapolis, MN: University of Minnesota Press

adolescence. In essence, maturation relates biological age to calendar age, with individuals classified as an early, average, or late maturing.

As shown in Scammon's curves, the reproductive system and resulting hormones—namely, testosterone (boys) and estrogen (girls)—develop slowly during the **pre-pubertal** period. Although youth are categorized as pre-pubertal during this time, there is still variation in growth and maturation. However, this variation widens more dramatically as youth enter puberty and the adolescent growth spurt. **Figure 21.5** shows the classic adolescent growth spurt where the change in height is expressed on a yearly basis, as centimeters of height gained in 1 year (cm/year).

PRE-PUBERTAL →

Relating to or in the period preceding puberty.

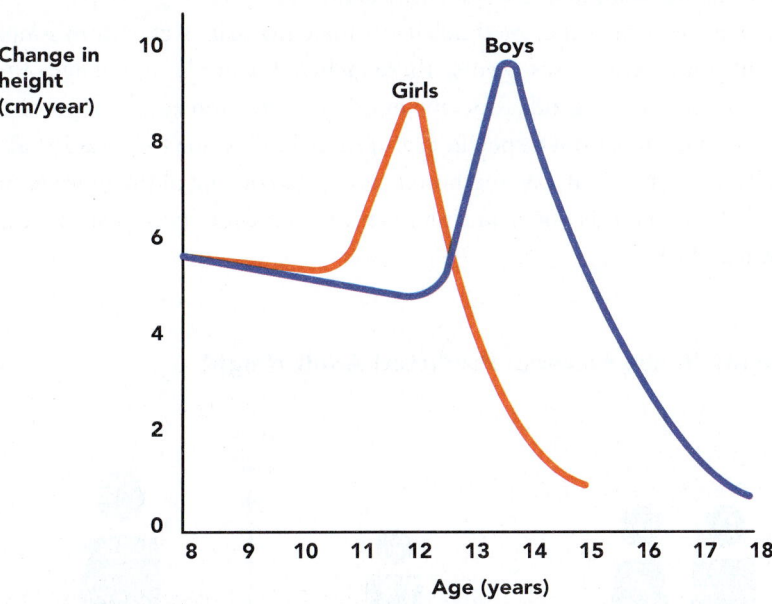

FIGURE 21.5 Adolescent Growth Spurt in Height

While variable, the onset of puberty typically occurs around age 10 for girls and age 12 for boys. The adolescent spurt is marked by the maximum growth in height, or peak height velocity, and the corresponding age at peak height velocity (APHV), which can be used as an indicator of maturity status.

On average, APHV is 12 years of age in girls and 14 years of age in boys, but, again, may occur earlier or later in some individuals. As mentioned, the APHV can be used as an indicator of maturity status, with individuals classified as early, average (or on time), or late maturing. Here, the plus or minus 1 rule is used. That is, if the average APHV is age 14 for boys, then those who attain PHV within ±1 year (13.0 to 15.0) are deemed average maturing. Those boys who attain APHV prior to age 13.0 are early maturers, and those who attain it after 15.0 years of age are late maturers. The same rule applies to females, though the APHV is 2 years earlier for each category (**Table 21.2**).

TABLE 21.2 Classification of Boys and Girls as Early, Average, or Late Maturing Based on the Age at Peak Height Velocity

	Early Maturing	Average or On Time	Late Maturing
Boys	Before age 13.0	Ages 13.0 to 15.0	After age 15.0
Girls	Before age 11.0	Ages 11.0 to 13.0	After age 13.0

PRACTICAL ASSESSMENT OF MATURITY

Two other methods are used to assess biological maturation: bone age and secondary sex characteristics. However, bone age requires exposure to radiation in a clinical setting and the expertise of someone familiar with the methods of assessing skeletal maturation. Similarly, the assessment of secondary sex characteristics (pubic hair in boys and girls; breast development in girls and genital development in boys), often referred to as Tanner stages, has limitations related to the invasive nature and social acceptability of the assessment. Likewise, there are limitations to the determination of APHV, which requires routine measurements (every 4 to 6 or 12 months) over many years, and most coaches, parents, and athletes want to know maturity status now.

Fortunately, there are other methods to estimate maturity status from simple, one-time anthropometric assessments. These include the prediction of age of peak height velocity, which is a gender-specific multiple-regression equation predicting how far an individual is from a specific maturational milestone (Mirwald et al., 2002). Additionally, the Khamis–Roche method is thought to be one of the more accurate height prediction methods not requiring the measurement of bone age (Roche et al., 1975) (**Figure 21.6**).

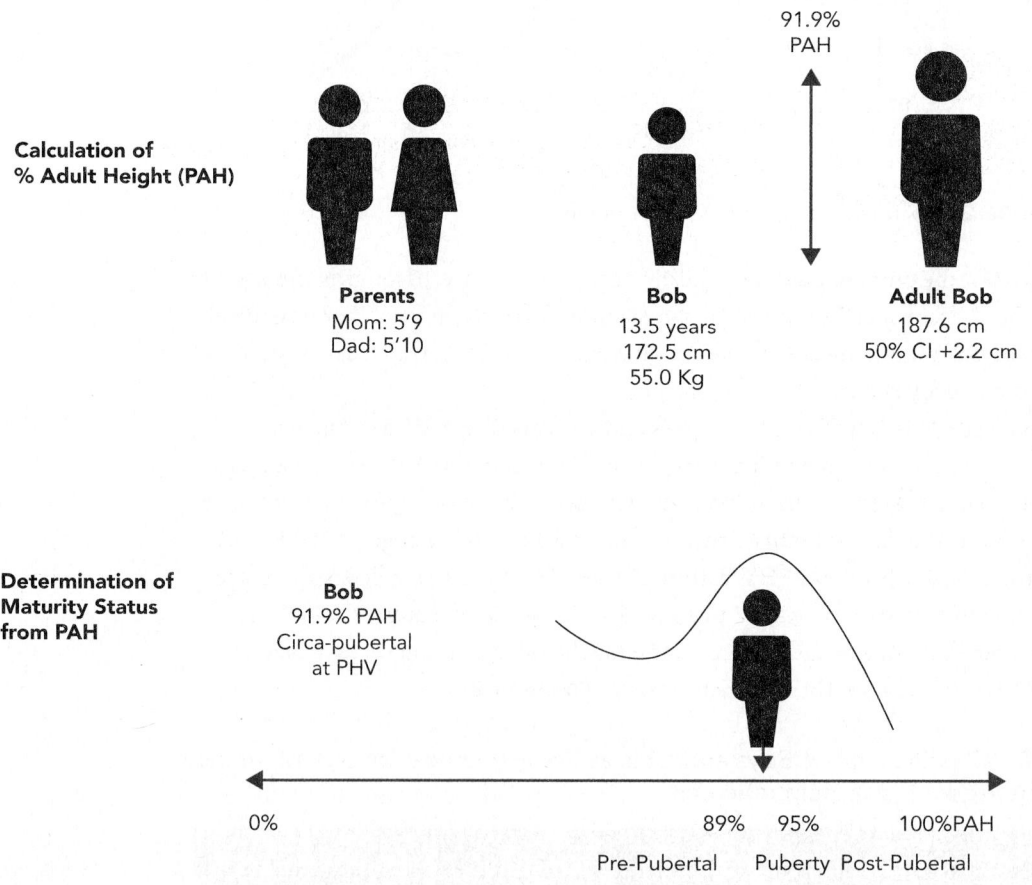

FIGURE 21.6 Khamis–Roche Method for Predicting Adult Height

Data from Roche, A. F., Wainer, H., & Thissen, D. (1975). Predicting adult stature for individuals. Monographs in paediatrics, 3, 1–114 Seefeldt, V. (1980). Developmental motor patterns. Implications for elementary school physical education. In C. H. Nadeau, W. R. Halliwell, K. M. Newell, & G. C. Roberts (Eds.). Psychology of Motor Behavior and Sport, 314–323. Champaign, IL: Human Kinetics.

It is vital that the Sports Performance Coach first understands the system of normal growth and maturation before considering training methodologies and their effectiveness. Much like a surgeon needs to understand anatomy and physiology before operating on a patient or a gardener needs to understand the soil and environment before choosing appropriate plants, the Sports Performance Coach who works with growing and maturing children and adolescents should understand the age- and maturity-related physical and behavioral changes that occur when designing, implementing, and evaluating training programs.

LESSON 2: AN OVERVIEW AND SYNTHESIS OF LONG-TERM ATHLETIC DEVELOPMENT

AN OVERVIEW AND SYNTHESIS OF LTAD

Given the gaps and shortcomings of the current approaches to youth sports training, the long-term athlete (or athletic) development model provides a framework for optimal health and performance by engaging all youth in physical activity/training programs that promote athleticism, physical fitness, and psychosocial well-being. Long-term athlete (or athletic) development has been an elusive and nebulous concept defined in many ways, but is perhaps captured best in the following definition: Long-term athlete development is the habitual development of athleticism over time with the goal of improving health, fitness, and physical performance, reducing injury risk, and developing confidence and competence in all youth (Lloyd et al., 2016).

Before moving ahead, two important points of clarification are in order. First, the LTAD model is not solely a pathway for competitive elite young athletes to reach the Olympics, college sports, or professional sports levels. Instead, youth of all ages, abilities, and aspirations, irrespective of whether they are involved in organized sport or engage in recreational physical activity, should participate in programs that promote both physical fitness and psychosocial well-being. In other words, LTAD is a holistic model designed to encourage a healthy relationship with physical activity throughout the lifespan for everybody.

Second, **athleticism** is merely a combination of health- and skill-related physical fitness that includes the ability to repeatedly perform a range of movements with precision and confidence in a variety of environments, which require competent levels of motor skills, strength, power, speed, agility, balance, coordination, and endurance (Myer et al., 2011; Lloyd et al., 2016). **Table 21.3** includes specific fundamental movement skills in all planes that should be included in the development of general athleticism. These can be categorized into locomotor, stability, and manipulative skills. Furthermore, these skills can be expressed through other physical qualities. It is hard to argue against fundamental movement skills and general athleticism for all youth.

ATHLETICISM →

The ability to repeatedly perform a range of movements with precision and confidence in a variety of environments, which require competent levels of motor skills, strength, power, speed, agility, balance, coordination, and endurance.

TABLE 21.3 Fundamental Movement Skills

Locomotor	Stability	Manipulative
Walking	Balancing	Throwing
Running	Landing	Catching
Hopping	Turning	Striking
Skipping	Twisting	Kicking
Bounding	Bending	Dribbling
Leaping	Stretching	Bouncing
Jumping	Extending	Pushing
Galloping	Hanging	Carrying
Sliding	Bracing	Trapping
Dodging		Collecting

LTAD ORIGINS AND USE

The notion of LTAD has grown in popularity over the past two decades. Like other strength and conditioning training methodologies (e.g., periodization, plyometrics), LTAD was conceptualized and implemented in the Eastern European Bloc countries in the mid-20th century. Along the lines of the LTAD model, these countries employed a systematic approach to the training of young athletes that included a daily routine that created a healthy balance between physical and mental exertion and relaxation based on age and experience.

✔ CHECK IT OUT

In the former Soviet Union, the Ready for Labour and Defence program, also known as the GTO, was the national physical culture training program introduced in 1931. This program was aimed at citizens of all ages and focused on earning badges for passing physical tests and participating in physical education programs (Ulyanova et al., 2019). In addition, school-age children who excelled in fitness testing were selected and placed into sports schools. By the late 1980s, there were approximately 6,000 sports schools in Russia serving more than 2 million student athletes. During this time frame, the Soviets also dominated international competition, placing first or second in the medal counts in both the summer and winter Olympiads from 1952 to 1992 (Benson, n.d.).

Two former Eastern European sport scientists, Tudor Bompa and Istvan Balyi, introduced the LTAD framework to the world (Bayli et al., 2014). Besides the concept of periodization, Bompa popularized the concept of **multilateral development**, which suggests the importance of young children developing a variety of fundamental skills to help them become good general athletes before they start training in a specific sport (Bompa, 2000).

Balyi et al. (2014) popularized a four-stage model of training, which included FUNdamentals, Training to Train, Training to Compete, and Training to Win. This model was then further developed into the current model in 2005. To learn more about the current Canadian LTAD model (**Figure 21.7**), see Sport for Life (2022).

> **MULTILATERAL →
> DEVELOPMENT**
>
> Exposure to a variety of fundamental skills to help youth develop general athleticism.

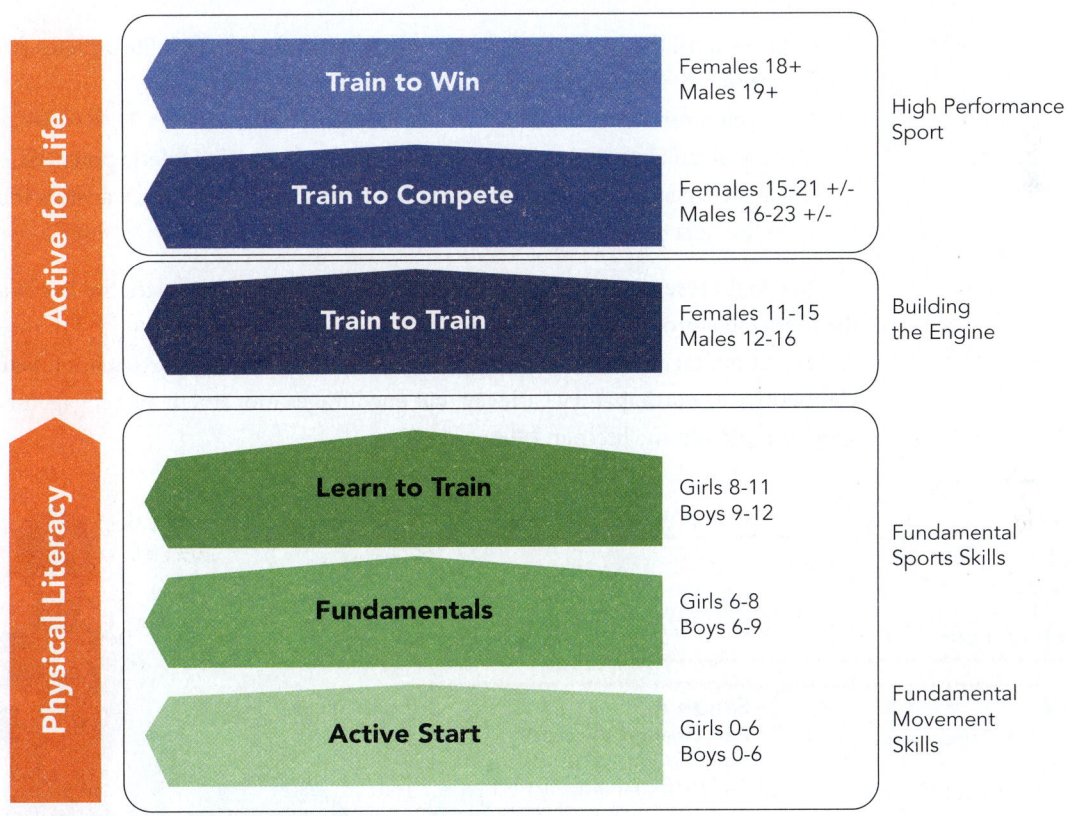

FIGURE 21.7 Canadian Sport for Life Physical Literacy

Data from Sport for Life. (2022). Long-Term Development Stages: A clear path to better sport, greater health, and higher achievement. Retrieved from https://sportforlife.ca/long-term-development/

THE AMERICAN DEVELOPMENTAL MODEL

In 2014, the United States Olympic and Paralympic Committee, in collaboration with multiple sports' national governing bodies, created the American Development Model (ADM) as an LTAD framework to promote healthy lifestyles and quality sport experiences for American youth (Team USA, 2022; United States Olympic and Paralympic Committee, 2016). Like other LTAD frameworks, the ADM also serves as an outline for coaches and personal fitness trainers to encourage greater participation in physical activity and sport and to increase the talent pool of available athletes for the Olympic and Paralympic Games.

ADM Key Principles

To help keep more youth involved in sport, the ADM suggests that quality sport experiences should incorporate five key principles:

1. Universal access to create opportunity for all athletes
2. Developmentally appropriate activities that emphasize motor and foundational skills
3. Multi-sport participation
4. Fun, engaging, and progressively challenging atmosphere
5. Quality coaching at all age level

In support of these five key principles and to create early positive experiences for all athletes, the ADM aims to achieve the following outcomes:

1. Grow both the general athlete population and the pool of elite athletes from which future U.S. Olympians and Paralympians are selected
2. Develop fundamental skills that transfer between sports
3. Provide an appropriate avenue to fulfill an individual's athletic potential
4. Create a generation that loves sport and physical activity and transfers that passion to the next generation

The ADM resembles other LTAD frameworks in that it organizes the five stages of the model in a progressive and developmental manner. The stages start with discovery and fundamental aspects of movement and ultimately lead the participant toward a competitive or participatory pathway that encourages movement and engagement with sport throughout the lifespan (**Figure 21.8**).

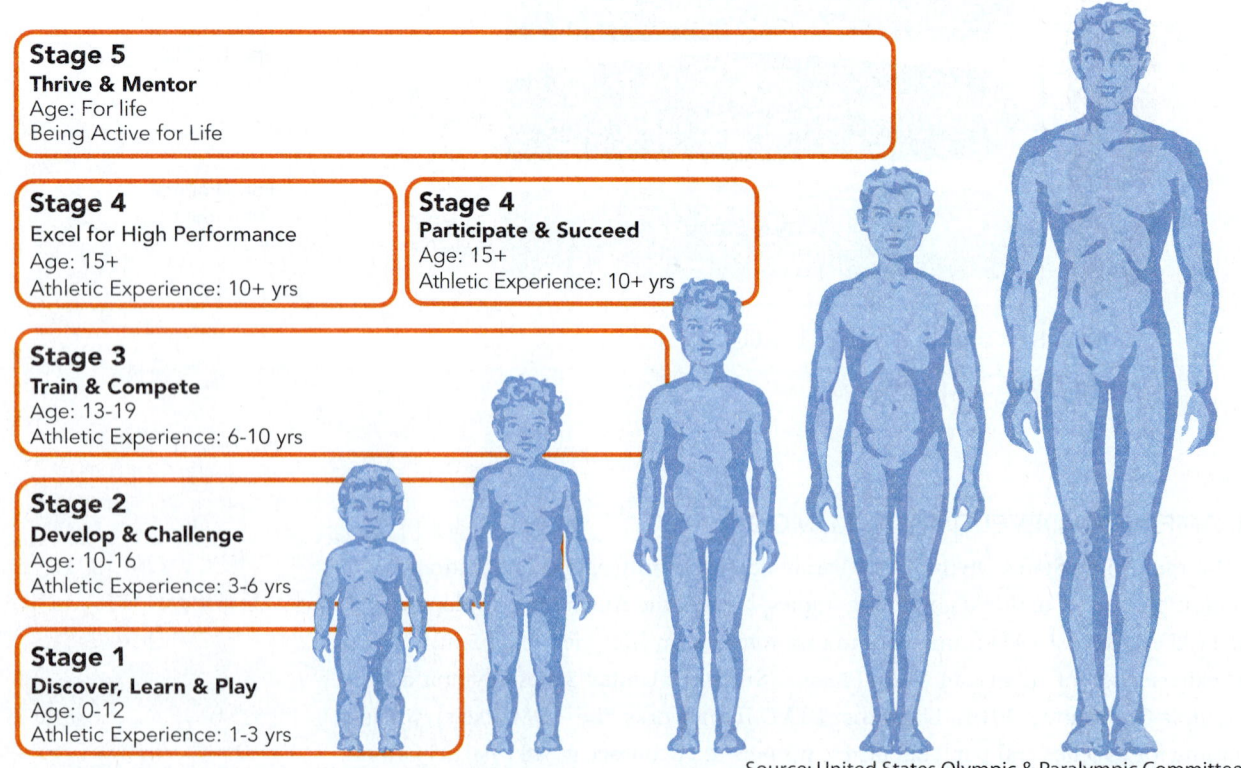

Stage 5
Thrive & Mentor
Age: For life
Being Active for Life

Stage 4
Excel for High Performance
Age: 15+
Athletic Experience: 10+ yrs

Stage 4
Participate & Succeed
Age: 15+
Athletic Experience: 10+ yrs

Stage 3
Train & Compete
Age: 13-19
Athletic Experience: 6-10 yrs

Stage 2
Develop & Challenge
Age: 10-16
Athletic Experience: 3-6 yrs

Stage 1
Discover, Learn & Play
Age: 0-12
Athletic Experience: 1-3 yrs

Source: United States Olympic & Paralympic Committee

FIGURE 21.8 Stages to a Better Sport Experience

Based on United States Olympic and Paralympic Committee. (2016). *American development model: Rebuilding athletes in America*. Retrieved from https://cdn3.sportngin .com/attachments/document/8c8b-2311769/USOC_ADM_Brochure_2016.pdf

THE 10 PILLARS OF LTAD AND THE YOUTH PHYSICAL DEVELOPMENT MODEL

As the Balyi model gained popularity globally, it also drew criticism from a group of academics. In 2011, a paper published in the *Journal of Sports Sciences* (Ford et al., 2011) called attention to a number of issues with the model. In particular, the critics questioned the theoretical model of "windows of opportunity," which are proposed critical periods or ages in which certain training can accelerate and enhance physical development. For example, it was proposed that for boys, the first speed training window occurs between the ages of 7 and 9 years, and the second occurs between the ages of 13 and 16 years. However, this theoretical model is based on the naturally occurring developmental trajectories for a range of fitness attributes, such as strength, jumping ability, speed, and aerobic fitness (i.e., normal growth and maturation), and lacks supportive evidence from a sufficient number of experimental training studies. In contrast, it has been shown that all fitness attributes are trainable across childhood and adolescence (Ford et al., 2011; Lloyd et al., 2016; Van Hooren & De Ste Croix, 2020)—a view that is embraced in the Youth Physical Development Model (**Figure 21.9**).

The seminal paper by Ford et al. (2011) catalyzed the establishment of the 10 pillars of LTAD outlined in the National Strength and Conditioning Association's position statement (Lloyd et al., 2016). The core principle of this position statement is that youth, irrespective of their age, abilities, and aspirations, should participate in LTAD programs that foster physical fitness and psychosocial well-being. The central tenet of LTAD invariably remains the health and well-being of the child. This journey toward physical literacy ought to commence in early childhood, primarily focusing on the development of fundamental movement skills (FMS), motor competence (MC), sport-specific skills (SSS), and muscular strength. The program should incorporate various activities, games, and sports that encourage and enhance a wide spectrum of motor skills (Lloyd et al., 2016).

The LTAD program should be systematically progressed and individualized using a range of training modes that enhance both health- and skill-related components of fitness and reduce the risk of injury. Importantly, the LTAD pathways should accommodate the highly individualized and nonlinear nature of the growth and development of youth. Moreover, qualified professionals and sound pedagogical approaches are fundamental to the success of LTAD programs. Practitioners should also incorporate relevant monitoring and assessment tools to evaluate the LTAD strategy.

The composite Youth Physical Development Model provides a flexible blueprint from which coaches can work to promote a holistic approach to the development of all youth. The model develops most, if not all, components of fitness throughout childhood and adolescence, albeit focusing on some aspects more than others at various stages (as opposed to the idea of windows of opportunity). For example, the model shows that a 12- to 13-year-old boy should primarily focus their training on strength, power, speed, agility, and sport-specific skill development, with a reduced focus on hypertrophy, mobility, fundamental movement skill, and endurance and metabolic conditioning.

Although most Sports Performance Coaches will not train preschool-age youth, this phase of development is still important to subsequent youth training. Youth should be introduced to movement and unstructured deliberate play during early childhood (age 2 to 5 years), as this is a crucial phase for the exploration and learning of a broad range of fundamental movement skills masked in fun-based learning environments (e.g., playground, backyard, daycare, swimming pool). Indeed, the fundamental movement skills are the building blocks of participation and enjoyment of physical activity, games, and sports. Just as a lack of reading literacy in early childhood can have far-reaching

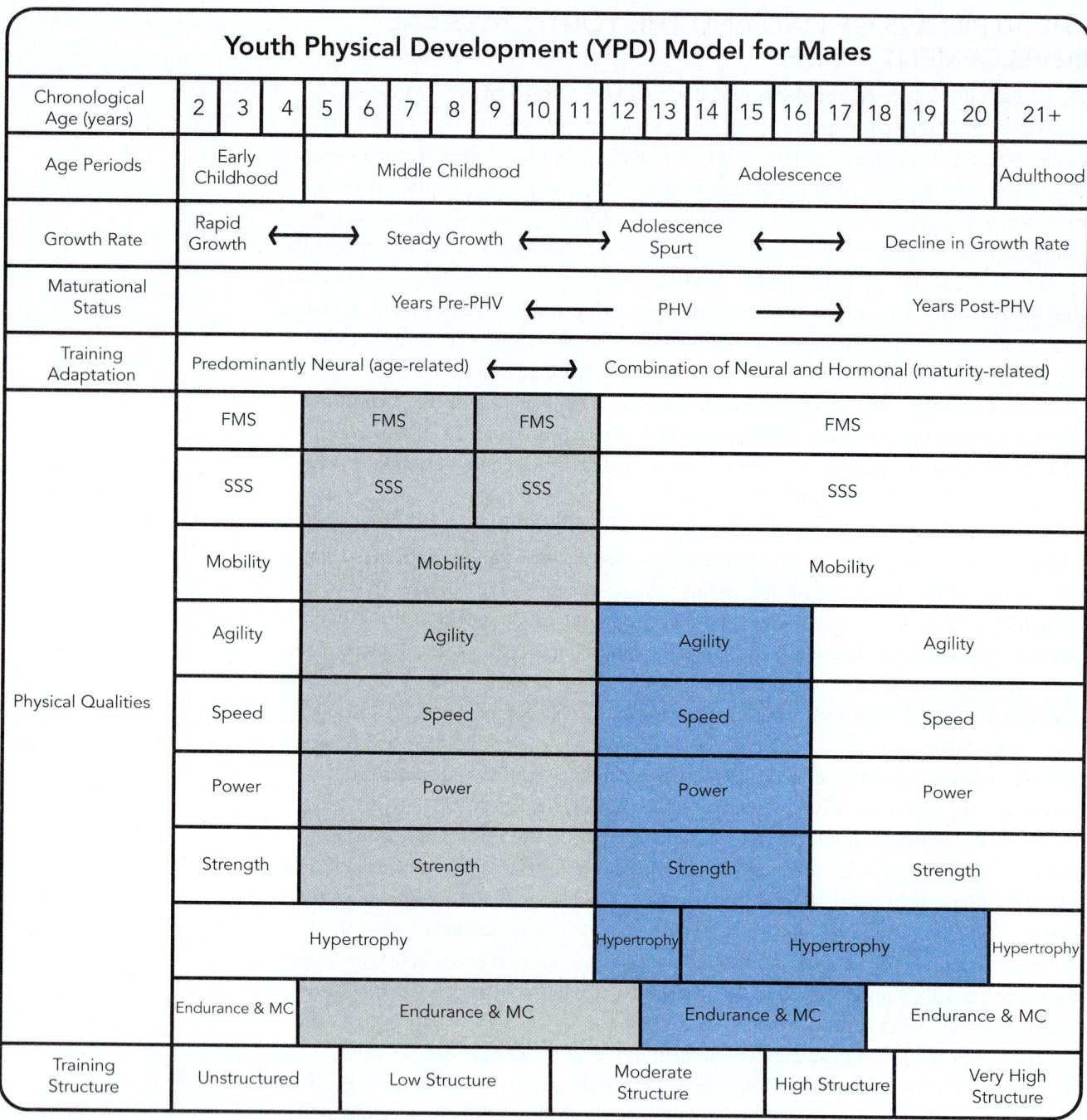

FIGURE 21.9A The Youth Physical Development Model

Data from Lloyd, R. S., & Oliver, J. L. (2012, June). The youth physical development model: A new approach to long-term athletic development. *Strength and Conditioning Journal, 34*(3): 61–72. https://doi.org/10.1519/SSC.0b013e31825760ea

consequences, so can physical illiteracy. As building blocks, fundamental movement skills such as walking, throwing, and balancing provide the foundation for other movements, such as playing soccer (running and kicking), gymnastics (balancing and bending), and the triple jump (running, jumping, and landing). If the fundamental movements are not nurtured and guided, the child will have less confidence and competence in movement ability, leading to a negative spiral of engagement in physical activity, exercise, and sports participation (Gao & Wang, 2019).

In mid-childhood to early adolescence or the elementary school years (age 5 to 12 years), children should be encouraged and allowed to sample or try a range of sports and

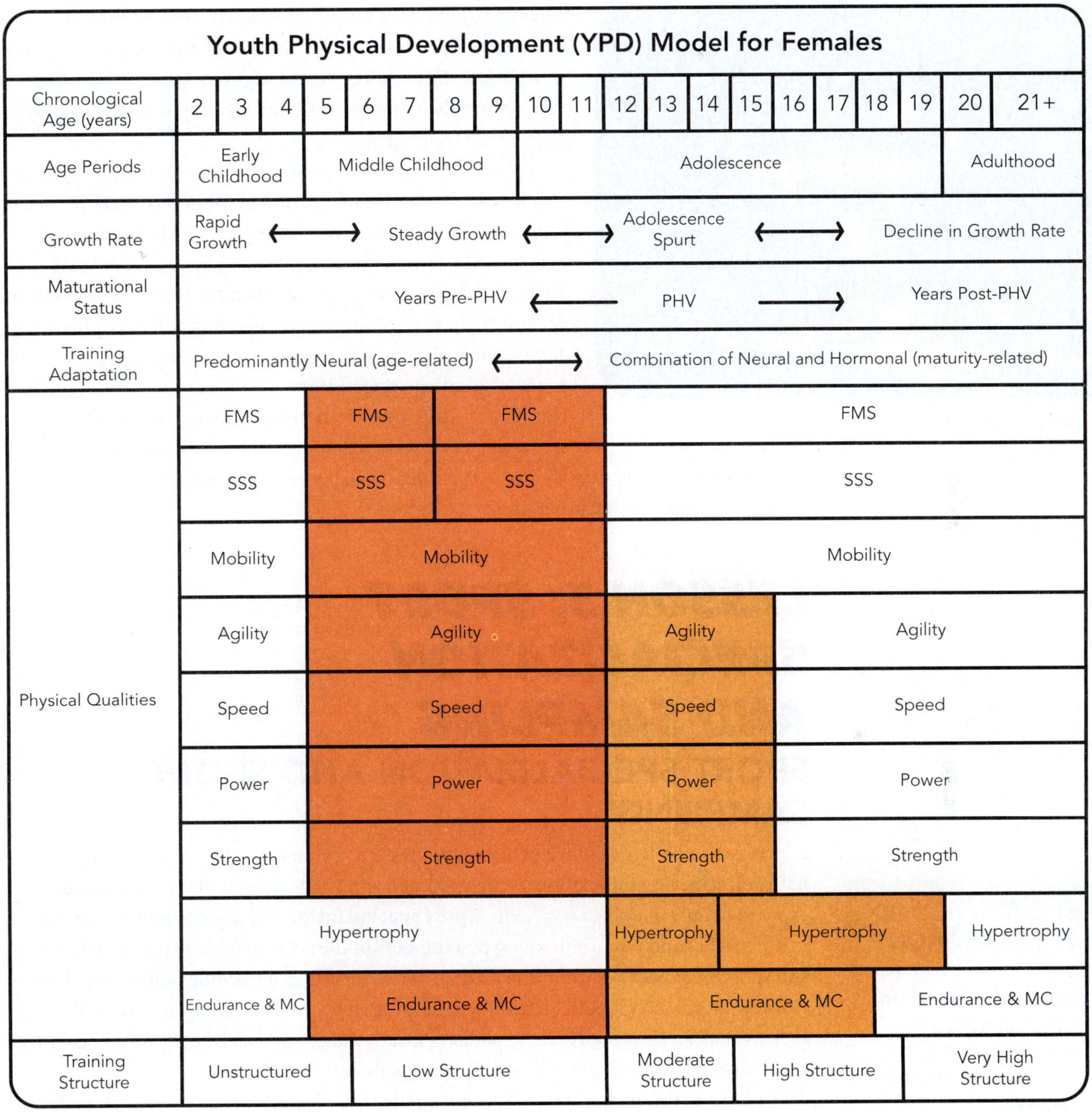

Youth Physical Development (YPD) Model for Females

Chronological Age (years)	2	3	4	5	6	7	8	9	10	11	12	13	14	15	16	17	18	19	20	21+
Age Periods	Early Childhood			Middle Childhood					Adolescence										Adulthood	
Growth Rate	Rapid Growth		⟷		Steady Growth			⟷			Adolescence Spurt			⟷			Decline in Growth Rate			
Maturational Status						Years Pre-PHV				⟵		PHV			⟶		Years Post-PHV			
Training Adaptation	Predominantly Neural (age-related)					⟷		Combination of Neural and Hormonal (maturity-related)												
Physical Qualities	FMS			FMS			FMS				FMS									
	SSS			SSS			SSS				SSS									
	Mobility			Mobility							Mobility									
	Agility			Agility							Agility				Agility					
	Speed			Speed							Speed				Speed					
	Power			Power							Power				Power					
	Strength			Strength							Strength				Strength					
	Hypertrophy										Hypertrophy		Hypertrophy				Hypertrophy			
	Endurance & MC		Endurance & MC								Endurance & MC					Endurance & MC				
Training Structure	Unstructured			Low Structure							Moderate Structure			High Structure			Very High Structure			

Lloyd, R. S., & Oliver, J. L. (2012)

FIGURE 21.9B The Youth Physical Development Model

Data from Lloyd, R. S., & Oliver, J. L. (2012, June). The youth physical development model: A new approach to long-term athletic development. *Strength and Conditioning Journal, 34*(3): 61–72. https://doi.org/10.1519/SSC.0b013e31825760ea

activities that assist in the further development and mastery of the fundamental movement and sport skills. Toward the latter part of this phase, they can be introduced to a more structured training environment that trains all fitness attributes in an integrated way. According to the Youth Physical Development Model, all fitness attributes are trainable at this age and the introduction of resistance training, which includes learning a variety of exercises using bodyweight, free weights, and other implements, is recommended (Lloyd, Oliver, et al., 2014). Perhaps more importantly, the focus should be on fun and

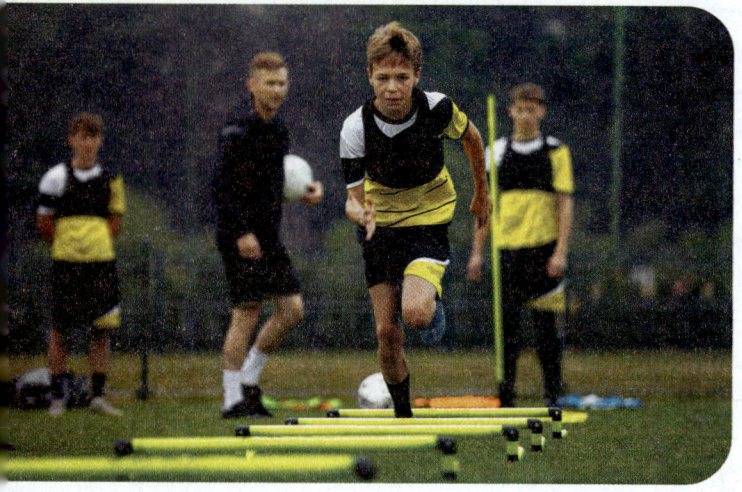

© Matimix/Shutterstock

enhancing the young person's self-worth and self-esteem. In essence, the aim is to build competent and confident movers. In addition, the program should begin to empower youth to take responsibility for learning and training so that they have a stake in the training process.

Adolescence (middle school and high school, age 13 to 18-plus years) is a dynamic period of life and is often the "make it or break it" point for many young athletes. Unfortunately, 70% to 80% of youth drop out of sports by age 15 (Merkel, 2013). In addition, this is a time when physical activity levels in general begin to decline precipitously. Regardless of whether an adolescent is playing recreational or performance-based sports, or merely participating in a fitness program, it is important to continue to foster peer relationships among youth, enhance self-esteem, and seek to empower them. Athletes in the performance pathway may choose to specialize in a sport and also begin to follow a highly structured sport-specific program.

LESSON 3: SPORT SPECIALIZATION AND SAMPLING
SPORT SPECIALIZATION AND SPORT SAMPLING

Exposure to a variety of movement experiences is a key aspect of the LTAD framework; however, achieving this exposure can be limited and challenging if the young athlete is exposed to only one sport or activity. **Sport specialization** is a topic of interest among many coaches and physical training practitioners in the areas of athletic performance and sport medicine (Waldron et al., 2019). Various national governing bodies (e.g., USA Hockey, USA Soccer, USA Lacrosse), youth sport club administrators, coaches, and parents at all levels of sport often ponder what advantages or disadvantages may occur by enabling children to follow one specific sport pathway.

In general, this interest arises due to the potential of acquiring and refining higher levels of overall sporting ability, technical skill, tactics, and mental preparation during earlier stages of development (Waldron et al., 2019). Alternatively, **sport sampling**, also known as multi-sport participation or multilateral development, is the practice of encouraging an individual to learn and participate in more than one sport or recreational activity over the span of 1 year (Carder et al., 2020). Sport sampling likely should occur over a period of several years and across key developmental stages, both physical and emotional, during childhood and adolescence.

Although the specialization and sampling pathways may not be alike in practice, the Sports Performance Coach and personal fitness trainer should understand the focus and direction of each approach to fully understand and appreciate what role either pathway may have on the organization of athletic development, athletic success, and physical activity throughout the lifespan.

SPORT SPECIALIZATION →

Intense technical or physical training in a single sport to the exclusion of all other sports.

SPORT SAMPLING →

Participation in two (nonsimultaneous) or more sports over the period of a year.

SPORT SPECIALIZATION

Specialized athlete development involves intensive, deliberate, and focused approaches toward organizing and structuring practice and competition for high-level success. Although the origins of sport specialization are not precisely known, this practice likely dates to the Olympiads of ancient Greece. During these periods, young males and females were exposed to a variety of physical and mental challenges in preparation and participation for various physical contests that emphasized health, civic duty, and preparation for battle (Demirel & Yildiran, 2013).

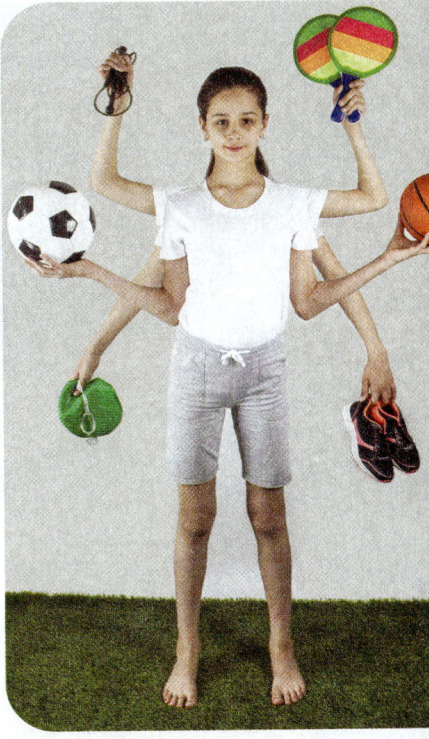

© Ksravik93/Shutterstock

Today, as a highly structured and regimented approach to achieve sporting success, sport specialization is being adopted by many schools and youth sport organizations throughout the United States. Indeed, it is not uncommon for youth sport administrators and coaches to promote a dedicated training approach that starts in early childhood and continues through late childhood and into adolescence (Normand et al., 2017). In addition to sport skill and physical training, implementation of other services may be encouraged, including but not limited to nutrition education and mental skills training. Ultimately, the aim of this training approach is to develop a very skilled and physically prepared child or adolescent athlete who performs at a high level of ability relative to their developmental stage.

A popular opinion among the coaches and parents who are involved in these programs is that the child will be able to sustain their advanced abilities through adolescence and become a candidate for participation among select or elite-level programs that offer opportunities to practice and compete on the regional or national stage (Normand et al., 2017). Other potential incentives may include opportunities for international competition, an intercollegiate athletic scholarship, or other forms of financial assistance. Coaches, parents, and youth athletes should recognize that the path to intercollegiate sport participation at all National Collegiate Athletic Association levels (Division I through III) from high school is very selective, with only a small percentage of male or female high school athletes participating at the intercollegiate level.

To date, in regard to intercollegiate or elite-level sports, there is little supporting evidence for the idea that specializing in one sport at an early age will lead to long-term success that continues into adulthood (LaPrade et al., 2016). In fact, several studies suggest just the opposite: Participation in multiple sports may produce athletes who are better suited to long-term success at elite levels of sport (Côté & Vierimaa, 2014). There are, of course, some potential exceptions, which can lead to confusion among performance coaches, personal fitness trainers, and parents. Thus, it is important to examine the practice of early versus late specialization with greater detail.

The introduction of organized physical training for sport is an essential consideration during athlete development and is often a point of contention and misunderstanding. Youth sport administrators, coaches, and parents—many of whom are volunteers—may not have a background in human growth and maturation. As a result, they typically use chronological age or educational grade level as an indicator of when it is appropriate for youth to start an intensive, deliberate, and structured physical preparation program for one sport. Compared to chronological age and educational grade level, biological markers of growth and maturation such as peak height and weight velocity are actually better indicators of the physical preparedness needed to initiate a specific athlete development program (Eisenmann et al., 2020).

In general, human growth tends to correspond with the various stages of the LTAD framework. For the Sports Performance Coach, understanding the variability of physical and emotional growth and maturation is essential because it raises important

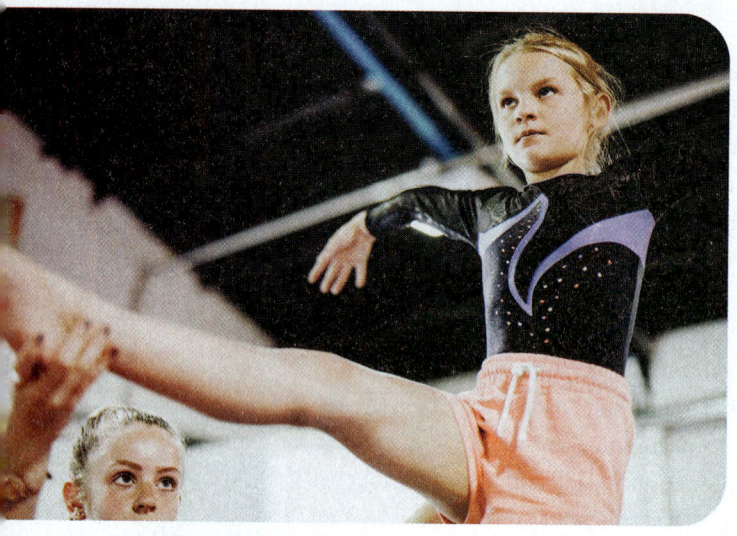

© Rawpixel.com/Shutterstock

considerations and suggests the need for accommodations that may influence the quality of programming for athletic success.

Because specialized youth athlete development is generally categorized as either early or late, knowledge and assessment of various biological maturation markers can provide guidance for the timing and prescription of several training variables, including the frequency, intensity, and volume of training (Lloyd, Oliver, et al., 2014). Simply using chronological age does not provide enough insight into the timing and rate of various biological and anthropometric changes that can influence safe and effective program design.

EARLY SPECIALIZATION

Early specialization is generally defined as participation in one sport for at least 8 months out of the year (often year-round) that occurs prior to the age of 12 (LaPrade et al., 2016). Athletes who specialize early are typically pre-pubertal and have not experienced the onset of their peak height and peak weight velocity, which becomes a key programming consideration. Physical changes to the human body because of human growth and maturation—called anthropometric changes—result in increases in stature (height), limb segment length, circumference, and body mass (both muscle and fat tissue). Anthropometric changes must be taken into consideration during training because changes to the physical dimensions of limbs and body segments also create changes to the inertial properties of the limbs, which in turn can affect limb velocities, acceleration, and whole-body movement in general (McGinnis, 2013).

Although anthropometric changes are a consideration for all sports, they are especially critical for sports or activities that require whole-body rotations, such as gymnastics, figure skating, diving, and other aerial or acrobatic activities (Kliethermes et al., 2021). Control of limbs and body segments is important for success in these types of activities, as scoring is heavily dependent on coordination of the limbs to perform these movements with great precision and balance. Complex aerial and acrobatic skills require a tremendous investment in time, practice, and competition for mastery to occur. The main point here is that the timing and rate of peak height and peak weight velocity can have an important influence on the learning of movements in general and of sport skills specifically (Lloyd, Oliver, et al., 2014).

In combination, the timing and rate of physical growth and the time needed to master complex aerial and acrobatic movements influence the scenario where it is favorable to start specialized skill and sport training early (pre-pubertal). This earlier approach to specialization allows for the central nervous system to make the proprioceptive and sensorimotor corrections needed to acquire complex aerial and acrobatic skills (Latash, 2008). In addition, mastery of these types of skills at an earlier age with refined sensorimotor ability enables the young athlete to adapt and regulate movement patterns that can be affected by changes in anthropometric features that occur later with the onset of peak height and weight velocity (Hewett et al., 2016).

LATE SPECIALIZATION

In contrast to sports that must consider the effect of anthropometric changes on skill acquisition and performance during earlier stages of athletic development, some sports are heavily dependent on the expression of muscular strength and power. In addition, muscular strength and power contribute to other important athletic abilities, including speed and agility. Increases in strength and power are due to significant increases in circulating androgenic (e.g., testosterone) and growth hormones that contribute to an increase in muscle (Lloyd, Oliver, et al., 2014). Although muscular strength and power are important attributes at any age, they become most apparent in puberty and during the post-pubertal years, after peak height and weight velocity are achieved. As a result, for sports that are heavily dependent on muscular strength, power, speed, and agility, it is not as important to emphasize the training of these abilities during the earlier stages of the LTAD framework.

Although strength-building exercises can be encouraged, there should be greater emphasis on acquiring fundamental movement skills and general movement ability during the earlier stages of training for some sports. Thus, sports that require greater focus on strength and power are referred to as **late specialization** sports. Because the anthropometric changes from growth and maturation are not immediately critical to long-term success, sports that typically fall under the late specialization label are generally team-oriented, racquet, or combative types of activities (Kliethermes et al., 2021).

Ultimately, the Sports Performance Coach should understand the variability in timing and growth rate and maturation, as this knowledge is an important tool that can help the coach evaluate young athletes and adjust their programming for athletic development. This is especially true for young athletes who are introduced to new movement experiences, skills, sports, and perhaps different sport positions with different physical demands or needs depending on their early or late maturation status (**Figure 21.10**).

> **LATE → SPECIALIZATION**
>
> The identification and participation in one sport, typically after the age of 12 or the initiation of peak height and weight velocity. As they are often preceded by the sampling of many sports or movement activities, team sports are generally characterized as late specialization sports.

Sport Specialization

	Early Specialization Sports	Late Specialization Sports
Characteristics	Artistic and Acrobatic Sports	Team sports; Combatives; Racquet sports
Examples	• Gymnastics • Figure skating • Diving	• Soccer • Baseball • Wrestling • Tennis

FIGURE 21.10 Sport Specialization

DELIBERATE PRACTICE VERSUS DELIBERATE PLAY

It is also important to consider the structure and nature of practice. **Deliberate practice** is a focused and demanding approach in which coaches dedicate more time and resources to one sport (Myer et al., 2016). This approach includes a high training frequency and a greater volume of intensive and repetitive physical training with the hope of achieving early mastery of sport skills, tactics, and physical preparation (**Figure 21.11**). Deliberate practice is especially common with the early specialization pathway and does not offer youth athletes much input regarding the organization of practice or the training environment.

> **DELIBERATE → PRACTICE**
>
> Focused, intensive, and high-frequency training approach with the intent of achieving mastery of sport skills, tactics, and physical preparation.

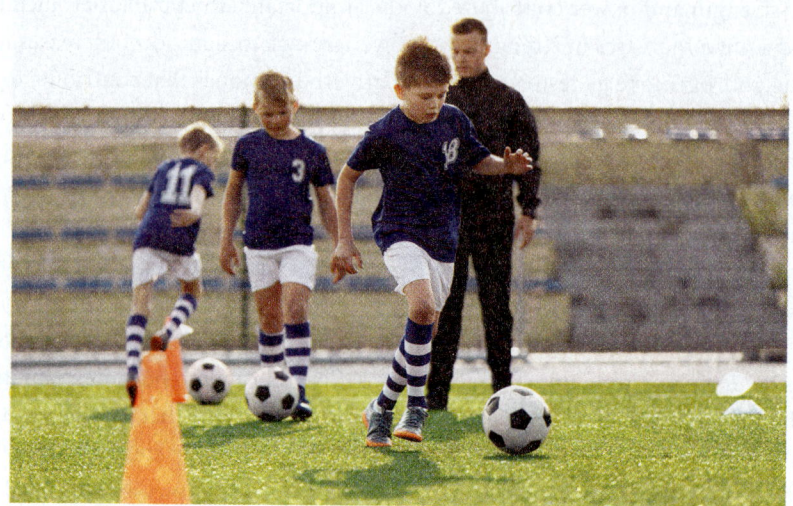

FIGURE 21.11 Deliberate Practice Environment
© Matimix/Shutterstock

In contrast, **deliberate play** is a coaching approach that offers a greater variety of movement experiences, which can vary on a continuum from free to structured (Côté & Vierimaa, 2014). This approach does not generally include a high frequency or volume of any single form of physical training. It also differs from deliberate practice in that there is no need to master a particular movement or skill at an early developmental stage. With deliberate play, Sports Performance Coaches can create learning conditions in which the youth athlete can experiment and use expressive movement actions in response to the training environment.

In deliberate play, modified rules, boundaries, barriers, equipment, and environments can be used at the liberty of the coach or trainer to allow the training setting to guide skill development or to allow movements to emerge from the setting that has been created. Meanwhile, youth athletes are encouraged to interact and overcome movement problems as they are encountered and to use spontaneous creativity (**Figure 21.12**) to help develop and refine movement abilities or related sport skills.

Because youth exhibit varying degrees of socioemotional and cognitive maturity, another valuable outcome of deliberate play is the element of fun (**Table 21.4**). Several

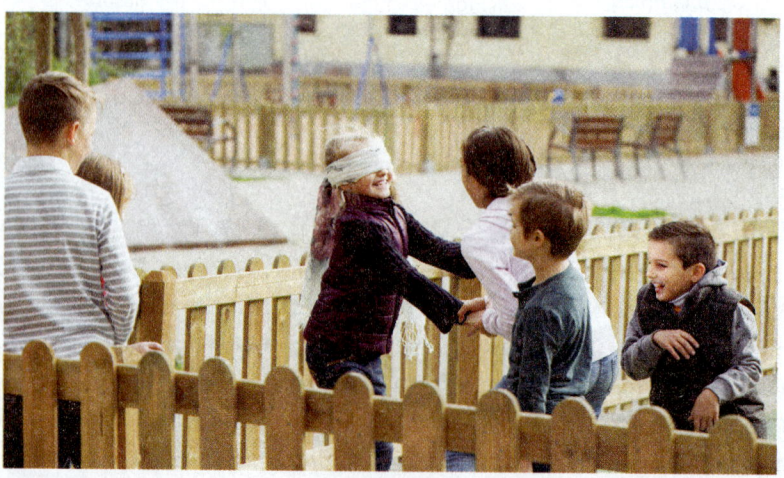

FIGURE 21.12 Deliberate Play Environment
© BearFotos/Shutterstock

TABLE 21.4   Deliberate Play Versus Deliberate Practice

Deliberate Play	Deliberate Practice
Fun and enjoyable	Not necessarily enjoyable
Flexible in structure	Structured with definite rules
No adult involvement needed	Adult involvement
Performed in multiple environments	Specialized environment
Pretend and few or no rules	Serious approach
No particular goal or specific objective	Has a definite aim or purpose

studies have found that for young athletes, movement that allows for self-discovery and expression without the pressure of a specific outcome is more enjoyable, giving the young athlete greater motivation to participate in the activity on a regular basis (Post et al., 2017). Although physical, emotional, and cognitive development may not mature simultaneously during childhood, it is generally understood that the development of these characteristics will progressively evolve from a very immature and playful state to one that embraces greater challenges and competition with quality coaching. Thus, for young athletes, instead of following a highly structured training routine, it is best to mix unstructured, semi-structured, or structured play or game conditions that can challenge the young athlete, yet also make the training experience enjoyable. This is important in the long-term development of youth athletes, as it also helps to avoid the high-frequency, redundant, and repetitive movement experiences that can lead to overuse injury, psychological burnout, or both (Jayanthi et al., 2019).

Another consideration concerning deliberate practice and deliberate play is their impact on multilateral development. The late specialization pathway allows for more time to be spent on new and diverse movement experiences or physical activities, including forms of play and simple games. These play opportunities complement sport training and are ideal at the earlier stages of athletic development, as they can become a proving ground for youth to explore and use a trial-and-error approach at attempting to learn new movements and movement corrections (Myer et al., 2016). Play-like activities and games utilize fundamental movement patterns from earlier stages of development that can be readily transferred to other sports. Over time, this multilateral experimentation can yield the competence and the confidence needed to learn more complex sport-specific patterns and skills by improving perceptual and spatial awareness of the many movement possibilities that exist among team, racket, or combative sports.

SPORT SAMPLING

As the young athlete matures, play should be encouraged to refine movement and sport skills; however, there will also be greater emphasis on games and competitive sport experiences. Although sport coaches may feel the need to have young athletes focus on one sport to excel, evidence supports encouraging athletes to participate in multiple sports throughout a given year (Valasek et al., 2019). This practice is called sport sampling, also known as sport diversification or multi-sport participation.

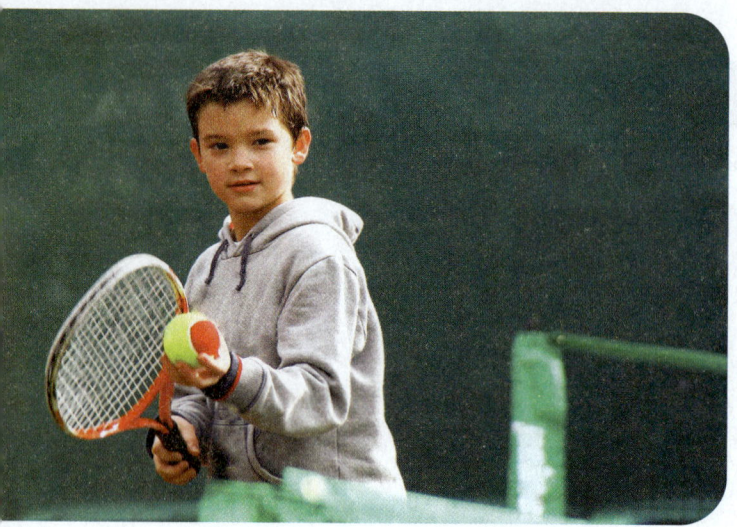

Sport sampling does not promote participating in multiple sports at the same time; instead, as one sport season is completed, it is followed by a different sport and the start of a new season (Myer et al., 2016). With a sampling approach, a multi-sport athlete might potentially always be in-season; therefore, monitoring the frequency and volume of training while ensuring appropriate rest and recovery is important to prevent overuse injury and psychological burnout. Depending on the athlete's developmental stage, other aspects of physical training (e.g., strength and power training, speed, agility) may be built into the program, and these activities can compound the stress and fatigue that will come from participating in multiple sports year-round.

SPORT SAMPLING'S INFLUENCE ON DEVELOPMENT AND PERFORMANCE

In regard to athletic development, Sports Performance Coaches must clearly understand the potential outcomes of following a single- versus multi-sport pathway. Either approach could bring success to an athlete, but there is no guarantee. Therefore, any decision regarding best practice should be made with the best interest of the athlete in mind.

Like deliberate play, sport sampling provides exposure to a diverse set of movements and sport skills. Multiple sport experiences enrich the sensorimotor system and improve perceptual-motor abilities that contribute to sport skill and tactical success (Güllich et al., 2022).

Although skills and tactics are unique to every sport, some general patterns of movement and strategy can be transferable from one sport to another (Strafford et al., 2018). These include common action characteristics (e.g., acceleration, deceleration, lowered center of gravity, force absorption, force generation, change of direction) and tactical features (e.g., chase, evade, dodge, find space).

Sport sampling can also challenge the sensorimotor complex of the young athlete with different competitive environments (e.g., playing surface, equipment, boundaries, space, or rules). For team, racquet, and combative sports, considerations based on skills, tactics, and environment are particular aspects that separate the early and late specialization approaches. An essential feature of late specialization is progressive long-term exposure to varied movement experiences throughout the developmental stages of the LTAD framework. Late specialization is an approach that provides ample opportunities to acquire, develop, and refine those perceptual motor abilities that ease the transition from fundamental to specific, and can encourage athletes to develop the confidence needed for lifelong participation in sport and physical activity.

OVERUSE INJURY

An **overuse injury** is best described as damage or trauma to a region of the body that occurs because of repetitive use over time without adequate opportunity for rest or recovery (Valovich McLeod et al., 2011). This kind of injury could be compounded if young athletes are spending additional time with skill and performance coaches outside of the time spent with their sport coach.

Whether an athlete follows an early or late specialization pathway, poor management of the frequency, volume, and intensity of training can lead to chronic discomfort and, in some cases, to potential risk for catastrophic injury. Sport, skill, and performance coaches

OVERUSE INJURY →

Chronic discomfort or trauma to tissues of the body that occurs as a result of high-volume, repetitive use without adequate opportunity for rest or recovery from training or competition.

should always have open lines of communication and monitor their young athletes to ensure opportunities for adequate rest and recovery are in place. If an early specialization approach is not critical, sport sampling and deliberate play offer opportunities to reduce the frequency and volume of repetitive movement patterns in practice and during competition (Myer et al., 2016). In addition, other forms of skill training or physical preparation that complement athletic development can be distributed over longer phases or periods of training to decrease physical or even psychological stress.

LOWER-EXTREMITY INJURY

Muscular co-contraction provides joint stability and injury resilience from ligament injury to the lower extremities. Although ankle sprains are the most common lower-extremity injury, noncontact anterior cruciate ligament (ACL) injuries are among the most catastrophic. Athletes become more resilient to a noncontact ACL injury when the muscle groups that surround the knee joint, chiefly the knee extensors and flexors, contract simultaneously to provide the necessary joint stability when absorbing force (Hewett et al., 2016). Exposing the young athlete to multiple sport experiences will create landing, cutting, and change-of-direction situations involving different environmental conditions and different playing surfaces. This type of movement diversity during the early developmental stages of the LTAD framework allows the sensorimotor system to become enriched, so that it can provide the dynamic knee joint stability needed for protection during practice and competition (Leventer et al., 2015). Ultimately, sport sampling can play a key role in improving proprioception, position sense, and perceptual motor ability that not only improves performance, but also reduces the incidence and severity of lower-extremity injuries (McGuine et al., 2017).

PSYCHOLOGICAL BURNOUT

Psychological burnout is a concern associated with an early sport specialization pathway. Because burnout can lead to a lack of participation in sport and physical activity, it is important to recognize the causes, signs, and symptoms of athlete burnout and for performance coaches and personal fitness trainers to take steps to prevent this condition (**Figure 21.13**).

> ### PSYCHOLOGI- →
> ### CAL BURNOUT
>
> Condition characterized by emotional and physical exhaustion from excessive physical training and competition. Signs and symptoms include, but are not limited to, fatigue, anxiety, a reduced sense of accomplishment with performance below expectations, and a devalued sense of sport whereby an athlete does not care for the sport anymore.

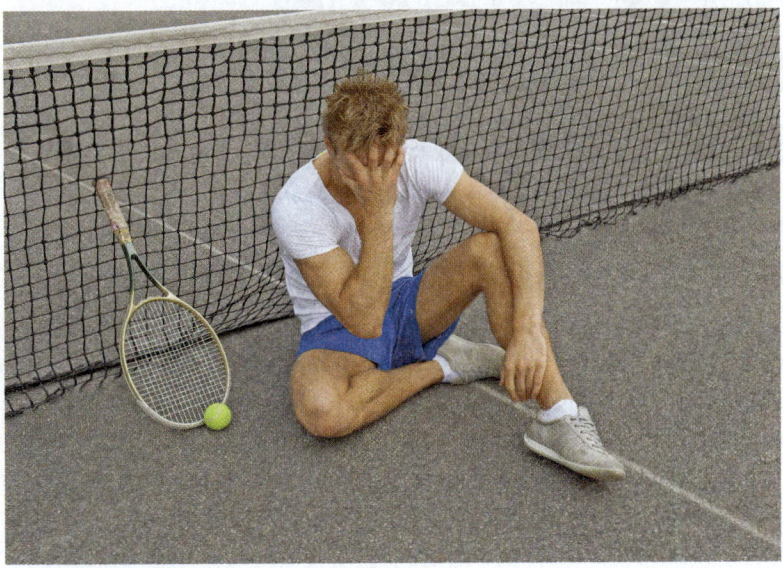

FIGURE 21.13 Psychological Burnout
© Studio Light and Shade/Shutterstock

Physical and mental exhaustion generally occurs when an athlete is exposed to a high frequency and volume of training or competition over a short period of time without opportunities for appropriate rest and recovery (Markati et al., 2019). For an athlete to be physically and mentally prepared for upcoming training sessions or competitions, optimal rest and methods of recovery are essential and a fundamental component of structured training and proper periodization.

In addition to the physical demands of sport preparation, greater competitiveness, parental involvement, and higher performance expectations can place a significant amount of emotional stress on the young athlete. It is important to recognize that young athletes are not "miniature adults." In turn, when possible, it has been suggested that coaches discourage early sport specialization prior to the age of 12 (LaPrade et al., 2016). Youth, in general, do not exhibit the physical maturity or emotional understanding needed to handle the physical and psychological demands often placed on them by deliberate practice or commitment to one sport.

Compared to their peers who follow the sport sampling approach, adolescent athletes who follow an early specialization path exhibit higher rates of participation dropout and greater incidence of psychological burnout (Giusti et al., 2020). Too much time dedicated to sport and performance training coupled with parental pressure can lead to a lack of enjoyment for sport and emotional exhaustion when there is less time for personal activities or socializing with peers (Witt & Dangi, 2018).

Young athletes thrive both physically and emotionally when they have an opportunity to achieve a healthy sport–school life balance (Côté & Vierimaa, 2014). Therefore, coaches, parents, and athletes should communicate and work together to create developmentally appropriate training environments that offer deliberate play as part of the training structure, require less parent involvement, and increase opportunities for input and feedback from the athlete (Morano et al., 2020).

LESSON 4: YOUTH ATHLETE PROGRAM DESIGN: ALIGNING THE LTAD FRAMEWORK AND NASM'S OPT™ MODEL

YOUTH ATHLETE PROGRAM DESIGN

Sports Performance Coaches need to apply youth training principles and the LTAD framework as part of clearly written programs that meet the needs of each youth athlete. Program design for youth entails turning the specific principles of youth growth and development into a long-term plan. The dual goals of youth sports performance are improving performance and embracing a physically active lifestyle that will endure throughout childhood and adolescence well into adulthood. The Sports Performance Coach needs to meet every youth at their level, whether the youth participant is just starting their journey, transitioning to elite performance, or anywhere in between, to encourage them to become the best version of themselves.

APPLICATION OF THE LTAD FRAMEWORK TO PROGRAM DESIGN

LTAD can be thought of as the framework of ideas, information, and principles that guide programming for aspiring athletes of all ages and abilities. One important note is that the LTAD framework goes beyond simply creating an exercise program; Sports Performance Coaches need to promote motor skill development and mastery, especially during the formative years as described in the LTAD models. Motor skills then need to be reinforced during late childhood and throughout adolescence and even into adulthood. As has been previously described in this chapter, youth are a heterogeneous population, with varying stages of growth and development, maturity, and readiness to participate in structured training programs.

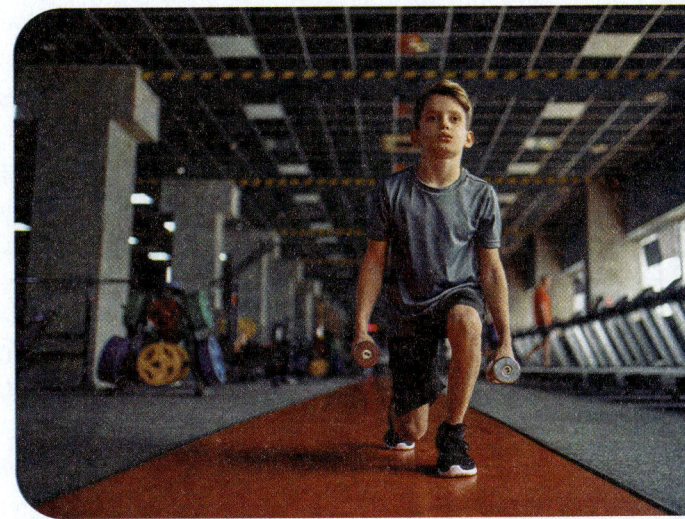

© Nomad_Soul/Shutterstock

The YPD Model was created as an evidence-based approach to inclusion of the 10 physical attributes across childhood and adolescence (Lloyd & Oliver, 2012). These 10 physical attributes include not only fundamental motor skills, but also sport-specific skills, mobility, agility, speed, power, strength, hypertrophy, and endurance and metabolic conditioning (**Figure 21.14**). It is imperative, therefore, that a variety of movements and exercises are introduced. Basic movement patterns help Sports Performance Coaches classify exercises for appropriate selection in the exercise program. There are many ways to classify these movements, such as the 10 fundamental exercise patterns (hinge, squat, lunge, horizontal push, horizontal pull, vertical push, vertical pull, brace, rotate, and carry), six load vectors, or the 10 key movements that form the foundation for movement in the LTAD framework (Lloyd et al., 2022).

 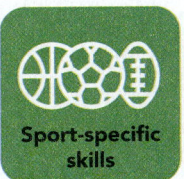  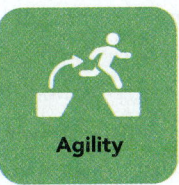 

Motor skills | Sport-specific skills | Mobility | Agility | Speed

10 Physical Attributes Across Childhood and Adolescence

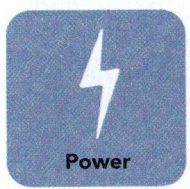 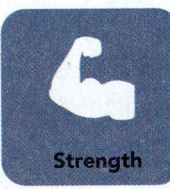 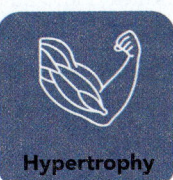  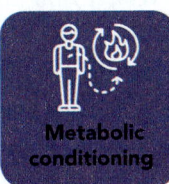

Power | Strength | Hypertrophy | Endurance | Metabolic conditioning

FIGURE 21.14 Physical Attributes Across Childhood and Adolescence

Data from Lloyd, R. S., & Oliver, J. L. (2012, June). The youth physical development model: A new approach to long-term athletic development. *Strength and Conditioning Journal, 34*(3): 61–72. https://doi.org/10.1519/SSC.0b013e31825760ea

To clarify the terminology, fundamental movement patterns are broad movement skills that can be built on to enhance overall movement—for example, learning to run, learning to kick, and then learning how to kick while running, as in soccer. Fundamental exercise patterns are the specific joint movements of exercises, such as squatting, lunging, and pressing.

In addition to fundamental movement and exercise patterns, other foundational movement patterns such as swimming, riding a bike, and treading water should be considered to broaden the scope of movement skills to promote LTAD (Hulteen et al., 2018). NASM's Optimal Performance Training™ (OPT™) Model advocates for fundamental exercise patterns specific to exercise prescription (squat, hip hinge, upper-body push, upper-body pull, press, and multiplanar and rotational movement). Thus, Sports Performance Coaches should incorporate exercise-specific fundamental patterns into the program design that are a mix of fundamental motor skills from the categories of object control, locomotion, and body awareness (Sutton, 2021). Sports Performance Coaches working with youth athletes should focus on developing a diverse movement base to support future exercises, activities, and sports in an intentional, structured, systematic process throughout childhood and adolescence.

According to Seefeldt's (1980) **proficiency barrier**, if fundamental motor task milestones are not reached by roughly 10 years of age, the child is less likely to become an expert mover. Stodden et al. (2013) investigated whether the proficiency barrier impacted physical activity and found that a **spiral of engagement** existed for physical activity. That is, a positive spiral of engagement exists when youth develop high motor competence over time, which fosters greater levels of physical activity, higher perceived motor competence, and increased physical fitness; a negative spiral of engagement exists when youth do not develop high motor competence over time, leading to reduced levels of physical activity, lower perceived motor competence, and lower levels of physical fitness (Gao & Wang, 2019). It is incumbent upon the Sports Performance Coach to ensure that the sessions with young athletes are fun, are engaging, and hold their attention.

PERIODIZATION AND PROGRAM DESIGN

A planned, systematic process for youth to develop the 10 physical attributes and foundational movement skills is fundamental to youth program design. Periodization establishes a systematic approach to program design that varies the amount and type of stress placed on the body to produce adaptation, promote improved performance, and reduce the risk of injury (Sutton, 2021).

Planned progressions of stages of periodization also enable the Sports Performance Coach to meet each youth athlete at their current level of development, fitness, and interest. This helps every youth athlete to achieve more than they could on their own, owing only to natural improvements in strength and endurance due to the growth and maturation process. Goals for youth should be more process-oriented, focusing on developing the 10 attributes across childhood and adolescence, developing healthy habits that will carry over throughout adulthood, and integrating health and physical fitness along their physical literacy journey. Sports Performance Coaches should match the periodization and program design for youth clients to the unique developmental and performance goals of each aspiring athlete.

PROGRAM DESIGN: THE LTAD FRAMEWORK AND NASM'S OPT MODEL

In developing programs for youth athletes, adopting a structured, scientific, and age-appropriate approach is crucial. This is where the OPT Model plays an instrumental role. This model provides a systematic, evidence-based, and periodized approach to athletic training and performance enhancement.

PROFICIENCY → BARRIER

The reduced ability to advance past the fundamental movement stage to the specialized skills phase, due to not attaining a certain level of mastery of fundamental movements; a barrier to later attaining skill mastery of specialized skills, such as those needed for sporting excellence.

SPIRAL OF → ENGAGEMENT

Variables within a feedback loop that are positive and continually positively influence the outcome (positive spiral of engagement) or are negative and continually hinder the outcome (negative spiral of engagement).

For youth athletes, it is especially critical to align this model with the key phases of LTAD, with training programs being specifically designed with the developmental stages of young athletes in mind. The OPT Model and the LTAD framework can be powerful tools for constructing training programs that evolve with the athlete as they grow, mature, and enhance their skills.

The LTAD framework offers a roadmap for athletic development punctuated by distinct phases, each targeting specific aspects of a young athlete's growth and maturation. These phases can be aligned with the OPT Model's structure, albeit with some adjustments considering the specific needs of youth athletes. For instance, more time is often spent in the general preparation phase of periodization with youth athletes than would typically be the case for adults. This phase focuses on building a broad fitness base and developing fundamental movement skills, setting the stage for more advanced training as athletes mature.

The key pillars of LTAD that need to be applied to program design are summarized in **Table 21.5** (Lloyd et al., 2016).

TABLE 21.5 Key Pillars for Successful Long-Term Athletic Development

Pillar	Description
1	Accommodate the highly individualized and nonlinear nature of the growth and development of youth.
2	Engage in LTAD programs that promote both physical fitness and psychosocial well-being, regardless of age, ability, and aspirations.
3	Enhance physical fitness from early childhood, with a primary focus on motor skill and muscular strength development.
4	Adopt an early sampling approach (i.e., sample various sports and physical activities) that promotes and enhances a broad range of motor skills.
5	Ensure the health and well-being of the child, above all else.
6	Participate in physical conditioning that helps reduce the risk of injury to ensure the child's ongoing participation in LTAD programs.
7	Provide all youth with a range of training modes to enhance both health-related and skills-related components of fitness.
8	Use relevant monitoring and assessment tools as part of a long-term physical development strategy.
9	Systematically progress and individualize training programs for successful long-term athletic development.
10	Include qualified professionals and sound pedagogical approaches.

Data from Lloyd, R. S., Cronin, J. B., Faigenbaum, A. D., Haff, G. G., Howard, R., Kraemer, W. J., Micheli, L. J., Myer, G. D., & Oliver, J. L. (2016). National strength and conditioning association position statement on long-term athletic development. *Journal of Strength and Conditioning Research, 30*(6), 1491–1509. https://doi.org/10.1519/JSC.0000000000001387

ACUTE TRAINING VARIABLES

All periodized training programs seek to optimally manipulate the acute training variables within the periodization phases. The Sports Performance Coach should consider how the acute training variables relate to youth-specific adaptations.

Repetitions

The best way to ensure quality resistance training repetitions for youth is to perform the movement first without added weight. For conditioning exercises, the sports performance specialist should watch for quality movement that improves over time and provide adequate rest between sets to ensure quality movement.

Set

The beginning youth athlete will begin with one set per exercise. The set will then be adjusted according to youth training guidelines (Lloyd, Faigenbaum, et al., 2014).

Training Intensity

While 1 to 5RM testing conducted following proper protocols has been shown to be safe and effective for children (Faigenbaum et al., 2003), maximal strength testing may *not* be appropriate for children and adolescents with little to no experience with the exercise being tested or poor motor ability for performing the exercise. Instead, it is recommended to focus on form and technique until testing can be implemented to measure strength rather than technique. Subjective measures, such as the **OMNI scale** (Pfeiffer et al., 2002) (**Figure 21.15**) and the visual scale (Faigenbaum et al., 2004) have been shown to be more appropriate for use in children than the **Borg scale**. To guard against overtraining

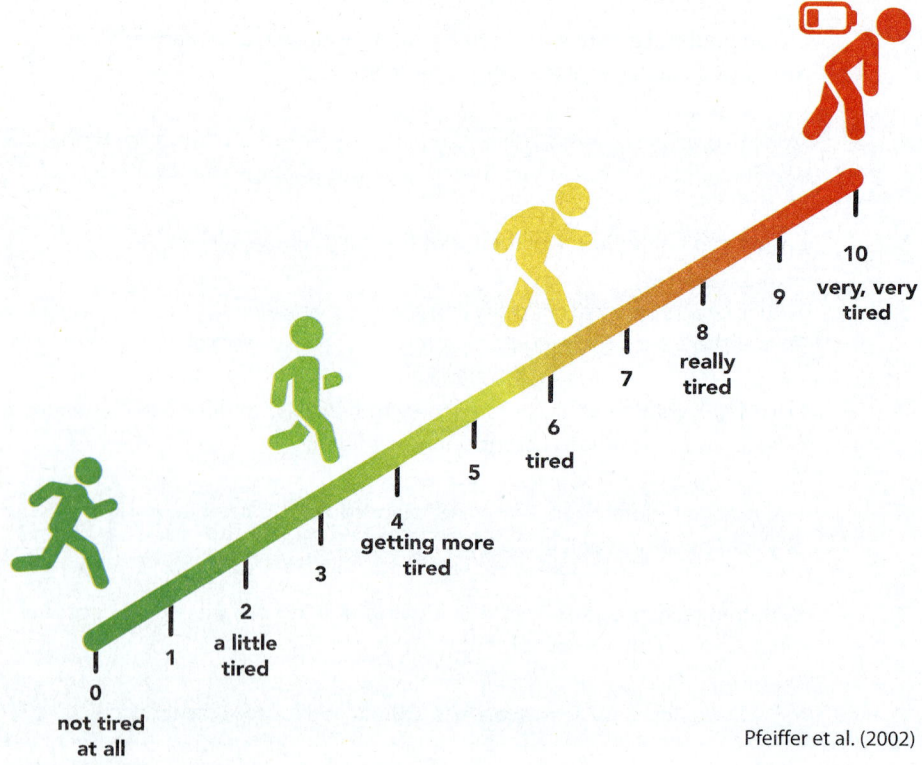

Pfeiffer et al. (2002)

FIGURE 21.15 OMNI Scale

Data from Pfeiffer, K. A., Pivarnik, J. M., Womack, C. J., Reeves, M. J., & Malina, R. M. (2002, Dec.). Reliability and validity of the Borg and OMNI rating of perceived exertion scales in adolescent girls. *Medicine & Science in Sports & Exercise, 34*(12): 2057–2061. https://doi.org/10.1097/00005768-200212000-00029

duration, the Borg CR100 scale has been shown to be a valid measure of the internal workload (Naidu et al., 2019).

Traditional calculations of intensity for cardiovascular fitness do not work well in youth populations (Machado & Denadai, 2011). Sports Performance Coaches can measure aerobic fitness using submaximal field tests to predict maximal values, such as the 1.5-mile run and the Yo-Yo Intermittent Test. For testing groups of children or adolescent athletes, the Yo-Yo Intermittent Test—Level 1 has shown excellent validity (Ahler et al., 2012) as has the Andersen test (Andersen et al., 2008). A review of fitness tests for youth found the 1.5-mile run showed only moderate validity (Castro-Piñero et al., 2010). Intensity in regard to cardiovascular fitness should consider the validity of the testing protocol for the age group and the athlete's relative level of interest in cardiovascular exercise.

Repetition Tempo

Research on tempo for resistance training for pre-pubertal youth suggests that Sports Performance Coaches should design programs with a tempo that matches the present motor skill ability of the youth. The terms *slow*, *moderate*, and *fast tempo* are subjective measures based on the youth athlete's proficiency in the movement or exercise.

Training Volume

Training volume includes not only the exercise performed under the qualified supervision of the Sports Performance Coach, but also the time spent in practice and sports competition plus the amount of time spent in other activities, whether additional sports teams or programs, specific coaching such as sport-position coaching, and time spent in physical education, recess, and other activity. Monitoring total training volume is often not done, however, as each trainer, coach, and teacher traditionally monitors only their aspect of training volume.

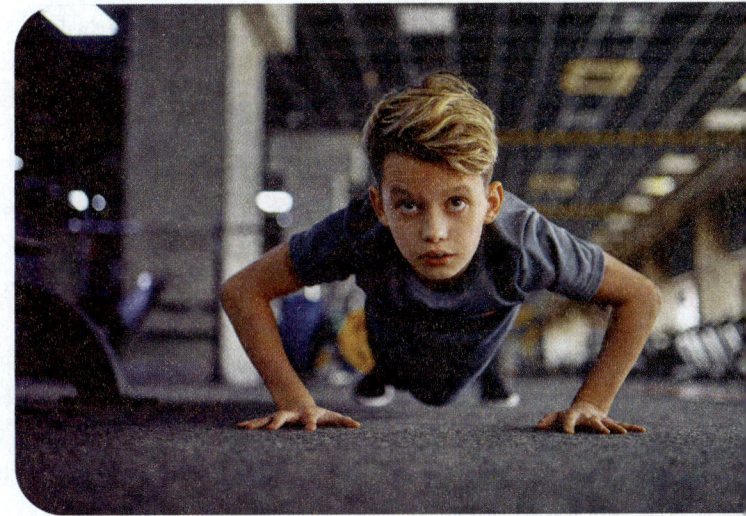

© Nomad_Soul/Shutterstock

The Sports Performance Coach can take the lead in monitoring training volume to ensure that the most appropriate training program is implemented based on the total training volume. Volume is often considered in terms of overall load, which includes both the internal load (internal responses to the training load, such as individual characteristics, training status, health, nutrition, and psychological status, measured by rate of perceived exertion [RPE], and heart rate response) and the external load (external measures of the load, including the physical work prescribed in the training plan). The external load may incorporate the work completed, velocity generated, total distance covered in bursts or in total, accelerations, or metabolic power components (Bourdon et al., 2017; Impellizzeri et al., 2019).

Internal and external loads must be considered within the context of the exercise or sport; there is not one gold standard of measurement that applies across all domains. Thus, careful consideration must be given to what is measured (Howard, 2022).

Rest Interval

Performance is typically the goal addressed by the training program, rather than fatigue of the metabolic system. For this reason, it is important to carefully monitor training sessions to ensure that the correct exercise technique is maintained for every exercise and every set. Several factors affect the amount of time required to recover between sets, such as training experience, intensity of the exercise, general fitness level, interindividual differences,

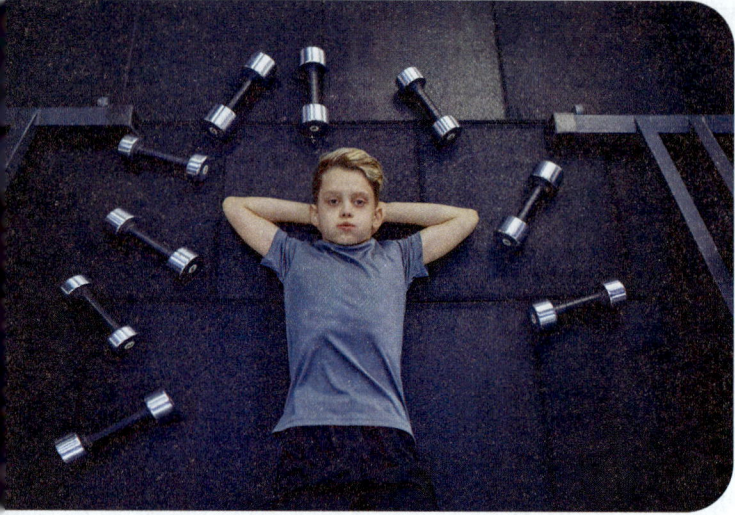

and recoverability (Hecksteden et al., 2015). Children tend to recover more quickly from resistance training exercise and high-intensity bouts than adults do, but within-session recovery always needs to be monitored.

Training Frequency

All activity must be considered in regard to training frequency, such as sports, play, physical education, and sports performance training. Participation in a quality strength and conditioning program is paramount to support motor competence and confidence, self-efficacy, development of healthful habits, and increased performance with reduced risk of injury. The strength and conditioning program should always be included in the LTAD program and never sacrificed for more sports practice and game play.

INTEGRATIVE NEUROMUSCU-LAR TRAINING (INT) →

A comprehensive training strategy that incorporates general (fundamental movements) and specific (skill-related) strength and conditioning activities designed to enhance health and skill-related fitness.

Training Duration

Training duration must be considered within the context of the training program's intensity and volume and should be considered from two perspectives: (1) the length (minutes and seconds) of each workout from start to finish and (2) the amount of time (days, weeks, months, or years) spent in one phase or period of training. For youth, the workout duration should match the level of interest, physical activity and fitness, and program goal. The magic notion of a 60-minute session is not always appropriate if the youth does not have the work capacity to complete the work. Instead, it is practical to start off gradually with bouts of at least 10 minutes, attempting to accumulate 60 minutes throughout the day. Likewise, a 3-hour sports practice is beyond the capability of many youths.

To balance the duration of exercise sessions with other activities, it is important to note the recommendations that practice and game time in hours should not exceed the youth's age in years (an 8-year-old should not train more than 8 hours per week, for example), and that the youth should take a break in a sport and in the annual plan of sports participation (Jayanthi et al., 2019). In the context of traditional periodization and the OPT Model, most of the time will be spent in developing and mastering fundamental skills and integrating muscle strength.

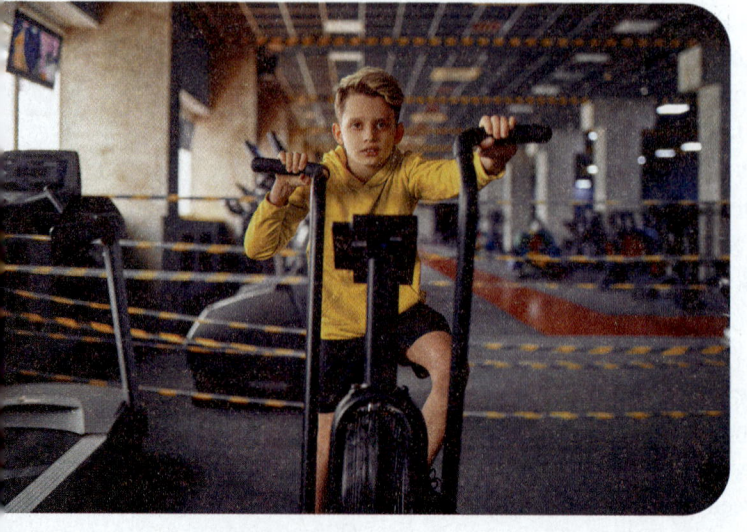

Exercise Selection

As Sports Performance Coaches are not only developing essential skills for youth but also introducing them to the complete library of exercises, it is important to follow a sensible progression when doing so. Exercises should be selected from the 10 fitness attributes (Lloyd & Oliver, 2012) across childhood and adolescence. Exercises for muscle strength are customarily classified as total-body, multi-joint, or single-joint. It is important to develop all three types of exercises using a variety of implements as well as bodyweight.

When considering the importance of acute training variables related to youth athletes, the OPT Model, with its integrated approach to program design, aligns with the LTAD and **Integrative Neuromuscular Training (INT)** models. More specific information on the importance of introducing various movement patterns, training techniques, and training stimuli to youth athletes is included in the Developmental Stage and Muscular Performance graph in Appendix E.

Specifically, the OPT Model considers the primary components of overall health and well-being of youth—namely, cardiovascular fitness, muscle strength, muscle endurance, and flexibility. It is important that these variables be integrated with fundamental movement skills as well as more skill-related movements such as agility, speed, and plyometrics. The OPT Model includes appropriate progressions across three levels: stabilization, strength, and power. These three levels are broken down into six phases (**Figure 21.16**):

- Phase 1: Stabilization endurance training, which now also includes focus on fundamental movement skills
- Phase 2: Strength endurance training
- Phase 3: Muscular development training
- Phase 4: Maximal strength training
- Phase 5: Power training
- Phase 6: Maximal power

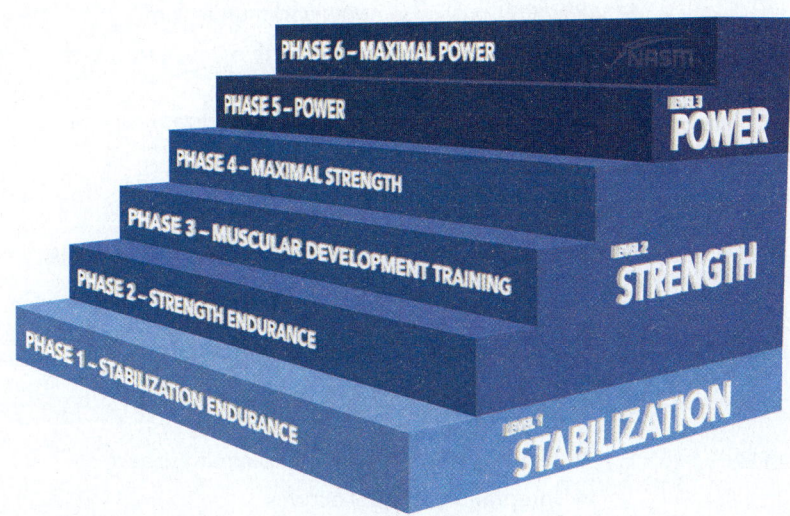

FIGURE 21.16 NASM's OPT™ Model

Although all phases might not be appropriate for youth athletes, the Sports Performance Coach can use the model as a general guide to attain the 10 fitness attributes recommended for children and adolescents. **Table 21.6** is a handy reference for Sports Performance Coaches seeking to apply the INT approach within the OPT Model.

THE YPD MODEL AND NASM'S OPT MODEL

The focus of the stabilization phase for youth should be on developing motor skill mastery and physical capacity as well as continued desire to participate in physical activity and exercise with confidence and competence. In a traditional periodization model, the stabilization phase can be thought of as similar to the general physical preparation phase, where the goal is to become more proficient and efficient in coping with the physical and metabolic changes and demands that will be required throughout the periodization (Bompa & Buzzichelli, 2019; Bompa & Haff, 2009). As youth athletes continue to develop stabilization and improve functional movements throughout childhood and adolescence, it is important to include stabilization exercises in each session and in all phases of the OPT Model.

TABLE 21.6 Principal Methodological Parameters to Develop the Different Components of INT

INT Component	Methodological Parameters for Tasks
Dynamic stability	• Balance training on a stationary supporting surface and static base of support
Lower-limb dynamic stability	• Balance training on a stationary surface under perturbations of different characteristics
Core dynamic stability	• Balance training that includes dynamic actions (SSS) • Balance training on the knees (stimulus focused on trunk and hip muscle stabilizers by not bearing the weight directly on the feet)
Coordination	• Development of appropriate strength capacity to perform FMS and SSS • Functional overload • Variety of movements and multitasking • Unanticipated reactions with sound technique
Strength	• Development of appropriate strength capacity to perform FMS and SSS • Functional overload
Plyometric training	• Development of stretch–shortening cycle ability, focusing on elastic energy and reflexive-muscle activity mechanisms • Ensuring proper movement mechanics (e.g., avoiding knee valgus or emphasizing soft landing)
Speed/agility	• Development of skills at maximum speed • Integration of COD actions • Training closely related coordination
Resistance to fatigue	• Development of skills under fatigue conditions • Stimulus-provoking cardiovascular, metabolic, and neuromuscular fatigue resistance

COD = changes of direction; FMS = fundamental movement skills; SSS = sport-specific skills.
Source: Fort-Vanmeerhaeghe et al. (2016).

The **YPD Model** (**Figure 21.17**) provides an excellent template from which to design a program that develops all physical attributes while adopting the OPT Model to provide fitness or sports performance professionals. It offers the latitude to go up and down the stairs, stopping at different steps, and moving to various heights, depending on the athlete's **development age** (chronological, biological, and training), goals, needs, and activities (Sutton, 2021).

One important distinction between the adult and youth versions of the OPT Model is that, rather than create optimal levels of stabilization and control, the focus is on

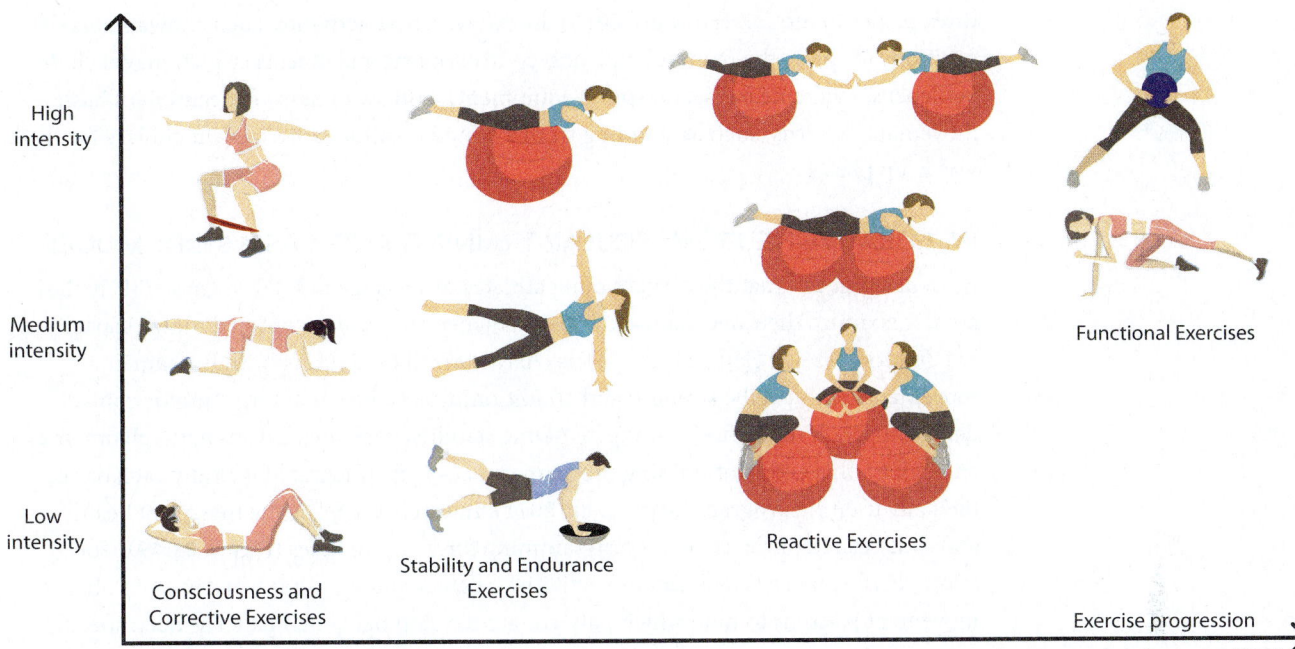

FIGURE 21.17 YPD Model

Based on Fort-Vanmeerhaeghe, A., Romero-Rodríguez, D., Lloyd, R., Kushner, A. M., & Myer, G. (2016, Aug.). Integrative neuromuscular training in youth athletes. Part II: Strategies to prevent injuries and improve performance. *Strength and Conditioning Journal.* 38(4): 9–27. https://doi.org/10.1519/SSC.0000000000000234

developing competency (and confidence) in a wide range of skills over a much longer period that include all fitness attributes, including stabilization strength and postural control (**Figure 21.18**). In one version of the daily exercise template (Appendix E: OPT Daily Exercise Template), the training of fitness attributes is distributed across the program. Note that this template groups core and balance as activation, and plyometric and SAQ as skill development for youth athletes.

During the warm-up, the progression should focus on movements that improve stability and balance from unstable to stable. Next, increase stability in one, two, and then

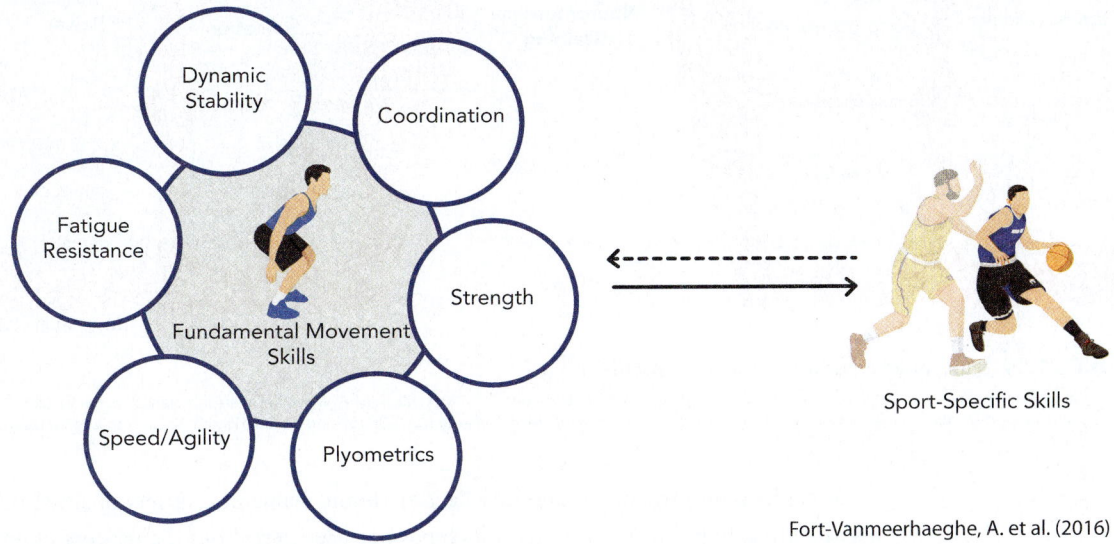

Fort-Vanmeerhaeghe, A. et al. (2016)

FIGURE 21.18 Strategies for Preventing Injuries

Based on Fort-Vanmeerhaeghe, A., Romero-Rodríguez, D., Lloyd, R., Kushner, A. M., & Myer, G. (2016, Aug.). Integrative neuromuscular training in youth athletes. Part II: Strategies to prevent injuries and improve performance. *Strength & Conditioning Journal.* 38(4): 9–27. https://doi.org/10.1519/SSC.0000000000000234

three planes of motion (Howard, 2018). Body awareness activities, such as awareness of positions in space, the manipulation and control of external objects (which may include kettlebells, medicine balls, and sports equipment), and awareness of execution of basic movement patterns, such as standing from a seated position, are excellent choices for the warm-up phase.

INTEGRATIVE NEUROMUSCULAR TRAINING AND NASM'S OPT MODEL

Evidence suggests that the earlier young athletes can engage in INT, the more likely they are to maximize their neuromuscular performance and achieve optimal motor capacity in adulthood (Myer et al., 2011). INT is characterized by training both fundamental movements and specific strength and conditioning activities that target motor control deficits through resistance training, dynamic stability, core-focused strength, plyometrics, and agility; this excellent training program can easily be integrated into any category of the daily training program (Myer et al., 2011). In essence, INT is the merger of health and skill-related physical fitness programming for youth athletes (**Figure 21.19**). The Sports Performance Coach can use activities, such as games, as informal ways to observe movement patterns to note which patterns are developing, which patterns need specific cueing and instruction, and which patterns are nearing mastery. In the activation and skill development phase, continued development of motor patterns through the fundamental movement patterns of squat, hinge, push, pull, press, and multiplanar and rotational movement in alignment with the athletic motor skill competencies is essential.

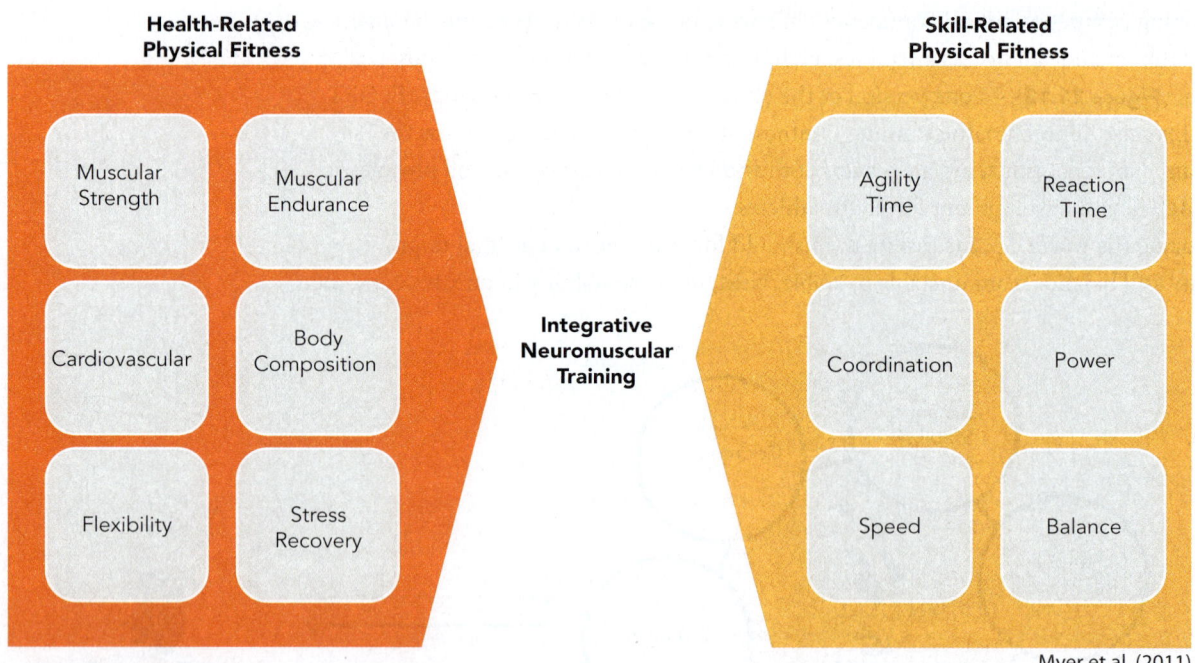

FIGURE 21.19 Integrative Neuromuscular Training (INT)

Based on Myer, G. D., Faigenbaum, A. D., Ford, K. R., Best, T. M., Bergeron, M. F., & Hewett, T. E. (2011, May–June). When to initiate integrative neuromuscular training to reduce sports-related injuries and enhance health in youth? *Current Sports Medicine Reports, 10*(3): 155–166. https://doi.org/10.1249/jsr.0b013e31821b1442

Specific to movement or exercise selection, being stable in a variety of situations is essential to skill mastery. Although much has been written about the process of moving from stable to unstable surfaces, the goal for most youth is to be as stable as possible in a variety of settings, on a variety of stable surfaces, in a variety of ways. As described in this chapter, physical literacy encompasses youth athletes' development of skills and abilities in activities and sports of interest as they grow. When building a young athlete's movement vocabulary, Sports Performance Coaches need to find the movements that resonate with each athlete and build on the success of that movement by introducing other movements that support it.

For example, most movement recommendations suggest that bodyweight exercises should come first; once the correct technique is established, they can then be weighted. The push-up is often cited as one of those movements. Youth athletes with overweight or obesity are not likely to experience movement success with this exercise, yet they could easily develop the proper technique with a movement that supports bodyweight (a suspension trainer, for example) or the use of lighter weights for upper-body pushing movements. Without knowing the progressions and regressions throughout the growth process, personal trainers could inflict more harm than good.

The training prescription, therefore, should help young movers establish movement competencies and use them to solve movement problems. Key elements of a Modified Model for Children and Early Adolescents can be found in Appendix E.

The INT approach has been studied and applied to physical education classes (Faigenbaum et al., 2011) and sports such as basketball (Howard, 2014), netball (Hopper et al., 2017), and football (soccer) (Panagoulis et al., 2020). Using soccer as an example, the Sports Performance Coach would assess the movement abilities of the young players such as when they are learning a new skill. For example, youth may struggle when combining the motor skills of running and kicking the ball. INT training would, therefore, include running without the ball, kicking without running, and finally running and kicking simultaneously. Once the athlete demonstrates competence, they would then perform running with the ball, kicking, and adding constraints to advance the skill under a variety of conditions. Such constraints could include adding a teammate (i.e., a coach or even a parent) and performing five passes before shooting on the goal. The INT training session also needs to include the components of health-related fitness (e.g., muscle strength, muscle power, muscle endurance, cardiovascular endurance, and flexibility), skills fitness (e.g., agility, balance, coordination, speed, power, and reactive ability), and sports fitness (e.g., applied motor skills in a sports context).

INT sessions are dosed in a balanced, age-related progression to improve any neuromotor deficiencies, increase overall health and skills fitness, and progress relevant sports skills. Lloyd et al. (2022) found that a program design frequency of two INT sessions per week was more beneficial than one session. The earlier that Sports Performance Coaches implement training programs for youth athletes that focus on the whole child's development, including motor proficiency, muscle strength, and plyometrics, the more likely those athletes are to achieve and extend their motor potential.

For adolescent soccer players who progressed though the stages of INT from an early age, the INT program can focus on mastering and refining motor skills and further developing core strength, the hamstrings' eccentric strength, the hip/knee musculature, and dynamic stability (Panagoulis et al., 2020). If adolescents have not engaged in early INT interventions, they should be assessed for motor skill deficiencies as well as strength, power, speed, and agility. The principle of training age applies across childhood and adolescence for INT, and the Sports Performance Coach should ensure that each activity is progressed appropriately. Lack of INT training can lead to poor postural control, which affects the ability to stop, cut, and change direction. Stopping, cutting, and changing direction are key predictors of injury in sports (Gabbett, 2010). Lack of muscle strength can predict poor mechanics of movement; for this reason, it is important to include strength training as part of INT programs at all levels of athletic participation.

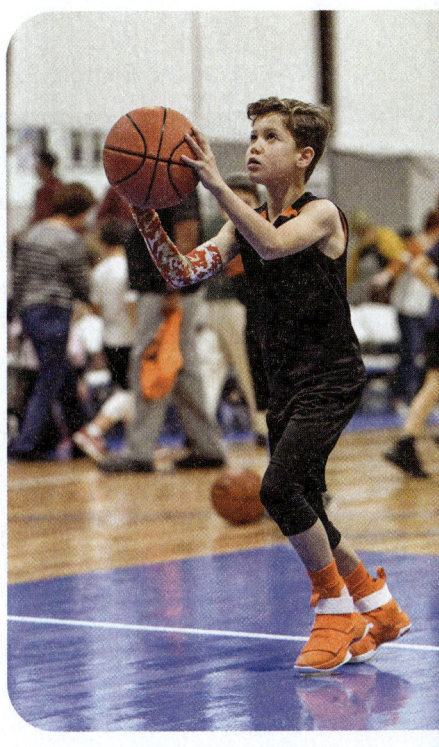

THE STRENGTH PHASE AND THE POWER PHASE

Muscle strength is linked to fundamental motor skills, making it critical to the success of LTAD programs. Movements that develop strength and power should be included throughout childhood and adolescence training, rather than during just one period or training phase. However, movement quality is still the most valuable feature, and additional resistance, or velocity, should not be added until the desired movement quality is achieved (e.g., technique before load). Recommendations for the acute training variables specific to youth resistance training can be found in Appendix E (adapted from Bracko, 2017; Faigenbaum et al., 2009; Lloyd, Faigenbaum, et al., 2014).

Sports-specific fitness skills such as sprinting and dodging are fun for youth athletes. So, while traditional periodized models include three stages, the progression for children and adolescents should be within and across the stages to take advantage of the trainability of all 10 fitness attributes in childhood and adolescence. Sports Performance Coaches should understand how best to program for youth based on their individual needs and how the OPT Model can progress them systematically and safely.

SAMPLE PROGRAMS

The Sports Performance Coach can choose from many programs when working with youth. The key is identifying the appropriate ages of the athlete (chronological, biological, and training) and matching the program goals to the young athlete's abilities. Rather than adopting an existing program, find the movements that the young athlete can complete successfully and build on those successes. The following examples illustrate two approaches to program design for youth athletes.

PRE-PEAK HEIGHT VELOCITY ATHLETE

Table 21.7 describes a sample two-times-per-week program for a 10-year-old who has been training for 6 months (Howard, 2018).

TABLE 21.7 Sample Exercise Program: 2 Days per Week

Pre-Peak Height Velocity Athlete	Day 1	Day 2
Warm-up	Walk–march–skip progressions (30 seconds × 2)	Obstacle course: Hopscotch to cones, forward rolls, hula hoop, cone zig zag, medicine ball slam (1 kg), and jump rope (20 seconds each, 40-second rest)
Activation, skill development, and resistance training	Coach pick*: 15 air squats (bodyweight) Athlete pick*: 20-yd shuttles × 3 with 2 minutes rest Coach pick: Hip hinge with 4-kg kettlebell Athlete pick: Leg press 0.5 × bodyweight Coach pick: Suspension trainer push/pull, 12 each superset × 2 supersets	Hip bridge, can openers, suspension training squats, medicine ball lateral rotations, mountain climbers, and kettlebell Romanian deadlifts (1 circuit to start)
Game	Athlete pick: Gaga	

POST-PEAK HEIGHT VELOCITY ATHLETE

Table 21.8 shows a sample three-times-per-week program for a 14-year-old youth softball athlete (Howard, 2018).

TABLE 21.8   Sample Exercise Program: 3 Days per Week

Pre-Peak Height Velocity Athlete	Day 1	Day 2	Day 3
Warm-up and activation	Triple extension 5 × 3 with 15-lb bar	Warm-up and activation	Warm-up, activation, and skill development
Resistance training	Core: Front squat 5 × 5 (65% 1RM) Push press 3 × 5 (50% 1RM) Romanian deadlift 3 × 8 (5-lb kettlebell in each hand) Accessory: Gluteal/hamstrings raise 3 × 8 IYT 2 × 10 (2-lb dumbbell) Push-ups, as many reps as possible	Power: High shrug pulls 3 × 3 (65% 1RM) Standing broad jumps × 3 (1-min rest between jumps) Core: Step-ups 5 × 5 (bodyweight) Incline press 5 × 5 (25% bodyweight) Trap bar deadlift 5 × 5 (10-lb kettlebells) Accessory: Pull-ups, as many reps as possible Lateral band walks light band × 30 seconds each way	Power: Jump shrugs 3 × 3 (20% bodyweight) Vertical jumps 3 × 5 each hand One-leg hops × 10 Resistance training Core: Back squats 5 × 3 (75% 1RM) Landmine one-arm press 3 × 5 (45-lb bar) One-leg Romanian deadlift 3 × 10 (10-lb kettlebell in hand on side being activated) Accessory: Pallof press 2 × 12 (medium weight band) Medicine ball rotation against the wall 3 × 5 (3 kg) Mountain climbers 30 seconds × 3

1RM: one-repetition maximum.

SUMMARY

The long-term athlete development (LTAD) model provides a framework for the Sports Performance Coach to engage all youth in the pursuit of optimal health, athleticism, physical fitness, and psychosocial well-being. Through the implementation of developmentally appropriate physical training programs for youth, LTAD can trigger a path to help promote physical activity throughout the lifespan. Insight into important principles related to growth, maturation, the central tenets of LTAD, and various program design principles will enable the Sports Performance Coach to have the tools needed to design safe and effective training programs for youth. Further, an understanding of the distinction and balance between sport specialization and sport sampling is essential to help increase youth participation in sport and physical activity, while at the same time helping to reduce the incidence of overuse injury and psychological burnout. Finally, the LTAD framework, when combined with quality and informed coaching, offers the opportunity to provide the necessary connections, competence, and confidence for youth of all abilities to pursue sport and physical activity in fun and nurturing environments.

KEY TAKEAWAYS

- Long-term athlete development is the habitual development of athleticism over time with the goal of improving health- and skill-related components of fitness, movement and sport skills, physical performance, and resilience to injury.
- Long-term athletic development provides a structured and progressive approach that introduces various modes of training and acute training variables that can enhance and enable positive psychosocial development, confidence, and competence in all youth.
- The Sports Performance Coach should understand and consider basic principles of normal growth, maturation, and development when designing, implementing, and evaluating training programs for youth.
- Specializing in one sport at a young age does not necessarily translate into long-term success in that sport in adolescence or adulthood. Individual growth and maturation are important indicators as to whether a child should follow an early or late specialization pathway.
- Sport sampling can expose the youth athlete to diverse movement experiences that can improve overall perceptual-motor ability and facilitate the transfer of general patterns of movement from one sport to another.
- Long-term athlete development provides a developmentally appropriate framework that can assist in the prevention of chronic overuse injury and psychological burnout.
- The phases of NASM's OPT Model align with the INT approach to create developmentally appropriate youth training programs.
- All physical attributes are trainable across childhood and adolescence, as demonstrated in the Youth Physical Development Model.

REFERENCES

Ahler, T., Bendiksen, M., Krustrup, P., & Wedderkopp, N. (2012). Aerobic fitness testing in 6- to 9-year-old children: Reliability and validity of a modified Yo-Yo IR1 test and the Andersen test. *European Journal of Applied Physiology, 112*(3), 871–876. https://doi.org/10.1007/s00421-011-2039-4

Andersen, L. B., Andersen, T. E., Andersen, E., & Anderssen, S. A. (2008). An intermittent running test to estimate maximal oxygen uptake: The Andersen test. *Journal of Sports Medicine and Physical Fitness, 48*(4), 434–437.

Aspen Institute. (2017). *State of play 2017: Trends and developments.* https://www.aspeninstitute.org/wp-content/uploads/2017/12/FINAL-SOP2017-report.pdf

Aspen Institute. (2021). *Youth sports facts: Participation rates.* Aspen Institute Project Play https://www.aspenprojectplay.org/youth-sports-facts/participation-rates

Balyi, I., Way, R., & Higgs, C. (2014). *Long-term athlete development.* Human Kinetics.

Benson, T. (n.d.). *The role of sports in the Soviet Union.* https://blogs.bu.edu/guidedhistory/russia-and-its-empires/tyler-benson/

Bompa, T. O. (2000). *Total training for young champions.* Human Kinetics.

Bompa, T. O., & Buzzichelli, C. A. (2019). *Periodization training for sports* (6th ed.). Human Kinetics.

Bompa, T. O., & Haff, G. (2009). *Periodization theory and methodology of training* (5th ed.). Human Kinetics.

Bourdon, P. C., Cardinale, M., Murray, A., Gastin, P., Kellmann, M., Varley, M. C., Gabbett, T. J., Coutts, A. J., Burgess, D. J., Gregson, W., & Cable, N. T. (2017). Monitoring athlete training loads: Consensus statement. *International Journal of Sports Physiology and Performance, 12*(suppl 2), S2161–S2170. https://doi.org/10.1123/IJSPP.2017-0208

Bracko, M. (2017). Getting young athletes off to a strong start. *American Fitness Magazine, 35*(2), 14–17.

Carder, S. L., Giusti, N. E., Vopat, L. M., Tarakemeh, A., Baker, J., Vopat, B. G., & Mulcahey, M. K. (2020). The concept of sport sampling versus sport specialization: Preventing youth athlete injury: A systematic review and meta-analysis. *American Journal of Sports Medicine, 48*(11), 2850–2857. https://doi.org/10.1177/0363546519899380

Castro-Piñero, J., Artero, E. G., España-Romero, V., Ortega, F. B., Sjöström, M., Suni, J., & Ruiz, J. R. (2010). Criterion-related validity of field-based fitness tests in youth: A systematic review. *British Journal of Sports Medicine, 44*(13), 934–943. https://doi.org/10.1136/bjsm.2009.058321

Centers for Disease Control and Prevention. (2017, June). *Clinical growth charts.* https://www.cdc.gov/growthcharts/clinical_charts.htm

Centers for Disease Control and Prevention. (2024, January 8). *Physical activity for children: An overview.* https://www.cdc.gov/physical-activity-basics/guidelines/children.html?CDC_AAref_Val=https://www.cdc.gov/physicalactivity/basics/children/index.htm

Côté, J., & Vierimaa, M. (2014). The developmental model of sport participation: 15 years after its first conceptualization. *Science & Sports, 29*(suppl), S63–S69. https://doi.org/10.1016/j.scispo.2014.08.133

Demirel, D. H., & Yildiran, I. (2013). The philosophy of physical education and sport from ancient times to the enlightenment. *European Journal of Educational Research, 2*(4), 191–202. https://doi.org/10.12973/eu-jer.2.4.191

Eisenmann, J. C., Till, K., & Baker, J. (2020). Growth, maturation and youth sports: Issues and practical solutions. *Annals of Human Biology, 47*(4), 324–327. http://doi.org/10.1080/03014460.2020.1764099

Faigenbaum, A. D., Farrell, A., Fabiano, M., Radler, T., Naclerio, F., Ratamess, N. A., Kang, J., & Myer, G. D. (2011). Effects of integrative neuromuscular training on fitness performance in children. *Pediatric Exercise Science, 23*(4), 573–584. https://doi.org/10.1123/pes.23.4.573

Faigenbaum, A. D., Kraemer, W. J., Blimkie, C. J. R., Jeffreys, I., Micheli, L. J., Nitka, M., & Rowland, T. W. (2009). Youth resistance training: Updated position statement paper from the National Strength and Conditioning Association. *Journal of Strength and Conditioning Research, 23*(5 suppl), S60–S79. https://doi.org/10.1519/JSC.0b013e31819df407

Faigenbaum, A. D., Milliken, L. A., Cloutier, G., & Westcott, W. L. (2004). Perceived exertion during resistance exercise by children. *Perceptual and Motor Skills, 98*(2), 627–637. https://doi.org/10.2466/pms.98.2.627-637

Faigenbaum, A. D., Milliken, L. A., & Westcott, W. L. (2003). Maximal strength testing in healthy children. *Journal of Strength and Conditioning Research, 17*(1), 162–166. https://journals.lww.com/nsca-jscr/abstract/2003/02000/maximal_strength_testing_in_healthy_children.25.aspx

Faigenbaum, A. D., Rebullido, T. R., & MacDonald, J. P. (2018). Pediatric inactivity triad: A risky PIT. *Current Sports Medicine Reports, 17*(2), 45–47. https://doi.org/10.1249/JSR.0000000000000450

Ford, P., De Ste Croix, M., Lloyd, R., Meyers, R., Moosavi, M., Oliver, J., Till, K., & Williams, C. (2011). The long-term athlete development model: Physiological evidence and application. *Journal of Sports Sciences, 29*(4), 389–402. https://doi.org/10.1080/02640414.2010.536849

Fort-Vanmeerhaeghe, A., Romero-Rodríguez, D., Lloyd, R., Kushner, A. M., & Myer, G. (2016). Integrative neuromuscular training in youth athletes. Part II: Strategies to prevent injuries and improve performance. *Strength and Conditioning Journal, 38*(4), 9–27. https://doi.org/10.1519/SSC.0000000000000234

Gabbett, T. J. (2010). The development and application of an injury prediction model for noncontact, soft-tissue injuries in elite collision sport athletes. *Journal of Strength and Conditioning Research, 24*(10), 2593–2603. https://doi.org/10.1519/JSC.0b013e3181f19da4

Gao, Z., & Wang, R. (2019). Children's motor skill competence, physical activity, fitness, and health promotion. *Journal of Sport and Health Science, 8*(2), 95–97. https://doi.org/10.1016/j.jshs.2018.12.002

Giusti, N. E., Carder, S. L., Vopat, L., Baker, J., Tarakemeh, A., Vopat, B., & Mulcahey, M. K. (2020). Comparing burnout in sport-specializing versus sport-sampling adolescent athletes: A systematic review and meta-analysis. *Orthopaedic Journal of Sports Medicine, 8*(3), 2325967120907579. https://doi.org/10.1177/2325967120907579

Güllich, A., Macnamara, B. N., & Hambrick, D. Z. (2022). What makes a champion? Early multidisciplinary practice, not early specialization, predicts world-class performance. *Perspectives on Psychological Science, 17*(1), 6–29. https://doi.org/10.1177/1745691620974772

Hecksteden, A., Kraushaar, J., Scharhag-Rosenberger, F., Theisen, D., Senn, S., & Meyer, T. (2015). Individual response to exercise training—A statistical perspective. *Journal of Applied Physiology, 118*(12), 1450–1459. https://doi.org/10.1152/japplphysiol.00714.2014

Hewett, T. E., Myer, G. D., Ford, K. R., Paterno, M. V., & Quatman, C. E. (2016). Mechanisms, prediction, and prevention of ACL injuries: Cut risk with three sharpened and validated tools. *Journal of Orthopaedic Research, 34*(11), 1843–1855. https://doi.org/10.1002/jor.23414

Hopper, A., Haff, E. E., Barley, O. R., Joyce, C., Lloyd, R. S., & Haff, G. G. (2017). Neuromuscular training improves movement competency and physical performance measures in 11–13-year-old female netball athletes. *Journal of Strength & Conditioning Research, 31*(5), 1165–1176. https://doi.org/10.1519/JSC.0000000000001794

Howard, R. (2014). Integrative neuromuscular training for youth basketball players. *NSCA Coach, 3*(1), 44–45.

Howard, R. (2018). The ABCs of long-term athletic development. *NSCA Coach, 4*(2), 36–39.

Howard, R. (2022). A closer look at the 10 pillars of LTAD: The programming pillars of LTAD for strength and conditioning professionals: Part 1. *NSCA Coach, 8*(3), 14–21.

Hulteen, R. M., Morgan, P. J., Barnett, L. M., Stodden, D. F., & Lubans, D. R. (2018). Development of foundational movement skills: A conceptual model for physical activity across the lifespan. *Sports Medicine, 48*(7), 1533–1540. https://doi.org/10.1007/s40279-018-0892-6

Impellizzeri, F. M., Marcora, S. M., & Coutts, A. J. (2019). Internal and external training load: 15 years on. *International Journal of Sports Physiology and Performance, 14*(2), 270–273. https://doi.org/10.1123/ijspp.2018-0935

Janssen, I., & LeBlanc, A. G. (2010). Systematic review of the health benefits of physical activity and fitness in school-aged children and youth. *International Journal of Behavioral Nutrition and Physical Activity, 7*, 40. https://doi.org/10.1186/1479-5868-7-40

Jayanthi, N. A., Post, E. G., Laury, T. C., & Fabricant, P. D. (2019). Health consequences of youth sport specialization. *Journal of Athletic Training, 54*(10), 1040–1049. https://doi.org/10.4085/1062-6050-380-18

Kann, L., McManus, T., Harris, W. A., Shanklin, S. L., Flint, K. H., Queen, B., Lowry, R., Chyen, D., Whittle, L., Thornton, J., Lim, C., Bradford, D., Yamakawa, Y., Leon, M., Brener, N., & Ethier, K. A. (2018). Youth risk behavior surveillance—United states, 2017. *MMWR. Surveillance Summaries, 67*(8), 1–114. https://doi.org/10.15585/mmwr.ss6708a1

Katzmarzyk, P. T., Denstel, K. D., Beals, K., Carlson, J., Crouter, S. E., McKenzie, T. L., Pate, R. R., Sisson, S. B., Staiano, A. E., Stanish, H., Ward, D. S., Whitt-Glover, M., & Wright, C. (2018). Results from the United States 2018 report card on physical activity for children and youth. *Journal of Physical Activity and Health, 15*(S2), S422–S424. https://doi.org/10.1123/jpah.2018-0476

Kliethermes, S. A., Marshall, S. W., LaBella, C. R., Watson, A. M., Brenner, J. S., Nagle, K. B., Jayanthi, N., Brooks, N. A., Tenforde, A. S., Herman, D. C., DiFiori, J. P., & Beutler, A. I. (2021). Defining a research agenda for youth sport specialisation in the USA: The AMSSM Youth Early Sport Specialization Summit. *British Journal of Sports Medicine, 55*(3), 135–143. https://doi.org/10.1136/bjsports-2020-102699

LaPrade, R. F., Agel, J., Baker, J., Brenner, J. S., Cordasco, F. A., Côté, J., Engebretsen, L., Feeley, B. T., Gould, D., Hainline, B., Hewett, T. E., Jayanthi, N., Kocher, M. S., Myer, G. D., Nissen, C. W., Philippon, M. J., & Provencher, M. T. (2016). AOSSM early sport specialization consensus statement. *Orthopaedic Journal of Sports Medicine, 4*(4), 2325967116644241. https://doi.org/10.1177/2325967116644241

Latash, M. L. (2008). *Neurophysiological basis of movement* (2nd ed.). Human Kinetics.

Leventer, L., Dicks, M., Duarte, R., Davids, K., & Araújo, D. (2015). Emergence of contact injuries in invasion team sports: An ecological dynamics rationale. *Sports Medicine, 45*(2), 153–159. https://doi.org/10.1007/s40279-014-0263-x

Lloyd, R. S., Cronin, J. B., Faigenbaum, A. D., Haff, G. G., Howard, R., Kraemer, W. J., Micheli, L. J., Myer, G. D., Oliver, J. L. (2016). National Strength and Conditioning Association position statement on long-term athletic development. *Journal of Strength and Conditioning Research, 30*(6), 1491–1509. https://doi.org/10.1519/JSC.0000000000001387

Lloyd, R. S., Dobbs, I. J., Wong, M. A., Moore, I. S., & Oliver, J. L. (2022). Effects of training frequency during a 6-month neuromuscular training intervention on movement competency, strength, and power in male youth. *Sports Health, 14*(1), 57–68. https://doi.org/10.1177/19417381211050005

Lloyd, R. S., Faigenbaum, A. D., Stone, M. H., Oliver, J. L., Jeffreys, I., Moody, J. A., Brewer, C., Pierce, K. C., McCambridge, T. M., Howard, R., Herrington, L., Hainline, B., Micheli, L. J., Jacques, R., Kraemer, W. J., McBride, M. G., Best, T. M., Chu, D. A., Alvar, B. A., & Myer, G. D. (2014). Position statement on youth resistance training: The 2014 International Consensus. *British Journal of Sports Medicine, 48*(7), 498–505. https://doi.org/10.1136/bjsports-2013-092952

Lloyd, R. S., & Oliver, J. L. (2012). The Youth Physical Development model: A new approach to long-term athletic development. *Strength and Conditioning Journal, 34*(3), 61–72. https://doi.org/10.1519/SSC.0b013e31825760ea

Lloyd, R. S., Oliver, J. L., Faigenbaum, A. D., Myer, G. D., & De Ste Croix, M. B. A. (2014). Chronological age vs. biological maturation: Implications for exercise programming in youth. *Journal of Strength and Conditioning Research, 28*(5), 1454–1464. https://doi.org/10.1519/JSC.0000000000000391

Machado, F. A., & Denadai, B. S. (2011). Validity of maximum heart rate prediction equations for children and adolescents. *Arquivos Brasileiros de Cardiologia, 97*(2), 136–140. https://doi.org/10.1590/s0066-782x2011005000078

Markati, A., Psychountaki, M., Kingston, K., Karteroliotis, K., & Apostolidis, N. (2019). Psychological and situational determinants of burnout in adolescent athletes. *International Journal of Sport and Exercise Psychology, 17*(5), 521–536. https://doi.org/10.1080/1612197X.2017.1421680

McGinnis, P. M. (2013). *Biomechanics of sport and exercise* (3rd ed.). Human Kinetics.

McGuine, T. A., Post, E. G., Hetzel, S. J., Brooks, M. A., Trigsted, S., & Bell, D. R. (2017). A prospective study on the effect of sport specialization on lower extremity injury rates in high school athletes. *American Journal of Sports Medicine, 45*(12), 2706–2712. https://doi.org/10.1177/0363546517710213

Merkel, D. L. (2013). Youth sport: Positive and negative impact on young athletes. *Open Access Journal of Sports Medicine, 4,* 151–160. https://doi.org/10.2147/OAJSM.S33556

Mirwald, R. L., Baxter-Jones, A. D., Bailey, D. A., & Beunen, G. P. (2002). An assessment of maturity from anthropometric measurements. *Medicine & Science in Sports & Exercise, 34*(4), 689–694. https://doi.org/10.1097/00005768-200204000-00020

Morano, M., Bortoli, L., Ruiz, M. C., & Robazza, C. (2020). Psychobiosocial states as mediators of the effects of basic psychological need satisfaction on burnout symptoms in youth sport. *International Journal of Environmental Research and Public Health, 17*(12), 4447. https://doi.org/10.3390/ijerph17124447

Myer, G. D., Faigenbaum, A. D., Ford, K. R., Best, T. M., Bergeron, M. F., & Hewett, T. E. (2011). When to initiate integrative neuromuscular training to reduce sports-related injuries and enhance health in youth? *Current Sports Medicine Reports, 10*(3), 155–166. https://doi.org/10.1249/jsr.0b013e31821b1442

Myer, G. D., Jayanthi, N., DiFiori, J. P., Faigenbaum, A. D., Kiefer, A. W., Logerstedt, D., & Micheli, L. J. (2016). Sports specialization, Part II: Alternative solutions to early sport specialization in youth athletes. *Sports Health, 8*(1), 65–73. https://doi.org/10.1177/1941738115614811

Naidu, S. A., Fanchini, M., Cox, A., Smeaton, J., Hopkins, W. G., & Serpiello, F. R. (2019). Validity of session rating of perceived exertion assessed via the CR100 scale to track internal load in elite youth football players. *International Journal of Sports Physiology and Performance, 14*(3), 403–406. https://doi.org/10.1123/ijspp.2018-0432

National Federation of State High School Associations. (2019). *Participation in high school sports registers first decline in 30 years.* https://nfhs.org/articles/participation-in-high-school-sports-registers-first-decline-in-30-years/

Normand, J. M., Wolfe, A., & Peak, K. (2017). A review of early sport specialization in relation to the development of a young athlete. *International Journal of Kinesiology & Sports Science, 5*(2), 37–42. https://journals.aiac.org.au/index.php/IJKSS/article/view/3433

Panagoulis, C., Chatzinikolaou, A., Avloniti, A., Leontsini, D., Deli, C. K., Draganidis, D., Stampoulis, T., Oikonomou, T., Papanikolaou, K., Rafailakis, L., Kambas, A., Jamurtas, A. Z., & Fatouros, I. G. (2020). In-season integrative neuromuscular strength training improves performance of early-adolescent soccer athletes. *Journal of Strength and Conditioning Research, 34*(2), 516–526. https://doi.org/10.1519/jsc.0000000000002938

Pfeiffer, K. A., Pivarnik, J. M., Womack, C. J., Reeves, M. J., & Malina, R. M. (2002). Reliability and validity of the Borg and OMNI rating of perceived exertion scales in adolescent girls. *Medicine & Science in Sports & Exercise, 34*(12), 2057–2061. https://doi.org/10.1097/00005768-200212000-00029

Post, E. G., Trigsted, S. M., Riekena, J. W., Hetzel, S., McGuine, T. A., Brooks, M. A., & Bell, D. R. (2017). The association of sport specialization and training volume with injury history in youth athletes. *American Journal of Sports Medicine, 45*(6), 1405–1412. https://doi.org/10.1177/0363546517690848

Roche, A. F., Wainer, H., & Thissen, D. (1975). Predicting adult stature for individuals. *Monographs in Paediatrics, 3,* 1–114.

Seefeldt, V. (1980). Developmental motor patterns: Implications for elementary school physical education. In C. H. Nadeau, W. R. Halliwell, K. M. Newell, & G. C. Roberts (Eds.), *Psychology of motor behavior and sport* (pp. 314–323). Human Kinetics.

Sport for Life. (2022). *Long-term development stages: A clear path to better sport, greater health, and higher achievement.* https://sportforlife.ca/long-term-development/

Strafford, B. W., van der Steen, P., Davids, K., & Stone, J. A. (2018). Parkour as a donor sport for athletic development in youth team sports: Insights through an ecological dynamics lens. *Sports Medicine–Open, 4,* 21. https://doi.org/10.1186/s40798-018-0132-5

Stodden, D. F., True, L. K., Langendorfer, S. J., & Gao, Z. (2013). Associations among selected motor skills and health-related fitness: Indirect evidence for Seefeldt's proficiency barrier in young adults? *Research Quarterly for Exercise and Sport, 84*(3), 397–403. https://doi.org/10.1080/02701367.2013.814910

Sutton, B. G. (Ed.). (2021). *NASM essentials of personal fitness training* (7th ed.). Jones & Bartlett Learning.

Team USA. (2022). *About the U.S. Olympic & Paralympic Committee.* https://www.teamusa.org/About-the-USOPC/Coaching-Education/American-Development-Model

Ulyanova, S., Fisheva, A., & Sosnina, M. (2019). Gto concept: Design and implementation in USSR in late 1920s–early 1930s. *European Proceedings of Social and Behavioural Sciences, Professional Culture of the Specialist of the Future.* https://doi.org/10.15405/epsbs.2018.12.02.201

United States Olympic and Paralympic Committee. (2016). *American development model: Rebuilding athletes in America*. https://cdn3.sportngin.com/attachments/document/8c8b-2311769/USOC_ADM_Brochure_2016 .pdf

Valasek, A. E., Young, J. A., Huang, L., Singichetti, B., & Yang, J. (2019). Age and sex differences in overuse injuries presenting to pediatric sports medicine clinics. *Clinical Pediatrics, 58*(7), 770–777. https://doi.org /10.1177/0009922819837360

Valovich McLeod, T. C., Decoster, L. C., Loud, K. J., Micheli, L. J., Parker, J. T., Sandrey, M. A., & White, C. (2011). National Athletic Trainers' Association position statement: Prevention of pediatric overuse injuries. *Journal of Athletic Training, 46*(2), 206–220. https://doi.org/10.4085/1062-6050-46.2.206

Van Hooren, B., & De Ste Croix, M. (2020). Sensitive periods to train general motor abilities in children and adolescents: Do they exist? A critical appraisal. *Strength and Conditioning Journal, 42*(6), 7–14. https://doi .org/10.1519/SSC.0000000000000545

Waldron, S., DeFreese, J. D., Register-Mihalik, J., Pietrosimone, B., & Barczak, N. (2019). The costs and benefits of early sport specialization: A critical review of literature. *Quest, 72*(1), 1–18. http://dx.doi.org/10.1080 /00336297.2019.1580205

Witt, P. A., & Dangi, T. B. (2018). Why children/youth drop out of sports. *Journal of Park and Recreation Administration, 36*(3), 191–199. https://doi.org/10.18666/JPRA-2018-V36-I3-8618

SECTION 6

NUTRITION AND SUPPLEMENTATION

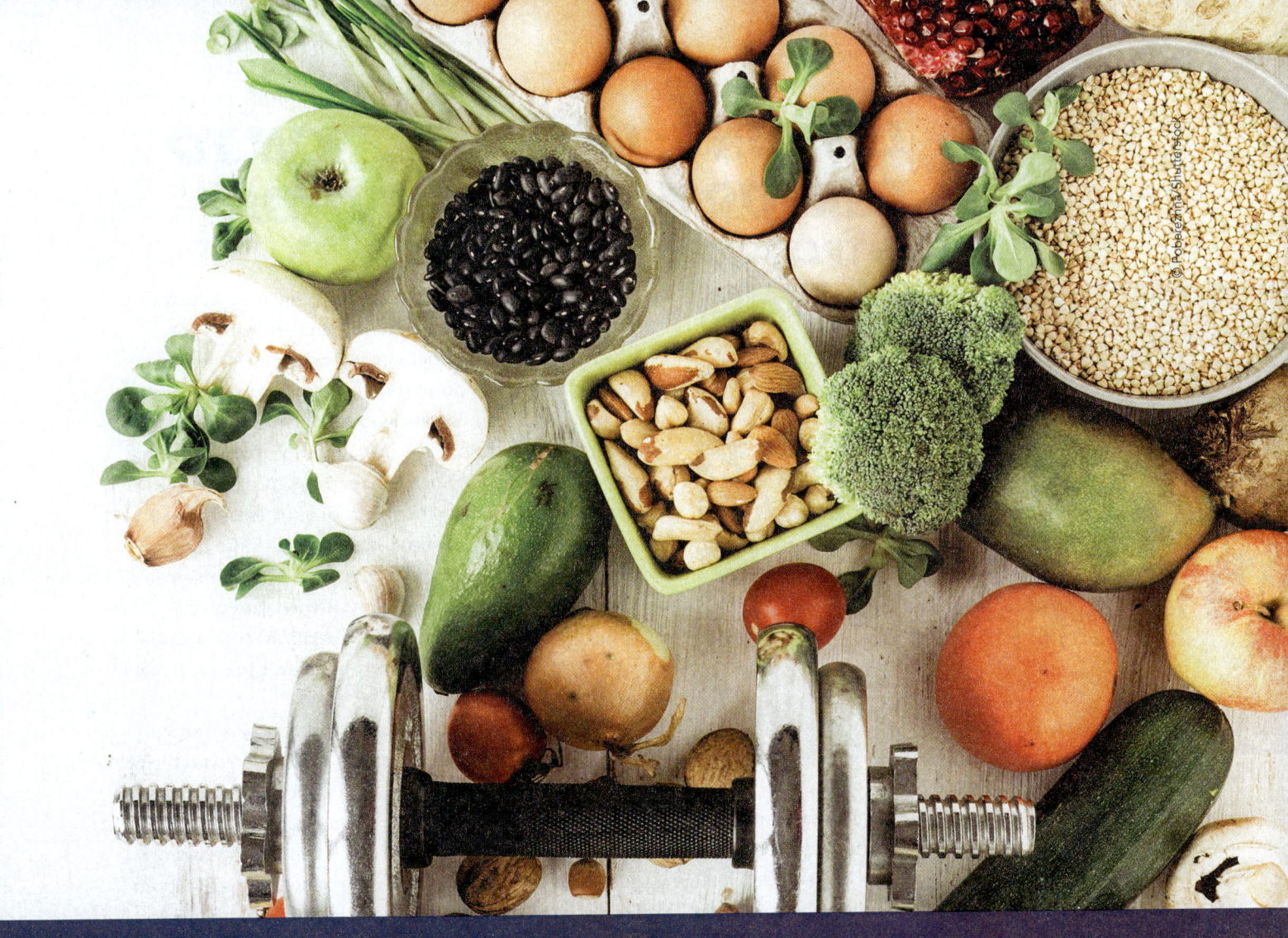

PERFORMANCE NUTRITION

LEARNING OBJECTIVES

Upon completion of this chapter, the Sports Performance Coach will be able to:

- **Explain** the limits of nutritional advice under the scope of practice.
- **Identify** macronutrients and micronutrients and their functions in relation to performance.
- **Describe** pre- and post-exercise nutrition strategies.
- **Identify** signs of dehydration and methods for preventing dehydration.
- **Describe** the basics of a nutritional assessment.

LESSON 1: INTRODUCTION TO PERFORMANCE NUTRITION
INTRODUCTION

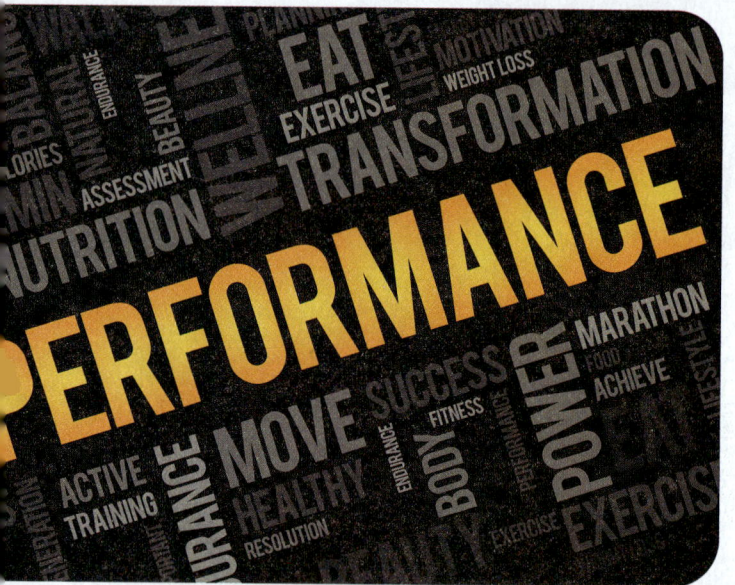

© Dizain/Shutterstock

Nutrition for athletes has an interesting dynamic. Athletes often do not think about nutrition when their habits are adequate for their level of activity. But when their nutrition is off, it can shift their mindset from performing to enduring. A sound nutritional plan is critical to supporting the demands of training and competition. The field of performance nutrition is growing quickly. The practice of performance nutrition involves taking the core components of nutrition—that is, ingestion, digestion, absorption, and uptake into target tissues—and using them in a strategic manner to enhance training, performance, and recovery. A wide variety of disciplines fall under the umbrella of performance nutrition; thus, many methods are employed and many goals are targeted to maximize potential results.

Traditional professional roles in sports, such as strength and conditioning coaching, have a lot in common with the field of nutrition. For instance, just as with exercise, prescription, timing, dosage, frequency, and recovery are all critical components of a well-designed nutritional plan. These aspects of nutrition help athletes build and maintain strength, increase speed, delay fatigue, and minimize the risk of both injury and exercise-induced immune problems, all while reducing recovery time so the athlete optimally progresses. Whether the individual is a strength athlete, an endurance athlete, or a person who casually exercises, there are key opportunities within the realm of performance nutrition that can benefit all.

Sports Performance Coaches must be well versed in the fundamentals of performance nutrition because nutritional needs and questions arise in virtually all roles. A sound nutrition plan is essential for achieving *and* maintaining optimal athletic performance (Spriet, 2019). Relevant specialists within the field include healthcare professionals such as medical doctors (MD), physical therapists (PT), **dietitian nutritionists (RD/RDN)**, and licensed nutrition specialists, such as **certified dietitian nutritionists (CDN)** and **licensed nutritionists (LN)**. These certifications and licenses all require formal higher education with a minimum of a bachelor's degree, and all require adherence to their specific scopes of practice, which are discussed in more detail in **Table 22.1**.

The longest-standing and most widely recognized nutrition specialty that is legally qualified to practice nutrition is the RD/RDN. The RD/RDN credential is widely recognized throughout the United States. This credential requires a bachelor's degree from an approved program and, as of January 1, 2024, requires a master's degree for new applicants. Another certification, the certified nutrition specialist (CNS), requires training of similar rigor to the RD/RDN, but many states do not allow for pathways to licensure outside of the RD/RDN option, which renders the CNS certification unsuitable for licensure in those states. It is critical that individuals who want to pursue nutrition understand the pathways for training, the requirements for certification, and the laws of their state that govern practice. **Table 22.2** outlines the educational requirements for the RD/RDN and CNS.

DIETITIAN NUTRITIONIST (RD/RDN) →

A health professional with specialized training in the use of diet and nutrition to keep the body healthy as well as addressing disease and engaging in medical nutrition therapy.

CERTIFIED DIETITIAN NUTRITIONIST (CDN) →

A registered dietitian who provides safe, effective, evidence-based nutrition services for health, fitness, and athletic performance.

TABLE 22.1 Health Professionals and Their Credentials

Health Professional	Credentials
Doctor of medicine	MD
Physical therapist	PT
Registered dietitian/registered dietitian nutritionist	RD/RDN
Certified dietitian nutritionist/licensed nutritionist	CDN/LN (state certified or licensed dietitian/nutritionist)

LICENSED NUTRITIONIST (LN) →

A healthcare professional who is licensed to perform nutrition counseling and provide nutrition education.

TABLE 22.2 Educational and Professional Requirements for the RD/RDN and CNS Certifications

Certification	Required Degree	Supervised Practice Program	National Exam	Continuing Education (CE)
RD/RDN	Have a bachelor's degree from a university or college accredited by the Accreditation Council for Education in Nutrition and Dietetics (ACEND). A master's degree is required for new applicants as of January 1, 2024.	Complete a 6- to 12- month ACEND-accredited supervised practice program at a healthcare facility, community agency, or a food service corporation combined with undergraduate or graduate studies.	Must pass a national exam in addition to completing their supervised practice to receive credentials.	Must complete appropriate CE requirements to maintain an active credential.
CNS	Have either a master of science or doctoral degree in a field of nutrition or a related field from a regionally accredited college or university in the United States, or its foreign equivalent. Or Have a doctoral degree in a field of clinical health care from a regionally accredited college or university in the United States, or its foreign equivalent.	Complete 1,000 hours of supervised practice by a CNS board-approved supervisor. The hours focus on personalized nutrition assessment and interpretation; nutrition intervention, education, counseling, and ongoing care; and personalized nutrition monitoring and evaluation.	Must pass a national exam in addition to completing their supervised practice to receive credentials.	Must complete appropriate CE requirements to maintain an active credential.

Adapted from the websites for the Academy of Nutrition and Dietetics (Registered Dietitian Nutritionist Fact Sheet, n.d.) and the American Nutrition Association (Nutritionists & Health Professionals | American Nutrition Association, n.d.).

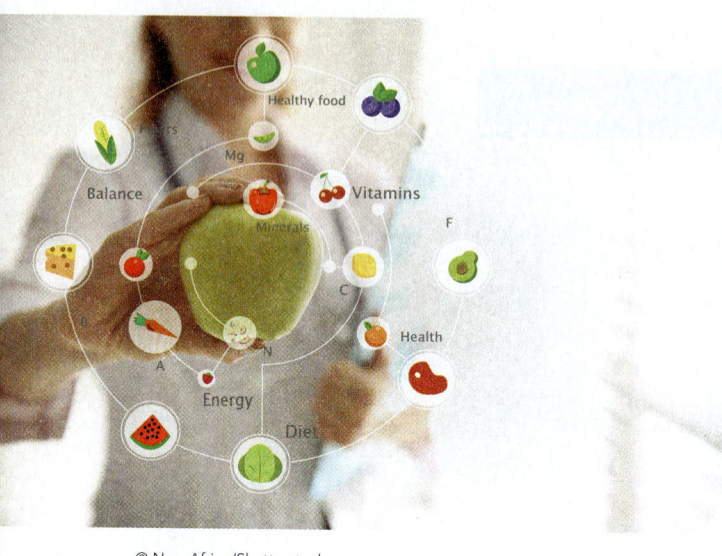

Additional training opportunities exist beyond the CNS and RD/RDN that, while not providing a clear path to licensure, are relevant to Sports Performance Coaches. Specialist in sports dietetics (CSSD) is a rigorous board certification in sports nutrition open only to RD/RDNs who have been licensed for at least 2 years and completed at least 2,000 hours of sports nutrition dietetics. This certification does not confer an additional scope of practice, but it is well respected and can potentially open many career doors once it is earned.

Table 22.3 lists common credentials that indicate individuals have completed formal training in the field of nutrition. These credentials are subject to individual state regulations that determine whether the individual can directly apply their knowledge with clients. Similar standards exist for nutrition credentials in Canada, the United Kingdom, and other nations.

TABLE 22.3 Nutrition Credentials and Qualifications

Nutrition Credential	Description
Registered dietitian/ registered dietitian nutritionist (RD/RDN)	Nationally recognized and credentialed in nutrition by the Commission on Dietetic Registration (CDR). Scope of practice ranges from clinical nutrition to community, food service, and nutrition education. Although nationally recognized, some states might still require RDs to obtain state licensure prior to practicing independently or in a clinical or medical setting.
Certification as a specialist in sports dietetics (CSSD)	A certification for registered dietitians who have extensive practice experience (2,000-plus hours) in the field of sports nutrition.
Certified dietitian/ nutritionist (CDN) or licensed dietitian/ nutritionist (LD/LDN)	State-certified or -licensed nutritionist. Licensed to practice nutrition in the certifying/licensing state. This licensure might be legally required in some states, for both RDs and non-RDs, to provide any nutrition counseling.
Certified nutrition specialist (CNS)	Certified by the Board for Certification of Nutrition Specialists. This certification qualifies individuals for licensure as a CDN or LD/LDN in some states.

Additional professionals, including personal trainers, strength and conditioning coaches, health coaches, and group fitness class instructors, will likely find themselves being asked questions by their clients about how diet affects their goals and active lifestyles. In fact, these professionals are often the first people approached with such questions. Before engaging on nutritional topics, each practitioner needs to understand the scope of practice of their field.

Always check the laws of the state or country before using terms such as "nutritionist" or "dietitian" as professional identification. In many regions, these terms are protected and can be used only by those individuals who meet specific requirements as defined in scope of practice laws. Many certifications contain "nutritionist" in the title—but earning such a certification does not necessarily give one the legal right to call themselves a nutritionist and rarely confers the legal right to practice nutrition. The website https://www.nutritioned.org/state-requirements/ is a useful but unofficial resource for learning about state laws on nutrition practice.

SCOPE OF PRACTICE AND PERFORMANCE NUTRITION

The term **scope of practice** refers to the range of activities that a professional is qualified and permitted to undertake. The scope of practice defines the procedures, actions, and processes that a healthcare practitioner is permitted to undertake in keeping with the terms of their professional license (Schuiling & Slager, 2000). It is important to understand that exceeding one's scope of practice has several consequences, including disciplinary action from the relevant medical board if licensed, legal action by the state, and risk of lawsuits in civil court. The scope of practice for the field of nutrition is regulated at the state level. While some states' laws are vague, many states have extensive laws that explain the process required to become licensed to practice nutrition. These laws also provide a framework for defining the scope of practice by spelling out the details that dictate how each profession can practice. Defining the role and scope of a Sports Performance Coach is important, because it provides a clear framework that the coach can work within and ensure they are not exposing themselves or their clients to unnecessary risks or liabilities.

⚠ **CRITICAL**

Sports Performance Coaches must review the details of their specific state's laws before discussing nutrition with their athletes, as these laws vary to a great extent. When coaching athletes on performance nutrition, it is also important to consult the American Nutrition Association: https://theana.org/advocate. Any person who gives nutritional advice outside of their legal scope, as defined by their state's guidelines, is breaking the law.

State laws clearly differentiate between **medical nutrition therapy (MNT)** and **non-medical lifestyle-oriented nutrition** with regard to providing nutrition advice and coaching as a performance enhancement specialist. MNT typically involves the diagnosis and treatment of medical conditions and is restricted to individuals who have adequate scope of practice for that therapy (e.g., registered dietitians or medical doctors). Sports Performance Coaches often do not have the required scope of practice for MNT and

SCOPE OF PRACTICE →

A term used to describe the skills, actions, procedures, and processes that a qualified individual is permitted to undertake, usually under a professional governing body accreditation and/or law.

MEDICAL NUTRITION THERAPY (MNT) →

The diagnosis and treatment of medical conditions, restricted to individuals who have adequate scope of practice for that therapy.

NON-MEDICAL LIFESTYLE-ORIENTED NUTRITION →

Education and coaching around lifestyle-based changes that improve the overall nutrition habits of an individual.

must use caution when discussing treatment or diagnosis. For instance, when working with an obese client, a non-medical practitioner can share basic nutrition ideas and food-preparation tips that support a healthy lifestyle, but they cannot prescribe a detailed diet to treat the client's obesity.

SPORTS PERFORMANCE COACHES ROLE IN PERFORMANCE NUTRITION

The role of a Sports Performance Coach largely focuses on the following areas:

- Physical assessment
- Programming of appropriate exercise and training based on the client's goals
- Nutrition coaching, including education on energy and nutrient balance, healthy eating patterns, hydration strategies, and goal-based nutrition guidance

Because nutrition is an integral part of a successful performance program, athletes seeking performance-related services are likely to request guidance on their diet and nutrition. Unless a Sports Performance Coach holds additional relevant credentials, providing athletes with specific dietary or nutritional supplement recommendations is outside their scope of practice. They can, however, provide education in the following areas (Kruskall, 2019):

- Principles of healthy nutrition and food preparation
- Food to include in the normal daily diet
- Essential nutrients needed by the body
- Recommended amounts of essential nutrients
- Actions of nutrients on the body
- Effects of deficiencies or excesses of nutrients
- Food and supplements that are good sources of essential nutrients

The Sports Performance Coach might also help athletes identify which dietary factors are contributing to poor performance, educate them on how metabolism relates to performance, explain how nutrition needs change based on exercise, and guide athletes toward more appropriate choices that better support their goals. However, if an athlete has a health condition that requires specific dietary modifications, such as diabetes, hypertension, or cardiovascular disease, or if an athlete requests the provision of specific meal plans, the Sports Performance Coach must refer them to a qualified nutrition or medical professional for further guidance and counseling. Such a referral ensures that the athlete benefits from the expertise provided by the appropriate professionals qualified in their areas of practice and respects the scope of practice for both professions.

Table 22.4 outlines the scope of practice specific to performance nutrition and identifies the types of services that the Sports Performance Coach might or might not provide.

DOMESTIC VERSUS INTERNATIONAL REGULATIONS

Much of this content centers on laws and practice regulations specific to the United States. However, the Sports Performance

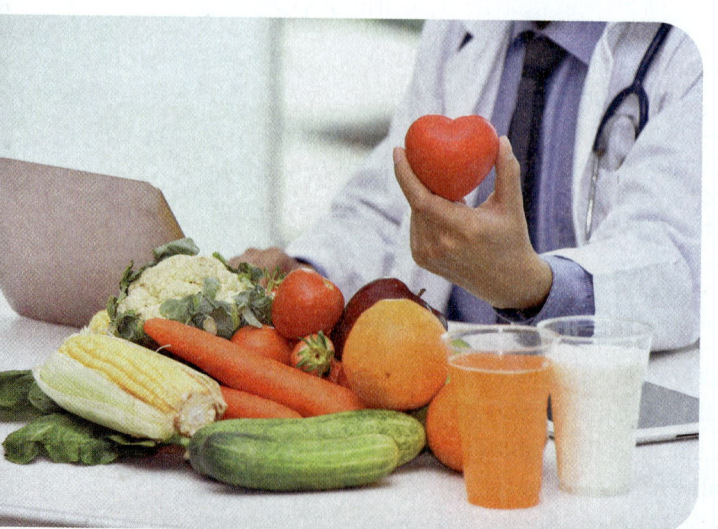

© Supavadee butradee/Shutterstock

TABLE 22.4 Nutrition Credentials and Qualifications for the Sports Performance Coach

Within Scope of Practice	Outside Scope of Practice (unless qualified in the applicable discipline)
Maintain a fitness log of the client's anthropometrics.	Order or interpret lab work.
Obtain a general diet history to review overall eating behavior and food choices and guide the client toward healthier food choices.	Provide a meal plan to the client.
Demonstrate food preparation methods.	Prescribe a therapeutic diet.
Review the importance of overall energy (calorie) balance and its effect on weight management.	Provide specific calorie recommendations or diagnose calorie-related conditions such as relative energy deficiency in sport (RED-S) or the female athlete triad.
Review factors that influence body weight, including social, lifestyle, and dietary habits.	Recommend supplements for weight gain or loss.
Review the actions of nutrients on the body.	Diagnose specific nutrient deficiencies.
Review the guidelines for recommended quantities of essential nutrients.	Recommend specific nutrient intake amounts.
Review how macronutrients impact performance and recovery.	Provide specific macronutrient recommendations.
Review the importance of hydration and the role of electrolytes.	Design a specific hydration protocol for the client.
Discuss pre-, intra-, and post-exercise nutrition for performance and recovery.	Design a specific nutrition plan for pre-, intra-, and post-exercise nutrition.

Coach needs to take similar precautions outside of the United States as well. Many countries have licensure laws that establish scopes of practice related to nutrition or dietetics. The European Federation of the Associations of Dietitians (EFAD) identifies several different dietetics-related fields across Europe, including clinical dietitians, food service dietitians, and public health or community dietitians. For those outside of the United States, the website for the International Confederation of Dietetic Associations is a good resource. In Canada, the aptly named Dietitians of Canada is the best resource. The concepts in this chapter provide background information that will enable sports professionals to take an informed approach to determining their scope and identifying their opportunities for practice.

LESSON 2: ENERGY
ENERGY BALANCE

ENERGY →

In the context of human performance, the power derived from utilizing physical or chemical resources, especially to provide light and heat or to work machines.

The first concepts that form the foundation of sports nutrition are **energy** and **energy balance**. In the context of human performance, energy is defined as power derived from the utilization of physical or chemical resources, especially to provide light and heat or to work machines. Translating this to nutrition and human performance, energy is the conversion of chemical energy, in the form of food, into mechanical energy, in the form of human movement. Energy balance is the relationship between energy intake from food and drink and energy output—the energy expended in a given time frame, usually thought of over the span of a given day (**Figure 22.1**). In the human body, energy is found in the form of chemical energy, called **calories**. All chemical energy that humans utilize comes from the food they consume.

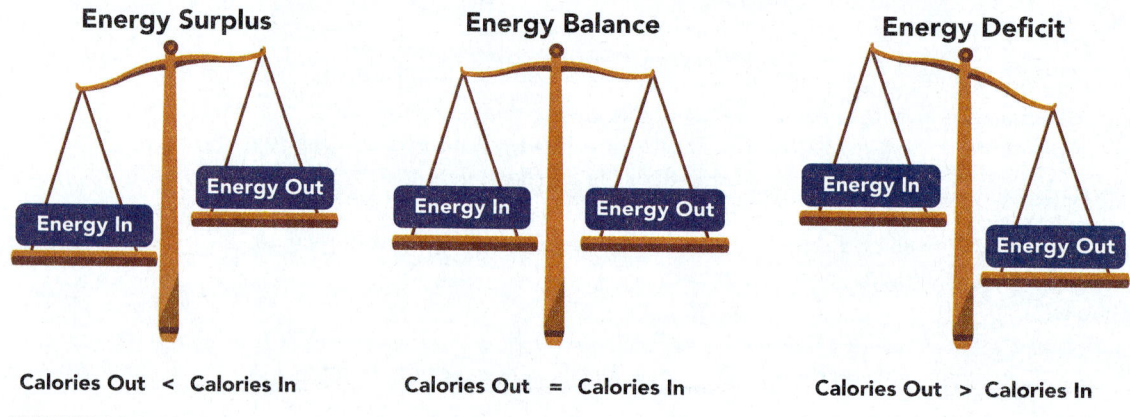

FIGURE 22.1 Energy Balance and Expenditure

ENERGY BALANCE →

The relationship between energy intake from food and drink and energy output.

In essence, energy balance refers to the state of the balance of energy going into and out of the human body. The body can be in one of three energy balance states: in balance, in surplus, or in deficit.

DEFINING CALORIE AND THE KILOCALORIE

Calories are the unit commonly used to quantify energy in food and how energy is expended during movement. A calorie (lowercase "c") is the unit used to quantify the transfer of energy from food to either storage in the body or mechanical work, such as movement. Formally, a calorie is the amount of energy required to raise the temperature of 1 gram of water by exactly 1°C. This is a very small amount of energy, so for the sake of practicality, either of the interchangeable terms Calorie (uppercase "C") or **kilocalorie (kcal)** is more commonly used. One Calorie is 1,000 calories.

CALORIE →

The amount of energy required to raise the temperature of 1 gram of water by exactly 1°C.

🤖 GETTING TECHNICAL

The terms "calorie" and "Calorie" are often used interchangeably. To further confuse matters, "calorie" is capitalized when it is used at the beginning of a sentence. Always understand which unit is being discussed. More often than not, Calorie is the intended term. In the rest of this book, anytime the word "calorie" is used, it implies the kilocalorie—or 1,000 calories—unless otherwise stated.

LAW OF THERMODYNAMICS

As the human body functions to transform one type of energy (e.g., chemical) into other types of energy (e.g., chemical, heat, mechanical), the laws of physics can be applied to energy in the human body. One of the core concepts to understand regarding nutrition is the **first law of thermodynamics**. This law states that within a closed system, energy is neither created nor destroyed. Any energy that enters the system must be used, stored, or excreted. The phrase **"calories in, calories out" (CICO)** is a simplified description of this process (**Figure 22.2**). On the surface, it seems as if it would be a simple matter to track Calories for the purpose of gaining, losing, or maintaining weight. However, the concepts that govern intake and usage, storage, and excretion are complex.

**KILOCALORIE →
(KCAL)**

1,000 calories.

**FIRST LAW →
OF THERMO-
DYNAMICS**

Within a closed system, energy is neither created nor destroyed.

**CALORIES IN, →
CALORIES OUT
(CICO)**

A way of stating the first law of thermodynamics in the context of human metabolism.

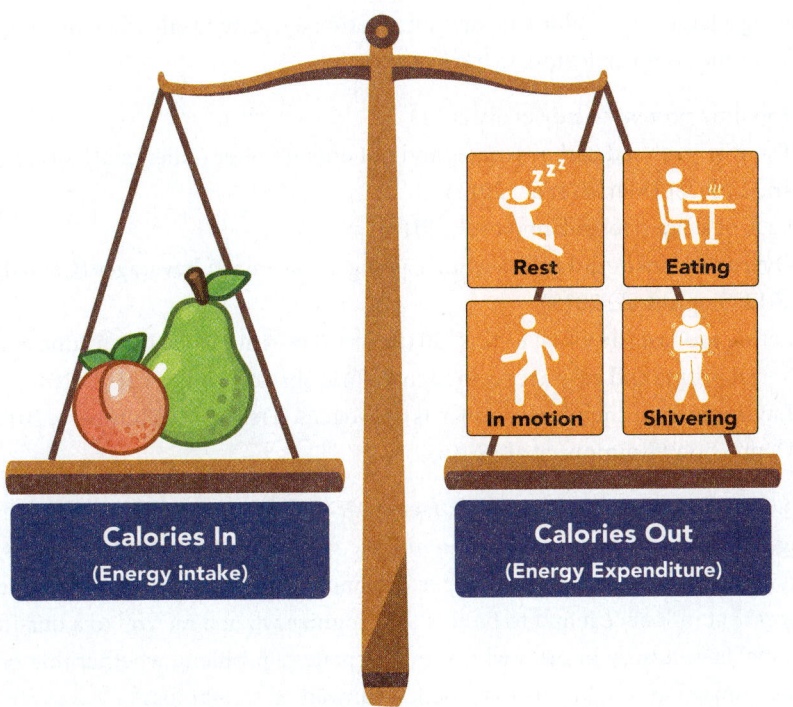

The Energy Balance Equation

Rest   Eating

In motion   Shivering

Calories In
(Energy intake)

Calories Out
(Energy Expenditure)

FIGURE 22.2 The Energy Balance Equation

CALORIES IN (ENERGY INTAKE)

The "calories in" side of the energy equation appears simple enough: It is the number of calories consumed. However, in practice, accurately quantifying this intake is difficult, mostly because measurements of calories in food tend to be imprecise. For example, packaged foods may differ meaningfully (hundreds of calories) from their stated nutrient and calorie counts, and homemade meals are subject to measurement errors during preparation. In addition, humans often drastically underestimate how many calories they consume (Jumpertz et al., 2013; Lichtman et al., 2010). Similarly, portion sizes in the real world are often measured by scoops and handfuls—and these estimates are often inaccurate (Hernández et al., 2006). All of these issues make the exact tracking of caloric intake difficult.

The ability of the average person to accurately estimate calorie intake is quite poor. Some studies show that people often underestimate their calorie intake by as much as 50%, which means that some people's estimates are off by 1,000 kilocalories per day (Berezovikova et al., 2021; Carlsen et al., 2010; de Vries et al., 1994; Headrick et al., 2013; Lichtman et al., 2010).

Not only is quantifying difficult, but human behavior surrounding eating is complicated as well. For example, the desire to eat is driven by many factors, including both the need to meet energy requirements and to enjoy food. While the primary driver is to satisfy energy needs as perceived by the brain, other intake-related factors do not directly relate to a true physiological need to maintain energy balance. This is exemplified by ordering a large, high-calorie dessert after eating a hearty meal. The following are a few examples of the complex factors that drive appetite:

- Too little protein (Leidy et al., 2011)
- Too many refined carbohydrates and not enough fiber (Aller et al., 2011)
- Too little fat (Martin et al., 2011)
- Lack of sleep (Hogenkamp et al., 2013)
- Over-intake of liquid calories, such as sugar-sweetened beverages (Cassady et al., 2012; Singh et al., 2015)
- Eating too fast (de Graaf & Kok, 2010; Ferriday et al., 2015; Maruyama et al., 2008)
- Social norms and easy access to high-calorie snacks (Njike et al., 2016)
- Environmental chemicals known as obesogens (Heindel & Blumberg, 2019)
- Depression (Simmons et al., 2016)

To summarize, a variety of complex factors drive food intake and there are serious challenges involved in measuring that intake accurately. Despite these challenges, quantifying caloric intake is critical to performance. Thus, it is important to understand the factors that influence it and to be able to recognize when a referral to a qualified professional is necessary in cases where intake creates a problem, whether that problem is a surplus (unwanted weight gain) or a deficit (unwanted weight loss).

TOTAL DAILY ENERGY EXPENDITURE (TDEE) →

The full sum of all energy expended in a given day by the human body.

RESTING METABOLIC RATE (RMR) →

The rate of energy expenditure at rest.

✓ **CHECK IT OUT**

In addition to appetite, cultural factors play a key role in regulating food intake, including parental role models, gender roles, habits of peer groups, being sedentary, food costs, and socioeconomic status (Chatham & Mixer, 2020; Vizcarra et al., 2019). Hormones such as leptin, ghrelin, and insulin play a role as well, but much of that is driven by the food choices that influence appetite. Attempts to simplify appetite and weight gain to hormones such as insulin have failed in recent well-designed studies (Gardner et al., 2018; Hall et al., 2021). Collectively, these factors shed light on why traditional dietary advice to "eat less" is complicated and often too general to benefit persons who struggle with overeating or obesity.

CALORIES OUT (ENERGY EXPENDITURE)

The "calories out" side of the energy equation has four key components that are referred to as **total daily energy expenditure (TDEE)**. TDEE consists of two main types of energy expenditure: resting energy expenditure and non-resting energy expenditure. Resting energy expenditure is often called the **resting metabolic rate (RMR)** or **basal metabolic rate (BMR)**. This is the energy required to maintain normal body function while at rest. Non-resting energy expenditure is all the energy a body expends moving and digesting food.

The non-resting energy expenditure is broken down into three main components:

- **Thermic effect of food (TEF)**: The energy a body spends digesting and absorbing the food it consumes.
- **Non-exercise activity thermogenesis (NEAT)**: The energy a body spends moving around during the day that is not from formal, structured exercise.
- **Thermic effect of activity (TEA)**: The energy that a body spends to engage in formal, structured exercise or sporting events.

It is important that the Sports Performance Coach has a working understanding of the components of energy expenditure because each component can affect the client's energy needs (**Table 22.5**). While BMR is fairly immutable, some aspects can vary substantially and have large effects on total energy needs (**Figure 22.3**). For example, an athlete might expend a lot of energy during training, but then be very sedentary for the rest of the day,

BASAL METABOLIC RATE (BMR) →

The metabolic rate (caloric expenditure) of the body at rest.

THERMIC EFFECT OF FOOD (TEF) →

The energy a body spends digesting and absorbing the food it consumes.

NON-EXERCISE ACTIVITY THERMOGENESIS →

The energy a body spends moving around during the day that is not from formal, structured exercise.

THERMIC EFFECT OF ACTIVITY →

The energy that a body spends to engage in formal, structured exercise or sporting events.

TABLE 22.5 Total Daily Energy Expenditure Components

Component	Definition
Total daily energy expenditure (TDEE)	All of the energy expended daily, including resting energy expenditure and non-resting energy expenditure.
Resting metabolic rate (RMR)	The energy required to maintain normal body function while at rest; usually 60% to 75% of daily energy.
Thermic effect of food (TEF)	The increase in energy that occurs several hours after eating food. It includes the digestion, absorption, metabolization, and uptake/storage in body tissue, which usually accounts for about 10% of daily energy.
Thermic effect of activity (TEA), also known as physical activity (PA)	All energy expended in excess of RMR and TEF; usually ranges from 15% to 30% of total daily energy. Elite athletes can stretch this as high as 50%.
Non-exercise activity thermogenesis (NEAT)	A component of TEA, but typically includes only involuntary actions such as fidgeting and shivering. Some sources include other non-exercise activities in this category, such as walking to work or typing.

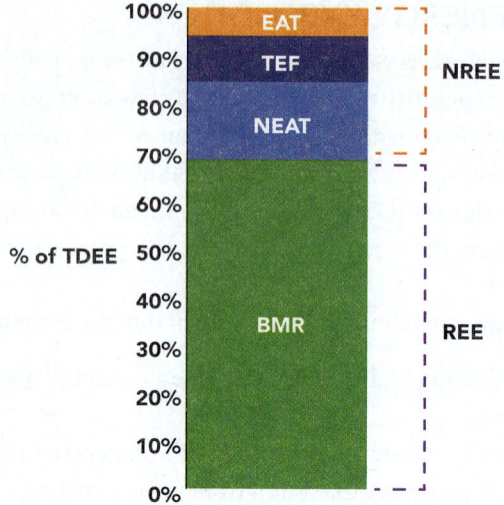

FIGURE 22.3 Energy Expenditure

EAT: exercise activity thermogenesis; NREE: non-resting energy expenditure; REE: resting energy expenditure.

which can lower their total energy needs by about 15%. Conversely, athletes might engage in a limited training volume, but their NEAT is incredibly high due to their occupation, so their energy needs might be 15% to 20% higher than expected.

ENERGY AVAILABILITY

It is critical for individuals who have performance goals to ensure there is enough energy available to perform the work necessary. Energy availability is defined as the amount of dietary energy available to sustain physiological function after subtracting the energetic cost of exercise (Areta et al., 2013; Areta et al., 2021). Unfortunately, athletes are far more likely than one would think to be in a state of low energy availability (LEA) because they often do not eat and drink enough to sustain their activity (Burke, 2001; Maughan et al., 1997; Ziegler et al., 2002). Some evidence also indicates that an athlete's knowledge of nutrition is related to their likelihood of maintaining an adequate energy balance (Magee et al., 2020).

📋 COACH'S CORNER

LEA is one of the key components underlying the female athlete triad and relative energy deficiency in sport (RED-S). These overlapping conditions can have serious implications for sex hormones, immunity, bone density, and many other areas of health. As a Sports Performance Coach, it is important to pay attention to an athlete's energy needs and keep an eye out for LEA among clients.

Figure 22.4A illustrates the health consequences of RED-S with an expanded concept of the female athlete triad to acknowledge a wider range of outcomes and the application to male athletes. **Figure 22.4B** depicts the potential performance effects of RED-S.

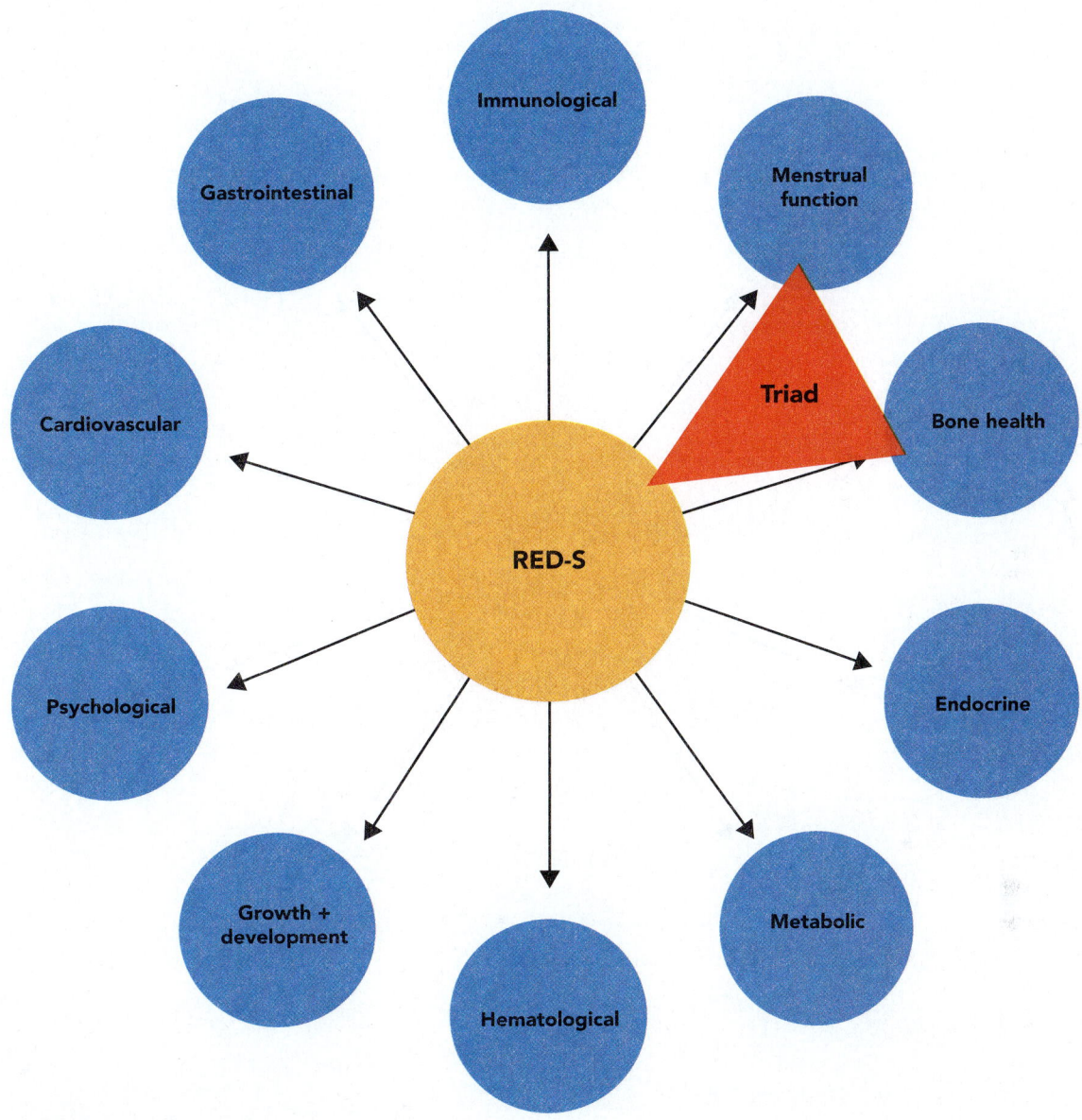

FIGURE 22.4A Relative Energy Deficiency in Sports

Reproduced from Mountjoy, M.et al. IOC consensus statement on relative energy deficiency in sport (RED-S): 2018 update. British Journal of Sports Medicine. 2018 Jun;52(11):687–697. doi: 10.1136/bjsports-2018-099193. PMID: 29773536.

ENERGY PRODUCTION

A meaningful understanding of how the body uses food as fuel requires a dive into biochemistry. Calories translate into the ability to perform work. For our purposes here, the focus of that work is exercise, which can be viewed as mechanical energy. Where nutrition meets physiology is at the transformation of chemical energy (derived from food) into mechanical energy (movement). This transformation of chemical energy has many variables, and one of the most important is speed. Just as is in the sport of cycling, sometimes you need as much speed as possible for a race. But other times, such as for an activity like a recovery ride, speed is a secondary consideration.

In the human body, three main sets of chemical reactions, known as energy systems, produce energy in the form of adenosine triphosphate (ATP). Which system the body uses to produce energy at any given moment is based on a number of factors: the rate at which the body needs ATP (energy) produced, the total amount of ATP the body needs, and

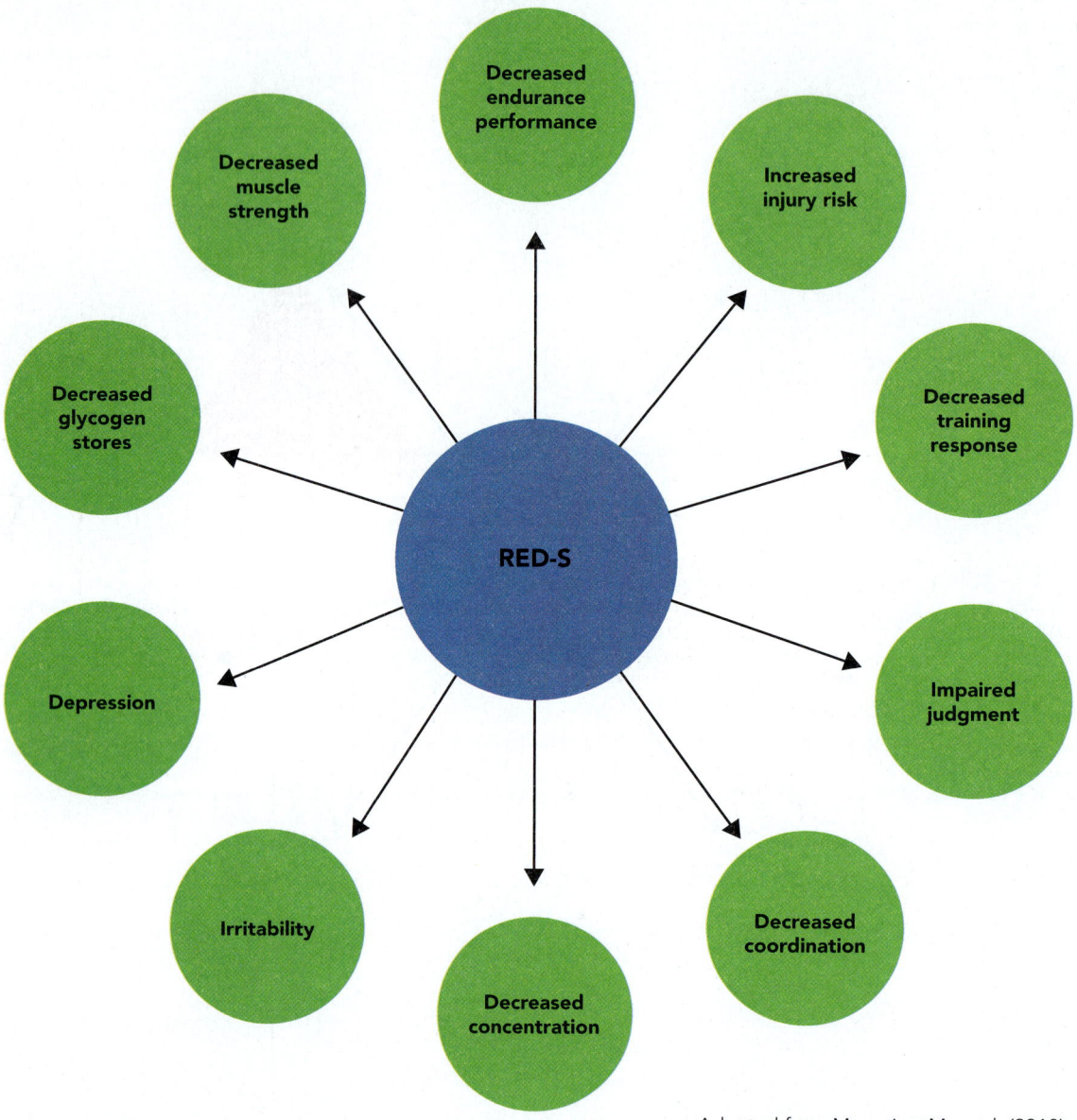

Adapted from Mountjoy, M. et al. (2018).

FIGURE 22.4B Relative Energy Deficiency in Sports

Reproduced from Mountjoy, M.et al. IOC consensus statement on relative energy deficiency in sport (RED-S): 2018 update. British Journal of Sports Medicine. 2018 Jun;52(11):687–697. doi: 10.1136/bjsports-2018-099193. PMID: 29773536.

the amount of chemicals that are available for the reaction to use. The rate at which ATP is produced is the most common way to think about and differentiate the three energy systems (**Figure 22.5**):

- ATP-PCr/phosphagen is a short-lived, rapid-acting energy system that provides an initial energy burst while the other energy systems get started. This process does not require oxygen; hence, it is called anaerobic.
- Glycolysis uses either a fast and efficient form of stored glucose called glycogen or circulating blood glucose. It cannot maintain its peak output for long. It is also anaerobic.
- Oxidative phosphorylation uses carbohydrates, fats, and (to a lesser degree) proteins to generate energy that the body can sustain for much longer periods. This process requires oxygen; hence, it is called aerobic.

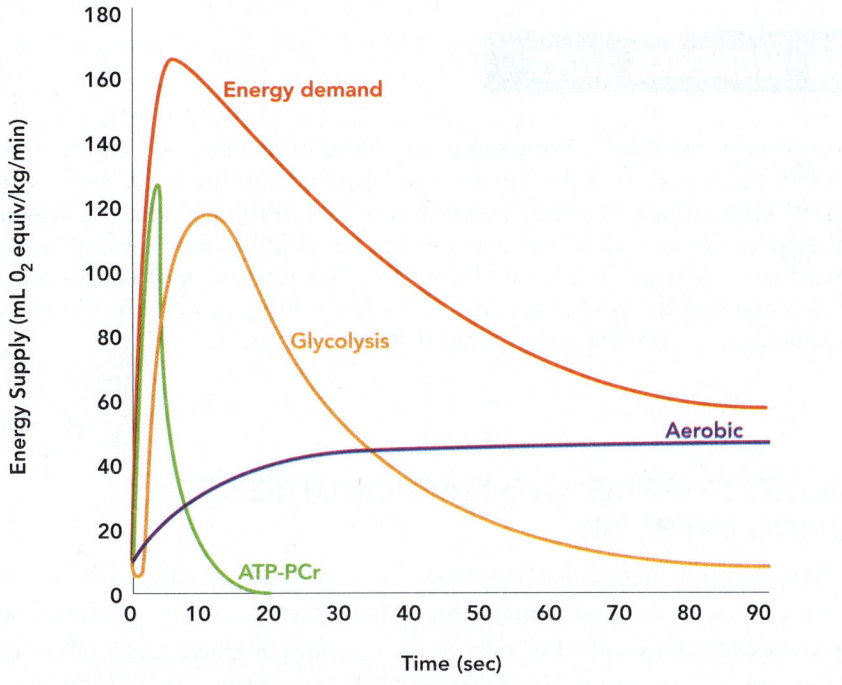

FIGURE 22.5 Energy Systems Contribution to Cycling Sprints

Contribution of energy systems during 90 seconds of all-out cycling effort of six trained male cyclists.

Reproduced from Gastin, P. B. (2001). Energy system interaction and relative contribution during maximal exercise. *Sports Medicine, 31*(10), 725–741.

Quick and forceful muscle contractions require fast access to energy, demonstrated in the spikes in the curves in Figure 22.5. There is a trade-off between the speed of ATP production for any given system of energy production and the amount of ATP it can provide (i.e., the fastest methods provide energy for the shortest durations). At the point at which the speed of ATP use outpaces the supply of ATP, there is a decrease in the amount of work the body can do. This is reflected in the energy demand curve, which quickly begins to slope down as the phosphocreatine system and glycolysis taper off.

Thus, speed is one factor that determines which energy systems provide most of the energy for exercise. Another factor is the availability of the substrates that fuel the chemical reactions. Each of the energy systems has different substrates that fuel it (**Table 22.6**).

TABLE 22.6 Substrates That Fuel Energy Systems

Phosphocreatine/phosphagen system	• Creatine phosphate • ADP
Glycolysis	• Glucose
Aerobic/oxidative system	• Glucose • Fatty acids • Amino acids*

*Amino acids are used sparingly under energy-sufficient conditions and contribute minimally to overall energy production in most circumstances.

ENERGY SYSTEMS AND MACRONUTRIENTS DURING EXERCISE

The three energy systems utilize substrates to convert chemical energy into mechanical energy for exercise; these nutrients are found in the form of creatine phosphate, glucose, fatty acids, and amino acids. The body creates creatine phosphate, and it is not considered a major source of energy because it can provide only approximately 10 to 30 seconds of energy production. Essentially, this means that the body utilizes the three macronutrients (carbohydrates, fats, and proteins) to produce most of the energy during exercise. However, which nutrients the body uses during exercise vary substantially based on two major factors: the intensity and duration of the exercise. For the Sports Performance Coach, it is critical to understand how the body utilizes nutrients that are derived from food consumed to fuel different types of exercise.

The best way to understand how the body fuels exercise is to examine how the body shifts to and from the types of nutrients (carbohydrates and fats) and the sources of those nutrients (from the blood or stored in tissue) as exercise intensity increases or as duration increases (Romijn et al., 1993) (**Figure 22.6**). At rest and at low levels of intensity, the body utilizes primarily fatty acids and small amounts of glucose from the blood circulation and some fatty acids stored in muscle tissue to fuel the body's energy requirements. As exercise intensity increases to moderate intensity, the body shifts to utilizing more glucose from the blood, but also starts utilizing substantial amounts of glucose stored in the muscle in the form of glycogen. The body also starts more readily using fatty acids stored in the muscle tissue. As exercise intensity increases to an even higher level, the body starts to rely very heavily on stored glucose and glucose from the blood and utilizes fewer fatty acids.

In addition to exercise intensity, the duration of exercise affects the contribution of different nutrients to energy production, especially with moderate- to higher-intensity exercise. When an individual engages in moderate- to higher-intensity exercise, the stored nutrients begin to be depleted, as the body has finite stores of them. For example, when an individual engages in moderate- to higher-intensity exercise, they rely heavily on muscle glycogen and fatty acids stored in the muscle tissue. As exercise duration increases, the amount of those stores available drops and the body begins to utilize other sources of energy, specifically glucose and fatty acids from the blood circulation (Romijn et al., 1993). As such, the amount of glucose available to support more high-intensity work decreases, which results in decreased performance over time (**Figure 22.7**). This is one reason why people are unable to sustain high exercise intensity for long periods of time.

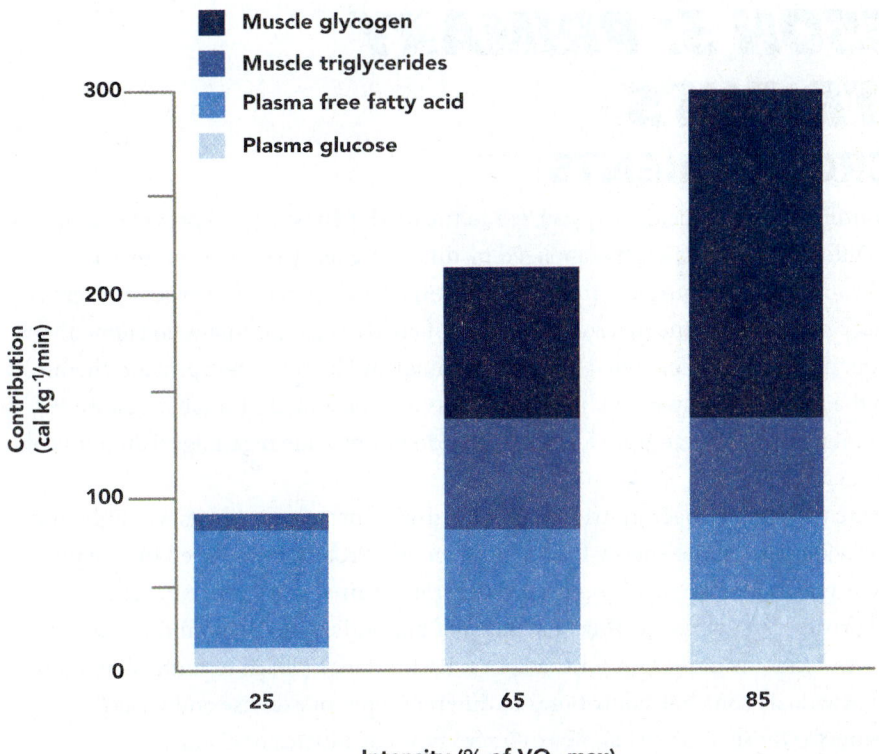

Adapted from Romijn, J. A. et al. (1993).

FIGURE 22.6 Exercise Intensity Effect on Energy Expenditure

Contributions of energy expenditure at varying levels of exercise intensity.

Romijn, J. A., Coyle, E. F., Sidossis, L. S., Gastaldelli, A., Horowitz, J. F., Endert, E., & Wolfe, R. R. (1993). Regulation of endogenous fat and carbohydrate metabolism in relation to exercise intensity and duration. *The American Journal of Physiology, 265*(3 Pt 1), E380–E391. Reprinted with permission.

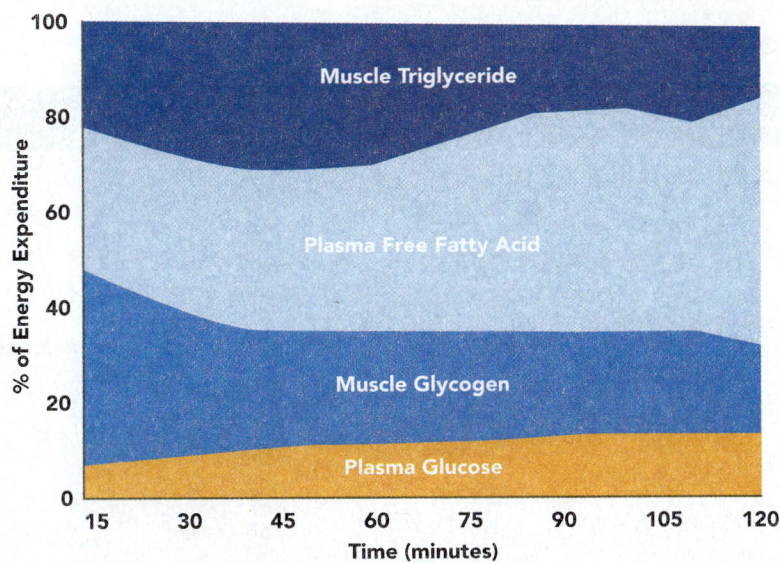

Adapted from Romijn, J. A. et al. (1993).

FIGURE 22.7 Substrate Contribution to Energy Production

Relative contribution of substrates to energy production during 120 minutes of exercise at 65% VO₂ max.

Romijn, J. A., Coyle, E. F., Sidossis, L. S., Gastaldelli, A., Horowitz, J. F., Endert, E., & Wolfe, R. R. (1993). Regulation of endogenous fat and carbohydrate metabolism in relation to exercise intensity and duration. *The American Journal of Physiology, 265*(3 Pt 1), E380–E391. Reprinted with permission.

LESSON 3: PRIMARY NUTRIENTS

MACRONUTRIENTS

The body utilizes the chemical energy stored in the food it consumes to provide energy for exercise. Different nutrients are metabolized by different energy systems; in turn, different nutrients from different sources in the body are utilized to fuel different types of exercise. The primary nutrients are the macronutrients, so named because humans consume them in larger quantities (approximately 10 or more grams) and because they provide chemical energy to the body. By comparison, micronutrients are consumed in smaller quantities, usually in milligram or microgram amounts, and do not provide meaningful amounts of chemical energy.

There are three main macronutrients: carbohydrates, proteins, and fats. Carbohydrates and fats provide most of the energy for fueling exercise. Protein, while used to provide energy, is primarily used to repair tissue and generate **amino acids** for important biological processes, such as creating enzymes and antibodies and maintaining chemical reactions. As such, it is important for the Sports Performance Coach to understand how the food individuals consume contributes to different types of exercise and what the requirements for those nutrients are for different types of athletes or clients.

> **AMINO ACID**
>
> An organic compound that contains a carboxyl group and an amino group and serves as the base unit of all proteins.

CARBOHYDRATES

Carbohydrates are a class of nutrients defined by their chemical structure, which consists of carbon, hydrogen, and oxygen; carbohydrates are also often referred to as sugars. Carbohydrates are classified according to the number of saccharide units they contain: monosaccharides, disaccharides, and polysaccharides (**Table 22.7**). They are primarily derived from plant sources such as fruits, grains, roots, and tubers.

TABLE 22.7 Classifications of Carbohydrates

Category	Types	Food Sources
Monosaccharides	Glucose Fructose Galactose	Honey Fruit Syrup Candy Sugar-sweetened beverages
Disaccharides	Sucrose Lactose Maltose	Table sugar Dairy Beer Cane sugar Root vegetables
Polysaccharides	Starch Fiber	Grains Tubers Vegetables

Carbohydrate—or more specifically glucose—is the substrate used for glycolysis, and serves as the fuel for the majority of the energy required for moderate- and high-intensity exercise. Glucose is found in two main forms in the human body: free glucose (blood sugar) and stored glucose (glycogen). The two major storage sites for glycogen are skeletal muscle and the liver. Due in part to its location, glycogen stored in skeletal muscle is used when muscles require carbohydrates for contraction and the body needs more glucose or needs glucose more quickly than can be absorbed from the blood. Glycogen stored in the liver is mainly used to maintain blood sugar levels, though it also provides some glucose for exercise. Although the exact amounts of glucose utilization and the source of where it comes from—blood glucose versus glycogen—vary based on the athlete's training status and where the glycogen is stored, glycogen can generally fuel about 2 hours of exercise, depending on the intensity of the exercise (Bob Murray, 2018; Coyle, 1995). The higher the exercise intensity, the more quickly glycogen is depleted, and the higher carbohydrate intake needs to be.

The differing utilization of carbohydrates as an energy source based on the intensity and duration or volume of exercise indicates that the carbohydrate requirements for athletes vary depending largely on those two key variables. **Table 22.8** lists general daily carbohydrate recommendations based on athletic intensity and duration.

TABLE 22.8 Daily Carbohydrate Intake Recommendations (Grams per Kilogram of Body Weight)

Exercise Intensity/Volume	Weight-Based Carbohydrate Recommendation	Sport/Event Example
Low-intensity or skill-based activities	3–5 g/kg	Table tennis Archery Golf
Moderate-intensity exercise lasting less than 1 hour	5–7 g/kg	Track and field Weight lifting
Moderate- to high-intensity exercise lasting 1–3 hours	6–10 g/kg	Cross-country running Endurance running Cycling Swimming Basketball Soccer Football Tennis
Moderate- to high-intensity exercise lasting more than 4 hours	10–12 g/kg	Triathlon Marathon Long-distance cycling

Data from Jeukendrup, A. & Gleeson, M. (2018). *Sport nutrition* (3rd ed.). Champaign, IL: Human Kinetics.

These amounts must be fine-tuned based on performance and feedback of the athlete. For intense endurance exercise lasting longer than 90 minutes, it is possible to load or super-compensate glycogen stores in the days leading up to an event. This is achieved by tapering the intensity of training in the days preceding the competition while consuming 10 to 12 g/kg of carbohydrates spread throughout the day for 2 days before the competition (Burke et al., 2018). Many athletes also eat a lower-fiber diet for 3 days before an event to reduce the contents of their bowels on race day.

The role of glycogen storage and needs-based intake underscores how the availability of carbohydrates affects the outcome of most competitions. As such, in addition to daily carbohydrate requirements for meeting energy needs, it is important to understand how to address acute feeding of carbohydrates. For example, if an athlete enters competition with low glycogen stores, then feeding during competition is critical to success (Widrick et al., 1993). Many endurance and essentially all ultra-endurance events allow for feeding during the event. Depending on digestive tolerance, the body can typically utilize up to 60 grams of carbohydrate per hour (Jeukendrup & Jentjens, 2000).

Generally, it is best to space the carbohydrate consumption throughout the hour. Athletes who become accustomed to this level of intake can work up to even higher amounts by mixing their carbohydrate sources. Those bodies can utilize up to 100 grams per hour when mixing glucose and fructose in a 2-to-1 ratio (Jentjens et al., 2004; Trommelen et al., 2017). However, this quantity of carbohydrate intake might cause gastrointestinal issues in many athletes. It is best to slowly increase the dosage during training, which has the effect of training the body to tolerate these high amounts (Jeukendrup, 2017; Jeukendrup & Jentjens, 2000).

✔ CHECK IT OUT

Traditional wisdom indicates that an athlete should not consume carbohydrates in the hour before training or competition due to fear of hypoglycemia. Studies confirm that not only is hypoglycemia from pre-event carbohydrate timing rare, but there can even be a performance *benefit* from consuming as little as 22 grams of carbohydrate in that period. In the rare case that an athlete becomes symptomatic from pre-race carbohydrates, they can consume them either 5 minutes before competition or during warm-up (Jeukendrup & Gleeson, 2018).

Endurance athletes must start with these general guidelines for fueling during exercise based on the duration of activity in minutes. Dosages are listed in grams per hour (g/h) and need to be consumed in 15- to 20-minute increments during the hour rather than all at once (**Figure 22.8**).

Fueling strategies during exercise require advanced planning so the athlete has access to the necessary nutrients. Planning is also necessary for the period following exercise to ensure adequate preparation for the next training session, as glycogen takes time to replenish. If the next session is at least 24 hours later, there is no need to deviate from the normal carbohydrate guidance in Table 22.8. For athletes who plan to train sooner (e.g., swimmers, who often train twice a day), carbohydrates must be consumed over a 2-hour period immediately after exercise at a rate of 1.2 to 1.5 g/kg per hour. Half of the dose

Recommended Carb Intake Based on Exercise Duration

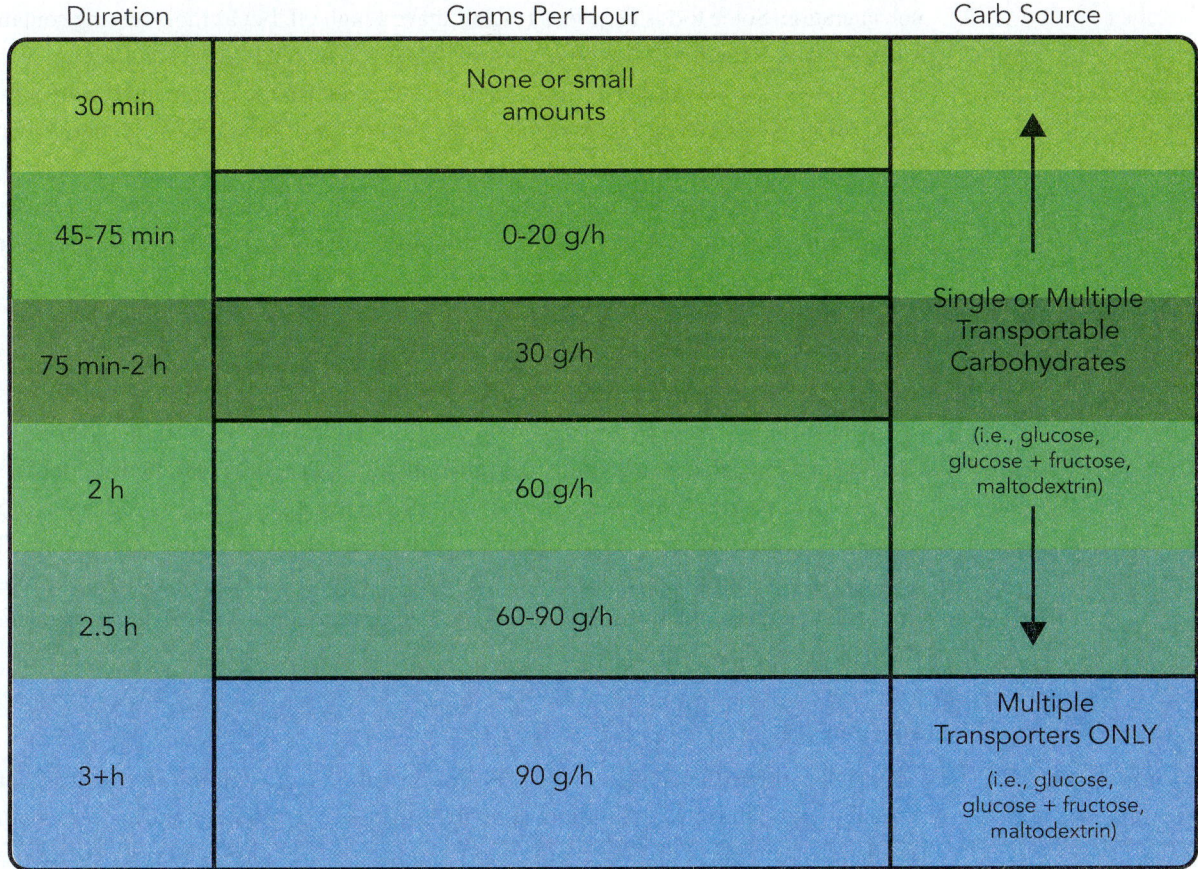

Duration	Grams Per Hour	Carb Source
30 min	None or small amounts	↑ Single or Multiple Transportable Carbohydrates
45-75 min	0-20 g/h	
75 min-2 h	30 g/h	
2 h	60 g/h	(i.e., glucose, glucose + fructose, maltodextrin)
2.5 h	60-90 g/h	↓
3+h	90 g/h	Multiple Transporters ONLY (i.e., glucose, glucose + fructose, maltodextrin)

FIGURE 22.8 General Guidelines for Fueling During Exercise

needs to be consumed every 30 minutes for a total of four doses. The rate of glycogen synthesis sharply declines after this 2-hour window.

GLYCEMIC INDEX AND PERFORMANCE NUTRITION

The **glycemic index (GI)** ranks foods based on how much they increase blood glucose over the 2-hour period after ingestion. Though the numbers vary in different studies, the ranking is typically based on how much a food portion containing 50 grams of carbohydrates raises blood glucose as compared to consuming 50 grams of pure glucose. The GI scores food on a scale from 0 to 100. Foods are considered to have a low GI if they have scores in the range of 0 to 55. Some examples include apples, peanuts, lentils, and most vegetables. Moderate-GI foods have scores ranging from 56 to 69 and include sweet potatoes, white and wild rice, and pineapple. Finally, foods are considered to have a high GI if they have scores of 70 to 100. Some examples include white potatoes, instant oatmeal, white bagels, and popcorn.

As discussed earlier, glycogen resynthesis is an important aspect of recovery for sports nutrition, especially when individuals are performing multiple training sessions or competition events in the same day. The ingestion of high-GI foods produces the best results for this purpose. The advantage of higher-GI foods disappears after the first 24 hours, at which point complex carbohydrates appear to perform as well or even better. Sugar-sweetened beverages are a poor choice for recovery because they often contain high levels of fructose that the liver must process, which significantly delays muscle glycogen synthesis.

> **GLYCEMIC INDEX (GI)**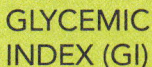
>
> A system of scoring foods that is based on the effect the food has on blood sugar levels.

GLYCEMIC INDEX VERSUS GLYCEMIC LOAD

A major shortcoming of the GI is that its formula does not take portion sizes into consideration. Some foods (e.g., watermelon) have a high GI, but a single serving contains far fewer than 50 grams of carbohydrates, so the GI's predicted effect on blood glucose is overstated. Issues like this led to the development of a refined measurement, the **glycemic load (GL)**. The GL is based on the amount of carbohydrates found in a single serving of a food. By factoring in serving size, the GL corrects for foods such as watermelon. Watermelon has a GL of approximately 4, which falls in the low range of 0 to 10. Medium-GL foods have a score between 11 and 19. Bananas are in this range. High-GL foods have a score of 20 or higher. White breads such as bagels are classic examples of high-GL foods.

GLYCEMIC INDEX AND PERFORMANCE

There has been much discussion around how the GI should be used in the context of sports nutrition. Some sources suggest that low-GI foods must be consumed before exercise to allow for sustained glucose availability during exercise, and high-GI foods must be consumed post-exercise to speed up recovery and glycogen synthesis. However, there is no clear evidence that these strategies provide meaningful benefits or improvements. The strongest evidence indicates that the total amount of carbohydrates ingested is the most important factor and that their GI scores have minimal impact on overall performance (Donaldson et al., 2010).

PROTEIN

Although carbohydrates often garner the most attention from endurance athletes, protein typically commands the attention of strength and power athletes. Unlike for carbohydrates and fat, the key role of protein is not energy production, but rather a more structural role. This is important because the body's daily protein requirements are not based on energy needs, but instead on how much body mass the athlete needs to maintain.

Protein contains not only carbon, hydrogen, and oxygen (as carbohydrates do), but also nitrogen (which carbohydrates lack). Protein molecules are made up of one or more amino acids. Amino acids all share a common structure of five different structures: a central carbon, a carboxyl group (organic acid—COOH), a hydrogen, an amino group (NH_2), and a side chain (R group). The first four components are the same for all amino acids, but the side chain varies—it is what makes each amino acid different (**Figure 22.9**). For example, the amino acid leucine has a large, branched structure for its side group, whereas glycine has a singular hydrogen atom as its side group. Amino acids are bonded

<aside>
GLYCEMIC LOAD (GL) →

A measure of how rapidly and how high a food raises blood sugar relative to the actual amount of food consumed.
</aside>

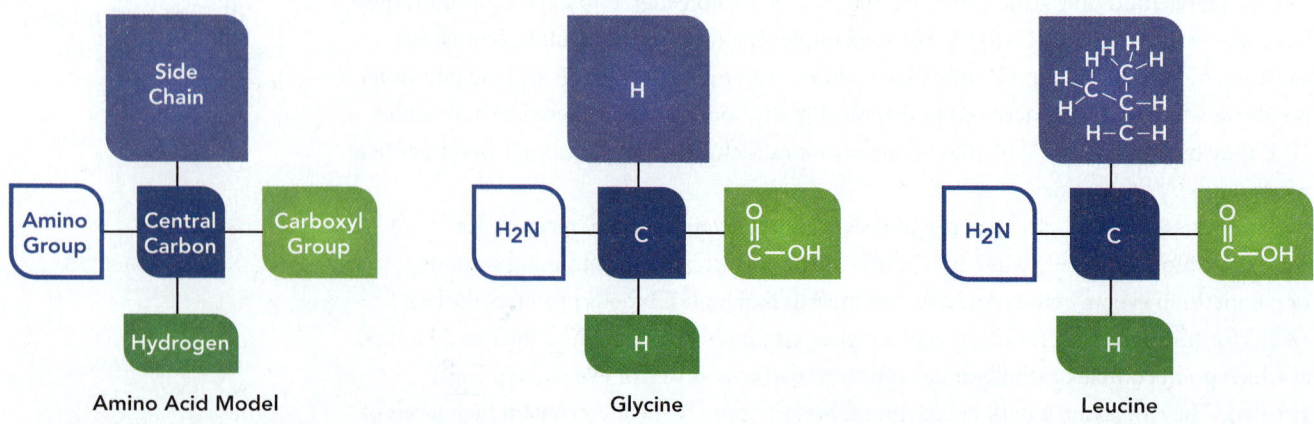

Amino Acid Model Glycine Leucine

FIGURE 22.9 Structure of Amino Acids

together from one carboxyl group to the next amino group by a peptide bond, which makes them stable molecules.

Sports Performance Coaches must have a thorough understanding of the relationship between amino acids and protein. Amino acids are what the human body utilizes for specific functions and what the body needs to derive from food (**Table 22.9**).

TABLE 22.9 The Functions of Protein in the Body

- Serves as a component of enzymes, which speed up chemical reactions in cells
- Serves as a component of many hormones, which help with communication and signaling in cells to facilitate processes such as muscle protein synthesis
- Serves as a structural component of skin, nails, hair, muscle, and connective tissue
- Serves as a component of key immune system molecules
- Helps regulate fluid and electrolyte balance
- Provides a small source of energy under normal conditions, and a larger source of energy during long-term stressors such as starvation

Data from Dunford, M., & Doyle, J.A. (2022). Nutrition for sport & exercise (5th Ed.).

▣ GETTING TECHNICAL

While protein and amino acids are consumed as part of the diet, approximately 85% of the amino acid pool in the body comes from skeletal muscle in a catabolic process known as muscle protein breakdown (Biolo et al., 1994). In essence, food-derived amino acids are recycled by the body continuously, indicating that protein intake over time matters just as much as acute protein intake.

One of the concepts at the heart of protein metabolism in the human body centers on how proteins are made of amino acids. **Anabolism** is the process of taking smaller pieces, such as individual amino acids, and combining them to make larger structures, such as muscle tissue. The opposite process—the breakdown of larger structures, such as muscle tissue, into smaller pieces, such as amino acids—is known as **catabolism**.

Anabolism and catabolism are important processes for the Sports Performance Coach to understand because they are central to protein metabolism for human performance. Anabolism is the process that fosters muscle growth and maintains muscle mass. Under most circumstances, athletes need to either maintain or build muscle. So, Sport Performance Coaches must be sure that **muscle protein synthesis (MPS)**, the anabolic process of making muscle tissue from amino acids, can keep pace with or exceed **muscle protein breakdown (MPB)**, the catabolic process of breaking down muscle tissue into individual amino acids.

The Sports Performance Coach must consider several aspects of protein intake when providing nutrition education to their clients, but the most important component is daily protein intake. The most effective way to ensure a client meets their protein intake requirements is to consume adequate protein based on their body mass (weight), their goal (e.g., building or maintaining lean mass), and their primary form of exercise (**Table 22.10**).

ANABOLISM

The process of taking smaller pieces, such as individual amino acids, and combining them to make larger structures, such as muscle tissue.

CATABOLISM

The breakdown of larger structures, such as muscle tissue, into smaller pieces, such as amino acids.

MUSCLE PROTEIN SYNTHESIS (MPS) →

The anabolic process of making muscle tissue from amino acids.

MUSCLE PROTEIN BREAKDOWN (MPB) →

The catabolic process of breaking down muscle tissue into individual amino acids.

The protein recommendations for athletes are considerably higher than the recommended daily intake (RDI) of 0.8 g/kg for the general population.

TABLE 22.10 Guidelines for Protein Intake

Goal or Population	Target Protein Amount in g/kg of Body Weight
Building and maintaining muscle mass	1.4–2.0 g/kg (Jäger et al., 2017)
Build muscle while in an energy surplus but limit fat gain	1.6 g/kg is the most needed for building muscle, but up to 2.2 g/kg limits fat gain (Leaf & Antonio, 2017; Morton et al., 2018)
Endurance athletes	1.2–1.6 g/kg and adequate calories are critical to avoid catabolizing muscle for energy (Houltham & Rowlands, 2014; Kato et al., 2016)
Overweight or obese adults	1.1–1.6 g/kg (Kim et al., 2016; Wycherley et al., 2012)

✔ CHECK IT OUT

Lean athletes in a caloric deficit are more susceptible to losing lean body mass (LBM) because it makes up a higher percentage of their body composition. The higher end of the recommended intake ranges is recommended for these athletes (Heymsfield et al., 2011).

🤖 GETTING TECHNICAL

There is ample evidence supporting higher intakes, but a question of safety arises in such cases. Notably, physicians are commonly concerned about kidney damage due to high protein intakes. Fortunately, numerous studies, including a recent large meta-analysis, concluded that high protein levels do not impair kidney function in healthy adults (Devries et al., 2018). However, protein intake is a serious issue in people with chronic kidney disease, so if a client has established kidney disease, protein recommendations must be set by their physician.

PROTEIN TIMING AND MEAL SIZES

After the daily protein requirements are being met consistently and the protein sources are high quality and meet the amino acids requirements, the Sports Performance Coach and the athlete might be interested in adjusting protein intake timing to optimize recovery. Two major considerations must be addressed by the Sports Performance Coach in this context. The first is how quickly the athlete needs to consume protein after a training session or performance. The second is how the athlete spaces their protein intake throughout the day.

Research has confirmed the existence of a period immediately post-workout, known as the post-workout window, during which muscle tissue is more sensitive to nutrients and takes up greater amounts of amino acids. However, resistance exercise actually sensitizes skeletal muscle to the effects of protein and amino acids for up to 24 hours. As such, timing is not as critical as long as protein targets are met, and protein intake is divided throughout the day—though there is no detriment to consuming protein within a short time frame of training or exercise (Jäger et al., 2017; Schoenfeld et al., 2013).

How an athlete consumes protein throughout the day to optimize muscle growth and recovery is best understood by examining two key variables. The first is the optimal amount in a given meal; the second is how those meals are spaced throughout the day.

With regard to the optimal meal size, current evidence suggests that the law of diminishing returns applies. Through a series of studies, it has been shown that as protein intake increases, the anabolic response increases but at a smaller rate. For example, consuming 20 grams of protein is more effective at stimulating muscle protein synthesis than consuming 10 grams, and consuming 40 grams is more effective than consuming 20 grams (Macnaughton et al., 2016). Furthermore, studies show that consuming 70 grams is also slightly more effective than consuming 40 grams (Kim et al., 2016). However, there are diminishing returns as protein intake goes up; that is, consuming 40 grams does not necessarily provide 100% increases in protein synthesis compared to consuming 20 grams, and consuming 70 grams does not provide 75% increases compared to consuming 40 grams. The optimal, practical intake for most clients and athletes falls somewhere in the 20 grams to 40 grams per meal range (**Figure 22.10**).

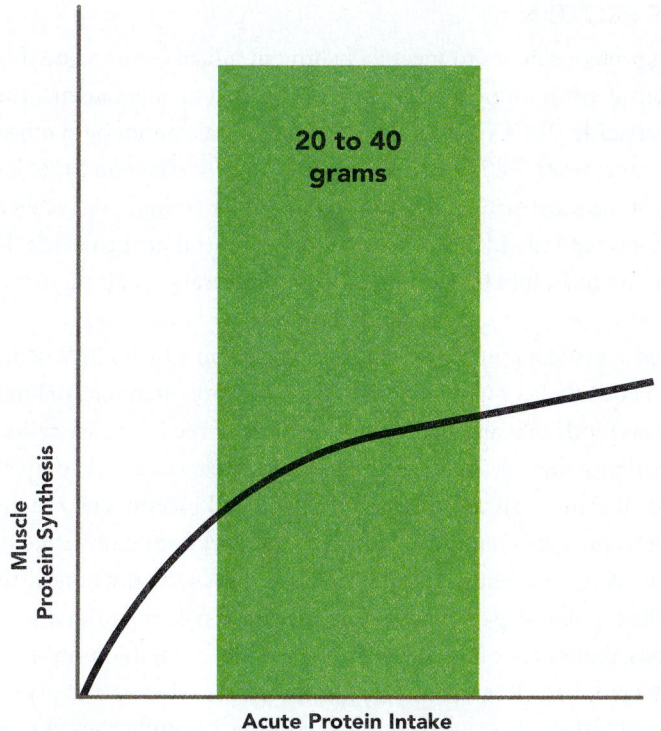

FIGURE 22.10 Practical Protein Intake per Meal

In addition to optimizing the amount of protein per meal, research shows how best to allocate protein intake throughout the day. Research has examined the practices of consuming protein in small amounts frequently throughout the day (small feedings every hour or two), in fewer meals but larger amounts (two meals with very large protein intakes), or in evenly spaced out meals with protein intake divided evenly among the meals (Areta et al., 2013; Kim et al., 2016). Current evidence suggests that evenly spaced-out meals with protein intake divided roughly equally between meals is the optimal approach.

📋 COACH'S CORNER

Intuitively, one might think that because training in a fasted state increases the amount of protein used for energy, eating protein before or during exercise reduces the risk of negative outcomes on MPS. However, athletes should instead focus on their normal protein intake ranges relative to their activity levels.

👍 HELPFUL HINT

Older athletes require more protein to achieve the same level of MPS, so they must target the higher end of each range (Barkoukis, 2016; Burd et al., 2013).

ESSENTIAL AMINO ACIDS (EAAs) →

Amino acids that are necessary for bodily functions but cannot be synthesized by the body and must be obtained in the diet.

NON-ESSENTIAL AMINO ACIDS →

Amino acids that the body can manufacture.

COMPLETE PROTEINS →

Foods that contain all nine of the essential amino acids.

INCOMPLETE PROTEINS →

Foods that are missing one or more of the nine essential amino acids.

SOURCES OF PROTEIN

When choosing protein sources to meet daily protein intake recommendations, it is important to consider the amino acid content of the food or supplement. There are nine **essential amino acids (EAAs)**—that is, amino acids that cannot be synthesized by the body and must come from food or drink. Due to its robust effect on MPS, leucine is often considered one of the most critical EAAs when muscular strength or recovery is the goal. It is also important that individuals consume **non-essential amino acids**; however, the human body can manufacture these amino acids if necessary and if there is sufficient dietary protein.

Food sources of protein are often categorized based on which kinds of amino acid they consist of. Foods that contain all nine of the EAAs are often referred to as **complete proteins**, whereas foods that are missing one or more of the EAAs are called **incomplete proteins**. Animal proteins, including dairy and eggs, are considered complete proteins; in contrast, almost all plant-derived proteins are considered incomplete proteins.

When athletes consume an omnivorous diet and meet their daily protein requirements, the likelihood of being deficient in specific amino acids is virtually nonexistent. However, athletes who utilize a plant-based diet have an increased risk of amino acid deficiencies because plant-based diets are often lower in leucine, lysine, methionine, isoleucine, threonine and tryptophan (Rogerson, 2017). Appropriate selections of plant-based protein sources can provide adequate sources, but they must be carefully chosen to ensure the athlete is receiving adequate intake of each amino acid.

FATS

Fats, like carbohydrates, are composed of carbon, hydrogen, and oxygen atoms. However, fats are structurally different than carbohydrates, such that they are not considered sugar molecules. They represent a much larger class of chemical structures found in the human body. Fat serves as the key fuel for metabolism during mild to moderate exercise and at rest. Fats are found in both plant and animal food sources. In addition to serving as a fuel source for activity, fat plays a key role in the following processes:

- Elasticity of cells
- Nervous system function
- Hormone production
- Stabilization of body temperature
- Absorption of fat-soluble vitamins

TYPES OF FAT

Many different types of fats can be found in the human body. The fats that are pertinent to the discussion of sports nutrition are **fatty acids (FA)**—specifically triacylglycerols, which are the main storage form for fats in the human body, in both adipose tissue and within muscles. Fatty acids are the fundamental building blocks of fat, which are broadly classified as **saturated fats (SFA)** or **unsaturated fats**. A detailed chart of types of fats can be found in Appendix E.

Saturated fats are synthesized by the body and are also found in many animal foods (e.g., beef), whole dairy products (e.g., butter and cream), and tropical oils (e.g., coconut and palm oil). These fats are often solid at room temperature. Unsaturated fats are

FATTY ACIDS (FA)

Carboxylic acids that function as the building blocks of fats in the human body.

SATURATED FATS (SFA)

A type of fat that has all of its carbons fully linked with hydrogen atoms.

UNSATURATED FATS →

A type of fat that has one or more carbons without a hydrogen atom and at least one double bond.

MONO-UNSATURATED FAT (MUFA) →

A type of fat that has one carbon without a hydrogen atom and one double bond.

POLY-UNSATURATED FAT (PUFA) →

A type of fat that has two or more carbons without a hydrogen atom and two or more double bonds.

LINOLEIC ACID →

A short-chain omega-6 fatty acid.

ALPHA-LINOLENIC ACID →

A short-chain omega-3 fatty acid derived from plants.

INTRA-MUSCULAR TRIGLYCERIDES →

A storage form of fatty acids that is found in skeletal muscles.

further categorized as either monosaturated or polyunsaturated. **Monounsaturated fats (MUFAs)** are found in almonds, avocados, canola oil, and olive oil. **Polyunsaturated fats (PUFAs)** are found in vegetable and fish oils. Unsaturated fats are often liquid at room temperature.

ESSENTIAL FATTY ACIDS

PUFAs are further subdivided into three groups: omega-3, omega-6, and omega-9. There are two essential fatty acids (EFAs) that must be consumed as part of the diet because they cannot be manufactured by the body: **linoleic acid** (an omega-6), which is found in vegetable oils, and **alpha-linolenic acid (ALA)** (an omega-3), which is found in fatty fish, seed oils, and leafy greens. Fish and algae sources of omega-3 fatty acids are high in eicosatetraenoic acid (EPA) and docosahexaenoic acid (DHA). These are considered conditionally EFAs because they are necessary for optimal functioning; specifically, EPA and DHA are involved in key biological processes such as inflammation, are part of the cell membrane structure, and act as signaling molecules. The recommended intake of omega-3 fatty acids is approximately 1.1 to 1.6 grams per day (the equivalent of one serving of cold-water fatty fish), and the intake of omega-6 fatty acids is approximately 12 to 17 grams per day (the equivalent of 2 to 3 ounces of nuts or seeds).

> ### 🤖 GETTING TECHNICAL
>
> Studies on EPA and DHA supplementation in athletes have resulted in somewhat inconsistent but generally positive results, especially in amateurs and when used over a longer term (more than 8 weeks) (Mickleborough, 2013; Thielecke & Blannin, 2020). Some evidence indicates that EPA and DHA supplementation might be helpful in reducing the brain damage sustained from traumatic brain injury and in reducing delayed-onset muscle soreness (DOMS) after eccentric exercise. However, there is little evidence that they improve performance (Maughan et al., 2018).

While fats are considered an essential nutrient, there is no clear minimum fat requirement for either health or performance outcomes. Fats are generally considered the remaining source of energy after protein and carbohydrate requirements are met, especially for athletes. As such, most guidelines are based on the current evidence around how best to structure a diet for athletes while consuming enough fats to prevent potential health issues.

The guidelines for fat intake for athletes recommend around 1.0 g/kg, which falls within the Dietary Reference Intake (DRI) range for fat of 20% to 35% of total calories, and the American College of Sports Medicine's recommendation of no less than 20% of total calories for athletes (Thomas et al., 2016). This requirement could increase to up to 2.0 g/kg in endurance athletes to replace **intramuscular triglycerides** (Horvath et al., 2000). According to the U.S. Department of Agriculture (USDA) guidelines, saturated fat should account for no more than 10% of the diet, while trans fats need to be restricted as much as possible (Snetselaar et al., 2021).

Guidelines for fat intake differ from those for protein and carbohydrate intake, because protein and carbohydrate intakes increase based on specific performance and body composition goals. The choice of the right amount of dietary fat for athletes is often centered on consuming only enough to avoid bodily damage. Many athletes prioritize carbohydrates and protein and consume fat only in amounts necessary to maintain caloric targets. Consuming too little fat can have negative consequences, however. The fat-soluble vitamins A, D, E, and K are found in fat-containing foods, and their absorption requires a small amount of fat. A chronic low-fat diet might not adequately replenish stores of fat, such as intramuscular triglycerides that are depleted during endurance and ultra-endurance events (Coyle et al., 2001). This could be particularly problematic for female athletes because they have higher levels of intramuscular triglycerides and rely more heavily on intramuscular triglycerides for submaximal exercise compared to males, so a fat deficit might impair their performance (Tate & Holtz, 1998; Volek et al., 2006). Furthermore, due to the caloric density of fat relative to protein and carbohydrates, reductions in dietary fat can result in the unintended under-consumption of calories.

> 👍 **HELPFUL HINT**
>
> The risk of a chronic low-fat diet not replenishing intramuscular triglycerides is very similar to how a low-carbohydrate diet does not adequately replenish muscle glycogen.

LESSON 4: MICRONUTRIENTS AND HYDRATION
MICRONUTRIENTS

Although macronutrients get most of the attention in discussions of performance nutrition, micronutrients are also essential components of a healthy diet and optimal human performance. Micronutrients do not directly provide energy, but they do play key roles in numerous systems affecting energy production, the immune system, tissue health, hormone and **neurotransmitter** functioning, the manufacturing of new cells and proteins, and the management of **oxidative stress**.

VITAMINS AND MINERALS

Micronutrients are classified into two categories: **vitamins** and **minerals** (**Table 22.11**). Vitamins are small, organic compounds required in small quantities, usually less than a

TABLE 22.11 Micronutrients: Vitamins Versus Minerals

Vitamins	Fat-soluble	A, D, E, K
	Water-soluble	B_1, B_2, B_3, B_5, B_6, B_7, B_9, B_{12}, C
Minerals	Major minerals	Calcium, chloride, magnesium, phosphorus, potassium, sodium, sulfur
	Trace minerals	Iron, manganese, copper, iodine, zinc, cobalt, fluoride, selenium

NEURO-TRANSMITTER →

A chemical substance used to communicate signals within the nervous system.

OXIDATIVE STRESS →

An imbalance between oxidants and antioxidants in the human body.

VITAMINS →

Small, organic compounds required in small quantities (usually less than a gram) that must be consumed in the diet because they cannot be manufactured by the body (with some exceptions).

MINERALS →

Inorganic substances required in small quantities (usually less than a gram) that must be consumed in the diet because they cannot be manufactured by the body.

WATER-SOLUBLE →

The ability for something to be dissolved in water.

FAT-SOLUBLE →

The ability for something to be dissolved in lipids.

gram, and must be consumed in the diet because they cannot be manufactured by the body (with some exceptions). Minerals are inorganic substances that, similar to vitamins, are required in small quantities, also usually less than a gram, and must be consumed in the diet because they cannot be manufactured by the body.

Vitamins are further classified based on whether they are **water-soluble** or **fat-soluble**. Water-soluble vitamins are not stored in body tissue (e.g., muscle or adipose tissue); fat-soluble vitamins are. The fat-soluble vitamins are vitamins A, D, E, and K; the water-soluble vitamins are the B-complex vitamins and vitamin C.

Minerals are further classified based on whether they are considered major minerals or trace minerals. Major minerals are those that are needed in quantities greater than 100 milligrams per day, whereas trace minerals are those that are needed in quantities less than 100 milligrams per day.

VITAMINS AND MINERALS IN SPORTS PERFORMANCE

Along with the increased energy needs that come with increased energy expenditure from exercise, micronutrient needs increase as well. For example, roughly 56% of athletes have insufficient levels of vitamin D (Farrokhyar et al., 2015), as many as 30% of female athletes have insufficient levels of iron (Parks et al., 2017), and an estimated 10% to 40% of athletes who do not supplement their diets with vitamins have insufficient levels of vitamin A and most of the B-complex vitamins (Parks et al., 2017; Wardenaar et al., 2017). These deficiencies appear not just in athletes, but also in the general population who might be considering utilizing a performance nutrition–based approach.

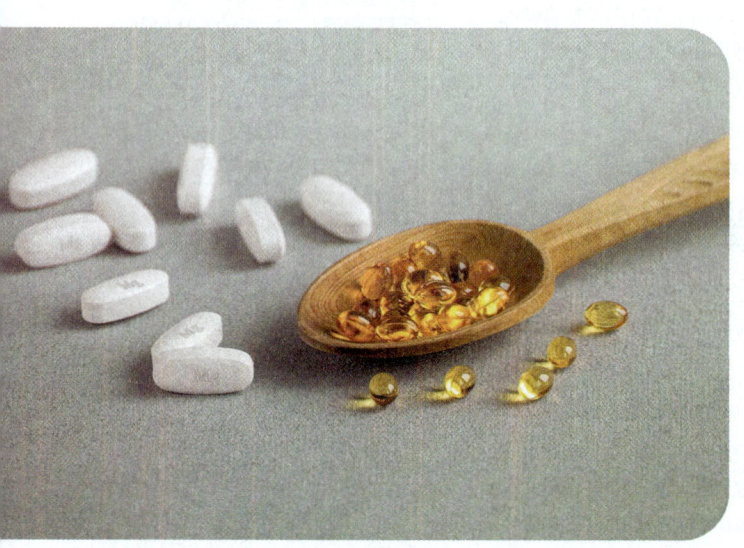

© Sergey Neanderthalec/Shutterstock

Despite data showing that many athletes are deficient in one or more vitamins or minerals, very little evidence supports the idea that over-the-counter supplements, such as a standard multivitamin, address any potential issues that might arise from those deficiencies. However, three strategies can make a difference (**Figure 22.11**). First, the athlete must eat enough food to meet their energy demands. Second, the athlete must focus on foods that have a high ratio of nutrients to calories, a concept known as **nutrient density**. Third, if overt deficiencies are observed and confirmed through blood tests, the athlete must see a medical professional for targeted micronutrient therapy that can help correct overt deficiencies.

NUTRIENT DENSITY →

The ratio of high-quality nutrients to calories in food.

ANTIOXIDANTS →

Nutrients that function in the human body to reduce oxidative stress.

 COACH'S CORNER

Nutrient density is an important concept in nutrition as it relates to how many nutrients (e.g., vitamins and minerals) the food has per unit (e.g., gram) consumed. Generally speaking, foods like fruits, vegetables, and animal products (e.g., meat, dairy, eggs) have greater nutrient density than processed foods (e.g., processed cereal products and processed oils).

| **Eat enough foods to meet energy demands** | **Eat foods with a high ratio of nutrients to calories** | **Refer out to a medical professional for targeted micronutrient therapy** |

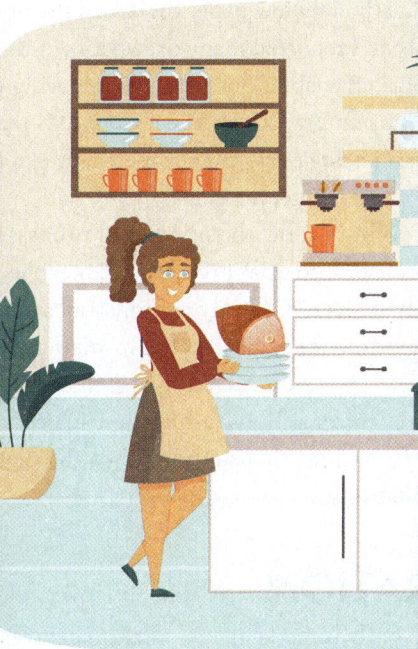
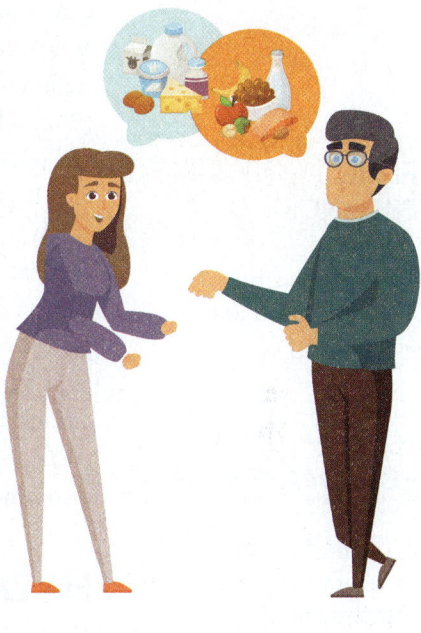

FIGURE 22.11 Strategies for Addressing Potential Issues

ANTIOXIDANTS

Other types of nutrients have drawn a great deal of interest and attention owing to their relation to health and performance, especially **antioxidants**. Antioxidants are nutrients that function in the human body to reduce oxidative stress. Nutrients such as vitamins E and C, selenium, **carotenoids**, and **flavonoids** are established antioxidants and play an important role in addressing oxidative stress. An understanding of antioxidants' role is important for Sport Performance Coaches due to the fact that exercise increases VO_2 by up to 20 times compared to resting values, which results in as much as a 200-fold increase in oxygen usage (Sen, 1995). This increase in oxygen utilization contributes to oxidative stress in skeletal muscle, which is associated with muscle damage and impaired muscle function. Many studies have examined antioxidants and found that they can prevent or reduce oxidative stress and reduce muscle damage (Jakeman & Maxwell, 1993; Nakhostin-Roohi et al., 2008). Although its name might make it sound like a negative process, oxidative stress actually plays a role in the healthy function of cells.

Regular training causes adaptations to elevated oxidant levels in a process known as **hormesis**. Those adaptations include beneficial changes to mitochondria (mitohormesis) (Ristow & Zarse, 2010) and make the body resistant to future oxidative challenges (Peternelj & Coombes, 2011). Researchers have studied the interaction of exercise and supplemental antioxidants in an effort to determine whether the process of trying to reduce oxidative stress has negative consequences. One study found that

CAROTENOIDS →

A class of nutrients that are pigments; they are often yellow, orange, or red.

FLAVONOIDS →

A class of phytonutrients that are pigments; they are found in plants.

HORMESIS →

A characteristic of biological systems that involves the response to stressors in a dose–response manner.

high doses of vitamin C for several days after exercise delayed muscle recovery (Close et al., 2006). Another study found that a mixture of antioxidant nutrients hindered the recovery of muscle damage following a 1000-meter kayak race. A third study found that supplementation with vitamins C and E inhibited the sensitizing effect that exercise has on insulin; it also negatively impacted the body's post-exercise adaptation to antioxidant defenses. Finally, a review paper discussed the findings of 23 studies on supplemental antioxidants and reported many drawbacks of their use. These included stunting of training-induced adaptations such as interfering with insulin signaling and vasodilation (Peternelj & Coombes, 2011). The challenge is that research papers are limited in scope and scientists testing performance metrics are not able to investigate all the potential drawbacks of these interventions.

At this point in time, the number of processes found to be impaired in current exercise-related antioxidant research makes the intake of supplemental antioxidants a risky endeavor, even if a study demonstrates benefit in a specific performance metric. None of the evidence indicates that meals rich in antioxidant-containing foods need to be avoided. However, current research on using those foods, such as blueberries or tart cherry juice, to boost athletic performance is inconsistent. Thus, while they are beneficial options that support a healthy diet, it is difficult to make specific recommendations.

HYDRATION

The human body is made up of approximately 60% water. That water is critical not only for sustaining life, but also for maintaining optimal performance. In the context of performance, water plays two major roles: facilitating energy-producing reactions (e.g., carbohydrate and fat metabolism) and maintaining core body temperature. As such, it is important that the Sport Performance Coach understands hydration and can effectively educate athletes on proper hydration strategies.

> ### 🤖 GETTING TECHNICAL
>
> Water is also important in other key aspects of human physiology that relate to performance. For example, water transports nutrients to tissues, aids in lubricating joints, and cushions the heart, lungs, and eyes.

MAINTAINING FLUID BALANCE

The goal in regard to hydration status is to maintain **fluid balance**, specifically of body water. Similar to the concept of energy balance, fluid balance reflects the relationship between fluid loss and fluid gain. **Euhydration** is a state in which fluid loss and gain are matched, whereas **hyperhydration** is a state in which fluid gain is greater than fluid loss and **hypohydration** is a state in which fluid loss is greater than fluid gain. The term **dehydration** is often used interchangeably with *hypohydration*; in reality, dehydration refers to the process of losing body water, whereas hypohydration refers to the state of hydration.

FLUID BALANCE →

The relationship between fluid loss and fluid gain.

EUHYDRATION →

A state of fluid balance in which fluid loss matches fluid gain.

HYPER-HYDRATION →

A state of fluid balance in which fluid gain is greater than fluid loss.

HYPO-HYDRATION →

A state of fluid balance in which fluid loss is greater than fluid gain.

DEHYDRATION →

The process of losing body water.

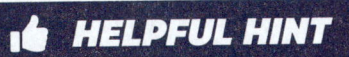
Hypohydration Versus Dehydration
Hypohydration is a state of hydration. Dehydration is the process that leads from euhydration to hypohydration.

HYDRATION AND EVAPORATIVE COOLING

Muscles at work generate heat during exercise, which causes body temperature to rise. If the skin temperature exceeds the temperature of the air, the skin cools through the process of sweat evaporation. Sweating itself does not cause cooling; instead, the evaporation of sweat is responsible for the transfer of heat. If the outside temperature is warmer than the skin, the body gains heat. Humidity exerts a strong influence on this process by limiting the amount of evaporation that occurs. If humidity reaches 100%, sweat does not evaporate, but rather falls off the body or accumulates in clothing, resulting in an increase in body temperature. Additionally, if an individual begins to run low on body water (hypohydration), their ability to regulate their core body temperature is impaired, increasing their risk of hyperthermia.

Dehydration is a well-known phenomenon in sports, yet athletes continue to suffer its effects. Dehydration impacts performance through the following mechanisms:

- Decrease in blood volume
- Reduced skin blood flow
- Reduced sweat rate
- Reduced heat dissipation
- Core temperature elevation
- Higher rate of muscle glycogen use

GETTING TECHNICAL

Any fluid lost through a means other than sweating, including sweat removed with a towel, has no cooling effect. This process is exacerbated by clothing that is not well ventilated; such clothing prevents the airflow that enables evaporation. For this reason, team sports like American football, with its bulky equipment and uniforms, present much different challenges than individual sports like tennis, which do not have specific clothing and equipment requirements. After an athlete starts to sweat, their body progressively dehydrates. As that happens, both the rate of skin blood flow and the rate of sweating eventually decrease, which causes an increase in body temperature. This vicious cycle can ultimately lead to fatigue, heat injury, hospitalization, and even death.

MONITORING HYDRATION WITH WEIGHT

It is wise to get in the habit of checking body weight first thing in the morning after the first urination. Ideally, urine will be pale in color. Large deviations in body weight and darker-colored urine indicate dehydration. After exercise, for each kilogram (2.2 pounds) of body weight lost, 1.5 L (0.4 gallon) of fluid needs to be consumed with the addition of 500 to 700 mg/L of sodium. This ratio allows for complete rehydration within 6 hours (Jeukendrup & Gleeson, 2018).

An athlete needs to consume about 500 mL (17 ounces) of water approximately 2 hours before exercise (American College of Sports Medicine et al., 2000). This allows time for gastric emptying and elimination. The flavor and temperature of the fluid can affect an athlete's ability to drink frequently, so the athlete needs to choose a cool-temperature, palatable flavor. If exercise is less than 45 minutes in duration, there is often no need for fluid replacement until after it ends. During exercise, the athlete needs to consume 120 to 180 mL (4 to 6 ounces) of fluid every 15 to 20 minutes. If exercise lasts at least an hour, the athlete will benefit from the addition of carbohydrates and 500 to 700 mg/L of sodium to promote fluid retention and prevent **hyponatremia**.

Currently available sports drinks are a good option if they are not overly concentrated. Concentrations of carbohydrate exceeding 8% and drinks with a high amount of fructose can cause gastrointestinal upset and need to be avoided unless the athlete has a history of success with the mixture. One challenge with sports drinks is that they tend to contain far less sodium than recommended, so check the label and consider adding additional sodium if needed.

HYPO-NATREMIA →

A state of having lower than normal levels of sodium present in the bloodstream.

Urine color

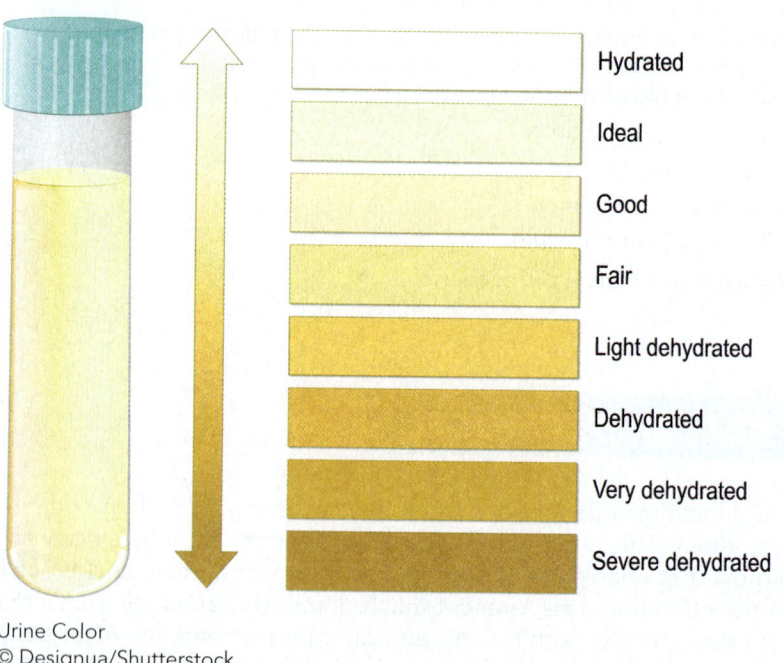

- Hydrated
- Ideal
- Good
- Fair
- Light dehydrated
- Dehydrated
- Very dehydrated
- Severe dehydrated

Urine Color
© Designua/Shutterstock

DEHYDRATION AND HYPONATREMIA SYMPTOMS

Regular exercisers must be familiar with the warning signs of hypohydration so they can act before the condition evolves into heat illness. Thirst and fatigue are often the first signs, followed by flushed skin and muscle cramps. As the condition progresses, the athlete might experience dizziness, chills, headache, nausea, and vomiting. Rehydration, shade, and potentially medical care need to be sought immediately. Heat illness can be a life-threatening condition.

Hyponatremia, also known as water intoxication, arises when excess fluids are consumed without adequate sodium. This condition is possible with consumption of water alone, but it is much more common in athletes who lose sodium in sweat and replace it with plain water. Endurance and ultra-endurance athletes are at the greatest risk for hyponatremia due to the duration of their events. The symptoms are similar to severe dehydration and include headache, vomiting, fatigue, confusion, and swollen hands and feet (McDermott et al., 2017).

📋 COACH'S CORNER

If an endurance athlete exercises for longer than 3 hours and uses a sports drink to meet both fuel (carbohydrates) and hydration needs, the amount of fluid required to meet the recommended 90 grams of carbohydrates per hour will result in hyperhydration. Thus, the athlete needs to consider taking food and drink together if a carbohydrate-containing exercise fluid is used. Exercise duration, intensity, and environment impact fluid and fuel needs differently. To avoid mistakes that might negatively impact performance, an athlete should plan their fueling and hydration strategy prior to training or competition.

DEVELOPING A HYDRATION PLAN

The goal for any hydration plan is for the athlete to (1) arrive at their workout well hydrated, (2) replace fluids as necessary before hypohydration impacts performance, and (3) replace fluids after exercise to reach euhydration. **Table 22.12** shows common hydration strategies for before, during, and after exercise.

TABLE 22.12 Hydration Strategies

Before exercise	Consume water regularly throughout the day, especially before exercise; 500 mL (17 oz) before exercise is encouraged.
	Assess your hydration status by checking your urine color and checking fasting body weight.
	Bring water with you to your exercise/training session or performance.
During exercise	Consume 120–180 mL (4–6 oz) of fluid every 15–20 minutes.
	Utilize thirst as a signal for drinking.
	If engaging in hard exercise, take a systematic approach to hydration.
	Include additional electrolytes to replace lost electrolytes during hard or extended-duration sessions.
	Utilizing flavored beverages may assist in consuming more liquid.
After exercise	For each kilogram (2.2. lb) of body weight lost, 1.5 L (0.4 gal) of fluid. should be consumed—again, with the addition of 500–700 mg/L of sodium.
	Water, milk, and recovery drinks can all be used to replace fluid.

Ideally, hydration during a sporting event will allow the athlete to avoid hyperhydration and maintain fluid intake at no more than 2% to 3% of their body mass. A 2% loss is equivalent to 1.5 L (0.4 gallon) of water for a 70-kg (154-pound) athlete (McDermott et al., 2017). To put that into perspective, strenuous exercise in the heat can induce sweating rates of 2 to 3 L per hour (0.5 to 0.8 gallon per hour), and the maximal fluid intake rate is 1 to 1.5 L per hour (33.8 to 50.7 ounces per hour) due to how fast fluid exits the stomach (Sawka & Coyle, 1999). In practice, that number is probably at the low end of the range for intense exercise, because gastric emptying slows at intensities greater than 70% VO_2 max (Horner et al., 2015). The body then acquires water from elsewhere in the body, including from blood, extracellular fluid, and glycogen, but even after factoring those sources of water, an athlete can still enter a state of hypohydration.

📋 COACH'S CORNER

Exercise has an antidiuretic effect, which means athletes can consume up to, and perhaps more than, 300 mg/day of caffeine without any noticeable impact on urine output. Females have a stronger diuretic effect and might have to experiment with a dosage that works for them (Zhang et al., 2015).

👍 HELPFUL HINT

Athletes participating in sports like running and cycling often derive benefit from a reduction in weight. Consuming water, carrying fluids on their bike (for cyclists), or carrying fluids in a pack or bottle (for runners) adds weight that can impact the athlete's performance. In some situations, hypohydration is mild enough that, if the athlete can tolerate the discomfort, there are performance gains from not hydrating. The amount of fluid consumed or carried needs to be tailored to the heat, intensity, hydration state, and remaining workload. Skipping that final fueling station or dumping the contents of a water bottle can sometimes make a positive difference in performance as long as it is done safely.

LESSON 5: INTRODUCTION TO ASSESSING ATHLETE NUTRITION

DIETARY ASSESSMENT: THE BASICS

Assessing an athlete's nutrition needs and their current nutrition behaviors is one of the most important parts of the nutrition coaching component for a Sports Performance Coach. Nutrition and dietary assessments are beneficial and essential tools because they objectively measure athletes' behavior related to their goals. The Sports Performance Coach needs to use these assessments at the beginning of any coaching relationship to establish a baseline, in the middle of the coaching relationship to measure and assess progress, and at the end to determine changes and establish metrics around the success of the programs that the coach and the athlete engaged in together.

The best method for performing a dietary assessment depends on the coach and athlete, as well as the situation in which the coaching relationship is occurring. There are several industry standard approaches and tools that the Sports Performance Coach might consider using, including the Food Frequency Questionnaire, 24-hour dietary recall, and diet records and food journals.

FOOD FREQUENCY QUESTIONNAIRE

The **Food Frequency Questionnaire (FFQ)** is a tool used in research or clinical settings to assess food habits and patterns at a high level. The FFQ is most famously used in the National Health and Nutrition Examination Survey (NHANES) research study. It relies on a preset list of foods and collects data for a long period of time, typically 7 to 30 days, but is sometimes used to assess food behaviors over a period of several years. It is a good choice for estimating a typical diet, but is better suited to institutional settings than to individual athletes and coaches. The FFQ is not very accurate at an individual level, and it lacks details that are required when working with clients on an individual basis. The full Food Frequency Questionnaire can be found in Appendix E.

24-HOUR DIETARY RECALL

Another method of dietary assessment is the **24-hour dietary recall**. This method involves talking with a client and asking them to recall everything they ate and drank the previous day. This assessment technique is simpler than the FFQ but is subject to errors, such as people forgetting snacks or misjudging quantities of food. The 24-hour recall method can also be significantly biased based on how the interviewer asks questions, when they ask questions, and which types of questions they ask. This approach might be more appropriate in an individual coaching setting because it can provide more details than an FFQ. A 24-Hour Dietary Recall worksheet can be found in Appendix E.

DIET RECORDS/FOOD JOURNALS

A **diet record (food journal)** involves real-time tracking of an individual's food on paper, an app, or a computer. In today's digital world, several high-quality tools have been developed with accurate databases that enable individuals to effectively log the types of foods they consume and the nutrient contents of those foods. One strength of this approach is the convenience of an app or other technology, which allows people to enter the specific quantities of each food or drink consumed during a meal or snack. The user can scan items with barcodes with a cell phone camera to add the item to their log. These apps allow the user to easily select frequently eaten foods again in the future. After the user enters their portion sizes, the app calculates the estimated calorie count, macronutrient ratios, and select micronutrients. Any meal that a user does not enter can be written down, added later, or estimated at the end of the day, much as with the 24-hour dietary recall. The diet record is often the recommended tool when working directly with athletes because it allows the coach and client to have a real-time understanding of the exact types, amounts, and timing of the foods the athlete is consuming. A Diet Record Worksheet can be found in Appendix E.

Regardless of the method used, the Sports Performance Coach needs to thoroughly explain the assessments and encourage the athlete to be as honest and accurate as possible and to ask questions if anything is unclear. **Table 22.13** compares the various types of dietary assessments.

DIETARY ASSESSMENT IN PRACTICE

When conducting a dietary assessment, the Sports Performance Coach must remember that the overarching goal when utilizing any assessment tool is to capture enough

---

FOOD FREQUENCY QUESTION-NAIRE (FFQ) →

A survey questionnaire that utilizes a preset list of foods and asks about the frequency of consumption.

24-HOUR DIETARY RECALL →

A method of dietary assessment that involves talking with a client and asking them to recall everything they ate and drank on the previous day.

DIET RECORD (FOOD JOURNAL) →

A method of dietary assessment involving real-time tracking of an individual's food on paper, an app, or a computer.

TABLE 22.13 Dietary Assessments: Strengths and Weaknesses

Dietary Assessment	Description	Strengths	Weaknesses
Food Frequency Questionnaire (FFQ)	Athletes report whether they consumed a variety of foods and beverages over the past 12 months, identifying them as rarely, sometimes, or consistently used, along with an estimated portion size.	Useful for estimating long-term food and beverage habits. Provides estimates of foods and beverages consumed with high frequencies. Low burden on the client.	Can inaccurately capture foods that are culturally specific. Restricted to items that are specifically listed in the instrument. Subjective reporting of frequencies might not be accurate for a 12-month recall.
24-hour dietary recall	Athletes recall their past 24 hours of food and beverage intake, including what was consumed, at what time, where, and why it was consumed.	Provides detailed information of the previous day's total dietary intake. Low burden on the client.	Does not account for day-to-day intake variations. Not recommended for individuals who have trouble with memory. Items can easily be forgotten. Needs to follow an average day of eating and avoid holidays, vacations, and weekends.
Diet record/ food journal	All foods and beverages are recorded by the client as they are consumed, usually over several days.	Provides detailed information on all food and beverages consumed, along with portion size description, calories, protein, carbohydrates, and fats. Provides good estimates of total nutrient intake. Little reliance on memory if it is filled out as foods are consumed. Captures average days along with outliers like weekends and holidays.	Can be labor intensive to maintain as days of recording increase. Can potentially cause people to change their habits while recording their intake. Users must be competent in estimating portion sizes for accurate information.

variations in the diet to get a representative picture of intake. As such, when performing a dietary assessment, the Sports Performance Coach needs to collect data consistently over multiple days. It can also help to do repeat assessments a few weeks apart to ensure that the days captured in the initial assessment truly reflect an athlete's habits.

Body weight is another key metric because it is a good proxy for energy balance. Measuring body weight after urinating in the morning is helpful to see if there is an energy surplus, deficit, or balance. Stable weight over several days suggests energy balance, weight loss indicates a deficit, and weight gain indicates a surplus (**Figure 22.12**).

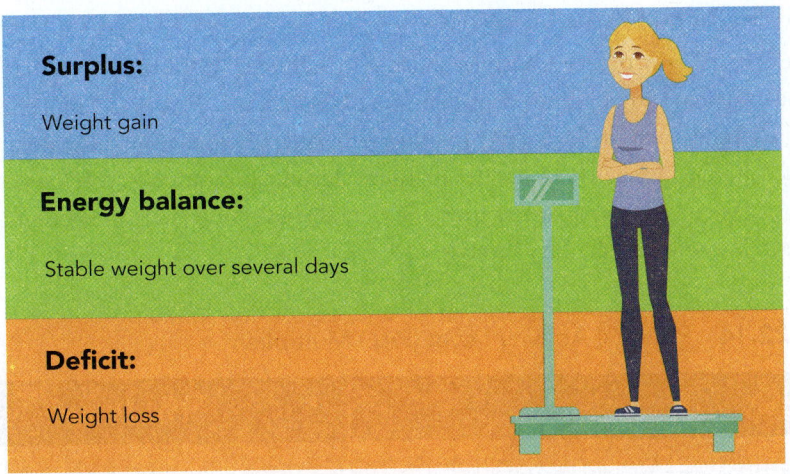

FIGURE 22.12 Measuring Body Weight for Energy Balance

DETERMINING ENERGY NEEDS

The first principle that a Sports Performance Coach needs to consider when assessing and determining the nutrition recommendations for an athlete is their energy needs. If an athlete has too little energy, they are unlikely to perform at their peak capacity and have an increased risk of getting sick or injured. If an athlete has too much energy, they might gain unnecessary body weight, which could impair their performance or increase their risk of chronic diseases. As such, it is important for the Sports Performance Coach to accurately estimate and then test the energy needs of the athlete because energy requirements vary substantially between individuals. For example, the energy requirements can differ by as much as 2,000 kcal a day for a triathlete who trains 6 to 8 hours a day, 5 days a week, and a recreational team sports athlete who trains 2 or 3 days a week, for an hour at a time, and competes once a week.

There are two primary ways for a Sports Performance Coach to determine the energy needs of an athlete: estimate them using validated estimating equations or track the athlete's current intake and adjust it based on any changes in body weight. Using an equation to estimate caloric requirements is the most common method because it can be done immediately, and the process takes significantly less work on the athlete's part. However, the advantage it offers in speed is offset by poorer accuracy, as any calculations done with equations are never entirely accurate on an individual level. Conversely, an athlete manually tracking their intake and body weight is not only a slower process but also involves a learning curve that can be frustrating or difficult, especially when the athlete has no experience with this process.

If the Sports Performance Coach opts to utilize estimating equations, there are two steps that they need to follow to get the best starting point:

1. Determine the athlete's basal metabolic rate (BMR) using one of the estimating equations.
2. Adjust the athlete's BMR for daily activity.

ESTIMATE BMR

The Sports Performance Coach can utilize several published estimating equations for BMR. One of the most commonly used options is the Mifflin–St. Jeor equation, which takes into consideration the athlete's age, height, and body mass:

Men: BMR = (10 × weight in kg) + (6.25 × height in cm) − (5 × age in years) + 5

Women: BMR = (10 × weight in kg) + (6.25 × height in cm) − (5 × age in years) − 161

ADJUST FOR PHYSICAL ACTIVITY

After the Sports Performance Coach establishes the athlete's BMR, they need to take additional physical activities into consideration (**Table 22.14**). This is accomplished by applying a physical activity level (PAL) multiplier. Generally speaking, individuals who are considered athletes are active or greater on the scale, but some athletes who have sedentary jobs and engage in more skill-based sports (e.g., golf) have total energy expenditures that are more in line with a sedentary lifestyle.

TABLE 22.14 Physical Activity Level (PAL) Multiplier

Category	PAL Value
Sedentary or light activity lifestyle	1.40–1.69
Active or moderately active lifestyle	1.70–1.99
Vigorous or vigorously active lifestyle	2.00–2.40

DETERMINING MACRONUTRIENT REQUIREMENTS

After a Sports Performance Coach determines an athlete's energy needs, it is time to determine how those calories should be divided among the different macronutrients. Determining macronutrient requirements for performance nutrition is different from the process for general nutrition or nutrition for weight loss because athletes have more specific requirements for macronutrients than other populations. An appropriate way to determine the appropriate macronutrient levels is by finding the protein and carbohydrate requirements for an individual based on their sport and training volume and then filling in the remaining calories from fats. **Table 22.15** highlights weight-based protein and carbohydrate recommendations based on sport and training volume.

The best way to understand macronutrient needs is to work through an example. Imagine you have a client named Roberto. Roberto is a 5 feet 9 inches (175 cm), 165-pound (75-kg), 32-year-old male marathon runner who trains 5 days per week, approximately 2 to 3 hours per session, but has a sedentary job as an accountant. Roberto has a healthy body weight, but wants to ensure that he has enough energy to effectively train and recover. Here is how to work out his energy and nutrient needs based on the recommendations and proposed process.

Step 1: Determine BMR
    Men: BMR = $(10 \times 75 \text{ kg}) + (6.25 \times 175) - (5 \times 32) + 5 = 1{,}689$ kcal
Step 2: Adjust for physical activity
    Using a PAL of 2.0, Roberto's total energy needs is $(1{,}689 \times 2.0) = 3{,}380$ kcal.
Step 3: Set protein and carbohydrate requirements
    Roberto is an endurance athlete who falls on the higher end of the protein requirements, so his protein is set at 1.6 g/kg, which is 120 grams of protein, or 480 calories from protein.
        Roberto's training volume is moderate to high intensity at 1 to 3 hours, so his carbohydrate requirements are approximately 6 g/kg, or 450 grams of carbohydrates. This is 1,800 calories from carbohydrates.

TABLE 22.15 Weight-Based Protein and Carbohydrate Recommendations Based on Sport and Training Volume

Protein Recommendations	
Sport Type	**Protein Intake Range (g/kg)**
Endurance	1.2–1.6
Strength and power	1.6–2.0
Team sports	1.4–1.8
Injury	2–2.4
Aged (40–80 years)	1.6–2.0
Aged (> 80 years)	2–2.4
Carbohydrate Recommendations	
Training Volume	**Carbohydrate Intake Range (g/kg)**
Low intensity or skill-based activities	3–5
Moderate exercise ≤ 1 hour	5–7
Moderate to high intensity 1–3 hours	6–10
Moderate to high intensity ≥ 4 hours	10–12

Determining his fat intake is a matter of filling in his remaining calories from fats:

3,380 kcal – 480 protein kcal – 1,800 carbohydrate kcal = 1,100 kcal from fat.

1,100 kcal/9 kcal per gram = 122 grams of fat.

These basic steps and guidelines can be followed to determine starting points for macronutrient intakes. The coach and athlete need to work together to make adjustments based on personal preferences and feedback from the athlete and their training performance.

MICRONUTRIENT CONSIDERATIONS BASED ON DIETARY PRINCIPLES

In addition to addressing macronutrient requirements, nutrition coaches work with clients to provide education around food choices to help them meet their micronutrient requirements. It can be difficult to provide clear, detailed instructions to athletes that will ensure they meet micronutrient requirements. However, helping clients understand the core principles and building habits around those principles can help them satisfy their micronutrient needs.

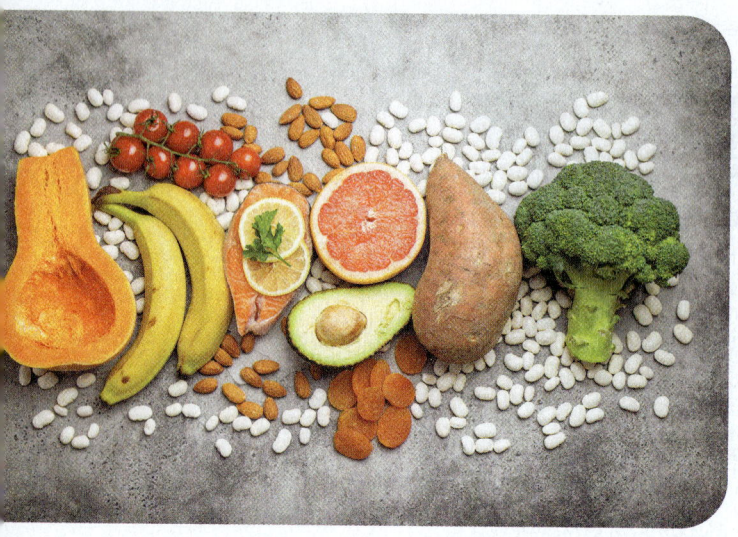
© Elena Eryomenko/Shutterstock

One of the first principles is to focus the diet on nutrient-dense foods. These foods have high levels of nutrients per gram of food consumed. Foods often considered nutrient-dense include fruits, vegetables, nuts, seeds, eggs, fish, and lean meats. These foods provide very high levels of vitamins and minerals per gram and per unit of energy. Basing a diet on these foods can help athletes successfully meet their nutrient requirements.

Another principle is to limit processed food intake. Although some athletes need to consume processed foods due to unusually high calorie needs, most need to keep their processed food intake to a small percentage of their diet. The main reason for this is that, with the exception of fortified foods, most processed foods contain very few micronutrients.

The last principle is to eat a varied diet, which is often colloquialized as "eat the rainbow." Oftentimes, foods of different colors contain different micronutrients, and eating a variety of them helps an athlete consume a broad base of micronutrients. Thus, when structuring dietary patterns, it is important to eat a variety of foods over the course of a week or month, whenever possible.

SPECIFIC GOAL EXAMPLES

In addition to meeting energy needs and optimizing performance through nutrition, the Sports Performance Coach might work with athletes on specific goals that could require specific nutrition strategies. Specifically, some athletes might want to add muscle mass, and others might need to lose body mass. Each approach requires different strategies and tactics.

MUSCLE GAIN STRATEGIES

Gaining muscle, or lean mass, requires two specific things: sending the body the correct signals to trigger muscle growth and a calorie surplus. The nutrition component of coaching for sports performance focuses on calorie surplus. In addition to there being a calorie surplus, it is important that the Sports Performance Coach understands what an appropriate calorie surplus is and what type of nutrients need to make up that surplus.

Determining the correct calorie surplus requires striking a balance to ensure that the athlete is maximizing their body's ability to add lean muscle tissue while simultaneously minimizing how much adipose tissue (fat tissue) gets added along with lean muscle tissue. Recent evidence suggests that the ideal calorie surplus ranges between 300 and 500 calories per day above energy balance (weight stable) (Slater et al., 2019). In addition to having a smart calorie surplus, the sources of those calories might affect whether the calories go to lean mass or fat mass. There are limited data on this topic, but most evidence suggests that focusing on protein and carbohydrates as the source of surplus calories is more likely to favor lean mass accumulation over fat mass accumulation (Horton et al., 1995; Minehira et al., 2004; Slater et al., 2019).

If an athlete were to apply these nutrition strategies with the goal of muscle gain, **Table 22.16** shows what it might look like for an 80-kg (176-pound) male who is weight stable at an intake of 3,100 calories.

TABLE 22.16 Example: Muscle Gain Strategies

Selections	What Does It Look Like?
Calorie	Building muscle mass is easiest in a surplus. In this case, a 500-calorie surplus was chosen with a final goal of 3,600 calories. There appears to be an advantage to adding a couple of snacks in addition to three daily meals when eating in a surplus.
Protein	A 2.2-g/kg intake of protein was chosen for weight gain while minimizing fat, which is 176 grams of protein (2.2 × 80). Total calories from protein = 704 (176 × 4).
Carbohydrate	Based on exercise intensity and duration, 7-g/kg intake of carbohydrate was chosen, which is 560 grams of carbohydrate (7 × 80). Total calories from carbohydrate = 2,240 (560 × 4).
Total	The goal was 3,600 calories, which allows 800 calories (3,600 − 2,800) for fat. This equals 22% calories available for fat (800 / 3600), which fits the 20% to 35% recommendation.

FAT LOSS STRATEGIES

Some athletes require bodyweight loss for their sport. This loss could be needed to meet a weight class for competition or for improving power-to-weight ratios in sports such as cycling. In ideal cases, this weight loss needs be targeted toward fat loss. As with lean mass gains, it is important for the Sports Performance Coach to consider the magnitude of the energy deficit required to lose body mass as well as which macronutrients should be reduced to meet the decreased energy requirements.

Current evidence-based guidelines recommend a modest deficit of around 250 to 500 calories per day for most athletes (Thomas et al., 2016). Furthermore, it is important that athletes continue to meet the necessary protein requirements to maintain lean mass and to ensure that they are consuming enough carbohydrates to fuel the work they are doing during training and competition. As such, most of the calorie reduction comes from lowering fat calories first and carbohydrate and protein calories second.

Calorie restriction can come with many challenges, one of which is how to control appetite during periods when an athlete is consuming less food. The Sports Performance Coach must consider the various factors that affect appetite, keeping the following recommendations in mind:

- Focus on complex carbohydrates that include adequate fiber and fewer simple sugars.
- Avoid sugar-sweetened beverages.
- Maintain a normal sleep pattern with enough total sleep per night.
- Eat slowly. Chewing food well is a good trick to encourage slower eating.
- Avoid environments that encourage higher-calorie feedings, such as all-you-can-eat buffets.

Table 22.17 is an example in which fat loss is the goal. In this case, the athlete is an 80-kg (176-pound) male who is weight stable at an intake of 3,100 calories.

As a final note, there is a common misconception that exercise of low to medium intensity is better for fat loss because this intensity burns the highest percentage of fat for fuel. It is important to look at longer time frames when evaluating fat oxidation and fat loss from exercise. As an example, one study of high-intensity interval training compared

TABLE 22.17 Example: Fat Loss Strategies

Selections	What Does It Look Like?
Calorie	A negative energy balance is best for fat loss. In this case, a 500-calorie deficit was chosen with a final goal of 2,600 calories.
Protein	A 1.6-g/kg intake of protein was chosen for weight gain while minimizing fat. That is 128 grams of protein (1.6 × 80). Total calories from protein = 512 (128 × 4).
Carbohydrate	Based on exercise intensity and duration, a 5-g/kg intake of carbohydrate was chosen. That is 400 grams of carbohydrate (5 × 80). Total calories from carbohydrate = 1,600 (400 × 4).
Total	The 1,600 calories from carbohydrate + 512 calories from protein equals 2,112 total calories. The goal was 2,600 calories, which leaves 488 calories (2,600 − 2,112) from fat. That comes out to 18.8% fat (488/2,600), which is lower than the recommended 20% to 35%. This is very close, and many athletes would still use this macronutrient distribution. If interpreting the guidelines literally, either protein needs to be reduced, carbohydrates need be reduced, or calories need to be increased until fat reaches 20% of calories.

to lower-intensity endurance training found that for the same number of calories burned, the higher-intensity training resulted in more fat loss while also achieving a larger long-term (longer than 24 hours) effect on fat burning (Tremblay et al., 1994). There are pros and cons to all forms of exercise, and fat loss is within reach whether exercise burns fat or carbohydrates.

LESSON 6: COMMON SPORTS DIETS

POPULAR DIETS FOR PERFORMANCE NUTRITION

Much like the broader field of nutrition, performance nutrition is strongly influenced by media, culture, and professional athletes and celebrities. Over the past several decades, several different diets have been popularized as effective tools for achieving optimal performance or hacking the body into achieving never-before-seen levels of achievement. These diets include the ketogenic diet, the paleo diet, and plant-based/vegan diets.

KETOGENIC DIET FOR PERFORMANCE

Ketogenic diets aim to have the individual reach a state of nutritional ketosis, primarily through carbohydrate restriction. People have a variety of reasons for choosing a ketogenic diet. This section focuses on increases in athletic performance. Evaluating the potential performance effects of a ketogenic diet requires a quick review of current evidence.

First, a 2018 study looked at strength, endurance, and high-intensity interval training outcomes for participants on a ketogenic diet versus a high-carbohydrate diet (McSwiney et al., 2018). The researchers documented several performance benefits for the ketogenic-diet group, but further review revealed a major limitation. The ketogenic-diet group lost over seven times more weight, 11.25 pounds, than the high-carbohydrate-diet group. It is difficult to interpret the performance benefits of an intervention when a key metric like weight shows such drastic differences. Six other trials found ketogenic diets impaired exercise performance (Burke et al., 2017; Burke et al., 2020; Burke et al., 2021; Fleming et al., 2003; Whitfield et al., 2021; Wroble et al., 2019).

In terms of how studies are conducted, it is common for studies of ketogenic diets to use **time to exhaustion (TTE)** as a determination of the effectiveness of the intervention. Unfortunately, that might not be a good measure for endurance performance (Faude et al., 2017; McLellan et al., 1995)—after all, sporting events do not generally require the competitor to continue at a low steady-state intensity until they fail from exhaustion. Results from actual competition are a much better metric.

The application of ketogenic diets in sports that appears the most promising involves competitions where circumstances make it difficult to ingest enough carbohydrates to complete the event, such as ultra-endurance running events, or where ingestion of carbohydrates induces nausea. In regard to nausea, the Sports Performance Coach and athlete must first troubleshoot the cause in case the issue can be resolved without having to restrict performance-enhancing carbohydrate intake (Wilson, 2019). Nausea might occur for many reasons during exercise:

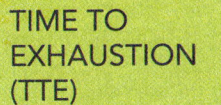

TIME TO EXHAUSTION (TTE) →

The time remaining before a specific level of work (power or intensity) can no longer be maintained.

- Catecholamine secretion (such as adrenaline)
- Hypohydration
- Heat stress
- Hyponatremia
- Altitude exposure
- Excessive food or fluid consumption
- Overly concentrated beverages
- Pre-exercise intake of fatty or protein-rich foods (especially consumed near exercise)
- Prolonged fasting
- Various supplements (caffeine, sodium bicarbonate, ketones)
- Certain drugs (antibiotics, opioids)
- Stomach infections
- Anxiety related to competition

Ultimately, the evidence does not support endurance performance gains as the main reason for pursuing a ketogenic diet. Lower-intensity events are less likely to be negatively impacted by adoption of this diet.

PALEO DIET FOR PERFORMANCE

The premise behind a paleo diet is to follow a dietary pattern that mimics pre-agriculture human society by limiting consumption of grains, legumes, most processed foods, and dairy. There are many ways to implement a paleo diet, so it is difficult to definitively state how the fundamental diet affects performance nutrition.

The hallmark of a paleo diet is the list of foods that it excludes, which is one of its potential shortcomings. The exclusion of foods such as white potatoes, dairy products, most grains, sugar, and legumes (peanuts, lentils, peas, beans) poses a potential threat to adequate intake of the nutrients

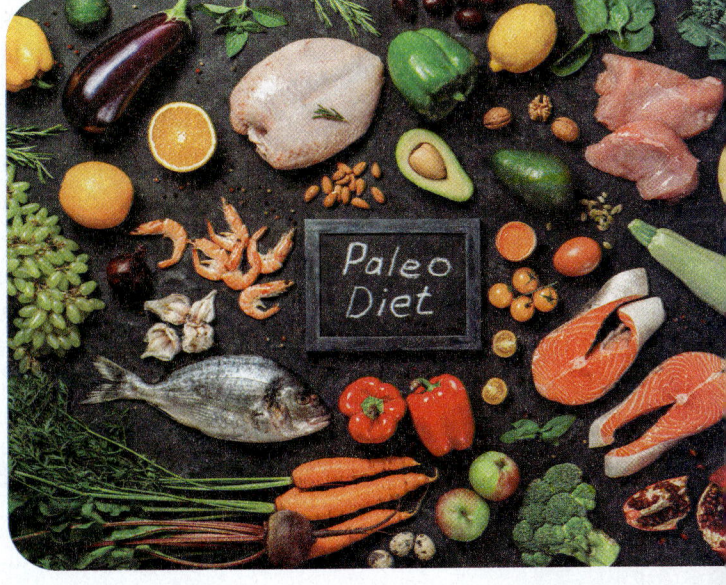

© Fascinadora/Shutterstock

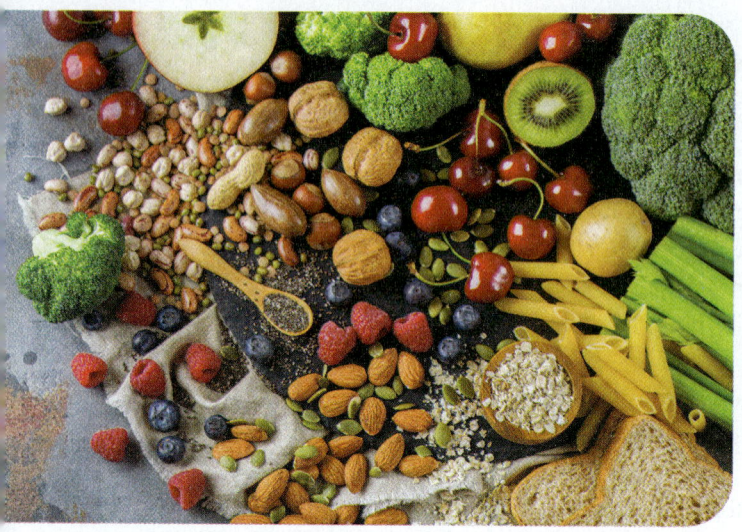
© Antonina Vlasova/Shutterstock

found in those foods—namely, calcium, dietary fiber, resistant starch, and more generally carbohydrates (a full list is provided in the Paleo Diet Exclusions in Appendix E). Additionally, if the dietary restrictions are not well implemented, they can result in the diet being too low in calories to support vigorous activity. A dietary assessment is critical to evaluate the energy and macronutrient balance of an athlete's diet. If the implementation leads to high fat and low carbohydrate consumption, then the advice regarding ketogenic diets applies, as do the energy and carbohydrate requirements. However, if a paleo diet is well composed, there is no reason from a performance perspective for an athlete to avoid it.

VEGAN DIET FOR PERFORMANCE

Vegan diets exclude all animal products, including meat, eggs, seafood, fish, dairy products, and honey. Those exclusions put vegans at risk of having low intakes of protein, creatine, carnitine, the amino acid leucine, the omega-3 fatty acids EPA and DHA, iron, calcium, vitamin D, iodine, zinc, and vitamin B_{12} (Appleby & Key, 2016; Clarys et al., 2014; Craig, 2009). A vegan diet is similar to a paleo diet in that it is defined by what it excludes. Because the very things vegans avoid—animal products—are dense in calories, one risk of a vegan diet is the failure to meet the energy needs of active individuals.

Another challenge is that plant-based protein sources have higher concentrations of antinutrients, such as trypsin inhibitors, phytates, and tannins, which inhibit the digestion and absorption of protein (Sarwar Gilani et al., 2012). These compounds are partially eliminated through cooking, but because plants are lower in leucine, any additional challenges incrementally limit the anabolic potential of the diet.

A careful and well-rounded, calorie-dense diet complete with supplementation of nutrients in which an individual is deficient can enable any athlete at any level to successfully follow a vegan diet. Vegan protein powders are an especially good resource because they bypass the issue of antinutrients and the dosage can be tailored to match the leucine amounts needed by athletes (van Vliet et al., 2015). It is important to note that many of the nutrients potentially deficient in a vegan diet cannot be easily tested to determine their adequacy—specifically, calcium, carnosine, creatine, and iodine as well as EPA and DHA.

The Sports Performance Coach must monitor the athlete's food intake for nutrient sufficiency to find which nutrients need to be supplemented. Creatine, for example, is not found in any plant foods. It is synthesized in the liver, but vegans and vegetarians have lower levels than omnivores (Kaviani et al., 2020).

The Sports Performance Coach must also consider the potential drawbacks and shortcomings of a vegan or plant-based diet and work with athletes to ameliorate any of those drawbacks and shortcomings. There have been many successful vegan strength, power, and endurance athletes over the years, which is a testament to the fact that this diet can be a successful option when approached with care.

SUMMARY

Nutrition is pivotal in human performance, as it provides the energy necessary to fuel the body's movement and activity. This energy, which is stored as chemical energy in food, is transformed into mechanical energy via human metabolism, a process crucial for all forms of physical exertion.

Given this central role of nutrition, Sports Performance Coaches must have a solid grasp of the fundamentals of performance nutrition. They should understand how different types of nutrients support training, performance, and recovery. In this context, educating athletes about their energy requirements and metabolism relative to their specific sports becomes an integral part of the coaching process.

When diving into performance nutrition, Sports Performance Coaches must pay close attention to their scope of practice. The laws defining this scope can vary regionally and should be thoroughly reviewed by each professional. Coaches are primarily responsible for discussing and providing guidelines on nutrition. However, providing specific in-depth nutrition advice or personalized meal planning might fall outside a coach's purview and be better handled by a registered dietitian or other certified nutrition professionals. Coaches must acknowledge their limitations and responsibly refer athletes to qualified professionals when the situation calls for it.

Effective coaching in performance nutrition relies on a thorough understanding of each athlete's unique energy and nutrient needs based on their specific sport and training load. Energy balance, the concept of calories as a measure of energy in food, the components of energy expenditure, and the factors influencing energy need all come into play here. A comprehensive plan that adapts to the ever-changing needs of day-to-day and month-to-month training is vital to achieving peak mental and physical performance. Moreover, coaches should be aware of the influence of media and popular diets on performance nutrition and employ various tools for assessing an athlete's nutrition needs and behaviors. The appropriate levels of macronutrients (carbohydrates, proteins, and fats) and micronutrients are also vital for fueling exercise and supporting overall health. This balancing act should be part of the conversation with athletes about their dietary habits and choices.

KEY TAKEAWAYS

- Energy balance is important for maintaining weight, body composition, and general health.
- Macronutrient and micronutrient intake that meets the demands of training and recovery is a fundamental requirement to make progress as an athlete.
- Protein recommendations range from approximately 1.6 g/kg to 2.2 g/kg per day, with endurance athletes falling at the lower end of that continuum and strength/power athletes falling at the higher end.
- Carbohydrate recommendations range from 3 to 12 g/kg per day based on the type of training and the volume of training an athlete engages in.
- Hydration is a pivotal component of success. Strategies for food and drink need to be planned in advance to accommodate optimal pre-, intra-, and post-workout intake.
- Replacing fluid following competition includes consuming 20 to 180 mL (4 to 6 ounces) of fluid every 15 to 20 minutes during competition, and 1.5 L (0.4 gallon) of fluid after competition for every 1 kg of body weight lost during competition, all with the addition of 500 to 700 mg/L of sodium (Jeukendrup & Gleeson, 2018).
- When an athlete needs to gain or lose weight, it is important that they identify the correct calorie changes. When attempting to gain lean body mass (muscle tissue), they need to set calorie surplus targets at 300 to 500 kcal per day. When attempting to lose fat mass, they need to set calorie deficit targets at 250 to 500 kcal per day.
- The success or failure of any diet is sensitive to its ability to provide necessary calories and nutrients, as well as the level of difficulty of implementing the diet. Athletes and coaches need to approach restrictive diets with care.

REFERENCES

Aller, E. E. J. G., Abete, I., Astrup, A., Martinez, J. A., & van Baak, M. A. (2011). Starches, sugars and obesity. *Nutrients, 3*(3), 341–369.

American College of Sports Medicine, American Dietetic Association, & Dietitians of Canada. (2000). Joint position statement: Nutrition and athletic performance. American College of Sports Medicine,

American Dietetic Association, and Dietitians of Canada. *Medicine & Science in Sports & Exercise, 32*(12), 2130–2145.

Appleby, P. N. & Key, T. J. (2016). The long-term health of vegetarians and vegans. *Proceedings of the Nutrition Society, 75*(3), 287–293.

Areta, J. L., Burke, L. M., Ross, M. L., Camera, D. M., West, D. W. D., Broad, E. M., Jeacocke, N. A., Moore, D. R., Stellingwerff, T., Phillips, S. M., Hawley, J. A., & Coffey, V. G. (2013). Timing and distribution of protein ingestion during prolonged recovery from resistance exercise alters myofibrillar protein synthesis. *Journal of Physiology, 591*(9), 2319–2331.

Areta, J. L., Taylor, H. L., & Koehler, K. (2021). Low energy availability: History, definition and evidence of its endocrine, metabolic and physiological effects in prospective studies in females and males. *European Journal of Applied Physiology, 121*(1), 1–21.

Barkoukis, H. (2016). Nutrition recommendations in elderly and aging. *Medical Clinics of North America, 100*(6), 1237–1250.

Berezovikova, I., Denisova, D., & Shcherbakova, L. (2021). Underestimation of energy intake in overweight Siberian adolescents. *European Journal of Public Health, 31*(suppl 3). https://doi.org/10.1093/eurpub/ckab165.559

Biolo, G., Gastaldelli, A., Zhang, X. J., & Wolfe, R. R. (1994). Protein synthesis and breakdown in skin and muscle: A leg model of amino acid kinetics. *American Journal of Physiology, 267*(3 pt 1), E467–E474. https://doi.org/10.1152/ajpendo.1994.267.3.E467

Bob Murray, C. R. (2018). Fundamentals of glycogen metabolism for coaches and athletes. *Nutrition Reviews, 76*(4), 243.

Burd, N. A., Gorissen, S. H., & van Loon, L. J. C. (2013). Anabolic resistance of muscle protein synthesis with aging. *Exercise and Sport Sciences Reviews, 41*(3), 169–173.

Burke, L. M. (2001). Energy needs of athletes. *Canadian Journal of Applied Physiology/Revue Canadienne de Physiologie Appliquee, 26*(suppl), S202–S219.

Burke, L. M., Hawley, J. A., Jeukendrup, A., Morton, J. P., Stellingwerff, T., & Maughan, R. J. (2018). Toward a common understanding of diet–exercise strategies to manipulate fuel availability for training and competition preparation in endurance sport. *International Journal of Sport Nutrition and Exercise Metabolism, 28*(5), 451–463. https://doi.org/10.1123/ijsnem.2018-0289

Burke, L. M., Ross, M. L., Garvican-Lewis, L. A., Welvaert, M., Heikura, I. A., Forbes, S. G., Mirtschin, J. G., Cato, L. E., Strobel, N., Sharma, A. P., & Hawley, J. A. (2017). Low carbohydrate, high fat diet impairs exercise economy and negates the performance benefit from intensified training in elite race walkers. *Journal of Physiology, 595*(9), 2785–2807.

Burke, L. M., Sharma, A. P., Heikura, I. A., Forbes, S. F., Holloway, M., McKay, A. K. A., Bone, J. L., Leckey, J. J., Welvaert, M., & Ross, M. L. (2020). Crisis of confidence averted: Impairment of exercise economy and performance in elite race walkers by ketogenic low carbohydrate, high fat (LCHF) diet is reproducible. *PLoS One, 15*(6), e0234027.

Burke, L. M., Whitfield, J., Heikura, I. A., Ross, M. L. R., Tee, N., Forbes, S. F., Hall, R., McKay, A. K. A., Wallett, A. M., & Sharma, A. P. (2021). Adaptation to a low carbohydrate high fat diet is rapid but impairs endurance exercise metabolism and performance despite enhanced glycogen availability. *Journal of Physiology, 599*(3), 771–790.

Carlsen, M. H., Lillegaard, I. T. L., Karlsen, A., Blomhoff, R., Drevon, C. A., & Andersen, L. F. (2010). Evaluation of energy and dietary intake estimates from a food frequency questionnaire using independent energy expenditure measurement and weighed food records. *Nutrition Journal, 9*(1), 1–9.

Cassady, B. A., Considine, R. V., & Mattes, R. D. (2012). Beverage consumption, appetite, and energy intake: What did you expect? *American Journal of Clinical Nutrition, 95*(3), 587–593.

Chatham, R. E. & Mixer, S. J. (2020). Cultural influences on childhood obesity in ethnic minorities: A qualitative systematic review. *Journal of Transcultural Nursing: Official Journal of the Transcultural Nursing Society, 31*(1), 87–99.

Clarys, P., Deliens, T., Huybrechts, I., Deriemaeker, P., Vanaelst, B., De Keyzer, W., Hebbelinck, M., & Mullie, P. (2014). Comparison of nutritional quality of the vegan, vegetarian, semi-vegetarian, pesco-vegetarian and omnivorous diet. *Nutrients, 6*(3), 1318–1332.

Close, G. L., Ashton, T., Cable, T., Doran, D., Holloway, C., McArdle, F., & MacLaren, D. P. M. (2006). Ascorbic acid supplementation does not attenuate post-exercise muscle soreness following muscle-damaging exercise but may delay the recovery process. *British Journal of Nutrition, 95*(5), 976–981.

Coyle, E. F. (1995). Substrate utilization during exercise in active people. *American Journal of Clinical Nutrition, 61*(4 suppl), 968S–979S.

Coyle, E. F., Jeukendrup, A. E., Oseto, M. C., Hodgkinson, B. J., & Zderic, T. W. (2001). Low-fat diet alters intramuscular substrates and reduces lipolysis and fat oxidation during exercise. *American Journal of Physiology, Endocrinology and Metabolism, 280*(3), E391–E398.

Craig, W. J. (2009). Health effects of vegan diets. *American Journal of Clinical Nutrition, 89*(5), 1627S–1633S.

de Graaf, C., & Kok, F. J. (2010). Slow food, fast food and the control of food intake. *Nature Reviews. Endocrinology, 6*(5), 290–293.

de Vries, J. H., Zock, P. L., Mensink, R. P., & Katan, M. B. (1994). Underestimation of energy intake by 3-d records compared with energy intake to maintain body weight in 269 nonobese adults. *American Journal of Clinical Nutrition, 60*(6), 855–860. https://doi.org/10.1093/ajcn/60.6.855

Devries, M. C., Sithamparapillai, A., Brimble, K. S., Banfield, L., Morton, R. W., & Phillips, S. M. (2018). Changes in kidney function do not differ between healthy adults consuming higher- compared with lower- or normal-protein diets: A systematic review and meta-analysis. *Journal of Nutrition, 148*(11), 1760–1775. https://doi.org/10.1093/jn/nxy197

Donaldson, C. M., Perry, T. L., & Rose, M. C. (2010). Glycemic index and endurance performance. *International Journal of Sport Nutrition and Exercise Metabolism, 20*(2), 154–165.

Dunford, M., & Doyle, J. A. (2022). *Nutrition for sport and exercise* (5th ed.). Cengage.

Farrokhyar, F., Tabasinejad, R., Dao, D., Peterson, D., Ayeni, O. R., Hadioonzadeh, R., & Bhandari, M. (2015). Prevalence of vitamin D inadequacy in athletes: A systematic review and meta-analysis. *Sports Medicine, 45*(3), 365–378.

Faude, O., Hecksteden, A., Hammes, D., Schumacher, F., Besenius, E., Sperlich, B., & Meyer, T. (2017). Reliability of time-to-exhaustion and selected psycho-physiological variables during constant-load cycling at the maximal lactate steady-state. *Applied Physiology, Nutrition, and Metabolism/Physiologie Appliquee, Nutrition et Metabolisme, 42*(2), 142–147.

Ferriday, D., Bosworth, M. L., Lai, S., Godinot, N., Martin, N., Martin, A. A., Rogers, P. J., & Brunstrom, J. M. (2015). Effects of eating rate on satiety: A role for episodic memory? *Physiology & Behavior, 152*(pt B), 389–396.

Fleming, J., Sharman, M. J., Avery, N. G., Love, D. M., Gómez, A. L., Scheett, T. P., Kraemer, W. J., & Volek, J. S. (2003). Endurance capacity and high-intensity exercise performance responses to a high fat diet. *International Journal of Sport Nutrition and Exercise Metabolism, 13*(4), 466–478.

Gardner, C. D., Trepanowski, J. F., Del Gobbo, L. C., Hauser, M. E., Rigdon, J., Ioannidis, J. P. A., Desai, M., & King, A. C. (2018). Effect of low-fat vs. low-carbohydrate diet on 12-month weight loss in overweight adults and the association with genotype pattern or insulin secretion: The DIETFITS randomized clinical trial. *Journal of the American Medical Association, 319*(7), 667–679.

Gastin, P. B. (2001). Energy system interaction and relative contribution during maximal exercise. *Sports Medicine, 31*(10), 725–741.

Hall, K. D., Guo, J., Courville, A. B., Boring, J., Brychta, R., Chen, K. Y., Darcey, V., Forde, C. G., Gharib, A. M., Gallagher, I., Howard, R., Joseph, P. V., Milley, L., Ouwerkerk, R., Raisinger, K., Rozga, I., Schick, A., Stagliano, M., Torres, S., … Chung, S. T. (2021). Effect of a plant-based, low-fat diet versus an animal-based, ketogenic diet on ad libitum energy intake. *Nature Medicine, 27*(2), 344–353.

Headrick, L. B., Rowe, C. C., Kendall, A. R., Zitt, M. A., Bolton, D. L., & Langkamp-Henken, B. (2013). Adults in all body mass index categories underestimate daily energy requirements. *Journal of Nutrition Education and Behavior, 45*(5), 460–465.

Heindel, J. J. & Blumberg, B. (2019). Environmental obesogens: Mechanisms and controversies. *Annual Review of Pharmacology and Toxicology, 59*, 89–106.

Hernández, T., Wilder, L., Kuehn, D., Rubotzky, K., Moser-Veillon, P., Godwin, S., Thompson, C., & Wang, C. (2006). Portion size estimation and expectation of accuracy. *Journal of Food Composition and Analysis, 19*, S14–S21. https://doi.org/10.1016/j.jfca.2006.02.010

Heymsfield, S. B., Thomas, D., Nguyen, A. M., Peng, J. Z., Martin, C., Shen, W., Strauss, B., Bosy-Westphal, A., & Muller, M. J. (2011). Voluntary weight loss: Systematic review of early phase body composition changes: Early phase weight loss. *Obesity Reviews, 12*(5), e348–e361. https://doi.org/10.1111/j.1467-789X.2010.00767.x

Hogenkamp, P. S., Nilsson, E., Nilsson, V. C., Chapman, C. D., Vogel, H., Lundberg, L. S., Zarei, S., Cedernaes, J., Rångtell, F. H., Broman, J.-E., Dickson, S. L., Brunstrom, J. M., Benedict, C., & Schiöth, H. B. (2013). Acute sleep deprivation increases portion size and affects food choice in young men. *Psychoneuroendocrinology, 38*(9), 1668–1674.

Horner, K. M., Schubert, M. M., Desbrow, B., Byrne, N. M., & King, N. A. (2015). Acute exercise and gastric emptying: A meta-analysis and implications for appetite control. *Sports Medicine, 45*(5), 659–678.

Horton, T. J., Drougas, H., Brachey, A., Reed, G. W., Peters, J. C., & Hill, J. O. (1995). Fat and carbohydrate overfeeding in humans: Different effects on energy storage. *American Journal of Clinical Nutrition, 62*(1). https://doi.org/10.1093/ajcn/62.1.19

Horvath, P. J., Eagen, C. K., Fisher, N. M., Leddy, J. J., & Pendergast, D. R. (2000). The effects of varying dietary fat on performance and metabolism in trained male and female runners. *Journal of the American College of Nutrition, 19*(1), 52–60.

Houltham, S. D., & Rowlands, D. S. (2014). A snapshot of nitrogen balance in endurance-trained women. *Applied Physiology, Nutrition, and Metabolism, 39*(2), 219–225. https://doi.org/10.1139/apnm-2013-0182

Jäger, R., Kerksick, C. M., Campbell, B. I., Cribb, P. J., Wells, S. D., Skwiat, T. M., Purpura, M., Ziegenfuss, T. N., Ferrando, A. A., Arent, S. M., Smith-Ryan, A. E., Stout, J. R., Arciero, P. J., Ormsbee, M. J., Taylor, L. W., Wilborn, C. D., Kalman, D. S., Kreider, R. B., Willoughby, D. S., ... Antonio, J. (2017). International Society of Sports Nutrition position stand: Protein and exercise. *Journal of the International Society of Sports Nutrition, 14*. https://doi.org/10.1186/s12970-017-0177-8

Jakeman, P., & Maxwell, S. (1993). Effect of antioxidant vitamin supplementation on muscle function after eccentric exercise. *European Journal of Applied Physiology and Occupational Physiology, 67*(5), 426–430.

Jentjens, R. L. P. G., Moseley, L., Waring, R. H., Harding, L. K., & Jeukendrup, A. E. (2004). Oxidation of combined ingestion of glucose and fructose during exercise. *Journal of Applied Physiology, 96*(4), 1277–1284.

Jeukendrup, A. E. (2017). Training the gut for athletes. *Sports Medicine, 47*(suppl 1), 101–110.

Jeukendrup, A., & Gleeson, M. (2018). *Sport nutrition* (3rd ed.). Human Kinetics.

Jeukendrup, A. E., & Jentjens, R. (2000). Oxidation of carbohydrate feedings during prolonged exercise: Current thoughts, guidelines and directions for future research. *Sports Medicine, 29*(6), 407–424.

Jumpertz, R., Venti, C. A., Le, D. S., Michaels, J., Parrington, S., Krakoff, J., & Votruba, S. (2013). Food label accuracy of common snack foods. *Obesity, 21*(1), 164–169. https://doi.org/10.1002/oby.20185

Kato, H., Suzuki, K., Bannai, M., & Moore, D. R. (2016). Protein requirements are elevated in endurance athletes after exercise as determined by the indicator amino acid oxidation method. *PLoS One, 11*(6), e0157406. https://doi.org/10.1371/journal.pone.0157406

Kaviani, M., Shaw, K., & Chilibeck, P. D. (2020). Benefits of creatine supplementation for vegetarians compared to omnivorous athletes: A systematic review. *International Journal of Environmental Research and Public Health, 17*(9), 3041. https://doi.org/10.3390/ijerph17093041

Kim, I.-Y., Schutzler, S., Schrader, A., Spencer, H. J., Azhar, G., Ferrando, A. A., & Wolfe, R. R. (2016). The anabolic response to a meal containing different amounts of protein is not limited by the maximal stimulation of protein synthesis in healthy young adults. *American Journal of Physiology-Endocrinology and Metabolism, 310*(1), E73–E80.

Kruskall, L.G. (2019). Nutrition and the exercise professional's scope of practice. *American College of Sports Medicine* (ACSM). https://www.acsm.org/blog-detail/acsm-certified-blog/2019/09/09/nutrition-scope-of-practice

Leaf, A., & Antonio, J. (2017). The effects of overfeeding on body composition: The role of macronutrient composition: A narrative review. *International Journal of Exercise Science, 10*(8), 1275–1296.

Leidy, H. J., Tang, M., Armstrong, C. L. H., Martin, C. B., & Campbell, W. W. (2011). The effects of consuming frequent, higher protein meals on appetite and satiety during weight loss in overweight/obese men. *Obesity, 19*(4), 818–824. https://doi.org/10.1038/oby.2010.203

Lichtman, S. W., Pisarska, K., Berman, E. R., Pestone, M., Dowling, H., Offenbacher, E., Weisel, H., Heshka, S., Matthews, D. E., & Heymsfield, S. B. (2010). Discrepancy between self-reported and actual caloric intake and exercise in obese subjects. *New England Journal of Medicine, 327*, 1893–1898. https://doi.org/10.1056/NEJM199212313272701

Macnaughton, L. S., Wardle, S. L., Witard, O. C., McGlory, C., Hamilton, D. L., Jeromson, S., Lawrence, C. E., Wallis, G. A., & Tipton, K. D. (2016). The response of muscle protein synthesis following whole-body resistance exercise is greater following 40 g than 20 g of ingested whey protein. *Physiological Reports, 4*(15), e12893. https://doi.org/10.14814/phy2.12893

Magee, M. K., Lockard, B. L., Zabriskie, H. A., Schaefer, A. Q., Luedke, J. A., Erickson, J. L., Jones, M. T., & Jagim, A. R. (2020). Prevalence of low energy availability in collegiate women soccer athletes. *Journal of Functional Morphology and Kinesiology, 5*(4). https://doi.org/10.3390/jfmk5040096

Martin, C. K., Rosenbaum, D., Han, H., Geiselman, P. J., Wyatt, H. R., Hill, J. O., Brill, C., Bailer, B., Miller, B. V. 3rd, Stein, R., Klein, S., & Foster, G. D. (2011). Change in food cravings, food preferences, and appetite during a low-carbohydrate and low-fat diet. *Obesity, 19*(10), 1963–1970.

Maruyama, K., Sato, S., Ohira, T., Maeda, K., Noda, H., Kubota, Y., Nishimura, S., Kitamura, A., Kiyama, M., Okada, T., Imano, H., Nakamura, M., Ishikawa, Y., Kurokawa, M., Sasaki, S., & Iso, H. (2008). The joint impact on being overweight of self reported behaviours of eating quickly and eating until full: Cross sectional survey. *British Medical Journal, 337*, a2002.

Maughan, R. J., Burke, L. M., Dvorak, J., Larson-Meyer, D. E., Peeling, P., Phillips, S. M., Rawson, E. S., Walsh, N. P., Garthe, I., Geyer, H., Meeusen, R., van Loon, L. J. C., Shirreffs, S. M., Spriet, L. L., Stuart, M., Vernec, A.,

Currell, K., Ali, V. M., Budgett, R. G., ... Engebretsen, L. (2018). IOC consensus statement: Dietary supplements and the high-performance athlete. *British Journal of Sports Medicine, 52*(7), 439–455.

Maughan, R. J., Leiper, J. B., & Shirreffs, S. M. (1997). Factors influencing the restoration of fluid and electrolyte balance after exercise in the heat. *British Journal of Sports Medicine, 31*(3), 175–182.

McDermott, B. P., Anderson, S. A., Armstrong, L. E., Casa, D. J., Cheuvront, S. N., Cooper, L., Kenney, W. L., O'Connor, F. G., & Roberts, W. O. (2017). National Athletic Trainers' Association position statement: Fluid replacement for the physically active. *Journal of Athletic Training, 52*(9), 877–895.

McLellan, T. M., Cheung, S. S., & Jacobs, I. (1995). Variability of time to exhaustion during submaximal exercise. *Canadian Journal of Applied Physiology/Revue Canadienne de Physiologie Appliquee, 20*(1), 39–51.

McSwiney, F. T., Wardrop, B., Hyde, P. N., Lafountain, R. A., Volek, J. S., & Doyle, L. (2018). Keto-adaptation enhances exercise performance and body composition responses to training in endurance athletes. *Metabolism: Clinical and Experimental, 81*, 25–34.

Mickleborough, T. D. (2013). Omega-3 polyunsaturated fatty acids in physical performance optimization. *International Journal of Sport Nutrition and Exercise Metabolism, 23*(1), 83–96.

Minehira, K., Vega, N., Vidal, H., Acheson, K., & Tappy, L. (2004). Effect of carbohydrate overfeeding on whole body macronutrient metabolism and expression of lipogenic enzymes in adipose tissue of lean and overweight humans. *International Journal of Obesity, 28*(10), 1291–1298. https://doi.org/10.1038/sj.ijo.0802760

Morton, R. W., Murphy, K. T., McKellar, S. R., Schoenfeld, B. J., Henselmans, M., Helms, E., Aragon, A. A., Devries, M. C., Banfield, L., Krieger, J. W., & Phillips, S. M. (2018). A systematic review, meta-analysis and meta-regression of the effect of protein supplementation on resistance training–induced gains in muscle mass and strength in healthy adults. *British Journal of Sports Medicine, 52*(6), 376–384. https://doi.org/10.1136/bjsports-2017-097608

Mountjoy, M., Sundgot-Borgen, J., Burke, L., Ackerman, K. E., Blauwet, C., Constantini, N., Lebrun, C., Lundy, B., Melin, A., Meyer, N., Sherman, R., Tenforde, A. S., Torstveit, M. K., & Budgett, R. (2018). International Olympic Committee (IOC) consensus statement on relative energy deficiency in sport (RED-S): 2018 update. *International Journal of Sport Nutrition and Exercise Metabolism, 28*(4), 316–331. https://doi.org/10.1123/ijsnem.2018-0136

Nair, K. S., Halliday, D., & Griggs, R. C. (1988). Leucine incorporation into mixed skeletal muscle protein in humans. *American Journal of Physiology-Endocrinology and Metabolism, 254*, E208–E213.

Nakhostin-Roohi, B., Babaei, P., Rahmani-Nia, F., & Bohlooli, S. (2008). Effect of vitamin C supplementation on lipid peroxidation, muscle damage and inflammation after 30-min exercise at 75% VO_2max. *Journal of Sports Medicine and Physical Fitness, 48*(2), 217–224.

Njike, V. Y., Smith, T. M., Shuval, O., Shuval, K., Edshteyn, I., Kalantari, V., & Yaroch, A. L. (2016). Snack food, Satiety, and weight. *Advances in Nutrition, 7*(5), 866–878.

Parks, R. B., Hetzel, S. J., & Brooks, M. A. (2017). Iron deficiency and anemia among collegiate athletes: A retrospective chart review. *Medicine and Science in Sports and Exercise, 49*(8), 1711–1715.

Peternelj, T.-T. & Coombes, J. S. (2011). Antioxidant supplementation during exercise training: Beneficial or detrimental? *Sports Medicine, 41*(12), 1043–1069.

Ristow, M., & Zarse, K. (2010). How increased oxidative stress promotes longevity and metabolic health: The concept of mitochondrial hormesis (mitohormesis). *Experimental Gerontology, 45*(6), 410–418.

Rogerson, D. (2017). Vegan diets: Practical advice for athletes and exercisers. *Journal of the International Society of Sports Nutrition, 14*, 36.

Romijn, J. A., Coyle, E. F., Sidossis, L. S., Gastaldelli, A., Horowitz, J. F., Endert, E., & Wolfe, R. R. (1993). Regulation of endogenous fat and carbohydrate metabolism in relation to exercise intensity and duration. *American Journal of Physiology, 265*(3 pt 1), E380–E391.

Sarwar Gilani, G., Wu Xiao, C., & Cockell, K. A. (2012). Impact of antinutritional factors in food proteins on the digestibility of protein and the bioavailability of amino acids and on protein quality. *British Journal of Nutrition, 108*(suppl 2), S315–S332.

Sawka, M. N., & Coyle, E. F. (1999). Influence of body water and blood volume on thermoregulation and exercise performance in the heat. *Exercise and Sport Sciences Reviews, 27*, 167–218.

Schoenfeld, B. J., Aragon, A. A., & Krieger, J. W. (2013). The effect of protein timing on muscle strength and hypertrophy: A meta-analysis. *Journal of the International Society of Sports Nutrition, 10*(1), 1–13.

Schuiling, K. D., & Slager, J. (2000). Scope of practice: Freedom within limits. *Journal of Midwifery & Women's Health, 45*(6), 465–471. https://doi.org/10.1016/s1526-9523(00)00070-2

Sen, C. K. (1995). Oxidants and antioxidants in exercise. *Journal of Applied Physiology, 79*(3), 675–686.

Simmons, W. K., Burrows, K., Avery, J. A., Kerr, K. L., Bodurka, J., Savage, C. R., & Drevets, W. C. (2016). Depression-related increases and decreases in appetite: Dissociable patterns of aberrant activity in reward and interoceptive neurocircuitry. *American Journal of Psychiatry, 173*(4), 418–428.

Singh, G. M., Micha, R., Khatibzadeh, S., Lim, S., Ezzati, M., Mozaffarian, D., & Global Burden of Diseases Nutrition and Chronic Diseases Expert Group (NutriCoDE). (2015). Estimated global, regional, and national disease burdens related to sugar-sweetened beverage consumption in 2010. *Circulation, 132*(8), 639–666.

Slater, G. J., Dieter, B. P., Marsh, D. J., Helms, E. R., Shaw, G., & Iraki, J. (2019). Is an energy surplus required to maximize skeletal muscle hypertrophy associated with resistance training. *Frontiers in Nutrition, 6*. https://doi.org/10.3389/fnut.2019.00131

Snetselaar, L. G., de Jesus, J. M., DeSilva, D. M., & Stoody, E. E. (2021). Dietary guidelines for Americans, 2020–2025: Understanding the scientific process, guidelines, and key recommendations. *Nutrition Today, 56*(6), 287–295.

Spriet, L. L. (2019). Performance nutrition for athletes. *Sports Medicine, 49*(suppl 1), 1.

Tate, C. A., & Holtz, R. W. (1998). Gender and fat metabolism during exercise: A review. *Canadian Journal of Applied Physiology/Revue Canadienne de Physiologie Appliquee, 23*(6), 570–582.

Thielecke, F., & Blannin, A. (2020). Omega-3 fatty acids for sport performance: Are they equally beneficial for athletes and amateurs? A narrative review. *Nutrients, 12*(12), 3712. https://doi.org/10.3390/nu12123712

Thomas, D. T., Erdman, K. A., & Burke, L. M. (2016). American College of Sports Medicine joint position statement: Nutrition and athletic performance. *Medicine & Science in Sports & Exercise, 48*(3), 543–568. https://doi.org/10.1249/MSS.0000000000000852

Tremblay, A., Simoneau, J.-A., & Bouchard, C. (1994). Impact of exercise intensity on body fatness and skeletal muscle metabolism. *Metabolism, 43*(7), 814–818. https://doi.org/10.1016/0026-0495(94)90259-3

Trommelen, J., Fuchs, C. J., Beelen, M., Lenaerts, K., Jeukendrup, A. E., Cermak, N. M., & van Loon, L. J. C. (2017). Fructose and sucrose intake increase exogenous carbohydrate oxidation during exercise. *Nutrients, 9*(2). https://doi.org/10.3390/nu9020167

van Vliet, S., Burd, N. A., & van Loon, L. J. C. (2015). The skeletal muscle anabolic response to plant–versus animal–based protein consumption. *Journal of Nutrition, 145*(9), 1981–1991.

Vizcarra, M., Palomino, A. M., Iglesias, L., Valencia, A., Gálvez Espinoza, P., & Schwingel, A. (2019). Weight matters: Factors influencing eating behaviors of vulnerable women. *Nutrients, 11*(8), 1809. https://doi.org/10.3390/nu11081809

Volek, J. S., Forsythe, C. E., & Kraemer, W. J. (2006). Nutritional aspects of women strength athletes. *British Journal of Sports Medicine, 40*(9), 742–748.

Wardenaar, F., Brinkmans, N., Ceelen, I., Van Rooij, B., Mensink, M., Witkamp, R., & De Vries, J. (2017). Micronutrient intakes in 553 Dutch elite and sub-elite athletes: Prevalence of low and high intakes in users and non-users of nutritional supplements. *Nutrients, 9*(2). https://doi.org/10.3390/nu9020142

Whitfield, J., Burke, L. M., McKay, A. K. A., Heikura, I. A., Hall, R., Fensham, N., & Sharma, A. P. (2021). Acute ketogenic diet and ketone ester supplementation impairs race walk performance. *Medicine & Science in Sports & Exercise, 53*(4), 776–784.

Widrick, J. J., Costill, D. L., Fink, W. J., Hickey, M. S., McConell, G. K., & Tanaka, H. (1993). Carbohydrate feedings and exercise performance: Effect of initial muscle glycogen concentration. *Journal of Applied Physiology, 74*(6), 2998–3005.

Wilson, P. B. (2019). "I think I'm gonna hurl": A narrative review of the causes of nausea and vomiting in sport. *Sports, 7*(7), 162. https://doi.org/10.3390/sports7070162

Wroble, K. A., Trott, M. N., Schweitzer, G. G., Rahman, R. S., Kelly, P. V., & Weiss, E. P. (2019). Low-carbohydrate, ketogenic diet impairs anaerobic exercise performance in exercise-trained women and men: A randomized-sequence crossover trial. *Journal of Sports Medicine and Physical Fitness, 59*(4), 600–607.

Wycherley, T. P., Moran, L. J., Clifton, P. M., Noakes, M., & Brinkworth, G. D. (2012). Effects of energy-restricted high-protein, low-fat compared with standard-protein, low-fat diets: A meta-analysis of randomized controlled trials. *American Journal of Clinical Nutrition, 96*(6), 1281–1298. https://doi.org/10.3945/ajcn.112.044321

Zhang, Y., Coca, A., Casa, D. J., Antonio, J., Green, J. M., & Bishop, P. A. (2015). Caffeine and diuresis during rest and exercise: A meta-analysis. *Journal of Science and Medicine in Sport/Sports Medicine Australia, 18*(5), 569–574.

Ziegler, P. J., Jonnalagadda, S. S., Nelson, J. A., Lawrence, C., & Baciak, B. (2002). Contribution of meals and snacks to nutrient intake of male and female elite figure skaters during peak competitive season. *Journal of the American College of Nutrition, 21*(2), 114–119.

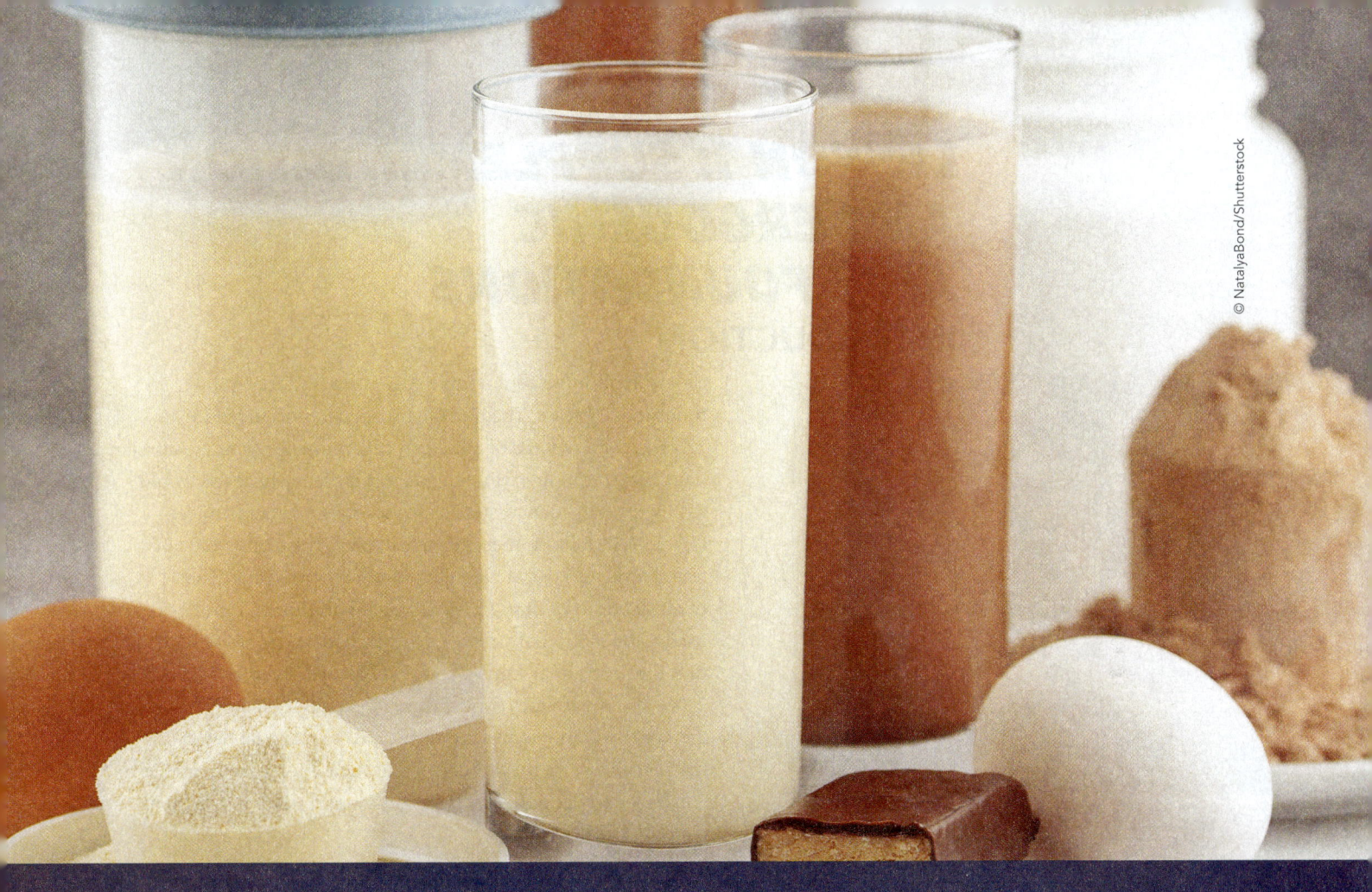

© NatalyaBond/Shutterstock

SUPPLEMENTATION AND ERGOGENIC AIDS

CHAPTER TWENTY-THREE

LEARNING OBJECTIVES

Upon completion of this chapter, the Sports Performance Coach will be able to:

- **Explain** a food-first approach for supporting an athlete's nutrition needs.

- **Evaluate** the risks and benefits of common supplement options.

- **Assess** the athlete's need for supplementation using a thorough decision-making process.

- **Identify** the supplements appropriate in supporting an athlete's nutrition priorities and needs.

- **Identify** appropriate application strategies for various supplements.

LESSON 1: SUPPLEMENTATION AND ERGOGENIC AIDS FOUNDATIONS

INTRODUCTION

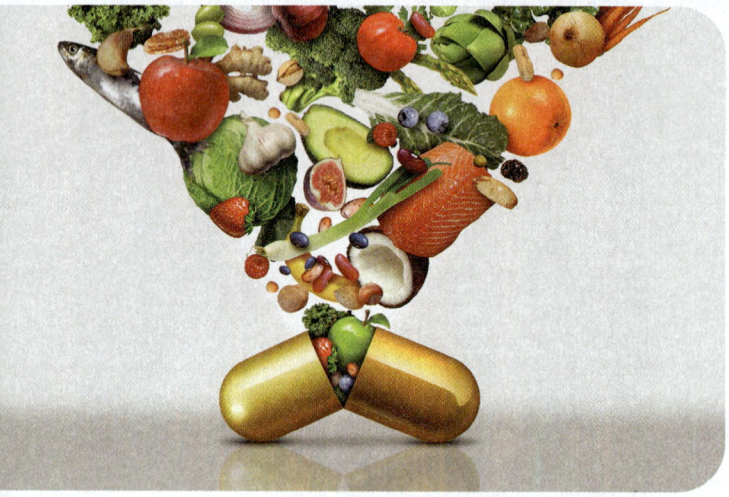

© Lightspring/Shutterstock

The search for the competitive edge dates back several thousands of years. The first Olympic games occurred in 776 B.C., and records of athletes' preparation for their events cite their consumption of different substances they believed would aid their performance, such as seeds and even hallucinogens (Silver, 2001). From then through 1968, Olympians were not tested for drugs despite athletes admitting to doping. That practice began as early as 1904, when marathoner Tom Hicks used a concoction of strychnine, brandy, and egg white to help him finish the final 4 miles and win his race (Kremenik et al., 2006). Today, athletes continue to use strategies involving dietary supplements and ergogenic aids to facilitate better performance, and they often consult their Sports Performance Coach for advice and direction on how and when to use them.

DIETARY SUPPLEMENTS AND ERGOGENIC AIDS

Although the terms are sometimes used interchangeably when discussing products taken to improve performance or body composition, dietary supplements and ergogenic aids are actually different. A **dietary supplement** is defined by the U.S. Food and Drug Administration (FDA) as any product taken by mouth that contains a dietary ingredient. A dietary ingredient might include vitamins, minerals, botanicals, amino acids, or enzymes, either alone or in combination (FDA, 1994).

The word *ergogenic* is composed of two parts: *ergo*, meaning "work," and *genic*, meaning "to generate." Thus, an **ergogenic aid** is something that helps to generate work. In the field of physics, work is the product of force and distance. An ergogenic aid is anything that helps to generate force or cover a distance. Ergogenic aids are not limited to nutrition, and can include mechanical, physiological, pharmacologic, and psychological aids as well, some of which might be relevant to the Sports Performance Coach in addition to nutritional ergogenic aids. The five types of ergogenic aids are highlighted in **Figure 23.1**. Some ergogenic aids are classified as being more than one type of ergogenic aid. For example, alcohol is both a legal pharmacologic drug (although its use is illegal in competition) and a psychological aid because it can help calm nerves. As an example of a mechanical ergogenic aid, swimmers wear specialized suits to help them reduce their friction in the water and improve the efficiency of each stroke—and ultimately finish the race faster. Although other types of ergogenic aids exist and might be relevant to a Sports Performance Coach, this chapter focuses on nutritional ergogenic aids.

COMMON USES FOR SUPPLEMENTS

Athletes use nutritional supplements for various reasons. A recent survey conducted by the Council for Responsible Nutrition (2018) reported that 75% of adults in the United States use at least one dietary supplement. The most common reason cited for supplement use is

---

DIETARY SUPPLEMENT →

A product other than tobacco that is intended to supplement the diet that bears or contains one or more of the following dietary ingredients: vitamin; mineral; herb or other botanical; amino acid; dietary supplement that increases the total dietary intake; or a concentrate, metabolite, constituent, extract, or combination of any previously described ingredient.

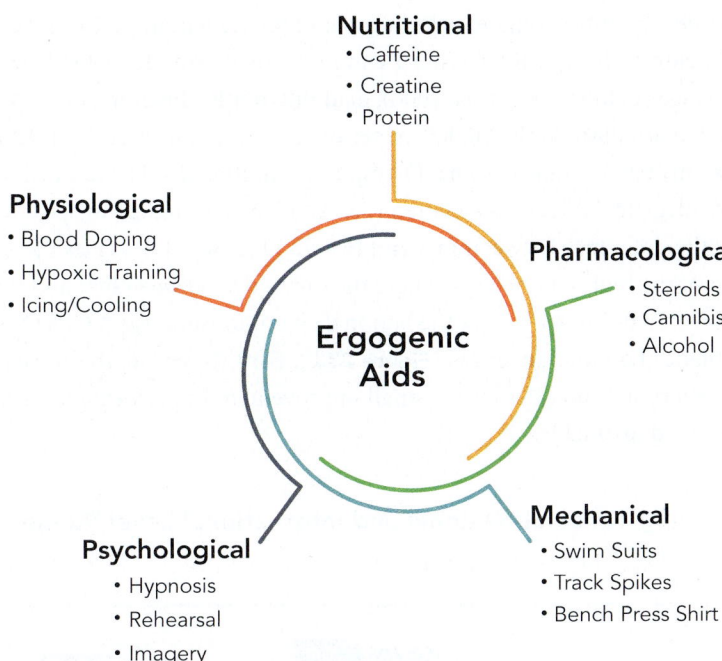

Nutritional
- Caffeine
- Creatine
- Protein

Physiological
- Blood Doping
- Hypoxic Training
- Icing/Cooling

Ergogenic Aids

Pharmacological
- Steroids
- Cannibis
- Alcohol

Psychological
- Hypnosis
- Rehearsal
- Imagery

Mechanical
- Swim Suits
- Track Spikes
- Bench Press Shirt

FIGURE 23.1 Ergogenic Aids

ERGOGENIC AID →

A dietary supplement that might enhance performance or body composition; also referred to as a performance supplement.

overall wellness. Other common reasons for supplement use among the general population include weight management, immune health, beauty, energy, and to fill nutrient gaps. More specific reasons vary by age group, and athletes represent their own unique group.

Athletes place a greater emphasis on the ergogenic aid category of dietary supplements. A higher percentage of the athletic population appears to use supplements, and this share is increasing. A 1994 poll of more than 10,000 athletes found that 46% of college athletes and 59% of elite athletes use dietary supplements (Sobal & Marquart, 1994). By comparison, a 2017 analysis of 553 elite and sub-elite athletes that observed that 97% had used dietary supplements at least once, and 85% had used them in the past month (Wardenaar et al., 2017). Dietary supplement use appears to be influenced by the sport and training volume in some athletes. Lun et al. (2012) found that 67% of elite Canadian athletes use dietary supplements when their training volume is low (less than 5 hours per week) versus 95% when their training volume is high (more than 25 hours per week). In some sports, the dietary supplement usage rate is 100%.

A survey investigating motivations for dietary supplement use reported that most (81%) athletes use dietary supplements to enhance performance and to stay healthy, while 52% use supplements to support their immune system, 43% to support their diet, and 19% for medical issues (Parnell et al., 2015). Another study reported that, relative to their usage rates, few athletes fully understand the full picture of supplement use (Petkova et al., 2018). Despite 81% to 100% of athletes using dietary supplements, just 68% understood there are health risks associated with dietary supplement use. Importantly, most athletes (77%) reported they follow the instructions of their sports dietitian. The current utilization rates and gaps in knowledge highlight the need for the Sports Performance Coach to understand which dietary supplements are safe and efficacious.

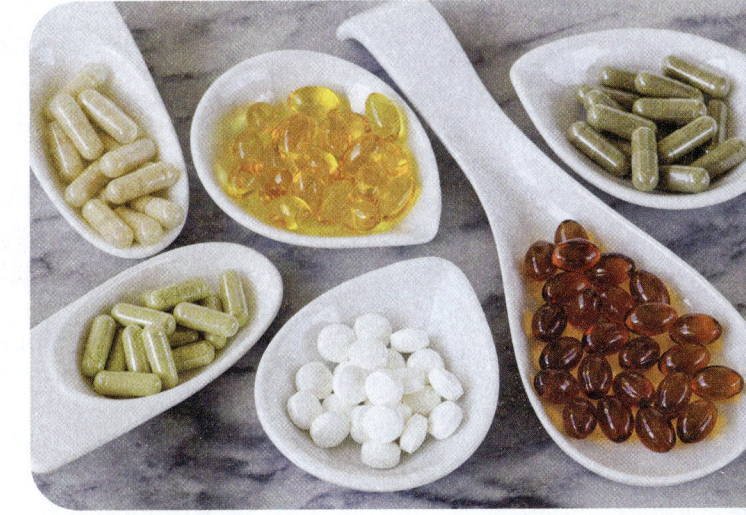

© Pat_Hastings/Shutterstock

As competition becomes tougher, even a small improvement in performance is meaningful. In elite cyclists, as little as a 0.5% improvement in performance can be a worthwhile change (Paton & Hopkins, 2006). Said differently, the difference between first place and twelfth place in the 10,000-meter men's running final at the 2012 London Olympics was only 0.66% (International Olympic Committee, 2021). Contrast that with the National Collegiate Athletic Association (NCAA) Division 1 2021 men's 10,000-meter results, where the difference between first and twelfth place was 1.3% (Flash Results, 2021), and the results at the high school level, where the difference between first and twelfth place for the boys 5,000-meter race at the national championship was 2.67% (National Scholastic Athletics Foundation, 2021) (**Figure 23.2**). For this reason, the attractiveness of supplementation that can offer even a small improvement in performance is both understandable and justifiable.

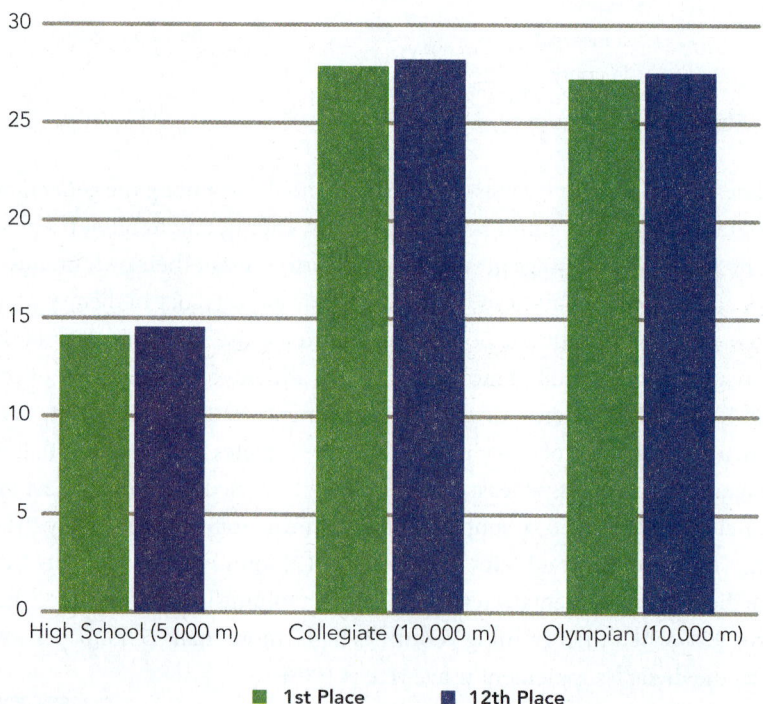

Finishing Times of National and International Level Runners

■ 1st Place   ■ 12th Place

FIGURE 23.2 Difference Between First and Twelfth Place Among Athletes

Data from National Scholastic Athletics Foundation. (2021). 2021 The Nike Outdoor Nationals. https://theoutdoornationals.runnerspace.com/eprofile.php?do=info&event_id=14188

⚠ **CRITICAL**

There are some supplements that athletes might require or decide to utilize to improve performance that must be referred out to a licensed healthcare professional. For example, iron supplementation needs to be administered under the supervision of a physician.

THIRD-PARTY VERIFICATION

When dietary supplements make the news, it is typically for unbecoming reasons, such as adulteration or contamination. This viewpoint has contributed to the notion that dietary supplements are unregulated, which is not true. The supplement industry in developed countries *is* a regulated industry. However, it is a more loosely regulated industry than, for example, the pharmaceutical industry. One of the major differences between industries like the supplement industry and the pharmaceutical industry is that pharmaceuticals require preapproval from the FDA *before* they can enter the market. In contrast, the supplement industry is regulated post-facto by the FDA, which is responsible for taking action against any adulterated or misbranded dietary supplement product *after* it reaches the market (FDA, 2019).

After a dietary supplement is on the market, government agencies visit supplement manufacturing facilities for audits, purchase products from the market and test them, review company websites for misuse of claims, and take other actions to regulate dietary supplements. When viewed through the lens of potential harm to a consumer, it makes sense that larger companies are the most intensely scrutinized. This does not mean that being manufactured by a big brand with high name recognition guarantees the safety of a dietary supplement. Indeed, although governing agencies' attention is focused on these firms, smaller companies and bad actors can, either knowingly or unknowingly, produce products that are noncompliant or dangerous.

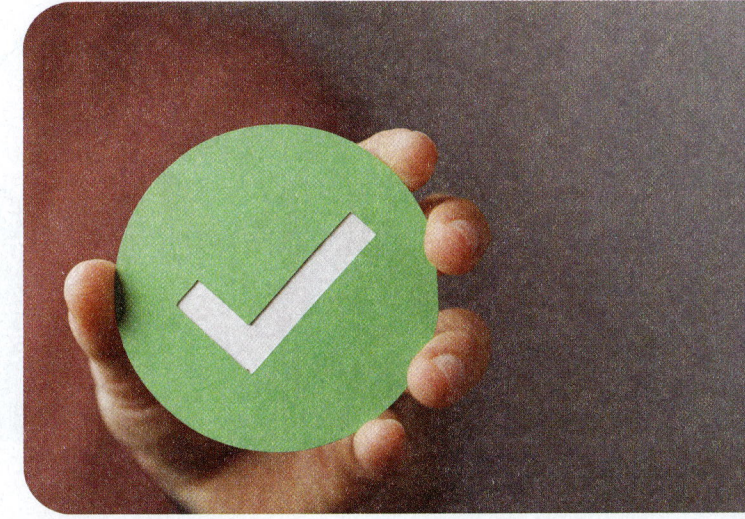

© Wirestock Creators/Shutterstock

In many cases, smaller dietary supplement companies (i.e., those with lower overall revenues) do not invest heavily in quality control and might unknowingly sell products containing a contaminated ingredient. In other cases, firms may deliberately mislabel and sell adulterated products. It is these sorts of cases that often get publicized.

This risk has led to the creation of third-party verification companies, which test and verify that dietary supplements meet certain safety criteria. The criteria differ from one certifying body to another.

Some major certifiers are NSF International, NSF International Certified for Sport, Informed Choice, Informed Sport, USP (United States Pharmacopeia), and BSCG (Banned Substances Control Group) Certified Drug Free. NSF International, NSF International Certified for Sport, and Informed Choice have a sport certification that caters to athletes by testing for **banned substances**. NSF International Certified for Sport is recognized by the U.S. Anti-Doping Agency as well as several North American professional sports organizations. In the case of Major League Baseball, individual clubs are permitted to provide and recommend dietary supplements that are NSF International Certified for Sport, and other leagues might set similar policies.

All of the independent verification services check that the products are produced in a facility that adheres to current good manufacturing practices (cGMP) and that tests for contamination, which means testing for bacteria, heavy metals, pesticides, and other contaminants. Those that provide label content testing check the product to ensure the ingredients listed on the label are present in the product at the quantities specified. Most important to the athlete, NSF International Certified for Sport, Informed Choice,

> **BANNED SUBSTANCES** →
>
> Dietary supplements that are prohibited from use in a specific sport or sport league. Banned supplements might not be illegal or banned at all times during the year.

Informed Sport, and BSCG Certified Drug Free test against the "prohibited list" developed by the World Anti-Doping Agency (WADA) as well as other substances prohibited by different organizations. Fitness professionals and athletes can look for the logos for guidance on which third-party testing was conducted.

> ⚠ **CRITICAL**
>
> Know which certifications mean the product is tested for banned substances. Just because a product is tested and certified does not guarantee it is 100% risk-free.

WORLD ANTI-DOPING AGENCY AND NATIONAL COLLEGIATE ATHLETIC ASSOCIATION

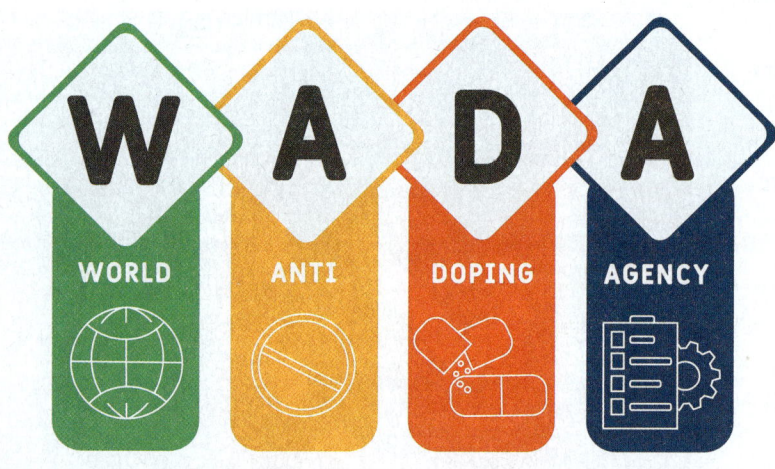

© Kozhedub_nc/Shutterstock

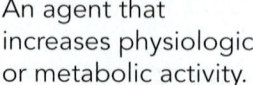

STIMULANT →

An agent that increases physiologic or metabolic activity.

The International Olympic Committee established WADA in 1999 to monitor and prevent the use of performance-enhancing substances in Olympic sports. This organization also serves to harmonize anti-doping rules across different countries. Every year on October 1, WADA updates and publishes its prohibited list at www.wada-ama.org. After the list's publication in October, athletes must conform with it by the start of the following year.

A committee consisting of the International Olympic Committee and representatives sent by national governments determines which substances make the list. Country- or region-specific work is delegated to national or regional anti-doping organizations that are compliant with WADA's code.

The drug testing program established by the NCAA tests student athletes for performance-enhancing drugs and masking agents year-round, as well as for **stimulants** and recreational drugs during championships. The individual colleges and universities that are members of the NCAA might test student athletes on their own schedule in addition to the NCAA's testing. The NCAA has not published an approved list of dietary supplements, and it prohibits the provision of dietary supplements to student athletes. Institutions can provide food and food-similar supplements such as carbohydrate, protein, and electrolyte bars or beverages, but they cannot provide dietary supplements such as creatine. Student athletes might choose to use other dietary supplements of their own volition, but they are responsible for all positive drug tests.

The prohibited-substances lists from WADA and NCAA are not perfectly harmonized; although they largely overlap, some substances are present on one but not the other. It is important to know which list applies to which athlete or if both apply, such as in the case of a student athlete who also qualifies to compete in the Olympics in their sport. Likewise, it is important when using permissible dietary supplements to choose trusted brands that the Sports Performance Coach and athlete are confident do not contain banned substances by looking for a third-party verification or by other means (**Figure 23.3**).

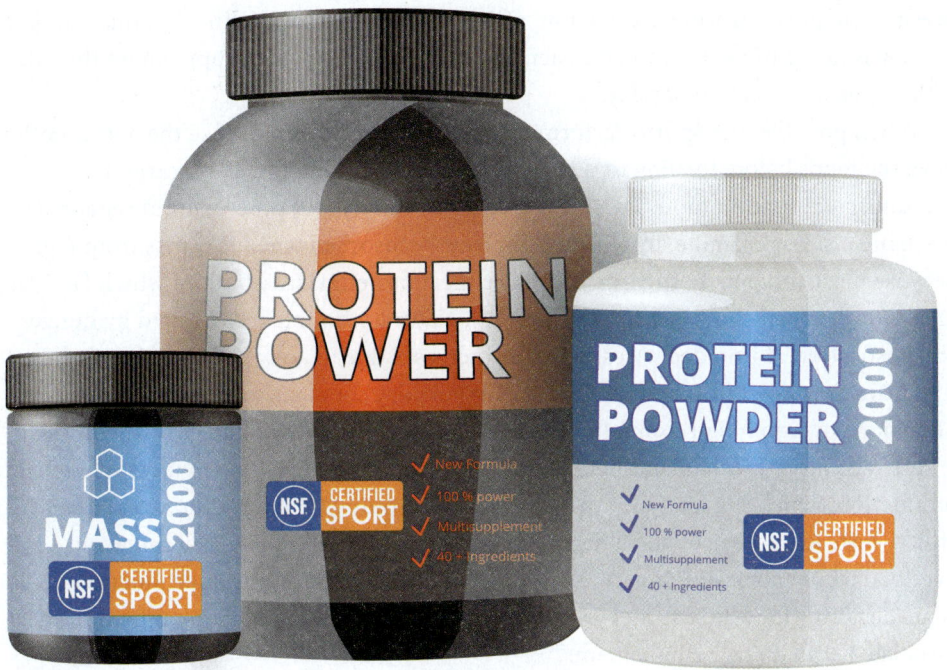

FIGURE 23.3 Third-Party Verification Logos

FOOD-FIRST APPROACH

Dietary supplements are, as the name suggests, intended to supplement the human diet. They are not intended to be a first line of defense or first choice to address nutritional needs. For supplement ingredients that are found in biologically meaningful amounts in foods, it is preferable for the athlete to work those foods into the diet rather than turn to supplements first. In some cases, however, supplementation might be the only viable option, such as to obtain optimal doses of creatine or beta-alanine.

Foods inherently contain many nutrients, including well-known macronutrients and micronutrients, in addition to lesser-known **phytonutrients** or constituents that might confer benefits to health and performance. Consuming foods classified as "empty calories" while taking a variety of dietary supplements to meet nutritional needs is a situation that an individual can improve by using a food-first approach. Athletes and Sports Performance Coaches can use the National Institutes of Health's Fact Sheets for Professionals to find food sources and even some dietary supplements rich in various vitamins and minerals.

Supplementation is a solution for cases in which it is difficult to consume enough food to obtain necessary quantities of vitamins, minerals, or other components. For example, diets that reduce or eliminate animal protein might require supplementation with vitamin B_{12}. Vitamin D deficiency is quite prevalent among athletes, and supplementing the vitamin might be the best way to address deficiencies because food sources of vitamin D are relatively sparse.

More sport-specific ergogenic aids, such as creatine and beta-alanine, as well as other non-nutrient dietary supplements, are present in food items in very low concentrations. In these cases, it might not be possible to ingest enough of the specific foods to produce the desired effect. Beef products are rich in creatine, containing approximately 1 gram of creatine per pound of meat. However, for healthy adults,

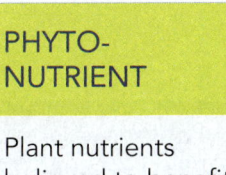

PHYTO-
NUTRIENT

Plant nutrients believed to benefit human health.

HEME

A type of iron found in animal foods.

HEPCIDIN

A protein that regulates iron levels in the body by slowing iron uptake.

TOXICITY

Accumulation of too much of a vitamin or mineral within the body, resulting in illness or other symptoms.

research supports creatine use at a rate of 5 grams per day, and eating 5 pounds of beef per day is not feasible. It is much easier, and far less expensive, to supplement the diet with 5 grams of creatine per day.

When possible, the Sports Performance Coach needs to emphasize the consumption of whole foods before turning to dietary supplements. In many cases, nutrient amounts coming from foods are self-regulated by satiety and other natural regulatory mechanisms. For example, iron is most efficiently absorbed when it comes from meat because meat contains **heme** iron as well as meat protein factor, both of which facilitate greater iron absorption (Jackson et al., 2016). Natural iron intake is limited by hunger, and absorption of iron decreases as intake increases due to an inhibitory protein called **hepcidin** that slows iron uptake. When using dietary supplements, however, it is possible to overdo it. For example, acutely increasing iron intake can overwhelm the body's regulatory mechanisms because the body does not have time to increase hepcidin production, which can lead to iron **toxicity** or poisoning (Chang & Rangan, 2011). If an athlete instead chooses to add a daily serving of meat to their diet, they can avoid acute overload while increasing iron intake and allowing time for hepcidin production, if it is needed. This food-first strategy also avoids the adulteration and contamination risks associated with dietary supplements.

📋 COACH'S CORNER

Athletes can fall into the trap of utilizing supplements to cover up a low-quality diet, especially when they have high energy requirements.

LESSON 2: ASSESSING NUTRIENT NEEDS
DETERMINING NUTRITION PRIORITIES

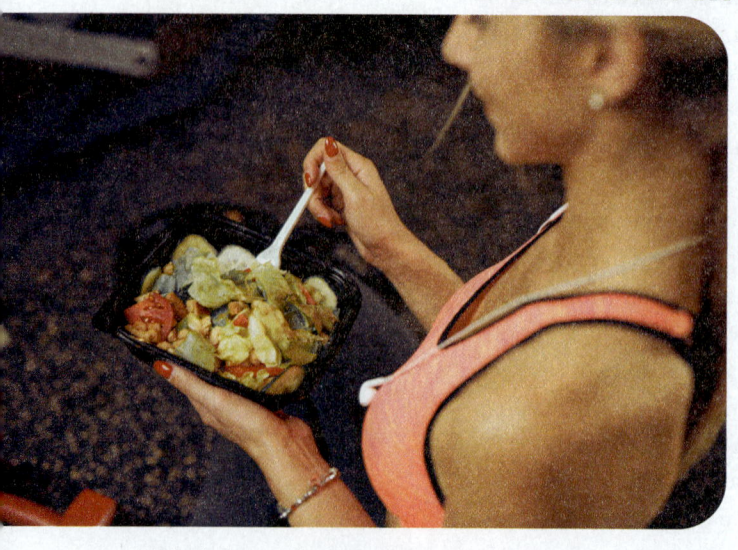

© Milan Ilic Photographer/Shutterstock

Before evaluating dietary supplements for an athlete to use, the Sports Performance Coach must determine the athlete's macronutrient needs. Using a food-first approach, an athlete is likely to meet their micronutrient needs if they have no dietary restrictions. If the athlete has dietary restrictions, take care to identify potential insufficiencies and incorporate foods that address potential gaps. Then analyze the athlete's diet and specific needs and consider supplementation to address gaps or ergogenic aids for nutrient timing or convenience. The Sports Performance Coach can help determine whether the athlete needs a dietary supplement or whether such a supplement would offer a high reward-to-risk ratio by knowing the athlete's needs, identifying which dietary supplements are effective for different desirable outcomes, and weighing the costs and benefits.

Always be mindful of your scope of practice. Refer the athlete out to, or work with, a registered dietitian if you suspect the athlete has a nutrient deficiency.

UNCOVERING NEEDS

In every scenario, the Sports Performance Coach and the athlete need to have a great idea of which attributes of performance the athlete needs to be successful in their sport or to achieve their goals. Long-distance runners need great endurance, and sprinters need excellent power and speed. Understanding the needs of the sport is the first step toward determining whether supplementation is useful.

The nutritional needs and related supplements for every individual sport can be broadly categorized into one of three groups according to the sport's energy demands or bioenergetics: phosphagen, anaerobic, and aerobic. Athletes participating in short-duration, maximal-effort sports such as weightlifting, a 100-meter sprint, and shotput rely on the phosphagen system; athletes participating in brief but intense sports such as middle-distance runs, swimming, and hockey primarily rely on the anaerobic system; and athletes participating in extended-duration sports such as long-distance endurance events and soccer primarily rely on the aerobic system.

Athletes whose sport aligns with the phosphagen energy system are likely interested in maximizing their phosphagen energy storage, such as with creatine supplementation. These athletes want large, powerful muscles that do not need a high level of endurance or mitochondria, and they want to optimize their power output and strength. In addition to supplementing creatine to increase phosphate levels, these athletes might also be interested in supplementing with protein and amino acids (to support muscle size), caffeine (to confer benefits to strength and power), and other dietary supplements that achieve similar outcomes.

Athletes in anaerobically oriented sports can benefit from the same strategies used by athletes who participate in phosphagen energy system–dominant sports. They also benefit from having adequate carbohydrate availability to fuel the anaerobic energy system and beta-alanine to buffer the lactic acid product of anaerobic metabolism. Likewise, athletes in aerobically oriented sports can benefit from lactate management and adequate carbohydrate availability. These athletes are much more likely to use and benefit from energy replacement during exercise due to the length and energy demands of their sport. They might need electrolyte replacement due to sweating, and they are very likely to benefit from caffeine supplementation.

In addition to energy needs, some sports offer other opportunities to benefit from a dietary supplement. Team sports often require reacting to what the other team does, and doing so as fast as possible is likely to yield a better result. Therefore, a dietary supplement that enhances attention and reaction time could enhance sports performance. Some athletes might be very skilled but suffer game-day anxiety; a dietary supplement that helps manage stress could be an option.

Some athletes might have nutrient needs that are not being met. These nutrient deficiencies may manifest differently, depending on which type of nutrient is in short supply. Treating true nutrient deficiencies is beyond the scope of the Sports Performance Coach. Thus, if a nutrient deficiency is thought to be present, the Sports Performance Coach must refer the athlete to a registered dietitian or healthcare professional.

In most cases, the question is whether the dietary supplement will meet the goals and performance needs of the sport. To understand if, when, and how a supplement might achieve those ends, the Sports Performance Coach needs to look for evidence.

EVALUATING EVIDENCE

Although the existence versus absence of published studies on a dietary supplement does not determine its efficacy, evaluating peer-reviewed published research is currently the best way to determine the potential benefit or detriment of a supplement to an athlete. When using research to examine the evidence regarding any dietary supplementation, fitness professionals must consider the hierarchy of scientific evidence (**Figure 23.4**). At the bottom level are case studies, which are observations of a single person. These types of studies are more common in the medical literature on rare diseases, but they are atypical in dietary supplement research. Case studies are often considered starting points for forming an educated opinion on a topic, but do not contain enough evidence for readers to be fully informed on a supplement or intervention. Ideally, research on dietary supplements will be conducted in the form of randomized controlled trials. Then, when enough trials have been performed, systematic reviews and meta-analyses using those randomized controlled trials will be carried out to ensure a very high quality of evidence. However, reviews and meta-analyses are not available for all dietary supplements.

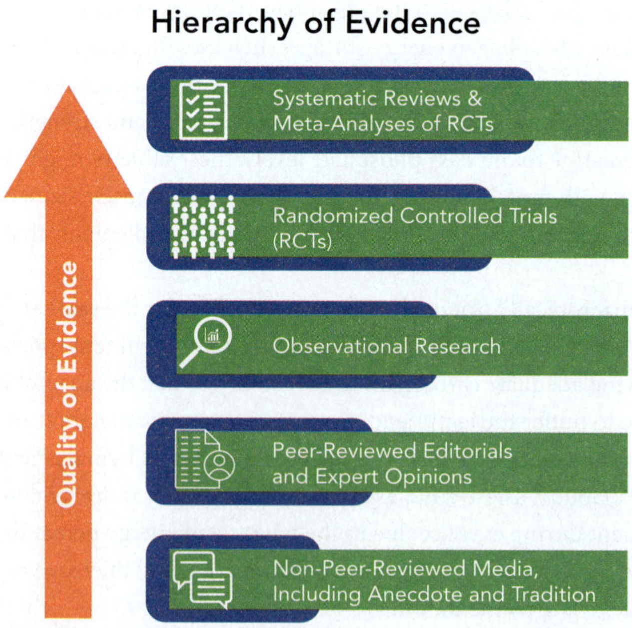

Hierarchy of Evidence

FIGURE 23.4 Hierarchy of Evidence

Sources such as Pubmed and Google Scholar are excellent resources for finding primary evidence, reviews, and meta-analyses that can indicate whether a dietary supplement is worthwhile to use. When searching for information on a new topic, it is good practice for the Sports Performance Coach to find a review or meta-analysis first, then read additional reports on specific randomized controlled trials.

To find applicable information, it can help to form a PICOT question. A PICOT question considers the population sample, intervention, comparison or control, outcome, and time frame (**Figure 23.5**). The population sample is the type of athlete or their specific sport. If a specific sport has not been investigated, find evidence from a sport with similar demands. For example, a long-distance runner is more similar to a long-distance cyclist than they are to a sprinter. The intervention needs to include the dietary supplement in question. In most cases, it is best if the dietary supplement is evaluated alongside a placebo as the comparison. Think about which outcomes need to be known—maximal strength, power output, lactate threshold, or another attribute? Then determine the time frame of supplementation. Dietary supplements might work acutely with a single dose, or they might require time to take effect. Consider the point in a training macro-cycle when the effectiveness of the supplement can be evaluated.

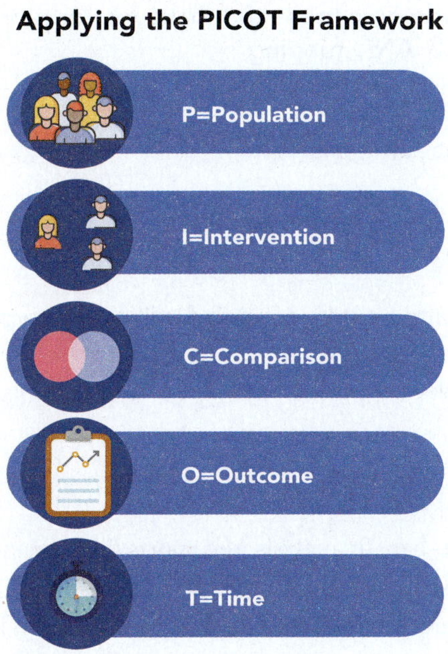

Applying the PICOT Framework

P=Population

I=Intervention

C=Comparison

O=Outcome

T=Time

FIGURE 23.5 PICOT Framework

After the Sports Performance Coach identifies all five of these components, they can write the PICOT question. For example, in collegiate football players (P), does preseason (T) creatine consumption (I) versus a placebo (C) improve 225-pound bench press repetition to failure performance (O) (**Figure 23.6**)? Then, look for research that has investigated this question.

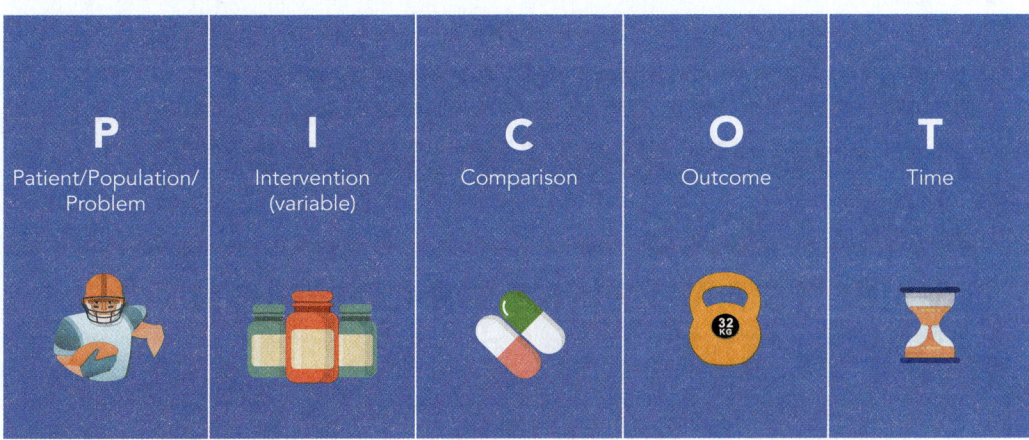

| **P** | **I** | **C** | **O** | **T** |
| Patient/Population/Problem | Intervention (variable) | Comparison | Outcome | Time |

FIGURE 23.6 Writing the Question Example: Collegiate Football

Pick any dietary supplement ingredient you are curious about. Search for the name of the ingredient, one or two keywords, and the word "supplement" in Google Scholar. Scan the titles and see if you have the results you need. If not, use advanced search techniques, such as the following:

1. Quotation marks
   - A word or phrase enclosed in quotation marks tells Google to return results with that word or phrase.
   - Example: caffeine supplement "time trial"
2. AND
   - Use AND to refine search results to include only those that have two or more key terms.
   - Example: caffeine supplement "time trial" AND running
3. OR
   - Use OR to find one thing or another.
   - Example: coffee OR caffeine supplement "time trial"
4. Minus sign
   - Use the minus sign to eliminate certain words from appearing.
   - Example: caffeine supplement -preworkout
5. Allintitle
   - Use this command to greatly reduce results after becoming familiar with typical publication titles.
   - Example: Allintitle: "caffeine supplementation"

COST–BENEFIT ANALYSIS

Prior to conducting a cost–benefit analysis, the Sports Performance Coach should establish that the food-first approach is not feasible or reasonable, the dietary supplement of interest is legal, and there is evidence of its safety and efficacy. Finally, weigh the costs and benefits need against each other to determine whether supplementation is worthwhile.

If the supplement has demonstrated efficacy and the athlete or sponsor determines that the efficacy is worth the financial cost without violating NCAA or other rules, it is likely acceptable for the athlete to use the product. If safety concerns arise, weigh those as well as the financial costs and safety risks against the potential usefulness of the product. Ultimately, the final decision is the athlete's, and the Sports Performance Coach's responsibility is to present the costs, risks, and benefits. A Dietary Supplement Use Decision Tree can be found in Appendix E.

LESSON 3: OVERVIEW OF SUPPLEMENT BENEFITS AND RISKS
BENEFITS AND RISKS OF COMMON SUPPLEMENTS

Supplements come with a myriad of potential benefits and risks. On the positive side, they can provide a convenient way to ensure optimal intake of vital nutrients, potentially improving athletic performance, supporting muscle recovery, and enhancing overall health.

Some supplements offer targeted benefits such as boosting energy, enhancing focus, or aiding muscle growth and repair. However, not all supplements are without risk. Overuse, interactions with other substances, or consumption of poor-quality or contaminated products can lead to adverse health effects. Athletes must understand that supplements are not a substitute for a balanced diet and regular exercise, and these substances should be used under the supervision of a healthcare professional to mitigate their potential risks.

Hundreds of potential dietary supplements are available for an athlete to take. Some are more common than others. Although it is still prudent to independently investigate their risks and benefits, some dietary supplements are clearly worth discussing.

HEALTH-BASED SUPPLEMENTS

Dietary supplements are divided into two broad categories based on their purpose: health or performance. Although performance supplements might be the first to come to mind for athletes, health-based supplements are more common overall and compose a larger share of the market.

Health-based supplements include vitamins, minerals, omega-3 fatty acids, probiotics, and more. Among all supplement users, at least 70% take a multivitamin for overall health and wellness (Council for Responsible Nutrition, 2018). Health is directly tied to performance, and an athlete in poor health is unlikely to perform well. Thus, while it is tempting to focus on ergogenic aids, it is important to make sure the athlete establishes a base of good health prior to adding ergogenic aids to the mix.

✔ CHECK IT OUT

Research demonstrates that multivitamins and mineral supplements effectively address common nutrient deficiencies (Bailey et al., 2012; Blumberg et al., 2017). Analysis of nearly 11,000 U.S. adults' diets showed that frequent use of these supplements largely eradicates nutrient inadequacy, except for vitamin D, calcium, and magnesium (Blumberg et al., 2017). Thus, a daily multivitamin and mineral supplement tailored to individual needs represent a practical nutritional approach. Additional supplementation is necessary to fulfill the daily requirements for minerals such as calcium, magnesium, and iron, as well as other vital nutrients such as vitamin D and the omega-3 fatty acids DHA and EPA. Supplements are not a substitute for a healthy diet but can aid the athlete in reaching the recommended nutrient levels, potentially supporting healthy aging.

WATER-SOLUBLE VITAMINS

The water-soluble vitamins (**Figure 23.7**) are vitamin C and the B-complex vitamins (B_1, B_2, B_3, B_5, B_6, B_7, B_9, and B_{12}). Compared to fat-soluble vitamins, water-soluble vitamins are more transient within the body because they can be absorbed efficiently through water and excreted in the urine while not being stored in fat. Vitamins come in different forms, and more often than not, water-soluble vitamins are found in dietary supplements as their active form.

Vitamins

FIGURE 23.7 Water-Soluble Vitamins

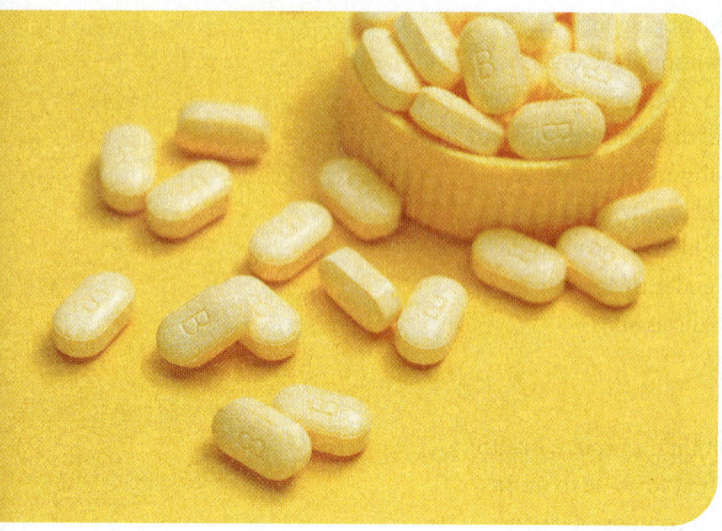
© Jinning Li/Shutterstock

Vitamin C

The active form of vitamin C is L-ascorbic acid. Vitamin C's primary functions include collagen synthesis, immune function, glutathione synthesis, and protein metabolism. Mega-dosing vitamin C has become a somewhat common practice in society owing to the belief that it helps resist and recover from colds. The body is efficient at removing excess vitamin C, so toxicity is rarely a concern. Even when it is taken in amounts 200 times the recommended daily value, body levels of vitamin C increase to only four times their normal levels (Padayatty et al., 2004). However, gastrointestinal distress is a potential adverse effect of large-dose vitamin C supplementation.

The immune effects of vitamin C and other supplements in athletes are often examined in terms of upper respiratory tract infection (URTI)—that is, the common cold—including its characteristics and presence. Increasing vitamin C intake in athletes might reduce the incidence, severity, and duration of colds by as much as 50% (Constantini et al., 2011; Peters et al., 1993). These effects are typically observed in athletes competing or training outdoors for sports with a large aerobic demand, so the results might be less robust in those competing indoors or with a low aerobic component.

The B Vitamins

The B-complex vitamins have numerous functions. As a group, they are significantly involved in energy metabolism. Although a nutrition facts or supplement facts label might list the name of the B vitamin or the number, all B vitamins have a written name as well as a number (**Table 23.1**). B-vitamin toxicity has been observed only for niacin, vitamin B_6, and folate. In the case of niacin and vitamin B_6, very high doses are sometimes found in sports supplements. Excess niacin can produce mild side effects that include flushing and nausea (MacKay et al., 2012; Minto et al., 2017). Vitamin B_6 toxicity is unlikely, but the side effects are more serious, including progressive sensory neuropathy (numbness or tingling of the hands and feet), ataxia (nerve damage, resulting in impaired coordination),

TABLE 23.1 B-Complex Vitamins by Number and Name

Number	Name
B_1	Thiamin
B_2	Riboflavin
B_3	Niacin
B_5	Pantothenic acid
B_6	Pyridoxine
B_7	Biotin
B_9	Folate
B_{12}	Cobalamin

sensitivity to light, and skin lesions (abnormal skin growth or appearance) (Bendich & Cohen, 1990; Gdynia et al., 2008; Morris et al., 2008; Perry et al., 2004).

When athletes are already consuming adequate amounts of B vitamins, additional supplementation is unlikely to benefit their performance (Haymes, 1991). Deficiencies in just one B vitamin at a time have not shown a negative effect on performance. However, insufficient intake of multiple B vitamins has, and their replacement through supplementation might help reverse that effect (Clarkson, 1993). Even so, increased need due to exercise is thought to be made up for by diet. The Sports Performance Coach likely does not need to look for B-vitamin insufficiencies in athletes because many staple foods are fortified with these vitamins and they are present in many dietary supplements.

FAT-SOLUBLE VITAMINS

There are four fat-soluble vitamins: A, D, E, and K. As the name implies, these vitamins are absorbed with, and stored in, fat (**Figure 23.8**). With that understanding, it is easy to comprehend why fat-soluble vitamins are more likely to present a risk for toxicity; these vitamins accumulate in the body more easily than water-soluble vitamins do.

Vitamins

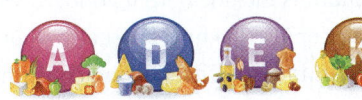

FIGURE 23.8 Fat-Soluble Vitamins

Vitamin A

Vitamin A is usually found in the form of beta-carotene. However, **beta-carotene** is not a vitamin so much as it is a **provitamin**—a precursor to vitamin A. In addition to beta-carotene, alpha-carotene and beta-cryptoxanthin are other forms of provitamin A that can be found in dietary supplements. Other carotenoids, such as lutein, lycopene, and zeaxanthin, do not contribute to vitamin A levels. The most **biologically active** form of vitamin A is retinol, which can be supplemented as a retinyl ester.

Vitamin A toxicity is possible and is characterized by dizziness, headache, reduced bone density, coma, congenital birth defects, and death (Trumbo et al., 2001). Vitamin A levels have not been observed to be insufficient in athletes and are unlikely to modulate performance (van Erp-Baart et al., 1989). The Sports Performance Coach likely does not need to suspect vitamin A insufficiency in athletes.

Vitamin D

Vitamin D is important for bone health, immune modulation, and skeletal muscle function. Although both ergocalciferol (D_2) and cholecalciferol (D_3) can increase blood vitamin D levels, vitamin D_3 is more efficacious at doing so (Armas et al., 2004). Taking too much vitamin D can cause weight loss, excessive urination, and **heart arrhythmias**, and when taken together with calcium at high doses, kidney stones and tissue calcification (*Dietary Reference Intakes for Calcium and Vitamin D*, 2011). The **tolerable upper limit** is 4,000 IU *daily (Dietary Reference Intakes for Calcium and Vitamin D*, 2011).

Vitamin D has wide-ranging benefits. In terms of its more direct benefits for athletics, vitamin D might improve a number of areas of human performance, including oxygen consumption, recovery, sprint and jump performance, and testosterone in men. Recovery from exercise is enhanced by 4,000 IU daily vitamin D supplementation in recreationally trained individuals (Barker et al., 2013). In professional athletes, intakes of 5,000 and

BETA-CAROTENE →

The red-orange pigment found in vegetables and fruits that is converted to vitamin A in the body.

PROVITAMIN →

A compound that can be converted to a vitamin.

BIOLOGICALLY ACTIVE →

The form in which a vitamin must be to exert an effect within the body.

HEART ARRHYTHMIA →

An irregular heartbeat.

TOLERABLE UPPER LIMIT →

The greatest quantity of a vitamin or mineral that might be consumed in a day without risk of an adverse health effect.

6,000 IU of this vitamin improve power output and VO_2 max, respectively (Close et al., 2013; Jastrzębska et al., 2016). One study of professional football players in a sunny area in Spain measured in October and February reported that 64% and 7%, respectively, were deficient in vitamin D, further suggesting that its supplementation might have utility, particularly during the winter months (Galan et al., 2012).

The Endocrine Society and the Institute of Medicine do not agree on optimal vitamin D intakes; their recommendations, relative to each other, support higher or lower quantities. As evident by the studies using supplements of 4,000 to 6,000 IU per day, the ergogenic effects of vitamin D are observed at doses greater than the tolerable upper limit. Although adequate levels might be achieved with or without supplementation, performance or recovery enhancement seems more likely to occur with high-dose vitamin D intake achieved by supplementation (Dahlquist et al., 2015). However, the Sports Performance Coach might incur liability if they recommend the athlete exceed the tolerable upper limit for any vitamin or mineral.

Vitamin E

Vitamin E is an antioxidant vitamin that plays roles in vascular health, cancer, and **immunodeficiencies** (*Dietary Reference Intakes for Vitamin C, Vitamin E, Selenium, and Carotenoids*, 2000). The E vitamins include both tocopherols and tocotrienols. The biologically active form is alpha-tocopherol, which is usually—but not always—the source found in dietary supplements. Vitamin E toxicity via food consumption has not been reported, but high levels of vitamin E from supplementation have been associated with excessive bleeding due to its role in inhibiting **platelet aggregation** (Owen & Dewald, 2021).

Vitamin E most likely does not have an effect on exercise performance. In two studies examining elite endurance athletes and two studies in recreationally trained individuals, researchers consistently failed to observe an improvement in performance markers (Keong et al., 2006; McAnulty et al., 2005; Patil et al., 2009; Rokitzki et al., 1994). However, two of these studies (one each by training status) did find an improvement in oxidation status, suggesting vitamin E functioned effectively as an antioxidant. The Sports Performance Coach is unlikely to encounter poor vitamin E status in athletes.

Vitamin K

Vitamin K works with vitamin D to support bone health and, independently, blood clotting. Vitamin K is also very unlikely to reach toxic levels in the body, but it should not be taken with anticoagulant drugs, such as warfarin.

Vitamin K's role in bone health is relevant for exercising individuals who might have a low vitamin K status. While these results might also be typical of non-athletes, female athletes with vitamin K deficiency who took supplements of 10 mg/day vitamin K were observed to have improved bone formation markers, suggesting a net positive shift in bone formation (Craciun et al., 1998). Indeed, a meta-analysis on vitamin K for preventing fractures found that in all but one study, vitamin K was associated with a reduced risk of fractures. The one study that did not observe the reduced risk featured an athletic population sample, whereas the other studies were carried out in various special populations (Cockayne et al., 2006).

MINERALS

Minerals are inorganic, natural substances that are important to human nutrition. There are 16 **essential** minerals, of which 14 appear on nutrition and supplement fact labels: calcium, iron, phosphorus, iodine, magnesium, zinc, selenium, copper, manganese, chromium, molybdenum, chloride, sodium, and potassium.

IMMUNO-DEFICIENCY →

A weakened immune system.

PLATELET AGGREGATION →

An accumulation of blood cells prior to a clot.

ESSENTIAL →

A nutrient that must be obtained in the diet because the body is incapable of producing the nutrient on its own.

Sodium

Of particular importance in sport are the electrolyte minerals, primarily sodium and potassium. By proxy, chloride is often found in electrolyte supplements because salt (sodium chloride) is the primary ingredient used to deliver sodium. Sometimes potassium chloride is used for the same reason. Sodium deserves special attention for athletes, as prolonged exercise can produce a condition known as hyponatremia, or low blood sodium. This can also be caused by drinking plain water without added sodium. Symptoms of hyponatremia include nausea, headache, confusion, and fatigue. In very serious cases, hyponatremia can cause brain swelling and death.

Sodium is often overconsumed, and potassium is often underconsumed. In the United States, 99% of the population consumes more sodium than is recommended, but only 5% have the recommended intake of potassium (Cogswell et al., 2012). These numbers cannot be uniformly applied to athletes or anyone with a high sweat rate. Because sweat rates vary based on the type and intensity of exercise, broad recommendations cannot be made. In general, 300 to 600 mg of additional sodium is needed per hour of exercise that induces subjectively high sweating (Vitale & Getzin, 2019).

✔ CHECK IT OUT

People with saltier sweat can be visually identified by allowing sweat to dry on dark clothes before washing. Salty sweat on clothes forms a white ring around the edge of the sweat when dry. This white ring is sodium.

📋 COACH'S CORNER

For endurance events, athletes need to avoid water losses in excess of 2% bodyweight, which can compromise performance. One strategy is to develop a personalized hydration plan based on the athlete's own sweat rate, approximate sodium loss per liter (L) of sweat, and anticipated finish time. Here is one example using an anticipated completion time of 3 hours for a 60-kg (132-pound) athlete with a sweat rate of 4 liters per hour and an average sodium loss of 500 mg per liter.

Maximum fluid needs are sweat rate times duration divided by number of 15-minute segments in the total duration of the event.

1. 4 liter per hour × 3 hours / 12 = 0.35 liter per 15 minutes
2. Minimum fluid needs are to prevent loss of no more than 2% bodyweight and are related to the maximum need.
   - 60 kg × 0.02 = 1.2 kg or 1.2 liter
   - 4 × 3 – 1.2 = 3 liter
   - 3 liter / 12 = 0.25 liter per 15 minutes
3. To replace the necessary sodium, add 500 mg of sodium to each pound of fluid.
   - 1 pound of fluid = 2.2 liter
   - 500 mg of sodium in every 2.2 liter of fluid
   - 227 mg of sodium per liter of fluid

In this example, fluid needs are 0.25 – 0.35 liter per 15 minutes, and each liter needs to contain 227 mg of sodium. You can modify the example to accommodate athletes with different needs (Ayotte & Corcoran, 2018).

Iron

Iron's major function is in the formation of hemoglobin, which carries oxygen in the blood and therefore directly impacts aerobic exercise performance. Athletes' iron needs are 30% to 70% greater than those of the general population (*Dietary Reference Intakes for Vitamin C, Vitamin E, Selenium, and Carotenoid*, 2000). Iron deficiencies range from 20% to 50% in female athletes and from 4% to 50% in male athletes, with the greater rates of deficiency being observed in endurance athletes (Hinton, 2014). In those who are deficient, restoring iron levels to the normal range improves performance (Celsing et al., 1986; Pedlar et al., 2018; Woodson et al., 1978).

Iron needs to be supplemented under supervision of a physician, as it increases the risk for toxicity as well as **adverse events**, including **serious adverse events**. The Sports Performance Coach should consider close examination of an athlete's diet if they display lethargic symptoms or pale color, especially in young women participating in endurance sports. If their iron intake is found to be low, suggest dietary modification or refer the athlete to a registered dietitian or physician if adverse events are a risk.

Calcium

Calcium plays a crucial role in bone health, alongside vitamin D and vitamin K. For purposes of bone health, the Sports Performance Coach needs to be aware of female athletes who display habits consistent with the female athlete triad: disordered eating, amenorrhea, and **osteoporosis** (Kunstel, 2005). Average calcium intake among Division 1-A women is approximately 400 mg below the adequate level for the general population, and athletes might require even more calcium (Clarkson & Haymes, 1995; Leachman Slawson et al., 2001). Lack of calcium is a contributor to stress fractures (Chen et al., 2013). Individuals with calcium deficiency might need a more comprehensive diet assessment and can be referred to a registered dietitian or medical professional. There are no reports of calcium improving athletic performance, and one study has indicated calcium has no effect on aerobic exercise performance (Heffernan et al., 2019).

Magnesium

Magnesium is another of the more common mineral supplements that might be consumed in isolation. Frank magnesium deficiency to the extent that it causes complications is uncommon. However, about 50% of the U.S. population consumes less than the estimated average requirement (DiNicolantonio et al., 2018). Due to loss of this mineral in sweat and urine, athletes have a 10% to 20% greater magnesium requirement, and intakes of less than 260 mg (males) and 220 mg (females) per day might cause a deficiency (Nielsen & Lukaski, 2006).

Low magnesium levels can trigger muscle cramps, particularly in the legs, and involuntary contractions; increasing magnesium intake can prevent both of these symptoms (Garrison et al., 2012). Athletes competing in weight class–restricted sports are at greater risk of deficiency due to weight manipulation. Only limited evidence supports magnesium supplementation for improving performance, though most athletes have an inadequate intake. Therefore, it is probable that magnesium supplementation is unlikely to produce an ergogenic effect if it is not correcting a deficiency or inadequate intake (Volpe, 2015). Similar to the case for iron and calcium, the Sports Performance Coach can perform a dietary analysis to observe mineral intake levels and decide whether diet optimization is necessary or whether the athlete needs to be referred to a registered dietitian or physician.

ADVERSE EVENT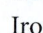

Any unfavorable medical occurrence associated with the use of a dietary supplement.

SERIOUS ADVERSE EVENT →

Any adverse event that results in any life-threatening situation, inpatient hospitalization, persistent incapacity of a person's ability to conduct a normal life, a congenital anomaly, reproductive harm, or death.

OSTEOPO-ROSIS →

A condition of reduced bone mineral density that increases risk of fracture.

Iodine

Iodine is the primary mineral used to form thyroid hormones. In the early 1900s, iodine was added to salt to prevent goiters. Iodine deficiency is now uncommon in developed countries, but it still affects more than 2 billion people worldwide (Peterson, 2000). Low iodine levels can lead to reduced cognitive ability, and iodine deficiency is the most common cause of preventable cognitive disability. Excess iodine consumption can cause an underactive thyroid gland, but it takes very high doses to cause toxicity. Toxicity is manifested as nausea, weak pulse, coma, and vomiting (Trumbo et al., 2001). There is no research showing iodine has a direct relevance to sports performance (Heffernan et al., 2019).

Zinc

Zinc deficiency is rare, and it is difficult to ascertain its prevalence. Evaluation of eight elite swimmers suggested that, on average, they could be borderline deficient, but prevalence was not determined (Giolo De Carvalho et al., 2012). Individuals who are vegetarian or vegan, and women who are pregnant are more likely to have insufficient zinc intake (Institute of Medicine, 2001). Exercise does not appear to alter zinc status, but rather redistributes the body's existing zinc stores between muscle, liver, and other cells (Chu & Samman, 2014). Athletes low in zinc have reduced power output and a reduced lactate threshold (Chu & Samman, 2014; Micheletti et al., 2001). One study observed an improvement in oxygen consumption with zinc supplementation (Saeedy et al., 2016), and others reported improved testosterone status in men with such supplementation (Cinar et al., 2017; Neek et al., 2011). However, other studies suggest zinc does not have a direct effect on performance (Davison et al., 2016; Khaled et al., 1999).

Chromium

Chromium deficiency and toxicity has not been observed in healthy individuals. In those with diabetes or prediabetes, chromium supplementation has been shown in some studies to improve glucose regulation (Costello et al., 2019). Because of its potential insulin-modulating effects, chromium has been suggested in media reports to improve muscle hypertrophy and performance. However, scientific studies on the subject do not support this use case (Campbell et al., 1999; Campbell et al., 2002; Davis et al., 2000; Hallmark et al., 1996; Joseph et al., 1999; Livolsi et al., 2001; Walker et al., 1998).

Selenium, copper, manganese, and molybdenum are unlikely to be found outside of multivitamins unless prescribed by a physician under unusual circumstances.

OMEGA-3

Omega-3 acids are a type of unsaturated fatty acid. The omega-3 terminology refers to the location of the first double bond in the carbon chain, which is located on the third carbon. There are three types of omega-3 acids: **eicosapentaenoic acid (EPA)**, **docosahexaenoic acid (DHA)**, and alpha-linolenic acid (ALA). EPA and DHA are usually referred to as fish oil, as fish are the most abundant source of these fatty acids. However, they can also be sourced from shellfish, such as krill and oysters. ALA is a plant source of omega-3, and it is found primarily in nuts and seeds. EPA and DHA are of greater relevance, as they are the biologically active forms, whereas only about 10% of ALA is converted to EPA in the body (Gerster, 1998; Wang et al., 2006).

Fish oil is best known for its role in heart health. It is effective in reducing triglycerides and inflammatory markers while increasing high-density lipoprotein (HDL) cholesterol (Dangardt et al., 2010; Wei & Jacobson, 2011; Zulyniak et al., 2013). DHA, in particular, is beneficial for brain health. It might be of direct relevance to athletes competing in

---

OMEGA-3 →

Polyunsaturated fats; eicosapentaenoic acid (EPA), docosahexaenoic acid (DHA), and alpha-linolenic acid (ALA).

EICOSA-PENTAENOIC ACID (EPA) →

An omega-3 fatty acid derived from animals, usually a marine animal.

DOCOSAHEX-AENOIC ACID (DHA) →

An omega-3 fatty acid derived from animals, usually a marine animal.

contact sports, as supplementing with DHA has been observed to ward off brain trauma by protecting against hypoxia (Mayurasakorn et al., 2011; Oliver et al., 2016). Furthermore, fish oil might improve recovery from exercise, possibly by attenuating inflammation, as well as components of performance (e.g., VO$_2$ max), but these effects have not been reliably observed to translate into improved performance (e.g., in time trials) in athletes (Lewis et al., 2020; Thielecke & Blannin, 2020). A reliable improvement in mood from fish oil supplementation has been reported across various sports, including rugby, soccer, recreational athletics, and karate (Lewis et al., 2020).

It is likely that most athletes can benefit from fish oil supplementation in terms of their health. Athletes participating in contact sports can be recommended to take fish oil to help prevent or delay negative effects of concussion, especially if there is a high likelihood of concussion (e.g., in American football and combat sports). Because fish oil might improve maximal oxygen consumption and is unlikely to impair performance, athletes benefiting from greater aerobic capacity might also be interested in supplementing with fish oil.

PROBIOTICS AND PREBIOTICS

Probiotics are the bacteria that make up the body's microbiome. Prebiotics are usually a fiber that the bacteria can ferment and feed on to proliferate. Attention to the human body's microbiome and the popularity of probiotic and prebiotic supplements have grown sharply over the past decade. Although some things are known in this area, there remains much more to learn. Some of the key benefits of probiotics include promotion of gut health and immune function. However, research supports several other specific functions, such as improvements in heart and brain health.

Probiotics refer to an entire group of bacteria. However, dietary supplements typically provide only a few, often very specific types of probiotics. They are named according to their genus and species, which might be familiar terms, and they often have further subspecies and strain designations. This terminology can get confusing, as it is possible that only specific strains within a species are relevant for a particular outcome. This is important to keep in mind when reading the literature on probiotics, because different strains of the same species of bacteria can have different effects. Essentially, they are a different bacterium altogether.

Because probiotic effects are strain-specific, it is important to understand that even within the same species of a bacterium, different strains of that species can be responsible for health or ergogenic effects, whereas others are not effective or have unknown efficacy. **Table 23.2** clarifies this distinction for the case of *Lactobacillus helveticus* versus *Lactobacillus helveticus* La L10.

TABLE 23.2 Probiotic Strains and Effect

Genus	Species	Subspecies	Strain Designation	Effect
Lactobacillus	*helveticus*	LAFTI	L10	Improved immunity in athletes
Lactobacillus	*helveticus*	Not available	Not available	Unknown

As it relates to the athlete and sports performance, the microbiome of different individuals of various health statuses also differs. In specific athletes, the microbiome may even change between an athlete's chosen sports (Jäger et al., 2019; O'Donovan et al., 2020). To date, prebiotic research in athletes has mostly focused on probiotic and prebiotic co-ingestion, though studies are few in number (Calero et al., 2020). Currently, the scientific literature supports probiotic use for outcomes such as gut health and immunity, but it is equivocal regarding the effects of probiotics on performance. In both cases, it appears that any potential effect is highly dependent on the specific strain of probiotic consumed. Therefore, athletes interested in obtaining the benefits of probiotics should not look for just "a probiotic," but rather strains of probiotics that can produce the desired effect.

Furthermore, probiotics are measured in colony-forming units (CFU) rather than by mass or volume. Because probiotics are living creatures, the amount of CFU gradually declines with time. If the label of the dietary supplement being evaluated includes a disclaimer with the phrase "at the time of bottling" (or something similar) in reference to the dose of probiotics, you can rest assured there will be fewer CFU in the product at the time of consumption than are listed on the supplement facts panel. Be aware of the efficacious dose and the expiration date of the product.

🤖 GETTING TECHNICAL

The effects of probiotics are often strain-specific. Supplementing with *L. acidophilus* LAFTI10, *L. fermentum* VRI-003, *L. casei* Shirota, *L. fermentum* PCC, *B. animalis lactis* BI-04, or *L. helveticus* Lafti L10 in isolation, or with others in combination, has shown efficacy for improving immunological function, which might include reduced severity or incidence of URTI in athletes (Jäger et al., 2019). However, many other strains have been tested for similar outcomes and have failed to show an effect. *B. breve* BR03 + *S. thermophilus* FP4, *L. plantarum* TWK, and several multi-strain combinations improve at least one parameter of performance. However, the majority of strains have failed to demonstrate an ergogenic effect (Jäger et al., 2019).

DIGESTIVE ENZYMES

The term *digestive enzymes* refers to any enzyme that assists in the breakdown of food or macronutrients. Broadly, digestive enzymes include lipases or proteases for lipids and proteins, respectively. They can also be amylase, maltase, sucrase, and lactase for carbohydrates. Most digestive enzyme supplements focus on lipase or protease because carbohydrate digestion is not a common issue, with the exception of fiber and lactose. Lactase, in particular, is added to some dairy products (e.g., Lactaid milk) as well as being available as a dietary supplement for individuals who have difficulty digesting lactose (milk sugar); it is effective for correcting lactose malabsorption (Lami et al., 1988).

Proteases are the most relevant to athletic populations. Some have been independently studied and shown to improve amino acid absorption when co-ingested with protein. Specifically, combining a protease with whey protein consumed at rest significantly increases absorption of total and all but four individual amino acids (Oben et al., 2008). In theory, increasing amino acid absorption might enhance the benefits of amino acid and protein supplements, but more research is needed to determine the true benefit of protease supplementation on performance and recovery.

LESSON 4: UNDERSTANDING PERFORMANCE SUPPLEMENTATION

PERFORMANCE SUPPLEMENTATION CONSIDERATIONS AND APPLICATIONS

Performance supplementation for athletes is a nuanced area, which is aimed at maximizing athletic performance while maintaining overall health. It involves carefully selecting and applying dietary supplements tailored to individual athletic needs, goals, and physiological parameters. This process demands a thorough understanding of each supplement's benefits, appropriate timing, dosages, and potential side effects. Additionally, it considers factors such as the athlete's sport, training regimen, dietary habits, and individual metabolic responses. Crucially, it underscores the importance of quality control, ensuring products are free from harmful contaminants and comply with legal and ethical guidelines. Hence, performance supplementation is not just about taking a pill or powder; it is about a comprehensive, evidence-based approach to augmenting athletic performance and health.

In the prior lesson, some of the health-based supplements and their benefits and risks were discussed. In this lesson, we take a deeper dive into the benefits and risks of common performance supplements.

ERGOGENIC AIDS

Of primary interest to athletes in the dietary supplement world are ergogenic aids. Ergogenic aids improve an athlete's ability to perform work. An astounding number of dietary supplements are touted as ergogenic aids, but only a few ingredients have been rigorously tested and substantiated as effective. The Sports Performance Coach needs to work with athletes to provide safe and effective supplementation that can help improve their physical attributes without causing undue harm or risk of harm. To do so, it is critical to know which are effective, at what dose, and what the common side effects and adverse events can be.

PROTEIN AND AMINO ACIDS

Amino acids are the building blocks of proteins. Therefore, dietary supplements that are whole proteins, essential amino acids (EAA), or **branched-chain amino acids (BCAA)**, despite being marketed differently and presented as unique products, share very similar functionality (**Table 23.3**). Briefly, all three types of products augment muscle size and recovery by increasing rates of muscle protein synthesis (MPS) (Hirsch et al., 2021; Hormoznejad et al., 2019; Howatson et al., 2012; Vieillevoye et al., 2010). However, the hypertrophic effects of BCAA supplementation are limited to older-adult populations (Komar et al., 2015).

Protein

Protein powders are available as protein concentrates (80% protein) or isolates (90% protein). The remaining 10% to 20% of these powders is composed of moisture, calcium, ash, carbohydrate (lactose), and fat. Unless the individual has a strong need to tightly control carbohydrate and fat intake, a protein concentrate is the most cost-effective

---

BRANCHED-CHAIN AMINO ACIDS (BCAA) →

The three essential amino acids (leucine, isoleucine, and valine) that are abundant in skeletal muscle tissue; named for their branch-like structure.

TABLE 23.3 Amino Acid Classification

Essential	Nonessential
Histidine	Alanine
Lysine	Arginine
Methionine	Glutamine
Phenylalanine	Asparagine
Threonine	Cysteine
Tryptophan	Glutamic acid
Branched-chain amino acids	Aspartic acid
Valine	Glycine
Leucine	Proline
Isoleucine	Serine
	Threonine

strategy to increase protein without increasing intake of other macronutrients. Popular for use in the post-workout "window of opportunity," any high-quality protein source performs about equally to a whey protein shake for muscle growth and recovery, such as a meal with beef, chicken, fish, or pork, as long as they are leaner pieces—fat slows digestion, and protein shakes often have very little fat. Moreover, the post-exercise window is larger than believed, at about 2 hours. As there is no good reason *not* to consume protein shortly after exercise, the athlete should keep in mind that protein timing yields no productive results when total daily protein intake is equal (Schoenfeld et al., 2013), and post-exercise is an opportunity to contribute to total daily protein intake.

Protein supplements provide a liquid alternative to solid protein choices, and they are a convenient option for increasing total daily protein intake. They are beneficial for increasing muscle size and strength when diets are low or moderate in protein intake (e.g., less than 1.6 g/kg/day) in healthy individuals (Morton et al., 2018). This is also likely true to some degree in resistance-trained individuals. However, when total daily protein intake is not controlled, any beneficial effects can be attributed only to total protein, rather than being viewed as unique effects of the supplemental protein (Naclerio & Larumbe-Zabala, 2016).

Essential Amino Acids

EAAs function similarly to protein when athletes are consuming 3.5 g, but not 1.9 g of leucine (Pasiakos et al., 2011). These amino acids might be supplemented in place of protein

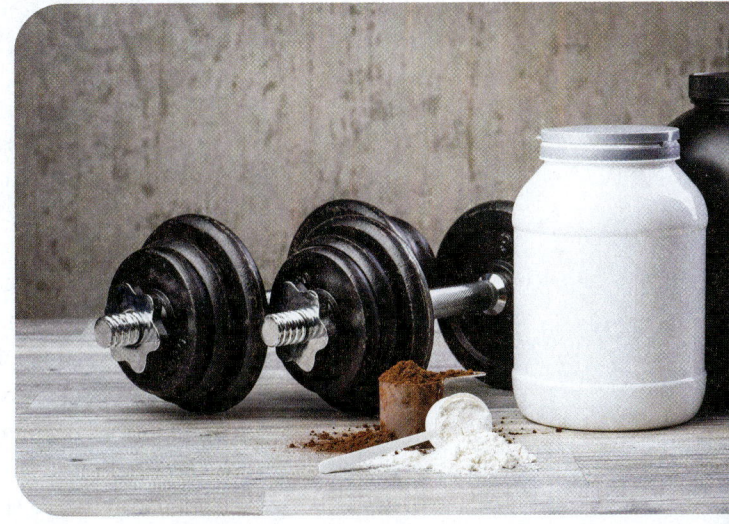

© Room 76/Shutterstock

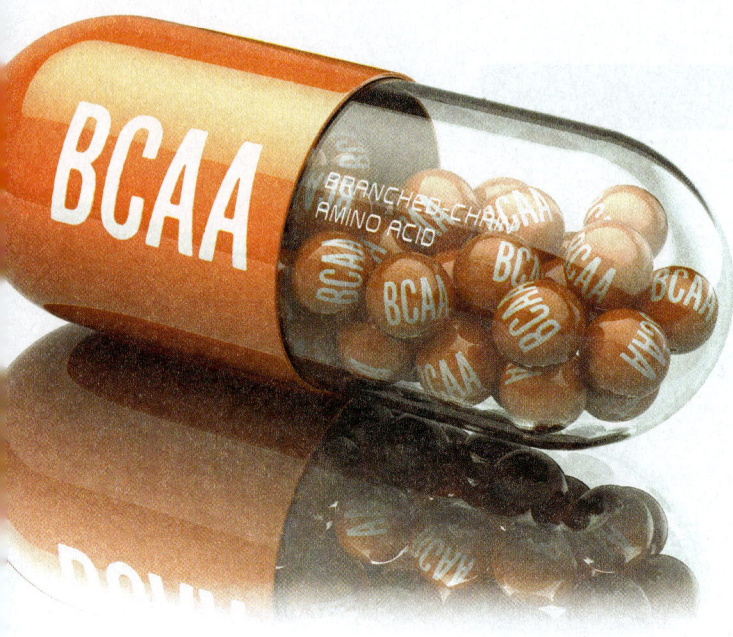

© Maxx-Studio/Shutterstock

for a comparable increase in muscle protein synthesis for athletes needing fewer calories, with aversion to allergens, who adhere to a special diet, and for a reduced potential for gastric distress (Wilkinson et al., 2018).

Branched-Chain Amino Acids

During exercise, there is evidence that BCAA supplementation can reduce muscle damage and improve performance, possibly by serving as a fuel substrate in the Kreb's cycle. A meta-analysis of eight randomized controlled trials found that BCAA supplementation reduced delayed-onset muscle soreness (DOMS) (Fedewa et al., 2019). Regarding endurance-type performance, studies have produced mixed findings, with some reporting an effect and others not (Greer et al., 2011; Kephart et al., 2015; Portier et al., 2008). Most studies do not support the use of BCAA for improving muscle strength and hypertrophy (Plotkin et al., 2021).

The Sports Performance Coach can use supplemental protein powders to help athletes achieve their total daily protein intake (**Table 23.4**). EAAs might be a viable substitute for whole proteins in situations where a rich, thick drink is unpalatable or nauseating. However, these situations are most likely limited to extended bouts of exercise or competition that do not allow breaks for regular food consumption. BCAAs might help manage soreness, but they are unlikely to outperform EAAs or protein in this regard.

TABLE 23.4   Protein and Amino Acid Effects on Lean Mass and DOMS

Supplement Type	Effect on Lean Mass	Effect on DOMS
Whole protein	Increases	Decreases
EAA	Increases	Decreases
BCAA	No effect (Plotkin et al., 2021)	Decreases
Leucine	No effect (Plotkin et al., 2021)	No effect

For all effects, it is assumed that the individual is healthy, younger than the age of 65, engaged in a resistance training program, and consuming adequate calories and protein.

Collagen

Collagen is a type of protein that has recently gained popularity as a dietary supplement. Its benefits are primarily related to skin and joint health. Collagen supplements might be beneficial for reducing joint pain, as collagen proteins form cartilage, tendons, and joints (Clark et al., 2008; Khatri et al., 2021; Zdzieblik et al., 2017; Zdzieblik et al., 2021). The provision of collagen peptides in the form of supplements supplies the peptides and amino acids necessary for forming these unique connective tissues.

Undenatured type II collagen benefits both individuals with diagnosed osteoarthritis and those without joint pain aside from during physical activity.

Forty milligrams taken daily improves outcomes versus placebo, and in one study compared to the commonly used joint supplements glucosamine and chondroitin as well (Lugo et al., 2013; Lugo et al., 2016). Another study evaluating 10 grams of hydrolyzed collagen in athletes for 24 weeks found the supplement improved both subjective (self-reported) and objective (physician-evaluated) joint relief (Clark et al., 2008).

As a protein source for daily recovery, collagen is likely inferior to whey and other high-quality animal proteins because collagen has a lower leucine content (Khatri et al., 2021; Oikawa et al., 2020). However, it might have efficacy in recovery from injury or joint discomfort.

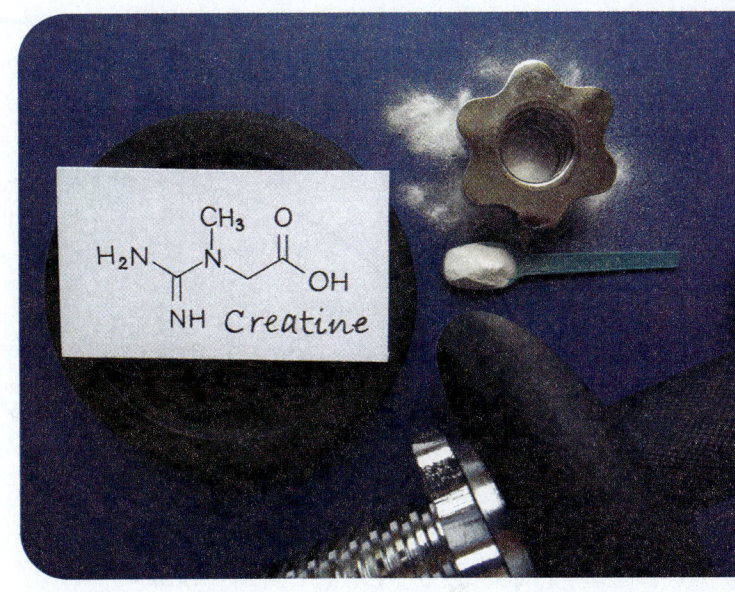

© Danijela Maksimovic/Shutterstock

CREATINE

Creatine is one of the most well-researched and strongly substantiated ergogenic aids available. It is best known for enhancing muscle size and strength gains. It does so by increasing fatigue resistance to short, high-intensity activities, such as resistance training and sprinting. Thus, part of how creatine works is to enable the athlete to push the physical limits on work capacity and increase training volume, thereby creating more of a stimulus for adaptation.

Mechanism of Action

The human body naturally produces creatine at a rate of about 1 gram per day from the amino acids methionine, arginine, and glycine. Creatine is stored in the muscles and functions to replenish ATP by holding on to **phosphagen** until ATP is transformed into ADP or AMP, then rephosphorylating them to ATP, so it can continue to power muscular contractions (**Figure 23.9**). This helps to extend the ability of the phosphagen energy system to serve as the primary energy system for about 5 extra seconds, or a 50% increase. This can manifest during exercise as the ability to perform extra repetitions with the same weight or sustaining power output during a sprint for a longer duration than without creatine (Volek et al., 1997).

In addition to muscle tissue, creatine is found in the brain, and supplementation increases brain stores as well. Because creatine supports the phosphagen energy system, it might help prevent or delay the damage that can occur from ischemic brain injuries by supplying brain cells with ATP so they stay alive with a limited supply of nutrients. Early research in this area suggested that creatine supplementation can prevent damage in brain areas following trauma (Adcock et al., 2002). Although it is beyond the scope of the Sports Performance Coach to advise anyone on the treatment of traumatic brain injury, creatine primarily has a preventive role in this area. Given its relatively low financial cost and well-supported ability to improve exercise capacity, creatine is a good choice to supplement anyway. With the potential added benefit of reducing the severity of brain injury, it can be considered for athletes participating in contact sports (Kreider & Stout, 2021).

Forms

Creatine comes in many different forms. However, most of these are simply marketing ploys, and none has demonstrated superiority to **creatine monohydrate** (Fazio et al., 2021; Jäger et al., 2011). From a molecular perspective, creatine monohydrate contains

---

CREATINE →

A molecule made from amino acids and used as a dietary supplement to facilitate ATP regeneration for improved training capacity, strength, power, and muscle mass.

PHOSPHAGEN →

A high-energy molecule that releases energy when its bonds are broken.

CREATINE → MONOHYDRATE

The most common, and likely most effective, form of creatine available as a dietary supplement.

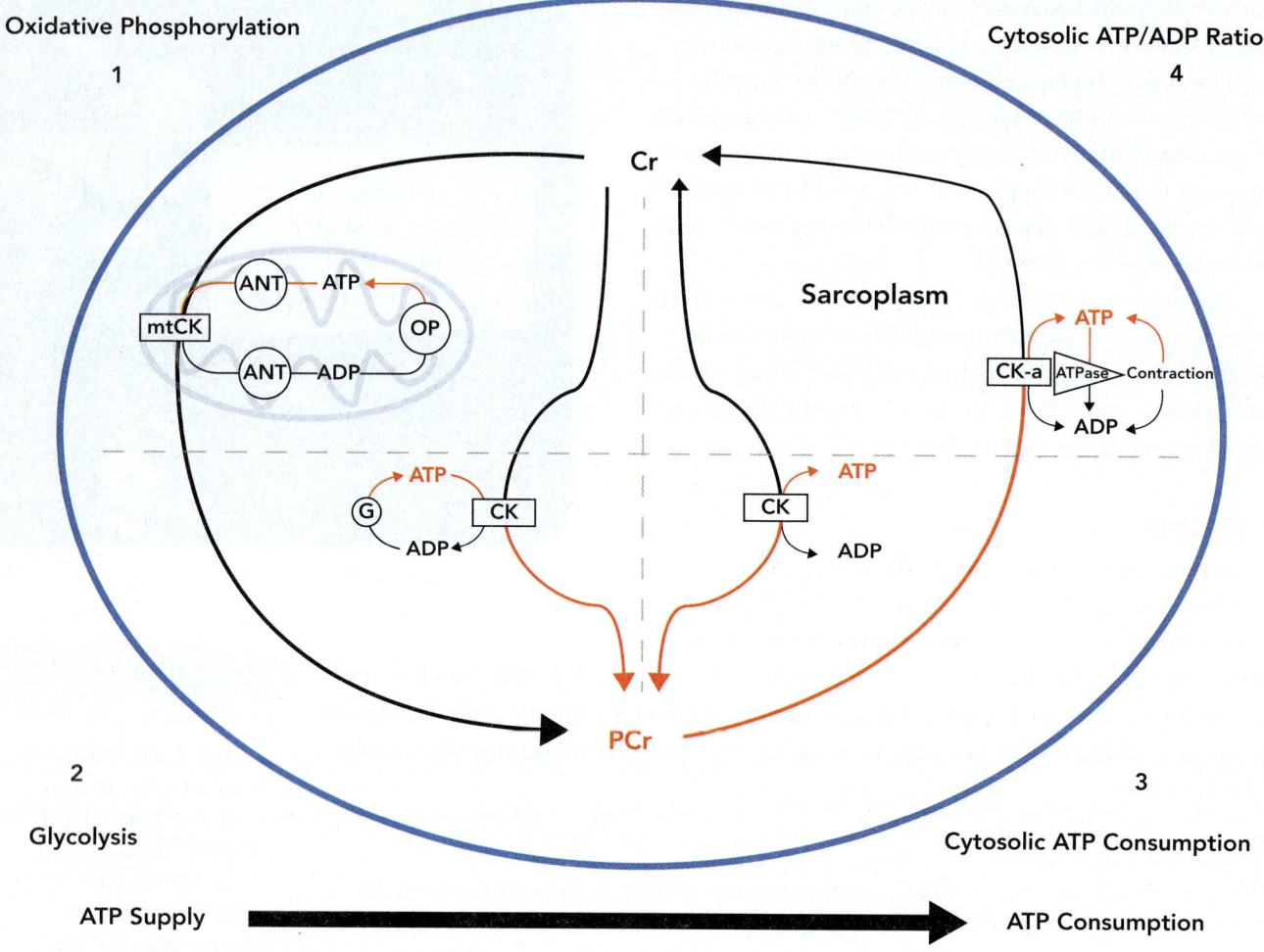

FIGURE 23.9 The Role of Creatine in ATP Energy Production

the greatest concentration of pure creatine (87.9%) among the many different forms of creatine, such as creatine ethyl ester (82.4%), creatine alpha-ketoglutarate (creatine AKG; 53.8%), and creatine gluconate (40.2%) (**Table 23.5**). Data on bioavailability and impact on muscle creatine stores are lacking for many of the various forms. However, creatine monohydrate appears to be better for loading muscle creatine stores and shows less conversion to its metabolite, creatinine, compared to creatine ethyl ester (Spillane et al., 2009). Although creatine monohydrate has frequently been shown to improve muscular strength, power, and size, alternative forms of creatine collectively demonstrate inconsistent efficacy as an ergogenic aid versus placebo (Fazio et al., 2021).

Dosing

Most research has investigated and supports a dose of 5 grams per day. The 5 gram per day dose is popular among athletes participating in strength and power sports as well as bodybuilding, for which it is known to be effective (Branch, 2003; Law et al., 2009; Rawson & Volek, 2003). Creatine supplementation has also been shown to be effective for improving oxygen consumption and glycogen resynthesis and has minor effects on endurance improvement (Ayoama et al., 2003; Graef et al., 2009; van Loon et al., 2004). Because water is stored along with creatine, a common side effect of creatine supplementation is weight gain, which at least during the first few weeks of

TABLE 23.5 Creatine Monohydrate Supplementation Efficiency Comparison

Form of Creatine	Creatine Content (Percentage)
Creatine monohydrate	87.9
Creatine ethyl ester	82.4
Creatine malate (3:1)	74.7
Creatine citrate (3:1)	66
Creatine pyruvate (2:1)	60
Creatine a-ketoglutarate	53.8
Creatine oroate (3:1)	45.8
Creatine gluconate	40.2

supplementation is predominately water weight. While this is not body fat gain, a heavier body can be problematic for athletes participating in weight class–restricted sports and endurance athletes, as it decreases their efficiency of movement. As an alternative to the 5 grams dose, 3 grams per day (or 0.03 g/kg bodyweight) might be effective while not producing a significant weight gain (Rawson et al., 2011).

Loading and Timing

Creatine is loaded into muscle cells. Many different **loading** strategies have been researched. Creatine does not need to be loaded at the onset of supplementation, although this does speed up full saturation of the muscle tissue so creatine can start working sooner than it would without loading (Kreider et al., 2017). One common loading strategy is to use 20 grams per day for 1 week, then shift to a daily maintenance dose of 5 grams (**Figure 23.10**). It is possible that creatine consumed after exercise enhances skeletal muscle loading, though this finding has not been replicated (Antonio & Ciccone, 2013). Otherwise, timing of creatine intake might be of little consequence.

Finally, creatine does not need to be cycled. It was once believed that chronic creatine supplementation would compromise **endogenous** production, but that idea has since been disproven (Kreider et al., 2017; Rawson et al., 2004).

Side Effects

Contrary to media reports, the scientific literature has not shown creatine to have many adverse side effects. The most common side effect is weight gain, which can be a function of water retention or increased lean mass. Creatine has not been found to alter any of a wide variety of blood markers over a 21-month period in Division I collegiate American football players (Kreider et al., 2003). Some of the confusion about creatine's effects on the kidneys is attributable to creatinine, which is used as a marker of kidney damage and might prompt a false-positive diagnosis. Long-term supplementation of creatine has not been found to alter either kidney or liver function in athletes (Mayhew et al., 2002; Poortmans & Francaux, 1999).

LOADING (NUTRITION) →

The practice of using large doses of a supplement to saturate muscle tissues or other body stores prior to resorting to a smaller, maintenance dose.

ENDOGENOUS →

Produced or synthesized within an organism.

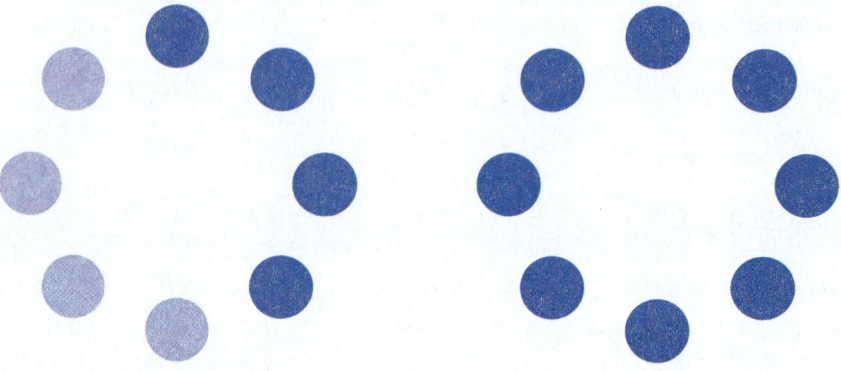

Creatine Loading

A common loading strategy is to use 20 g per day for 1 week prior to a daily maintenance dose of 5 grams.

Loading Phase
20-30 grams per
day for 5-7 days

Maintenance Phase
3-5 grams per
day to maintain

FIGURE 23.10 Creatine Loading

CAFFEINE (STIMULANTS)

Stimulants are a class of psychoactive compounds that alter nervous system activity and generally result in improved or accelerated physical and mental bodily functions. Caffeine is a very common food component and dietary supplement. It is present in coffee, tea, soda, pre-workout beverages, fat burners, energy drinks and shots, and even gum. Of all the dietary supplements, caffeine is probably the one athletes are already familiar with, using it to reduce the feeling of being tired. For many, that includes caffeine consumption as a regular part of their daily routine, whether for exercise or not.

Coffee and tea remain the most used caffeine-delivery beverages. On average, each person consumes 236 cups of tea and 132 cups of coffee per year (Technavio, 2021).

Stimulants, including caffeine, increase physiological and metabolic activity. Caffeine as an ergogenic aid is primarily used to provide a sensation of energy, for aerobic endurance, and to increase metabolic rate.

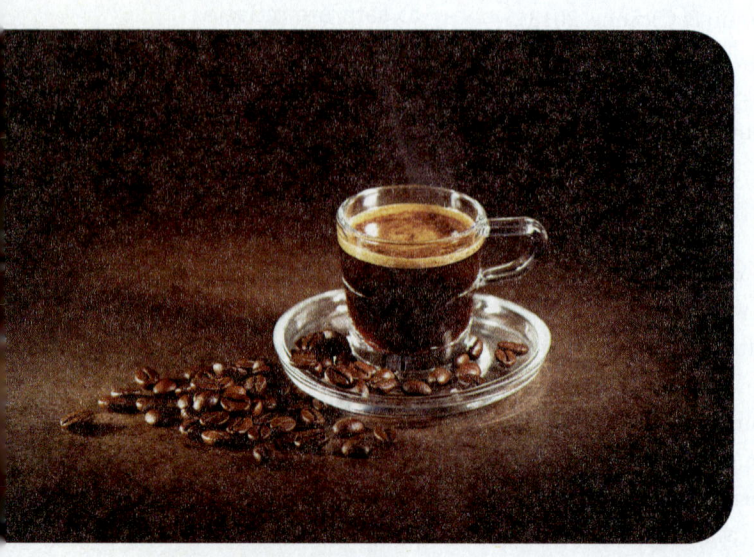

© DUSAN ZIDAR/Shuttertstock

> **ADRENALINE** →
>
> Also known as epinephrine; a hormone that excites bodily processes, increasing alertness and cell metabolism.

Caffeine in dietary supplements is most often found as caffeine anhydrous, a highly concentrated, nearly pure form of caffeine. Caffeine might also be supplemented as caffeine citrate or dicaffeine malate, or derived from natural sources such as green coffee beans, green tea, or guarana. Optimal caffeine dosing is about 3 to 6 mg/kg of bodyweight (1.4 to 2.7 mg/lb) consumed about 1 hour prior to exercise (Goldstein et al., 2010). Exceeding 6 mg/kg increases the potential for adverse events and performance-impairing effects. Most individuals respond well to caffeine, but 5% to 15% are genetically averse to the benefits of caffeine and do not have a positive experience (Pickering & Kiely, 2018).

By chemically blocking receptors that produce the sense of tiredness, caffeine increases wakefulness, attention, and focus. Caffeine also releases **adrenaline**; the adrenaline increases the person's metabolic rate, leading to more energy being metabolized (Clark et al., 2020). This aspect of caffeine supplementation is responsible for its popularity as a fat burner (adrenaline releases lipids from body fat storage) as well as a potential mechanism of action: improving pain tolerance.

Although it was previously thought to be a result of fatty acid mobilization, which could then be used as fuel substrate, the ergogenic effects of caffeine are now hypothesized to be primarily due to improved neurotransmission, arousal, and pain tolerance, as the body does not utilize most of the free fatty acids (Astrup et al., 1990; Davis & Green, 2009; Graham, 2001). This allows an athlete to push a little longer or harder than without caffeine. Regardless of the true mechanism, caffeine has consistently demonstrated improvements in endurance performance, with improvements in responders being measured in the range of 5% to 9% (Paton et al., 2010; Schneiker et al., 2006).

By increasing metabolic rate, lipolysis, and satiety, caffeine might enhance weight loss (Astrup et al., 1990; Tabrizi et al., 2019; Tremblay et al., 1988). However, it might need to be combined with other ingredients, such as green tea or ephedra, for this effect to occur, as caffeine tolerance might blunt the long-term effects (Astrup et al., 1992; Tabrizi et al., 2019; Westerterp-Plantenga et al., 2005).

Secondary to its effects on endurance performance, caffeine has a small effect in improving strength endurance, maximal strength, and power output. Two meta-analyses have found caffeine to be effective for improving upper-body (but not lower-body) maximal strength (Ferreira et al., 2021; Grgic et al., 2018). One of those studies also evaluated strength endurance (measured as repetitions to failure at a submaximal load), finding that caffeine has a positive effect on upper-body and lower-body strength endurance. It was also suggested that 5 mg/kg was the only effective dose for this outcome (Ferreira et al., 2021), and that the effects might be less pronounced in trained individuals (Grgic et al., 2018). Finally, caffeine was found to improve power in the form of both a vertical jump (Grgic et al., 2018) and anaerobic power output during a cycle ergometry test (Grgic, 2018).

The Sports Performance Coach must use caution when recommending stimulants, including caffeine. The Road to Caffeine found in Appendix E visually explains the ergogenic effect of caffeine on performance. Other commonly encountered stimulants, such as yohimbe, higenamine, hordenine, and octopamine, are associated with adverse events or mislabeling, or are on the FDA's advisory list (Cohen et al., 2016). The latter means they are on their way to being prohibited in the United States, meaning they are not considered dietary supplements. As of 2021, the FDA had sent warning letters to some dietary supplement companies that use ingredients on the advisory list.

BANNED SUPPLEMENTS AND PRACTICES

Because dietary supplements' route to the market is left mostly unchecked until they are investigated by a regulating body, the Sports Performance Coach must consider several issues prior to educating athletes on their use. First, consider whether the dietary supplement is effective for the intended purpose by looking for studies from reputable sources (e.g., peer-reviewed papers) or position papers from reputable organizations (e.g., International Society of Sports Nutrition). If the product is determined to be effective, consider whether it is legal and safe to use.

In addition, give special consideration to athletes who might be restricted by a regulating body, such as the NCAA

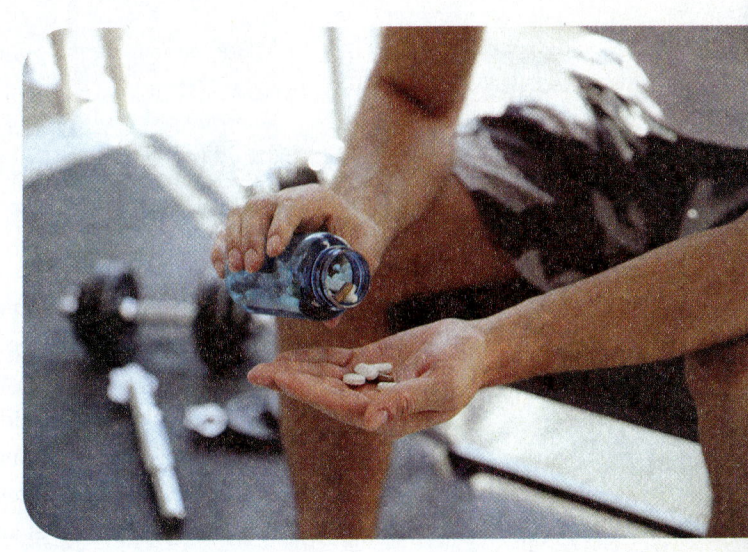

© New Africa/Shutterstock

or WADA. Just because a dietary supplement is legal, that does not mean it is always permitted in a sport. In some cases, a dietary supplement or other substance might be prohibited only during certain phases of the competitive year or during competition. Moreover, prescriptions that an athlete might be using under the supervision of their physician might need to be submitted for exemption depending on the regulating organization.

STEROIDS

Anabolic androgenic steroids (AAS), or just steroids, are an example of an ergogenic aid that is not a dietary supplement. Steroids are either a hormone or derived from a hormone, usually **testosterone**. They are used primarily for increasing strength and muscle mass while facilitating body fat reduction. Some side effects of steroids are permanent, such as hair loss, whereas others are transient, occurring only while someone is using steroids, such as aggression (Hoffman & Ratamess, 2006). **Table 23.6** lists common side effects of steroids.

TABLE 23.6 Side Effects of Steroid Use

Men	Women
Acne	Development of masculine features
Loss of head hair	Increased body and facial hair
Gynecomastia (development of breasts)	Deepening of voice
Irritability and aggression	Irritability and aggression
Altered sex drive (increased or decreased)	Altered sex drive (increased or decreased)
Sleeplessness	Fluid retention
Testicular atrophy	Menstruation irregularities
Decreased sperm count	Breast atrophy
Worsened cholesterol profiles	Clitoral enlargement
Prostate enlargement	Acne

Briefly, AAS function by mimicking the effects of testosterone at the androgen receptor. Some compounds are more androgenic, producing male secondary sex characteristics, whereas others are more anabolic. AAS shut down natural testosterone production, which explains why these steroids are commonly used alongside testosterone. Upon cessation of the supplementation, natural testosterone levels take time to return to normal. During this phase, the user often loses much, or all, of their progress made while using AAS depending on their diet and training practices. Although the Sports Performance Coach can recommend that athletes not use AAS, some athletes do so anyway. In these cases, it is strongly recommended they discuss their use of AAS with a medical doctor to help manage side effects and monitor for any adverse events.

Dietary supplements that contain banned substances typically do not say so on the label. Rather, banned substances are present in the product without being listed on the label to provide the user with a desired effect, such as strength, that the user attributes to the listed ingredients while unaware they are using something much more potent. These types of products are usually, but not always, sold at retail locations and not online—perhaps a result of the FDA's purchases of such products from websites (e.g., Amazon) for random testing. An analysis of more than 600 dietary supplements in 13 countries found an average adulteration rate of 14.8%, with the United States ranking as number 4 in terms of the most frequently adulterated products (18.8%) (Geyer et al., 2008). The greatest adulteration rate was found in the Netherlands (25.8%). A more recent review found weight loss and bodybuilding supplements to be frequently adulterated—on average, 33.9% of the time across 14 studies and 19.4% of the time across six studies (Geyer et al., 2008; Rocha et al., 2016). In some cases, this is intentional. At other times, it is unintentional and could be due to a variety of reasons, such as cross-contamination, lack of testing, or not properly qualifying ingredient suppliers. It is best practice to recommend only dietary supplements from brands that have their products tested by a reputable third party.

EPHEDRA

Ephedra is an example of a once-legal dietary supplement that was later banned by the FDA (in 2004). The active component of ephedra, ephedrine, is an alkaloid that is a bronchodilator. It is still used today in prescription and over-the-counter medication for relief of asthma, respiratory tract infections, and low blood pressure.

Ephedra was a very popular weight-loss ingredient while it was legal. It was often used alongside caffeine and aspirin (in the form of either salicin in white willow bark or over-the-counter aspirin), and the resultant effects were highly potent. In one study that did not feature any attempt to change lifestyle (e.g., diet and exercise), ephedrine, caffeine, and white willow bark supplementation for 12 weeks produced a 1.57 kg greater weight loss (2.2 kg versus 0.5 kg) and 1.7 cm greater reduction in waist circumference (Coffey et al., 2004). In a study that featured a lifestyle intervention—namely, a reduced-calorie diet—for just 8 weeks plus ephedrine with caffeine, both groups lost weight (10.1 kg and 8.4 kg, treatment and placebo, respectively), but the treatment group lost 4.5 kg more body fat while preserving 2.8 kg more fat-free mass (Astrup et al., 1992).

Prior to the FDA banning ephedra, it was already prohibited for use in the Olympics and by other sports organizations, as it was determined to pose undue risk. In 2002, there were more than 10,000 reported ephedra poisonings, and between 2001 and 2004, there were 21 deaths from this cause (Zell-Kanter et al., 2015). Other side effects of ephedra use include hypertension, cardiac arrythmia, heart attack, seizure, and stroke.

> **EPHEDRA** →
>
> A plant-sourced alkaloid with metabolism-enhancing effects. It is an illegal supplement in the United States and European Union.

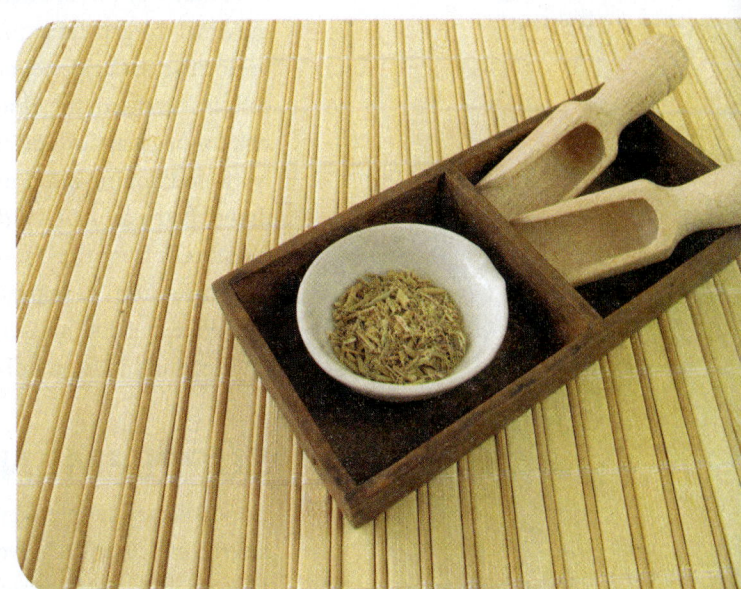

© Heike Rau/Shutterstock

DHEA

Dehydroepiandrosterone (DHEA) is a precursor to testosterone (and estrogen) that is still considered a legal dietary supplement in the United States. However, it is included on WADA's prohibited substances list. Because DHEA can be

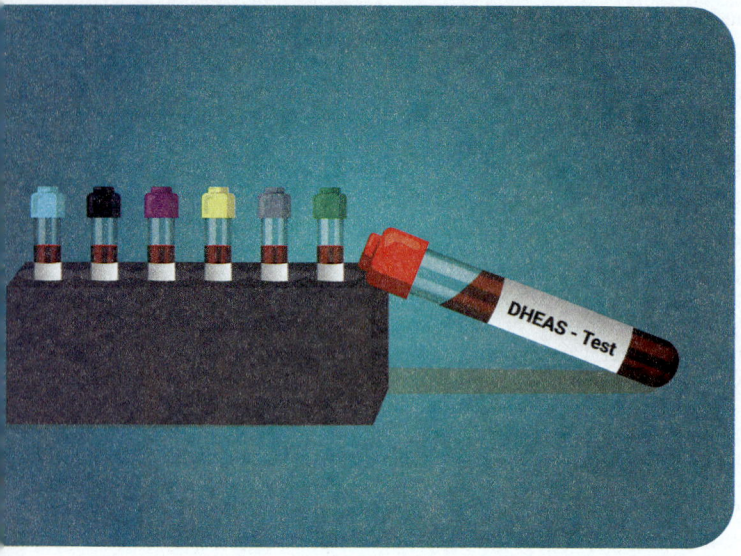

© Innovative Creation/Shutterstock

converted to testosterone in the body, it is supplemented with the expectation that it will increase testosterone levels, with such elevated levels functioning similarly to AAS.

A recent meta-analysis of 42 publications on DHEA supplementation found that this product does increase testosterone levels (Li et al., 2020). However, the magnitude of effect is much larger for women than for men. First, consider that the normal physiologic range for testosterone is 280 to 1100 ng/dL in men and 15 to 70 ng/dL in women. The study found a weighted mean difference of 31 ng/dL in women versus 21 ng/dL in men. Now, consider that testosterone used as an AAS often increases testosterone levels above 1100 ng/dL to produce the supraphysiological effects for which it is known. Thus, it is clear that DHEA supplementation does not really produce steroid-like effects.

DHEA supplementation has not been noted to produce negative results or adverse events. A review featuring 28 studies in men and 63 studies in women reported no significant adverse events or negative side effects, and in all trials, supplementation either produced no effect or had a positive effect on at least one dependent variable (Traish et al., 2011). Nonetheless, for athletes who adhere to WADA, NCAA, or other regulations, use of DHEA is not currently permitted.

BLOOD DOPING AND EPO

Aerobic exercise is a very oxygen-demanding activity. Oxygen that is needed in the muscle tissues to support ATP production is transported in the blood on the hemoglobin in red blood cells. The use of erythropoietin (EPO) and practice of blood doping are two ways that endurance athletes might increase their oxygen-carrying capacity by increasing red blood cell mass in the bloodstream.

EPO is protein that is naturally produced by the body to stimulate red blood cell production. **Exogenous** use serves the same function, but it can produce supraphysiological levels. Due to the nature of the techniques conflicting with ethics, few studies of this application are available. However, EPO has been shown to increase maximal oxygen consumption by as much as 16.6% and translate to a 5% improvement in performance (Bejder et al., 2019; Heuberger et al., 2013). Because the number of red blood cells is increased, the blood becomes more viscous (thicker). This increases the person's risk for heart attack and stroke, chest pain, hypertension, and autoimmune disorders.

Blood doping is a process by which the athlete has one to two pints of their own blood drawn (such as in a blood donation). The blood is centrifuged to separate the solid red blood cells from the liquid component, and the red blood cells are saved until the day prior to competition. At that point, they are reinjected into the athlete, thereby increasing their red blood cell count. A visual explanation of the effect of blood doping on performance can be found in Appendix E.

| EXOGENOUS → |
| Coming from outside the body. |

SUPPLEMENTATION APPLICATION

Use of dietary supplements can vary from supplement to supplement. For many, their desired effects are achieved, at least in part, by consistent consumption. For others, consumption can be timed relative to exercise, and taken with or without food. Still others might be used situationally. For example, fat-soluble vitamins might be better absorbed when consumed with a fat-containing meal compared to a low-fat meal or just water (Jeanes et al., 2004). Moreover, large doses of vitamins or minerals, like those used in supplementation, can cause nausea. This nausea can be reduced by taking supplements with a meal.

Some vitamins and minerals impact each other's absorption. For example, vitamin C can increase iron absorption, but decrease vitamin B_{12} absorption (Clarkson, 1993; Schmid et al., 1996). The effects they have on one another are typically not of concern. In selected cases beyond the scope of the Sports Performance Coach, some vitamin or mineral supplementation might be contraindicated. Therefore, it must be known if the athlete is using any medications or is prescribed a vitamin or mineral supplement prior to adding dietary supplements to their routine.

Co-ingestion of some dietary supplements with sugar might increase their bioavailability. Creatine is one such example. In one study, taking 5 grams of creatine monohydrate with an additional 18 grams of dextrose increased creatine retention from 61% to 80% over 3 days (Greenwood et al., 2003). However, it is not clear whether this practice yields any additional performance benefit beyond the loading phase.

Endurance and team sport exercise can deplete carbohydrates at a rate of 30 to 60 grams per hour and by as much as 90 grams per hour during ultra-endurance events (Jeukendrup, 2014). Therefore, during events lasting longer than about 2 hours (when stores are depleted to an extent that can compromise performance), replacing oxidized carbohydrate at the corresponding rate is recommended. **Figure 23.11** offers general

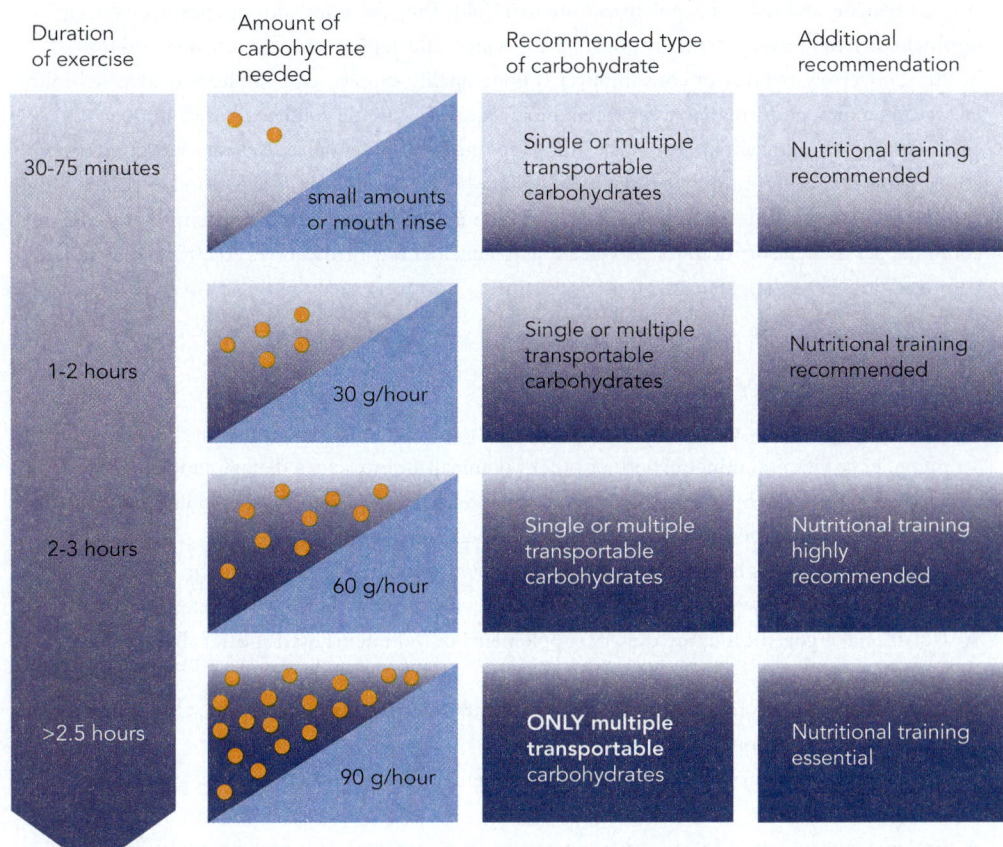

FIGURE 23.11 Use of Carbohydrate Supplementation During Exercise

Reproduced from Jeukendrup, A. (2014). A step towards personalized sports nutrition: carbohydrate intake during exercise. *Sports Medicine, 44* Suppl 1, S25-33. https://doi.org/10.1007/s40279-014-0148-z

guidance on carbohydrate supplementation type and quantity during exercise relative to exercise volume.

For each dietary supplement recommended to an athlete, consider whether that dietary supplement's efficacy is influenced by co-ingestion with food, medication, or other dietary supplements as well as timing of the dietary supplement near exercise.

SUMMARY

Athletes have been seeking performance enhancement for centuries, from ancient Olympians consuming seeds and hallucinogens to present-day athletes using dietary supplements and ergogenic aids. As defined by the FDA, dietary supplements contain dietary ingredients, including vitamins, minerals, botanicals, amino acids, or enzymes. Despite frequent negative news about contamination or adulteration, the supplement industry is regulated, albeit more loosely than the pharmaceutical industry. Importantly, supplements are not intended to replace a balanced diet but rather to supplement it, especially in cases where achieving optimal doses of certain nutrients (e.g., creatine or beta-alanine) from food alone is challenging.

Before recommending dietary supplements, a Sports Performance Coach should assess the athlete's macronutrient needs. If an athlete's diet is well balanced and without restrictions, they will likely meet their micronutrient needs from food alone. In case of dietary restrictions, it is crucial to identify potential nutrient gaps and recommend appropriate foods or supplements. Sports Performance Coaches can play a vital role in determining whether an athlete requires a dietary supplement or an ergogenic aid based on their specific needs and the cost–benefit analysis of the potential supplements.

The benefits and risks of supplements are manifold. They can offer convenience in ensuring optimal nutrient intake, potentially boost performance, and support muscle recovery and overall health. Conversely, overuse or consumption of poor-quality supplements can lead to adverse health effects. Therefore, performance supplementation requires a careful, evidence-based approach, considering each supplement's benefits, timing, dosages, and potential side effects, along with the athlete's specific sport, training regimen, and dietary habits. Timing and the method of consumption can also vary among different supplements, and interactions between specific vitamins and minerals could impact their absorption. It's also essential to consider any medications an athlete may take before adding dietary supplements to their routine.

KEY TAKEAWAYS

- Dietary supplements are products taken by mouth that contain one or more of the following ingredients: vitamin; mineral; herb or other botanical; amino acid; a dietary supplement used to supplement the diet by increasing total dietary intake; or a concentrate, metabolite, constituent, extract, or combination of any previously described ingredient.
- Dietary supplements in the United States are regulated by the U.S. Food and Drug Administration. However, supplements are not reviewed prior to being marketed and sold.
- Nutritional ergogenic aids are dietary supplements or food items used specifically to enhance performance.
- Dietary supplements might produce adverse events. Such events might be due to the supplement itself or contamination of the supplement.
- Prior to using a dietary supplement, athletes are encouraged to use a food-first approach to nutrition.
- Protein supplements are a convenient method to increase total daily protein intake. However, they are not a replacement for good nutrition.
- Creatine is effective at a daily dose of 3 to 5 grams.
- Caffeine is effective at a dose of 3 to 6 mg/kg bodyweight

- Banned substances might or might not be illegal substances. Athletes must check with their sport's governing organization (e.g., NCAA) prior to consuming a dietary supplement, and the athlete is responsible for any substance found in their body.
- The Sports Performance Coach can help establish athletes' nutritional needs and important performance attributes. Based on that information, dietary supplements efficacious for meeting those needs can be considered for use after risk assessment.

REFERENCES

Adcock, K. H., Nedelcu, J., Loenneker, T., Martin, E., Wallimann, T., & Wagner, B. P. (2002). Neuroprotection of creatine supplementation in neonatal rats with transient cerebral hypoxia-ischemia. *Developmental Neuroscience, 24*(5), 382–388. https://doi.org/10.1159/000069043

Antonio, J., & Ciccone, V. (2013). The effects of pre versus post workout supplementation of creatine monohydrate on body composition and strength. *Journal of the International Society of Sports Nutrition, 10*(1), 36. https://doi.org/10.1186/1550-2783-10-36

Armas, L. A. G., Hollis, B. W., & Heaney, R. P. (2004). Vitamin D_2 is much less effective than vitamin D_3 in humans. *Journal of Clinical Endocrinology and Metabolism, 89*(11), 5387–5391. https://doi.org/10.1210/jc.2004-0360

Astrup, A., Breum, L., Toubro, S., Hein, P., & Quaade, F. (1992). The effect and safety of an ephedrine/caffeine compound compared to ephedrine, caffeine and placebo in obese subjects on an energy restricted diet: A double blind trial. *International Journal of Obesity and Related Metabolic Disorders, 16*(4), 269–277. https://www.ncbi.nlm.nih.gov/pubmed/1318281

Astrup, A., Toubro, S., Cannon, S., Hein, P., Breum, L., & Madsen, J. (1990). Caffeine: A double-blind, placebo-controlled study of its thermogenic, metabolic, and cardiovascular effects in healthy volunteers. *American Journal of Clinical Nutrition, 51*(5), 759–767. https://doi.org/10.1093/ajcn/51.5.759

Ayoama, R., Hiruma, E., & Sasaki, H. (2003). Effects of creatine loading on muscular strength and endurance of female softball players. *Journal of Sports Medicine and Physical Fitness, 43*(4), 481–487. https://www.ncbi.nlm.nih.gov/pubmed/14767409

Ayotte, D., & Corcoran, M. P. (2018). Individualized hydration plans improve performance outcomes for collegiate athletes engaging in in-season training. *Journal of the International Society of Sports Nutrition, 15*(1), 27. https://doi.org/10.1186/s12970-018-0230-2

Bailey, R. L., Fulgoni, V. L., Keast, D. R., & Dwyer, J. T. (2012). Examination of vitamin intakes among US adults by dietary supplement use. *Journal of the Academy of Nutrition and Dietetics, 112*(5), 657–663. https://doi.org/10.1016/j.jand.2012.01.026

Barker, T., Schneider, E. D., Dixon, B. M., Henriksen, V. T., & Weaver, L. K. (2013). Supplemental vitamin D enhances the recovery in peak isometric force shortly after intense exercise. *Nutrition & Metabolism, 10*(1), 69. https://doi.org/10.1186/1743-7075-10-69

Bejder, J., Breenfeldt Andersen, A., Solheim, S. A., Gybel-Brask, M., Secher, N. H., Johansson, P. I., & Nordsborg, N. B. (2019). Time trial performance is sensitive to low-volume autologous blood transfusion. *Medicine & Science in Sports & Exercise, 51*(4), 692–700. https://doi.org/10.1249/MSS.0000000000001837

Bendich, A., & Cohen, M. (1990). Vitamin B_6 safety issues. *Annals of the New York Academy of Sciences, 585,* 321–330. https://doi.org/10.1111/j.1749-6632.1990.tb28064.x

Blumberg, J. B., Frei, B. B., Fulgoni, V. L., Weaver, C. M., & Zeisel, S. H. (2017). Impact of frequency of multi-vitamin/multi-mineral supplement intake on nutritional adequacy and nutrient deficiencies in U.S. adults. *Nutrients, 9*(8). https://doi.org/10.3390/nu9080849

Branch, J. D. (2003). Effect of creatine supplementation on body composition and performance: A meta-analysis. *International Journal of Sport Nutrition and Exercise Metabolism, 13*(2), 198–226. https://doi.org/10.1123/ijsnem.13.2.198

Calero, C. D. Q., Rincón, E. O., & Marqueta, P. M. (2020). Probiotics, prebiotics and synbiotics: Useful for athletes and active individuals? A systematic review. *Beneficial Microbes, 11*(2), 135–149. https://doi.org/10.3920/BM2019.0076

Campbell, W. W., Joseph, L. J. O., Anderson, R. A., Davey, S. L., Hinton, J., & Evans, W. J. (2002). Effects of resistive training and chromium picolinate on body composition and skeletal muscle size in older women. *International Journal of Sport Nutrition and Exercise Metabolism, 12*(2), 125–135. https://doi.org/10.1123/ijsnem.12.2.125

Campbell, W. W., Joseph, L. J. O., Davey, S. L., Cyr-Campbell, D., Anderson, R. A., & Evans, W. J. (1999). Effects of resistance training and chromium picolinate on body composition and skeletal muscle in older men. *Journal of Applied Physiology, 86*(1), 29–39. https://doi.org/10.1152/jappl.1999.86.1.29

Celsing, F., Blomstrand, E., Werner, B., Pihlstedt, P., & Ekblom, B. (1986). Effects of iron deficiency on endurance and muscle enzyme activity in man. *Medicine & Science in Sports & Exercise*, *18*(2), 156–161. https://www.ncbi.nlm.nih.gov/pubmed/3702642

Chang, T. P.-Y., & Rangan, C. (2011). Iron poisoning: A literature-based review of epidemiology, diagnosis, and management. *Pediatric Emergency Care*, *27*(10), 978–985. https://doi.org/10.1097/PEC.0b013e3182302604

Chen, Y.-T., Tenforde, A. S., & Fredericson, M. (2013). Update on stress fractures in female athletes: Epidemiology, treatment, and prevention. *Current Reviews in Musculoskeletal Medicine*, *6*(2), 173–181. https://doi.org/10.1007/s12178-013-9167-x

Chu, A., & Samman, S. (2014). Zinc homeostasis in exercise: Implications for physical performance. *Vitamins & Minerals*, *3*(3), 40–42. https://doi.org/10.4172/vms.1000e132

Cinar, V., Talaghir, L. G., Akbulut, T., Turgut, M., & Sankaya, M. (2017). The effects of the zinc supplementation and weight trainings on the testosterone levels. *Human Sport Medicine*, *17*(4), 58–63. https://doi.org/10.14529/hsm170407

Clark, K. L., Sebastianelli, W., Flechsenhar, K. R., Aukermann, D. F., Meza, F., Millard, R. L., Deitch, J. R., Sherbondy, P. S., & Albert, A. (2008). 24-week study on the use of collagen hydrolysate as a dietary supplement in athletes with activity-related joint pain. *Current Medical Research and Opinion*, *24*(5), 1485–1496. https://doi.org/10.1185/030079908x291967

Clark, N. W., Wells, A. J., Coker, N. A., Goldstein, E. R., Herring, C. H., Starling-Smith, T. M., Varanoske, A. N., Panissa, V. L. G., Stout, J. R., & Fukuda, D. H. (2020). The acute effects of thermogenic fitness drink formulas containing 140 mg and 100 mg of caffeine on energy expenditure and fat metabolism at rest and during exercise. *Journal of the International Society of Sports Nutrition*, *17*(1), 10. https://doi.org/10.1186/s12970-020-0341-4

Clarkson, P. M. (1993). Nutritional needs in hot environments: Applications for military personnel in field operations. In *Field operations*. National Academies Press. https://www.ncbi.nlm.nih.gov/books/NBK236216/

Clarkson, P. M., & Haymes, E. M. (1995). Exercise and mineral status of athletes: Calcium, magnesium, phosphorus, and iron. *Medicine and Science in Sports and Exercise*, *27*(6), 831–843. https://www.ncbi.nlm.nih.gov/pubmed/7658944

Close, G. L., Russell, J., Cobley, J. N., Owens, D. J., Wilson, G., Gregson, W., Fraser, W. D., & Morton, J. P. (2013). Assessment of vitamin D concentration in non-supplemented professional athletes and healthy adults during the winter months in the UK: Implications for skeletal muscle function. *Journal of Sports Sciences*, *31*(4), 344–353. https://doi.org/10.1080/02640414.2012.733822

Cockayne, S., Adamson, J., Lanham-New, S., Shearer, M. J., Gilbody, S., & Torgerson, D. J. (2006). Vitamin K and the prevention of fractures: Systematic review and meta-analysis of randomized controlled trials. *Archives of Internal Medicine*, *166*(12), 1256–1261. https://doi.org/10.1001/archinte.166.12.1256

Coffey, C. S., Steiner, D., Baker, B. A., & Allison, D. B. (2004). A randomized double-blind placebo-controlled clinical trial of a product containing ephedrine, caffeine, and other ingredients from herbal sources for treatment of overweight and obesity in the absence of lifestyle treatment. *International Journal of Obesity*, *28*(11), 1411–1419. https://doi.org/10.1038/sj.ijo.0802784

Cogswell, M. E., Zhang, Z., Carriquiry, A. L., Gunn, J. P., Kuklina, E. V, Saydah, S. H., Yang, Q., & Moshfegh, A. J. (2012). Sodium and potassium intakes among US adults: NHANES 2003–2008. *American Journal of Clinical Nutrition*, *96*(3), 647–657. https://doi.org/10.3945/ajcn.112.034413

Cohen, P. A., Wang, Y.-H., Maller, G., DeSouza, R., & Khan, I. A. (2016). Pharmaceutical quantities of yohimbine found in dietary supplements in the USA. *Drug Testing and Analysis*, *8*(3–4), 357–369. https://doi.org/10.1002/dta.1849

Constantini, N. W., Dubnov-Raz, G., Eyal, B.-B., Berry, E. M., Cohen, A. H., & Hemilä, H. (2011). The effect of vitamin C on upper respiratory infections in adolescent swimmers: A randomized trial. *European Journal of Pediatrics*, *170*(1), 59–63. https://doi.org/10.1007/s00431-010-1270-z

Costello, R. B., Dwyer, J. T., & Merkel, J. M. (2019). Chromium supplements in health and disease. In *The Nutritional Biochemistry of Chromium (III)* (pp. 219-249). Elsevier. https://doi.org/10.1016/B978-0-444-64121-2.00007-6

Council for Responsible Nutrition. (2018). *New data reaffirm trust and confidence in industry, reveal modern trends and habits of American consumers*. https://www.crnusa.org/newsroom/new-data-reaffirm-trust-and-confidence-industry-reveal-modern-trends-and-habits-american

Craciun, A. M., Wolf, J., Knapen, M. H., Brouns, F., & Vermeer, C. (1998). Improved bone metabolism in female elite athletes after vitamin K supplementation. *International Journal of Sports Medicine*, *19*(7), 479–484. https://doi.org/10.1055/s-2007-971948

Dahlquist, D. T., Dieter, B. P., & Koehle, M. S. (2015). Plausible ergogenic effects of vitamin D on athletic performance and recovery. *Journal of the International Society of Sports Nutrition*, *12*(1), 1–12.

Dangardt, F., Osika, W., Chen, Y., Nilsson, U., Gan, L.-M., Gronowitz, E., Strandvik, B., & Friberg, P. (2010). Omega-3 fatty acid supplementation improves vascular function and reduces inflammation in obese adolescents. *Atherosclerosis*, *212*(2), 580–585. https://doi.org/10.1016/j.atherosclerosis.2010.06.046

Davis, J. K., & Green, J. M. (2009). Caffeine and anaerobic performance. *Sports Medicine*, *39*(10), 813–832. https://doi.org/10.2165/11317770-000000000-00000

Davis, J. M., Welsh, R. S., & Alerson, N. A. (2000). Effects of carbohydrate and chromium ingestion during intermittent high-intensity exercise to fatigue. *International Journal of Sport Nutrition and Exercise Metabolism*, *10*(4), 476–485. https://doi.org/10.1123/ijsnem.10.4.476

Davison, G., Marchbank, T., March, D. S., Thatcher, R., & Playford, R. J. (2016). Zinc carnosine works with bovine colostrum in truncating heavy exercise–induced increase in gut permeability in healthy volunteers. *American Journal of Clinical Nutrition*, *104*(2), 526–536. https://doi.org/10.3945/ajcn.116.134403

Dietary reference intakes for calcium and vitamin D. (2011). National Academies Press. https://doi.org/10.17226/13050

Dietary reference intakes for vitamin C, vitamin E, selenium, and carotenoids. (2000). National Academies Press. https://doi.org/10.17226/9810

DiNicolantonio, J. J., O'Keefe, J. H., & Wilson, W. (2018). Subclinical magnesium deficiency: A principal driver of cardiovascular disease and a public health crisis. *Open Heart*, *5*(1), e000668. https://doi.org/10.1136/openhrt-2017-000668

Fazio, C., Elder, C. L., & Harris, M. M. (2021). Efficacy of alternative forms of creatine supplementation on improving performance and body composition in healthy subjects. *Journal of Strength and Conditioning Research*, *36*(9), 2663–2670. https://doi.org/10.1519/JSC.0000000000003873

Fedewa, M. V., Spencer, S. O., Williams, T. D., Becker, Z. E., & Fuqua, C. A. (2019). Effect of branched-chain amino acid supplementation on muscle soreness following exercise: A meta-analysis. *International Journal for Vitamin and Nutrition Research*, *89*(5–6), 348–356. https://doi.org/10.1024/0300-9831/a000543

Ferreira, T. T., da Silva, J. V. F., & Bueno, N. B. (2021). Effects of caffeine supplementation on muscle endurance, maximum strength, and perceived exertion in adults submitted to strength training: A systematic review and meta-analyses. *Critical Reviews in Food Science and Nutrition*, *61*(15), 2587–2600. https://doi.org/10.1080/10408398.2020.1781051

Flash Results. (2021). *Men 10,000 meter*. https://dt8v5llb2dwhs.cloudfront.net/Outdoor/2021/008-1_compiled.htm

Galan, F., Ribas, J., Sánchez-Martinez, P. M., Calero, T., Sánchez, A. B., & Muñoz, A. (2012). Serum 25-hydroxyvitamin D in early autumn to ensure vitamin D sufficiency in mid-winter in professional football players. *Clinical Nutrition*, *31*(1), 132–136. https://doi.org/10.1016/j.clnu.2011.07.008

Garrison, S. R., Allan, G. M., Sekhon, R. K., Musini, V. M., & Khan, K. M. (2012). Magnesium for skeletal muscle cramps. *Cochrane Database of Systematic Reviews*, *9*, CD009402. https://doi.org/10.1002/14651858.CD009402.pub2

Gdynia, H.-J., Müller, T., Sperfeld, A.-D., Kühnlein, P., Otto, M., Kassubek, J., & Ludolph, A. C. (2008). Severe sensorimotor neuropathy after intake of highest dosages of vitamin B_6. *Neuromuscular Disorders*, *18*(2), 156–158. https://doi.org/10.1016/j.nmd.2007.09.009

Gerster, H. (1998). Can adults adequately convert alpha-linolenic acid (18:3n-3) to eicosapentaenoic acid (20:5n-3) and docosahexaenoic acid (22:6n-3)? *International Journal for Vitamin and Nutrition Research*, *68*(3), 159–173. https://www.ncbi.nlm.nih.gov/pubmed/9637947

Geyer, H., Parr, M. K., Koehler, K., Mareck, U., Schänzer, W., & Thevis, M. (2008). Nutritional supplements cross-contaminated and faked with doping substances. *Journal of Mass Spectrometry*, *43*(7), 892–902. https://doi.org/10.1002/jms.1452

Giolo De Carvalho, F., Rosa, F. T., Miguel Suen, V. M., Freitas, E. C., Padovan, G. J., & Marchini, J. S. (2012). Evidence of zinc deficiency in competitive swimmers. *Nutrition*, *28*(11–12), 1127–1131. https://doi.org/10.1016/j.nut.2012.02.012

Goldstein, E. R., Ziegenfuss, T., Kalman, D., Kreider, R., Campbell, B., Wilborn, C., Taylor, L., Willoughby, D., Stout, J., Graves, B. S., Wildman, R., Ivy, J. L., Spano, M., Smith, A. E., & Antonio, J. (2010). International Society of Sports Nutrition position stand: Caffeine and performance. *Journal of the International Society of Sports Nutrition*, *7*(1), 5. https://doi.org/10.1186/1550-2783-7-5

Graef, J. L., Smith, A. E., Kendall, K. L., Fukuda, D. H., Moon, J. R., Beck, T. W., Cramer, J. T., & Stout, J. R. (2009). The effects of four weeks of creatine supplementation and high-intensity interval training on cardiorespiratory fitness: A randomized controlled trial. *Journal of the International Society of Sports Nutrition*, *6*, 18. https://doi.org/10.1186/1550-2783-6-18

Graham, T. E. (2001). Caffeine and exercise. *Sports Medicine*, *31*(11), 785–807. https://doi.org/10.2165/00007256-200131110-00002

Greenwood, M., Kreider, R. B., Earnest, C. P., Rasmussen, C., & Almada, A. L. (2003). Differences in creatine retention among three nutritional formulations of oral creatine supplements. *Journal of Exercise Physiology*, *6*(2), 37–43.

Greer, B. K., White, J. P., Arguello, E. M., & Haymes, E. M. (2011). Branched-chain amino acid supplementation lowers perceived exertion but does not affect performance in untrained males. *Journal of Strength and Conditioning Research*, *25*(2), 539–544. https://doi.org/10.1519/JSC.0b013e3181bf443a

Grgic, J. (2018). Caffeine ingestion enhances Wingate performance: A meta-analysis. *European Journal of Sport Science*, *18*(2), 219–225. https://doi.org/10.1080/17461391.2017.1394371

Grgic, J., Trexler, E. T., Lazinica, B., & Pedisic, Z. (2018). Effects of caffeine intake on muscle strength and power: A systematic review and meta-analysis. *Journal of the International Society of Sports Nutrition*, *15*(1), 11. https://doi.org/10.1186/s12970-018-0216-0

Hallmark, M. A., Reynolds, T. H., DeSouza, C. A., Dotson, C. O., Anderson, R. A., & Rogers, M. A. (1996). Effects of chromium and resistive training on muscle strength and body composition. *Medicine & Science in Sports & Exercise*, *28*(1), 139–144. https://doi.org/10.1097/00005768-199601000-00025

Haymes, E. M. (1991). Vitamin and mineral supplementation to athletes. *International Journal of Sport Nutrition and Exercise Metabolism*, *1*(2), 146–169. https://doi.org/10.1123/ijsn.1.2.146

Heffernan, S., Horner, K., De Vito, G., & Conway, G. (2019). The role of mineral and trace element supplementation in exercise and athletic performance: A systematic review. *Nutrients*, *11*(3), 696. https://doi.org/10.3390/nu11030696

Heuberger, J. A. A. C., Cohen Tervaert, J. M., Schepers, F. M. L., Vliegenthart, A. D. B., Rotmans, J. I., Daniels, J. M. A., Burggraaf, J., & Cohen, A. F. (2013). Erythropoietin doping in cycling: Lack of evidence for efficacy and a negative risk–benefit. *British Journal of Clinical Pharmacology*, *75*(6), 1406–1421. https://doi.org/10.1111/bcp.12034

Hinton P. S. (2014). Iron and the endurance athlete. *Applied Physiology, Nutrition, and Metabolism*, *39*(9), 1012–1018. https://doi.org/10.1139/apnm-2014-0147

Hirsch, K. R., Greenwalt, C. E., Saylor, H. E., Gould, L. M., Harrison, C. H., Brewer, G. J., Blue, M. N. M., Ferrando, A. A., Huffman, K. M., Mayer-Davis, E. J., Ryan, E. D., & Smith-Ryan, A. E. (2021). High-intensity interval training and essential amino acid supplementation: Effects on muscle characteristics and whole-body protein turnover. *Physiological Reports*, *9*(1), e14655. https://doi.org/10.14814/phy2.14655

Hoffman, J. R., & Ratamess, N. A. (2006). Medical issues associated with anabolic steroid use: Are they exaggerated? *Journal of Sports Science & Medicine*, *5*(2), 182–193. https://www.ncbi.nlm.nih.gov/pubmed/24259990

Hormoznejad, R., Zare Javid, A., & Mansoori, A. (2019). Effect of BCAA supplementation on central fatigue, energy metabolism substrate and muscle damage to the exercise: A systematic review with meta-analysis. *Sport Sciences for Health*, *15*(2), 265–279. https://doi.org/10.1007/s11332-019-00542-4

Howatson, G., Hoad, M., Goodall, S., Tallent, J., Bell, P. G., & French, D. N. (2012). Exercise-induced muscle damage is reduced in resistance-trained males by branched chain amino acids: A randomized, double-blind, placebo controlled study. *Journal of the International Society of Sports Nutrition*, *9*(1), 20. https://doi.org/10.1186/1550-2783-9-20

Institute of Medicine (US) Panel on Micronutrients. (2001). *Dietary reference intakes for vitamin a, vitamin k, arsenic, boron, chromium, copper, iodine, iron, manganese, molybdenum, nickel, silicon, vanadium, and zinc*. National Academies Press (US). http://www.ncbi.nlm.nih.gov/books/NBK222310/

International Olympic Committee. (2021). *London 2012: Athletics 10000m men results*. https://olympics.com/en/olympic-games/london-2012/results/athletics/10000m-men

Jackson, J., Williams, R., McEvoy, M., MacDonald-Wicks, L., & Patterson, A. (2016). Is higher consumption of animal flesh foods associated with better iron status among adults in developed countries? A systematic review. *Nutrients*, *8*(2), 89. https://doi.org/10.3390/nu8020089

Jäger, R., Mohr, A. E., Carpenter, K. C., Kerksick, C. M., Purpura, M., Moussa, A., Townsend, J. R., Lamprecht, M., West, N. P., Black, K., Gleeson, M., Pyne, D. B., Wells, S. D., Arent, S. M., Smith-Ryan, A. E., Kreider, R. B., Campbell, B. I., Bannock, L., Scheiman, J., … Antonio, J. (2019). International Society of Sports Nutrition position stand: Probiotics. *Journal of the International Society of Sports Nutrition*, *16*(1), 1–44. https://doi.org/10.1186/s12970-019-0329-0

Jäger, R., Purpura, M., Shao, A., Inoue, T., & Kreider, R. B. (2011). Analysis of the efficacy, safety, and regulatory status of novel forms of creatine. *Amino Acids*, *40*(5), 1369–1383. https://doi.org/10.1007/s00726-011-0874-6

Jastrzębska, M., Kaczmarczyk, M., & Jastrzębski, Z. (2016). Effect of vitamin D supplementation on training adaptation in well-trained soccer players. *Journal of Strength and Conditioning Research*, *30*(9), 2648–2655. https://doi.org/10.1519/JSC.0000000000001337

Jeanes, Y. M., Hall, W. L., Ellard, S., Lee, E., & Lodge, J. K. (2004). The absorption of vitamin E is influenced by the amount of fat in a meal and the food matrix. *British Journal of Nutrition, 92*(4), 575–579. https://doi.org/10.1079/bjn20041249

Jeukendrup, A. (2014). A step towards personalized sports nutrition: Carbohydrate intake during exercise. *Sports Medicine, 44*(suppl 1), S25–S33. https://doi.org/10.1007/s40279-014-0148-z

Joseph, L. J., Farrell, P. A., Davey, S. L., Evans, W. J., & Campbell, W. W. (1999). Effect of resistance training with or without chromium picolinate supplementation on glucose metabolism in older men and women. *Metabolism: Clinical and Experimental, 48*(5), 546–553. https://doi.org/10.1016/s0026-0495(99)90048-3

Keong, C. C., Singh, H. J., & Singh, R. (2006). Effects of palm vitamin E supplementation on exercise-induced oxidative stress and endurance performance in the heat. *Journal of Sports Science & Medicine, 5*(4), 629–639. https://www.ncbi.nlm.nih.gov/pubmed/24357959

Kephart, W. C., Wachs, T. D., Thompson, R. M., Mobley, C. B., Fox, C. D., McDonald, J. R., Ferguson, B. S., Young, K. C., Nie, B., Martin, J. S., Company, J. M., Pascoe, D. D., Arnold, R. D., Moon, J. R., & Roberts, M. D. (2015). Ten weeks of branched chain amino acid supplementation improves select performance and immunological variables in trained cyclists. *Journal of the International Society of Sports Nutrition, 12*(S1), P20. https://doi.org/10.1186/1550-2783-12-S1-P20

Khaled, S., Brun, J. F., Cassanas, G., Bardet, L., & Orsetti, A. (1999). Effects of zinc supplementation on blood rheology during exercise. *Clinical Hemorheology and Microcirculation, 20*(1), 1–10. https://www.ncbi.nlm.nih.gov/pubmed/11185677

Khatri, M., Naughton, R. J., Clifford, T., Harper, L. D., & Corr, L. (2021). The effects of collagen peptide supplementation on body composition, collagen synthesis, and recovery from joint injury and exercise: a systematic review. *Amino Acids*. https://doi.org/10.1007/s00726-021-03072-x

Komar, B., Schwingshackl, L., & Hoffmann, G. (2015). Effects of leucine-rich protein supplements on anthropometric parameter and muscle strength in the elderly: A systematic review and meta-analysis. *Journal of Nutrition, Health & Aging, 19*(4), 437–446. https://doi.org/10.1007/s12603-014-0559-4

Kreider, R. B., Kalman, D. S., Antonio, J., Ziegenfuss, T. N., Wildman, R., Collins, R., Candow, D. G., Kleiner, S. M., Almada, A. L., & Lopez, H. L. (2017). International Society of Sports Nutrition position stand: Safety and efficacy of creatine supplementation in exercise, sport, and medicine. *Journal of the International Society of Sports Nutrition, 14*, 18. https://doi.org/10.1186/s12970-017-0173-z

Kreider, R. B., Melton, C., Rasmussen, C. J., Greenwood, M., Lancaster, S., Cantler, E. C., Milnor, P., & Almada, A. L. (2003). Long-term creatine supplementation does not significantly affect clinical markers of health in athletes. *Molecular and Cellular Biochemistry, 244*(1–2), 95–104. https://www.ncbi.nlm.nih.gov/pubmed/12701816

Kreider, R. B., & Stout, J. R. (2021). Creatine in health and disease. *Nutrients, 13*(2). https://doi.org/10.3390/nu13020447

Kremenik, M., Onodera, S., Nagao, M., Yuzuki, O., & Yonetani, S. (2006). A historical timeline of doping in the Olympics (Part 1 1896–1968). *Kawasaki Journal of Medical Welfare, 12*(1), 19–28.

Kunstel, K. (2005). Calcium requirements for the athlete. *Current Sports Medicine Reports, 4*(4), 203–206. https://doi.org/10.1097/01.csmr.0000306208.56939.01

Lami, F., Callegari, C., Tatali, M., Graziano, L., Guidetti, C., Miglioli, M., & Barbara, L. (1988). Efficacy of addition of exogenous lactase to milk in adult lactase deficiency. *American Journal of Gastroenterology, 83*(10), 1145–1149. https://www.ncbi.nlm.nih.gov/pubmed/3138908

Law, Y. L. L., Ong, W. S., GillianYap, T. L., Lim, S. C. J., & Von Chia, E. (2009). Effects of two and five days of creatine loading on muscular strength and anaerobic power in trained athletes. *Journal of Strength and Conditioning Research, 23*(3), 906–914. https://doi.org/10.1519/JSC.0b013e3181a06c59

Leachman Slawson, D., McClanahan, B. S., Clemens, L. H., Ward, K. D., Klesges, R. C., Vukadinovich, C. M., & Cantler, E. D. (2001). Food sources of calcium in a sample of African-American an Euro-American collegiate athletes. *International Journal of Sport Nutrition and Exercise Metabolism, 11*(2), 199–208. https://doi.org/10.1123/ijsnem.11.2.199

Lewis, N. A., Daniels, D., Calder, P. C., Castell, L. M., & Pedlar, C. R. (2020). Are there benefits from the use of fish oil supplements in athletes? A systematic review. *Advances in Nutrition, 11*(5), 1300–1314. https://doi.org/10.1093/advances/nmaa050

Li, Y., Ren, J., Li, N., Liu, J., Tan, S. C., Low, T. Y., & Ma, Z. (2020). A dose-response and meta-analysis of dehydroepiandrosterone (DHEA) supplementation on testosterone levels: Perinatal prediction of randomized clinical trials. *Experimental Gerontology, 141*, 111110. https://doi.org/10.1016/j.exger.2020.111110

Livolsi, J. M., Adams, G. M., & Laguna, P. L. (2001). The effect of chromium picolinate on muscular strength and body composition in women athletes. *Journal of Strength and Conditioning Research, 15*(2), 161–166. https://www.ncbi.nlm.nih.gov/pubmed/11710399

Lugo, J. P., Saiyed, Z. M., & Lane, N. E. (2016). Efficacy and tolerability of an undenatured type II collagen supplement in modulating knee osteoarthritis symptoms: A multicenter randomized, double-blind, placebo-controlled study. *Nutrition Journal, 15*, 14. https://doi.org/10.1186/s12937-016-0130-8

Lugo, J. P., Saiyed, Z. M., Lau, F. C., Molina, J. P. L., Pakdaman, M. N., Shamie, A. N., & Udani, J. K. (2013). Undenatured type II collagen (UC-II®) for joint support: A randomized, double-blind, placebo-controlled study in healthy volunteers. *Journal of the International Society of Sports Nutrition, 10*(1), 48. https://doi.org/10.1186/1550-2783-10-48

Lun, V., Erdman, K. A., Fung, T. S., & Reimer, R. A. (2012). Dietary supplementation practices in Canadian high-performance athletes. *International Journal of Sport Nutrition and Exercise Metabolism, 22*(1), 31–37. https://doi.org/10.1123/ijsnem.22.1.31

MacKay, D., Hathcock, J., & Guarneri, E. (2012). Niacin: Chemical forms, bioavailability, and health effects. *Nutrition Reviews, 70*(6), 357–366. https://doi.org/10.1111/j.1753-4887.2012.00479.x

Mayhew, D. L., Mayhew, J. L., & Ware, J. S. (2002). Effects of long-term creatine supplementation on liver and kidney functions in American college football players. *International Journal of Sport Nutrition and Exercise Metabolism, 12*(4), 453–460. https://doi.org/10.1123/ijsnem.12.4.453

Mayurasakorn, K., Williams, J. J., Ten, V. S., & Deckelbaum, R. J. (2011). Docosahexaenoic acid: Brain accretion and roles in neuroprotection after brain hypoxia and ischemia. *Current Opinion in Clinical Nutrition and Metabolic Care, 14*(2), 158–167. https://doi.org/10.1097/MCO.0b013e328342cba5

McAnulty, S. R., McAnulty, L. S., Nieman, D. C., Morrow, J. D., Shooter, L. A., Holmes, S., Heward, C., & Henson, D. A. (2005). Effect of alpha-tocopherol supplementation on plasma homocysteine and oxidative stress in highly trained athletes before and after exhaustive exercise. *Journal of Nutritional Biochemistry, 16*(9), 530–537. https://doi.org/10.1016/j.jnutbio.2005.02.001

Micheletti, A., Rossi, R., & Rufini, S. (2001). Zinc status in athletes: Relation to diet and exercise. *Sports Medicine, 31*(8), 577–582. https://doi.org/10.2165/00007256-200131080-00002

Minto, C., Vecchio, M. G., Lamprecht, M., & Gregori, D. (2017). Definition of a tolerable upper intake level of niacin: A systematic review and meta-analysis of the dose-dependent effects of nicotinamide and nicotinic acid supplementation. *Nutrition Reviews, 75*(6), 471–490. https://doi.org/10.1093/nutrit/nux011

Morris, M. S., Picciano, M. F., Jacques, P. F., & Selhub, J. (2008). Plasma pyridoxal 5′-phosphate in the US population: The National Health and Nutrition Examination Survey, 2003–2004. *American Journal of Clinical Nutrition, 87*(5), 1446–1454. https://doi.org/10.1093/ajcn/87.5.1446

Morton, R. W., Murphy, K. T., McKellar, S. R., Schoenfeld, B. J., Henselmans, M., Helms, E., Aragon, A. A., Devries, M. C., Banfield, L., Krieger, J. W., & Phillips, S. M. (2018). A systematic review, meta-analysis and meta-regression of the effect of protein supplementation on resistance training-induced gains in muscle mass and strength in healthy adults. *British Journal of Sports Medicine, 52*(6), 376–384. https://doi.org/10.1136/bjsports-2017-097608

Naclerio, F., & Larumbe-Zabala, E. (2016). Effects of whey protein alone or as part of a multi-ingredient formulation on strength, fat-free mass, or lean body mass in resistance-trained individuals: A meta-analysis. *Sports Medicine, 46*(1), 125–137. https://doi.org/10.1007/s40279-015-0403-y

National Scholastic Athletics Foundation. (2021). *2021: The Nike Outdoor Nationals.* https://theoutdoornationals.runnerspace.com/eprofile.php?do=info&event_id=14188

Neek, L. S., Gaeini, A. A., & Choobineh, S. (2011). Effect of zinc and selenium supplementation on serum testosterone and plasma lactate in cyclist after an exhaustive exercise bout. *Biological Trace Element Research, 144*(1–3), 454–462. https://doi.org/https://doi.org/10.1007/s12011-011-9138-2

Nielsen, F. H., & Lukaski, H. C. (2006). Update on the relationship between magnesium and exercise. *Magnesium Research, 19*(3), 180–189. https://www.ncbi.nlm.nih.gov/pubmed/17172008

Oben, J., Kothari, S. C., & Anderson, M. L. (2008). An open label study to determine the effects of an oral proteolytic enzyme system on whey protein concentrate metabolism in healthy males. *Journal of the International Society of Sports Nutrition, 5*, 10. https://doi.org/10.1186/1550-2783-5-10

O'Donovan, C. M., Madigan, S. M., Garcia-Perez, I., Rankin, A., O' Sullivan, O., & Cotter, P. D. (2020). Distinct microbiome composition and metabolome exists across subgroups of elite Irish athletes. *Journal of Science and Medicine in Sport, 23*(1), 63–68. https://doi.org/10.1016/j.jsams.2019.08.290

Oikawa, S. Y., Kamal, M. J., Webb, E. K., McGlory, C., Baker, S. K., & Phillips, S. M. (2020). Whey protein but not collagen peptides stimulate acute and longer-term muscle protein synthesis with and without resistance exercise in healthy older women: A randomized controlled trial. *American Journal of Clinical Nutrition, 111*(3), 708–718. https://doi.org/10.1093/ajcn/nqz332

Oliver, J. M., Jones, M. T., Kirk, K. M., Gable, D. A., Repshas, J. T., Johnson, T. A., Andréasson, U., Norgren, N., Blennow, K., & Zetterberg, H. (2016). Effect of docosahexaenoic acid on a biomarker of head trauma in

American football. *Medicine & Science in Sports & Exercise, 48*(6), 974–982. https://doi.org/10.1249/MSS.0000000000000875

Owen, K. N., & Dewald, O. (2021). Vitamin E toxicity. *StatPearls*. https://www.ncbi.nlm.nih.gov/pubmed/33232043

Padayatty, S. J., Sun, H., Wang, Y., Riordan, H. D., Hewitt, S. M., Katz, A., Wesley, R. A., & Levine, M. (2004). Vitamin C pharmacokinetics: Implications for oral and intravenous use. *Annals of Internal Medicine, 140*(7), 533–537. https://doi.org/10.7326/0003-4819-140-7-200404060-00010

Parnell, J. A., Wiens, K., & Erdman, K. A. (2015). Evaluation of congruence among dietary supplement use and motivation for supplementation in young, Canadian athletes. *Journal of the International Society of Sports Nutrition, 12*(1), 49. https://doi.org/10.1186/s12970-015-0110-y

Pasiakos, S. M., McClung, H. L., McClung, J. P., Margolis, L. M., Andersen, N. E., Cloutier, G. J., Pikosky, M. A., Rood, J. C., Fielding, R. A., & Young, A. J. (2011). Leucine-enriched essential amino acid supplementation during moderate steady state exercise enhances postexercise muscle protein synthesis. *American Journal of Clinical Nutrition, 94*(3), 809–818. https://doi.org/10.3945/ajcn.111.017061

Patil, S. M., Chaudhuri, D., & Dhanakshirur, G. B. (2009). Role of alpha-tocopherol in cardiopulmonary fitness in endurance athletes, cyclists. *Indian Journal of Physiology and Pharmacology, 53*(4), 375–379. https://www.ncbi.nlm.nih.gov/pubmed/20509332

Paton, C. D., & Hopkins, W. G. (2006). Variation in performance of elite cyclists from race to race. *European Journal of Sport Science, 6*(1), 25–31. https://doi.org/10.1080/17461390500422796

Paton, C. D., Lowe, T., & Irvine, A. (2010). Caffeinated chewing gum increases repeated sprint performance and augments increases in testosterone in competitive cyclists. *European Journal of Applied Physiology, 110*(6), 1243–1250. https://doi.org/10.1007/s00421-010-1620-6

Pedlar, C. R., Brugnara, C., Bruinvels, G., & Burden, R. (2018). Iron balance and iron supplementation for the female athlete: A practical approach. *European Journal of Sport Science, 18*(2), 295–305. https://doi.org/10.1080/17461391.2017.1416178

Perry, T. A., Weerasuriya, A., Mouton, P. R., Holloway, H. W., & Greig, N. H. (2004). Pyridoxine-induced toxicity in rats: A stereological quantification of the sensory neuropathy. *Experimental Neurology, 190*(1), 133–144. https://doi.org/10.1016/j.expneurol.2004.07.013

Peters, E. M., Goetzsche, J. M., Grobbelaar, B., & Noakes, T. D. (1993). Vitamin C supplementation reduces the incidence of postrace symptoms of upper-respiratory-tract infection in ultramarathon runners. *American Journal of Clinical Nutrition, 57*(2), 170–174. https://doi.org/10.1093/ajcn/57.2.170

Peterson, S. (2000). *Controlling iodine deficiency disorders: Studies for program management in sub-Saharan Africa* [Doctoral dissertation]. https://www.diva-portal.org/smash/get/diva2:165973/FULLTEXT01.pdf

Petkova, E., Ivanov, K., Ivanova, S., & Gueorguiev, T. (2018). The use of dietary supplements by professional athletes. *Biomedical Research, 29*(9), 1953–1955.

Pickering, C., & Kiely, J. (2018). Are the current guidelines on caffeine use in sport optimal for everyone? Inter-individual variation in caffeine ergogenicity, and a move towards personalised sports nutrition. *Sports Medicine, 48*(1), 7–16. https://doi.org/10.1007/s40279-017-0776-1

Plotkin, D. L., Delcastillo, K., Van Every, D. W., Tipton, K. D., Aragon, A. A., & Schoenfeld, B. J. (2021). Isolated leucine and branched-chain amino acid supplementation for enhancing muscular strength and hypertrophy: A narrative review. *International Journal of Sport Nutrition and Exercise Metabolism, 31*(3), 292–301. https://doi.org/10.1123/IJSNEM.2020-0356

Poortmans, J. R., & Francaux, M. (1999). Long-term oral creatine supplementation does not impair renal function in healthy athletes. *Medicine & Science in Sports & Exercise, 31*(8), 1108–1110. https://doi.org/10.1097/00005768-199908000-00005

Portier, H., Chatard, J. C., Filaire, E., Jaunet-Devienne, M. F., Robert, A., & Guezennec, C. Y. (2008). Effects of branched-chain amino acids supplementation on physiological and psychological performance during an offshore sailing race. *European Journal of Applied Physiology, 104*(5), 787–794. https://doi.org/10.1007/s00421-008-0832-5

Rawson, E. S., Persky, A. M., Price, T. B., & Clarkson, P. M. (2004). Effects of repeated creatine supplementation on muscle, plasma, and urine creatine levels. *Journal of Strength and Conditioning Research, 18*(1), 162–167. https://journals.lww.com/nsca-jscr/abstract/2004/02000/effects_of_repeated_creatine_supplementation_on.24.aspx

Rawson, E. S., Stec, M. J., Frederickson, S. J., & Miles, M. P. (2011). Low-dose creatine supplementation enhances fatigue resistance in the absence of weight gain. *Nutrition, 27*(4), 451–455. https://doi.org/10.1016/j.nut.2010.04.001

Rawson, E. S., & Volek, J. S. (2003). Effects of creatine supplementation and resistance training on muscle strength and weightlifting performance. *Journal of Strength and Conditioning Research, 17*(4), 822–831. https://journals.lww.com/nsca-jscr/abstract/2003/11000/effects_of_creatine_supplementation_and_resistance.31.aspx

Rocha, T., Amaral, J. S., & Oliveira, M. B. P. P. (2016). Adulteration of dietary supplements by the illegal addition of synthetic drugs: A review. *Comprehensive Reviews in Food Science and Food Safety, 15*(1), 43–62. https://doi.org/10.1111/1541-4337.12173

Rokitzki, L., Logemann, E., Huber, G., Keck, E., & Keul, J. (1994). Alpha-tocopherol supplementation in racing cyclists during extreme endurance training. *International Journal of Sport Nutrition, 4*(3), 253–264. https://doi.org/10.1123/ijsn.4.3.253

Saeedy, M., Bijeh, N., & Moazzami, M. (2016). The effect of six weeks of high-intensity interval training with and without zinc supplementation on aerobic power and anaerobic power in female futsal players. *International Journal of Applied Exercise Physiology, 5*(1), 1–10.

Schmid, A., Jakob, E., Berg, A., Russmann, T., König, D., Irmer, M., & Keul, J. (1996). Effect of physical exercise and vitamin C on absorption of ferric sodium citrate. *Medicine & Science in Sports & Exercise, 28*(12), 1470–1473. https://doi.org/10.1097/00005768-199612000-00005

Schneiker, K. T., Bishop, D., Dawson, B., & Hackett, L. P. (2006). Effects of caffeine on prolonged intermittent-sprint ability in team-sport athletes. *Medicine & Science in Sports & Exercise, 38*(3), 578–585. https://doi.org/10.1249/01.mss.0000188449.18968.62

Schoenfeld, B. J., Aragon, A. A., & Krieger, J. W. (2013). The effect of protein timing on muscle strength and hypertrophy: A meta-analysis. *Journal of the International Society of Sports Nutrition, 10*(1), 53. https://doi.org/10.1186/1550-2783-10-53

Silver, M. D. (2001). Use of ergogenic aids by athletes. *Journal of the American Academy of Orthopaedic Surgeons, 9*(1), 61–70. https://doi.org/10.5435/00124635-200101000-00007

Sobal, J., & Marquart, L. F. (1994). Vitamin/mineral supplement use among athletes: A review of the literature. *International Journal of Sport Nutrition, 4*(4), 320–334. https://doi.org/10.1123/ijsn.4.4.320

Spillane, M., Schoch, R., Cooke, M., Harvey, T., Greenwood, M., Kreider, R., & Willoughby, D. S. (2009). The effects of creatine ethyl ester supplementation combined with heavy resistance training on body composition, muscle performance, and serum and muscle creatine levels. *Journal of the International Society of Sports Nutrition, 6*(1), 6. https://doi.org/10.1186/1550-2783-6-6

Tabrizi, R., Saneei, P., Lankarani, K. B., Akbari, M., Kolahdooz, F., Esmaillzadeh, A., Nadi-Ravandi, S., Mazoochi, M., & Asemi, Z. (2019). The effects of caffeine intake on weight loss: A systematic review and dose-response meta-analysis of randomized controlled trials. *Critical Reviews in Food Science and Nutrition, 59*(16), 2688–2696. https://doi.org/10.1080/10408398.2018.1507996

Technavio. (2021). *Tea market analysis APAC, Europe, North America, South America, Middle East and Africa, US, China, India, Japan, UK: Size and forecast 2024–2028.* https://www.technavio.com/report/tea-market-industry-analysis

Thielecke, F., & Blannin, A. (2020). Omega-3 fatty acids for sport performance: Are they equally beneficial for athletes and amateurs? A narrative review. *Nutrients, 12*(12). https://doi.org/10.3390/nu12123712

Traish, A. M., Kang, H. P., Saad, F., & Guay, A. T. (2011). Dehydroepiandrosterone (DHEA)-A precursor steroid or an active hormone in human physiology (CME). *Journal of Sexual Medicine, 8*(11), 2960–2982. https://doi.org/10.1111/j.1743-6109.2011.02523.x

Tremblay, A., Masson, E., Leduc, S., Houde, A., & Després, J.-P. (1988). Caffeine reduces spontaneous energy intake in men but not in women. *Nutrition Research, 8*(5), 553–558. https://doi.org/10.1016/S0271-5317(88)80077-0

Trumbo, P., Yates, A. A., Schlicker, S., & Poos, M. (2001). Dietary reference intakes: Vitamin A, vitamin K, arsenic, boron, chromium, copper, iodine, iron, manganese, molybdenum, nickel, silicon, vanadium, and zinc. *Journal of the Academy of Nutrition and Dietetics, 101*(3), 294–301. https://doi.org/10.1016/S0002-8223(01)00078-5

U.S. Food and Drug Administration. (1994). *Dietary Supplement Health and Education Act of 1994: Technical Report 1.* https://ods.od.nih.gov/About/DSHEA_Wording.aspx

U.S. Food and Drug Administration. (2019). *Dietary supplements.* https://www.fda.gov/food/dietary-supplements

van Erp-Baart, A. M. J., Saris, W. H. M., Binkhorst, R. A., Vos, J. A., & Elvers, J. W. H. (1989). Nationwide survey on nutritional habits in elite athletes. Part II. Mineral and vitamin intake. *International Journal of Sports Medicine, 10*(suppl 1), S11–S16. https://doi.org/10.1055/s-2007-1024948

van Loon, L. J. C., Murphy, R., Oosterlaar, A. M., Cameron-Smith, D., Hargreaves, M., Wagenmakers, A. J. M., & Snow, R. (2004). Creatine supplementation increases glycogen storage but not GLUT-4 expression in human skeletal muscle. *Clinical Science, 106*(1), 99–106. https://doi.org/10.1042/CS20030116

Vieillevoye, S., Poortmans, J. R., Duchateau, J., & Carpentier, A. (2010). Effects of a combined essential amino acids/carbohydrate supplementation on muscle mass, architecture and maximal strength following heavy-load training. *European Journal of Applied Physiology, 110*(3), 479–488. https://doi.org/10.1007/s00421-010-1520-9

Vitale, K., & Getzin, A. (2019). Nutrition and supplement update for the endurance athlete: Review and recommendations. *Nutrients, 11*(6), 1289. https://doi.org/10.3390/nu11061289

Volek, J. S., Kramer, W. J., Bush, J. A., Boetes, M., Incledon, T., Clark, K. L., & Lynch, J. M. (1997). Creatine supplementation enhances muscular performance during high-intensity resistance exercise. *Journal of the Academy of Nutrition and Dietetics, 97*(7), 765–770. https://doi.org/10.1016/S0002-8223(97)00189-2

Volpe, S. L. (2015). Magnesium and the athlete. *Current Sports Medicine Reports, 14*(4), 279–283. https://doi.org/10.1249/JSR.0000000000000178

Walker, L. S., Bemben, M. G., Bemben, D. A., & Knehans, A. W. (1998). Chromium picolinate effects on body composition and muscular performance in wrestlers. *Medicine & Science in Sports & Exercise, 30*(12), 1730–1737. https://doi.org/10.1097/00005768-199812000-00012

Wang, C., Harris, W. S., Chung, M., Lichtenstein, A. H., Balk, E. M., Kupelnick, B., Jordan, H. S., & Lau, J. (2006). *N*-3 Fatty acids from fish or fish-oil supplements, but not alpha-linolenic acid, benefit cardiovascular disease outcomes in primary- and secondary-prevention studies: A systematic review. *American Journal of Clinical Nutrition, 84*(1), 5–17. https://doi.org/10.1093/ajcn/84.1.5

Wardenaar, F. C., Ceelen, I. J. M., Van Dijk, J.-W., Hangelbroek, R. W. J., Van Roy, L., Van der Pouw, B., De Vries, J. H. M., Mensink, M., & Witkamp, R. F. (2017). Nutritional supplement use by Dutch elite and sub-elite athletes: Does receiving dietary counseling make a difference? *International Journal of Sport Nutrition and Exercise Metabolism, 27*(1), 32–42. https://doi.org/10.1123/ijsnem.2016-0157

Wei, M. Y., & Jacobson, T. A. (2011). Effects of eicosapentaenoic acid versus docosahexaenoic acid on serum lipids: A systematic review and meta-analysis. *Current Atherosclerosis Reports, 13*(6), 474–483. https://doi.org/10.1007/s11883-011-0210-3

Westerterp-Plantenga, M. S., Lejeune, M. P. G. M., & Kovacs, E. M. R. (2005). Body weight loss and weight maintenance in relation to habitual caffeine intake and green tea supplementation. *Obesity Research, 13*(7), 1195–1204. https://doi.org/10.1038/oby.2005.142

Wilkinson, D. J., Bukhari, S. S. I., Phillips, B. E., Limb, M. C., Cegielski, J., Brook, M. S., Rankin, D., Mitchell, W. K., Kobayashi, H., Williams, J. P., Lund, J., Greenhaff, P. L., Smith, K., & Atherton, P. J. (2018). Effects of leucine-enriched essential amino acid and whey protein bolus dosing upon skeletal muscle protein synthesis at rest and after exercise in older women. *Clinical Nutrition, 37*(6 pt A), 2011–2021. https://doi.org/10.1016/j.clnu.2017.09.008

Woodson, R. D., Wills, R. E., & Lenfant, C. (1978). Effect of acute and established anemia on O_2 transport at rest, submaximal and maximal work. *Journal of Applied Physiology: Respiratory, Environmental and Exercise Physiology, 44*(1), 36–43. https://doi.org/10.1152/jappl.1978.44.1.36

Zdzieblik, D., Brame, J., Oesser, S., Gollhofer, A., & König, D. (2021). The influence of specific bioactive collagen peptides on knee joint discomfort in young physically active adults: A randomized controlled trial. *Nutrients, 13*(2), 523. https://doi.org/10.3390/nu13020523

Zdzieblik, D., Oesser, S., Gollhofer, A., & König, D. (2017). Improvement of activity-related knee joint discomfort following supplementation of specific collagen peptides. *Applied Physiology, Nutrition, and Metabolism, 42*(6), 588–595. https://doi.org/10.1139/apnm-2016-0390

Zell-Kanter, M., Quigley, M. A., & Leikin, J. B. (2015). Reduction in ephedra poisonings after FDA ban. *New England Journal of Medicine, 372*(22), 2172–2174. https://doi.org/10.1056/NEJMc1502505

Zulyniak, M. A., Perreault, M., Gerling, C., Spriet, L. L., & Mutch, D. M. (2013). Fish oil supplementation alters circulating eicosanoid concentrations in young healthy men. *Metabolism: Clinical and Experimental, 62*(8), 1107–1113. https://doi.org/10.1016/j.metabol.2013.02.004

APPENDIX A

SPORT-SPECIFIC ASSESSMENT AND PROGRAM STRATEGIES

BASEBALL

Note: For the purposes of this content, baseball programming will be a methodology shared across pitchers and position players. Although a case can be made for different programming strategies between pitchers and position players, clinical implementation has proven that the same OPT™ program can have tremendous impacts on injury prevention and performance enhancement for both pitchers and position players due to the overall demands of the sport.

Demands of the Sport (Gambetta, 1999)	
General information	• 4.3–4.4 seconds: Sprint time from home plate to first base • 3.6 seconds or less: Sprint time to steal from first base to second base • 9 minutes: Average time spent on defense for a half inning
Pitchers	• Starting pitcher: 6⅓ innings pitched per game • Nine-inning game: A pitcher will go nine innings 15% of all starts • Average number of pitches per inning: 15 • Average fastball velocity (first inning): 87 mph
Catchers	• Total throws: 221 • Throws from standing position: 89 • Throws from knees: 76 • Total sprints: 15 @ 30 yards/2 @ 5 yards • Total squat movements: 238 • Time on defense: 1 hour 40 minutes 50 seconds per game

SUGGESTED ASSESSMENTS FOR BASEBALL

Assessment Type	Assessment Method
Transitional assessments	• Overhead squat • Single-leg squat • Split squat • Star excursion balance test
Mobility assessments (if needed)	• Foot and ankle testing • Lumbo-pelvic-hip complex testing • Shoulder and spine testing
Dynamic movement assessments	• Drop jump assessment • Shark skill test • Davies test • Triple crossover hop test
Aerobic test (choose one of the following)	• 12-minute run test • 1.5-mile run test • Beep test
Anaerobic test	• 300-yard shuttle run
Muscular endurance assessments	• Push-up test • Pull-up test • Curl-up test

Assessment Type	Assessment Method
Muscular strength assessments	• 1–5 RM bench press • 1–5 RM squat • Nordic hamstring lower test
Power assessments	• Vertical jump test (double-leg) • Vertical jump test (single-leg) • Rotational medicine ball throw test (left and right)
Speed assessments (Norms may not exist for the following tests. Use these as objective measures of improvement over time.)	• 30-yard sprint test • Timed: Home to first base • Timed: Home to second base • Timed: Home to third base
Agility assessments	• LEFT (lower-extremity functional test) • 5–10–5 (pro agility test)

OFF-SEASON GOALS AND CONSIDERATIONS FOR BASEBALL

Goals	Considerations

• Physical and mental reconditioning
• Correcting impaired movement patterns based on results of transitional postural assessments
• Improving:
  • Range of motion, joint stability, and muscle strength and endurance
  • Cardiorespiratory endurance (aerobic/anaerobic)
  • Total-body stabilization, strength, and power
• Increasing:
  • Arm and shoulder strength and stability
  • Speed, agility, and quickness (position players)
	• Planning and programming will be based on assessment, client goals, and the demand of the sport.
	• A systematic off-season plan will incorporate integrated training including:
	  • Core training
	  • Balance training
	  • Plyometric training
	  • Speed, agility, and quickness training
	  • Integrated resistance training
	  • Cardiorespiratory training combined with a proper nutrition plan to maximize training and recovery
	• An off-season training schedule will be developed by working backward from the commencement of spring training/season to allow for maximum injury prevention and performance gains without the athlete overtraining.
	• Performance programs will be modified appropriately, from a volume and exercise standpoint, to accommodate baseball-specific activities to avoid overtraining and maximize results. The athlete will continue to increase baseball skill activities.

SAMPLE OFF-SEASON OPT BASEBALL PLAN (OCTOBER–FEBRUARY)

Level	Phase	JAN Off-Season (4)	FEB Off-Season (5)	MAR Pre-Season (4)	APR In-Season (5)	MAY–SEP In-Season	OCT Off-Season (1)	NOV Off-Season (2)	DEC Off-Season (3)
Corrective							X		
Stabilization	1		X					X	
Strength	2		X						X
	3								
	4								
Power	5	X	X						
	6								

SAMPLE OFF-SEASON WEEKLY OPT BASEBALL SCHEDULE

Month 1: 3 days/week

	MON	TUE	WED	THU	FRI	SAT	SUN
OPT Phase	Corrective	OFF	Corrective	OFF	Corrective	OFF	OFF

Month 2: 3 days/week

	MON	TUE	WED	THU	FRI	SAT	SUN
OPT Phase	Stabilization Endurance	OFF	Stabilization Endurance	OFF	Stabilization Endurance	OFF	OFF

Month 3: 4 days/week

	MON	TUE	WED	THU	FRI	SAT	SUN
OPT Phase	Corrective	OFF	Corrective	OFF	Corrective	OFF	OFF
Other	Conditioning	Conditioning			Conditioning		

Month 4: 5 days/week

	MON	TUE	WED	THU	FRI	SAT	SUN
OPT Phase	Stabilization Endurance	OFF	Stabilization Endurance	OFF	Stabilization Endurance	OFF	OFF
Other		Conditioning		Conditioning			

Month 5: 5 days/week

	MON	TUE	WED	THU	FRI	SAT	SUN
OPT Phase	Corrective	OFF	Corrective	OFF	Corrective	OFF	OFF
Other		Conditioning		Conditioning			

Conditioning = cardio training and/or sport-specific drills.

SAMPLE OFF-SEASON OPT BASEBALL PROGRAMS

Corrective Exercise Training

Inhibit	Sets	Reps	Time
Myofascial Rolling			
Tensor fascia latae	1		30 sec
IT band	1		30 sec
Thoracic spine	1		30 sec
Lats	1		30 sec
LENGTHEN	**Sets**	**Reps**	**Time**
Gastrocnemius stretch	1		30 sec
Supine piriformis stretch	1		30 sec
Posterior shoulder stretch	1		30 sec
Lat stretch	1		30 sec

(continues)

(continued)

ACTIVATE	Sets	Reps	Tempo	Intensity	Rest
Side-lying hip abduction	2	10	4/2/1		0 sec
Floor bridge	2	10	4/2/1		0 sec
Standing shoulder external rotation	2	10	4/2/1		0 sec
Bent-over DB cobra	2	10	4/2/1		90 sec

INTEGRATE		Sets	Reps	Tempo	Intensity	Rest
Back	Single-leg cable row	2	10	4/2/1	60%	0 sec
Shoulders	Single-leg shoulder scaption	2	10	4/2/1	60%	90 sec

PHASE 1: STABILIZATION ENDURANCE TRAINING

WARM-UP	Sets	Reps	Time
Myofascial Rolling			
Tensor fascia latae	1		30 sec
Piriformis	1		30 sec
Lats	1		30 sec
Static Stretching			
Gastrocnemius stretch	1		30 sec
Supine piriformis stretch	1		30 sec
Posterior shoulder stretch	1		30 sec

Dynamic Stretching	Sets	Reps	Tempo	Rest
Lunge with rotation	1	10	Moderate	0 sec
Medicine ball woodchop	1	10	Moderate	0 sec

CORE AND BALANCE	Sets	Reps	Tempo	Rest
Quadruped arm opposite-leg raise	2	15	4/2/1	0 sec
Floor bridge	2	15	4/2/1	0 sec
Single-leg MB lift and chop	2	15	4/2/1	60 sec

PLYOMETRICS		Sets	Reps	Tempo		Rest
Box jump with stabilization		2	10	Hold landing		50 sec
SPEED/AGILITY/QUICKNESS		**Sets**	**Reps**	**Tempo**		**Rest**
Speed ladder: Four exercises		2				60 sec
RESISTANCE		**Sets**	**Reps**	**Tempo**	**Intensity**	**Rest**
Total body	Step-up, balance to overhead press	2	15	4/2/1	65%	0 sec
Chest	SL suspension chest press	2	15	4/2/1	65%	0 sec
Back	Single-leg cable row	2	15	4/2/1	65%	0 sec
Shoulders	Single-leg scaption	2	15	4/2/1	65%	0 sec
Legs	Single-leg Romanian deadlift	2	15	4/2/1	65%	90 sec
COOL-DOWN						
Myofascial rolling and static stretching						

PHASE 2: STRENGTH ENDURANCE

WARM-UP	Sets	Reps	Time
Myofascial Rolling			
IT band	1		30 sec
Thoracic spine	1		30 sec
Lats	1		30 sec
Active Stretching			
Standing adductor stretch	1	10	
Standing hip flexor stretch	1	10	
Floor lat stretch	1	10	

(continues)

(continued)

WARM-UP				
Dynamic Stretching	**Sets**	**Reps**	**Tempo**	**Rest**
Multiplanar lunge with reach	1	10	Moderately fast	0 sec
Squat to overhead reach	1	10	Moderately fast	0 sec

CORE AND BALANCE				
Sets	**Reps**	**Tempo**	**Rest**	
Cable rotation	2	10	1/1/1	0 sec
Cable chop	2	10	1/1/1	0 sec
Single-leg squat touchdown	2	10	1/1/1	60 sec

PLYOMETRICS				
Sets	**Reps**	**Tempo**	**Rest**	
Cone jumps: Side to side	3	10	Repeating	0 sec
Power step-ups	3	10	Repeating	60 sec

SPEED/AGILITY/QUICKNESS				
Sets	**Reps**	**Distance**	**Rest**	
Speed ladder: Six exercises	2			60 sec
T-drill	4		10 yd	60 sec

RESISTANCE		**Sets**	**Reps**	**Tempo**	**Intensity**	**Rest**
Total body	Optional					
Chest	1. Incline DB press	3	8	2/0/2	80%	0 sec
	2. Cable chest press		12	4/2/1	50%	
Back	1. Seated lat pull-down	3	8	2/0/2	80%	0 sec
	2. Single-leg cable row		12	4/2/1	50%	
Shoulders	1. Seated overhead DB press	3	8	2/0/2	80%	0 sec
	2. Bent-over DB combo II		12	4/2/1	50%	
Legs	1. Barbell squats	3	8	2/0/2	80%	0 sec
	2. Side lunge to balance		12	4/2/1	50%	60 sec

COOL-DOWN
Myofascial rolling and static stretching

PHASE 5: POWER TRAINING

WARM-UP		Sets	Reps	Time
Myofascial Rolling				
Tensor fascia latae		1		30 sec
Piriformis		1		30 sec
Lats		1		30 sec
Dynamic Warm-up (Some athletes may still require static stretching prior to dynamic warm-up.)				
Lateral tube walking		1	10	0 sec
Lunge w/rotation		1	10	0 sec
Push-up w/rotation		1	10	0 sec
Iron cross		1	10	0 sec
Russian twist		1	10	60 sec

CORE, BALANCE, AND PLYOMETRICS	Sets	Reps	Tempo	Rest
No CORE, BALANCE, AND PLYOMETRICS (incorporated into dynamic warm-up and resistance training)				

SPEED/AGILITY/QUICKNESS	Sets	Reps	Distance	Rest
Speed ladder: Six exercises	2			60 sec
T-drill	4		10 yd	60 sec

RESISTANCE		Sets	Reps	Tempo	Intensity	Rest
Total body	Optional					
Chest	Incline DB press	3	5	Controlled	85%	0 sec
	Rotational chest pass		10	Explosive	2% of BW	2 min
Back	Seated cable row	3	5	Controlled	85%	0 sec
	MB soccer throw		10	Explosive	2% of BW	2 min
Shoulders	Shoulder press machine	3	5	Controlled	85%	0 sec
	Overhead MB throw		10	Explosive	2% of BW	2 min
Legs	Barbell squat	3	5	Controlled	85%	0 sec
	Ice skater		10	Explosive	2% of BW	3 min

COOL-DOWN
Myofascial rolling and static stretching

PRE-SEASON GOALS AND CONSIDERATIONS FOR BASEBALL

Goals	Considerations

• Correcting impaired movement patterns based on results of pre-season assessments
• Maintaining:
  • Physical health (decrease chance of injury for participation in practice and games, and optimal performance within such activities)
  • Range of motion, joint stability, and muscle strength and endurance
  • Cardiorespiratory endurance (aerobic/anaerobic)
  • Total-body stabilization, strength, and power
  • Speed, agility, and quickness (position players)
	• A systematic pre-season plan that transitions the athlete from performance enhancement to injury prevention and maintenance of off-season gains will be developed. This transition should be implemented with the consideration that the athlete's sport participation level is increasing dramatically from what they have become used to in the off-season. The proper recovery and conditioning should be applied during this time of increased activity.
	• Consider the exercise volume of injury prevention and performance training based on the athlete's increased activity level.

SAMPLE PRE-SEASON OPT BASEBALL PLAN (MARCH)

Level	Phase	JAN Off-Season	FEB Off-Season	MAR Pre-Season (1)	APR In-Season	MAY–SEP In-Season	OCT Off-Season	NOV Off-Season	DEC Off-Season
Corrective				X					
Stabilization	1			X					
Strength	2			X					
	3								
	4								
Power	5								
	6								

SAMPLE PRE-SEASON WEEKLY OPT BASEBALL SCHEDULE

Month 1

	MON	TUE	WED	THU	FRI	SAT	SUN
OPT Phase	Strength Endurance	Corrective	OFF	Stabilization Endurance	Corrective	OFF	OFF
Other	Game	Game	Game		Game	Game	

SAMPLE PRE-SEASON OPT BASEBALL PROGRAMS

Corrective Exercise Training

INHIBIT	Sets	Reps	Time
Myofascial Rolling			
Tensor fascia latae	1		30 sec
Piriformis	1		30 sec
Lats	1		30 sec

LENGTHEN	Sets	Reps	Time
Gastrocnemius stretch	1		30 sec
Supine biceps femoris stretch	1		30 sec
Standing pec stretch	1		30 sec
Floor lat stretch	1		30 sec

ACTIVATE	Sets	Reps	Tempo	Intensity	Rest
Single-leg calf raise	2	10	4/2/1		0 sec
Standing shoulder external rotation	2	10	4/2/1		0 sec
Bent-over DB combo I	2	10	4/2/1		0 sec

INTEGRATE		Sets	Reps	Tempo	Intensity	Rest
Back	Single-leg, single-arm cable row	2	12	4/2/1	60%	0 sec
Shoulders	Single-leg, single-arm scaption	2	12	4/2/1	60%	90 sec

PHASE 1: STABILIZATION ENDURANCE TRAINING

WARM-UP	Sets	Reps	Time
Myofascial Rolling			
Tensor fascia latae	1		30 sec
Piriformis	1		30 sec
Lats	1		30 sec

(continues)

(*continued*)

WARM-UP			Sets	Reps	Time
Static Stretching					
Gastrocnemius stretch			1		30 sec
Supine biceps femoris stretch			1		30 sec
Posterior shoulder stretch			1		30 sec
Dynamic Stretching		Sets	Reps	Tempo	Rest
Lunge with rotation		1	10	Moderate	0 sec
Medicine ball woodchop		1	10	Moderate	0 sec

CORE AND BALANCE	Sets	Reps	Tempo	Rest
Side iso-abs with hip abduction	2	15	4/2/1	0 sec
Floor cobra	2	15	4/2/1	0 sec
Single-leg balance reach	2	15	4/2/1	60 sec

PLYOMETRICS	Sets	Reps	Tempo	Rest
No PLYOMETRICS because of increased activity				

SPEED/AGILITY/QUICKNESS	Sets	Reps	Distance	Rest
No SAQ because of on-field drills and conditioning				

RESISTANCE		Sets	Reps	Tempo	Intensity	Rest
Total body	Optional	2	15	4/2/1	65%	0 sec
Chest	Push-up: Feet in suspension	2	15	4/2/1	65%	0 sec
Back	Single-leg suspension row	2	15	4/2/1	65%	0 sec
Shoulders	Single-leg scaption	2	15	4/2/1	65%	0 sec
Legs	Step-up to balance: Transverse plane	2	15	4/2/1	65%	90 sec

COOL-DOWN
Myofascial rolling and static stretching

PHASE 2: STRENGTH ENDURANCE TRAINING

WARM-UP		Sets	Reps		Time
Myofascial Rolling					
Piriformis		1			30 sec
Adductors		1			30 sec
Thoracic spine		1			30 sec
Active Stretching					
Gastrocnemius stretch		1	10		
Standing adductor stretch		1	10		
Standing pec stretch		1	10		

Dynamic Stretching		Sets	Reps	Tempo	Rest
Multiplanar lunge with reach		1	10	Moderately fast	0 sec
Squat to overhead reach		1	10	Moderately fast	0 sec

CORE AND BALANCE		Sets	Reps	Tempo	Rest
Cable crunch		2	10	1/1/1	0 sec
Back extension		2	10	1/1/1	0 sec
Step-up to balance: Transverse plane		2	10	1/1/1	60 sec

PLYOMETRICS		Sets	Reps	Tempo	Rest
No PLYOMETRICS because of increased activity					

SPEED/AGILITY/QUICKNESS		Sets	Reps	Distance	Rest
No SAQ because of on-field drills and conditioning					

RESISTANCE		Sets	Reps	Tempo	Intensity	Rest
Total body	Optional					
Chest	Machine chest press	3	12	2/0/2	70%	0 sec
	Push-up: Feet in suspension		8	4/2/1		

(continues)

(continued)

RESISTANCE		Sets	Reps	Tempo	Intensity	Rest
Back	Seated cable row	3	12	2/0/2	70%	0 sec
	Back extension		8	4/2/1		
Shoulders	Standing overhead press	3	12	2/0/2	70%	0 sec
	SL DB scaption		8	4/2/1		
Legs	Forward DB lunge	3	12	2/0/2	70%	0 sec
	Single-leg squat		8	4/2/1		60 sec
COOL-DOWN						
Myofascial rolling and static stretching						

IN-SEASON GOALS AND CONSIDERATIONS FOR BASEBALL

Goals	Considerations

• Maintaining:
  • Range of motion, joint stability, and muscle strength and endurance
  • Cardiorespiratory endurance (aerobic/anaerobic)
  • Total-body stabilization, strength, and power
  • Speed, agility, and quickness (position players)
  • Arm and shoulder strength
• Establishing with the athlete a communication process for monitoring in-season maintenance and a plan that works based on what the athlete needs, wants, and will have the capability to do while playing baseball
	• Assessments and testing, to ensure program considerations are being made to prevent overuse injuries and maintain performance levels, will be performed.
	• Impaired movement patterns with exercise strategies being implemented will be attended to.
	• A systematic in-season maintenance plan will be developed that allows the athlete to minimize decreases in performance and chance of injury over a long season with repetitive sport movement patterns (hitting and throwing).
	• The exercise volume of injury prevention, and performance training based on the athlete's increased travel and activity level, will be considered.

IN-SEASON OPT BASEBALL PLAN (APRIL–SEPTEMBER)

Level	Phase	JAN – FEB	MAR	APR	MAY	JUNE	JUL	AUG	SEPT	OCT– DEC
		Off-Season	Pre-Season	In-Season (1)	In-Season (2)	In-Season (3)	In-Season (4)	In-Season (5)	In-Season (6)	Off-Season
Corrective				X	X	X	X	X	X	
Stabilization	1			X	X	X	X	X	X	
Strength	2			X	X	X	X	X	X	
	3									
	4									
Power	5									
	6									

SAMPLE IN-SEASON WEEKLY OPT BASEBALL SCHEDULE

Any Month

	MON	TUE	WED	THU	FRI	SAT	SUN
OPT Phase	Strength Endurance	OFF	Corrective	OFF	Stabilization Endurance	Corrective	OFF
Other	Game	Game	Game		Game	Game	Game

SAMPLE IN-SEASON OPT BASEBALL PROGRAM

Corrective Exercise Training

INHIBIT	Sets	Reps	Time
Myofascial Rolling			
Tensor fascia latae	1		30 sec
Piriformis	1		30 sec
Lats	1		30 sec

(continues)

(continued)

LENGTHEN	Sets	Reps	Time
Gastrocnemius stretch	1		30 sec
Supine biceps femoris stretch	1		30 sec
Standing pec stretch	1		30 sec
Floor lat stretch	1		30 sec

ACTIVATE		Sets	Reps	Tempo	Intensity	Rest
Single-leg hip extension		1	15	4/2/1		0 sec
Floor bridge		1	15	4/2/1		0 sec
SL bent-over DB cobra		1	15	4/2/1		90 sec

INTEGRATE		Sets	Reps	Tempo	Intensity	Rest
Total body	Cable squat to row	3	10	4/2/1	60%	0 sec
Total body	Side lunge, curl to overhead press: Single-arm	3	10	4/2/1	60%	90 sec

PHASE 1: STABILIZATION ENDURANCE TRAINING

WARM-UP	Sets	Reps	Time
Myofascial Rolling			
Tensor fascia latae	1		30 sec
Piriformis	1		30 sec
Lats	1		30 sec
Static Stretching			
Gastrocnemius stretch	1		30 sec
Standing adductor stretch	1		30 sec
Standing pec stretch	1		30 sec

WARM-UP		Sets	Reps	Time
Dynamic Stretching	Sets	Reps	Tempo	Rest
Lunge with rotation	1	10	Moderate	0 sec
Medicine ball woodchop	1	10	Moderate	0 sec
CORE AND BALANCE	Sets	Reps	Tempo	Rest
Side iso-abs	2	15	4/2/1	0 sec
Floor bridge: Single-leg	2	15	4/2/1	0 sec
Single-leg balance reach	2	15	4/2/1	60 sec
PLYOMETRICS	Sets	Reps	Tempo	Rest
Multiplanar hop with stabilization box jump-down	2	10	Hold landing	60 sec

RESISTANCE		Sets	Reps	Tempo	Intensity	Rest
Total body	Cable squat to row	2	15	4/2/1	65%	0 sec
Chest	Suspension push-up: Feet in straps	2	15	4/2/1	65%	0 sec
Back	SL bent-over DB Cobra	2	15	4/2/1	65%	0 sec
Shoulders	Single-leg cable lift	2	15	4/2/1	65%	0 sec
Legs	Step-up to balance: Frontal plane	2	15	4/2/1	65%	90 sec

COOL-DOWN
Myofascial rolling and static stretching

BASKETBALL

Note: For the purposes of this content, the basketball programming will be a methodology shared across "bigs" (centers and forwards) and "smalls" (guards). Through years of clinical application of the OPT™ Model with basketball players, from youth leagues through the professional association, there has not been a need to treat the athletes differently from a strength and conditioning aspect. At a fundamental level, all positions on the court experience the same movement patterns and energy expenditure demands; therefore, we will focus on how the OPT Model can be used for all basketball positions alike. If the Sports Performance Coach needs to modify the model based on the athlete's needs, then it is very appropriate to do so based on the assessment process and the goals set for the athlete.

GENERAL INFORMATION (MCCLAY ET AL., 1994A, 1994B)

Demands of the Sport	
Jumps classification	• Low: A shot or unchallenged rebound • Medium: Most rebounds, defending jump shots, and a jump shot • High: Maximal or near maximal as would occur with a dunk, blocked shot, or challenged jump shot
Jumps in a game	• Low: 30% • Medium: 45% • High: 25%
Average number of jumps per game: 70	• Guards: 55 • Centers: 83 • Forward: 72

Ground reaction forces	• Running:
	  • Vertical: 3 × body weight (BW)
	  • Anterior/posterior: 0.5 × BW
	  • Mediolateral: 0.25 × BW
	• Vertical forces:
	  • Starting: 0.8 × BW
	  • Lay-up landing: 8.9 × BW
	  • Stopping: 2.7 × BW
	  • Cutting: 3.0 × BW
	• Anterior/posterior forces:
	  • Stopping: 1.3 × BW
	• Mediolateral direction:
	  • Shuffling: 1.4 × BW

ACTIVITY INFORMATION (GAMBETTA, 1999)

Demands of the Sport	
Total game time (professional): 48 minutes	• 4 × 12-minute quarters • 15-minute halftime • 2 minutes between quarters
Activity type	• Walking or standing: 4 minutes • Jogging: 4 minutes • Running: 4 minutes • Sprinting: 3 minutes • Shuffling (low to medium intensity): 9 minutes • Shuffling (high intensity): 2 minutes • Jumping: 41 seconds

Demands of the Sport	
Movement	• While the ball is in play, a change in movement category happens every 2 seconds • There are 1,000 different movements during a game • 28% of all court time is spent in strenuous exertion • Intense activity occurs for 13–14 seconds at a time • 105 intense activities per game, every 21 seconds • 31% of the game is devoted to side-to-side movements (66% of these movements are intense efforts) • Individual shuffle movements are 1–4 seconds in duration • Sprints are 1–5 seconds in duration

SUGGESTED ASSESSMENTS FOR BASKETBALL

Assessment Type	Assessment Method
Transitional postural assessments	• Overhead squat test • Single-leg squat test • Split squat • Star excursion balance test
Mobility assessments (if needed)	• Foot and ankle testing • Lumbo-pelvic-hip complex testing • Shoulder and spine testing
Dynamic movement assessments	• Drop jump • Shark skill test • Davies test • Triple crossover hop test
Aerobic test (choose one of the following)	• Beep test • Yo-yo intermittent recovery test
Anaerobic test	• 300-yard shuttle run
Muscular endurance assessment	• Push-up test • Pull-up test • Curl-up test
Muscular strength assessment	• 1–5 RM bench press • 1–5 RM squat • Nordic hamstring lower test

(continues)

(continued)

Assessment Type	Assessment Method

Power assessments	• Vertical jump test
	  • Double-leg
	  • Single-leg
	  • 15-foot approach (single- or two-leg)
	• Horizontal broad jump (single-leg)
	• Medicine ball soccer throw
	• Rotational medicine ball throw test (left and right)

Speed assessments (Norms may not exist for the following tests. Use these as objective measures of improvement over time.)	• 40-yard sprint test • ¾ court sprint (baseline to farthest from the throw line)
Agility assessments	• LEFT (lower-extremity functional test) • 5–10–5 (pro agility test) • 5–0–5 test

OFF-SEASON GOALS AND CONSIDERATIONS FOR BASKETBALL

Goals	Considerations

• Physical and mental reconditioning
• Correcting impaired movement patterns based on results of transitional postural assessments
• Improving range of motion, joint stability, and muscle strength and endurance
  • Typical areas of focus for enhanced flexibility or range of motion include ankle dorsiflexion, hip internal rotation, rectus femoris, and lats.
  • Typical areas of focus for enhanced strengthening include gluteus medius, pectineus, gluteus maximus, posterior tibialis, medial gastrocnemius, and core musculature.
• Improving:
  • Cardiorespiratory endurance (aerobic/anaerobic)
  • Total-body stabilization, strength, and power
• Increasing reaction time, speed, agility, and quickness
	• Planning and programming will be based on assessment, client goals, and the demands of the sport.
	• A systematic off-season plan will incorporate integrated training, including:
	  • Core training
	  • Balance training
	  • Plyometric training
	  • Speed, agility, and quickness training
	  • Integrated resistance training
	  • Cardiorespiratory training combined with a proper nutrition plan to maximize training and recovery
	• An off-season training schedule will be developed by working backward from the commencement of the pre-season to allow for maximum injury prevention and performance gains without the athlete overtraining.
	• Opportunities for appropriate rest will be provided between workouts.
	• Considerations will include:
	  • Basketball conditioning will be as like the game as possible.

Goals	Considerations
	• Although the game of basketball is a very dynamic activity, many basketball players enter the off-season having diminished stabilization mechanisms that must be trained and reconditioned. • Performance programs will be modified appropriately, from a volume and exercise standpoint, to accommodate basketball-specific activities to avoid overtraining and maximize results. The athlete will continue to increase basketball skill activities as the off-season progresses.

SAMPLE OFF-SEASON OPT BASKETBALL PLAN (MAY–SEPTEMBER)

Level	Phase	JAN	FEB	MAR–APR	MAY	JUN	JUL	AUG	SEP	OCT	NOV–DEC
		In-Season	In-Season	In-Season	Off-Season (1)	Off-Season (2)	Off-Season (3)	Off-Season (4)	Off-Season (5)	Pre-Season	In-Season
Corrective					X						
Stabilization	1					X			X		
Strength	2						X		X		
	3										
	4										
Power	5		X					X	X		
	6										

SAMPLE OFF-SEASON WEEKLY OPT BASKETBALL SCHEDULE

Month 1: 3 days/week

	MON	TUE	WED	THU	FRI	SAT	SUN
OPT Phase	Corrective	OFF	Corrective	OFF	Corrective	OFF	OFF

Month 2: 3 days/week

	MON	TUE	WED	THU	FRI	SAT	SUN
OPT Phase	Stabilization Endurance	OFF	Stabilization Endurance	OFF	Stabilization Endurance	OFF	OFF
Other	On-court conditioning				On-court conditioning		

Month 3: 5 days/week

	MON	TUE	WED	THU	FRI	SAT	SUN
OPT Phase	Stabilization Endurance Total body	OFF	Stabilization Endurance Upper body	OFF	Stabilization Endurance Lower body	OFF	OFF
Other		On-court conditioning		On-court conditioning			

Month 4: 5 days/week

	MON	TUE	WED	THU	FRI	SAT	SUN
OPT Phase	Power	OFF	Power	OFF	Power	OFF	OFF
Other	On-court conditioning	On-court conditioning		On-court conditioning			

Month 5: 5 days/week

	MON	TUE	WED	THU	FRI	SAT	SUN
OPT Phase	Strength Endurance		Stabilization Endurance		Power	OFF	OFF
Other		On-court conditioning		On-court conditioning			

SAMPLE OFF-SEASON OPT BASKETBALL PROGRAMS

Corrective Exercise Training

INHIBIT	Sets	Reps	Time
Myofascial Rolling			
Calves	1		30 sec
IT band	1		30 sec
Tensor fascia latae	1		30 sec
LENGTHEN	Sets	Reps	Time
Gastrocnemius stretch	1		30 sec
Soleus	1		30 sec
Supine biceps femoris stretch	1		30 sec

ACTIVATE	Sets	Reps	Tempo	Intensity	Rest
Posterior tibialis strengthening	2	12	4/2/1		0 sec
Single-leg calf raise	2	12	4/2/1		0 sec
Single-leg hip adduction: Pectineus	2	12	4/2/1		0 sec
Single-leg hip abduction: Gluteus medius	2	12	4/2/1		90 sec

INTEGRATE		Sets	Reps	Tempo	Intensity	Rest
Total body	Step-up, balance to overhead press	2	12	4/2/1	60%	90 sec

PHASE 1: STABILIZATION ENDURANCE TRAINING

WARM-UP	Sets	Reps	Time
Myofascial Rolling			
Tensor fascia latae	1		30 sec
Piriformis	1		30 sec
Static Stretching			
Gastrocnemius stretch	1		30 sec
Kneeling hip flexor stretch	1		30 sec
Standing biceps femoris stretch	1		30 sec

Dynamic Stretching	Sets	Reps	Tempo	Rest
Lunge with rotation	1	10	Moderate	0 sec
Medicine ball woodchop	1	10	Moderate	0 sec

CORE AND BALANCE	Sets	Reps	Tempo	Rest
Side iso-ab	2	15	4/2/1	0 sec
Floor bridge	2	15	4/2/1	0 sec
Single-leg balance reach	2	15	4/2/1	60 sec

(continues)

(continued)

PLYOMETRICS	Sets	Reps	Tempo	Rest
Box jump-down with stabilization	2	8	Hold landing	60 sec

SPEED/AGILITY/QUICKNESS	Sets	Reps	Tempo	Rest
Speed ladder: Six exercises	2			60 sec

RESISTANCE		Sets	Reps	Tempo	Intensity	Rest
Total body	Step-up, balance to overhead press: Sagittal plane	2	15	4/2/1	65%	0 sec
Chest	Cable chest press	2	15	4/2/1	65%	0 sec
Back	Single-leg cable row	2	15	4/2/1	65%	0 sec
Shoulders	Single-leg lateral raise	2	15	4/2/1	65%	0 sec
Legs	Single-leg Romanian deadlift	2	15	4/2/1	65%	90 sec

COOL-DOWN
Myofascial rolling and static stretching

PHASE 2: STRENGTH ENDURANCE TRAINING

WARM-UP	Sets	Reps	Time
Myofascial Rolling			
IT band	1		30 sec
Piriformis	1		30 sec
Calf	1		30 sec
Active Stretching			
Standing adductor stretch	1	10	
Standing hip flexor stretch	1	10	
Floor lat stretch	1	10	

Dynamic Stretching	Sets	Reps	Tempo	Rest
Multiplanar lunge	1	10	Moderately fast	0 sec
Squat to overhead reach	1	10	Moderately fast	0 sec

CORE AND BALANCE		Sets	Reps	Tempo	Rest
Knee-ups		2	12	1/1/1	0 sec
Back extension		2	12	1/1/1	0 sec
Single-leg squat touchdown		2	12	1/1/1	60 sec
PLYOMETRICS		**Sets**	**Reps**	**Tempo**	**Rest**
Power step-ups		2	8	Repeating	0 sec
Butt kicks		2	8	Repeating	60 sec
SPEED/AGILITY/QUICKNESS		**Sets**	**Reps**	**Tempo**	**Rest**
Speed ladder: Six exercises		2			60 sec
Box drill		6			30 sec
LEFT test		2			60 sec

RESISTANCE		Sets	Reps	Tempo	Intensity	Rest
Total body	Optional					
Chest	Machine press	3	8	2/0/2	75%	0 sec
	Cable chest press		12	4/2/1	55%	
Back	Seated lat pull-down	3	8	2/0/2	75%	0 sec
	Standing cable row: alternating arm		12	4/2/1	55%	
Shoulders	Standing lateral raise	3	8	2/0/2	75%	0 sec
	SL DB press		12	4/2/1	55%	
Legs	Barbell squats	3	8	2/0/2	75%	60 sec
	Side lunge to balance		12	4/2/1	55%	

COOL-DOWN

Myofascial rolling and static stretching

PHASE 5: POWER TRAINING

WARM-UP		Sets	Reps	Time
Myofascial Rolling				
Calf		1		30 sec
Tensor fascia latae		1		30 sec
Piriformis		1		30 sec
Dynamic Warm-up (Some athletes may still require static stretching prior to the dynamic warm-up.)				
Lateral tube walking		1	10	0 sec
Prisoner squats		1	10	0 sec
Multiplanar lunge		1	10	0 sec
Leg swings: Front to back		1	10	0 sec
Leg swings: Side to side		1	10	0 sec
MB rotations		1	10	0 sec
Russian twist		1	10	0 sec
Multiplanar hop to stabilization		1	10	60 sec

CORE AND BALANCE	Sets	Reps	Tempo	Rest
No CORE AND BALANCE (incorporated into dynamic warm-up)				

PLYOMETRICS	Sets	Reps	Tempo	Rest
No PLYOMETRICS (incorporated into dynamic warm-up)				

SPEED/AGILITY/QUICKNESS	Sets	Reps	Tempo	Rest
Speed ladder: Eight exercises	1			60 sec
Box drill	4			15 sec
T-drill	4			25 sec
Shuttle: Six lengths of basketball court	2			60 sec

RESISTANCE		Sets	Reps	Tempo	Intensity	Rest
Total body	DB squat, curl to overhead press	3	5	Controlled	85%	0 sec
	DB snatch		10	Explosive	45%	2 min
Chest	DB chest press	3	5	Controlled	85%	0 sec
	Cable chest press		10	Explosive	2% of BW	2 min
Back	Seated lat pull-down	3	5	Controlled	85%	0 sec
	Standing cable row: alternating arm		10	Explosive	2% of BW	2 min
Shoulders	Incorporated in total-body exercises					
Legs	Barbell squat	3	5	Controlled	85%	0 sec
	Squat jump		10	Explosive of BW		3 min

COOL-DOWN

Myofascial rolling and static stretching

PRE-SEASON GOALS AND CONSIDERATIONS FOR BASKETBALL

Goals	Considerations

• Correcting impaired movement patterns based on results of pre-season assessments
• Maintaining:
  • Physical health (decreases chance of injury for participation in practice and games, and optimal performance within such activities)
  • Range of motion, joint stability, and muscle strength and endurance
  • Cardiorespiratory endurance (aerobic/anaerobic)
  • Total-body stabilization, strength, and power
  • Speed, agility, and quickness
	• A systematic pre-season plan that transitions the athlete from performance enhancement to injury prevention and maintenance of off-season gains will be developed. This transition should be implemented with the consideration that the athlete's sport participation level is increasing dramatically from what they have become used to in the off-season.
	• Proper recovery and conditioning should be applied during this time of increased activity.
	• Consider the exercise volume of injury prevention and performance training based on the athlete's increased activity level.

SAMPLE PRE-SEASON OPT BASKETBALL PLAN (OCTOBER)

Level	Phase	JAN In-Season	FEB In-Season	MAR In-Season	APR In-Season	MAY–SEP Off-Season	OCT Pre-Season (1)	NOV In-Season	DEC In-Season
Corrective							X		
Stabilization	1						X		
Strength	2						X		
	3								
	4								
Power	5								
	6								

SAMPLE PRE-SEASON WEEKLY OPT BASKETBALL SCHEDULE

Month 1

	MON	TUE	WED	THU	FRI	SAT	SUN
OPT Phase	Strength Endurance Upper body	OFF	Corrective	OFF	Stabilization Endurance Lower body	OFF	OFF
Other		Game			Game		

SAMPLE PRE-SEASON OPT BASKETBALL PROGRAMS

Corrective Exercise Training

INHIBIT	Sets	Reps	Time
Myofascial Rolling			
Tensor fascia latae	1		30 sec
IT band	1		30 sec
Adductors	1		30 sec
LENGTHEN	Sets	Reps	Time
Gastrocnemius stretch	1		30 sec
Supine biceps femoris stretch	1		30 sec

LENGTHEN	Sets	Reps	Time
Standing adductor stretch	1		30 sec
Kneeling hip flexor stretch	1		30 sec

ACTIVATE	Sets	Reps	Tempo	Intensity	Rest
Side-lying hip abduction	2	10	4/2/1		0 sec
Suspension bridge	2	10	4/2/1		90 sec

INTEGRATE	Sets	Reps	Tempo	Intensity	Rest
Single-leg squat	2	12	4/2/1	60%	90 sec

PHASE 1: STABILIZATION ENDURANCE TRAINING (LOWER BODY)

WARM-UP	Sets	Reps	Time
Myofascial Rolling			
Tensor fascia latae	1		30 sec
Piriformis	1		30 sec
Thoracic spine	1		30 sec
Static Stretching			
Gastrocnemius stretch	1		30 sec
Standing adductor stretch	1		30 sec
Standing biceps femoris stretch	1		30 sec

Dynamic Stretching	Sets	Reps	Tempo	Rest
Lunge with rotation	1	10	Moderate	0 sec
Medicine ball woodchop	1	10	Moderate	0 sec

CORE AND BALANCE	Sets	Reps	Tempo	Rest
Side iso-ab	2	15	4/2/1	0 sec
Floor bridge: Single-leg	2	15	4/2/1	0 sec
Single-leg balance reach	2	15	4/2/1	60 sec

(continues)

(continued)

PLYOMETRICS	Sets	Reps	Tempo	Rest
Squat jump with stabilization	2	10	Hold landing	60 sec

SPEED/AGILITY/QUICKNESS	Sets	Reps	Distance	Rest
No SAQ because of on-court drills and conditioning				

RESISTANCE		Sets	Reps	Tempo	Intensity	Rest
Total body	Step-up, balance to overhead press: SA	2	15	4/2/1	65%	0 sec
Legs	Single-leg Romanian deadlift	2	15	4/2/1	65%	0 sec
	Single-leg calf raise					
	Lunge to balance: Frontal plane	2	15	4/2/1	65%	90 sec

COOL-DOWN
Myofascial rolling and static stretching

PHASE 2: STRENGTH ENDURANCE TRAINING (UPPER BODY)

WARM-UP	Sets	Reps	Time
Myofascial Rolling			
Thoracic spine	1		30 sec
Lats	1		30 sec
Active Stretching			
Floor lat stretch	1	10	
Standing pec stretch	1	10	

Dynamic Stretching	Sets	Reps	Tempo	Rest
Rotation med ball throw	1	10	Moderately fast	0 sec
Med ball back extension throw	1	10	Moderately fast	0 sec

CORE AND BALANCE	Sets	Reps	Tempo	Rest
No CORE AND BALANCE due to lack of time (core/balance type exercises incorporated in resistance training)				

PLYOMETRICS		Sets	Reps	Tempo	Rest
No PLYOMETRICS because of increased activity					

SPEED/AGILITY/QUICKNESS		Sets	Reps	Distance	Rest
No SAQ because of on-court drills and conditioning					

RESISTANCE		Sets	Reps	Tempo	Intensity	Rest
Chest	Bench press	3	12	2/0/2	70%	0 sec
	Push-up: Feet in suspension		8	4/2/1		
Back	Seated cable row	3	12	2/0/2	70%	0 sec
	SL cable pull-down		8	4/2/1		
Shoulders	Standing overhead press	3	12	2/0/2	70%	0 sec
	SL DB scaption		8	4/2/1		

COOL-DOWN
Myofascial rolling and static stretching

IN-SEASON GOALS AND CONSIDERATIONS FOR BASKETBALL

Goals	Considerations
• Maintaining: • Range of motion, joint stability, and muscle strength and endurance • Cardiorespiratory endurance (aerobic/anaerobic) • Total-body stabilization, strength, and power • Speed, agility, and quickness (position players) • Arm and shoulder strength • Establishing with the athlete a communication process for monitoring in-season maintenance, and a plan that works based on what the athlete needs, wants, and will have the capability to do while playing basketball	• Assessments and testing to ensure program considerations are being made to prevent overuse injuries and maintain performance levels will be performed. • Impaired movement patterns with exercise strategies being implemented will be attended to. • Additional conditioning, for athletes who may not get the same type of on-the-court minutes during games as others, will be considered. • Athletes, who may get limited to no play time during games, will be considered for progression to the strength and power phases of the OPT Model to offset the lack of on-court power/explosive movements that they are missing due to lack of playing time. • Coaching styles and their practice routines will be assessed, and workouts will be adjusted accordingly in-season. Adjustments to avoid overtraining and undertraining are important. • A systematic in-season maintenance plan will be developed that allows the athlete to minimize decreases in performance and chance of injury over a long season with repetitive sport movement patterns. • The exercise volume of injury prevention, and performance training based on the athlete's increased travel and activity level, will be considered.

IN-SEASON OPT BASKETBALL PLAN (NOVEMBER–APRIL)

Level	Phase	JAN In-Season (3)	FEB In-Season (4)	MAR In-Season (5)	APR In-Season (6)	MAY–SEP Off-Season	OCT Pre-Season	NOV In-Season (1)	DEC In-Season (2)
Corrective		X	X	X	X			X	X
Stabilization	1	X	X	X	X			X	X
Strength	2	X	X	X	X			X	X
	3								
	4								
Power	5								
	6								

SAMPLE IN-SEASON WEEKLY OPT BASKETBALL SCHEDULE

Any Month

	MON	TUE	WED	THU	FRI	SAT	SUN
OPT Phase	Strength Endurance Upper body	OFF	Corrective	Corrective	Stabilization Endurance	OFF	Corrective
Other	Game			Game		Game	

SAMPLE IN-SEASON OPT BASKETBALL PROGRAM

Corrective Exercise Training

INHIBIT	Sets	Reps	Time
Myofascial Rolling			
Tensor fascia latae	1		30 sec
Piriformis	1		30 sec
Lats	1		30 sec

LENGTHEN	Sets	Reps	Time
Gastrocnemius stretch	1		30 sec
Standing biceps femoris stretch	1		30 sec
Kneeling hip flexor stretch	1		30 sec
Floor lat stretch	1		30 sec

ACTIVATE	Sets	Reps	Tempo	Intensity	Rest
Single-leg calf raise	1	15	4/2/1		0 sec
Single-leg hip extension	1	15	4/2/1		0 sec
Suspension bridge	1	15	4/2/1		90 sec

INTEGRATE	Sets	Reps	Tempo	Intensity	Rest
Total-body cable squat to row	3	10	4/2/1	60%	90 sec

PHASE 1: STABILIZATION ENDURANCE TRAINING

WARM-UP	Sets	Reps	Time
Myofascial Rolling			
Tensor fascia latae	1		30 sec
Piriformis	1		30 sec
IT band	1		30 sec
Static Stretching			
Gastrocnemius stretch	1		30 sec
Standing biceps femoris stretch	1		30 sec
Kneeling hip flexor stretch	1		30 sec
Supine piriformis stretch	1		30 sec

Dynamic Stretching	Sets	Reps	Tempo	Rest
Lunge with rotation	1	10	Moderate	0 sec
Prisoner squats to calf raise	1	10	Moderate	0 sec

(continues)

(continued)

CORE AND BALANCE	Sets	Reps	Tempo	Rest
Side iso-abs	3	12	4/2/1	0 sec
Floor cobra	3	12	4/2/1	0 sec
Single-leg lift and chop	3	12	4/2/1	60 sec

PLYOMETRICS	Sets	Reps	Tempo	Rest
No PLYOMETRICS because of increased activity				

SPEED/AGILITY/QUICKNESS
No SAQ because of on-court drills and conditioning

RESISTANCE		Sets	Reps	Tempo	Intensity	Rest
Total body	Cable squat to row	3	12	4/2/1	70%	0 sec
Chest	Suspension SL chest press	3	12	4/2/1	70%	0 sec
Back	Incorporated in total-body exercise					
Shoulders	Single-leg overhead DB press	3	12	4/2/1	70%	0 sec
Legs	Lunge to balance: Frontal plane	3	12	4/2/1	70%	60 sec

COOL-DOWN
Myofascial rolling and static stretching

PHASE 2: STRENGTH ENDURANCE TRAINING (UPPER BODY)

WARM-UP	Sets	Reps	Time
Myofascial Rolling			
Piriformis	1		30 sec
Adductor	1		30 sec
Thoracic spine	1		30 sec
Active Stretching			
Gastrocnemius stretch	1	10	
Standing adductor stretch	1	10	
Standing pec stretch	1	10	

WARM-UP

Dynamic Stretching	Sets	Reps	Tempo	Rest
Multiplanar lunge with reach	1	10	Moderately fast	0 sec
Modified push up to rotation	1	10	Moderately fast	0 sec

CORE AND BALANCE	Sets	Reps	Tempo	Rest
Cable chop	3	10	1/1/1	0 sec
Single-leg squat	3	10	1/1/1	60 sec

PLYOMETRICS	Sets	Reps	Tempo	Rest
No PLYOMETRICS because of increased activity				

SPEED/AGILITY/QUICKNESS	Sets	Reps	Distance	Rest
No SAQ because of on-court drills and conditioning				

RESISTANCE		Sets	Reps	Tempo	Intensity	Rest
Chest	Incline DB press	2	10	2/0/2	75%	0 sec
	Cable chest press		10	4/2/1	60%	
Back	Seated cable row	2	10	2/0/2	75%	0 sec
	SL lat pull-down		10	4/2/1	60%	
Shoulders	Seated DB scaption	2	10	2/0/2	75%	0 sec
	SL SA DB press		10	4/2/1	60%	

COOL-DOWN

Myofascial rolling and static stretching

PHASE 2: STRENGTH ENDURANCE TRAINING

WARM-UP	Sets	Reps	Time
Myofascial Rolling			
Tensor fascia latae	1		30 sec
IT band	1		30 sec
Lats	1		30 sec

(continues)

(continued)

WARM-UP	Sets	Reps	Time
Active Stretching			
Gastrocnemius stretch	1	10	
Standing adductor stretch	1	10	
Standing pec stretch	1	10	

Dynamic Stretching	Sets	Reps	Tempo	Rest
Multiplanar lunge with reach	1	10	Moderate	0 sec
Squat to overhead reach	1	10	Moderate	0 sec

CORE AND BALANCE	Sets	Reps	Tempo	Rest
Reverse crunch	3	10	1/1/1	0 sec
Back extension	3	10	1/1/1	0 sec
Turning step-up to balance	3	10	1/1/1	60 sec

PLYOMETRICS	Sets	Reps	Tempo	Rest
Front power step-up	3	10	Repeating	60 sec

SPEED/AGILITY/QUICKNESS	Sets	Reps	Distance	Rest
Speed ladder: Six exercises	2			60 sec

RESISTANCE		Sets	Reps	Tempo	Intensity	Rest
Total body	Optional					
Chest	Incline DB press	2	10	2/0/2	75%	0 sec
	Cable chest press		10	4/2/1	60%	
Back	Seated cable row	2	10	2/0/2	75%	0 sec
	SL lat pull-down		10	4/2/1	60%	
Shoulders	Seated DB scaption	2	10	2/0/2	75%	0 sec
	SL SA DB press		10	4/2/1	60%	
Legs	Deadlift	2	10	2/0/2	75%	60 sec
	Reverse lunge to balance		10	4/2/1	60%	

COOL-DOWN
Myofascial rolling and static stretching

FOOTBALL

Note: The Sports Performance Coach will focus on the design and assessment of a program for football players that considers the demands of the sport, the movement patterns, and the physical conditioning required for the sport. In the case of a performance program for football players, both skill position players and linemen can be treated separately with individual programs for each. However, in this section, we will explore football as a sport without a tremendous amount of specificity to the multiple positions and the various types of training that can be implemented with each.

NASM has implemented the OPT™ Model with multiple ability levels (high school, college, combine prep, and NFL) and a variety of positions within football, and has had

Demands of the Sport	
General Information	**Specific Information (Gambetta, 1999)**

• Activity characterized by high-intensity, intermittent movement with physical contact
 	
• High-intensity movement followed by active rest periods after each play
 	
• For the most part, all movement occurs from a completely stationary start position
 	
• Aerobic and anaerobic energy systems important to cardiorespiratory conditioning
 	
• Change of direction includes stopping, backward running, lateral movement, and engaging in physical activity while in a stationary position
 	
• Players wear equipment that adds 15–20 pounds of additional load, which they carry throughout the game
 	
• Frequent body contact (player to player) that adds additional stress to the body
	• Duration of game: 60 minutes (4 × 15-minute quarters)
	• *Team A Offense:*
	  • Plays per game: 74.7 (plays per quarter: 18.7)
	  • Drives per game: 13.3 (drives per quarter: 3.3)
	  • Yards per drive: 24
	  • Plays per drive: 5.6 (Each play averages: 5.0 seconds of work; 26.8 seconds of relief)
	  • Runs per drive: 2.3%–41.5% (Each run averages: 4.3 seconds of work; 27.9 seconds of relief)
	  • Passes per drive: 3.3%–58.5% (Each play averages: 5.5 seconds of work; 26.0 seconds of relief)
	• *Team B Offense:*
	  • Plays per game: 64.7 (plays per quarter: 16.2)
	  • Drives per game: 12.3 (drives per quarter: 3.1)
	  • Yards per drive: 29
	  • Plays per drive: 5.3 (Each play averages: 5.0 seconds of work; 36.4 seconds of relief)
	  • Runs per drive: 3.0%–57.2% (Each run averages: 4.4 seconds of work; 36.1 seconds of relief)
	  • Passes per drive: 2.3%–42.8% (Each play averages: 5.8 seconds of work; 36.8 seconds of relief)

Position Specific Metrics				
	Total Yards	Total Time (min)	Avg. Yd/Play	Avg. Sec/Play
OL	484	3.54	6.05	2.67
RB	732	3.30	9.15	2.48
WR	1,224	4.03	15.3	3.0

success with correcting movement imbalances, preventing injury, and improving performance (speed, agility, quickness, strength, power). A football player of any skill and ability will receive tremendous benefits by following the application guidelines and techniques presented.

Consider that within football and the training progression that takes place, each position can be treated similarly in the early phases. The program then becomes more specific to the individual, their position, conditioning, and the demands and skills necessary to excel in that position. The progression does not happen quickly, but it does occur over the course of an off-season or structured strength and conditioning program.

SUGGESTED ASSESSMENTS FOR FOOTBALL

Assessment Type	Assessment Method
Transitional postural assessments	• Overhead squat test • Single-leg squat test • Split squat • Star excursion balance test
Mobility assessments (if needed)	• Foot and ankle testing • Lumbo-pelvic-hip complex testing • Shoulder and spine testing
Dynamic movement assessments	• Drop jump • Shark skill test • Davies test • 6-meter timed hop test
Aerobic test (choose one of the following)	• 12-minute run test • 1.5-mile run test • Beep test
Anaerobic test	• 300-yard shuttle run
Muscular endurance assessments	• Push-up test • Pull-up test • Curl-up test
Muscular strength assessments	• Grip strength • 1–5 RM bench press • 1–5 RM squat • 1–5 RM deadlift • Nordic hamstring lower test
Power assessments	• Vertical jump test (double-leg) • Horizontal broad jump (single-leg) • Rotational medicine ball throw test (left and right) • Power clean assessment
Speed assessments	• 40-yard sprint test
Agility assessments	• LEFT (lower-extremity functional test) • 5–10–5 (pro agility test)

OFF-SEASON GOALS AND CONSIDERATIONS FOR FOOTBALL

Goals	Considerations

• Physical and mental reconditioning
• Reconditioning from the physical contact and additional stress placed on the body
• Correcting impaired movement patterns based on results of transitional postural assessments
• Improving
  • Range of motion, joint stability, and muscle strength and endurance
  • Cardiorespiratory endurance (aerobic/anaerobic)
  • Total-body stabilization, strength, and power
  • Speed, agility, and quickness
• Increasing lean body mass and size
	• Planning and programming will be based on assessment, client goals, and the demands of the sport.
	• A systematic off-season plan will incorporate integrated training, including:
	  • Core training
	  • Balance training
	  • Power training
	  • Speed, agility, and quickness training
	  • Integrated resistance training
	  • Cardiorespiratory training combined with a proper nutrition plan to maximize training and recovery
	• Opportunities for appropriate rest between workouts will be provided.
	• An off-season training schedule, that works backward from the commencement of the pre-season, will be developed to allow for maximum injury prevention and performance gains without the athlete overtraining.
	• Conditioning for football will be as similar to the game as possible.
	• Circuit-based training, and conditioning utilizing cardio machines and exercises incorporating ground reaction forces when designing a conditioning program, will be considered.

SAMPLE OFF-SEASON OPT FOOTBALL PLAN (JANUARY–JUNE)

Level	Phase	JAN Off-Season (1)	FEB Off-Season (2)	MAR Off-Season (3)	APR Off-Season (4)	MAY Off-Season (5)	JUN Off-Season (6)	JUL Pre-Season	AUG Pre-Season	SEP–DEC In-Season
Corrective		X								
Stabilization	1	X								
Strength	2		X				X			
	3			X						
	4				X		X			
Power	5					X	X			
	6									

SAMPLE OFF-SEASON WEEKLY OPT FOOTBALL SCHEDULE

Month 1: 3 days/week

	MON	TUE	WED	THU	FRI	SAT	SUN
OPT Phase	Corrective	OFF	Stabilization Endurance	OFF	Corrective	OFF	OFF

Month 2: 3 days/week

	MON	TUE	WED	THU	FRI	SAT	SUN
OPT Phase	Strength Endurance Back, biceps, legs	OFF	Strength Endurance Chest, shoulders, triceps	OFF	Strength Endurance Total body	OFF	OFF

Month 3: 4 days/week

	MON	TUE	WED	THU	FRI	SAT	SUN
OPT Phase	Muscular Development Chest, shoulders, triceps	Muscular Development Back, biceps, legs	OFF	Muscular Development Chest, shoulders, triceps	Muscular Development Back, biceps, legs	OFF	OFF
Other	Conditioning				Conditioning		

Month 4: 5 days/week

	MON	TUE	WED	THU	FRI	SAT	SUN
OPT Phase	Maximal Strength Chest	Maximal Strength Legs	Maximal Strength Back	Maximal Strength Shoulders	Maximal Strength Total body, arms	OFF	OFF
Other	Conditioning		Conditioning		Conditioning		

Month 5: 4 days/week

	MON	TUE	WED	THU	FRI	SAT	SUN
OPT Phase	Power	Power	OFF	Power	Power	OFF	OFF
Other	Conditioning	Conditioning		Conditioning	Conditioning		

Month 6: 5 days/week

	MON	TUE	WED	THU	FRI	SAT	SUN
OPT Phase	Maximal Strength	OFF	Strength Endurance	OFF	Power	OFF	OFF
Other		Conditioning		Conditioning			

SAMPLE OFF-SEASON OPT FOOTBALL PROGRAMS

Corrective Exercise Training

INHIBIT	Sets	Reps	Time
Myofascial Rolling			
IT band	1		30 sec
Adductor	1		30 sec
Tensor fascia latae	1		30 sec

LENGTHEN	Sets	Reps	Time
Gastrocnemius stretch	1		30 sec
Supine biceps femoris stretch	1		30 sec
Kneeling hip flexor stretch	1		30 sec
Floor lat stretch	1		30 sec

ACTIVATE		Sets	Reps	Tempo	Intensity	Rest
Single-leg calf raise		3	10	4/2/1		0 sec
Side-lying hip abduction		3	10	4/2/1		0 sec
SL bent-over cobra		3	10	4/2/1		60 sec

INTEGRATE		Sets	Reps	Tempo	Intensity	Rest
Total body	Cable squat to row	3	10	4/2/1	60%	60 sec

PHASE 1: STABILIZATION ENDURANCE TRAINING

WARM-UP		Sets	Reps	Time
Myofascial Rolling				
Tensor fascia latae		1		30 sec
IT band		1		30 sec
Piriformis		1		30 sec
Static Stretching				
Gastrocnemius stretch		1		30 sec
Kneeling hip flexor stretch		1		30 sec
Standing adductor stretch		1		30 sec
Floor lat stretch		1		30 sec

Dynamic Stretching	Sets	Reps	Tempo	Rest
Lunge with rotation	1	10	Moderate	0 sec

CORE AND BALANCE	Sets	Reps	Tempo	Rest
Side iso-ab	3	12	4/2/1	0 sec
Suspension bridge	3	12	4/2/1	0 sec
Single-leg balance reach	3	12	4/2/1	60 sec

PLYOMETRICS	Sets	Reps	Tempo	Rest
Box jump-down with stabilization	3	10	Hold landing	60 sec

SPEED/AGILITY/QUICKNESS	Sets	Reps	Tempo	Rest
Speed ladder: Six exercises	2			60 sec

RESISTANCE		Sets	Reps	Tempo	Intensity	Rest
Total body	Single-leg squat touchdown to overhead press	3	15	4/2/1	65%	0 sec
Chest	Suspension chest press	3	15	4/2/1	65%	0 sec
Back	Suspension row	3	15	4/2/1	65%	0 sec

RESISTANCE		Sets	Reps	Tempo	Intensity	Rest
Shoulders	Single-leg PNF	3	15	4/2/1	65%	0 sec
Legs	Lunge to balance: Frontal plane	3	12	4/2/1	65%	90 sec

COOL-DOWN
Myofascial rolling and static stretching

PHASE 2: STRENGTH ENDURANCE TRAINING (BACK, BICEPS, LEGS)

WARM-UP		Sets	Reps	Time
Myofascial Rolling				
IT band		1		30 sec
Piriformis		1		30 sec
Lats		1		30 sec
Active Stretching				
Standing adductor stretch		1	10	
Standing hip flexor stretch		1	10	
Supine biceps femoris stretch		1	10	

Dynamic Stretching	Sets	Reps	Tempo	Rest
Squat to overhead reach	1	10	Moderately fast	0 sec

CORE AND BALANCE	Sets	Reps	Tempo	Rest
Reverse crunches	2	10	1/1/1	0 sec
Back extension	2	10	1/1/1	0 sec
Single-leg Romanian deadlift	2	10	1/1/1	60 sec

PLYOMETRICS	Sets	Reps	Tempo	Rest
Repeat box jumps	2	10	Repeating	0 sec
Tuck jumps	2	10	Repeating	60 sec

(continues)

(continued)

SPEED/AGILITY/QUICKNESS		Sets	Reps	Tempo		Rest
Speed ladder: Six exercises		3				60 sec

RESISTANCE		Sets	Reps	Tempo	Intensity	Rest
Total body	Optional					
Back	Pull-ups	3	8	2/0/2	80%	0 sec
	SL bent-over cable row		12	4/2/1	50%	
Biceps	Barbell curls	3	8	2/0/2	80%	0 sec
	Single-leg DB curl		12	4/2/1	50%	
Legs	Barbell squats	3	8	2/0/2	80%	60 sec
	Side lunge to balance		12	4/2/1	50%	

COOL-DOWN
Myofascial rolling and static stretching

PHASE 2: STRENGTH ENDURANCE TRAINING (CHEST, SHOULDERS, TRICEPS)

WARM-UP	Sets	Reps	Time
Myofascial Rolling			
IT band	1		30 sec
Piriformis	1		30 sec
Lats	1		30 sec
Active Stretching			
Standing adductor stretch	1	10	
Standing hip flexor stretch	1	10	
Supine biceps femoris stretch	1	10	

Dynamic Stretching	Sets	Reps	Tempo	Rest
Forward lunge with scaption (no weight)	1	10	Moderately fast	0 sec

CORE AND BALANCE	Sets	Reps	Tempo	Rest
Knee-ups	2	10	1/1/1	0 sec
Cable lifts	2	10	1/1/1	0 sec
Step-up to balance: Frontal plane	2	10	1/1/1	60 sec
PLYOMETRICS	Sets	Reps	Tempo	Rest
Butt kickers	2	10	Repeating	0 sec
Tuck jumps	2	10	Repeating	60 sec
SPEED/AGILITY/QUICKNESS	Sets	Reps	Tempo	Rest
Speed ladder: Six exercises	3			60 sec

RESISTANCE		Sets	Reps	Tempo	Intensity	Rest
Chest	Bench press	3	8	2/0/2	80%	0 sec
	Stability ball push-ups		12	4/2/1	50%	
Shoulders	Seated military press	3	8	2/0/2	80%	0 sec
	Single-leg suspension Y's		12	4/2/1	50%	
Triceps	Triceps push-downs	3	8	2/0/2	80%	60 sec
	Single-leg suspension triceps extensions		12	4/2/1	50%	

COOL-DOWN
Myofascial rolling and static stretching

PHASE 3: MUSCULAR DEVELOPMENT TRAINING (CHEST, SHOULDERS, TRICEPS)

WARM-UP	Sets	Reps	Time
Myofascial Rolling			
Quadriceps/hip flexors	1		30 sec
Pecs	1		30 sec
Lats	1		30 sec

(continues)

(continued)

WARM-UP		Sets	Reps	Time
Active Stretching				
Gastrocnemius stretch		1	10	
Kneeling hip flexor stretch		1	10	
Ball lat stretch		1	10	
Standing pec stretch		1	10	

Dynamic Stretching	Sets	Reps	Tempo	Rest
MB woodchop throw	1	10	Moderately fast	0 sec
Reverse lunge to scaption (no weight)	1	10	Moderately fast	0 sec

CORE AND BALANCE	Sets	Reps	Tempo	Rest
Crunch with rotation	2	12	1/1/1	0 sec
Russian twists	2	12	1/1/1	0 sec
Lunge to balance: Sagittal plane	2	12	1/1/1	60 sec

PLYOMETRICS	Sets	Reps	Tempo	Rest
Power step-ups	2	10	Repeating	0 sec
Tuck jump	2	10	Repeating	60 sec

SPEED/AGILITY/QUICKNESS	Sets	Reps	Tempo	Rest
Speed ladder: Six exercises	3			60 sec

RESISTANCE		Sets	Reps	Tempo	Intensity	Rest
Chest	DB bench press	3	8	2/0/2	80%	1 min
Chest	Incline bench press	3	8	2/0/2	80%	1 min
Shoulders	Seated overhead barbell press	3	8	2/0/2	80%	1 min
Shoulders	Seated lateral raise	3	8	2/0/2	80%	1 min
Triceps	Triceps press-down	3	8	2/0/2	80%	1 min
Triceps	Triceps extension machine	3	8	2/0/2	80%	1 min

COOL-DOWN
Myofascial rolling and static stretching

PHASE 3: MUSCULAR DEVELOPMENT TRAINING (BACK, BICEPS, LEGS)

WARM-UP		Sets	Reps	Time
Myofascial Rolling				
IT band		1		30 sec
Piriformis		1		30 sec
Adductors		1		30 sec
Thoracic spine		1		30 sec
Active Stretching				
Gastrocnemius stretch		1	10	
Kneeling hip flexor stretch		1	10	
Standing adductor stretch		1	10	
Quadruped thoracic rotation		1	10	

Dynamic Stretching	Sets	Reps	Tempo	Rest
Forward lunge with rotation	1	10	Moderately fast	0 sec
Push-up to rotation	1	10	Moderately fast	0 sec

CORE AND BALANCE	Sets	Reps	Tempo	Rest
Cable chop	2	12	1/1/1	0 sec
Knee-ups with rotation	2	12	1/1/1	0 sec
Lunge to balance: Frontal plane	2	12	1/1/1	60 sec

PLYOMETRICS	Sets	Reps	Tempo	Rest
Lunge jumps	2	10	Repeating	0 sec
Power step-ups	2	10	Repeating	60 sec

SPEED/AGILITY/QUICKNESS	Sets	Reps	Tempo	Rest
No SAQ on this day				

(continues)

(continued)

RESISTANCE		Sets	Reps	Tempo	Intensity	Rest
Back	Seated lat pull-down	3	8	2/0/2	80%	1 min
Back	Seated cable row	3	8	2/0/2	80%	1 min
Biceps	Barbell curl	3	8	2/0/2	80%	1 min
Biceps	Seated DB curl	3	8	2/0/2	80%	1 min
Legs	Leg press	3	8	2/0/2	80%	1 min
Legs	Barbell Romanian deadlifts	3	8	2/0/2	80%	1 min
COOL-DOWN						
Myofascial rolling and static stretching						

PHASE 4: MAXIMAL STRENGTH TRAINING (TOTAL BODY)

WARM-UP	Sets	Reps	Time
Myofascial Rolling			
IT band	1		30 sec
Piriformis	1		30 sec
Calf	1		30 sec
Pecs	1		30 sec
Active Stretching			
Standing adductor stretch	1	10	
Standing hip flexor	1	10	
Floor lat stretch	1	10	
Standing pec stretch	1	10	

Dynamic Stretching	Sets	Reps	Tempo	Rest
Reverse lunge with overhead reach (spinal extension)	1	10	Moderately fast	0 sec
MB rotation chest throw	1	10	Moderately fast	0 sec
SL bent-over combo II	1	10	Moderately fast	0 sec

CORE AND BALANCE	Sets	Reps	Tempo	Rest
Cable rotations	2	12	1/1/1	0 sec
Cable lift and chop	2	12	1/1/1	0 sec
Lunge to balance: Transverse plane	2	12	1/1/1	60 sec

PLYOMETRICS	Sets	Reps	Tempo	Rest
No PLYOMETRICS on this day				

SPEED/AGILITY/QUICKNESS	Sets	Reps	Tempo	Rest
No SAQ on this day				

RESISTANCE		Sets	Reps	Tempo	Intensity	Rest
Chest	Bench press	4	5	1/0/1	85%	3 min
Back	Seated lat pull-down	4	5	1/0/1	85%	3 min
Shoulders	Seated overhead DB press	4	5	1/0/1	85%	3 min
Legs	Barbell squats	4	5	1/0/1	85%	3 min

COOL-DOWN
Myofascial rolling and static stretching

PHASE 5: POWER TRAINING

WARM-UP	Sets	Reps	Time
Myofascial Rolling			
Tensor fascia latae	1		30 sec
Piriformis	1		30 sec
Thoracic spine	1		30 sec
Lats	1		30 sec

(*continues*)

(continued)

WARM-UP		Sets	Reps	Time
Dynamic Warm-up (Some athletes may still require static stretching prior to dynamic warm-up.)				
Prisoner squats		1	10	0 sec
Multiplanar lunges		1	10	0 sec
Single-leg squat touchdown		1	10	0 sec
Push-up with rotation		1	10	0 sec
Leg swings: Front to back		1	10	0 sec
MB lift chop		1	10	0 sec
MB rotations		1	10	60 sec

CORE AND BALANCE	Sets	Reps	Tempo	Rest
No CORE AND BALANCE (incorporated into dynamic warm-up)				

PLYOMETRICS	Sets	Reps	Tempo	Rest
No PLYOMETRICS (incorporated into dynamic warm-up)				

SPEED/AGILITY/QUICKNESS	Sets	Reps	Tempo	Rest
Speed ladder: Six exercises	2			60 sec
Box drill	4			30 sec
T-drill	4			30 sec

RESISTANCE		Sets	Reps	Tempo	Intensity	Rest
Total body	Deadlift shrug to calf raise	4	5	1/0/1	85%	0 sec
	DB snatch		8	Explosive	4% of BW	2 min
Chest	Bench press	4	5	1/0/1	85%	0 sec
	Rotational chest press		8	Explosive	4% of BW	2 min
Shoulders	Incorporated in total-body exercises					
Legs	Barbell squats	4	5	1/0/1	85%	0 sec
	Squat jumps		8	Explosive		3 min

COOL-DOWN
Myofascial rolling and static stretching

PRE-SEASON GOALS AND CONSIDERATIONS FOR FOOTBALL

Goals	Considerations

• Correcting impaired movement patterns based on results of pre-season assessments
 • Maintaining:
  • Physical health (decreases the chance of injury for participation in practice and games and optimal performance within such activities)
  • Range of motion, joint stability, and muscle strength and endurance
  • Cardiorespiratory endurance (aerobic/anaerobic)
  • Total-body stabilization, strength, and power
	• A systematic pre-season plan that transitions the athlete from performance enhancement to injury prevention and maintenance of off-season gains will be developed. This transition should be implemented with the consideration that the athlete's sport participation level is increasing dramatically from what they have become used to in the off-season.
	 • Proper recovery and conditioning during this time of increased activity will be applied.
	 • Exercise volume of injury prevention and performance training based on the athlete's increased activity level will be considered.

SAMPLE PRE-SEASON OPT FOOTBALL PLAN (JULY–AUGUST)

Level	Phase	JAN-JUN Off-Season	JUL Pre-Season (1)	AUG Pre-Season (2)	SEP In-Season	OCT In-Season	NOV In-Season	DEC In-Season
Corrective			X	X				
Stabilization	1		X	X				
Strength	2		X	X				
	3		X	X				
	4							
Power	5							
	6							

SAMPLE PRE-SEASON WEEKLY OPT FOOTBALL SCHEDULE

Months 1 and 2

	MON	TUE	WED	THU	FRI	SAT	SUN
OPT Phase	Corrective	Strength Endurance Shoulders, legs	Muscular Development Chest, back	Corrective		Muscular Development Shoulders, legs	Strength Endurance Chest, back
Other		Game			Game		

SAMPLE PRE-SEASON OPT FOOTBALL PROGRAMS

Corrective Exercise Training

INHIBIT	Sets	Reps	Time
Myofascial Rolling			
Piriformis	1		30 sec
Tensor fascia latae	1		30 sec
Lats	1		30 sec

LENGTHEN	Sets	Reps	Time
Gastrocnemius stretch	1		30 sec
Floor lat stretch	1		30 sec
Standing psoas stretch	1		30 sec
Erector spinae stretch	1		30 sec

ACTIVATE		Sets	Reps	Tempo	Intensity	Rest
Prone iso-ab		2	12	4/2/1		0 sec
Suspension bridge		2	12	4/2/1		60 sec

INTEGRATE		Sets	Reps	Tempo	Intensity	Rest
Total body	Cable squat to row	2	12	4/2/1	60%	60 sec

PHASE 1: STABILIZATION ENDURANCE TRAINING

WARM-UP	Sets	Reps	Time
Myofascial Rolling			
Tensor fascia latae	1		30 sec
IT band	1		30 sec
Piriformis	1		30 sec
Lat/pecs	1		30 sec

WARM-UP		Sets	Reps		Time
Static Stretching					
Gastrocnemius stretch		1			30 sec
Kneeling hip flexor stretch		1			30 sec
Standing adductor stretch		1			30 sec
Floor lat stretch		1			30 sec
Dynamic Stretching		Sets	Reps	Tempo	Rest
Lunge with rotation		1	10	Moderate	0 sec
CORE AND BALANCE		Sets	Reps	Temp	Rest
Side iso-ab w/hip abduction		2	12	4/2/1	0 sec
SL bent-over DB cable		2	12	4/2/1	0 sec
Single-leg lift and chop		2	12	4/2/1	60 sec

PLYOMETRICS	Sets	Reps	Tempo	Rest
No PLYOMETRICS due to increased on-field activity				

SPEED/AGILITY/QUICKNESS	Sets	Reps	Distance	Rest
No SAQ because of on-field conditioning				

RESISTANCE		Sets	Reps	Tempo	Intensity	Rest
Total body	Optional					
Chest	Suspension push-up: Feet in straps	2	15	4/2/1	65%	0 sec
Back	Single-leg lat pull-down	2	15	4/2/1	65%	0 sec
Shoulders	Single-leg overhead DB press	2	15	4/2/1	65%	0 sec
Legs	Lunge to balance: Transverse plane	2	12 ea.	4/2/1	65%	90 sec

COOL-DOWN
Myofascial rolling and static stretching

PHASE 2: STRENGTH ENDURANCE TRAINING (CHEST, BACK)

WARM-UP		Sets	Reps		Time
Myofascial Rolling					
IT band		1			30 sec
Tensor fascia latae		1			30 sec
Pecs		1			30 sec
Thoracic spine		1			30 sec
Active Stretching					
Gastrocnemius stretch		1	10		
Kneeling hip flexor stretch		1	10		
Supine biceps femoris stretch		1	10		
Standing pec stretch		1	10		

Dynamic Stretching	Sets	Reps	Tempo	Rest
Bent-over scaption (bodyweight)	1	10	Moderately fast	0
Modified push-up with rotation	1	10	Moderately fast	0

CORE AND BALANCE	Sets	Reps	Tempo	Rest
Cable rotations	2	10	1/1/1	0 sec
Cable lift	2	10	1/1/1	0 sec
Step-up to balance: Frontal plane	2	10	1/1/1	60 sec

PLYOMETRICS	Sets	Reps	Tempo	Rest
No PLYOMETRICS because of increased on-field activity				

SPEED/AGILITY/QUICKNESS	Sets	Reps	Distance	Rest
No SAQ because of on-field conditioning				

RESISTANCE		Sets	Reps	Tempo	Intensity	Rest
Chest	Bench press	2	12	2/0/2	70%	0 sec
	Stability ball push-ups		8	4/2/1		

RESISTANCE		Sets	Reps	Tempo	Intensity	Rest
Back	Seated cable row	2	12	2/0/2	70%	0 sec
	SL bent-over DB cobra		8	4/2/1		
Chest	Incline bench press	2	12	2/0/2	70%	0 sec
	Cable chest press		8	4/2/1		
Back	Seated lat pull-down	2	12	2/0/2	70%	60 sec
	SL cable row		8	4/2/1		

COOL-DOWN						
Myofascial rolling and static stretching						

PHASE 2: STRENGTH ENDURANCE TRAINING (SHOULDERS, LEGS)

WARM-UP	Sets	Reps	Time
Myofascial Rolling			
Tensor fascia latae	1		30 sec
Piriformis	1		30 sec
Lats	1		30 sec
Active Stretching			
Gastrocnemius stretch	1	10	
Kneeling hip flexor stretch	1	10	
Supine biceps femoris stretch	1	10	
Standing pec stretch	1	10	

Dynamic Stretching	Sets	Reps	Tempo	Rest
Bent-over scaption (bodyweight)	1	10	Moderately fast	0
Modified push-up with rotation	1	10	Moderately fast	0

(*continues*)

(continued)

CORE AND BALANCE	Sets	Reps	Tempo	Rest
Knee-ups	2	10	1/1/1	0 sec
Back extension with rotation	2	10	1/1/1	0 sec
Single-leg Romanian deadlift	2	10	1/1/1	60 sec

PLYOMETRICS	Sets	Reps	Tempo	Rest
No PLYOMETRICS because of increased on-field activity				

SPEED/AGILITY/QUICKNESS	Sets	Reps	Distance	Rest
No SAQ because of on-field conditioning				

RESISTANCE		Sets	Reps	Tempo	Intensity	Rest
Shoulders	Shoulder press machine	2	12	2/0/2	70%	0 sec
	Suspension Y's		8	4/2/1		
Legs	Barbell squats	2	12	2/0/2	70%	0 sec
	SL squat		8	4/2/1		
Shoulders	Seated lateral raise	2	12	2/0/2	70%	0 sec
	SL DB scaption		8	4/2/1		
Legs	Barbell deadlift	2	12	2/0/2	70%	60 sec
	Step-up to balance		8	4/2/1		

COOL-DOWN	
Myofascial rolling and static stretching	

PHASE 3: MUSCULAR DEVELOPMENT TRAINING (CHEST, BACK)

WARM-UP	Sets	Reps	Time
Myofascial Rolling			
IT band	1		30 sec
Tensor fascia latae	1		30 sec
Thoracic spine	1		30 sec

WARM-UP		Sets	Reps	Time
Active Stretching				
Gastrocnemius stretch		1	10	
Kneeling hip flexor stretch		1	10	
Standing biceps femoris stretch		1	10	
Standing pec stretch		1	10	

Dynamic Stretching	Sets	Reps	Tempo	Rest
Bent-over combo I (bodyweight)	1	10	Moderately fast	0 sec
Push-up to rotation	1	10	Moderately fast	0 sec

CORE AND BALANCE	Sets	Reps	Tempo	Rest
Knee-ups	2	12	1/1/1	0 sec
Reverse hypers	2	12	1/1/1	0 sec
Single-leg squat	2	12	1/1/1	60 sec

PLYOMETRICS	Sets	Reps	Tempo	Rest
No PLYOMETRICS on this day				

SPEED/AGILITY/QUICKNESS	Sets	Reps	Tempo	Rest
No SAQ on this day				

RESISTANCE		Sets	Reps	Tempo	Intensity	Rest
Chest	Chest press machine	2	10	2/0/2	75%	0 min
Back	Lat pull-down	2	10	2/0/2	75%	1 min
Chest	Incline DB chest press	2	10	2/0/2	75%	0 min
Back	Seated cable row	2	10	2/0/2	75%	1 min
Chest	DB bench press	2	10	2/0/2	75%	0 min
Back	Pull-up	2	10	2/0/2	75%	1 min

COOL-DOWN
Myofascial rolling and static stretching

PHASE 3: MUSCULAR DEVELOPMENT TRAINING (SHOULDERS, LEGS)

WARM-UP		Sets	Reps		Time
Myofascial Rolling					
IT band		1			30 sec
Tensor fascia latae		1			30 sec
Thoracic spine		1			30 sec
Active Stretching					
Gastrocnemius stretch		1	10		
Kneeling hip flexor stretch		1	10		
Supine biceps femoris stretch		1	10		
Standing pec stretch		1	10		

Dynamic Stretching		Sets	Reps	Tempo	Rest
Bent-over combo II (bodyweight)		1	10	Moderately fast	0 sec
Reverse lunge with overhead reach		1	10	Moderately fast	0 sec

CORE AND BALANCE		Sets	Reps	Tempo	Rest
Back extension		2	12	1/1/1	0 sec
Reverse crunch		2	12	1/1/1	0 sec
Single-leg squat touchdown		2	12	1/1/1	90 sec

PLYOMETRICS		Sets	Reps	Tempo	Rest
No PLYOMETRICS on this day					

SPEED/AGILITY/QUICKNESS		Sets	Reps	Tempo	Rest
No SAQ on this day					

RESISTANCE		Sets	Reps	Tempo	Intensity	Rest
Shoulders	Shoulder press machine	2	10	2/0/2	75%	0 min
Legs	Lunge: Frontal plane	2	10	2/0/2	75%	1 min
Shoulders	Seated lateral raise	2	10	2/0/2	75%	0 min
Legs	Barbell squat	2	10	2/0/2	75%	1 min

RESISTANCE		Sets	Reps	Tempo	Intensity	Rest
Shoulders	Seated overhead barbell press	2	10	2/0/2	75%	0 min
Legs	Barbell Romanian deadlift	2	10	2/0/2	75%	1 min
COOL-DOWN						
Myofascial rolling and static stretching						

IN-SEASON GOALS AND CONSIDERATIONS FOR FOOTBALL

Goals	Considerations
• Maintaining: • Range of motion, joint stability, and muscle strength and endurance • Cardiorespiratory endurance (aerobic/anaerobic) • Total-body stabilization, strength, and power • Establishing with the athlete a communication process for monitoring in-season maintenance, and a plan that works based on what the athlete needs, wants, and will have the capability to do focusing on their job playing football	• Assessments and testing, to ensure program considerations are being made to prevent overuse injuries and maintain performance levels, will be performed. • Impaired movement patterns with exercise strategies being implemented will be attended to. • Additional conditioning, for athletes who may not get the same type of on-field practice or game minutes as others, will be considered. • A systematic in-season maintenance plan will be developed that allows the athlete to minimize decreases in performance and chance of injury over a long season with repetitive sport movement patterns and physical contact. • The exercise volume of injury prevention, and performance training based on the athlete's increased travel and activity level, will be considered.

IN-SEASON OPT FOOTBALL PLAN (SEPTEMBER–DECEMBER)

Level	Phase	JAN–JUN Off-Season	JULY Pre-Season	AUG Pre-Season	SEP In-Season (1)	OCT In-Season (2)	NOV In-Season (3)	DEC In-Season (4)
Corrective					X	X	X	X
Stabilization	1				X	X	X	X
Strength	2				X	X	X	X
	3							
	4							
Power	5							
	6							

SAMPLE IN-SEASON WEEKLY OPT FOOTBALL SCHEDULE

Any Month

	MON	TUE	WED	THU	FRI	SAT	SUN
OPT Phase	Rest	Stabilization Endurance	Corrective	Strength Endurance	Corrective	Stabilization Endurance	Corrective
Other	Game						

SAMPLE IN-SEASON OPT FOOTBALL PROGRAM

Corrective Exercise Training

INHIBIT	Sets	Reps	Time
Myofascial Rolling			
Calves	1		30 sec
IT band	1		30 sec
Tensor fascia latae	1		30 sec

LENGTHEN	Sets	Reps	Time
Gastrocnemius stretch	1		30 sec
Soleus stretch	1		30 sec
Supine biceps femoris stretch	1		30 sec

ACTIVATE		Sets	Reps	Tempo	Intensity	Rest
Floor bridge		2	12	4/2/1		0 sec
Single-leg calf raise		2	12	4/2/1		0 sec
INTEGRATE		Sets	Reps	Tempo	Intensity	Rest
Total body	Step-up, balance to overhead press	2	12	4/2/1	60%	60 sec

PHASE 1: STABILIZATION ENDURANCE TRAINING

WARM-UP		Sets	Reps	Time
Myofascial Rolling				
Tensor fascia latae		1		30 sec
IT band		1		30 sec
Piriformis		1		30 sec
Static Stretching				
Gastrocnemius stretch		1		30 sec
Kneeling hip flexor stretch		1		30 sec
Standing adductor stretch		1		30 sec
Floor lat stretch		1		30 sec

Dynamic Stretching	Sets	Reps	Tempo	Rest
Lunge with rotation	1	10	Moderate	0

CORE AND BALANCE	Sets	Reps	Tempo	Rest
Side iso-abs w/hip abduction	2	12	4/2/1	0 sec
SL bent-over cobra	2	12	4/2/1	0 sec
Single-leg lift and chop	2	12	4/2/1	60 sec

PLYOMETRICS, SPEED/AGILITY/QUICKNESS	Sets	Reps	Tempo	Rest
No PLYOMETRICS or SAQ due to increased on-field activity				

RESISTANCE		Sets	Reps	Tempo	Intensity	Rest
Total body	Optional					
Chest	Standing cable chest press	2	15	4/2/1	65%	0 sec
Back	Single-leg straight-arm pull-down	2	15	4/2/1	65%	0 sec
Shoulders	Suspension SL Y's	2	15	4/2/1	65%	0 sec
Legs	Lunge to balance: Sagittal plane	2	15	4/2/1	65%	90 sec

COOL-DOWN
Myofascial rolling and static stretching

PHASE 2: STRENGTH ENDURANCE TRAINING

WARM-UP		Sets	Reps	Time
Myofascial Rolling				
IT band		1		30 sec
Tensor fascia latae		1		30 sec
Lat/pec		1		30 sec
Active Stretching				
Gastrocnemius stretch		1	10	
Kneeling hip flexor stretch		1	10	
Supine biceps femoris stretch		1	10	
Standing pec stretch		1	10	

Dynamic Stretching	Sets	Reps	Tempo	Rest
Multiplanar lunge with reach	1	10	Moderately fast	0
Squat to overhead reach	1	10	Moderately fast	0

CORE AND BALANCE	Sets	Reps	Tempo	Rest
Long lever crunch	2	10	1/1/1	0 sec
Cable lift	2	10	1/1/1	0 sec
Step-up to balance: Frontal plane	2	10	1/1/1	60 sec

PLYOMETRICS	Sets	Reps	Tempo	Rest
No PLYOMETRICS because of increased on-field activity				

SPEED/AGILITY/QUICKNESS	Sets	Reps	Distance	Rest
No SAQ because of on-field drills and conditioning				

RESISTANCE		Sets	Reps	Tempo	Intensity	Rest
Total body	Optional					
Chest	DB bench press	3	12	2/0/2	70%	0 sec
	Push-up		8	4/2/1	70%	

RESISTANCE		Sets	Reps	Tempo	Intensity	Rest
Back	Seated lat pull-down	3	12	2/0/2	70%	0 sec
	Standing SA cable row		8	4/2/1	70%	
Shoulders	Shoulder press machine	3	12	2/0/2	70%	0 sec
	SL overhead DB press with SA		8	4/2/1	70%	
Legs	Leg press	3	12	2/0/2	70%	60 sec
	Lunge to balance		8	4/2/1	70%	

COOL-DOWN
Myofascial rolling and static stretching

GOLF

Note: Research has shown that golf-specific exercise programs improve strength, flexibility, and balance in golfers. Improvements in these areas result in increased upper-torso axial rotational velocity, which results in increased club-head speed, ball velocity, and driving distance (Lephart et al., 2007).

Better golfers possess unique physical characteristics that are important for greater proficiency. These characteristics have also been demonstrated to be modifiable through golf-specific training programs (Sell et al., 2007).

Implementing a progressive functional training program including flexibility, core, balance, and integrated resistance exercises has been shown to provide significant improvements in club-head speed and several components of functional fitness (Thompson et al., 2007). Golf may not look as physically demanding as other sports; however, the entire movement system must be functioning and trained to perform at the highest levels. Correcting muscle imbalances, increasing flexibility, and improving functional performance have been shown to improve a golfer's on-course results. The Sports Performance Coach should consider a progressive and systematic program for golfers looking to prevent overuse injury and improve play.

All programs should be designed based on an assessment that identifies the needs of the athlete, then strategically applies the assessment results to the training plan. The nature of golf, probably more than any other sport, is defined by one repetitive movement (i.e., the golf swing) and requires a blend of mobility and stability to properly execute the skill of the golf swing.

In many places, golf is a year-round activity and is not defined by a season (in-season/ off-season). Considering that many athletes play or practice year-round, and there is not a truly defined season for most, golf programming strategies will follow an undulating programming model. Because golf requires a unique blend of stabilization, strength, and power, an undulating model can address these needs within a shorter period. The Sports Performance Coach must understand the functional movement of the golf swing; however, any golf-specific instruction should be left to a trained golf-teaching professional.

- Golf is played by a wide range of age groups.
- Physical demands, regardless of age, are typically the same for each individual.
- This sport consists of repetitive movement patterns in the transverse plane.
- Golf can cause chronic musculoskeletal problems from repetitive movement patterns (Gosheger et al., 2003).
- Cardiorespiratory conditioning may not seem as important as in other sports; however, the average golfer walks between 4 and 5 miles per round, and endurance can become a factor in a golfer's performance.
- A proper golf-specific warm-up prior to play and practice has shown a significant increase in golfers' performance compared with not performing a warm-up (Fradkin et al., 2007). The Sports Performance Coach should consider designing a proper warm-up for a golfer beyond their strength and conditioning program. A proper warm-up that includes dynamic stretching has also been shown to reduce golf injuries and improve performance (Ehlert & Wilson, 2019).
- Golf requires a unique combination of stabilization, strength, and power throughout the entire human movement system and specifically in the spine, hips, and shoulders.
- Muscular imbalances throughout the human movement system, described as overactive muscles (tightness) and underactive muscles (weakness), can cause faulty movement patterns and can limit the golfer's ability to swing effectively.
- Flexibility has been shown to be the most important variable regarding performance and injury through clinical trials.

SUGGESTED ASSESSMENTS FOR GOLF

Assessment Type	Assessment Method
Transitional assessments	- Overhead squat - Single-leg squat - Split squat - Star excursion balance test
Mobility assessments (if needed)	- Foot and ankle testing - Lumbo-pelvic-hip complex testing - Shoulder and spine testing
Dynamic movement assessments	- Drop jump assessment - Shark skill test - Davies test
Aerobic test (choose one of the following)	- 12-minute run test - 1.5-mile run test - Beep test
Muscular endurance assessments	- Push-up test - Pull-up test - Curl-up test
Muscular strength assessments	- 1–5 RM bench press - 1–5 RM squat
Power assessments	- Rotational medicine ball throw test (left and right) - Power clean assessment

ANNUAL OPT GOLF PLAN (JANUARY–DECEMBER)

Level	Phase	JAN	FEB	MAR	APR	MAY	JUN	JUL	AUG	SEP	OCT	NOV	DEC
Corrective		X	X	X	X	X	X	X	X	X	X	X	X
Stabilization	1	X	X	X	X	X	X	X	X	X	X	X	X
Strength	2	X	X	X	X	X	X	X	X	X	X	X	X
	3												
	4												
Power	5	X	X	X	X	X	X	X	X	X	X	X	X
	6												

SAMPLE MONTHLY OPT GOLF SCHEDULE

Month 1

Week 1: 2 days/week

	MON	TUE	WED	THU	FRI	SAT	SUN
OPT Phase	Corrective	OFF	OFF	Stabilization Endurance	OFF	Warm-up	OFF
Other	Play						

Week 2: 3 days/week

	MON	TUE	WED	THU	FRI	SAT	SUN
OPT Phase	Strength Endurance	OFF	Corrective	Stabilization Endurance	OFF	Warm-up	OFF
Practice	Play						

Week 3: 2 days/week

	MON	TUE	WED	THU	FRI	SAT	SUN
OPT Phase	OFF	Corrective	OFF	Power	OFF	Warm-up	Warm-up
Other						Play	Play

Week 4: 3 days/week

	MON	TUE	WED	THU	FRI	SAT	SUN
OPT Phase	Strength Endurance	OFF	Stabilization	OFF	Warm-up	OFF	Corrective
Other	Play						

CORRECTIVE EXERCISE GOALS AND CONSIDERATIONS FOR GOLF

Goals	Considerations
• Correct impaired movement patterns and muscle imbalances based on movement assessment results • Improve: • Range of motion, joint stability, and muscle strength and endurance • Total-body stabilization • Consistently implement and perform the corrective program, due to the repetitive nature of the golf swing • Incorporate balance training to improve sensorimotor and proprioceptive skills	• Proper warm-up will be created that incorporates the corrective exercise program. • Evaluation of the assessment results and the physical demands of the swing will lead to a further understanding of which muscles must have the proper amount of range of motion throughout the golf swing.

SAMPLE OPT GOLF PROGRAMS

Corrective Exercise Training

INHIBIT	Sets	Reps	Time
Myofascial Rolling			
Tensor fascia latae	1		30 sec
Piriformis	1		30 sec
Lats	1		30 sec
Thoracic spine	1		30 sec
LENGTHEN	**Sets**	**Reps**	**Time**
Gastrocnemius stretch	1		30 sec
Standing biceps femoris stretch	1		30 sec
Supine piriformis stretch	1		30 sec
Floor lat stretch	1		30 sec

ACTIVATE	Sets	Reps	Tempo	Intensity	Rest
Side-lying hip abduction	2	12	4/2/1		0 sec
Standing hip adduction	2	12	4/2/1		0 sec
Quadruped arm opposite-leg raise	2	12	4/2/1		90 sec

INTEGRATE		Sets	Reps	Tempo	Intensity	Rest
Total body	Cable squat to row: Single-arm	2	12	4/2/1	60%	90 sec

STRENGTH AND CONDITIONING GOALS AND CONSIDERATIONS FOR GOLF

Goals	Considerations
• Continually correct and maintain impaired movement patterns based on assessment results • Maintain: • Physical health (decreased chance of injury for participation in practice/games, and optimal performance within such activities) • Range of motion, joint stability, and muscle strength/endurance • Cardiorespiratory endurance (aerobic) • Total-body stabilization, strength, and power • Incorporate the power phase into the program to improve velocity and rate of force production	• A systematic plan that implements an undulating programming model, integrating corrective exercise, stabilization, strength, and power, will be developed. • Understanding that the golf swing contains elements of stability, strength, and power will be essential. • Total training volume, including sport-specific training, must be considered.

PHASE 1: STABILIZATION ENDURANCE TRAINING

WARM-UP	Sets	Reps	Time
Myofascial rolling			
Tensor fascia latae	1		30 sec
Piriformis	1		30 sec
Thoracic spine	1		30 sec
Static Stretch			
Gastrocnemius stretch	1		30 sec
Supine piriformis stretch	1		30 sec

(continues)

(continued)

WARM-UP		Sets	Reps		Time
Static Stretch					
Floor lat stretch		1			30 sec
Erector spinae stretch		1			30 sec

Dynamic Stretch		Sets	Reps	Tempo	Rest
Lunge with rotation		1	10	Moderate	0 sec
MB woodchop		1	10	Moderate	0 sec

CORE AND BALANCE		Sets	Reps	Tempo	Rest
Side-iso-ab		2	12	4/2/1	0 sec
Suspension bridge		2	12	4/2/1	0 sec
Single-leg balance reach		2	12	4/2/1	60 sec

PLYOMETRICS		Sets	Reps	Tempo	Rest
Box jump with stabilization		2	6	Hold landing	60 sec

RESISTANCE		Sets	Reps	Tempo	Intensity	Rest
Total body	Optional					
Chest	Suspension push-up: Feet in straps	2	15	4/2/1	60%	0 sec
Back	SL bent-over cobra	2	15	4/2/1	60%	0 sec
Shoulders	Single-leg cable lift: Single-arm	2	15	4/2/1	60%	0 sec
Legs	Lunge to balance: Frontal plane	2	15	4/2/1	60%	90 sec

COOL-DOWN
Myofascial rolling and static stretching

PHASE 2: STRENGTH ENDURANCE TRAINING

WARM-UP		Sets	Reps		Time
Myofascial Rolling					
IT band		1			30 sec
Piriformis		1			30 sec
Lats		1			30 sec
Active Stretch					
Standing adductor stretch		1			30 sec
Supine biceps femoris stretch		1			30 sec
Kneeling hip flexor stretch		1			30 sec
Standing pec stretch		1			30 sec

Dynamic Stretch	Sets	Reps	Tempo	Rest
Multiplanar lunge with reach	1	10	Moderately fast	0 sec
Squat to overhead reach	1	10	Moderately fast	0 sec

CORE AND BALANCE	Sets	Reps	Tempo	Rest
Crunch with rotation	2	12	1/1/1	0 sec
Cable lift	2	12	1/1/1	0 sec
Step-up to balance: Transverse plane	2	12	1/1/1	60 sec

PLYOMETRICS	Sets	Reps	Tempo	Rest
Power step-up	2	8	Repeating	60 sec

RESISTANCE		Sets	Reps	Tempo	Intensity	Rest
Total body	Optional					
Chest	Incline DB chest press	2	12	2/0/2	70%	0 sec
	Cable chest press		8	4/2/1		
Back	Seated lat pull-down	2	12	2/0/2	70%	0 sec
	Single-leg cable row		8	4/2/1		

(continues)

(continued)

RESISTANCE		Sets	Reps	Tempo	Intensity	Rest
Shoulders	Seated overhead DB press	2	12	2/0/2	70%	0 sec
	SL scaption		8	4/2/1		
Legs	DB squats	2	12	2/0/2	70%	60 sec
	Side lunge to balance		8	4/2/1		

COOL-DOWN
Myofascial rolling and static stretching

PHASE 5: POWER TRAINING

WARM-UP	Sets	Reps	Time
Myofascial Rolling			
Tensor fascia latae	1		30 sec
Piriformis	1		30 sec
Lats	1		30 sec
Dynamic Warm-up (Some athletes may still require static stretching prior to dynamic warm-up.)			
Lateral tube walking	1	10	0 sec
Lunge with rotation	1	10	0 sec
Russian twist	1	10	60 sec

CORE AND BALANCE	Sets	Reps	Tempo	Rest
Cable rotation	2	12	Fast	0 sec
Cable lift	2	12	Fast	0 sec
Multiplanar hop with stabilization	2	12	Controlled	60 sec

RESISTANCE		Sets	Reps	Tempo	Intensity	Rest
Total body	Optional					
Chest	Incline DB press	3	5	1/0/1	85%	0 sec
	Rotational chest pass		10	Explosive	2% of BW	2 min

RESISTANCE		Sets	Reps	Tempo	Intensity	Rest
Back	Seated cable row	3	5	1/0/1	85%	0 sec
	Woodchop throw		10	Explosive	2% of BW	2 min
Shoulders	Seated overhead DB press	3	5	1/0/1	85%	0 sec
	Oblique MB throw		10	Explosive	2% of BW	2 min
Legs	DB squat	3	5	1/0/1	85%	0 sec
	Squat jump		10	Explosive	BW	2 min

COOL-DOWN
Myofascial rolling and static stretching

PRE-PRACTICE/PLAY WARM-UP GOALS AND CONSIDERATIONS FOR GOLF

Goals	Considerations

• Ensure:
    • Warm-up is multiplanar; it increases tissue temperature and elasticity, and activates muscles specific to the golf swing
    • Warm-up transitions from exercises directly into hitting golf balls, and should be implemented as part of the pre-practice or pre-play routine for each session
	• Corrective exercise programming and dynamic warm-up activities for a proper warm-up will be integrated.

WARM-UP AT COURSE (PRE-PRACTICE/PRE-PLAY)

STATIC STRETCH	Sets	Reps	Time
Gastrocnemius stretch	1		30 sec
Floor lat stretch	1		30 sec
Standing biceps femoris stretch	1		30 sec
Standing pec stretch	1		30 sec
Standing hip flexor stretch	1		30 sec
Erector spinae stretch	1		30 sec

(continues)

(continued)

DYNAMIC WARM-UP			
MB rotations	1	12	0 sec
Lunge with rotation	1	12	0 sec
MB flexion/extension (use golf club instead of MB)	1	12	0 sec
Single-leg Romanian deadlift	1	12	60 sec

HOCKEY

Note: The Sports Performance Coach will focus on position players within hockey and not specifically on the goaltending position. In the case of a performance program with hockey players, position players and goalies will receive tremendous benefits by following the application guidelines and techniques presented subsequently. The goaltending position is unique within the sport; however, the same basic fundamentals should be considered when analyzing movement patterns, the demands of the sport/position, and enhancing performance.

If the Sports Performance Coach needs to modify the model based on the athlete's needs, then it is very appropriate to do so based on the assessment process, the position's needs, and the goals set for the athlete. The Sports Performance Coach will focus on "off-ice" performance training to decrease injury and increase "on-ice" performance.

Demands of the Sport	
General Information	**Specific Information (Bangsbo et al., 2006)**
<ul><li>Activity characterized by high-intensity intermittent skating and rapid changes in velocity and duration</li><li>Aerobic and anaerobic energy systems are important to cardiorespiratory conditioning.</li><li>Movement is primarily skating forward without the puck; however, movement is rarely linear for more than a couple of strides. This should not be confused with lateral motion; turns can range from gradual to sharp, and therefore loading of the legs is rarely equal.</li><li>Change of direction includes stopping, backward skating, and some lateral movement.</li></ul>	<ul><li>Duration of game: 60 minutes (3 × 20-minute periods)</li><li>Player on ice (shift): 15–20 minutes; defensemen typically play more minutes than forwards</li><li>Duration of each shift: 30–80 seconds</li><li>Average shift length: 39 seconds</li><li>Recovery between shifts: 3–4 minutes</li><li>Work-to-rest ratio of 1:2 to 1:3</li><li>Brief periods of accelerated sprints while on the ice: 4–7 seconds</li><li>Frequent body contact (player-to-player, player-to-boards), which adds additional stress to the body</li></ul>

SUGGESTED ASSESSMENTS FOR HOCKEY

Assessment Type	Assessment Method
Transitional postural assessments	• Overhead squat test • Single-leg squat test • Split squat • Star excursion balance test
Mobility assessments (if needed)	• Foot and ankle testing • Lumbo-pelvic-hip complex testing • Shoulder and spine testing
Dynamic movement assessments	• Drop jump • Shark skill test • Davies test • Triple crossover hop test
Aerobic test (choose one of the following)	• 12-minute run test • 1.5-mile run test • Beep test
Anaerobic test	• 300-yard shuttle run
Muscular endurance assessments	• Push-up test • Pull-up test • Curl-up test
Muscular strength assessments	• Grip strength • 1–5 RM bench press • 1–5 RM squat • 1–5 RM deadlift
Power assessments	• Vertical jump test (double-leg) • Vertical jump test (single-leg) • Rotational medicine ball throw test (left and right)
Speed assessments	• 40-yard sprint test
Agility assessments	• T-test • 5–10–5 (pro agility test)

Goals	Considerations
• Physical and mental reconditioning • Reconditioning from the physical contact and additional stress placed on the body • Correcting impaired movement patterns based on results of transitional postural assessments • Improving • Range of motion, joint stability, and muscle strength and endurance • Cardiorespiratory endurance (aerobic/anaerobic) • Total-body stabilization, strength, and power • Speed, agility, and quickness • Increasing lean body mass and size • Determine, through assessment, demands-of-sport analysis and athlete goals, which plan and program should be created to achieve both the needs and the goals	• Planning and programming will be based on assessment, client goals, and the demands of the sport. • A systematic off-season plan will incorporate integrated training, including: • Core training • Balance training • Power training • Speed, agility, and quickness training • Integrated resistance training • Cardiorespiratory training combined with a proper nutrition plan to maximize training and recovery • Opportunities for appropriate rest between workouts will be provided. • An off-season training schedule, which works backward from the commencement of the pre-season, will be developed to allow for maximum injury prevention and performance gains without the athlete overtraining. • Conditioning for hockey will be as similar to the game demands as possible. • Off-ice conditioning utilizing cardio machines and exercises incorporating ground-reaction forces will be considered when designing a conditioning program.

Note: Annual programming and periodization is based on elite-level hockey schedules. Lower-level and younger athletes may play shortened seasons and, therefore, will have a longer off-season. Off-season programming should be adjusted in this case to progress the athlete at the proper pace to reach the pre-season in optimal condition.

SAMPLE OFF-SEASON OPT HOCKEY PLAN (MAY–AUGUST)

Level	Phase	JAN–APR In-Season	MAY Off-Season (1)	JUN Off-Season (2)	JUL Off-Season (3)	AUG Off-Season (4)	SEP Pre-Season	OCT In-Season	NOV In-Season	DEC In-Season
Corrective			X							
Stabilization	1		X			X				
Strength	2			X	X	X				
	3									
	4			X						
Power	5				X	X				
	6									

SAMPLE OFF-SEASON WEEKLY OPT HOCKEY SCHEDULE

Month 1: 3 days/week

	MON	TUE	WED	THU	FRI	SAT	SUN
OPT Phase	Stabilization Endurance	OFF	Corrective	OFF	Stabilization Endurance	OFF	OFF

Month 2: 4 days/week

	MON	TUE	WED	THU	FRI	SAT	SUN
OPT Phase	Strength Endurance Upper body	Corrective	Maximal Strength Total body	OFF	Strength Endurance Lower body	OFF	OFF

Month 3: 5 days/week

	MON	TUE	WED	THU	FRI	SAT	SUN
OPT Phase	Power	Conditioning	Strength Endurance	Conditioning	Power	OFF	OFF

Month 4: 5 days/week

	MON	TUE	WED	THU	FRI	SAT	SUN
OPT Phase	Strength Endurance	OFF	Stabilization Endurance	OFF	Power	OFF	OFF
Other		Conditioning	Conditioning	Conditioning			

SAMPLE OFF-SEASON OPT HOCKEY PROGRAMS

Corrective Exercise Training

INHIBIT	Sets	Reps	Time
Myofascial Rolling			
IT band	1		30 sec
Adductor	1		30 sec
Tensor fascia latae	1		30 sec
LENGTHEN	**Sets**	**Reps**	**Time**
Gastrocnemius stretch	1		30 sec
Supine biceps femoris stretch	1		30 sec

(continues)

(continued)

LENGTHEN			Sets	Reps	Time
Standing adductor stretch			1		30 sec
Standing psoas stretch			1		30 sec

ACTIVATE	Sets	Reps	Tempo	Intensity	Rest
Single-leg hip abduction	3	10	4/2/1		0 sec
Single-leg hip adduction	3	10	4/2/1		0 sec
SL bent-over cobra	3	10	4/2/1		60 sec

INTEGRATE	Sets	Reps	Tempo	Intensity	Rest
Total-body turning step-up to an overhead press: Single-arm	3	10	4/2/1	60%	60 sec

PHASE 1: STABILIZATION ENDURANCE TRAINING

WARM-UP			Sets	Reps	Time
Myofascial Rolling					
Tensor fascia latae			1		30 sec
Adductors			1		30 sec
Static Stretching					
Gastrocnemius stretch			1		30 sec
Kneeling hip flexor stretch			1		30 sec
Standing biceps femoris stretch			1		30 sec

Dynamic Stretching	Sets	Reps	Tempo	Rest
Lunge with rotation	1	10	Moderate	0 sec
MB woodchop	1	10	Moderate	0 sec

CORE AND BALANCE	Sets	Reps	Tempo	Rest
Quadruped arm opposite-leg raise	3	12	4/2/1	0 sec
Floor cobra	3	12	4/2/1	0 sec
Single-leg lift and chop	3	12	4/2/1	60 sec

PLYOMETRICS	Sets	Reps	Tempo	Rest
Box jump-down with stabilization	3	8	Hold landing	60 sec

SPEED/AGILITY/QUICKNESS	Sets	Reps	Tempo	Rest
Speed ladder: Six exercises	2			60 sec

RESISTANCE		Sets	Reps	Tempo	Intensity	Rest
Total body	Optional					
Chest	Cable chest press: Alternate arm	3	12	4/2/1	70%	0 sec
Back	Suspension SL row	3	12	4/2/1	70%	0 sec
Shoulders	Single-leg overhead DB press: Single-arm	3	12	4/2/1	70%	0 sec
Legs	Single-leg squat	3	12	4/2/1	70%	90 sec

COOL-DOWN
Myofascial rolling and static stretching

PHASE 2: STRENGTH ENDURANCE TRAINING

WARM-UP	Sets	Reps	Time
Myofascial Rolling			
IT band	1		30 sec
Piriformis	1		30 sec
Tensor fascia latae	1		30 sec
Active Stretching			
Standing adductor stretch	1	10	
Standing hip flexor stretch	1	10	
Floor lat stretch	1	10	

Dynamic Stretching	Sets	Reps	Tempo	Rest
Multiplanar lunge with MB wood chop	1	10	Moderately fast	0 sec

(continues)

(continued)

CORE AND BALANCE	Sets	Reps	Tempo	Rest
Cable lift	2	10	1/1/1	0 sec
Back extension	2	10	1/1/1	0 sec
Single-leg squat	2	10	1/1/1	60 sec

PLYOMETRICS	Sets	Reps	Tempo	Rest
Repeat squat jumps	3	10	Repeating	0 sec
Repeat box jumps	3	10	Repeating	60 sec

SPEED/AGILITY/QUICKNESS	Sets	Reps	Tempo	Rest
Speed ladder: Six exercises	2			60 sec
LEFT test	3			45 sec

RESISTANCE		Sets	Reps	Tempo	Intensity	Rest
Total body	Optional					
Chest	Incline DB press	3	8	2/0/2	80%	0 sec
	Cable chest press		12	4/2/1	50%	
Back	Seated lat pull-down	3	8	2/0/2	80%	0 sec
	Single-leg cable row		12	4/2/1	50%	
Shoulders	Seated overhead DB press		8	2/0/2	80%	0 sec
	Bent-over DB combo II		12	4/2/1	50%	
Legs	Barbell squats	3	8	2/0/2	80%	60 sec
	Side lunge to balance		12	4/2/1	50%	

COOL-DOWN
Myofascial rolling and static stretching

PHASE 4: MAXIMAL STRENGTH TRAINING

WARM-UP		Sets	Reps	Time
Myofascial Rolling				
IT band		1		30 sec
Piriformis		1		30 sec
Lats/pecs		1		30 sec
Active Stretching				
Standing adductor stretch		1	10	
Standing hip flexor stretch		1	10	
Floor lat stretch		1	10	

Dynamic Stretching	Sets	Reps	Tempo	Rest
"World's Greatest Stretch"	1	10	Controlled	0 sec

CORE AND BALANCE	Sets	Reps	Tempo	Rest
Cable rotations	2	12	1/1/1	0 sec
Cable lifts	2	12	1/1/1	0 sec
Step-up to balance: Frontal plane	2	12	1/1/1	90 sec

PLYOMETRICS	Sets	Reps	Tempo	Rest
No PLYOMETRICS on this day				

SPEED/AGILITY/QUICKNESS	Sets	Reps	Tempo	Rest
No SAQ on this day				

RESISTANCE		Sets	Reps	Tempo	Intensity	Rest
Total body	Barbell clean	4	5	Explosive	85%	3 min
Chest	Bench press	4	5	1/0/1	85%	3 min
Back	Done in total-body exercise					
Shoulders	Seated overhead barbell press	4	5	1/0/1	85%	3 min

(continues)

(continued)

RESISTANCE		Sets	Reps	Tempo	Intensity	Rest
Biceps	Seated DB curl	4	5	1/0/1	85%	3 min
Triceps	Supine triceps extensions	4	5	1/0/1	85%	3 min
Legs	Done in total-body exercise					
COOL-DOWN						
Myofascial rolling and static stretching						

PHASE 5: POWER TRAINING

WARM-UP	Sets	Reps	Time
Myofascial Rolling			
Tensor fascia latae	1		30 sec
Adductor	1		30 sec
Thoracic spine	1		30 sec
Dynamic Warm-up (Some athletes may still require static stretching prior to dynamic warm-up.)			
Lateral tube walking	1	10	0 sec
Prisoner squats	1	10	0 sec
Lunge with rotation	1	10	0 sec
Leg swings: Side to side	1	10	0 sec
MB lift and chop	1	10	0 sec
MB rotations	1	10	0 sec
Push-up with rotation	1	10	60 sec

CORE AND BALANCE	Sets	Reps	Tempo	Rest
No CORE AND BALANCE (incorporated into dynamic warm-up)				

PLYOMETRICS	Sets	Reps	Tempo	Rest
No PLYOMETRICS (incorporated into dynamic warm-up)				

SPEED/AGILITY/QUICKNESS	Sets	Reps	Tempo	Rest
Speed ladder: Six exercises	2			60 sec
T-drill	4			60 sec

RESISTANCE		Sets	Reps	Tempo	Intensity	Rest
Total body	Deadlift shrug to calf raise	4	4	1/0/1	90%	0 sec
	Push press		8	Explosive	4% of BW	2 min
Chest	Bench press	4	4	1/0/1	90%	0 sec
	Rotational chest press		8	Explosive	4% of BW	2 min
Back	Seated cable row	4	4	1/0/1	90%	0 sec
	Overhead MB throw		8	Explosive	4% of BW	2 min
Shoulders	Done in total-body exercises					
Legs	Barbell squats	4	4	1/0/1	90%	0 sec
	Power step-up		8	Explosive	4% of BW	3 min

COOL-DOWN
Myofascial rolling and static stretching

PRE-SEASON GOALS AND CONSIDERATIONS FOR HOCKEY

Goals	Considerations

• Correcting impaired movement patterns based on results of pre-season assessments
• Maintaining:
  • Physical health (decreases the chance of injury for participation in practice and games, and optimal performance within such activities)
  • Range of motion, joint stability, and muscle strength and endurance
  • Cardiorespiratory endurance (aerobic/anaerobic)
  • Total-body stabilization, strength, and power
	• A systematic pre-season plan that transitions the athlete from performance enhancement to injury prevention and maintenance of off-season gains will be developed. This transition should be implemented with the consideration that the athlete's sport participation level is increasing dramatically from what they have become used to in the off-season.
	• Proper recovery and conditioning, during this time of increased activity, will be applied.
	• Exercise volume of injury prevention. and performance training based on the athlete's increased activity level, will be considered.

SAMPLE PRE-SEASON OPT HOCKEY PLAN (SEPTEMBER)

Level	Phase	JAN–APR In-Season	MAY Off-Season	JUN Off-Season	JUL Off-Season	AUG Pre-Season (1)	SEP In-Season	OCT In-Season	NOV–DEC In-Season
Corrective								X	
Stabilization	1							X	
Strength	2							X	
	3								
	4								
Power	5								
	6								

SAMPLE PRE-SEASON WEEKLY OPT HOCKEY SCHEDULE

Month 1

	MON	TUE	WED	THU	FRI	SAT	SUN
OPT Phase	Strength Endurance	OFF	Corrective	OFF	Stabilization Endurance	OFF	Corrective
Other		Game		Game		Game	

SAMPLE PRE-SEASON OPT HOCKEY PROGRAMS

Corrective Exercise Training

INHIBIT	Sets	Reps	Time
Myofascial Rolling			
Tensor fascia latae	1		30 sec
IT band	1		30 sec
Adductors	1		30 sec

LENGTHEN			Sets	Reps	Time
Supine biceps femoris stretch			1		30 sec
Kneeling hip flexor stretch			1		30 sec
Standing adductor stretch			1		30 sec
Floor lat stretch			1		30 sec

ACTIVATE	Sets	Reps	Tempo	Intensity	Rest
Side-lying hip adduction	1	15	4/2/1		0 sec
Suspension bridge	1	15	4/2/1		90 sec

INTEGRATE		Sets	Reps	Tempo	Intensity	Rest
Total body	Squat, curl to overhead press	1	15	4/2/1	60%	90 sec

PHASE 1: STABILIZATION ENDURANCE TRAINING

WARM-UP			Sets	Reps	Time
Myofascial Rolling					
Tensor fascia latae			1		30 sec
Piriformis			1		30 sec
Static Stretching					
Standing adductor stretch			1		30 sec
Kneeling hip flexor stretch			1		30 sec
Posterior shoulder stretch			1		30 sec

Dynamic Stretching	Sets	Reps	Tempo	Rest
Lunge with rotation	1	10	Moderate	0 sec
MB wood chop	1	10	Moderate	0 sec

CORE AND BALANCE	Sets	Reps	Tempo	Rest
Side iso-ab with hip abduction	2	15	4/2/1	0 sec
Floor bridge: Single-leg	2	15	4/2/1	0 sec
Single-leg throw and catch	2	15	4/2/1	60 sec

(continues)

(continued)

PLYOMETRICS	Sets	Reps	Tempo	Rest
No PLYOMETRICS due to increased activity				

SPEED/AGILITY/QUICKNESS	Sets	Reps	Distance	Rest
No SAQ due to increased on-ice conditioning				

RESISTANCE		Sets	Reps	Tempo	Intensity	Rest
Total body	Cable squat to row	2	15	4/2/1	65%	0 sec
Chest	SL suspension chest press	2	15	4/2/1	65%	0 sec
Back	Done in total-body exercise					
Shoulders	Single-leg scaption	2	15	4/2/1	65%	0 sec
Legs	Single-leg Romanian deadlift	2	12 ea.	4/2/1	65%	90 sec

COOL-DOWN
Myofascial rolling and static stretching

PHASE 2: STRENGTH ENDURANCE TRAINING

WARM-UP	Sets	Reps	Time
Myofascial Rolling			
Tensor fascia latae	1		30 sec
Adductors	1		30 sec
Active Stretching			
Standing adductor stretch	1	10	
Kneeling hip flexor stretch	1	10	
Supine biceps femoris stretch	1	10	

Dynamic Stretching	Sets	Reps	Tempo	Rest
Multiplanar lunge with MB wood chop	1	10	Moderately fast	0 sec

CORE AND BALANCE	Sets	Reps	Tempo	Rest
Crunch with rotation	2	12	1/1/1	0 sec
Back extension	2	12	1/1/1	0 sec
Single-leg squat touchdown	2	10	1/1/1	60 sec

PLYOMETRICS		Sets	Reps	Tempo		Rest
No PLYOMETRICS due to increased activity						

SPEED/AGILITY/QUICKNESS		Sets	Reps	Distance		Rest
No SAQ due to on-ice conditioning						

RESISTANCE		Sets	Reps	Tempo	Intensity	Rest
Chest	Incline DB press	2	12	2/0/2	70%	0 sec
	Cable chest press		8	4/2/1		
Back	Bent-over row	2	12	2/0/2	70%	0 sec
	Single-leg cable pull-down		8	4/2/1		
Shoulders	Seated overhead DB press	2	12	2/0/2	70%	0 sec
	SL lateral raise		8	4/2/1		
Legs	Deadlift	2	12	2/0/2	70%	60 sec
	SL RDL		8	4/2/1		

COOL-DOWN
Myofascial rolling and static stretching

IN-SEASON GOALS AND CONSIDERATIONS FOR HOCKEY

Goals	Considerations

• Maintaining:
  • Range of motion, joint stability, and muscle strength and endurance
  • Cardiorespiratory endurance (aerobic/anaerobic)
  • Total-body stabilization, strength, and power
• Establishing with the athlete a communication process for monitoring in-season maintenance and a plan that works based on what the athlete needs, wants, and will have the capability to do focusing on their job playing hockey
	• Assessments and testing, to ensure program considerations are being made to prevent overuse injuries and maintain performance levels, will be performed.
	• Impaired movement patterns with exercise strategies being implemented will be attended to.
	• Additional conditioning, for athletes who may not get the same type of on-ice practice or game minutes as others, will be considered.
	• A systematic in-season maintenance plan will be developed that allows the athlete to minimize decreases in performance and chance of injury over a long season with repetitive sport movement patterns and physical contact.
	• The exercise volume of injury prevention, and performance training based on the athlete's increased travel and activity level, will be considered.

IN-SEASON OPT HOCKEY PLAN (OCTOBER–APRIL)

Level	Phase	JAN In-Season (4)	FEB In-Season (5)	MAR In-Season (6)	APR In-Season (7)	MAY–AUG Off-Season	SEP Pre-Season	OCT In-Season (1)	NOV In-Season (2)	DEC In-Season (3)
Corrective		X	X	X	X			X	X	X
Stabilization	1	X	X	X	X			X	X	X
Strength	2		X		X			X		X
	3									
	4	X		X					X	
Power	5									
	6									

SAMPLE IN-SEASON WEEKLY OPT HOCKEY SCHEDULE

Any Month

	MON	TUE	WED	THU	FRI	SAT	SUN
OPT Phase	Maximal strength	OFF	Corrective	OFF	Stabilization Endurance	OFF	Corrective
Other		Game		Game		Game	

SAMPLE IN-SEASON OPT HOCKEY PROGRAM

Corrective Exercise Training

INHIBIT	Sets	Reps	Time
Myofascial Rolling			
Tensor fascia latae	1		30 sec
Adductors	1		30 sec
Thoracic spine	1		30 sec

LENGTHEN		Sets	Reps	Time
Supine biceps femoris stretch		1		30 sec
Kneeling hip flexor stretch		1		30 sec
Standing adductor stretch		1		30 sec
Standing pec stretch		1		30 sec

ACTIVATE	Sets	Reps	Tempo	Intensity	Rest
Side-lying hip adduction	1	15	4/2/1		0 sec
Suspension bridge	1	15	4/2/1		0 sec
Single-leg extension	1	15	4/2/1		90 sec

INTEGRATE		Sets	Reps	Tempo	Intensity	Rest
Total body	Side lunge to overhead press	1	15	4/2/1	60%	90 sec

PHASE 1: STABILIZATION ENDURANCE TRAINING

WARM-UP	Sets	Reps	Time
Myofascial Rolling			
Tensor fascia latae	1		30 sec
Piriformis	1		30 sec
Static Stretching			
Gastrocnemius stretch	1		30 sec
Kneeling hip flexor stretch	1		30 sec
Posterior shoulder stretch	1		30 sec

Dynamic Stretching	Sets	Reps	Tempo	Rest
Lunge with rotation	1	10	Moderate	0 sec
MB wood chop	1	10	Moderate	0 sec

(continues)

(continued)

CORE AND BALANCE	Sets	Reps	Tempo	Rest
Prone iso-abs	2	15	4/2/1	0 sec
Bent-over SL cobra	2	15	4/2/1	0 sec
Single-leg balance reach	2	15	4/2/1	60 sec

PLYOMETRICS, SPEED/AGILITY/QUICKNESS	Sets	Reps	Tempo	Rest
No PLYOMETRICS or SAQ due to increased activity and on-ice conditioning				

RESISTANCE		Sets	Reps	Tempo	Intensity	Rest
Total body	Lunge, balance to overhead press	2	15	4/2/1	65%	0 sec
Chest	SL suspension chest press	2	15	4/2/1	65%	0 sec
Back	Single-leg cable row	2	15	4/2/1	65%	0 sec
Shoulders	Done in total-body exercise					
Legs	Step-up to balance: Transverse plane	2	15	4/2/1	65%	90 sec

COOL-DOWN
Myofascial rolling and static stretching

PHASE 2: STRENGTH ENDURANCE TRAINING

WARM-UP	Sets	Reps	Time
Myofascial Rolling			
Tensor fascia latae	1		30 sec
Thoracic spine	1		30 sec
Active Stretching			
Standing adductor stretch	1	10	
Standing hip flexor stretch	1	10	
Floor lat stretch	1	10	

WARM-UP				
Dynamic Stretching	**Sets**	**Reps**	**Tempo**	**Rest**
Multiplanar lunge with MB wood chop	1	10	Moderately fast	0 sec

CORE AND BALANCE				
Cable rotation	**Sets**	**Reps**	**Tempo**	**Rest**
Cable rotation	2	12	1/1/1	0 sec
Crunch	2	12	1/1/1	0 sec
Single-leg Romanian deadlift	2	12	1/1/1	60 sec

PLYOMETRICS	**Sets**	**Reps**	**Tempo**	**Rest**
No PLYOMETRICS because of increased activity				

SPEED/AGILITY/QUICKNESS	**Sets**	**Reps**	**Distance**	**Rest**
No SAQ because of on-ice conditioning				

RESISTANCE		**Sets**	**Reps**	**Tempo**	**Intensity**	**Rest**
Total body	Cable squat to row	2	12	2/0/2	70%	0 sec
	Step-up, balance to overhead press		8	4/2/1		
Chest	Incline bench press	2	12	2/0/2	70%	0 sec
	Push up		8	4/2/1		
Back	Done in total-body exercise					
Shoulders	Done in total-body exercise					
Biceps	Standing DB curl	2	12	2/0/2	70%	0 sec
Triceps	Standing suspension extension	2	12	4/2/1	70%	0 sec
Legs	Barbell squat	2	12	2/0/2	70%	60 sec
	SL RDL		8	4/2/1		

COOL-DOWN
Myofascial rolling and static stretching

PHASE 4: MAXIMAL STRENGTH TRAINING

WARM-UP	Sets	Reps	Time
Myofascial Rolling			
IT band	1		30 sec
Adductors	1		30 sec
Tensor fascia latae	1		30 sec
Active Stretching			
Standing adductor stretch	1	10	
Standing hip flexor stretch	1	10	
Standing pec stretch	1	10	
Floor lat stretch	1	10	

Dynamic Stretching	Sets	Reps	Tempo	Rest
"World's Greatest Stretch"	1	10	Controlled	0 sec

CORE AND BALANCE	Sets	Reps	Tempo	Rest
Knee-ups	2	12	1/1/1	0 sec
Back extension	2	12	1/1/1	0 sec
Step-up to balance	2	12	1/1/1	90 sec

PLYOMETRICS	Sets	Reps	Tempo	Rest
No PLYOMETRICS on this day				

SPEED/AGILITY/QUICKNESS	Sets	Reps	Distance	Rest
No SAQ on this day				

RESISTANCE		Sets	Reps	Tempo	Intensity	Rest
Total body	Deadlift shrug to calf raise	4	5	Explosive	85%	3 min
Chest	Bench press	4	5	Controlled	85%	3 min
Back	Seated cable row	4	5	Controlled	85%	3 min

RESISTANCE		Sets	Reps	Tempo	Intensity	Rest
Shoulders	Seated overhead barbell press	4	5	Controlled	85%	3 min
Legs	Barbell squat	4	5	Controlled	85%	3 min
COOL-DOWN						
Myofascial rolling and static stretching						

SOCCER

Note: For the purposes of this content, the Sports Performance Coach should focus on using the OPT™ Model with all players. Although the demands of soccer positions vary, the fundamental principles of integrated training will improve all positions' stability, strength, and power. The prevalence of lower-extremity injuries in soccer is a cause of concern for all sports coaches (Junge & Dvorak, 2004). Corrective exercise programs have shown promise in reducing certain injuries in a variety of demographics (Campa et al., 2019; Grooms et al., 2013; Mozafaripour et al., 2022).

If an individual needs to modify the model based on the athlete's needs, then it is very appropriate to do so based on the assessment process, the position's needs, and the goals set for the athlete. The Sports Performance Coach will focus on "off-field" performance training to decrease injury and increase "on-field" performance.

Demands of the Sport	
General Information	**Activity Information**
<ul><li>Less than 2% of the total distance covered during a game is with the ball.</li><li>The aerobic energy system predominates and is responsible for as much as 98% of the energy utilized (Bangsbo et al., 1991).</li><li>Matches are typically decided at the highest speeds, with the ATP-PCr and glycolytic systems being dominant.</li></ul>	<ul><li>Distance covered by a player in a match: 10–13 km (Mohr et al., 2003)</li><li>1,000–1,200 changes in locomotion patterns occur during a match; there is approximately one change every 4.5 seconds of play (Bangsbo, 1994b)</li><li>Activity pattern defined by running intensity/speed:<ul><li>Standing: 17.1% of total activity</li><li>Walking: 40.4% of total activity</li><li>Low-intensity running: 35.1% of total activity</li><li>High-intensity running: 8.1% of total activity</li><li>Sprinting: 0.7% of total activity</li></ul></li><li>Average sprint: 15 meters</li><li>Average one sprint every 90 seconds</li><li>Variations in all demands are position-specific and vary between matches</li><li>Higher-level players will cover more ground and spend more time at higher intensities than lower-level players (Gore, 2000)</li><li>Distance covered in the second half of play is typically less than that covered in the first half of play (Gore, 2000)</li></ul>

SUGGESTED ASSESSMENTS FOR SOCCER

Assessment Type	Assessment Method
Transitional postural assessments	• Overhead squat test • Single-leg squat test • Split squat • Star excursion balance test
Mobility assessments (if needed)	• Foot and ankle testing • Lumbo-pelvic-hip complex testing • Shoulder and spine testing
Dynamic movement assessments	• Drop jump • Shark skill test • Davies test • Triple cross-over hop test
Aerobic test (choose one of the following)	• 12-minute run test • 1.5-mile run test • Beep test • Yo-yo intermittent recovery test
Anaerobic test	• 300-yard shuttle run
Muscular endurance assessments	• Push-up test • Pull-up test • Curl-up test
Muscular strength assessments	• 1–5 RM bench press • 1–5 RM squat • Nordic hamstring lower test
Power assessments	• Vertical jump test (double-leg) • Vertical jump test (single-leg) • Rotational medicine ball throw test (left and right) • Medicine ball soccer throw
Speed assessments	• 40-yard sprint test • 10-yard sprint test
Agility assessments	• LEFT (lower-extremity functional test) • T-test • 5–10–5 (pro agility test)

OFF-SEASON GOALS AND CONSIDERATIONS FOR SOCCER

Goals	Considerations

• Physical and mental reconditioning
• Reconditioning from the physical contact and additional stress placed on the body
• Correcting impaired movement patterns based on results of transitional postural assessments
• Improve
  • Range of motion, joint stability, and muscle strength and endurance
  • Cardiorespiratory endurance (aerobic/anaerobic)
  • Total-body stabilization, strength, and power
• Increase
  • Reaction time, speed, agility, and quickness
  • Lean body mass and size
• Determine, through assessment, demands-of-sport analysis and athlete goals, which plan and program should be created to achieve both the needs and the goals
	• Planning and programming will be based on assessment, client goals, and the demands of the sport.
	• A systematic off-season plan will incorporate integrated training, including:
	  • Core training
	  • Balance training
	  • Power training
	  • Speed, agility, and quickness training
	  • Integrated resistance training
	  • Cardiorespiratory training combined with a proper nutrition plan to maximize training and recovery
	• Opportunities for appropriate rest between workouts will be provided.
	• An off-season training schedule, which works backward from the commencement of the pre-season, will be developed to allow for maximum injury prevention and performance gains without the athlete overtraining.
	• Conditioning for soccer will be as similar to the game demands as possible.
	  • Ground-reaction forces, starting and stopping, and change of direction will also be considered when designing a conditioning program.
	• Performance programs will be modified, from a volume and exercise standpoint, to accommodate specific activities to avoid overtraining and maximize results. The athlete will continue to increase soccer skill activities as the off-season progresses.

SAMPLE OFF-SEASON OPT SOCCER PLAN (JANUARY–JULY)

Level	Phase	JAN Off-Season (1)	FEB Off-Season (2)	MAR Off-Season (3)	APR Off-Season (4)	MAY Off-Season (5)	JUN Off-Season (6)	JUL Off-Season (7)	AUG Pre-Season	SEP–DEC In-Season
Corrective										
Stabilization	1		X			X		X		
Strength	2			X			X	X		
	3									
	4									
Power	5				X			X		
	6									

SAMPLE OFF-SEASON WEEKLY OPT SOCCER SCHEDULE

Month 1: 2 days/week

	MON	TUE	WED	THU	FRI	SAT	SUN
OPT Phase	Corrective	OFF	OFF	Corrective	OFF	OFF	OFF

Month 2: 2 days/week

	MON	TUE	WED	THU	FRI	SAT	SUN
OPT Phase	Stabilization Endurance	OFF	OFF	Stabilization Endurance	OFF	OFF	OFF

Month 3: 4 days/week

	MON	TUE	WED	THU	FRI	SAT	SUN
OPT Phase	Strength Endurance		OFF	Strength Endurance		OFF	OFF
Other		Conditioning			Conditioning		

Month 4: 4 days/week

	MON	TUE	WED	THU	FRI	SAT	SUN
OPT Phase	Power		OFF	Power		OFF	OFF
Other		Conditioning			Conditioning		

Month 5: 5 days/week

	MON	TUE	WED	THU	FRI	SAT	SUN
OPT Phase	Stabilization Endurance		Stabilization Endurance		Stabilization Endurance	OFF	OFF
Other		Conditioning		Conditioning			

Month 6: 5 days/week

	MON	TUE	WED	THU	FRI	SAT	SUN
OPT Phase	Strength Endurance	OFF	Strength Endurance	OFF	Strength Endurance	OFF	OFF
Other		Conditioning		Conditioning			

Month 7: 5 days/week

	MON	TUE	WED	THU	FRI	SAT	SUN
OPT Phase	Strength Endurance		Stabilization Endurance	Power	OFF	OFF	Other
Other	Conditioning		Conditioning				

SAMPLE OFF-SEASON OPT SOCCER PROGRAMS

Corrective Exercise Training

INHIBIT	Sets	Reps	Time
Myofascial Rolling			
Calves	1		30 sec
Tensor fascia latae	1		30 sec
IT band	1		30 sec
Adductors			

LENGTHEN	Sets	Reps	Time
Gastrocnemius stretch	1		30 sec
Soleus stretch	1		30 sec
Supine biceps femoris stretch	1		30 sec
Kneeling hip flexor stretch	1		30 sec
Standing adductor stretch	1		30 sec

ACTIVATE	Sets	Reps	Tempo	Intensity	Rest
Single-leg calf raise	2	12	4/2/1		0 sec
Single-leg hip adduction	2	12	4/2/1		0 sec
Single-leg hip abduction: Gluteus medius	2	12	4/2/1		0 sec
Floor bridge	2	12	4/2/1		90 sec

INTEGRATE	Sets	Reps	Tempo	Intensity	Rest
Cable squat to row	2	12	4/2/1	60%	0 sec

PHASE 1: STABILIZATION ENDURANCE TRAINING

WARM-UP		Sets	Reps	Time
Myofascial Rolling				
Tensor fascia latae		1		30 sec
Piriformis		1		30 sec
Static Stretching				
Gastrocnemius stretch		1		30 sec
Kneeling hip flexor stretch		1		30 sec
Standing biceps femoris stretch		1		30 sec

Dynamic Stretching	Sets	Reps	Tempo	Rest
Lunge with rotation	1	10	Moderate	0 sec
MB woodchop	1	10	Moderate	0 sec

CORE AND BALANCE	Sets	Reps	Tempo	Rest
Side iso-ab	1	15	4/2/1	0 sec
Floor bridge: Single-leg	1	15	4/2/1	0 sec
Single-leg balance reach	1	15	4/2/1	60 sec

PLYOMETRICS	Sets	Reps	Tempo	Rest
Squat jump with stabilization	1	6	Hold landing	60 sec

SPEED/AGILITY/QUICKNESS	Sets	Reps	Tempo	Rest
Speed ladder: Six exercises	2			60 sec

RESISTANCE		Sets	Reps	Tempo	Intensity	Rest
Total body	Lunge, balance to overhead press: Single-arm	1	20	4/2/1	60%	0 sec
Chest	Cable chest press: Alternate-arm	1	20	4/2/1	60%	0 sec
Back	SL bent-over DB cobra	1	20	4/2/1	60%	0 sec
Shoulders	Done in total-body exercise					

RESISTANCE		Sets	Reps	Tempo	Intensity	Rest
Biceps	Single-leg DB curl: Alternate-arm	1	20	4/2/1	60%	0 sec
Triceps	SL triceps extension	1	20	4/2/1	60%	0 sec
Legs	Single-leg squat	1	20	4/2/1	60%	90 sec
COOL-DOWN						
Myofascial rolling and static stretching						

PHASE 2: STRENGTH ENDURANCE TRAINING

WARM-UP	Sets	Reps	Time
Myofascial Rolling			
IT band	1		30 sec
Piriformis	1		30 sec
Calves	1		30 sec
Active Stretching			
Standing adductor stretch	1	10	
Standing hip flexor stretch	1	10	
Standing pec stretch	1	10	

Dynamic Stretching	Sets	Reps	Tempo	Rest
Multiplanar lunge with MB woodchop	1	10	Moderately fast	0
Squat to overhead reach	1	10	Moderately fast	0

CORE AND BALANCE	Sets	Reps	Tempo	Rest
Knee-ups	2	12	1/1/1	0 sec
Back extension with rotation	2	12	1/1/1	0 sec
Single-leg squat touchdown	2	12	1/1/1	60 sec

PLYOMETRICS	Sets	Reps	Tempo	Rest
Butt kicks	2	8	Repeating	0 sec
Cone hops: Side to side	2	8	Repeating	60 sec

(continues)

(continued)

SPEED/AGILITY/QUICKNESS		Sets	Reps	Tempo		Rest
Speed ladder: Six exercises		2				60 sec
LEFT test		2				60 sec

RESISTANCE		Sets	Reps	Tempo	Intensity	Rest
Total body	Optional					
Chest	Incline DB press	2	12	2/0/2	70%	0 sec
	Cable chest press: SA		8	4/2/1		
Back	Seated lat pull-down	2	12	2/0/2	70%	0 sec
	Single-leg cable row		8	4/2/1		
Shoulders	Seated overhead DB press		12	2/0/2	70%	0 sec
	SL scaption raise		8	4/2/1		
Legs	Barbell squats	3	12	2/0/2	70%	60 sec
	Side lunge to balance		8	4/2/1		

COOL-DOWN
Myofascial rolling and static stretching

PHASE 5: POWER TRAINING

WARM-UP	Sets	Reps	Time
Myofascial Rolling			
Calves	1		30 sec
Tensor fascia latae	1		30 sec
Adductors	1		30 sec
Dynamic Warm-up (Some athletes may still require static stretching prior to dynamic warm-up.)			
Lateral tube walking	1	10	0 sec
Prisoner squats	1	10	0 sec
Lunge with rotation	1	10	0 sec

WARM-UP		Sets	Reps	Time
Dynamic Warm-up (Some athletes may still require static stretching prior to dynamic warm-up.)				
Leg swings: Front to back		1	10	0 sec
Push-up with rotation		1	10	0 sec
Scorpion		1	10	0 sec
Multiplanar hop to stabilization		1	10	60 sec

CORE AND BALANCE		Sets	Reps	Tempo	Rest
No CORE AND BALANCE (incorporated into dynamic warm-up and resistance workout)					

PLYOMETRICS		Sets	Reps	Tempo	Rest
No PLYOMETRICS (incorporated into dynamic warm-up and resistance workout)					

SPEED/AGILITY/QUICKNESS		Sets	Reps	Tempo	Rest
Speed ladder: Eight exercises		1			60 sec
Box drill		4			30 sec

RESISTANCE		Sets	Reps	Tempo	Intensity	Rest
Total body	Lunge, curl to overhead press	3	5	1/0/1	85%	0 sec
	Overhead MB throw		10	Explosive	2% of BW	2 min
Chest	DB chest press	3	5	1/0/1	85%	0 sec
	Rotational chest press		10	Explosive	2% of BW	2 min
Back	Seated lat pull-down	3	5	1/0/1	85%	0 sec
	MB soccer throw		10	Explosive	2% of BW	2 min
Shoulders	Done in total-body exercises					
Legs	Barbell squat	3	5	1/0/1	85%	0 sec
	Power step-ups		10	Explosive	2% of BW	2 min

COOL-DOWN
Myofascial rolling and static stretching

PRE-SEASON GOALS AND CONSIDERATIONS FOR SOCCER

Goals	Considerations

• Correct impaired movement patterns based on results of pre-season assessments
• Maintain:
  • Physical health (decreases the chance of injury for participation in practice and games and ensures optimal performance within such activities)
  • Range of motion, joint stability, and muscle strength and endurance
  • Cardiorespiratory endurance (aerobic/anaerobic)
  • Total-body stabilization, strength, and power
	• A systematic pre-season plan that transitions the athlete from performance enhancement to injury prevention and maintenance of off-season gains will be developed. This transition should be implemented with the consideration that the athlete's sport participation level is increasing dramatically from what they have become used to in the off-season.
	• Proper recovery and conditioning, during this time of increased activity, will be applied.
	• Exercise volume of injury prevention, and performance training based on the athlete's increased activity level, will be considered.

SAMPLE PRE-SEASON OPT SOCCER PLAN (AUGUST)

Level	Phase	JAN–JUL Off-Season	AUG Pre-Season (1)	SEP–DEC In-Season
Corrective				
Stabilization	1		X	
Strength	2		X	
	3			
	4			
Power	5			
	6			

SAMPLE PRE-SEASON WEEKLY OPT SOCCER SCHEDULE

Month 1

	MON	TUE	WED	THU	FRI	SAT	SUN
OPT Phase	Stabilization Endurance	OFF	Strength Endurance	OFF	Corrective	OFF	Corrective
Other						Game	

SAMPLE PRE-SEASON OPT SOCCER PROGRAMS

Corrective Exercise Training

INHIBIT	Sets	Reps	Time
Myofascial Rolling			
Quads	1		30 sec
Tensor fascia latae	1		30 sec
IT band	1		30 sec
Adductors	1		30 sec
LENGTHEN	**Sets**	**Reps**	**Time**
Gastrocnemius stretch	1		30 sec
Supine piriformis stretch	1		30 sec
Supine biceps femoris stretch	1		30 sec
Kneeling hip flexor stretch	1		30 sec
Standing adductor stretch	1		30 sec

ACTIVATE	Sets	Reps	Tempo	Intensity	Rest
Side-lying hip adduction	3	10	4/2/1		0 sec
Single-leg hip abduction: Gluteus medius	3	10	4/2/1		60 sec

INTEGRATE		Sets	Reps	Tempo	Intensity	Rest
Total body	Side lunge to overhead press: Single-arm	3	10	4/2/1	60%	60 sec

PHASE 1: STABILIZATION ENDURANCE TRAINING

WARM-UP	Sets	Reps	Time
Myofascial Rolling			
Tensor fascia latae	1		30 sec
IT band	1		30 sec
Piriformis	1		30 sec

(continues)

(*continued*)

WARM-UP			Sets	Reps	Time
Static Stretching					
Gastrocnemius stretch			1		30 sec
Kneeling hip flexor stretch			1		30 sec
Standing hip flexor stretch			1		30 sec
Standing adductor stretch			1		30 sec
Floor lat stretch			1		30 sec

Dynamic Stretching	Sets	Reps	Tempo	Rest
Lunge with rotation	1	10	Moderate	0 sec
MB woodchop	1	10	Moderate	0 sec

CORE AND BALANCE	Sets	Reps	Tempo	Rest
Quadruped arm opposite-leg raise	2	15	4/2/1	0 sec
Floor bridge: Alternate-leg	2	15	4/2/1	0 sec
Single-leg lift and chop	2	15	4/2/1	60 sec

PLYOMETRICS	Sets	Reps	Tempo	Rest
No PLYOMETRICS due to increased activity				

SPEED/AGILITY/QUICKNESS	Sets	Reps	Distance	Rest
No SAQ due to increased activity				

RESISTANCE		Sets	Reps	Tempo	Intensity	Rest
Total body	Optional					
Chest	SL suspension chest press	2	15	4/2/1	65%	0 sec
Back	SL suspension row	2	15	4/2/1	65%	0 sec
Shoulders	Bent-over row DB combo I	2	15	4/2/1	65%	0 sec
Legs	Single-leg Romanian deadlift	2	15	4/2/1	65%	90 sec

COOL-DOWN
Myofascial rolling and static stretching

IN-SEASON GOALS AND CONSIDERATIONS FOR SOCCER

Goals	Considerations
<ul><li>Maintain:<ul><li>Range of motion, joint stability, and muscle strength and endurance</li><li>Cardiorespiratory endurance (aerobic/anaerobic)</li><li>Total-body stabilization, strength, and power</li></ul></li><li>Establish a communication process for monitoring in-season maintenance and a plan that works based on what the athlete needs, wants, and will have the capacity to do focusing on their job playing soccer</li></ul>	<ul><li>Assessments and testing, to ensure program considerations are being made to prevent overuse injuries and maintain performance levels, will be performed.</li><li>Impaired movement patterns with exercise strategies being implemented will be attended to.</li><li>Additional conditioning, for athletes who may not get the same type of on-field game minutes as others, will be considered.</li><li>A systematic in-season maintenance plan will be developed that allows the athlete to minimize a decrease in fitness and chances of injury over a long season with repetitive sport movement patterns.</li><li>The exercise volume of injury prevention, and performance training based on the athlete's increased travel and activity level, will be considered.</li></ul>

IN-SEASON OPT SOCCER PLAN (SEPTEMBER–DECEMBER)

Level	Phase	JAN–JUL Off-Season	AUG Pre-Season	SEP In-Season (1)	OCT In-Season (2)	NOV In-Season (3)	DEC In-Season (4)
Corrective				X	X	X	X
Stabilization	1			X	X	X	X
Strength	2			X	X	X	X
	3						
	4						
Power	5						
	6						

SAMPLE IN-SEASON WEEKLY OPT SOCCER SCHEDULE

Any Month

	MON	TUE	WED	THU	FRI	SAT	SUN
OPT Phase	Corrective	Strength Endurance	OFF	Corrective	Corrective	OFF	
Other					Game		Game

SAMPLE IN-SEASON OPT SOCCER PROGRAM

Corrective Exercise Training

INHIBIT	Sets	Reps	Time
Myofascial Rolling			
Quads	1		30 sec
Tensor fascia latae	1		30 sec
IT band	1		30 sec
Adductors	1		30 sec

LENGTHEN	Sets	Reps	Time
Gastrocnemius stretch	1		30 sec
Supine piriformis stretch	1		30 sec
Supine biceps femoris stretch	1		30 sec
Kneeling hip flexor stretch	1		30 sec
Standing adductor stretch	1		30 sec

ACTIVATE	Sets	Reps	Tempo	Intensity	Rest
Single-leg hip adduction	2	12	4/2/1		0 sec
Single-leg calf raise	2	12	4/2/1		60 sec

INTEGRATE		Sets	Reps	Tempo	Intensity	Rest
Total body	Side step-up, balance to overhead press	2	12	4/2/1	60%	60 sec

PHASE 1: STABILIZATION ENDURANCE TRAINING

WARM-UP	Sets	Reps	Time
Myofascial Rolling			
Tensor fascia latae	1		30 sec
IT band	1		30 sec
Piriformis	1		30 sec
Static Stretching			
Gastrocnemius stretch	1		30 sec
Kneeling hip flexor stretch	1		30 sec
Supine biceps femoris stretch	1		30 sec

WARM-UP			Sets	Reps	Time
Dynamic Stretching		Sets	Reps	Tempo	
Lunge with rotation		1	10	Moderate	0 sec
MB woodchop		1	10	Moderate	0 sec
CORE AND BALANCE		Sets	Reps	Tempo	Rest
Prone iso-ab		2	15	4/2/1	0 sec
Standing cable iso-rotation		2	15	4/2/1	0 sec
Single-leg rotation		2	15	4/2/1	60 sec
PLYOMETRICS, SPEED/AGILITY/QUICKNESS		Sets	Reps	Tempo	Rest
Box jump-up with stabilization		2	6	Controlled	60 sec

SPEED/AGILITY/QUICKNESS
No SAQ due to increased activity

RESISTANCE		Sets	Reps	Tempo	Intensity	Rest
Total body	Optional					
Chest	SL suspension chest press	2	15	4/2/1	65%	0 sec
Back	Single-leg cable row: Single-arm	2	15	4/2/1	65%	0 sec
Shoulders	Suspension Y's	2	15	4/2/1	65%	0 sec
Legs	SL squat	2	15	4/2/1	65%	90 sec

COOL-DOWN
Myofascial rolling and static stretching

PHASE 2: STRENGTH ENDURANCE TRAINING

WARM-UP	Sets	Reps	Time
Myofascial Rolling			
IT band	1		30 sec
Piriformis	1		30 sec
Thoracic spine	1		30 sec

(continues)

(continued)

WARM-UP		Sets	Reps		Time
Active Stretching					
Gastrocnemius		1	10		
Standing hip flexor stretch		1	10		
Standing adductor stretch		1	10		
Dynamic Stretching	Sets	Reps	Tempo		Rest
Multiplanar lunge with reach	1	10	Moderately fast		0 sec
Squat to overhead reach	1	10	Moderately fast		0 sec

CORE AND BALANCE	Sets	Reps	Tempo		Rest
Crunch with rotation	2	12	1/1/1		0 sec
Cable rotations	2	12	1/1/1		0 sec
Side step-up to balance	2	12	1/1/1		60 sec

PLYOMETRICS	Sets	Reps	Tempo		Rest
No PLYOMETRICS because of increased activity					

SPEED/AGILITY/QUICKNESS	Sets	Reps	Distance		Rest
No SAQ because of on-field conditioning					

RESISTANCE		Sets	Reps	Tempo	Intensity	Rest
Total body	Optional					
Chest	Incline DB press	3	10	2/0/2	75%	0 sec
	Suspension push-up: Feet in straps		10	4/2/1	60%	
Back	Seated cable row	3	10	2/0/2	75%	0 sec
	SL lat pull-down		10	4/2/1	60%	
Shoulders	Seated DB scaption	3	10	2/0/2	75%	0 sec
	SL SA DB press		10	4/2/1	60%	
Legs	Deadlift	3	10	2/0/2	75%	60 sec
	Reverse lunge to balance		10	4/2/1	60%	

COOL-DOWN
Myofascial rolling and static stretching

REFERENCES

Bangsbo, J. (1994a). *Fitness training in football: A scientific approach*. August Krogh Institute, University of Copenhagen.

Bangsbo, J. (1994b). The physiology of soccer: With special reference to intense intermittent exercise. *Acta Physiologica Scandinavica. Supplementum, 619*, 1–155.

Bangsbo, J., Mohr, M., & Krustrup, P. (2006). Physical and metabolic demands of training and match-play in the elite football player. *Journal of Sports Sciences, 24*(7), 665–674. https://doi.org/10.1080/02640410500482529

Bangsbo, J., Nørregaard, L., & Thorsø, F. (1991). Activity profile of competition soccer. *Canadian Journal of Sport Sciences/Journal Canadien des Sciences du Sport, 16*(2), 110–116.

Campa, F., Spiga, F., & Toselli, S. (2019). The effect of a 20-week corrective exercise program on functional movement patterns in youth elite male soccer players. *Journal of Sport Rehabilitation, 28*(7), 746–751. https://doi.org/10.1123/jsr.2018-0039

Ehlert, A., & Wilson, P. (2019). A systematic review of golf warm-ups: Behaviors, injury, and performance. *Journal of Strength and Conditioning Research, 33*(12), 3444-3462. https://doi.org/10.1519/JSC.0000000000003329

Fradkin, A. J., Cameron, P. A., & Gabbe, B. J. (2007). Is there an association between self-reported warm-up behaviour and golf related injury in female golfers? *Journal of Science and Medicine in Sport, 10*(1), 66–71. https://doi.org/10.1016/j.jsams.2006.04.001

Gambetta, V. (1999). *Building the complete athlete* (5th ed.). Gambetta Sports Training Systems.

Gosheger, G., Liem, D., Ludwig, K., Greshake, O., & Winkelmann, W. (2003). Injuries and overuse syndromes in golf. *American Journal of Sports Medicine, 31*(3), 438–443. https://doi.org/10.1177/03635465030310031901

Gore, C.J. (2000). *Physiological tests for elite athletes.* Human Kinetics.

Grooms, D. R., Palmer, T., Onate, J. A., Myer, G. D., & Grindstaff, T. (2013). Soccer-specific warm-up and lower extremity injury rates in collegiate male soccer players. *Journal of Athletic Training, 48*(6), 782–789. https://doi.org/10.4085/1062-6050-48.4.08

Junge, A., & Dvorak, J. (2004). Soccer injuries: A review on incidence and prevention. *Sports Medicine, 34*(13), 929–938. https://doi.org/10.2165/00007256-200434130-00004

Lephart, S. M., Smoliga, J. M., Myers, J. B., Sell, T. C., & Tsai, Y.-S. (2007). An eight-week golf-specific exercise program improves physical characteristics, swing mechanics, and golf performance in recreational golfers. *Journal of Strength and Conditioning Research, 21*(3), 860. https://journals.lww.com/nsca-jscr/abstract/2007/08000/an_eight_week_golf_specific_exercise_program.36.aspx

McClay, I. S., Robinson, J. R., Andriacchi, T. P., Frederick, E. C., Gross, T., Martin, P., Valiant, G., Williams, K. R., & Cavanagh, P. R. (1994a). A kinematic profile of skills in professional basketball players. *Journal of Applied Biomechanics, 10*(3), 205–221. https://doi.org/10.1123/jab.10.3.205

McClay, I. S., Robinson, J. R., Andriacchi, T. P., Frederick, E. C., Gross, T., Martin, P., Valiant, G., Williams, K. R., & Cavanagh, P. R. (1994b). A profile of ground reaction forces in professional basketball. *Journal of Applied Biomechanics, 10*(3), 222–236. https://doi.org/10.1123/jab.10.3.222

Mohr, M., Krustrup, P., & Bangsbo, J. (2003). Match performance of high-standard soccer players with special reference to development of fatigue. *Journal of Sports Sciences, 21*(7), 519–528. https://doi.org/10.1080/0264041031000071182

Mozafaripour, E., Seidi, F., Minoonejad, H., Bayattork, M., & Khoshroo, F. (2022). The effectiveness of the comprehensive corrective exercise program on kinematics and strength of lower extremities in males with dynamic knee valgus: A parallel-group randomized wait-list controlled trial. *BMC Musculoskeletal Disorders, 23*(1), 700. https://doi.org/10.1186/s12891-022-05652-8

Sell, T. C., Tsai, Y.-S., Smoliga, J. M., Myers, J. B., & Lephart, S. M. (2007). Strength, flexibility, and balance characteristics of highly proficient golfers. *Journal of Strength and Conditioning Research, 21*(4), 1166. https://journals.lww.com/nsca-jscr/abstract/2007/11000/strength,_flexibility,_and_balance_characteristics.31.aspx

Thompson, C. J., Cobb, K. M., & Blackwell, J. (2007). Functional training improves club head speed and functional fitness in older golfers. *Journal of Strength and Conditioning Research, 21*(1), 131–137. https://doi.org/10.1519/00124278-200702000-00024

PERCENT OF ONE-REP MAXIMUM (1RM) CONVERSION

Weight	30%	40%	50%	55%	60%	65%	70%	75%	80%	85%	90%
5	2	2	3	3	3	3	4	4	4	4	5
10	3	4	5	6	6	7	7	8	8	9	9
15	5	6	8	8	9	10	11	11	12	13	14
20	6	8	10	11	12	13	14	15	16	17	18
25	8	10	13	14	15	16	18	19	20	21	23
30	9	12	15	17	18	20	21	23	24	26	27
35	11	14	18	19	21	23	25	26	28	30	32
40	12	16	20	22	24	26	28	30	32	34	36
45	14	18	23	25	27	29	32	34	36	38	41
50	15	20	25	28	30	33	35	38	40	43	45
55	17	22	28	30	33	36	39	41	44	47	50
60	18	24	30	33	36	39	42	45	48	51	54
65	20	26	33	36	39	42	46	49	52	55	59
70	21	28	35	39	42	46	49	53	56	60	63
75	23	30	38	41	45	49	53	56	60	64	68
80	24	32	40	44	48	52	56	60	64	68	72
85	26	34	43	47	51	55	60	64	68	72	77
90	27	36	45	50	54	59	63	68	72	77	81
95	29	38	48	52	57	62	67	71	76	81	86
100	30	40	50	55	60	65	70	75	80	85	90
105	32	42	53	58	63	68	74	79	84	89	95
110	33	44	55	61	66	72	77	83	88	94	99
115	35	46	58	63	69	75	81	86	92	98	104
120	36	48	60	66	72	78	84	90	96	102	108
125	38	50	63	69	75	81	88	94	100	106	113

(continues)

Weight	30%	40%	50%	55%	60%	65%	70%	75%	80%	85%	90%
130	39	52	65	72	78	85	91	98	104	111	117
135	41	54	68	74	81	88	95	101	108	115	122
140	42	56	70	77	84	91	98	105	112	119	126
145	44	58	73	80	87	94	102	109	116	123	131
150	45	60	75	83	90	98	105	113	120	128	135
155	47	62	78	85	93	101	109	116	124	132	140
160	48	64	80	88	96	104	112	120	128	136	144
165	50	66	83	91	99	107	116	124	132	140	149
170	51	68	85	94	102	111	119	128	136	145	153
175	53	70	88	96	105	114	123	131	140	149	158
180	54	72	90	99	108	117	126	135	144	153	162
185	56	74	93	102	111	120	130	139	148	157	167
190	57	76	95	105	114	124	133	143	152	162	171
195	59	78	98	107	117	127	137	146	156	166	176
200	60	80	100	110	120	130	140	150	160	170	180
205	62	82	103	113	123	133	144	154	164	174	185
210	63	84	105	116	126	137	147	158	168	179	189
215	65	86	108	118	129	140	151	161	172	183	194
220	66	88	110	121	132	143	154	165	176	187	198
225	68	90	113	124	135	146	158	169	180	191	203
230	69	92	115	127	138	150	161	173	184	196	207
235	71	94	118	129	141	153	165	176	188	200	212
240	72	96	120	132	144	156	168	180	192	204	216
245	74	98	123	135	147	159	172	184	196	208	221
250	75	100	125	138	150	163	175	188	200	213	225

Weight	30%	40%	50%	55%	60%	65%	70%	75%	80%	85%	90%
255	77	102	128	140	153	166	179	191	204	217	230
260	78	104	130	143	156	169	182	195	208	221	234
265	80	106	133	146	159	172	186	199	212	225	239
270	81	108	135	149	162	176	189	203	216	230	243
275	83	110	138	151	165	179	193	206	220	234	248
280	84	112	140	154	168	182	196	210	224	238	252
285	86	114	143	157	171	185	200	214	228	242	257
290	87	116	145	160	174	189	203	218	232	247	261
295	89	118	148	162	177	192	207	221	236	251	266
300	90	120	150	165	180	195	210	225	240	255	270
305	92	122	153	168	183	198	214	229	244	259	275
310	93	124	155	171	186	202	217	233	248	264	279
315	95	126	158	173	189	205	221	236	252	268	284
320	96	128	160	176	192	208	224	240	256	272	288
325	98	130	163	179	195	211	228	244	260	276	293
330	99	132	165	182	198	215	231	248	264	281	297
335	101	134	168	184	201	218	235	251	268	285	302
340	102	136	170	187	204	221	238	255	272	289	306
345	104	138	173	190	207	224	242	259	276	293	311
350	105	140	175	193	210	228	245	263	280	298	315
355	107	142	178	195	213	231	249	266	284	302	320
360	108	144	180	198	216	234	252	270	288	306	324
365	110	146	183	201	219	237	256	274	292	310	329
370	111	148	185	204	222	241	259	278	296	315	333
375	113	150	188	206	225	244	263	281	300	319	338

(continues)

Weight	30%	40%	50%	55%	60%	65%	70%	75%	80%	85%	90%
380	114	152	190	209	228	247	266	285	304	323	342
385	116	154	193	212	231	250	270	289	308	327	347
390	117	156	195	215	234	254	273	293	312	332	351
395	119	158	198	217	237	257	277	296	316	336	356
400	120	160	200	220	240	260	280	300	320	340	360
405	122	162	203	223	243	263	284	304	324	344	365
410	123	164	205	226	246	267	287	308	328	349	369
415	125	166	208	228	249	270	291	311	332	353	374
420	126	168	210	231	252	273	294	315	336	357	378
425	128	170	213	234	255	276	298	319	340	361	383
430	129	172	215	237	258	280	301	323	344	366	387
435	131	174	218	239	261	283	305	326	348	370	392
440	132	176	220	242	264	286	308	330	352	374	396
445	134	178	223	245	267	289	312	334	356	378	401
450	135	180	225	248	270	293	315	338	360	383	405
455	137	182	228	250	273	296	319	341	364	387	410
460	138	184	230	253	276	299	322	345	368	391	414
465	140	186	233	256	279	302	326	349	372	395	419
470	141	188	235	259	282	306	329	353	376	400	423
475	143	190	238	261	285	309	333	356	380	404	428
480	144	192	240	264	288	312	336	360	384	408	432
485	146	194	243	267	291	315	340	364	388	412	437
490	147	196	245	270	294	319	343	368	392	417	441
495	149	198	248	272	297	322	347	371	396	421	446
500	150	200	250	275	300	325	350	375	400	425	450

Weight	30%	40%	50%	55%	60%	65%	70%	75%	80%	85%	90%
505	152	202	253	278	303	328	354	379	404	429	455
510	153	204	255	281	306	332	357	383	408	434	459
515	155	206	258	283	309	335	361	386	412	438	464
520	156	208	260	286	312	338	364	390	416	442	468
525	158	210	263	289	315	341	368	394	420	446	473
530	159	212	265	292	318	345	371	398	424	451	477
535	161	214	268	294	321	348	375	401	428	455	482
540	162	216	270	297	324	351	378	405	432	459	486
545	164	218	273	300	327	354	382	409	436	463	491
550	165	220	275	303	330	358	385	413	440	468	495
555	167	222	278	305	333	361	389	416	444	472	500
560	168	224	280	308	336	364	392	420	448	476	504
565	170	226	283	311	339	367	396	424	452	480	509
570	171	228	285	314	342	371	399	428	456	485	513
575	173	230	288	316	345	374	403	431	460	489	518
580	174	232	290	319	348	377	406	435	464	493	522
585	176	234	293	322	351	380	410	439	468	497	527
590	177	236	295	325	354	384	413	443	472	502	531
595	179	238	298	327	357	387	417	446	476	506	536
600	180	240	300	330	360	390	420	450	480	510	540
605	182	242	303	333	363	393	424	454	484	514	545
610	183	244	305	336	366	397	427	458	488	519	549
615	185	246	308	338	369	400	431	461	492	523	554
620	186	248	310	341	372	403	434	465	496	527	558
625	188	250	313	344	375	406	438	469	500	531	563

(continues)

Weight	30%	40%	50%	55%	60%	65%	70%	75%	80%	85%	90%
630	189	252	315	347	378	410	441	473	504	536	567
635	191	254	318	349	381	413	445	476	508	540	572
640	192	256	320	352	384	416	448	480	512	544	576
645	194	258	323	355	387	419	452	484	516	548	581
650	195	260	325	358	390	423	455	488	520	553	585
655	197	262	328	360	393	426	459	491	524	557	590
660	198	264	330	363	396	429	462	495	528	561	594
665	200	266	333	366	399	432	466	499	532	565	599
670	201	268	335	369	402	436	469	503	536	570	603
675	203	270	338	371	405	439	473	506	540	574	608
680	204	272	340	374	408	442	476	510	544	578	612
685	206	274	343	377	411	445	480	514	548	582	617
690	207	276	345	380	414	449	483	518	552	587	621
700	210	280	350	385	420	455	490	525	560	595	630
705	212	282	353	388	423	458	494	529	564	599	635
710	213	284	355	391	426	462	497	533	568	604	639
715	215	286	358	393	429	465	501	536	572	608	644
720	216	288	360	396	432	468	504	540	576	612	648
725	218	290	363	399	435	471	508	544	580	616	653
730	219	292	365	402	438	475	511	548	584	621	657
735	221	294	368	404	441	478	515	551	588	625	662
740	222	296	370	407	444	481	518	555	592	629	666
745	224	298	373	410	447	484	522	559	596	633	671
750	225	300	375	413	450	488	525	563	600	638	675
755	227	302	378	415	453	491	529	566	604	642	680

Weight	30%	40%	50%	55%	60%	65%	70%	75%	80%	85%	90%
760	228	304	380	418	456	494	532	570	608	646	684
765	230	306	383	421	459	497	536	574	612	650	689
770	231	308	385	424	462	501	539	578	616	655	693
775	233	310	388	426	465	504	543	581	620	659	698
780	234	312	390	429	468	507	546	585	624	663	702
785	236	314	393	432	471	510	550	589	628	667	707
790	237	316	395	435	474	514	553	593	632	672	711
795	239	318	398	437	477	517	557	596	636	676	716
800	240	320	400	440	480	520	560	600	640	680	720
805	242	322	403	443	483	523	564	604	644	684	725
810	243	324	405	446	486	527	567	608	648	689	729
815	245	326	408	448	489	530	571	611	652	693	734
820	246	328	410	451	492	533	574	615	656	697	738
825	248	330	413	454	495	536	578	619	660	701	743
830	249	332	415	457	498	540	581	623	664	706	747
835	251	334	418	459	501	543	585	626	668	710	752
840	252	336	420	462	504	546	588	630	672	714	756
845	254	338	423	465	507	549	592	634	676	718	761
850	255	340	425	468	510	553	595	638	680	723	765
855	257	342	428	470	513	556	599	641	684	727	770
860	258	344	430	473	516	559	602	645	688	731	774
865	260	346	433	476	519	562	606	649	692	735	779
870	261	348	435	479	522	566	609	653	696	740	783
875	263	350	438	481	525	569	613	656	700	744	788
880	264	352	440	484	528	572	616	660	704	748	792

(continues)

Weight	30%	40%	50%	55%	60%	65%	70%	75%	80%	85%	90%
885	266	354	443	487	531	575	620	664	708	752	797
890	267	356	445	490	534	579	623	668	712	757	801
895	269	358	448	492	537	582	627	671	716	761	806
900	270	360	450	495	540	585	630	675	720	765	810
905	272	362	453	498	543	588	634	679	724	769	815
910	273	364	455	501	546	592	637	683	728	774	819
915	275	366	458	503	549	595	641	686	732	778	824
920	276	368	460	506	552	598	644	690	736	782	828
925	278	370	463	509	555	601	648	694	740	786	833
930	279	372	465	512	558	605	651	698	744	791	837
935	281	374	468	514	561	608	655	701	748	795	842
940	282	376	470	517	564	611	658	705	752	799	846
945	284	378	473	520	567	614	662	709	756	803	851
950	285	380	475	523	570	618	665	713	760	808	855
955	287	382	478	525	573	621	669	716	764	812	860
960	288	384	480	528	576	624	672	720	768	816	864
965	290	386	483	531	579	627	676	724	772	820	869
970	291	388	485	534	582	631	679	728	776	825	873
975	293	390	488	536	585	634	683	731	780	829	878
980	294	392	490	539	588	637	686	735	784	833	882
985	296	394	493	542	591	640	690	739	788	837	887
990	297	396	495	545	594	644	693	743	792	842	891
995	299	398	498	547	597	647	697	746	796	846	896
1000	300	400	500	550	600	650	700	750	800	850	900

ONE-REP MAXIMUM (1RM) CONVERSION

Pounds	10 reps	9 reps	8 reps	7 reps	6 reps	5 reps	4 reps	3 reps	2 reps
5	7	6	6	6	6	6	6	5	5
10	13	13	13	12	12	11	11	11	11
15	20	19	19	18	18	17	17	16	16
20	27	26	25	24	24	23	22	22	21
25	33	32	31	30	29	29	28	27	26
30	40	39	38	36	35	34	33	32	32
35	47	45	44	42	41	40	39	38	37
40	53	52	50	48	47	46	44	43	42
45	60	58	56	55	53	51	50	49	47
50	67	65	63	61	59	57	56	54	53
55	73	71	69	67	65	63	61	59	58
60	80	77	75	73	71	69	67	65	63
65	87	84	81	79	76	74	72	70	68
70	93	90	88	85	82	80	78	76	74
75	100	97	94	91	88	86	83	81	79
80	107	103	100	97	94	91	89	86	84
85	113	110	106	103	100	97	94	92	89
90	120	116	113	109	106	103	100	97	95
95	127	123	119	115	112	109	106	103	100
100	133	129	125	121	118	114	111	108	105
105	140	135	131	127	124	120	117	114	111
110	147	142	138	133	129	126	122	119	116
115	153	148	144	139	135	131	128	124	121
120	160	155	150	145	141	137	133	130	126
125	167	161	156	152	147	143	139	135	132

Pounds	10 reps	9 reps	8 reps	7 reps	6 reps	5 reps	4 reps	3 reps	2 reps
130	173	168	163	158	153	149	144	141	137
135	180	174	169	164	159	154	150	146	142
140	187	181	175	170	165	160	156	151	147
145	193	187	181	176	171	166	161	157	153
150	200	194	188	182	176	171	167	162	158
155	207	200	194	188	182	177	172	168	163
160	213	206	200	194	188	183	178	173	168
165	220	213	206	200	194	189	183	178	174
170	227	219	213	206	200	194	189	184	179
175	233	226	219	212	206	200	194	189	184
180	240	232	225	218	212	206	200	195	189
185	247	239	231	224	218	211	206	200	195
190	253	245	238	230	224	217	211	205	200
195	260	252	244	236	229	223	217	211	205
200	267	258	250	242	235	229	222	216	211
205	273	265	256	248	241	234	228	222	216
210	280	271	263	255	247	240	233	227	221
215	287	277	269	261	253	246	239	232	226
220	293	284	275	267	259	251	244	238	232
225	300	290	281	273	265	257	250	243	237
230	307	297	288	279	271	263	256	249	242
235	313	303	294	285	276	269	261	254	247
240	320	310	300	291	282	274	267	259	253
245	327	316	306	297	288	280	272	265	258
250	333	323	313	303	294	286	278	270	263

(continues)

Pounds	10 reps	9 reps	8 reps	7 reps	6 reps	5 reps	4 reps	3 reps	2 reps
255	340	329	319	309	300	291	283	276	268
260	347	335	325	315	306	297	289	281	274
265	353	342	331	321	312	303	294	286	279
270	360	348	338	327	318	309	300	292	284
275	367	355	344	333	324	314	306	297	289
280	373	361	350	339	329	320	311	303	295
285	380	368	356	345	335	326	317	308	300
290	387	374	363	352	341	331	322	314	305
295	393	381	369	358	347	337	328	319	311
300	400	387	375	364	353	343	333	324	316
305	407	394	381	370	359	349	339	330	321
310	413	400	388	376	365	354	344	335	326
315	420	406	394	382	371	360	350	341	332
320	427	413	400	388	376	366	356	346	337
325	433	419	406	394	382	371	361	351	342
330	440	426	413	400	388	377	367	357	347
335	447	432	419	406	394	383	372	362	353
340	453	439	425	412	400	389	378	368	358
345	460	445	431	418	406	394	383	373	363
350	467	452	438	424	412	400	389	378	368
355	473	458	444	430	418	406	394	384	374
360	480	465	450	436	424	411	400	389	379
365	487	471	456	442	429	417	406	395	384
370	493	477	463	448	435	423	411	400	389
375	500	484	469	455	441	429	417	405	395

Pounds	10 reps	9 reps	8 reps	7 reps	6 reps	5 reps	4 reps	3 reps	2 reps
380	507	490	475	461	447	434	422	411	400
385	513	497	481	467	453	440	428	416	405
390	520	503	488	473	459	446	433	422	411
395	527	510	494	479	465	451	439	427	416
400	533	516	500	485	471	457	444	432	421
405	540	523	506	491	476	463	450	438	426
410	547	529	513	497	482	469	456	443	432
415	553	535	519	503	488	474	461	449	437
420	560	542	525	509	494	480	467	454	442
425	567	548	531	515	500	486	472	459	447
430	573	555	538	521	506	491	478	465	453
435	580	561	544	527	512	497	483	470	458
440	587	568	550	533	518	503	489	476	463
445	593	574	556	539	524	509	494	481	468
450	600	581	563	545	529	514	500	486	474
455	607	587	569	552	535	520	506	492	479
460	613	594	575	558	541	526	511	497	484
465	620	600	581	564	547	531	517	503	489
470	627	606	588	570	553	537	522	508	495
475	633	613	594	576	559	543	528	514	500
480	640	619	600	582	565	549	533	519	505
485	647	626	606	588	571	554	539	524	511
490	653	632	613	594	576	560	544	530	516
495	660	639	619	600	582	566	550	535	521
500	667	645	625	606	588	571	556	541	526

(continues)

Pounds	10 reps	9 reps	8 reps	7 reps	6 reps	5 reps	4 reps	3 reps	2 reps
505	673	652	631	612	594	577	561	546	532
510	680	658	638	618	600	583	567	551	537
515	687	665	644	624	606	589	572	557	542
520	693	671	650	630	612	594	578	562	547
525	700	677	656	636	618	600	583	568	553
530	707	684	663	642	624	606	589	573	558
535	713	690	669	648	629	611	594	578	563
540	720	697	675	655	635	617	600	584	568
545	727	703	681	661	641	623	606	589	574
550	733	710	688	667	647	629	611	595	579
555	740	716	694	673	653	634	617	600	584
560	747	723	700	679	659	640	622	605	589
565	753	729	706	685	665	646	628	611	595
570	760	735	713	691	671	651	633	616	600
575	767	742	719	697	676	657	639	622	605
580	773	748	725	703	682	663	644	627	611
585	780	755	731	709	688	669	650	632	616
590	787	761	738	715	694	674	656	638	621
595	793	768	744	721	700	680	661	643	626
600	800	774	750	727	706	686	667	649	632
605	807	781	756	733	712	691	672	654	637
610	813	787	763	739	718	697	678	659	642
615	820	794	769	745	724	703	683	665	647
620	827	800	775	752	729	709	689	670	653
625	833	806	781	758	735	714	694	676	658

Pounds	10 reps	9 reps	8 reps	7 reps	6 reps	5 reps	4 reps	3 reps	2 reps
630	840	813	788	764	741	720	700	681	663
635	847	819	794	770	747	726	706	686	668
640	853	826	800	776	753	731	711	692	674
645	860	832	806	782	759	737	717	697	679
650	867	839	813	788	765	743	722	703	684
655	873	845	819	794	771	749	728	708	689
660	880	852	825	800	776	754	733	714	695
665	887	858	831	806	782	760	739	719	700
670	893	865	838	812	788	766	744	724	705
675	900	871	844	818	794	771	750	730	711
680	907	877	850	824	800	777	756	735	716
685	913	884	856	830	806	783	761	741	721
690	920	890	863	836	812	789	767	746	726
695	927	897	869	842	818	794	772	751	732
700	933	903	875	848	824	800	778	757	737
705	940	910	881	855	829	806	783	762	742
710	947	916	888	861	835	811	789	768	747
715	953	923	894	867	841	817	794	773	753
720	960	929	900	873	847	823	800	778	758
725	967	935	906	879	853	829	806	784	763
730	973	942	913	885	859	834	811	789	768
735	980	948	919	891	865	840	817	795	774
740	987	955	925	897	871	846	822	800	779
745	993	961	931	903	876	851	828	805	784
750	1000	968	938	909	882	857	833	811	789

(continues)

Pounds	10 reps	9 reps	8 reps	7 reps	6 reps	5 reps	4 reps	3 reps	2 reps
755	1007	974	944	915	888	863	839	816	795
760	1013	981	950	921	894	869	844	822	800
765	1020	987	956	927	900	874	850	827	805
770	1027	994	963	933	906	880	856	832	811
775	1033	1000	969	939	912	886	861	838	816
780	1040	1006	975	945	918	891	867	843	821
785	1047	1013	981	952	924	897	872	849	826
790	1053	1019	988	958	929	903	878	854	832
795	1060	1026	994	964	935	909	883	859	837
800	1067	1032	1000	970	941	914	889	865	842
805	1073	1039	1006	976	947	920	894	870	847
810	1080	1045	1013	982	953	926	900	876	853
815	1087	1052	1019	988	959	931	906	881	858
820	1093	1058	1025	994	965	937	911	886	863
825	1100	1065	1031	1000	971	943	917	892	868
830	1107	1071	1038	1006	976	949	922	897	874
835	1113	1077	1044	1012	982	954	928	903	879
840	1120	1084	1050	1018	988	960	933	908	884
845	1127	1090	1056	1024	994	966	939	914	889
850	1133	1097	1063	1030	1000	971	944	919	895
855	1140	1103	1069	1036	1006	977	950	924	900
900	1200	1161	1125	1091	1059	1029	1000	973	947
905	1207	1168	1131	1097	1065	1034	1006	978	953
910	1213	1174	1138	1103	1071	1040	1011	984	958
915	1220	1181	1144	1109	1076	1046	1017	989	963

Pounds	10 reps	9 reps	8 reps	7 reps	6 reps	5 reps	4 reps	3 reps	2 reps
920	1227	1187	1150	1115	1082	1051	1022	995	968
925	1233	1194	1156	1121	1088	1057	1028	1000	974
930	1240	1200	1163	1127	1094	1063	1033	1005	979
935	1247	1206	1169	1133	1100	1069	1039	1011	984
940	1253	1213	1175	1139	1106	1074	1044	1016	989
945	1260	1219	1181	1145	1112	1080	1050	1022	995
950	1267	1226	1188	1152	1118	1086	1056	1027	1000
955	1273	1232	1194	1158	1124	1091	1061	1032	1005
960	1280	1239	1200	1164	1129	1097	1067	1038	1011
965	1287	1245	1206	1170	1135	1103	1072	1043	1016
970	1293	1252	1213	1176	1141	1109	1078	1049	1021
975	1300	1258	1219	1182	1147	1114	1083	1054	1026
980	1307	1265	1225	1188	1153	1120	1089	1059	1032
985	1313	1271	1231	1194	1159	1126	1094	1065	1037
990	1320	1277	1238	1200	1165	1131	1100	1070	1042
995	1327	1284	1244	1206	1171	1137	1106	1076	1047
1000	1333	1290	1250	1212	1176	1143	1111	1081	1053

SUMMARY OF ERGOGENIC AIDS AND RELATED SUBSTANCES*

Type of Supplement	Common Uses (Claims)	Typical Dosage**	Considerations Rating as Ergogenic Aid (1 to 5)***
5-Hydroxytryptophan (5-HTP)	Used to increase serotonin levels in the brain. These increases in serotonin may lead to reduced appetite and carbohydrate craving; promote sleep; reduce depression.	200–300 mg/day (for mental health-associated effects) 750–900 mg/day (for weight loss/appetite regulatory effects)	Minimal efficacy as an ergogenic aid. Primarily used as a tool to help reduce caloric intake by reducing carbohydrate cravings.[1,2] There appears to be minimal efficacy for sleep as well.[3] Its utilization as an antidepressant should be used under the direction of a licensed mental health professional. **Rating: 1**
Acetyl-L-carnitine (see also Carnitine)	Used to increase the shuttling of fatty acids into the mitochondria, which may improve exercise performance and accelerate recovery. Acetylated (acetyl-L-carnitine) passes the blood–brain barrier more effectively so it may provide enhanced brain function and lower depression among elderly population. Displays some antioxidant capacity.	500–2,000 mg/day	There appears to be very small to minimal clinically meaningful improvement in exercise capacity, performance, or recovery.[4,5] It does appear to provide some benefit in the reduction of oxidative stress and some markers of exercise-induced metabolic damage.[6–9] **Rating: 2**
Alpha-ketoglutarate	Alpha-ketoglutarate (AKG) is a carboxylated keto acid that helps create ATP, is involved in maintaining nitrogen balance, and produces glutamine. It is marketed as a tool to help reduce muscle protein breakdown and recover from surgery due to its anti-catabolic properties. It is also sold as an anti-aging supplement.	4–6 g/day (no consensus dosing currently available)	There is minimal research showing AKG is effective for improving exercise performance. The research is further muddled with many studies combining L-arginine with AKG.[10–13] There does appear to be evidence for its utilization in post-surgical settings to reduce muscle catabolism.[14] **Rating: 1**
Alpha-ketoisocaproate (KIC)	Alpha-ketoisocaproate (KIC) is a product of leucine metabolism. Given its connection to leucine, claims are often made that it reduces muscle protein catabolism and can reduce exercise-induced fatigue.	1.5–9 g/day	There is minimal research on KIC alone as an ergogenic aid. The studies that have been published show no effect on exercise performance.[15–17] **Rating: 1**

(continues)

Type of Supplement	Common Uses (Claims)	Typical Dosage**	Considerations Rating as Ergogenic Aid (1 to 5)***
Alpha-linolenic acid (ALA; also see DHA and EPA)	Alpha-linolenic acid (ALA) is a short-chain omega-3 fatty acid that increases blood levels of omega-3 fatty acids. Is found in both food sources and supplemental sources. Anti-inflammatory properties may help with recovery from exercise.	1.6 g/day (men), 1.1 g/day (women) Supplemented at 3–14 g/day	ALA supplementation has shown minimal benefit for exercise performance in humans. There is a small amount of evidence showing supplementation with ALA can reduce exercise-induced inflammation and potentially reduce declines in training performance. However, the evidence is limited and the effect size is small.[18,19] **Rating: 2**
Androstenedione	Precursor for testosterone; intended to increase testosterone, enhance muscle protein synthesis, and overall muscle growth.	0–300 mg/day (used in research)	Androstenedione increases estrogen but not testosterone in most individuals. Does not provide greater muscle growth or strength growth compared to placebo.[20–23] **Rating: 1**
Arginine	An amino acid that is often claimed to increase growth hormone and promote muscle protein synthesis. Through its conversion into nitric oxide (NO) can cause vasodilation and increase blood flow.	1–10 g/day Doses of 10 g or greater can result in gastrointestinal distress	The evidence suggests that arginine does result in increased growth hormone release at specific doses, but these results are short and are unlikely to impact skeletal muscle metabolism in a meaningful way.[24–26] Arginine does appear to cause small but unreliable increases in blood flow after supplementation.[27–30] **Rating: 2**
Beta-alanine	Beta-alanine is the rate-limiting amino acid for producing carnosine inside muscle cells. Carnosine acts primarily as an intracellular buffer and antioxidant.	2–5 g/day Requires 4-6 weeks of loading before effects are seen Doses may be taken in multiple small doses throughout the day to reduce paresthesia	Among one of the most effective ergogenic aids. When supplemented for 4-6 weeks, beta-alanine increases aerobic and anaerobic exercise capacity. Most studies show a ~2%-15% increase in performance, depending on type and duration of exercise.[31–33] It is most effective for high-intensity exercise that lasts 1-10 minutes.[34] **Rating: 4**

Type of Supplement	Common Uses (Claims)	Typical Dosage**	Considerations Rating as Ergogenic Aid (1 to 5)***
Beta-carotene	Beta-carotene is a precursor to vitamin A. It mainly functions as an antioxidant and is often claimed to prevent/reduce exercise-induced muscle soreness and enhance exercise recovery.	5–30 mg/day	There appears to be no measurable benefit for enhancing recovery or reducing exercise-induced muscle soreness.[35,36] **Rating: 1**
Beta-hydroxy-beta-methylbutyrate (HMB)	Beta-hydroxy-beta-methylbutyrate (HMB) is a metabolite of leucine that is used to help trigger muscle protein synthesis and reduce muscle protein breakdown.	1–6 g/day	The evidence on HMB in young, athletic populations is mixed. It may have a small benefit to muscle growth, with a slightly greater effect seen in trained individuals.[37–39] However, these results are not entirely supported by the literature.[40] The anti-catabolic effects of HMB are likely more pronounced among older individuals.[41–44] **Rating: 2**
Branched-chain amino acids (BCAA) (leucine, isoleucine, and valine)	BCAAs represent a subclass of amino acids that have effects on muscle growth and development. They play a role in activating muscle protein synthesis, reducing muscle protein breakdown, and may help reduce fatigue during longer, endurance type exercise.	3–20 g/day	As a supplement, BCAAs show minimal benefit for muscle growth or muscle protein breakdown, especially when individuals consume adequate BCAAs through diet.[45–47] There does appear to be some benefit to BCAA supplementation for fatigue during longer events, likely as a result of reducing glycogen utilization and increasing fat oxidation.[48–50] **Rating: 2.5**
Bromelain	Bromelain is a complex that contains a protein-digesting enzyme that can be absorbed by the body and function within the circulating blood. It helps digest protein in the stomach and once in the body functions as an anti-inflammatory agent.	200–2,000 mg/day (when used for digestive help, taken with a meal) 200–800 mg/day (when used as an anti-inflammatory)	There is minimal high-quality evidence available on bromelain. The limited research suggests it does have some benefit for reducing inflammation and inflammatory-related conditions, such as arthritis.[51] However, it does not appear to be as effective as NSAIDS like ibuprofen.[52] **Rating: 3**

(continues)

Type of Supplement	Common Uses (Claims)	Typical Dosage**	Considerations Rating as Ergogenic Aid (1 to 5)***
Caffeine	Caffeine acts as a central nervous system stimulant. It also alters substrate metabolism to increase fat mobilization. It is used as an ergogenic aid to increase strength and overall exercise capacity.	Ideal dose: 3–6 mg/kg body weight Minimal effective dose: 2 mg/kg body weight	Caffeine increases a wide range of exercise performance metrics, including: muscle endurance, muscle strength, anaerobic power, and aerobic endurance.[53–55] The effect of caffeine on fat metabolism is limited as most of the mobilized fat gets recycled.[56] Higher doses of caffeine do increase resting metabolic rate by ~50–100 kcal, which can provide a small benefit for weight loss.[57,58] **Rating: 4**
Capsaicin	Capsaicin is the molecule found in peppers that is responsible for the "spicy" sensation. It is used primarily as a weight loss aid but also may provide small benefits for exercise performance.	~1–12 mg/day dose of active capsaicin	There is some evidence that capsaicin can assist with weight loss through both reducing overall food intake and by slightly increasing metabolic rate.[59,60] Capsaicin may also provide small reductions in perceived fatigue during exercise, especially muscular endurance during resistance training.[61,62] **Rating: 3–4**
Carnitine (see also Acetyl-L-carnitine)	Used to increase the shuttling of fatty acids into the mitochondria, which may improve exercise performance and accelerate recovery. Acetylated (acetyl-L-carnitine) passes the blood–brain barrier more effectively so it may provide enhanced brain function and lower depression among elderly population. Displays some antioxidant capacity.	500–2,000 mg/day 1,000 mg/day	There appears to be very small to minimal clinically meaningful improvement in exercise capacity, performance, or recovery.[4,5] It does appear to provide some benefit in the reduction of oxidative stress and some markers of exercise-induced metabolic damage.[6–9] May benefit certain types of dementia; more research needed.[2,3] **Rating: 2**

Type of Supplement	Common Uses (Claims)	Typical Dosage**	Considerations Rating as Ergogenic Aid (1 to 5)***
Casein	Casein is a specific component of milk protein and differs from whey protein in both structure and absorption. Casein is digested slower than whey and is often considered a longer acting protein source	Utilized as a part of total dietary protein, dosage depends on dietary protein needs	Casein provides a slightly lower muscle protein synthesis response when directly compared to whey protein. However, the muscle protein synthesis of casein is longer in duration than whey protein.[63] In outcome-based studies, both whey and casein appear to provide similar results with regard to increasing strength and muscle mass.[64] **Rating: 3.5**
Chitosan	Chitosan is a compound that is derived from the shells of crustaceans (e.g., lobsters) and some fungi. It is marketed primarily as a "fat blocker" as it can lower total fat absorption.	0.5–5 g/day	Chitosan dose in the 2–3 grams per day range may result in modest (~1 kg) fat loss over the course of 3–4 months. However, these results may not be long term and it may interfere with the absorption of fat-soluble vitamins.[65] **Rating: 2**
Chondroitin sulfate (see also Glucosamine)	Chondroitin sulfate (CS) is a glycosaminoglycan found naturally in our cartilage tissue. Supplemental CS is believed to improve cartilage integrity, improve joint health, and help with osteoarthritis. It is often consumed alongside glucosamine sulfate.	800–1,200 mg/day	Chondroitin may provide a small benefit to joint space and osteoarthritis among some populations. However, the evidence is limited and it may not work for everyone.[66,67] **Rating: 2**
Chromium chloride Chromium nicotinate (chromium + niacin)	Chromium is a trace mineral that is involved in insulin signaling, the antioxidant system, and potentially body weight regulation.	200–1,000 mcg/day	Chromium supplementation can help improve insulin signaling/insulin resistance among people with type 2 diabetes or already established glucose regulation issues.[68–71] Chromium may provide a very small weight loss effect among adults with obesity or overweight, but the effect is small (~1 kg).[72] **Rating: 2**

(continues)

Type of Supplement	Common Uses (Claims)	Typical Dosage**	Considerations Rating as Ergogenic Aid (1 to 5)***
Chrysin	A flavonoid compound derived primarily from bee pollen. It is claimed to increase testosterone levels.	400–3,000 mg/day	Orally consumed chrysin appears to be ineffective due to the lack of absorption and the very low doses.[73] **Rating: Unknown**
Citrulline	Citrulline is an amino acid that is often used to increase blood flow due to its conversion to L-arginine and then nitric oxide. When supplemented in the form of citrulline malate, it may increase ATP production from the Krebs cycle.	3–8 g/day	Acute citrulline supplementation provides minimal benefit; however, chronic supplementation can increase power output and exercise capacity.[74–78] **Rating: 3**
Citrus aurantium—bitter orange (source of synephrine)	Citrus aurantium (CA) is utilized similarly to caffeine as a way to increase resting energy expenditure and enhance fat oxidation. The primary active compounds in CA are synephrine, octamine, and tyramine.	10–20 mg of active synephrine three times per day (currently available CA products are standardized to synephrine content)	CA results in small increases in metabolic rate (~50–65 kcal); however, these appear to disappear after weeks of supplementation.[79,80] There appears to be no meaningful improvement in exercise performance, however some people report elevated heart rate and blood pressure after consuming, especially when taken alongside caffeine.[81,82] **Rating: 1.5**
Coenzyme Q10 (ubiquinone)	Coenzyme Q10 (CoQ10) is a vitamin-like compound produced naturally by the body. It is found primarily in the mitochondria and utilized for energy production. Also functions as an antioxidant.	100–200 mg/day Higher doses (up to 1,200 mg) appear to be well tolerated	CoQ10 supplementation may increase exercise performance among people with heart failure but not among otherwise healthy individuals.[83] May help reduce the frequency and severity of migraines among some individuals.[84,85] **Rating: 2.5**
Cola nut (see Caffeine)	Herbal source of caffeine		
Conjugated linoleic acid (CLA)	CLA is a naturally occuring trans fat that is often utilized as a fat-loss supplement.	3–6.5 g/day	CLA appears to provide a very small benefit for weight loss above placebo. The effect appears to be ~1–2 pounds over a ~6–12 month time frame.[86,87] **Rating: 2**

Type of Supplement	Common Uses (Claims)	Typical Dosage**	Considerations Rating as Ergogenic Aid (1 to 5)***
Creatine	Creatine is a molecule found in the human body primarily in the form of creatine phosphate. It functions as a phosphate donor to create ATP in the phosphagen energy system. It is taken as a supplement to enhance exercise performance and for its neurocognitive benefits.	Loading dose: 0.3 g/kg body weight (~25 g/day) Maintenance dose: 0.03 g/kg body weight (~3–5 g/day)	Creatine has perhaps the largest body of scientific evidence to support its use as an ergogenic aid. Creatine supplementation increases muscle creatine content, strength, muscular endurance, anaerobic capacity, and lean mass as a result of higher training volumes.[88–91] **Rating: 4–5**
DHA (docosahexaenoic acid) (also see Alpha-linolenic acid and EPA)	DHA is a long-chain omega-3 fatty acid that may help lower blood lipids and improve the risk profile for many chronic diseases. DHA is one of the primary ingredients in fish oil and is researched as a combination of DHA and EPA.	200–400 mg/day; typically taken combined with EPA in fish or algae oil	There does not appear to be any meaningful improvement in exercise performance from DHA or fish oil supplementation. However, supplementation may reduce markers of exercise-induced damage and oxidative stress, which may reduce recovery times.[92–93] Fish oil's main benefits appear to stem from their ability to lower triglycerides and alter cholesterol levels among some individuals.[94] **Rating: 3**
DHEA (dehydro-epiandrosterone)	DHEA is a steroid-based hormone that is naturally produced by the adrenal glands and is a precursor to testosterone and estrogen. It is taken supplementally with the goal of increasing testosterone and lean body mass.	50–200 mg/day	DHEA moderately increases testosterone, more so in women than in men. The effects appear to be much smaller and less consistent among younger, trained individuals.[95,96] DHEA also raises estrogen in many cases. There is no evidence suggesting it actually benefits lean body mass.[97] It is also considered a banned substance by most professional sporting organizations and is tested for by WADA and USADA. **Rating: 1.5**

(continues)

Type of Supplement	Common Uses (Claims)	Typical Dosage**	Considerations Rating as Ergogenic Aid (1 to 5)***
EPA (eicosapentanoic acid) (also see Alpha-linolenic acid and DHA)	EPA is a long-chain omega-3 fatty acid that may help lower blood lipids and improve the risk profile for many chronic diseases. EPA is one of the primary ingredients in fish oil and is researched as a combination of DHA and EPA.	200–400 mg/day; typically taken combined with EPA in fish or algae oil	There does not appear to be any meaningful improvement in exercise performance from DHA or fish oil supplementation. However, supplementation may reduce markers of exercise-induced damage and oxidative stress, which may reduce recovery times.[92,93] Fish oil's main benefits appear to stem from their ability to lower triglycerides and alter cholesterol levels among some individuals.[94] **Rating: 3**
Ephedra (ma huang)	Ephedra is an herb that is utilized for weight loss, exercise performance, as well as the treatment of asthma and allergies. The primary active ingredient in ephedra is ephedrine (usually combined with a source of caffeine).	20–25 mg, taken three times a day (for total dosage of ~60–75 mg/day)	Ephedra has robust effects on metabolic rate, with average increases of ~5%–10% observed in many studies (~100–250 kcals per day).[98–100] These increases in metabolic rate often lead to reductions in body weight.[101–103] Ephedra is an enhancing supplement, with benefits being shown when it is consumed alongside caffeine.[104–106] There is substantial risk with ephedra, especially cardiovascular risk with there being an increased risk of stroke, myocardial infarction, and sudden death.[107] Currently, ephedra is not legal in the United States. **Rating: 3–4**
Ginkgo biloba (leaf extract standardized to 24% ginkgo flavonoid glycosides and 6% terpenes)	Ginkgo biloba is a herbal supplement that is utilized primarily to enhance cognitive function among older adults.	For acute benefits: Consume 120–250 mg within 4 hours of a task For chronic benefits: Consume ~120–360 mg/day, broken into three equal doses	Ginkgo biloba supplementation appears to convey consistent but very modest neurocognitive benefits, especially to older adults.[108–111] Given the potential for interactions with medications such as blood thinners, ginkgo biloba should be used with the approval of a medical professional. **Rating: 2.5**

Type of Supplement	Common Uses (Claims)	Typical Dosage**	Considerations Rating as Ergogenic Aid (1 to 5)***
Glucosamine	Glucosamine is a compound found in virtually all human tissues and occurs in high concentrations in cartilage. It is used alongside chondroitin sulfate to help with osteoarthritis. Only taken in combination with chondroitin.	General population: 1,500 mg/day Athletes: Upwards of 3,000 mg/day Can be spread out evenly across three doses	Glucosamine shows similar results as chondroitin sulfate, largely due to the co-ingestion. It appears to offer a consistent but modest benefit for the reduction of osteoarthritis-related symptoms.[112–114] **Rating: 2.5**
Glutamine	Glutamine is a conditionally essential amino acid that has increased utilization during periods of illness, trauma, or surgery. It is often used for a variety of purposes, such as gastrointestinal support, prevention of muscle wasting, post-exercise recovery, and immune system support.	2–20 g/day Doses above 0.75 g/kg body weight are not recommended	Glutamine supplementation does not provide any meaningful benefit for athletic populations with regard to building muscle mass or recovery. However, it can be helpful for reducing the likelihood of upper respiratory tract infections among athletes with high training volumes.[115,116] **Rating: 2**
Green tea extract	Green tea extract is a rich source of a phytochemical known as epigallocatechin gallate (EGCG) as well as caffeine. It is primarily utilized as a supplement for weight loss and general health.	~400–500 mg of EGCG required to see effects	Green tea extract has shown small yet inconsistent increases in fat oxidation and benefits for weight loss. These effects appear to be washed out when consumed alongside caffeine.[117–120] **Rating: 3**
HMB (hydroxymethylbutyrate or beta-hydroxy beta-methyl-butyrate)	Beta-hydroxy-beta-methylbutyrate (HMB) is a metabolite of leucine that is used to help trigger muscle protein synthesis and reduce muscle protein breakdown. Typically used to reduce protein degradation and promote muscle protein accretion during resistance training.	1–6 g/day	The evidence on HMB in young, athletic populations is mixed. It may have a small benefit to muscle growth, with a slightly greater effect seen in trained individuals.[37–39] However, these results are not entirely supported by the literature.[40] The anti-catabolic effects of HMB are likely more pronounced among older individuals.[41–44] **Rating: 2**

(continues)

Type of Supplement	Common Uses (Claims)	Typical Dosage**	Considerations Rating as Ergogenic Aid (1 to 5)***
HCA (hydroxycitric acid) (*Garcinia cambogia* is a natural source of HCA)	HCA is a fruit that is utilized for weight loss by inhibiting fatty acid synthesis, enhancing fat oxidation, and reducing appetite.	~500 mg/day	HCA appears to prevent fatty acid synthesis in rodents but does not appear to provide any meaningful effects in humans.[121] **Rating: 1**
Inositol	Inositol represents a group of molecules that are similar to glucose but are not processed like glucose. Inositol's primary effects are to improve insulin signaling and improve glucose control.	1–4 g/day	Inositol reliably improves insulin signaling and glucose control in humans. The results appear to be most robust among people with diabetes and women who are pregnant or have polycystic ovary syndrome (PCOS).[122–127] **Rating: 3.5**
Iron	Iron is considered an essential mineral and is involved primarily in the transportation of oxygen from the lungs to the rest of the body.	Variable, depends on iron status	Iron supplementation can enhance exercise performance in individuals with anemic and nonanemic iron deficiency; medical assessment of iron status and supervision of iron supplementation is advisable.[128–130] **Rating: 5 (if iron deficient)**
Leucine (L-leucine) (see Branched-chain amino acids)			
Lipoic acid (alpha-lipoic acid)	Lipoic acid is an antioxidant compound found primarily in the mitochondria and is often used in disease states like type 2 diabetes.	300–1,800 mg/day	Lipoic acid, specifically alpha-lipoic acid, has been shown to provide a small benefit on glucose metabolism, body weight reduction, and oxidative stress levels among people with obesity, overweight, and type 2 diabetes.[131–134] **Rating: TBD**
Ma huang (see Ephedra)			

Type of Supplement	Common Uses (Claims)	Typical Dosage**	Considerations Rating as Ergogenic Aid (1 to 5)***
Medium-chain triglycerides (MCTs)	MCTs are a type of triglyceride (fat) that is absorbed directly into the bloodstream, unlike longer chain triglycerides, which are transported through the lymph system first. They are often utilized to aid weight loss and increase endurance performance.	20–85 g/day Doses at the high end of range may cause steatorrhea in some individuals	Supplementation with MCTs may temporarily increase energy expenditure (for ~7–14 days) and potentially cause short-term accelerated weight loss.[135,136] However, over the long term these effects are likely to disappear.[137] While MCTs may alter substrate utilization and increase fatty acid oxidation, they are unlikely to provide meaningful improvements to overall athletic performance in higher-intensity endurance events.[138,139] **Rating: 2**
Pyruvate (pyruvic acid)	Pyruvate is produced naturally in our body as a result of glycolysis. Supplementation with pyruvate is often utilized as a way to increase ATP production from the Krebs cycle.	7–50 g/day (used in research) Pyruvate is poorly absorbed, and doses above 15 g may cause gastrointestinal distress	Pyruvate appears to be largely ineffective and no meaningful improvement in exercise has been noted consistently across the research literature.[140,141] **Rating: 1.5**
Sodium bicarbonate	Sodium bicarbonate ($NaHCO_3$) is found naturally in our bloodstream and is the main extracellular buffer in the human body. Supplementation with $NaHCO_3$ is often used as a way to enhance our natural buffering capacity and improve anaerobic performance. Sodium citrate can also be used as a similar supplement.	Sodium bicarbonate: 200–300 mg/kg body weight (60–150 minutes prior to exercise) Sodium citrate: 500 mg/kg body weight	Both chronic and acute supplementation with sodium bicarbonate can increase the buffering capacity for anaerobic performance. The magnitude of the benefit depends on the duration and overall intensity of the event, but improvements of 3%–10% are often observed.[142–145] **Rating: 4.5**

(continues)

Type of Supplement	Common Uses (Claims)	Typical Dosage**	Considerations Rating as Ergogenic Aid (1 to 5)***
Sodium chloride	Sodium chloride (salt) provides the body with the main extracellular electrolyte (sodium). Sodium is critical for maintaining osmolality status, especially during sweat-inducing exercise. Offsetting sodium losses through supplementation can help maintain performance.	Highly variable; depends on individual sweat rate and sodium loss in sweat	Sweat rates and sodium loss in sweat can vary greatly among athletes. Very heavy training can cause losses as much as 10,000 mg of sodium per day (~5 teaspoons of salt). Supplementation with salt can offset dehydration and decreases in osmolality that arise from prolonged sweating.[146,147] **Rating: 4**
Taurine	Taurine is considered a non-proteinogenic amino acid. Its primary functions include cardiovascular, brain, and retinal function. Taurine is primarily used to improve exercise performance among people with heart failure and may lower blood pressure.	1–6 g/day	Among individuals with heart failure, taurine may improve cardiac output and muscle endurance.[148,149] Taurine can also provide a small benefit for blood pressure among people with prehypertension.[150] There is limited evidence to support its use for improving exercise performance among otherwise healthy people. **Rating: 2**
Valine (see Branched-chain amino acids)			
Vanadyl sulfate (Vanadium)	Vanadium, often consumed as vanadyl sulfate, is primarily said to enhance control of blood sugar level. There is some speculation that it can enhance muscle development with strength training.	~100–150 mg/day	Vanadium (vanadyl sulfate) has been shown to provide a small reduction in glycated hemoglobin and improvement in insulin signaling among people with type 2 diabetes.[151,152] There is currently no evidence that it aids in exercise performance or enhances muscle growth.[153,154] **Rating: 1.5**

Type of Supplement	Common Uses (Claims)	Typical Dosage**	Considerations Rating as Ergogenic Aid (1 to 5)***
Zinc magnesium aspartate (ZMA)	Zinc magnesium aspartate, commonly referred to as ZMA, has been used as a tool to increase testosterone and muscle growth. It has also been utilized as a sleep aid.	Ingredient doses vary based on the custom formulation of the supplement manufacturer	The scientific literature does not support ZMA as an effective tool for increasing testosterone or improving training or accelerating muscle growth.[155–157] **Rating: 2**

*The information in this table is for instructional purposes only to describe the major purported uses of the components of dietary supplements. Many of these substances are powerful chemicals and should be used only with medical guidance and proper dosage. Caution is especially important for anyone using medication, for children, and for women during pregnancy and lactation.

**Typical dosages are based on current popular use and/or doses used in research. Safety issues may exist for some of these doses—even for nutrients. For many ergogenic aids, it is best to consult with a healthcare professional for dosage concerns related to an individual's goals and specific health status.

***Ratings of potential for efficacy for some or all of the claims based on current research perspectives and a certain amount of unavoidable subjective judgment: 5 = very good, 4 = good, 3 = fair, 2 = poor, 1 = very poor, ?, TBD, Unknown = not known, Depends = depends on conditions and purpose of use.

REFERENCES

1. Cangiano, C. *et al.* Effects of oral 5-hydroxy-tryptophan on energy intake and macronutrient selection in non-insulin dependent diabetic patients. *Int. J. Obes. Relat. Metab. Disord.* 22, (1998).

2. Cangiano, C. *et al.* Eating behavior and adherence to dietary prescriptions in obese adult subjects treated with 5-hydroxytryptophan. *Am. J. Clin. Nutr.* 56, (1992).

3. Sutanto, C. N. *et al.* The impact of 5-hydroxytryptophan supplementation on sleep quality and gut microbiota composition in older adults: A randomized controlled trial. *Clin. Nutr.* 43, (2024).

4. Mielgo-Ayuso, J. *et al.* Effect of acute and chronic oral l-carnitine supplementation on exercise performance based on the exercise intensity: A systematic review. *Nutrients* 13, (2021).

5. Vecchio, M., Chiaramonte, R., Testa, G. & Pavone, V. Clinical effects of L-carnitine supplementation on physical performance in healthy subjects, the key to success in rehabilitation: A systematic review and meta-analysis from the rehabilitation point of view. *J. Funct. Morphol. Kinesiol.* 6, (2021).

6. Fathizadeh, H. *et al.* The effects of L-carnitine supplementation on indicators of inflammation and oxidative stress: a systematic review and meta-analysis of randomized controlled trials. *J. Diabetes Metab. Disord.* 19, (2020).

7. Volek, J. S. *et al.* L-Carnitine L-tartrate supplementation favorably affects markers of recovery from exercise stress. *Am. J. Physiol. Endocrinol. Metab.* 282, (2002).

8. Bloomer, R. J. & Smith, W. A. Oxidative stress in response to aerobic and anaerobic power testing: Influence of exercise training and carnitine supplementation. *Res. Sports Med.* 17, (2009).

9. Cao, Y. *et al.* Single dose administration of L-carnitine improves antioxidant activities in healthy subjects. *Tohoku J. Exp. Med.* 224, (2011).

10. Gatterer, H. *et al.* Short-term supplementation with alpha-ketoglutaric acid and 5-hydroxymethylfurfural does not prevent the hypoxia induced decrease of exercise performance despite attenuation of oxidative stress. *Int. J. Sports Med.* 34, 1–7 (2013).

11. Wax, B., Kavazis, A. N., Webb, H. E. & Brown, S. P. Acute L-arginine alpha ketoglutarate supplementation fails to improve muscular performance in resistance trained and untrained men. *J. Int. Soc. Sports Nutr.* 9, 1–6 (2012).

12. Liu, Y. *et al.* Improved training tolerance by supplementation with α-Keto acids in untrained young adults: a randomized, double blind, placebo-controlled trial. *J. Int. Soc. Sports Nutr.* 9, 1–9 (2012).

13. Wax, B. *et al.* Effect of L-arginine alpha-ketoglutarate ingestion on muscular strength and endurance. *J. Strength Cond. Res.* 25, S111 (2011).

14. Wernerman, J., Hammarqvist, F. & Vinnars, E. Alpha-ketoglutarate and postoperative muscle catabolism. *Lancet* 335, 701–703 (1990).

15. Yarrow, J. F., Parr, J. J., White, L. J., Borsa, P. A. & Stevens, B. R. The effects of short-term alpha-ketoisocaproic acid supplementation on exercise performance: a randomized controlled trial. *J. Int. Soc. Sports Nutr.* 4, 2 (2007).

16. Sandstedt, S., Jorfeldt, L. & Larsson, J. Randomized, controlled study evaluating effects of branched chain amino acids and alpha-ketoisocaproate on protein metabolism after surgery. *Br. J. Surg.* 79, 217–220 (2005).

17. van Someren, K. A., Edwards, A. J. & Howatson, G. Supplementation with β-hydroxy-β-methylbutyrate (HMB) and α-ketoisocaproic acid (KIC) reduces signs and symptoms of exercise-induced muscle damage in man. *Int. J. Sport Nutr. Exerc. Metab.* 15, 413–424 (2005).

18. Isenmann, E., Trittel, L. & Diel, P. The effects of alpha lipoic acid on muscle strength recovery after a single and a short-term chronic supplementation - a study in healthy well-trained individuals after intensive resistance and endurance training. *J. Int. Soc. Sports Nutr.* 17, 1–13 (2020).

19. Cornish, S. M. C. & Chilibeck, P. D. C. Alpha-linolenic acid supplementation and resistance training in older adults. *Appl. Physiol. Nutr. Metab.* (2009).

20. King, D. S. *et al.* Effect of oral androstenedione on serum testosterone and adaptations to resistance training in young men: A randomized controlled trial. *JAMA* 281, 2020–2028 (1999).

21. Leder, B. Z. *et al.* Oral androstenedione administration and serum testosterone concentrations in young men. *JAMA* 283, (2000).

22. Pang, Q. *et al.* The effect of androstenedione supplementation on testosterone, estradiol, body composition, and lipid profile: a systematic review and meta-analysis of randomized controlled trials. *Hormones* 21, 545–554 (2022).

23. Catlin, D. H. *et al.* Trace contamination of over-the-counter androstenedione and positive urine test results for a nandrolone metabolite. *JAMA* 284, (2000).

24. Collier, S. R., Casey, D. P. & Kanaley, J. A. Growth hormone responses to varying doses of oral arginine. *Growth Horm. IGF Res.* 15, (2005).

25. Isidori, A., Lo Monaco, A. & Cappa, M. A study of growth hormone release in man after oral administration of amino acids. *Curr. Med. Res. Opin.* 7, (1981).

26. Marcell, T. J. *et al.* Oral arginine does not stimulate basal or augment exercise-induced GH secretion in either young or old adults. *J. Gerontol. A Biol. Sci. Med. Sci.* 54, (1999).

27. Fahs, C. A., Heffernan, K. S. & Fernhall, B. Hemodynamic and vascular response to resistance exercise with L-arginine. *Med. Sci. Sports Exerc.* 41, (2009).

28. Willoughby, D. S., Boucher, T., Reid, J., Skelton, G. & Clark, M. Effects of 7 days of arginine-alpha-ketoglutarate supplementation on blood flow, plasma L-arginine, nitric oxide metabolites, and asymmetric dimethyl arginine after resistance exercise. *Int. J. Sport Nutr. Exerc. Metab.* 21, (2011).

29. Schwedhelm, E. *et al.* Pharmacokinetic and pharmacodynamic properties of oral L-citrulline and L-arginine: impact on nitric oxide metabolism. *Br. J. Clin. Pharmacol.* 65, (2008).

30. Böger, R. H. *et al.* Restoring vascular nitric oxide formation by L-arginine improves the symptoms of intermittent claudication in patients with peripheral arterial occlusive disease. *J. Am. Coll. Cardiol.* 32, (1998).

31. Stout, J. R. *et al.* Effects of beta-alanine supplementation on the onset of neuromuscular fatigue and ventilatory threshold in women. *Amino Acids* 32, (2007).

32. Hoffman, J. R. *et al.* Short-duration beta-alanine supplementation increases training volume and reduces subjective feelings of fatigue in college football players. *Nutr. Res.* 28, (2008).

33. Zoeller, R. F., Stout, J. R., O'Kroy, J. A., Torok, D. J. & Mielke, M. Effects of 28 days of beta-alanine and creatine monohydrate supplementation on aerobic power, ventilatory and lactate thresholds, and time to exhaustion. *Amino Acids* 33, 505–510 (2006).

34. Saunders, B. *et al.* β-alanine supplementation to improve exercise capacity and performance: a systematic review and meta-analysis. *Br. J. Sports Med.* 51, (2017).

35. Yavari, A., Javadi, M., Mirmiran, P. & Bahadoran, Z. Exercise-induced oxidative stress and dietary antioxidants. *Asian J. Sports Med.* 6, (2015).

36. Sumida, S., Doi, T., Sakurai, M., Yoshioka, Y. & Okamura, K. Effect of a single bout of exercise and beta-carotene supplementation on the urinary excretion of 8-hydroxy-deoxyguanosine in humans. *Free Radic. Res.* 27, (1997).

37. Jówko, E. *et al.* Creatine and beta-hydroxy-beta-methylbutyrate (HMB) additively increase lean body mass and muscle strength during a weight-training program. *Nutrition* 17, 558–566 (2001).

38. Kraemer, W. J. *et al.* Effects of amino acids supplement on physiological adaptations to resistance training. *Med. Sci. Sports Exerc.* 41, (2009).

39. Gallagher, P. M., Carrithers, J. A., Godard, M. P., Schulze, K. E. & Trappe, S. W. Beta-hydroxy-beta-methylbutyrate ingestion, Part I: Effects on strength and fat free mass. *Med. Sci. Sports Exerc.* 32, (2000).

40. Jakubowski, J. S. *et al.* Supplementation with the Leucine Metabolite β-hydroxy-β-methylbutyrate (HMB) does not Improve Resistance Exercise-Induced Changes in Body Composition or Strength in Young Subjects: A Systematic Review and Meta-Analysis. *Nutrients* 12, (2020).

41. Lin, Z., Zhao, A. & He, J. Effect of β-hydroxy-β-methylbutyrate (HMB) on the muscle strength in the elderly population: A meta-analysis. *Frontiers in Nutrition* 9, (2022).

42. Phillips, S. M., Lau, K. J., D'Souza, A. C. & Nunes, E. A. An umbrella review of systematic reviews of β-hydroxy-β-methyl butyrate supplementation in ageing and clinical practice. *J. Cachexia Sarcopenia Muscle* 13, 2265–2275 (2022).

43. Na, C. R., Mm, A. G., de Almeida D, O. & Araujo, E. M. Q. Effects of beta-hydroxy-beta-methylbutyrate supplementation on elderly body composition and muscle strength: A review of clinical trials. *Ann. Nutr. Metab.* 77, (2021).

44. Wu, H. *et al.* Effect of beta-hydroxy-beta-methylbutyrate supplementation on muscle loss in older adults: a systematic review and meta-analysis. *Arch. Gerontol. Geriatr.* 61, (2015).

45. Wolfe, R. R. Branched-chain amino acids and muscle protein synthesis in humans: myth or reality? *J. Int. Soc. Sports Nutr.* 14, 1–7 (2017).

46. Kaspy, M. S., Hannaian, S. J., Bell, Z. W. & Churchward-Venne, T. A. The effects of branched-chain amino acids on muscle protein synthesis, muscle protein breakdown and associated molecular signalling responses in humans: an update. *Nutr. Res. Rev.* 1–14 (2023).

47. Kerksick, C. M. *et al.* The effects of protein and amino acid supplementation on performance and training adaptations during ten weeks of resistance training. *J. Strength Cond. Res.* 20, (2006).

48. Gualano, A. B. *et al.* Branched-chain amino acids supplementation enhances exercise capacity and lipid oxidation during endurance exercise after muscle glycogen depletion. *J. Sports Med. Phys. Fitness* 51, (2011).

49. Blomstrand, E., Hassmén, P., Ek, S., Ekblom, B. & Newsholme, E. A. Influence of ingesting a solution of branched-chain amino acids on perceived exertion during exercise. *Acta Physiol. Scand.* 159, (1997).

50. Wiśnik, P., Chmura, J., Ziemba, A. W., Mikulski, T. & Nazar, K. The effect of branched chain amino acids on psychomotor performance during treadmill exercise of changing intensity simulating a soccer game. *Appl. Physiol. Nutr. Metab.* 36, (2011).

51. Walker, A. F., Bundy, R., Hicks, S. M. & Middleton, R. W. Bromelain reduces mild acute knee pain and improves well-being in a dose-dependent fashion in an open study of otherwise healthy adults. *Phytomedicine* 9, (2002).

52. Faramarzi, M., Sadighi, M., Shirmohamadi, A., Kazemi, R. & Zohdi, M. Effectiveness of Bromelain in the control of postoperative pain after periodontal surgery: A crossover randomized clinical trial. *J. Adv. Periodontol. Implant. Dent.* 15, (2023).

53. Grgic, J. *et al.* Wake up and smell the coffee: caffeine supplementation and exercise performance—an umbrella review of 21 published meta-analyses. *Br. J. Sports Med.* 54, 681–688 (2020).

54. Guest, N. S. *et al.* International society of sports nutrition position stand: caffeine and exercise performance. *J. Int. Soc. Sports Nutr.* 18, 1–37 (2021).

55. Martins, G. L., Guilherme, J. P. L., Ferreira, L. H. B., de Souza-Junior, T. P. & Lancha, A. H., Jr. Caffeine and exercise performance: Possible directions for definitive findings. *Front. Sports Act. Living* 2, (2020).

56. Acheson, K. J. *et al.* Metabolic effects of caffeine in humans: lipid oxidation or futile cycling? *Am. J. Clin. Nutr.* 79, 40–46 (2004).

57. Dulloo, A. G., Geissler, C. A., Horton, T., Collins, A. & Miller, D. S. Normal caffeine consumption: influence on thermogenesis and daily energy expenditure in lean and postobese human volunteers. *Am. J. Clin. Nutr.* 49, (1989).

58. Astrup, A. *et al.* Caffeine: a double-blind, placebo-controlled study of its thermogenic, metabolic, and cardiovascular effects in healthy volunteers. *Am. J. Clin. Nutr.* 51, (1990).

59. Yoshioka, M. *et al.* Maximum tolerable dose of red pepper decreases fat intake independently of spicy sensation in the mouth. *Br. J. Nutr.* 91, (2004).

60. Ludy, M.-J., Moore, G. E. & Mattes, R. D. The effects of capsaicin and capsiate on energy balance: critical review and meta-analyses of studies in humans. *Chem. Senses* 37, 103–121 (2012).

61. Grgic, J. *et al.* Effects of capsaicin and capsiate on endurance performance: A meta-analysis. *Nutrients* 14, (2022).

62. Conrado de Freitas, M. *et al.* Acute capsaicin supplementation improves resistance training performance in trained men. *J. Strength Cond. Res.* 32, 2227–2232 (2018).

63. Boirie, Y. *et al.* Slow and fast dietary proteins differently modulate postprandial protein accretion. *Proc. Natl. Acad. Sci. U. S. A.* 94, (1997).

64. Wilborn, C. D. *et al.* The effects of pre- and post-exercise whey vs. casein protein consumption on body composition and performance measures in collegiate female athletes. *J. Sports Sci. Med.* 12, 74 (2013).

65. Huang, H., Liao, D., Zou, Y. & Chi, H. The effects of chitosan supplementation on body weight and body composition: a systematic review and meta-analysis of randomized controlled trials. *Crit. Rev. Food Sci. Nutr.* 60, (2020).

66. Zhu, X., Sang, L., Wu, D., Rong, J. & Jiang, L. Effectiveness and safety of glucosamine and chondroitin for the treatment of osteoarthritis: a meta-analysis of randomized controlled trials. *J. Orthop. Surg. Res.* 13, (2018).

67. Hochberg, M. C. Structure-modifying effects of chondroitin sulfate in knee osteoarthritis: an updated meta-analysis of randomized placebo-controlled trials of 2-year duration. *Osteoarthritis Cartilage* 18 Suppl 1, (2010).

68. Racek, J. *et al.* Influence of chromium-enriched yeast on blood glucose and insulin variables, blood lipids, and markers of oxidative stress in subjects with type 2 diabetes mellitus. *Biol. Trace Elem. Res.* 109, (2006).

69. Frauchiger, M. T., Wenk, C. & Colombani, P. C. Effects of acute chromium supplementation on postprandial metabolism in healthy young men. *J. Am. Coll. Nutr.* 23, (2004).

70. Suksomboon, N., Poolsup, N. & Yuwanakorn, A. Systematic review and meta-analysis of the efficacy and safety of chromium supplementation in diabetes. *J. Clin. Pharm. Ther.* 39, 292–306 (2014).

71. Zhao, F. *et al.* Effect of chromium supplementation on blood glucose and lipid levels in patients with type 2 diabetes mellitus: A systematic review and meta-analysis. *Biol. Trace Elem. Res.* 200, 516–525 (2021).

72. Tian, H. *et al.* Chromium picolinate supplementation for overweight or obese adults. *Cochrane Database Syst. Rev.* 2013, (2013).

73. Gambelunghe, C. *et al.* Effects of chrysin on urinary testosterone levels in human males. *J. Med. Food* 6, (2003).

74. Hwang, P. *et al.* Eight weeks of resistance training in conjunction with glutathione and L-Citrulline supplementation increases lean mass and has no adverse effects on blood clinical safety markers in resistance-trained males. *J. Int. Soc. Sports Nutr.* 15, (2018).

75. Trexler, E. T. *et al.* Acute effects of citrulline supplementation on high-intensity strength and power performance: A systematic review and meta-analysis. *Sports Med.* 49, (2019).

76. Gonzalez, A. M., Spitz, R. W., Ghigiarelli, J. J., Sell, K. M. & Mangine, G. T. Acute effect of citrulline malate supplementation on upper-body resistance exercise performance in recreationally resistance-trained men. *J. Strength Cond. Res.* 32, (2018).

77. Bailey, S. J. *et al.* l-Citrulline supplementation improves O_2 uptake kinetics and high-intensity exercise performance in humans. *J. Appl. Physiol.* 119, (2015).

78. Suzuki, T., Morita, M., Kobayashi, Y. & Kamimura, A. Oral L-citrulline supplementation enhances cycling time trial performance in healthy trained men: Double-blind randomized placebo-controlled 2-way crossover study. *J. Int. Soc. Sports Nutr.* 13, (2016).

79. Stohs, S. J. *et al.* Effects of p-synephrine alone and in combination with selected bioflavonoids on resting metabolism, blood pressure, heart rate and self-reported mood changes. *Int. J. Med. Sci.* 8, (2011).

80. Greenway, F. *et al.* Dietary herbal supplements with phenylephrine for weight loss. *J. Med. Food* 9, (2006).

81. Gutiérrez-Hellín, J. *et al.* Acute consumption of p-synephrine does not enhance performance in sprint athletes. *Appl. Physiol. Nutr. Metab.* 41, (2016).

82. Koncz, D., Tóth, B., Bahar, M. A., Roza, O. & Csupor, D. The safety and efficacy of citrus aurantium (bitter orange) extracts and p-synephrine: A systematic review and meta-analysis. *Nutrients* 14, (2022).

83. Lei, L. & Liu, Y. Efficacy of coenzyme Q10 in patients with cardiac failure: a meta-analysis of clinical trials. *BMC Cardiovasc. Disord.* 17, (2017).

84. Dahri, M., Tarighat-Esfanjani, A., Asghari-Jafarabadi, M. & Hashemilar, M. Oral coenzyme Q10 supplementation in patients with migraine: Effects on clinical features and inflammatory markers. *Nutr. Neurosci.* 22, (2019).

85. Shoeibi, A. *et al.* Effectiveness of coenzyme Q10 in prophylactic treatment of migraine headache: an open-label, add-on, controlled trial. *Acta Neurol. Belg.* 117, (2017).

86. Onakpoya, I. J., Posadzki, P. P., Watson, L. K., Davies, L. A. & Ernst, E. The efficacy of long-term conjugated linoleic acid (CLA) supplementation on body composition in overweight and obese individuals: a systematic review and meta-analysis of randomized clinical trials. *Eur. J. Nutr.* 51, (2012).

87. Namazi, N., Irandoost, P., Larijani, B. & Azadbakht, L. The effects of supplementation with conjugated linoleic acid on anthropometric indices and body composition in overweight and obese subjects: A systematic review and meta-analysis. *Crit. Rev. Food Sci. Nutr.* 59, 2720–2733 (2019).

88. Kreider, R. B. *et al.* International Society of Sports Nutrition position stand: safety and efficacy of creatine supplementation in exercise, sport, and medicine. *J. Int. Soc. Sports Nutr.* 14, 1–18 (2017).

89. Burke, R. *et al.* The effects of creatine supplementation combined with resistance training on regional measures of muscle hypertrophy: A systematic review with meta-analysis. *Nutrients* 15, (2023).

90. Wu, S.-H. *et al.* Creatine supplementation for muscle growth: A scoping review of randomized clinical trials from 2012 to 2021. *Nutrients* 14, (2022).

91. Brustovetsky, N., Brustovetsky, T. & Dubinsky, J. M. On the mechanisms of neuroprotection by creatine and phosphocreatine. *J. Neurochem.* 76, (2001).

92. Xin, G. & Eshaghi, H. Effect of omega-3 fatty acids supplementation on indirect blood markers of exercise-induced muscle damage: Systematic review and meta-analysis of randomized controlled trials. *Food Sci. Nutr.* 9, 6429 (2021).

93. Jakeman, J. R., Lambrick, D. M., Wooley, B., Babraj, J. A. & Faulkner, J. A. Effect of an acute dose of omega-3 fish oil following exercise-induced muscle damage. *Eur. J. Appl. Physiol.* 117, 575–582 (2017).

94. Wang, T. *et al.* Association between omega-3 fatty acid intake and dyslipidemia: A continuous dose-response meta-analysis of randomized controlled trials. *J. Am. Heart Assoc.* 12, (2023).

95. Li, Y. *et al.* A dose-response and meta-analysis of dehydroepiandrosterone (DHEA) supplementation on testosterone levels: perinatal prediction of randomized clinical trials. *Exp. Gerontol.* 141, (2020).

96. Merritt, P., Stangl, B., Hirshman, E. & Verbalis, J. Administration of dehydroepiandrosterone (DHEA) increases serum levels of androgens and estrogens but does not enhance short-term memory in post-menopausal women. *Brain Res.* 1483, (2012).

97. Baker, W. L., Karan, S. & Kenny, A. M. Effect of dehydroepiandrosterone on muscle strength and physical function in older adults: a systematic review. *J. Am. Geriatr. Soc.* 59, (2011).

98. Dulloo, A. G. & Miller, D. S. The thermogenic properties of ephedrine/methylxanthine mixtures: human studies. *Int. J. Obes.* 10, (1986).

99. Pasquali, R. *et al.* Effects of chronic administration of ephedrine during very-low-calorie diets on energy expenditure, protein metabolism and hormone levels in obese subjects. *Clin. Sci.* 82, (1992).

100. Molnár, D. Effects of ephedrine and aminophylline on resting energy expenditure in obese adolescents. *Int. J. Obes. Relat. Metab. Disord.* 17 Suppl 1, (1993).

101. Hackman, R. M. *et al.* Multinutrient supplement containing ephedra and caffeine causes weight loss and improves metabolic risk factors in obese women: a randomized controlled trial. *Int. J. Obes.* 30, (2006).

102. Pasquali, R. *et al.* Does ephedrine promote weight loss in low-energy-adapted obese women? *Int. J. Obes.* 11, (1987).

103. Boozer, C. N. *et al.* Herbal ephedra/caffeine for weight loss: a 6-month randomized safety and efficacy trial. *Int. J. Obes. Relat. Metab. Disord.* 26, (2002).

104. Magkos, F. & Kavouras, S. A. Caffeine and ephedrine: physiological, metabolic and performance-enhancing effects. *Sports Med.* 34, (2004).

105. Williams, A. D., Cribb, P. J., Cooke, M. B. & Hayes, A. The effect of ephedra and caffeine on maximal strength and power in resistance-trained athletes. *J. Strength Cond. Res.* 22, (2008).

106. Bell, D. G., Jacobs, I. & Ellerington, K. Effect of caffeine and ephedrine ingestion on anaerobic exercise performance. *Med. Sci. Sports Exerc.* 33, (2001).

107. Andraws, R., Chawla, P. & Brown, D. L. Cardiovascular effects of ephedra alkaloids: a comprehensive review. *Prog. Cardiovasc. Dis.* 47, (2005).

108. Ihl, R., Tribanek, M. & Bachinskaya, N. Efficacy and tolerability of a once daily formulation of Ginkgo biloba extract EGb 761® in Alzheimer's disease and vascular dementia: results from a randomised controlled trial. *Pharmacopsychiatry* 45, (2012).

109. Napryeyenko, O. & Borzenko, I. Ginkgo biloba special extract in dementia with neuropsychiatric features. A randomised, placebo-controlled, double-blind clinical trial. *Arzneimittelforschung* 57, (2007).

110. Wesnes, K., Simmons, D., Rook, M. & Simpson, P. A double-blind placebo-controlled trial of tanakan in the treatment of idiopathic cognitive impairment in the elderly. *Hum. Psychopharmacol.* 2, 159–169 (1987).

111. Snitz, B. E. *et al.* Ginkgo biloba for preventing cognitive decline in older adults: a randomized trial. *JAMA* 302, (2009).

112. Vlad, S. C., LaValley, M. P., McAlindon, T. E. & Felson, D. T. Glucosamine for pain in osteoarthritis: why do trial results differ? *Arthritis Rheum.* 56, (2007).

113. Wangroongsub, Y., Tanavalee, A., Wilairatana, V. & Ngarmukos, S. Comparable clinical outcomes between glucosamine sulfate-potassium chloride and glucosamine sulfate sodium chloride in patients with mild and moderate knee osteoarthritis: a randomized, double-blind study. *J. Med. Assoc. Thai.* 93, (2010).

114. Clegg, D. O. *et al.* Glucosamine, chondroitin sulfate, and the two in combination for painful knee osteoarthritis. *N. Engl. J. Med.* 354, (2006).

115. Castell, L. M. & Newsholme, E. A. Glutamine and the effects of exhaustive exercise upon the immune response. *Can. J. Physiol. Pharmacol.* 76, (1998).

116. Castell, L. M., Poortmans, J. R. & Newsholme, E. A. Does glutamine have a role in reducing infections in athletes? *Eur. J. Appl. Physiol. Occup. Physiol.* 73, (1996).

117. Asbaghi, O. *et al.* Effect of green tea on anthropometric indices and body composition in patients with type 2 diabetes mellitus: A systematic review and meta-analysis. *Complement. Med. Res.* 28, (2021).

118. Maki, K. C. *et al.* Green tea catechin consumption enhances exercise-induced abdominal fat loss in overweight and obese adults. *J. Nutr.* 139, (2009).

119. Wang, H. *et al.* Effects of catechin enriched green tea on body composition. *Obesity* 18, (2010).

120. Stendell-Hollis, N. R. *et al.* Green tea improves metabolic biomarkers, not weight or body composition: a pilot study in overweight breast cancer survivors. *J. Hum. Nutr. Diet.* 23, (2010).

121. Mattes, R. D. & Bormann, L. Effects of (-)-hydroxycitric acid on appetitive variables. *Physiol. Behav.* 71, (2000).

122. Özturan, A. *et al.* Effect of inositol and its derivatives on diabetes: a systematic review. *Crit. Rev. Food Sci. Nutr.* 59, (2019).

123. Miñambres, I., Cuixart, G., Gonçalves, A. & Corcoy, R. Effects of inositol on glucose homeostasis: Systematic review and meta-analysis of randomized controlled trials. *Clin. Nutr.* 38, (2019).

124. Unfer, V., Facchinetti, F., Orrù, B., Giordani, B. & Nestler, J. Myo-inositol effects in women with PCOS: a meta-analysis of randomized controlled trials. *Endocr. Connect.* 6, (2017).

125. Wei, J., Yan, J. & Yang, H. Inositol nutritional supplementation for the prevention of gestational diabetes mellitus: A systematic review and meta-analysis of randomized controlled trials. *Nutrients* 14, (2022).

126. Mashayekh-Amiri, S., Mohammad-Alizadeh-Charandabi, S., Abdolalipour, S. & Mirghafourvand, M. Myo-inositol supplementation for prevention of gestational diabetes mellitus in overweight and obese pregnant women: a systematic review and meta-analysis. *Diabetol. Metab. Syndr.* 14, (2022).

127. Motuhifonua, S. K., Lin, L., Alsweiler, J., Crawford, T. J. & Crowther, C. A. Antenatal dietary supplementation with myo-inositol for preventing gestational diabetes. *Cochrane Database Syst. Rev.* 2, (2023).

128. Solberg, A. & Reikvam, H. Iron status and physical performance in athletes. *Life* 13, (2023).

129. Rubeor, A., Goojha, C., Manning, J. & White, J. Does iron supplementation improve performance in iron-deficient nonanemic athletes? *Sports Health* 10, 400 (2018).

130. Šmid, A. N. *et al.* Effects of oral iron supplementation on blood iron status in athletes: A systematic review, meta-analysis and meta-regression of randomized controlled trials. *Sports Med.* 54, 1231–1247 (2024).

131. Porasuphatana, S. *et al.* Glycemic and oxidative status of patients with type 2 diabetes mellitus following oral administration of alpha-lipoic acid: a randomized double-blinded placebo-controlled study. *Asia Pac. J. Clin. Nutr.* 21, (2012).

132. Ziegler, D. *et al.* Efficacy and safety of antioxidant treatment with α-lipoic acid over 4 years in diabetic polyneuropathy: the NATHAN 1 trial. *Diabetes Care* 34, (2011).

133. Koh, E. H. *et al.* Effects of alpha-lipoic Acid on body weight in obese subjects. *Am. J. Med.* 124, (2011).

134. McNeilly, A. M. *et al.* Effect of α-lipoic acid and exercise training on cardiovascular disease risk in obesity with impaired glucose tolerance. *Lipids Health Dis.* 10, (2011).

135. White, M. D., Papamandjaris, A. A. & Jones, P. J. Enhanced postprandial energy expenditure with medium-chain fatty acid feeding is attenuated after 14 d in premenopausal women. *Am. J. Clin. Nutr.* 69, 883–889 (1999).

136. St-Onge, M.-P., Ross, R., Parsons, W. D. & Jones, P. J. H. Medium-chain triglycerides increase energy expenditure and decrease adiposity in overweight men. *Obes. Res.* 11, 395–402 (2003).

137. Mumme, K. & Stonehouse, W. Effects of medium-chain triglycerides on weight loss and body composition: a meta-analysis of randomized controlled trials. *J. Acad. Nutr. Diet.* 115, (2015).

138. Chapman-Lopez, T. J. & Koh, Y. The effects of medium-chain triglyceride oil supplementation on endurance performance and substrate utilization in healthy populations: A systematic review. *J. Obes. Metab. Syndr.* 31, 217 (2022).

139. Clegg, M. E. Medium-chain triglycerides are advantageous in promoting weight loss although not beneficial to exercise performance. *Int. J. Food Sci. Nutr.* 61, 653–679 (2010).

140. Morrison, M. A., Spriet, L. L. & Dyck, D. J. Pyruvate ingestion for 7 days does not improve aerobic performance in well-trained individuals. *J. Appl. Physiol.* 89, (2000).

141. Stone, M. H. *et al.* Effects of in-season (5 weeks) creatine and pyruvate supplementation on anaerobic performance and body composition in American football players. *Int. J. Sport Nutr.* 9, (1999).

142. Grgic, J., Grgic, I., Del Coso, J., Schoenfeld, B. J. & Pedisic, Z. Effects of sodium bicarbonate supplementation on exercise performance: an umbrella review. *J. Int. Soc. Sports Nutr.* 18, (2021).

143. Edge, J., Bishop, D. & Goodman, C. Effects of chronic NaHCO3 ingestion during interval training on changes to muscle buffer capacity, metabolism, and short-term endurance performance. *J. Appl. Physiol.* 101, (2006).

144. Driller, M. W., Gregory, J. R., Williams, A. D. & Fell, J. W. The effects of serial and acute NaHCO3 loading in well-trained cyclists. *J. Strength Cond. Res.* 26, (2012).

145. Price, M. J. & Simons, C. The effect of sodium bicarbonate ingestion on high-intensity intermittent running and subsequent performance. *J. Strength Cond. Res.* 24, (2010).

146. Del Coso, J. *et al.* Effects of oral salt supplementation on physical performance during a half-ironman: A randomized controlled trial. *Scand. J. Med. Sci. Sports* 26, 156–164 (2016).

147. Earhart, E. L., Weiss, E. P., Rahman, R. & Kelly, P. V. Effects of oral sodium supplementation on indices of thermoregulation in trained, endurance athletes. *J. Sports Sci. Med.* 14, 172 (2015).

148. Waldron, M., Patterson, S. D., Tallent, J. & Jeffries, O. The effects of an oral taurine dose and supplementation period on endurance exercise performance in humans: A meta-analysis. *Sports Med.* 48, (2018).

149. McGurk, K. A., Kasapi, M. & Ware, J. S. Effect of taurine administration on symptoms, severity, or clinical outcome of dilated cardiomyopathy and heart failure in humans: a systematic review. *Wellcome Open Res.* 7, (2022).

150. Sun, Q. *et al.* Taurine supplementation lowers blood pressure and improves vascular function in prehypertension: Randomized, double-blind, placebo-controlled study. *Hypertension* 67, (2016).

151. Cusi, K. *et al.* Vanadyl sulfate improves hepatic and muscle insulin sensitivity in type 2 diabetes. *J. Clin. Endocrinol. Metab.* 86, (2001).

152. Cohen, N. *et al.* Oral vanadyl sulfate improves hepatic and peripheral insulin sensitivity in patients with non-insulin-dependent diabetes mellitus. *J. Clin. Invest.* 95, (1995).

153. Clarkson, P. M. & Rawson, E. S. Nutritional supplements to increase muscle mass. *Crit. Rev. Food Sci. Nutr.* 39, (1999).

154. Kreider, R. B. Dietary supplements and the promotion of muscle growth with resistance exercise. *Sports Med.* 27, (1999).

155. Koehler, K., Parr, M. K., Geyer, H., Mester, J. & Schänzer, W. Serum testosterone and urinary excretion of steroid hormone metabolites after administration of a high-dose zinc supplement. *Eur. J. Clin. Nutr.* 63, (2009).

156. Gallagher, C. *et al.* Effects of supplementing zinc magnesium aspartate on sleep quality and submaximal weightlifting performance, following two consecutive nights of partial sleep deprivation. *Nutrients* 16, (2024).

157. Gholipour, B. A. *et al.* The effect of zinc supplementation on sleep quality of ICU nurses: A double blinded randomized controlled trial. *Workplace Health Saf.* 66, (2018).

APPENDIX E

HANDOUTS

CHAPTER 3

SPORTS MENTAL TOUGHNESS QUESTIONNAIRE (SMTQ)

Please indicate your agreement/disagreement with each of the following statements in relation to your involvement with participation in sports.

1. I can regain my composure if I have momentarily lost it.

   1   2   3   4

   (Not at All True)   (Very True)

2. I worry about performing poorly.

   1   2   3   4

   (Not at All True)   (Very True)

3. I am committed to completing the tasks I have to do.

   1   2   3   4

   (Not at All True)   (Very True)

4. I am overcome by self-doubt.

   1   2   3   4

   (Not at All True)   (Very True)

5. I have an unshakable confidence in my ability.

   1   2   3   4

   (Not at All True)   (Very True)

6. I have what it takes to perform well while under pressure.

   1   2   3   4

   (Not at All True)   (Very True)

7. I get angry and frustrated when things do not go my way.

   1   2   3   4

   (Not at All True)   (Very True)

8. I give up in difficult situations.

   1   2   3   4

   (Not at All True)   (Very True)

9. I get anxious about events I did not expect or cannot control.

   1   2   3   4

   (Not at All True)   (Very True)

10. I get distracted easily and lose my concentration.

    1   2   3   4

    (Not at All True)   (Very True)

11. I have qualities that set me apart from other competitors.

    1   2   3   4

    (Not at All True)   (Very True)

12. I take responsibility for setting myself challenging targets.

    1   2   3   4

    (Not at All True)   (Very True)

13. I view potential threats as positive opportunities.

    1   2   3   4

    (Not at All True)   (Very True)

14. Under pressure, I am able to make decisions with confidence and commitment.

    1   2   3   4

    (Not at All True)   (Very True)

SPORTS ANXIETY SCALE – 2
Reactions to Playing Sports

Many athletes get tense or nervous before or during games, meets, or matches. This happens even to pro athletes. Please read each question. Then, circle the number that says how you USUALLY feel before or while you compete in sports. There are no right or wrong answers. Please be as truthful as you can.

Before or while I compete in sports:	Not at All	A Little	Pretty Much	Very Much
1. It is hard to concentrate on the game.	1	2	3	4
2. My body feels tense.	1	2	3	4
3. I worry that I will not play well.	1	2	3	4
4. It is hard for me to focus on what I am supposed to do.	1	2	3	4
5. I worry that I will let others down.	1	2	3	4
6. I feel tense in my stomach.	1	2	3	4
7. I lose focus on the game.	1	2	3	4
8. I worry that I will not play my best.	1	2	3	4
9. I worry that I will play badly.	1	2	3	4
10. My muscles feel shaky.	1	2	3	4
11. I worry that I will mess up during the game.	1	2	3	4
12. My stomach feels upset.	1	2	3	4
13. I cannot think clearly during the game.	1	2	3	4
14. My muscles feel tight because I am nervous.	1	2	3	4
15. I have a hard time focusing on what my coach tells me.	1	2	3	4

Adapted from Smith et al. (2006).

SCORING

To calculate your score, add up all the numbers that were circled, then combine them using the following categories to get a score for each of the scales. Add up all results for the Trait Anxiety Score.

- **Somatic Score:** Add up questions 2, 6, 10, 12, 14
- **Worry Score:** Add up questions 3, 5, 8, 9, 11
- **Concentration Disruption:** 1, 4, 7, 13, 15

CHAPTER 7

2023 PAR-Q+

The Physical Activity Readiness Questionnaire for Everyone

The health benefits of regular physical activity are clear; more people should engage in physical activity every day of the week. Participating in physical activity is very safe for MOST people. This questionnaire will tell you whether it is necessary for you to seek further advice from your doctor OR a qualified exercise professional before becoming more physically active.

GENERAL HEALTH QUESTIONS

Please read the 7 questions below carefully and answer each one honestly: check YES or NO.	YES	NO
1) Has your doctor ever said that you have a heart condition ☐ OR high blood pressure ☐?	☐	☐
2) Do you feel pain in your chest at rest, during your daily activities of living, OR when you do physical activity?	☐	☐
3) Do you lose balance because of dizziness OR have you lost consciousness in the last 12 months? Please answer NO if your dizziness was associated with over-breathing (including during vigorous exercise).	☐	☐
4) Have you ever been diagnosed with another chronic medical condition (other than heart disease or high blood pressure)? PLEASE LIST CONDITION(S) HERE: _____	☐	☐
5) Are you currently taking prescribed medications for a chronic medical condition? PLEASE LIST CONDITION(S) AND MEDICATIONS HERE: _____	☐	☐
6) Do you currently have (or have had within the past 12 months) a bone, joint, or soft tissue (muscle, ligament, or tendon) problem that could be made worse by becoming more physically active? Please answer NO if you had a problem in the past, but it does not limit your current ability to be physically active. PLEASE LIST CONDITION(S) HERE: _____	☐	☐
7) Has your doctor ever said that you should only do medically supervised physical activity?	☐	☐

☑ **If you answered NO to all of the questions above, you are cleared for physical activity.**
Please sign the PARTICIPANT DECLARATION. You do not need to complete Pages 2 and 3.

▶ Start becoming much more physically active – start slowly and build up gradually.

▶ Follow Global Physical Activity Guidelines for your age (https://www.who.int/publications/i/item/9789240015128).

▶ You may take part in a health and fitness appraisal.

▶ If you are over the age of 45 yr and NOT accustomed to regular vigorous to maximal effort exercise, consult a qualified exercise professional before engaging in this intensity of exercise.

▶ If you have any further questions, contact a qualified exercise professional.

PARTICIPANT DECLARATION

If you are less than the legal age required for consent or require the assent of a care provider, your parent, guardian or care provider must also sign this form.

I, the undersigned, have read, understood to my full satisfaction and completed this questionnaire. I acknowledge that this physical activity clearance is valid for a maximum of 12 months from the date it is completed and becomes invalid if my condition changes. I also acknowledge that the community/fitness center may retain a copy of this form for its records. In these instances, it will maintain the confidentiality of the same, complying with applicable law.

NAME _____ DATE _____

SIGNATURE _____ WITNESS _____

SIGNATURE OF PARENT/GUARDIAN/CARE PROVIDER _____

🔴 **If you answered YES to one or more of the questions above, COMPLETE PAGES 2 AND 3.**

⚠️ **Delay becoming more active if:**

✓ You have a temporary illness such as a cold or fever; it is best to wait until you feel better.

✓ You are pregnant - talk to your health care practitioner, your physician, a qualified exercise professional, and/or complete the ePARmed-X+ at www.eparmedx.com before becoming more physically active.

✓ Your health changes - answer the questions on Pages 2 and 3 of this document and/or talk to your doctor or a qualified exercise professional before continuing with any physical activity program.

2023 PAR-Q+

FOLLOW-UP QUESTIONS ABOUT YOUR MEDICAL CONDITION(S)

1. Do you have Arthritis, Osteoporosis, or Back Problems?

If the above condition(s) is/are present, answer questions 1a-1c   If **NO** ☐ go to question 2

1a. Do you have difficulty controlling your condition with medications or other physician-prescribed therapies? (Answer **NO** if you are not currently taking medications or other treatments)   YES ☐ NO ☐

1b. Do you have joint problems causing pain, a recent fracture or fracture caused by osteoporosis or cancer, displaced vertebra (e.g., spondylolisthesis), and/or spondylolysis/pars defect (a crack in the bony ring on the back of the spinal column)?   YES ☐ NO ☐

1c. Have you had steroid injections or taken steroid tablets regularly for more than 3 months?   YES ☐ NO ☐

2. Do you currently have Cancer of any kind?

If the above condition(s) is/are present, answer questions 2a-2b   If **NO** ☐ go to question 3

2a. Does your cancer diagnosis include any of the following types: lung/bronchogenic, multiple myeloma (cancer of plasma cells), head, and/or neck?   YES ☐ NO ☐

2b. Are you currently receiving cancer therapy (such as chemotheraphy or radiotherapy)?   YES ☐ NO ☐

3. Do you have a Heart or Cardiovascular Condition? This includes Coronary Artery Disease, Heart Failure, Diagnosed Abnormality of Heart Rhythm

If the above condition(s) is/are present, answer questions 3a-3d   If **NO** ☐ go to question 4

3a. Do you have difficulty controlling your condition with medications or other physician-prescribed therapies? (Answer **NO** if you are not currently taking medications or other treatments)   YES ☐ NO ☐

3b. Do you have an irregular heart beat that requires medical management? (e.g., atrial fibrillation, premature ventricular contraction)   YES ☐ NO ☐

3c. Do you have chronic heart failure?   YES ☐ NO ☐

3d. Do you have diagnosed coronary artery (cardiovascular) disease and have not participated in regular physical activity in the last 2 months?   YES ☐ NO ☐

4. Do you currently have High Blood Pressure?

If the above condition(s) is/are present, answer questions 4a-4b   If **NO** ☐ go to question 5

4a. Do you have difficulty controlling your condition with medications or other physician-prescribed therapies? (Answer **NO** if you are not currently taking medications or other treatments)   YES ☐ NO ☐

4b. Do you have a resting blood pressure equal to or greater than 160/90 mmHg with or without medication? (Answer **YES** if you do not know your resting blood pressure)   YES ☐ NO ☐

5. Do you have any Metabolic Conditions? This includes Type 1 Diabetes, Type 2 Diabetes, Pre-Diabetes

If the above condition(s) is/are present, answer questions 5a-5e   If **NO** ☐ go to question 6

5a. Do you often have difficulty controlling your blood sugar levels with foods, medications, or other physician-prescribed therapies?   YES ☐ NO ☐

5b. Do you often suffer from signs and symptoms of low blood sugar (hypoglycemia) following exercise and/or during activities of daily living? Signs of hypoglycemia may include shakiness, nervousness, unusual irritability, abnormal sweating, dizziness or light-headedness, mental confusion, difficulty speaking, weakness, or sleepiness.   YES ☐ NO ☐

5c. Do you have any signs or symptoms of diabetes complications such as heart or vascular disease and/or complications affecting your eyes, kidneys, **OR** the sensation in your toes and feet?   YES ☐ NO ☐

5d. Do you have other metabolic conditions (such as current pregnancy-related diabetes, chronic kidney disease, or liver problems)?   YES ☐ NO ☐

5e. Are you planning to engage in what for you is unusually high (or vigorous) intensity exercise in the near future?   YES ☐ NO ☐

2023 PAR-Q+

6. **Do you have any Mental Health Problems or Learning Difficulties?** This includes Alzheimer's, Dementia, Depression, Anxiety Disorder, Eating Disorder, Psychotic Disorder, Intellectual Disability, Down Syndrome

If the above condition(s) is/are present, answer questions 6a-6b   If **NO** ☐ go to question 7

6a.	Do you have difficulty controlling your condition with medications or other physician-prescribed therapies? (Answer **NO** if you are not currently taking medications or other treatments)	YES ☐	NO ☐
6b.	Do you have Down Syndrome **AND** back problems affecting nerves or muscles?	YES ☐	NO ☐

7. **Do you have a Respiratory Disease?** This includes Chronic Obstructive Pulmonary Disease, Asthma, Pulmonary High Blood Pressure

If the above condition(s) is/are present, answer questions 7a-7d   If **NO** ☐ go to question 8

7a.	Do you have difficulty controlling your condition with medications or other physician-prescribed therapies? (Answer **NO** if you are not currently taking medications or other treatments)	YES ☐	NO ☐
7b.	Has your doctor ever said your blood oxygen level is low at rest or during exercise and/or that you require supplemental oxygen therapy?	YES ☐	NO ☐
7c.	If asthmatic, do you currently have symptoms of chest tightness, wheezing, laboured breathing, consistent cough (more than 2 days/week), or have you used your rescue medication more than twice in the last week?	YES ☐	NO ☐
7d.	Has your doctor ever said you have high blood pressure in the blood vessels of your lungs?	YES ☐	NO ☐

8. **Do you have a Spinal Cord Injury?** This includes Tetraplegia and Paraplegia

If the above condition(s) is/are present, answer questions 8a-8c   If **NO** ☐ go to question 9

8a.	Do you have difficulty controlling your condition with medications or other physician-prescribed therapies? (Answer **NO** if you are not currently taking medications or other treatments)	YES ☐	NO ☐
8b.	Do you commonly exhibit low resting blood pressure significant enough to cause dizziness, light-headedness, and/or fainting?	YES ☐	NO ☐
8c.	Has your physician indicated that you exhibit sudden bouts of high blood pressure (known as Autonomic Dysreflexia)?	YES ☐	NO ☐

9. **Have you had a Stroke?** This includes Transient Ischemic Attack (TIA) or Cerebrovascular Event

If the above condition(s) is/are present, answer questions 9a-9c   If **NO** ☐ go to question 10

9a.	Do you have difficulty controlling your condition with medications or other physician-prescribed therapies? (Answer **NO** if you are not currently taking medications or other treatments)	YES ☐	NO ☐
9b.	Do you have any impairment in walking or mobility?	YES ☐	NO ☐
9c.	Have you experienced a stroke or impairment in nerves or muscles in the past 6 months?	YES ☐	NO ☐

10. **Do you have any other medical condition not listed above or do you have two or more medical conditions?**

If you have other medical conditions, answer questions 10a-10c   If **NO** ☐ read the Page 4 recommendations

10a.	Have you experienced a blackout, fainted, or lost consciousness as a result of a head injury within the last 12 months **OR** have you had a diagnosed concussion within the last 12 months?	YES ☐	NO ☐
10b.	Do you have a medical condition that is not listed (such as epilepsy, neurological conditions, kidney problems)?	YES ☐	NO ☐
10c.	Do you currently live with two or more medical conditions?	YES ☐	NO ☐

PLEASE LIST YOUR MEDICAL CONDITION(S) AND ANY RELATED MEDICATIONS HERE: _____

_____

GO to Page 4 for recommendations about your current medical condition(s) and sign the PARTICIPANT DECLARATION.

Copyright © 2023 PAR-Q+ Collaboration   3/ 4
01-11-2022

2023 PAR-Q+

ENERGY DEMANDS OF SPORTS

Sport	Phosphagen System	Glycolytic System	Aerobic System
American football	High	Moderate	Low
Archery	High	Low	—
Baseball	High	Low	—
Basketball	High	Moderate to high	Low
Boxing	High	High	Moderate
Diving	High	Low	—
Fencing	High	Moderate	—
Field events (athletics)	High	—	—
Field hockey	High	Moderate	Moderate
Golf	High	—	Moderate
Gymnastics	High	Moderate	—
Ice hockey	High	Moderate	Moderate
Lacrosse	High	Moderate	Moderate
Marathon running	Low	Low	High
Mixed martial arts	High	High	Moderate
Powerlifting	High	Low	—
Rowing	Low	Moderate	High
Skiing:			
Cross-country	Low	Low	High
Downhill	High	High	Moderate
Soccer (football)	High	Moderate	Moderate
Strongman	High	Moderate to high	Low
Swimming:			
Short distance	High	Moderate	—
Long distance	Low	Moderate	High
Tennis	High	Moderate	Low

(continues)

(*continued*)

Sport	Phosphagen System	Glycolytic System	Aerobic System
Track (athletics):			
Sprints	High	Moderate	—
Middle distance	High	High	Moderate
Long distance	—	Moderate	High
Ultra-endurance	—	—	High
Volleyball	High	Moderate	—
Weightlifting	High	High	Moderate
Wrestling	High	Moderate	Low

OVERHEAD SQUAT ASSESSMENT OBSERVATIONAL FINDINGS RECORDING TEMPLATE

Checkpoint	Viewpoint	Movement Impairment	Result
Foot and ankle	Anterior	• Feet turn out	☐ Right ☐ Left ☐ Both
	Lateral	• Heel rise	☐ Right ☐ Left ☐ Both
	Posterior	• Excessive pronation	☐ Right ☐ Left ☐ Both
Knee	Anterior	• Valgus	☐ Right ☐ Left ☐ Both
		• Varus	☐ Right ☐ Left ☐ Both
	Lateral	• Knee dominance	☐ Right ☐ Left ☐ Both
Lumbo-pelvic-hip complex	Anterior or posterior	• Asymmetric weight shift	☐ Right ☐ Left
	Lateral	• Excessive anterior pelvic tilt	☐ Yes ☐ No
		• Excessive posterior pelvic tilt	☐ Yes ☐ No
		• Excessive forward trunk lean	☐ Yes ☐ No
Shoulders and thoracic spine	Anterior or posterior	• Scapular elevation	☐ Right ☐ Left ☐ Both
	Lateral	• Arms fall forward	☐ Right ☐ Left ☐ Both
Head and cervical spine	Lateral	• Excessive cervical extension/forward head	☐ Yes ☐ No

Right/Left/Both refers to the stance or forward leg when the impairment occurs. Mark ***Right*** or ***Left*** or ***Both*** based on the limb for which a movement impairment was observed. For asymmetric weight shift, mark the direction in which the shift occurred.

Checkpoint	Viewpoint	Movement Impairment	Result
MODIFICATIONS			
Heels elevated	Squat performance improves?	☐ Yes ☐ No	
Hands on hips	Squat performance improves?	☐ Yes ☐ No	

SINGLE-LEG SQUAT ASSESSMENT AND SPLIT SQUAT OBSERVATIONAL RECORDING TEMPLATE

Checkpoint	Viewpoint	Movement Impairment	Result
Foot and ankle	**Lateral**	• Heel rise	☐ Right ☐ Left ☐ Both
	Posterior	• Excessive pronation	☐ Right ☐ Left ☐ Both
Knee	**Anterior**	• Valgus	☐ Right ☐ Left ☐ Both
		• Varus	☐ Right ☐ Left ☐ Both
	Lateral	• Knee dominance	☐ Right ☐ Left ☐ Both
Lumbo-pelvic-hip complex	**Anterior**	• Asymmetric weight shift	☐ Right ☐ Left
		• Inward trunk rotation	☐ Right ☐ Left ☐ Both
		• Outward trunk rotation	☐ Right ☐ Left ☐ Both
	Lateral	• Excessive anterior rotation	☐ Yes ☐ No
		• Excessive posterior pelvic tilt	☐ Yes ☐ No
		• Excessive forward trunk lean	☐ Yes ☐ No

Right/Left/Both refers to the stance or forward leg when the impairment occurs. Mark *Right* or *Left* or *Both* based on the limb for which a movement impairment was observed. For asymmetric weight shift, mark the direction to which the shift occurs.

SPLIT SQUAT JUMP ASSESSMENT OBSERVATIONAL FINDINGS RECORDING TEMPLATE

Checkpoint	Viewpoint	Movement Impairment	Results
Foot and ankle	Lateral	• Heel rise (front foot)	☐ Right ☐ Left ☐ Both
	Posterior	• Excessive pronation	☐ Right ☐ Left ☐ Both
Knee	Anterior	• Valgus	☐ Right ☐ Left ☐ Both
		• Varus	☐ Right ☐ Left ☐ Both
	Lateral	• Knee dominance (front knee)	☐ Right ☐ Left ☐ Both
Lumbo-pelvic-hip complex	Anterior	• Asymmetric weight shift	☐ Right ☐ Left
		• Inward trunk rotation	☐ Right ☐ Left
		• Outward trunk rotation	☐ Right ☐ Left
	Lateral	• Excessive anterior pelvic tilt	☐ Yes ☐ No
		• Excessive posterior pelvic tilt	☐ Yes ☐ No
		• Excessive forward trunk lean	☐ Yes ☐ No

STAR EXCURSION BALANCE TEST OBSERVATIONAL RECORDING TEMPLATE

	Trial 1	Trial 2	Trial 3	Average Distance Score (Sum of trials / 3)	Normalized Score (distance / leg length × 100)	Movement Compensations
Right Leg						
Anterior						Yes or No
Posterolateral						Yes or No
Posteromedial						Yes or No
Left Leg						
Anterior						Yes or No
Posterolateral						Yes or No
Posteromedial						Yes or No

Movement Compensations:

DROP JUMP OBSERVATIONAL FINDINGS RECORDING TEMPLATE

Checkpoint	Viewpoint	Movement Impairment	Result
Foot and ankle	Anterior	● Excessive pronation	☐ Right ☐ Left ☐ Both
		● Feet turn out	☐ Right ☐ Left ☐ Both
		● Asymmetric contact/landing	☐ Right first ☐ Left first ☐ No
Knee	Anterior	● Valgus	☐ Right ☐ Left ☐ Both
		● Valgus	☐ Right ☐ Left ☐ Both
	Lateral	● Knee dominance	☐ Right ☐ Left ☐ Both
		● Stiff landing	☐ Yes ☐ No
Lumbo-pelvic-hip complex	Anterior	● Asymmetric weight shift	☐ Right ☐ Left
	Lateral	● Excessive anterior pelvic tilt	☐ Yes ☐ No
		● Excessive posterior pelvic tilt	☐ Yes ☐ No
		● Excessive forward trunk lean	☐ Yes ☐ No

Right/Left/Both refers to the stance or forward leg when the impairment occurs. Mark *Right* or *Left* or *Both* based on the limb for which a movement impairment was observed. For asymmetric weight shift, mark the direction in which the shift occurred.

MOBILITY SCREENING OBSERVATIONAL FINDINGS RECORDING TEMPLATE

Checkpoint	Screening Test	Overactive Shortened	Results
Foot and ankle	Ankle dorsiflexion	● Gastrocnemius/soleus	☐ Yes ☐ No
	First MTP extension	● Flexor hallucis longus	☐ Yes ☐ No
		● Knee dominance	☐ Yes ☐ No
Lumbo-pelvic-hip complex	Lumbar flexion and extension	● Rectus abdominis, internal obliques, and external obliques	☐ Yes ☐ No
	Hip extension, adduction, and knee flexion	● Restricted hip extension: psoas, rectus femoris	☐ Yes ☐ No
		● Restricted adduction: tensor fascia lata	☐ Yes ☐ No
		● Restricted knee flexion: rectus femoris	☐ Yes ☐ No

(continues)

(continued)

Checkpoint	Screening Test	Overactive Shortened	Results
	Hip abduction and external rotation	• Hip adductors	☐ Yes ☐ No
	Passive hip internal rotation	• Piriformis, quadratus femoris, and gluteus maximus	☐ Yes ☐ No
	Seated hip internal and external rotation	• Restricted internal rotation: piriformis, gemellus superior/inferior, obturator internus/externus, quadratus femoris, gluteus maximus	☐ Yes ☐ No
		• Restricted external rotation: tensor fascia lata, gluteus minimus/medius (anterior fibers), and hip adductors	☐ Yes ☐ No
Shoulder	Shoulder flexion	• Latissimus dorsi, teres major, and pectoralis major (lower fibers)	☐ Yes ☐ No
	Shoulder retraction	• Pectoralis minor	☐ Yes ☐ No
	Shoulder extension	• Anterior deltoid, pectoralis major (upper fibers), coracobrachialis, biceps brachii	☐ Yes ☐ No
	Shoulder internal rotation	• Teres minor and infraspinatus	☐ Yes ☐ No
	Shoulder external rotation	• Subscapularis, teres major, latissimus dorsi, and pectoralis major	☐ Yes ☐ No
Thoracic	Extension	• Rectus abdominis, internal obliques, and external obliques	☐ Yes ☐ No
	Rotation	• Rectus abdominis, internal obliques, external obliques, and erector spinae	☐ Yes ☐ No

SHARK SKILL TEST OBSERVATIONAL FINDINGS TEMPLATE

	Time	Faults (+ 0.10 per fault)	Total Time	Movement Compensations
Right				
Trial 1				Yes or No
Trial 2				Yes or No
Left				
Trial 1				Yes or No
Trial 2				Yes or No

DAVIES TEST OBSERVATIONAL FINDINGS TEMPLATE

Trial	Time	Repetitions (Touches)	Movement Compensations
1	15 seconds		Yes or No
2	15 seconds		Yes or No
3	15 seconds		Yes or No

Average Score: Trial 1 _____ + Trial 2 _____ + Trial 3 _____ /3 =

Movement compensations:

ASYMMETRIC PERFORMANCE TESTS OBSERVATIONAL FINDINGS TEMPLATE

	Trial 1	Trial 2	Trial 3	Average Distance Score (Sum of trials / 3)	Movement Compensations
Right Leg					
Single-leg hop test					Yes or No
Triple hop test					Yes or No
Triple crossover hop test					Yes or No
6-meter timed hop test					Yes or No
Left Leg					
Single-leg hop test					Yes or No
Triple hop test					Yes or No
Triple crossover hop test					Yes or No
6-meter timed hop test					Yes or No
Movement compensations:					

CHAPTER 8

MAXIMAL OXYGEN UPTAKE SCORE
MAXIMAL OXYGEN UPTAKE SCORE FOR MEN

HR	300 kpm/min	600 kpm/min	900 kpm/min	1,200 kpm/min	1,500 kpm/min	HR	300 kpm/min	600 kpm/min	900 kpm/min	1,200 kpm/min
120	2.2	3.5	4.8			148	2.4	3.2	4.3	5.4
121	2.2	3.4	4.7			149	2.3	3.2	4.3	5.4
122	2.2	3.4	4.6			150	2.3	3.2	4.2	5.3
123	2.1	3.4	4.6			151	2.3	3.1	4.2	5.2
124	2.1	3.3	4.5	6.0		152	2.2	3.1	4.1	5.2
125	2.0	3.2	4.4	5.9		153	2.2	3.0	4.1	5.2
126	2.0	3.1	4.3	5.8		154	2.2	3.0	4.0	5.1
127	2.0	3.1	4.2	5.7		155	2.1	3.0	4.0	5.1
128	2.0	3.0	4.2	5.6		156	2.1	2.9	4.0	5.0
129	1.9	3.0	4.2	5.6		157	2.1	2.9	3.9	5.0
130	1.9	2.9	4.1	5.5		158	2.1	2.9	3.9	4.9
131	1.9	2.9	4.0	5.4		159	2.1	2.8	3.8	4.9
132	1.8	2.9	4.0	5.3		160	2.1	2.8	3.7	4.8
133	1.8	2.8	3.9	5.3		161	2.0	2.8	3.7	4.8
134	1.8	2.8	3.9	5.2		162	2.0	2.8	3.7	4.7
135	1.7	2.8	3.8	5.1		163	2.0	2.8	3.6	4.6
136	1.7	2.7	3.8	5.0		164	2.0	2.8	3.6	4.6
137	1.7	2.7	3.7	5.0		165	2.0	2.7	3.6	4.5
138	1.6	2.7	3.7	4.9		166	1.9	2.7	3.5	4.5
139	1.6	2.6	3.6	4.8	6.0	167	1.9	2.7	3.5	4.5
140	1.6	2.6	3.6	4.8	5.9	168	1.9	2.6	3.4	4.4
141		2.6	3.5	4.7	5.9	169	1.9	2.6		4.3

HR	300 kpm/min	600 kpm/min	900 kpm/min	1,200 kpm/min	1,500 kpm/min	HR	300 kpm/min	600 kpm/min	900 kpm/min	1,200 kpm/min
142		2.5	3.5	4.6	5.8	170	1.8	2.6		4.3
143		2.5	3.4	4.6	5.7					
144		2.5	3.4	4.5	5.7					
145		2.4	3.4	4.5	5.6					
146		2.4	3.3	4.4	5.6					
147		2.4	3.3	4.4	5.5					

Adapted from Acevedo & Starks (2011).

MAXIMAL OXYGEN UPTAKE SCORE FOR WOMEN

HR	300 kpm/min	450 kpm/min	600 kpm/min	750 kpm/min	900 kpm/min	HR	300 kpm/min	450 kpm/min	600 kpm/min	750 kpm/min	900 kpm/min
120	2.6	3.4	4.1	4.8		146	1.6	2.2	2.6	3.2	3.7
121	2.5	3.3	4.0	4.8		147	1.6	2.1	2.6	3.1	3.6
122	2.5	3.2	3.9	4.7		148	1.6	2.1	2.6	3.1	3.6
123	2.4	3.1	3.9	4.7		149		2.1	2.6	3.0	3.5
124	2.4	3.1	3.8	4.6		150		2.0	2.5	3.0	3.5
125	2.3	3.0	3.7	4.5		151		2.0	2.5	3.0	3.4
126	2.3	3.0	3.6	4.4		152		2.0	2.5	2.9	3.4
127	2.2	2.9	3.5	4.3		153		2.0	2.4	2.9	3.3
128	2.2	2.8	3.5	4.2	4.8	154		2.0	2.4	2.8	3.3
129	2.2	2.8	3.4	4.1	4.8	155		1.9	2.4	2.8	3.2
130	2.1	2.7	3.4	4.0	4.7	156		1.9	2.3	2.8	3.2
131	2.1	2.7	3.4	4.0	4.6	157		1.9	2.3	2.8	3.2
132	2.0	2.7	3.3	3.9	4.5	158		1.8	2.3	2.7	3.1
133	2.0	2.6	3.2	3.8	4.4	159		1.8	2.2	2.7	3.1
134	2.0	2.6	3.9	3.8	4.4	160		1.8	2.2	2.6	3.0

(continues)

(continued)

HR	300 kpm/min	450 kpm/min	600 kpm/min	750 kpm/min	900 kpm/min	HR	300 kpm/min	450 kpm/min	600 kpm/min	750 kpm/min	900 kpm/min
135	2.0	2.6	3.2	3.7	4.3	161		1.8	2.2	2.6	3.0
136	1.9	2.5	3.1	3.6	4.2	162		1.8	2.2	2.6	3.0
137	1.9	2.5	3.0	3.6	4.2	163		1.7	2.2	2.6	2.9
138	1.8	2.4	3.0	3.5	4.1	164		1.7	2.1	2.5	2.9
139	1.8	2.4	2.9	3.5	4.0	165		1.7	2.1	2.5	2.9
140	1.8	2.4	2.8	3.4	4.0	166		1.7	2.1	2.5	2.8
141	1.8	2.3	2.8	3.4	3.9	167		1.6	2.1	2.4	2.8
142	1.7	2.3	2.8	3.3	3.9	168		1.6	2.0	2.4	2.8
143	1.7	2.2	2.7	3.3	3.8	169		1.6	2.0	2.4	2.8
144	1.7	2.2	2.7	3.2	3.8	170		1.6	2.0	2.4	2.7
145	1.6	2.2	2.7	3.2	3.7						

Adapted from Acevedo & Starks, 2011.

PERCENTILE RANKS FOR THE 12-MINUTE RUN

Percentile	Age in Years and Distance Run					
	20–29		30–39		40–49	
	km	miles	km	miles	km	miles
MEN						
90th	2.90	1.81	2.82	1.75	2.72	1.69
80th	2.78	1.73	2.67	1.66	2.57	1.60
70th	2.62	1.63	2.56	1.59	2.46	1.53
60th	2.54	1.58	2.48	1.54	2.40	1.49
50th	2.46	1.53	2.40	1.49	2.30	1.43
40th	2.37	1.47	2.32	1.44	2.22	1.38
30th	2.29	1.42	2.24	1.39	2.14	1.33

Percentile	Age in Years and Distance Run					
	20–29		30–39		40–49	
	km	miles	km	miles	km	miles
20th	2.20	1.37	2.14	1.33	2.06	1.28
10th	2.06	1.28	2.01	1.25	1.95	1.21
WOMEN						
90th	2.59	1.61	2.53	1.57	2.43	1.51
80th	2.46	1.53	2.40	1.49	2.27	1.41
70th	2.35	1.46	2.27	1.41	2.20	1.37
60th	2.27	1.41	2.19	1.36	2.11	1.31
50th	2.20	1.37	2.14	1.33	2.04	1.27
40th	2.12	1.32	2.04	1.27	1.96	1.22
30th	2.03	1.26	1.95	1.21	1.90	1.18
20th	1.95	1.21	1.88	1.17	1.82	1.13
10th	1.82	1.13	1.75	1.09	1.70	1.05

Adapted from Hoff & Triplett (2015).

1.5-MILE RUN TEST REFERENCE SCORES
Reference Scores for Men

Rating	Time to Complete 1.5-Mile Run				
	20–29 Years Old	30–39 Years Old	40–49 Years Old	50–59 Years Old	60–69 Years Old
Superior	8:22–9:10	8:49–9:31	9:02–9:47	9:31–10:27	10:09–11:20
Excellent	9:34–10:08	9:52–10:38	10:09–11:09	11:09–12:08	12:10–13:25
Good	10:49–11:27	11:09–11:49	11:52–12:25	12:53–13:53	14:33–15:20
Fair	11:58–12:29	12:25–12:53	13:05–13:50	14–33–15:14	16:19–17:19
Poor	13:08–13:58	13:48–14:33	14:33–15:32	16:16–17:30	18:39–20:13
Very poor	15:14–20:55	15:56–20:55	17:04–22:22	19:24–27:08	23:27–31:59

Data from Cooper Institute. (2007). Physical fitness assessments and norms for adults and law enforcement. Dallas, TX.

Reference Scores for Women

Rating	Time to Complete 1.5-Mile Run				
	20–29 Years Old	30–39 Years Old	40–49 Years Old	50–59 Years Old	60–69 Years Old
Superior	9:23–10:20	9:52–11:08	10:09–11:35	11:34–13:16	12:25–14:28
Excellent	10:59–11:56	11:43–12:53	12:25–13:38	13:58–15:14	15:32–16:46
Good	12:51–13:25	13:41–14:33	14:33–15:17	16:26–17:19	18:05–18:52
Fair	14:15–15:05	15:14–15:56	16:13–17:11	18:05–19:10	20:08–20:55
Poor	15:56–17:11	16:46–18:18	18:26–19:43	20:17–21:57	22:34–23:55
Very poor	18:39–25:17	20:13–25:10	21:52–27:55	23:55–30:34	26:32–33:05

Data from Cooper Institute (2007).

BEEP TEST SHUTTLE REFERENCE SCORES (AGED 9–17 YEARS)

Age (in years)	20-Meter Shuttle Run (Number of Laps) Percentiles by Age and Sex in 1,142,026 Children and Youth Aged 9–17 Years from 50 Countries Since 1981										
	P_5	P_{10}	P_{20}	P_{30}	P_{40}	P_{50}	P_{60}	P_{70}	P_{80}	P_{90}	P_{95}
Boys											
9	9	14	20	24	28	32	36	40	45	52	58
10	9	14	21	25	29	33	37	42	47	55	62
11	9	15	22	27	31	36	40	45	51	60	67
12	9	16	24	29	34	39	45	50	57	67	75
13	11	18	26	33	39	44	50	56	64	75	84
14	13	20	29	36	43	48	55	62	70	81	92
15	14	22	31	39	45	52	58	66	74	86	97
16	15	23	33	41	48	54	61	69	78	91	102
17	16	25	35	43	50	57	64	72	81	95	107

20-Meter Shuttle Run (Number of Laps) Percentiles by Age and Sex in 1,142,026 Children and Youth Aged 9–17 Years from 50 Countries Since 1981

Age (in years)	P_5	P_{10}	P_{20}	P_{30}	P_{40}	P_{50}	P_{60}	P_{70}	P_{80}	P_{90}	P_{95}
Girls											
9	8	12	17	21	24	26	29	33	36	42	47
10	7	11	17	21	24	27	30	34	38	44	49
11	6	11	16	21	24	28	31	35	40	46	52
12	5	10	16	21	25	28	32	36	41	48	54
13	5	10	17	21	25	29	33	37	42	50	56
14	5	10	17	21	25	29	33	38	43	50	57
15	5	10	17	21	26	30	34	38	44	51	58
16	5	10	17	21	26	30	34	39	44	52	59
17	5	11	17	21	26	30	35	39	45	53	60

Adapted from Tomkinson et al. (2017).

DESCRIPTIVE DATA RESULTS FOR YO-YO WITHIN VARIOUS SPORTS

Group, Sport, or Position	Number of Athletes	Yo-Yo IR1	
		Distance (m)	Distance (yd)
National soccer (men) (74)	18	2,260 ± 80	2,472 ± 87
National soccer (men) (74)	24	2,040 ± 60	2,231 ± 66
National rugby league (men) (4)	23	1,656 ± 403	1,811 ± 441
Semiprofessional rugby league (men) (4)	27	1,564 ± 415	1,710 ± 454
National soccer (women) (76)	17	1,224 ± 255	1,339 ± 279
National soccer (men) (76)	17	2,414 ± 456	2,640 ± 499
National junior soccer (women) (76)	17	826 ± 160	903 ± 175
National junior soccer (men) (76)	17	2,092 ± 260	2,287 ± 284

(continues)

(continued)

Group, Sport, or Position	Number of Athletes	Yo-Yo IR1	
		Distance (m)	Distance (yd)
Under 17 soccer (men) (76)	60	1,556 ± 478	1,702 ± 523
Under 16 rugby union (men) (85)	150	1,150 ± 403	1,258 ± 441
Under 14 elite basketball (men) (116)	15	1,100 ± 385	1,203 ± 421
Under 15 elite basketball (men) (116)	15	1,283 ± 461	1,403 ± 504
Under 17 elite basketball (men) (116)	17	1,412 ± 245	1,544 ± 268
Under 18 Gaelic football (men) (22)	265	1,465 ± 370	1,602 ± 405

The values listed are means ± standard deviation. The data are based on research studies and are descriptive, not normative. Use numbers for reference only.

PERCENTILE RANKS FOR 300-YARD SHUTTLE RUN FOR NCAA DIVISION I ATHLETES (TIME IN SECONDS)

Percentile	Baseball	Men's Basketball	Women's Basketball	Softball
90th	56.7	54.1	58.4	63.3
80th	58.9	55.1	61.8	65.1
70th	59.9	55.6	63.6	66.5
60th	61.3	56.3	64.7	67.9
50th	62.0	56.7	65.2	69.2
40th	63.2	57.2	65.9	71.3
30th	63.9	58.1	66.8	72.4
20th	65.3	58.9	68.1	74.6
10th	67.7	60.2	68.9	78.0

Adapted from Hoffman (2006).

UNITED STATES MAX GRIP STRENGTH SCORES

Sex	Age Group (years)	n	Mean (SE)	20th (SE)	40th (SE)	50th (SE)	60th (SE)	80th (SE)
Men	6–8	332	55.1 (1.1)	43.9 (0.8)	49.2 (1.4)	53.2 (1.4)	56.41 (1.7)	67.6 (1.6)
	9–11	282	82.3 (1.3)	65.8 (1.8)	76.8 (1.5)	81.0 (1.3)	84.0 (1.2)	95.3 (2.5)
	12–15	303	138.2 (3.6)	99.2 (3.4)	124. (6.1)	138.9 (5.0)	147.1 (3.9)	170.9 (3.6)
	16–19	290	187.7 (3.0)	163.9 (3.5)	180.3 (3.4)	187.9 (3.3)	194.3 (3.3)	209.7 (2.4)
	20–29	454	210.2 (2.7)	178.2 (4.1)	200.4 (3.1)	208.1 (2.4)	218.0 (3.9)	241.4 (3.9)
	30–39	411	216.4 (1.8)	184.7 (2.5)	209.5 (2.1)	16.1 (1.8)	224.6 (3.0)	245.3 (3.1)
	40–49	378	206.7 (2.7)	180.0 (2.5)	198.2 (3.1)	207.6 (2.9)	212.4 (3.1)	234.4 (3.3)
	50–59	372	194.0 (4.2)	161.9 (5.9)	188.1 (3.7)	195.0 (3.5)	203.3 (3.6)	220.2 (4.7)
	60–69	373	181.7 (4.2)	152.2 (5.6)	176.5 (5.1)	184.9 (3.6)	191.6 (2.8)	206.0 (5.2)
	70+	302	153.9 (1.8)	128.7 (3.4)	146.0 (2.7)	155.5 (2.2)	162.1 (2.8)	178.1 (2.8)
Women	6–8	281	50.4 (0.9)	39.9 (1.0)	45.6 (1.0)	48.6 (1.0)	51.4 (0.9)	59.7 (1.4)
	9–11	301	78.2 (1.2)	61.9 (1.4)	71.5 (1.6)	75.8 (1.1)	81.0 (1.5)	93.9 (2.0)
	12–15	292	112.2 (1.8)	95.7 (1.4)	105.1 (2.1)	109.3 (1.7)	114.2 (2.9)	128.5 (3.1)
	16–19	285	124.7 (2.2)	107.8 (2.5)	117.5 (2.4)	122.5 (2.2)	126.6 (2.3)	141.7 (4.9)
	20–29	412	131.8 (1.1)	112.7 (1.2)	125.9 (1.3)	130.3 (1.2)	135.8 (1.1)	148.4 (1.1)
	30–39	382	136.5 (1.4)	117.9 (1.5)	128.8 (2.1)	135.8 (1.7)	139.6 (1.5)	154.2 (1.9)
	40–49	392	132.9 (1.4)	114.5 (2.2)	125.2 (1.8)	132.9 (1.5)	138.1 (2.0)	154.1 (2.6
	50–59	401	123.4 (1.5)	106.9 (2.0)	117.7 (1.8)	121.5 (2.0)	128.0 (2.4)	141.7 (2.2)
	60–69	354	116.3 (1.3)	1003. (2.6)	114.0 (1.8)	117.1 (1.3)	119.7 (1.5)	131.2 (1.9)
	70+	300	95.0 (1.4)	76.7 (1.8)	88.4 (1.7)	93.0 (1.9)	100.2 (2.4)	113.7 (1.5)

Mean, Standard Error, and Percentile Distribution of Grip Strength (in Pounds) in U.S. Children and Adults by Sex and Age Group, 2011–2012

Maximal contraction on each hand over three trials was summed to yield combined grip strength (in pounds) used to identify the age- and sex-appropriate quintile and median.

United States max grip strength scores (adapted from Perna et al., 2016)

PERCENTILE BREAKDOWN OF VERTICAL JUMP HEIGHT BY 5-YEAR GROUPINGS

	Men				Women			
	21–25 Years Old (n = 312)		26–30 Years Old (n = 188)		21–25 Years Old (n = 182)		26–30 Years Old (n = 42)	
Percentile	in.	cm	in.	cm	in.	cm	in.	cm
95th	28.0	71.1	27.5	69.9	19.0	48.3	18.0	45.7
90th	26.5	67.3	26.0	66.0	17.0	43.2	17.5	44.5
85th	25.5	64.8	25.0	63.5	16.0	40.6	17.5	44.5
80th	25.0	63.5	24.0	61.0	16.0	40.6	16.0	40.6
75th	24.5	62.2	24.0	61.0	15.5	39.4	16.0	40.6
70th	24.0	61.0	23.5	59.7	15.0	38.1	15.5	39.4
65th	23.5	59.7	23.0	58.4	14.5	36.8	15.0	38.1
60th	23.0	58.4	22.5	57.2	14.5	36.8	14.5	36.8
55th	23.0	58.4	22.0	55.9	14.5	35.6	14.5	36.8
50th	22.5	57.2	22.0	55.9	14.0	35.6	14.0	35.6
45th	22.0	55.9	22.0	55.9	14.0	35.6	14.0	34.3
40th	21.5	54.6	21.5	54.6	14.0	34.3	13.5	34.3
35th	21.0	53.3	21.0	53.3	13.5	33.0	13.5	34.3
30th	20.5	52.1	20.5	52.1	13.0	33.0	13.5	31.8
25th	21.5	50.8	20.0	50.8	13.0	31.8	12.5	31.8
20th	21.0	48.3	19.5	49.5	12.5	30.5	12.5	29.2
15th	18.5	47.0	18.5	47.0	11.5	29.2	11.5	27.9
10th	18.0	45.7	17.5	44.5	11.0	27.9	11.0	27.9
5th	16.5	41.9	16.0	40.6	10.0	25.4	10.0	25.4

Adapted from Paterson & Paterson (2004).

HORIZONTAL JUMP REFERENCE SCORES FOR ELITE MALE AND FEMALE ATHLETES

Percentile	Males		Females	
	in.	cm	in.	cm
90th	133	339	115	293
80th	122	309	110	279
70th	116	294	104	264
60th	110	279	98	249
50th	104	264	92	234
40th	98	249	86	219
30th	92	234	80	204
20th	86	219	74	189
10th	80	204	69	174

Adapted from Hoff & Triplett (2015).

RANKINGS FOR STANDING LONG JUMP IN. 15- AND 16-YEAR-OLD ATHLETES

Category	Males		Females	
	In	cm	in	cm
Excellent	79	201	65	166
Above average	73	186	61	156
Average	69	176	57	146
Below average	65	165	53	135
Poor	<65	<165	<53	<135

POWER CLEAN PERCENTILE RANKINGS

	Female				Male									
	Basketball		Softball		Football 14–15 Year Old		Football 16–18 Year Old		Football NCAA Division I		Baseball		Basketball	
Percentile	lb	kg	lb	kg	lb	kg	lb	kg	lb	kg	lb	kg	lb	kg
90th	130	59	122	55	213	97	250	114	300	136	265	120	250	114
80th	124	56	115	52	195	89	235	107	280	127	239	109	235	107
70th	117	53	115	48	190	235	107	102	270	123	225	102	230	105
60th	112	51	106	45	86	225	102	101	261	119	216	98	220	100
50th	110	50	94	43	173	79	208	95	252	115	206	94	215	98
40thh	103	47	93	42	165	75	200	91	242	110	200	91	205	93
30th	96	44	88	40	161	73	183	83	232	105	190	86	195	89
20th	88	40	80	36	153	70	165	75	220	100	182	83	180	82
10th	77	35	71	32	141	64	145	66	205	93	162	74	162	74
Mean	106	48	97	44	176	80	204	93	252	115	210	95	209	95

MALE AND FEMALE YOUTH TENNIS PLAYERS REFERENCE VALUES

		Males (cm)	Females (cm)
Tennis (younger than age 14)	Needs improvement	<520	<520
	Average	520–540	520–538
	Good	540–602	538–570
	Excellent	>602	>570
Tennis (younger than age 14)	Needs improvement	<640	<610
	Average	640–670	610–646
	Good	670–729	646–710
	Excellent	>729	>710

		Males (cm)	Females (cm)
Tennis (younger than age 16)	Needs improvement	<890	<720
	Average	890–920	720–740
	Good	920–1004	740–810
	Excellent	>1004	>810
Tennis (younger than age 18)	Needs improvement	<1080	<810
	Average	1080–1140	810–830
	Good	1140–1260	830–940
	Excellent	>1260	>940

Fernandez-Fernandez et al. (2014).

PERCENTILE RANKS FOR 40-YARD (36.6-M) SPRINT TIMES IN MALE YOUTH

Percentile	12–13 Years Old	14–15 Years Old	16–18 Years Old
90th	5.41	5.02	4.76
80th	5.63	5.15	4.85
70th	5.77	5.24	4.90
60th	5.84	5.32	4.98
50th	5.97	5.46	5.10
40th	6.08	5.54	5.13
30th	6.25	5.78	5.21
20th	6.32	6.02	5.30
10th	6.64	6.08	5.46
Mean	5.99	5.54	5.09
SD	0.39	0.43	0.28
N	45	92	94

Adapted from Hoffman (2006).

SPEED TEST NORMS FOR VARIOUS SPORTS (IN SECONDS)

Population	Sex	10 Yards	30 Yards	40 Yards
Baseball NCAA Division I	M			
Baseball Major League	M		3.75 ± 0.11	
Basketball NCAA Division I	M		3.79 ± 0.19	4.81 ± 0.26
Field hockey*	F			6.37 ± 0.27
American football NCAA Division I	M			4.74 ± 0.3
Defensive line				4.85 ± 0.2
Linebackers				4.64 ± 0.2
Defensive backs				4.52 ± 0.2
Quarterbacks				4.70 ± 0.1
Running backs				4.53 ± 0.2
Wide receivers				4.48 ± 0.1
Offensive line				5.12 ± 0.2
Tight ends				4.78 ± 0.2
Football NFL draftees	M			4.81 ± 0.31
Lacrosse NCAA Division III	F			5.40 ± 0.16
Rugby*	M			5.32 ± 0.26
Rugby*	F	2.00 ± 0.11		6.45 ± 0.36
Soccer NCAA Division I	M	1.63 ± 0.08		4.87 ± 0.16
Soccer NCAA Division II	M			4.73 ± 0.18
Soccer NCAA Division III	F			5.34 ± 0.17
Tennis NCAA Division I	M	1.79 ± 0.03		5.02 ± 0.24
Volleyball Junior National*	F	1.90 ± 0.01		
Volleyball Junior National*	M	1.80 ± 0.02		

*Distance in meters instead of yards. Adapted from Hoffman (2006).

PERCENTILE RANKS FOR PRO-AGILITY TEST IN NCAA DIVISION I COLLEGE ATHLETES

Percentile	Women's Volleyball	Women's Basketball	Women's Softball	Men's Basketball	Men's Baseball	Men's Football
90th	4.75	4.65	4.88	4.22	4.25	4.21
80th	4.84	4.82	4.96	4.29	4.36	4.31
70th	4.91	4.86	5.03	4.35	4.41	4.38
60th	4.98	4.94	5.10	4.39	4.46	4.44
50th	5.01	5.06	5.17	4.41	4.50	4.52
40th	5.08	5.10	5.24	4.44	4.55	4.59
30th	5.17	5.14	5.33	4.48	4.61	4.66
20th	5.23	5.23	5.40	4.51	4.69	4.76
10th	5.32	5.36	5.55	4.61	4.76	4.89
Mean	5.03	5.02	5.19	4.41	4.53	4.54
SD	0.20	0.26	0.26	0.18	0.23	0.27
N	81	128	118	87	165	869

Table scores adapted from Hoffman (2006).

PRO-AGILITY RESULTS FOR COLLEGE FOOTBALL PLAYERS PARTICIPATING IN THE NFL

Percentile	DL	LB	DB	OL	QB	RB	TE	WR
90th	4.22	4.07	3.89	4.45	4.07	4.02	4.18	3.97
80th	4.32	4.13	3.96	4.53	4.12	4.14	4.21	4.03
70th	4.38	4.16	4.05	4.57	4.16	4.18	4.26	4.07
60th	4.41	4.21	4.07	4.61	4.20	4.22	4.31	4.10
50th	4.46	4.24	4.12	4.69	4.25	4.25	4.35	4.15
40th	4.52	4.28	4.18	4.77	4.33	4.31	4.39	4.20
30th	4.58	4.31	4.19	4.83	4.36	4.34	4.42	4.24
20th	4.68	4.41	4.21	4.93	4.38	4.38	4.46	4.26
10th	4.75	4.53	4.27	5.06	4.41	4.49	4.56	4.33

(continues)

(continued)

Percentile	DL	LB	DB	OL	QB	RB	TE	WR
Mean	4.48	4.26	4.11	4.74	4.26	4.26	4.35	4.15
SD	0.22	0.17	0.15	0.39	0.15	0.16	0.13	0.15
N	89	38	76	125	125	58	39	85

Table scores adapted from Hoffman (2006).

T-TEST REFERENCE SCORES AMONG DIFFERENT SPORTS

		Time (in seconds)
Group, Sport, or Position	**Number of Athletes**	**T-Test**
College students (women) (97)	34	11.92 ± 0.52
College students (men) (108)	52	10.08 ± 0.46
Recreational athletes (women) (108)	20	11.70 ± 0.67
Recreational athletes (men) (108)	24	10.31 ± 0.46
Junior national volleyball (men) (33)	14	9:90 ± 0.17
Junior national volleyball (women) (33)	15	10.33 ± 0.13
NCAA Division I college lacrosse (women) (49)	11	10.50 ± 0.60
High school volleyball (women) (98)	27	10.96 ± 0.58
NCAA Division I volleyball (women) (98)	26	10.65 ± 0.52
Recreational athletes (women) (86)	52	12.52 ± 0.90
Recreational athletes (men) (86)	58	10.49 ± 0.89
College athletes (women) (86)	56	10.94 ± 0.60
College athletes (women) (86)	47	9.94 ± 0.50

The values listed are means ± standard deviation. The data are based on research studies and are descriptive, not normative. Use numbers for reference only.

Table adapted from Haff & Triplett (2015).

CHAPTER 13

PROPER LINEAR SPRINT

Body Part	Motion Summary	Problem	Cause	Drills for Correction
Head	As an athlete initiates acceleration, the head must cast downward. This begins forward movement by slightly placing the head's weight in front of the body's center of gravity. As the athlete approaches maximal running speed, the head is raised to align with the body's vertical axis.	Improper flexion or extension at the head	Fatigue or poor execution of proper mechanics	The athlete maintains proper eye focus ahead or slightly downcast, depending on the specific acceleration or maximal speed drills.
Shoulders	Shoulders should create an exaggerated flexion and extension opposite the lower-body movement (hip flexion/extension). During acceleration, shoulder extension (driving elbows backward) should cease when the hands pass the buttocks posteriorly. Shoulder flexion should end as the hands rise above the forehead level. Proper, aggressive shoulder extension during acceleration and maximal speed aid in proper contralateral movements such as hip and shoulder flexion. Attempts should be made to minimize shoulder abduction and thoracic rotation, keeping the elbows close to the body. This results in the hands approaching but not crossing the body's vertical midline. As the athlete approaches maximal speed, shoulder flexion and extension maintain a high amount of force but movement at the shoulder joint decreases in range of motion. Each shoulder should flex until the hands are even with the nose. Forcible shoulder extension is maintained to move the elbows down and back.	Tight and elevated shoulders during running Movement of the hands across the midline during flexion and extension, causing excessive rotation of the upper body	Arm movement is too forced and not natural Lack of coordination of the contralateral hip and shoulder flexion/ extension and overcompensation for poor hip flexion	Standing arm swings; relaxed shoulders while marching or skipping Standing arm swings, A-skips, cycling B- skips, weighted arm swings, and proper technique focus during all drills

(continues)

(*continued*)

Body Part	Motion Summary	Problem	Cause	Drills for Correction
Shoulders (*continued*)	The role of arm action shifts from creating propulsive force during acceleration to facilitating the balance of the contralateral hip flexion during maximal speed. During acceleration and maximal speed, shoulders should stay relaxed and swing naturally.			
Elbows	Elbows should be bent at 90 degrees during shoulder flexion with fingers extended. During shoulder extension, the angle at the elbow may naturally open slightly but must close to 90 degrees once again during shoulder flexion. Wrists should remain neutral with the fingers extended. This movement pattern is maintained as the athlete approaches maximal speed.	Excessive flexion or extension	Poor neural patterning	Standing arm swings, marches, A-skips, cycling B-skips, weighted arm swings, and proper technique focus during all drills
Hips	During acceleration, due to contralateral shoulder extension, hip flexion should reach a point slightly below parallel to the ground. Hip extension should be explosive, yet the posterior movement of the thigh beyond the body's center of gravity should be minimized to less than 20 degrees. As the athlete approaches maximal running speed, hip flexion approaches 90 degrees. Hip extension should remain explosive, yet posterior movement past the body's center of gravity must still be minimized. The pelvis must stay neutral during acceleration and maximal speed.	Inadequate hip flexion Inability to produce adequate force during hip extension (ground push-off) Excessive lumbar extension throughout stride cycle	Poor neural patterning, weak hip flexors, and tight hip extensors Weak posterior chain, tight hip flexors, and inadequate ankle mobility Weak anterior core and glute muscles and tight hip flexors	Flexibility drills for gluteals and hamstrings, resisted knee drives, marches, A-skips, and 1/3/5 wall drill Mobility and flexibility drills for ankle and hip flexors; strength, power, and plyometric drills focusing on the triple extension of the ankle, knee, and hip; 1/3/5 wall drills; and resisted speed drills Core strengthening drills, hip flexor flexibility drills, 1/3/5 wall drills, resisted sprints, and planks

Body Part	Motion Summary	Problem	Cause	Drills for Correction
Knees	During the drive phase in acceleration, the knee is fully extended to allow for maximal hip extension with the foot slightly behind the center of mass. The knee then flexes as the hip flexes during the recovery phase, driving the heel directly up toward the buttocks and over the opposite knee. During maximal hip flexion, the knee is flexed, leaving the shin nearly parallel to the ground. As the hip begins to extend again, the knee can swing open to create an angle roughly 90 degrees with the shin before it is rapidly extended again during foot contact. As the athlete approaches maximal speed, the more perpendicular body angle to the ground allows for greater hip flexion and, therefore, higher knee and heel lift.	Knee height is too low during the running stride, not allowing for adequate stride length Knee adduction during the stance phase of the stride cycle	Inadequate hip flexion during the drive phase of the running stride Poor ankle mobility, weak abductor/external rotators, and tight adductors/internal rotators	Resisted knee drives, marches, A-skips, and resisted sprints Flexibility exercises for gastrocnemius/soleus/Achilles complex, lateral tube walking, single-leg balance drills, and single-leg strength drills
Ankle and heel	The ankle should remain dorsiflexed to allow for proper foot contact on the ball of the foot during the drive phase. At foot contact, the angle created between the shin and the foot should be close to 45 degrees, referred to as a positive shin angle. This allows the appropriate horizontal force to be applied in the posterior direction. As the foot comes off the ground during recovery, the heel is raised toward the buttocks to step over the opposite knee. The height of the heel is related to the height of the knee during hip flexion, so the heel's height begins relatively low during acceleration and increases as maximal speed is approached. Due to overcoming initial inertia during acceleration, the ground contact time of the foot is slightly greater than at maximal speed.	Inability to maintain dorsiflexion throughout stride cycle Foot contact time is too long, resulting in decreased stride rate	Improper coaching ("run on the toes"), weak tibialis anterior, and tight gastrocnemius/soleus/Achilles complex Inability to maintain dorsiflexion, improper backside mechanics, and foot contact too far in front of the center of gravity	Mobility and flexibility exercises for gastrocnemius/soleus/Achilles complex, reverse calf raises, A-skips, and 1/3/5 wall drills Reverse calf raises, A-skips, cycling B-skips, and assisted sprints

(continues)

(continued)

Body Part	Motion Summary	Problem	Cause	Drills for Correction
Ankle and heel (*continued*)	As maximal speed is approached, foot contact is still on the ball of the foot but is slightly higher toward the toes. The ankle remains dorsiflexed, but as the foot contact moves slightly to a point directly under or slightly in front of the body's center of gravity, the angle between the foot and shin becomes less acute. As a result, ground contact time for the foot is decreased as maximal speed is achieved.			
Body angle concerning the ground	The body angle should be about 45 degrees to the ground during initial acceleration, allowing maximal force to be created posteriorly. A straight line should be observed from the top of the head, down the spine, and through the extended rear leg. As the athlete approaches maximal speed, the body angle increases to near perpendicular to the ground. This allows the hips to continue to drive the body's center of gravity forward.	Improper body angle at a phase of running (i.e., acceleration versus maximal speed)	Improper coaching ("bend forward" or "stay low" while sprinting) or poor neural patterning	Core strengthening drills, planks, 1/3/5 wall drills, and resisted and assisted speed drills

CHAPTER 15

PHASES OF THE SNATCH

Kinetic Chain Checkpoint	Phase						
	Setup	First Pull	Transition	Second Pull	Pull-Under	Catch	Stand
Feet	Straight, about hip-width apart, weight distribution in the center of the foot to slightly toward the toes	Actively press feet into the ground	Actively press feet into the ground	Actively pressing to create plantar flexion	From the ball of the foot to the floor—a split second off the ground to reposition for the catch	Flat on floor wider than starting position	Flat on floor wider than starting position; weight evenly distributed; actively engaged
Knees	Over the middle of the foot (shins slightly inclined toward the bar), tracking with toes, below the level of the hips	Straighten/extend the knees, but not fully locked out	Straighten/extend the knees, but not fully locked out	Straighten/extend the knees	Flexing	Flexed, tracking over toes	Extending, tracking over toes
Lumbo-pelvic-hip complex	Hips above the level of the knees and lower than the level of the shoulders, low back in a neutral position (lordotic curve)	Remains in the setup position	Hips begin to extend	Hips extending	Flexing at hips	Flexed	Hips extending; low back neutral
Shoulders	Higher than hips, leaning over the bar	Remain in the setup position	Remain in the setup position	Elevating/shrugging and high pulling	Rapidly moving from abduction/internal rotation to abduction/external rotation	Flexion/external rotation	Full flexion/abduction/external rotation; actively engaged
Head	Neutral with the neck in slight extension (this helps maintain thoracic extension), eyes should be looking out in front rather than down	Remains in the setup position	Remains in the setup position	Remains in the setup position	Remains in the setup position	Remains in the setup position	Remains in the setup position

PHASES OF THE CLEAN

Kinetic Chain Checkpoint	Phase						
	Setup	First Pull	Transition	Second Pull	Pull-Under	Catch	Stand
Feet	Straight, about hip-width apart, weight distribution in the center of the foot to slightly toward the toes	Actively press feet into the ground	Actively press feet into the ground	Actively press to create plantar flexion	From the ball of the foot to the floor—a split second off the ground to reposition for the catch	Flat on floor wider than starting position	Flat on floor wider than starting position; weight evenly distributed; actively engaged
Knees	Over the middle of the foot (shins slightly inclined toward the bar), tracking with toes, below the level of the hips	Straighten/ extend the knees, but not fully locked out	Straighten/ extend the knees, but not fully locked out	Straighten/ extend the knees	Flexing	Flexed, tracking over toes	Extended, tracking over toes
Lumbo-pelvic-hip complex	Hips above the level of the knees and lower than the level of the shoulders, low back in a neutral position (lordotic curve)	Remains in the setup position	Hips begin to extend	Hips extending	Flexing at hips	Flexed	Hips extending; low back neutral
Shoulders	Higher than hips and over the bar	Remain in the setup position	Remain in the setup position	Elevating/ shrugging and high pulling	Rapidly moving from abduction and internal rotation to abduction and external rotation	Flexion/ external rotation	Full flexion/ abduction/ external rotation; actively engaged
Head	Neutral with the neck in slight extension (this helps maintain thoracic extension), eyes should be looking out in front rather than down	Remains in the setup position	Remains in the setup position	Remains in the setup position	Remains in the setup position	Remains in the setup position	Remains in the setup position

PHASES OF THE JERK

Kinetic Chain Checkpoint	Phase					
	Setup	**Dip**	**Drive**	**Push-Under**	**Catch**	**Stand**
Feet	Straight, about hip-width apart, weight distribution in the center of the foot	Actively press feet flat into the ground	Actively press to create plantar flexion	From the ball of the foot to the floor—a split second off the ground to reposition for the catch	**Push jerk:** flat on floor, wider than starting position **Split jerk:** front foot flat, shin vertical, back foot on the ball	**Push jerk:** stand **Split jerk:** front foot small step backward; back foot steps forward
Knees	Soft, tracking with toes	Short, quick bend, tracking over toes	Straighten/ extend the knees	Flexing	Both bent	Extend
Lumbo-pelvic-hip complex	Low back in a neutral position (lordotic curve)	Remain neutral and braced	Hip extending	Flexing at hip	Front hip flexed, back hip extended, low back neutral	Hips extend, low back neutral
Shoulders	Tall	Remain in the setup position	Elevating/ shrugging	Rapidly moving from flexion to full overhead flexion	Fully flexed	Remain in the setup position
Head	Neutral with the neck in slight flexion (this helps maintain thoracic extension), eyes should be looking out in front rather than down	Remains in the setup position	Remains in the setup position	Remains in the setup position	Remains in the setup position	Fully flexed

Consideration		Determination	Correction
Motor Learning (Cueing and Feedback)		• First, determine what are/were the performance client's impairment findings from the assessment process. • Is there any pain? If so, stop the lift and consider referring out. • Based on this information, determine if the performance client can get into the correct position(s) for the lift they are performing (i.e., maintain knee and spine alignment throughout motion).	1. Make sure the performance client is in proper kinetic chain alignment 2. Make sure the performance client is aware of the impairment(s) that are occurring 3. Provide specific cues and feedback to help the performance client maintain correct posture and alignment If this does not resolve the impairment, it may be more of a mobility or stability/strength issue.
Neuromuscular Control	**Mobility** (ROM)	• Is there any pain? If so, stop the lift and consider referring out. • Determine if the impairment happens at a specific point in the movement or from the beginning. In other words, is the performance client able to maintain correct posture and alignment to a certain point before the impairment(s) appear?	1. Make sure the exercise selected is appropriate for the performance client's current level of mobility 2. Makes sure the performance client has the proper kinetic chain alignment relative to the lift they are performing (i.e., feet wide enough properly turned, proper grip, elbows properly positioned, etc.) If this does not resolve the issue, it may be a stability/strength issue.
	Stability/Strength (Load)	• Is there any pain? If so, stop the lift and consider referring out. • Determine if the performance client was able to perform the lift at lighter loads with minimal to no impairment(s) and if the impairment occurs later in the set or after they are fatigued.	1. Make sure the load is appropriate for the performance client's current level of stability/strength 2. Increased loads require greater stability and strength to perform and can often make the performance client move into greater ROM, which they may not yet have 3. May need to change the number of reps or sets depending on when impairment occurs If this does not resolve the issue, it may be a combination of these elements.

CHAPTER 18

SAMPLE TRAINING WEEK
Sample Off-Season Training Week

Sunday	Monday	Tuesday	Wednesday	Thursday	Friday	Saturday
Rest	Back Squat 3 × 8 @ 75% 1RM	Bench Press 3 × 8 @ 75% 1RM	Conditioning 3 × 300 yd (2-min recovery)	Deadlift 3 × 8 @ 75% 1RM	Narrow-Grip Strict Press 3 × 8 @ 75% 1RM	Conditioning 4 × 200 yd (1-min recovery) 6 × 50 yds (30-sec recovery)
	Stiff-Leg Deadlift 3 × 10 @ 70% 1RM	Bent-Over Row 3 × 8 @ 75% 1RM		Front Squat 3 × 10 @ 70% 1RM	Lat Pull-Down 3 × 8 @ 75% 1RM	
	Belt Squat 3 × 8 @ 80% 1RM	Swiss Bar Neutral-Grip Bench Press 3 × 8 @ 70% 1RM		Leg Press 3 × 8 @ 80% 1RM	Wide Dumbbell Overhead Press 3 × 8 @ 70% 1RM	
	Box Step-Up 2 × 8 @ 70% 1RM	Neutral-Grip Low-Pulley Row 3 × 8 @ 70% 1RM		Barbell Lunges 2 × 8 @ 70% 1RM	Chin-Ups 2 × 5 @ 6RM 1 × reps to failure	
	Nordic Curls 2 × 8	Cable Machine Chops/Lifts 4 × 10 (1 set per side per direction)		Nordic Curls 2 × 8	Cable Machine Chops/Lifts 4 × 10 (1 set per side per direction)	
	Dumbbell-Loaded Cossack Squat 2 × 8			Dumbbell-Loaded Lateral Box Step-Up 2 × 8		

Note: This is a sample week that includes an upper-/lower-body split routine and metabolic conditioning. Later in the off-season, there would likely be a greater emphasis on power (e.g., plyometrics), as the program transitions toward the pre-season. The exercise selections are based on total-body strength covering fundamental movements but can be adapted to fit the needs of the sport or the specific strengths/weaknesses of the athlete. The progression each week could be a combination of load and/or volume.

SAMPLE PRE-SEASON TRAINING WEEK

Sunday	Monday	Tuesday	Wednesday	Thursday	Friday	Saturday
Rest	Power Clean 3 × 3 @ 85% 1RM	Bench Press 3 × 5 @ 85% 1RM	Conditioning 2 × (8 × 20 yd: 10 yd out and back) (15- sec recovery)	Back Squat 3 × 5 @ 85% 1RM	Narrow-Grip Strict Press 3 × 5 @ 85% 1RM	Conditioning 6 × 40 yd (25-sec recovery) 2 × (8 × 10 yd) (10-sec recovery)
	Front Squat 3 × 6 @ 80% 1RM	Bent-Over Row 3 × 5 @ 85% 1RM		Stiff-Leg Deadlift 3 × 6 @ 80% 1RM	Lat Pull-Down 3 × 6 @ 85% 1RM	
	Box Step-Up 2 × 8 @ 70% 1RM	Swiss Bar Neutral-Grip Bench Press 2 × 6 @ 80% 1RM		Dumbbell-Load Plyometric Lunges 2 × 8 1RM	Wide Dumbbell Overhead Press 2 × 8 @ 70% 1RM	
	Nordic Curls 2 × 8	Neutral-Grip Low-Pulley Row 2 × 6 @ 80% 1RM		Dumbbell-Loaded Lateral Box Step-Up 2 × 8	Chin-Ups 2 × 5 @ 6RM	

Note: This is a sample week that includes an upper-/lower-body split routine and anaerobic conditioning. The strength training begins to incorporate a much greater emphasis on power. Later in the pre-season, there would likely be an even greater shift toward power (e.g., added accessories like hex bar jump squats, landmine jerks) as the program transitions toward the in-season. The exercise selections are based on total-body strength covering fundamental movements but can be adapted to fit the needs of the sport or the specific strengths/weaknesses of the athlete. There is a slight reduction in volume to accommodate sport practices, likely occurring on most days of the week.

SAMPLE IN-SEASON TRAINING PROGRAM

Sunday	Monday	Tuesday	Wednesday	Thursday	Friday	Saturday
	Power Clean 3 × 3 @ 90% 1RM		Front Squat 3 × 3 @ 85% 1RM 3 × 3 Vertical Jump (performed as superset)	3 × 20-yd Flying Sprints (60-sec recovery)	Hex Bar Jump Squat 3 × 3 @ 85% 1RM	
	Back Squat 3 × 5 @ 85% 1RM	Small-Sided Games 4 × 4 min (3-min active recovery between games)	Barbell Hip Thrust 3 × 3 @ 85% 1RM 3 × 3 Broad Jump (performed as superset)	3 ×	Vertical or Broad Jump 3 × 3 Max Effort	
Rest						Game Day
	Bench Press 3 × 5 @ 85% 1RM		Single-Arm Dumbbell Push-Press 3 × 5		Zig-Zag Hops 2 × 10 yd	
	Bent-Over Row 3 × 5 @ 85% 1RM		Renegade Rows 3 × 5			

Note: This is a sample week that includes two total-body workouts and a lower-body pre-game potentiation workout. Maintaining strength is important, but translating that strength into power and athleticism is even more important during the in-season. The exercise selections are less varied and focus on core exercises with the most positive transfer (dependent on the sport). The metabolic conditioning will be more of a maintenance stimulus from games and other practice drills. Small-sided games are an efficient method of offering an opportunity for athletes to be metabolically challenged while still implementing technical and tactical aspects of the sport. During in-season training, the previously trained strength and power should be translated into speed work, which requires more recovery than metabolic conditioning to promote neurological adaptations.

CHAPTER 20

EMOTIONAL RESPONSES OF ATHLETES TO INJURY QUESTIONNAIRE

Athlete Identification No.:

1. List in order of preference the sports and activities you participate in:
   a.
   b.
   c.
   d.
2. Why do you participate in sports? (Value the following: 10 = high, 0 = low)

Self-discipline

| 0 | 1 | 2 | 3 | 4 | 5 | 6 | 7 | 8 | 9 | 10 |

Stress management

| 0 | 1 | 2 | 3 | 4 | 5 | 6 | 7 | 8 | 9 | 10 |

Competition

| 0 | 1 | 2 | 3 | 4 | 5 | 6 | 7 | 8 | 9 | 10 |

Personal improvement

| 0 | 1 | 2 | 3 | 4 | 5 | 6 | 7 | 8 | 9 | 10 |

Socialization

| 0 | 1 | 2 | 3 | 4 | 5 | 6 | 7 | 8 | 9 | 10 |

Outlet of aggression

| 0 | 1 | 2 | 3 | 4 | 5 | 6 | 7 | 8 | 9 | 10 |

Fitness

| 0 | 1 | 2 | 3 | 4 | 5 | 6 | 7 | 8 | 9 | 10 |

Weight management

| 0 | 1 | 2 | 3 | 4 | 5 | 6 | 7 | 8 | 9 | 10 |

Fun

| 0 | 1 | 2 | 3 | 4 | 5 | 6 | 7 | 8 | 9 | 10 |

Other (i.e., well-being)

| 0 | 1 | 2 | 3 | 4 | 5 | 6 | 7 | 8 | 9 | 10 |

3. Would you describe yourself as an athlete?

1	2	3	4	5
(Absolutely not)				(Absolutely yes)

4. When did your injury occur?

Date: _____   Circle one: Before season   Mid-season   End season

5. What specific goals do you have in your sport? Have they changed since the injury? If yes, how?

6. How have you been feeling emotionally since the injury?

7. Please rank how these emotions describe how you are feeling because of the injury. (12 = high, 0 = low)

_____ Helpless   _____ Tense   _____ Bored   _____ Depressed

_____ Angry   _____ Frustrated   _____ Shocked   _____ Discouraged

_____ Frightened   _____ Optimistic   _____ In Pain   _____ Relieved

_____ Other

8. Do you have any fears about returning to sport? If yes, what are they?

9. Are you a person motivated to exercise?

0	1	2	3	4	5	6	7	8	9	10
(Not at all)										(Extremely)

10. How well do you generally handle pain?

1	2	3	4	5
(Not at all)		(Somewhat)		(Very well)

11. Are you encouraged in sports by your significant other? Indicate using Yes or No.

Is this support: pressure   no support   just right

Who exerts most pressure?

_____ Self   _____ Family member   _____ Coach   _____ Other

12. Do you have a strong family support system or close friends who know about your injury?

Circle one: Yes   No

If yes, who are they (i.e., coach, parent, spouse, teammate, friend)?

13. What do you think is the most important thing necessary for your successful recovery?

14. Is the most important thing something you have power over?

1	2	3	4	5
(Not at all)		(Somewhat)		(Very much)

15. How optimistic are you about fully recovering from your injury?

1	2	3	4	5
(Not at all)		(Somewhat)		(Very much)

Source: Smith, A. M., Scott, S. G., O'Fallon, W. M., & Young, M. L. (1990). Emotional responses of athletes to injury. *Mayo Clinic Proceedings*, *65*(1), 38–50. https://doi.org/10.1016/s0025-6196(12)62108-9

INJURY-PSYCHOLOGICAL READINESS TO RETURN TO SPORT SCALE (I-PRRS)

Answer the following questions referring to your main sport prior to injury. For each question, circle the number between to indicate how you feel right now.

Overall confidence to play is	0	10	20	30	40	50	60	70	80	90	100
Confidence to play without pain is	0	10	20	30	40	50	60	70	80	90	100
Confidence to give 100% effort is	0	10	20	30	40	50	60	70	80	90	100
Confidence in injured body part to handle the demands of the situation is	0	10	20	30	40	50	60	70	80	90	100
Confidence in skill level/ability is	0	10	20	30	40	50	60	70	80	90	100
Confidence not to concentrate on the injury is	0	10	20	30	40	50	60	70	80	90	100

SCORING [sum of responses] ÷ 10 = _____

PSYCHOLOGICAL READINESS TO RETURN TO SPORT		
Low Confidence	**Moderate Confidence**	**Highest Confidence**
0–20	30–40	50–60

Key
0–20 = Low confidence
30–40 = Moderate confidence
50–60 = Complete confidence

Adapted from Glazer D. D. (2009). Development and preliminary validation of the Injury-Psychological Readiness to Return to Sport (I-PRRS) scale. *Journal of Athletic Training*, 44(2), 185–189. https://doi.org/10.4085/1062-6050-44.2.185

PROFILE OF MOOD STATES (POMS)

The following list includes words and statements that describe feelings. Circle the number that best describes how you feel right now by selecting the appropriate indicator:
0 = Not at all, 1 = A little, 2 = Moderately, 3 = Quite a lot, 4 = Extremely.

	Not at All	A Little	Moderately	Quite a Lot	Extremely
Tense	0	1	2	3	4
Angry	0	1	2	3	4
Worn out	0	1	2	3	4
Unhappy	0	1	2	3	4
Proud	0	1	2	3	4
Lively	0	1	2	3	4
Confused	0	1	2	3	4
Sad	0	1	2	3	4
Active	0	1	2	3	4
On edge	0	1	2	3	4
Grouchy	0	1	2	3	4
Ashamed	0	1	2	3	4
Energetic	0	1	2	3	4

(continues)

(continued)

	Not at All	A Little	Moderately	Quite a Lot	Extremely
Hopeless	0	1	2	3	4
Uneasy	0	1	2	3	4
Restless	0	1	2	3	4
Unable to concentrate	0	1	2	3	4
Fatigued	0	1	2	3	4
Competent	0	1	2	3	4
Annoyed	0	1	2	3	4
Discouraged	0	1	2	3	4
Resentful	0	1	2	3	4
Nervous	0	1	2	3	4
Miserable	0	1	2	3	4
Confident	0	1	2	3	4
Bitter	0	1	2	3	4
Exhausted	0	1	2	3	4
Anxious	0	1	2	3	4
Helpless	0	1	2	3	4
Weary	0	1	2	3	4
Satisfied	0	1	2	3	4
Bewildered	0	1	2	3	4
Furious	0	1	2	3	4
Full of pep	0	1	2	3	4
Worthless	0	1	2	3	4
Forgetful	0	1	2	3	4
Vigorous	0	1	2	3	4

	Not at All	A Little	Moderately	Quite a Lot	Extremely
Uncertain about things	0	1	2	3	4
Bushed	0	1	2	3	4
Embarrassed	0	1	2	3	4

Grove, J. R., & Prapavessis, H. (1992). Preliminary evidence for the reliability and validity of an abbreviated Profile of Mood States. *Sport Psychology, 23*(2), 93–109.

ACL RETURN TO SPORT AFTER INJURY

Answer the following questions referring to your main sport prior to injury. For each question, circle the number between the two descriptions to indicate how you feel right now relative to the two extremes.

1. Are you confident that you can perform at your previous level of sport participation?

   Not at all confident   0   10   20   30   40   50   60   70   80   90   100   Fully confident

2. Do you think you are likely to reinjure your knee by participating in your sport?

   Extremely likely   0   10   20   30   40   50   60   70   80   90   100   Not likely at all

3. Are you nervous about playing your sport?

   Extremely nervous   0   10   20   30   40   50   60   70   80   90   100   Not nervous at all

4. Are you confident that you could play your sport without concern for your knee?

   Not at all confident   0   10   20   30   40   50   60   70   80   90   100   Fully confident

5. Do you find it frustrating to have to consider your knee with respect to your sport?

   Extremely frustrating   0   10   20   30   40   50   60   70   80   90   100   Not at all frustrating

6. Are you fearful of reinjuring your knee by playing your sport?

   Extremely fearful   0   10   20   30   40   50   60   70   80   90   100   No fear at all

Adapted from Webster, K. E., & Feller, J. A. (2018). Development and validation of a short version of the anterior cruciate ligament return to sport after injury (ACL-RSI) scale. *Orthopaedic Journal of Sports Medicine, 6*(4), 2325967118763763. https://doi.org/10.1177/2325967118763763

SINGLE ASSESSMENT NUMERIC EVALUATION (SANE)

This assessment tool is designed to allow you to report the status of any body part with the intent to help determine needs focused on returning to full participation.

How would you rate your [shoulder] today as a percentage of normal? (0% to 100% scale, with 100% being normal)

Rate your _____ for function with 100% being normal.

Not normal   0   10   20   30   40   50   60   70   80   90   100   Normal

Adapted from Williams, G. N., Gangel, T. J., Arciero, R. A., Uhorchak, J. M., & Taylor, D. C. (1999). Comparison of the single assessment numeric evaluation method and two shoulder rating scales: Outcomes measures after shoulder surgery. *American Journal of Sports Medicine, 27*(2), 214–221. https://doi.org/10.1177/03635465990270021701

FUNCTIONAL ARM SCALE FOR THROWERS (FAST)

This questionnaire seeks to provide insight about how your arm (shoulder, upper arm, elbow, forearm, write, hand, fingers) feels. The questions aim at identifying how your arm condition affects your ability to throw and to function in sport and daily activities.

Answer the following questions based on your arm condition during the last week by circling the number for the appropriate response. If you did not engage in an activity in the past week, answer questions based on your estimate of how your arm condition would affect your ability to engage in the activity.

*Pitchers, make sure to complete the pitcher-specific section.

	Completely	Extremely	Moderately	Slightly	Not Satisfied at All
1. How satisfied are you with the way your arm is now functioning?	1	2	3	4	5
	None	Mild	Moderate	Severe	Extreme
2. How much pain do you have in your injured arm prior to your start, following your warm-up?	1	2	3	4	5
3. How much pain or discomfort do you have in your arm at night?	1	2	3	4	5
4. How much strength have you lost in your arm as a result of your arm injury?	1	2	3	4	5
5. How much pain or discomfort do you have in your arm with daily activities involving reaching?	1	2	3	4	5
6. How much pain or discomfort do you have in your arm if you use it for activities that last longer than 30 minutes?	1	2	3	4	5

	Not at All	Slightly	Moderately	Severely	Extremely
7. How much has your arm injury limited your ability to advance in baseball or softball?	1	2	3	4	5
8. How much have you modified your behavior to avoid making your arm injury worse?	1	2	3	4	5
9. Since your arm injury, do you have a more negative outlook on life?	1	2	3	4	5
10. How much does your arm injury interfere with things that are important, other than sports?	1	2	3	4	5
11. How stiff is your arm at night?	1	2	3	4	5
12. How much has your playing time gone down since the injury to your arm?	1	2	3	4	5
13. How much are you limited when lifting your arm overhead to get dressed?	1	2	3	4	5

	No, Not at All	Yes, Slightly	Yes, Moderately	Yes, Severely	Yes, Extremely
14. Has your enjoyment of life decreased since your arm injury?	1	2	3	4	5
15. Has your arm injury decreased how long you can continue throwing during a single practice or game?	1	2	3	4	5
16. Have your sports accomplishments decreased since your arm injury?	1	2	3	4	5
17. Has your life been more stressful because of your arm injury?	1	2	3	4	5

	Not at All	Slightly	Moderately	Severely	Unable to Throw
18. How much has your arm injury limited your ability to throw "long toss"?	1	2	3	4	5
19. How much has your throwing accuracy decreased since your arm injury?	1	2	3	4	5

(continues)

(continued)

	Not at All	Slightly	Moderately	Severely	Unable to Throw
20. How weak does your arm feel during throwing?	1	2	3	4	5
21. How painful is your arm during "game speed" throwing?	1	2	3	4	5
22. How painful is your arm during 50% to 75% effort throwing?	1	2	3	4	5

PITCHER MODULE (ALL PITCHERS MUST COMPLETE THIS SECTION)

The following questions are designed to determine the impact of a baseball/softball pitcher's arm injury on pitching-specific functional performance.

	Not at All	Slightly	Moderately	Severely	Unable to Perform
1. How much has your arm injury limited the speed of your pitches?	1	2	3	4	5
2. How much has your arm injury limited your ability to throw "bullpen" sessions?	1	2	3	4	5
3. How much has your arm injury limited your ability to "hit" your spots?	1	2	3	4	5
4. How limited is your ability to pitch your turn in the rotation?	1	2	3	4	5
5. How much have your overall pitching statistics been hurt since your arm injury?	1	2	3	4	5
6. How much has your pitch count decreased since your arm injury?	1	2	3	4	5
7. How much has your arm injury limited your ability to throw different types of pitches?	1	2	3	4	5
8. How much has your pitch count decreased since your arm injury?	1	2	3	4	5
9. Do you need more time to recover between outings since your arm injury?	1	2	3	4	5

Adapted from Sauers, E. L., Bay, R. C., Snyder Valier, A. R., Ellery, T., & Huxel Bliven, K. C. (2017). The Functional Arm Scale for Throwers (FAST): Part I: The design and development of an upper extremity region-specific and population-specific patient-reported outcome scale for throwing athletes. *Orthopaedic Journal of Sports Medicine, 5*(3), 2325967117698455. https://doi.org/10.1177/2325967117698455

INTERVAL THROWING PROGRAM

Phase 1 Program for Baseball Players*

45-ft Phase		60-ft Phase		90-ft Phase		120-ft Phase	
Step 1	a. Warm-up throwing b. 45 ft, 25 throws c. Rest 5–10 min d. Warm-up throwing e. 45 ft, 25 throws	Step 3	a. Warm-up throwing b. 60 ft, 25 throws c. Rest 5–10 min d. Warm-up throwing e. 60 ft, 25 throws	Step 5	a. Warm-up throwing b. 90 ft, 25 throws c. Rest 5–10 min d. Warm-up throwing e. 90 ft, 25 throws	Step 7	a. Warm-up throwing b. 120 ft, 25 throws c. Rest 5–10 min d. Warm-up throwing e. 120 ft, 25 throws
Step 2	a. Warm-up throwing b. 45 ft, 25 throws c. Rest 5–10 min d. Warm-up throwing e. 45 ft, 25 throws f. Rest 5–10 min g. Warm-up throwing h. 45 ft, 25 throws	Step 4	a. Warm-up throwing b. 60 ft, 25 throws c. Rest 5–10 min d. Warm-up throwing e. 60 ft, 25 throws f. Rest 5–10 min g. Warm-up throwing h. 60 ft, 25 throws	Step 6	a. Warm-up throwing b. 90 ft, 25 throws c. Rest 5–10 min d. Warm-up throwing e. 90 ft, 25 throws f. Rest 5–10 min g. Warm-up throwing h. 90 ft, 25 throws	Step 8	a. Warm-up throwing b. 120 ft, 25 throws c. Rest 5–10 min d. Warm-up throwing e. 120 ft, 25 throws f. Rest 5–10 min g. Warm-up throwing h. 120 ft, 25 throws

150-ft Phase		180-ft Phase					
Step 9	a. Warm-up throwing b. 150 ft, 25 throws c. Rest 5–10 min d. Warm-up throwing e. 150 ft, 25 throws	Step 11	a. Warm-up throwing b. 180 ft, 25 throws c. Rest 5–10 min d. Warm-up throwing e. 180 ft, 25 throws	Step 13	a. Warm-up throwing b. 180 ft, 25 throws c. Rest 5–10 min d. Warm-up throwing e. 180 ft, 25 throws f. Rest 5–10 min g. Warm-up throwing h. 180 ft, 25 throws i. Rest 5–10 min j. Warm-up throwing k. 15 throws, progressing from 120 to 90 ft	**Note:** All throws should be on an arc with a crow hop. Warm-up throws consist of 10–20 throws at approximately 30 ft. The throwing program should be performed every other day, 3 times per week, unless otherwise specified by a physician or rehabilitation specialist. Perform each step _____ times before progressing to the next step.	

(continues)

(continued)

150-ft Phase		180-ft Phase		Note	Return to respective position or progress to Step 14 below		
Step 10	a. Warm-up throwing b. 150 ft, 25 throws c. Rest 5–10 min d. Warm-up throwing e. 150 ft, 25 throws f. Rest 5–10 min g. Warm-up throwing h. 150 ft, 25 throws	Step 12	a. Warm-up throwing b. 180 ft, 25 throws c. Rest 5–10 min d. Warm-up throwing e. 180 ft, 25 throws f. Rest 5–10 min g. Warm-up throwing h. 180 ft, 25 throws				

Flat-Ground Throwing for Baseball Pitchers

Step 14	a. Warm-up throwing b. 60 ft 10–15 throws c. 90 ft, 10 throws d. 120 ft, 10 throws e. 60 ft, (flat-ground) using pitching mechanics, 20–30 throws	Step 15	a. Warm-up throwing b. 60 ft, 10–15 throws c. 90 ft, 10 throws d. 120 ft, 10 throws e. 60 ft, (flat-ground) using pitching mechanics, 20–30 throws f. 60–90 ft, 10–15 throws g. 60 ft, (flat-ground) using pitching mechanics, 20 throws

Progress to Phase 2: Throwing off the Mound

*45 ft = 13.7 m; 60 ft = 18.3 m; 90 ft = 27.4 m; 120 ft = 36.6 m; 150 ft = 45.7 m; 180 ft = 54.8 m.

INTERVAL THROWING PROGRAM, PHASE 2: THROWING OFF THE MOUND*‡

Stage 1: Fastballs Only

Step 1	a. Interval throwing[t] b. 15 throws, 50%
Step 2	a. Interval throwing[t] b. 30 throws, 50%
Step 3	a. Interval throwing[t] b. 45 throws, 50%
Step 4	a. Interval throwing[t] b. 60 throws, 50%

Stage 1: Fastballs Only	
Step 5	a. Interval throwing[t] b. 70 throws, 50%
Step 6	a. 45 throws, 50% b. 30 throws, 75%
Step 7	a. 30 throws, 50% b. 45 throws, 75%
Step 8	a. 10 throws, 50% b. 65 throws, 75%

Stage 2: Fastballs Only	
Step 9	a. 60 throws, 75% b. 15 throws, batting practice
Step 10	a. 50–60 throws, 75% b. 30 throws, batting practice
Step 11	a. 45–50 throws, 75% b. 45 throws, batting practice

Stage 3	
Step 12	a. 30 throws, 75% b. 15 throws, 50%, begin breaking balls c. 45–60 throws, batting practice, fastball only
Step 13	a. 30 throws, 75% b. 30 breaking balls, 75% c. 30 throws, batting practice
Step 14	a. 30 throws, 75% b. 60–90 throws, batting practice, gradually increase breaking balls
Step 15	a. Simulated game: progressing by 15 throws per workout (pitch count)

*Represents percentage effort.

‡ All throwing off the mound should be done in the presence of a pitching coach or sport biomechanist to stress proper throwing mechanics (use speed gun to aid in effort control).

† Use interval throwing 120-ft (36.6-m) phase as warm-up.

SHORT-DURATION INTERVAL THROWING PROGRAM*

Day 1	a. 45 ft, 30 throws b. 60 ft, 30 throws	Day 12	a. Rest
Day 2	a. 45 ft, 45 throws b. 60 ft, 45 throws	Day 13	a. 60 ft, 100 throws b. Bullpen pitching, fastballs only, 25 pitches, 75% effort
Day 3	a. 60 ft, 125 throws	Day 14	a. 45 ft, 50 throws b. 90 ft, 30 throws c. 120 ft, 20 throws d. 45 ft, 50 throws
Day 4	a. 60 ft, 85 throws b. 90 ft, 30 throws c. 60 ft, 20 throws	Day 15	a. 60 ft, 100 throws b. Bullpen pitching, fastballs and change-ups, 35 pitches, 80% effort
Day 5	a. Rest	Day 16	a. Rest
Day 6	a. 60 ft, 100 throws b. 90 ft, 30 throws c. 60 ft, 20 throws	Day 17	a. 60 ft, 100 throws b. Bullpen pitching, all pitches, 45 pitches, 100% effort
Day 7	a. 60 ft, 50 throws b. 90 ft, 50 throws c. 60 ft, 50 throws	Day 18	a. 45 ft, 50 throws b. 90 ft, 30 throws c. 120 ft, 20 throws d. 45 ft, 50 throws
Day 8	a. 60 ft, 50 throws b. 90 ft, 50 throws c. 120 ft, 25 throws d. 60 ft, 20 throws	Day 19	a. Simulated game, 25 pitches
Day 9	a. Rest	Day 20	a. 45 ft, 50 throws b. 90 ft, 30 throws c. 120 ft, 20 throws d. 45 ft, 50 throws
Day 10	a. 60 ft, 50 throws b. 90 ft, 20 throws c. 120 ft, 50 throws d. 60 ft, 20 throws	Day 21	a. Game, 25–35 pitches
Day 11	a. 60 ft, 50 throws b. 90 ft, 20 throws c. 120 ft, 60 throws d. 60 ft, 20 throws		

*45 ft = 13.7 m; 60 ft = 18.3 m; 90 ft = 27.4 m; 120 ft = 36.6 m.

OPT® CES PROGRAMMING TEMPLATE

CLIENT'S NAME: Jim
GOAL: Manage bilateral knee and foot soreness
PHASE:
DATE:

EXERCISE	SETS	REPS	TEMPO	REST	NOTES
FLEXIBILITY: Inhibit with self-myofascial rolling or other technique and lengthen with stretching techniques					
Gastrocnemius	1	30 sec			
Adductors	1	30 sec			
IT band/TFL	1	30 sec			
FLEXIBILITY: Inhibit with self-myofascial rolling or other technique and lengthen with stretching techniques					
Piriformis	1	30 sec			
Peroneals	1	30 sec			
ACTIVATION: Isolated strengthening, trunk postural control (core), balance (hip/knee/ankle integration)					
Anterior tibialis	1	12	Slow		
Gluteus medius	1	12	Slow		
Gluteus maximus	1	12	Slow		
INTEGRATION AND SKILL DEVELOPMENT: Integrated dynamic movement, SAQ, plyometrics, goal-specific prep					
Single-leg balance reach	1–2	12	Slow	30 sec	
Front step-up to balance	1–2	12	Slow	30 sec	
Multiplanar hop	1–2	12	Control	30 sec	

(continues)

(continued)

EXERCISE	SETS	REPS	TEMPO	REST	NOTES
RESISTANCE TRAINING: Specific to phase and goal					
CLIENT'S CHOICE: Single joint, additional core training, accessory movements, metabolic conditioning					
COOL-DOWN: Myofascial technique and static stretch					

OPT® CES PROGRAMMING TEMPLATE

CLIENT'S NAME: Maria

GOAL: Improve hip mobility; prevent ACL injury

PHASE:

DATE:

EXERCISE	SETS	REPS	TEMPO	REST	NOTES
FLEXIBILITY: Inhibit with self-myofascial rolling or other technique and lengthen with stretching techniques					
Gastrocnemius	1	30 sec			.
Adductors	1	30 sec			
IT band/TFL	1	30 sec			

EXERCISE	SETS	REPS	TEMPO	REST	NOTES
ACTIVATION: Isolated strengthening, trunk postural control (core), balance (hip/knee/ankle integration)					
Anterior tibialis	1–2	30 sec	Slow		
Gluteus medius	1–2	30 sec	Slow		
Gluteus maximus	1–2	30 sec	Slow		
INTEGRATION AND SKILL DEVELOPMENT: Integrated dynamic movement, SAQ, plyometrics, goal-specific prep					
Lateral tube walk	1–2	30 sec	Slow	30 sec	
Single-leg squat	1–2	30 sec	Slow	30 sec	
Ice skater hop	1–2	30 sec	Control	30 sec	
RESISTANCE TRAINING: Specific to phase and goal					

EXERCISE	SETS	REPS	TEMPO	REST	NOTES
CLIENT'S CHOICE: Single joint, additional core training, accessory movements, metabolic conditioning					
COOL-DOWN: Myofascial technique and static stretch					

CLIENT'S NAME: Mika

GOAL: Manage bilateral foot pain for runner

PHASE:

DATE:

EXERCISE	SETS	REPS	TEMPO	REST	NOTES
FLEXIBILITY: Inhibit with self-myofascial rolling or other technique and lengthen with stretching techniques					
Gastrocnemius	1	30 sec			
Peroneals	1	30 sec			
Adductors	1	30 sec			
IT band/TFL	1	30 sec			
Soleus	1	30 sec			
ACTIVATION: Isolated strengthening, trunk postural control (core), balance (hip/knee/ankle integration)					
Anterior tibialis	1–2	12			
Foot intrinsics	1–2	12			
Gluteus maximus	1–2	12			
EXERCISE	SETS	REPS	TEMPO	REST	NOTES
INTEGRATION AND SKILL DEVELOPMENT: Integrated dynamic movement, SAQ, plyometrics, goal-specific prep					
Single-leg Romanian deadlift	1–2	12			
Ball wall squat	1–2	12			
Multiplanar hop with stability	1–2	12			
RESISTANCE TRAINING: Specific to phase and goal					

EXERCISE	SETS	REPS	TEMPO	REST	NOTES
CLIENT'S CHOICE: Single joint, additional core training, accessory movements, metabolic conditioning					
COOL-DOWN: Myofascial technique and static stretch					

OPT® CES PROGRAMMING TEMPLATE

CLIENT'S NAME: Dave

GOAL: Manage low back pain; improve overall stability and mobility

PHASE:

DATE:

EXERCISE	SETS	REPS	TEMPO	REST	NOTES
FLEXIBILITY: Inhibit with self-myofascial rolling or other technique and lengthen with stretching techniques					
Gastrocnemius	1	30 sec			
IT band/TFL	1	30 sec			
FLEXIBILITY: Inhibit with self-myofascial rolling or other technique and lengthen with stretching techniques					
Piriformis	1	30 sec			
Rectus femoris	1	30 sec			
Hamstrings	1	30 sec			
ACTIVATION: Isolated strengthening, trunk postural control (core), balance (hip/knee/ankle integration)					
Gluteus medius	1–2	12			
Gluteus maximus	1–2	12			

(continues)

(continued)

EXERCISE	SETS	REPS	TEMPO	REST	NOTES
INTEGRATION AND SKILL DEVELOPMENT: Integrated dynamic movement, SAQ, plyometrics, goal-specific prep					
Ball wall squat	1–2	12	Slow	30 sec	
Ball prone cobra	1–2	12	Slow	30 sec	
Single-leg balance reach	1–2	12	Slow	30 sec	
Single-leg hip rotation	1–2	12	Slow	30 sec	
RESISTANCE TRAINING: Specific to phase and goal					
CLIENT'S CHOICE: Single joint, additional core training, accessory movements, metabolic conditioning					
COOL-DOWN: Myofascial technique and static stretch					

CHAPTER 21

DEVELOPMENTAL STAGE AND MUSCULAR PERFORMANCE

How young is too young to start training?

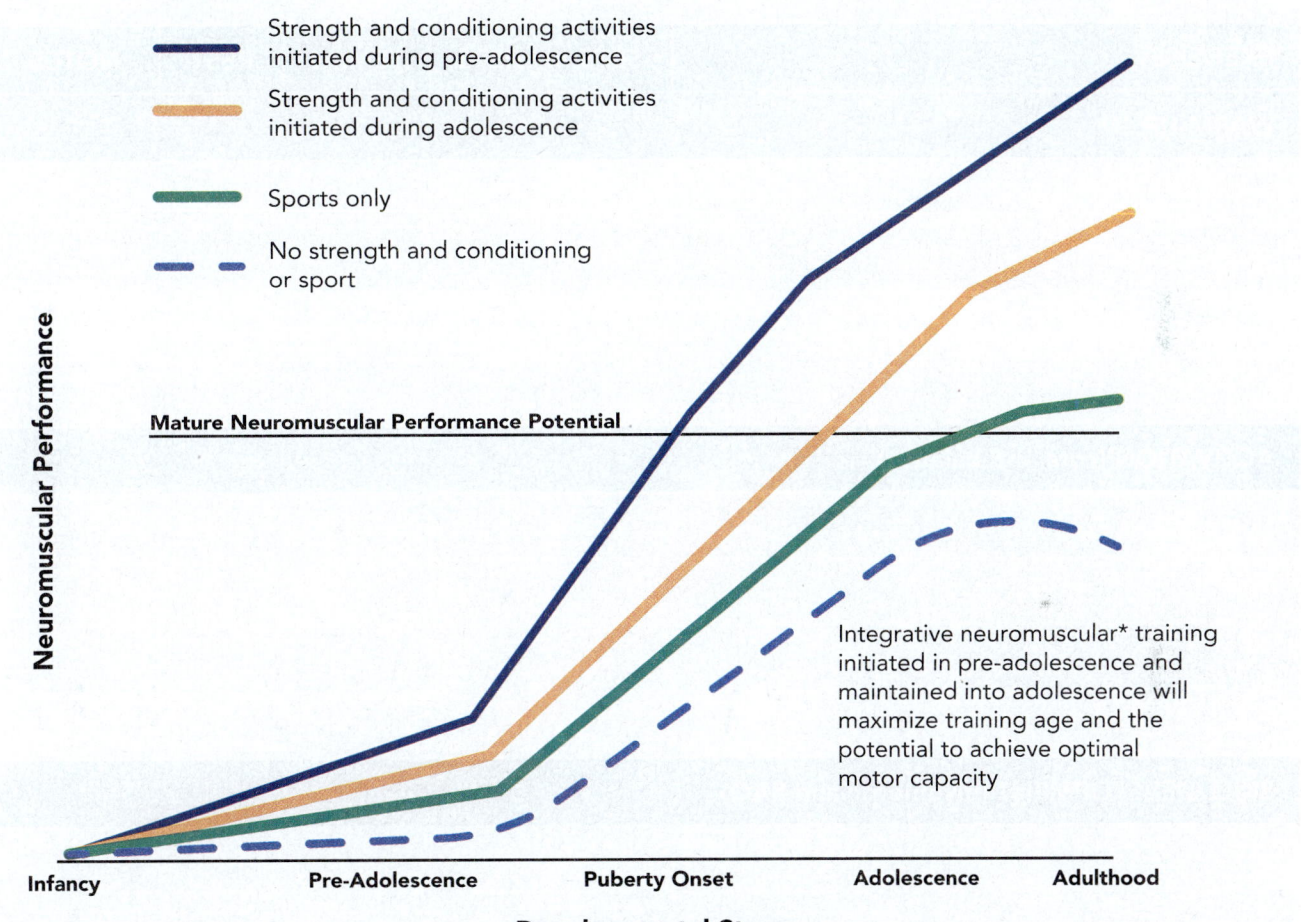

Legend:
- Strength and conditioning activities initiated during pre-adolescence
- Strength and conditioning activities initiated during adolescence
- Sports only
- No strength and conditioning or sport

Mature Neuromuscular Performance Potential

Integrative neuromuscular* training initiated in pre-adolescence and maintained into adolescence will maximize training age and the potential to achieve optimal motor capacity

Y-axis: Neuromuscular Performance

X-axis: Infancy — Pre-Adolescence — Puberty Onset — Adolescence — Adulthood

Developmental Stage

*Resistance training, dynamic stability exercises, core-focused training plyometric drills, and agility training

Adapted from Myer et al. (2013).

OPTIMUM PERFORMANCE TRAINING®

EXERCISE	SETS	REPS	TEMPO	REST	NOTES
CLIENT'S NAME:					
GOAL:					
PHASE:					
DATE:					
WARM-UP					
ACTIVATION (core and balance)					
SKILL DEVELOPMENT (plyometric and SAQ)					
RESISTANCE TRAINING					

EXERCISE	SETS	REPS	TEMPO	REST	NOTES
RESISTANCE TRAINING					
CLIENT'S CHOICE					
COOL-DOWN					

Coaching Tips:

MODIFIED MODEL FOR CHILDREN AND EARLY ADOLESCENTS

Goals/Focus	• General physical preparation
	    • Games (chase and be chased)
	    • Low structure
	    • One plane to two planes to three planes
	    • LTAD principles
	        • Include muscle-strengthening exercises with a variety of implements
	        • Focus on developing and improving fundamental movements
	• Improve overall cardiorespiratory and neuromuscular condition
	• Establish proper movement patterns and exercise technique
	• Address motor deficits

Adaptation	• 10 fitness attributes • Athletic motor skill competencies
Length of Phase	• Throughout childhood and adolescence

Method of Progression	• Motor skill competence followed by increasing complexity of motor skills and movement
	• Introduce all fitness attributes:
	    • Fundamental movement skills
	    • Sport-specific skills
	    • Strength
	    • Flexibility
	    • Core
	    • Balance
	    • Plyometric
	    • SAQ
	• Introduce all functional movements of exercise:
	    • Squat
	    • Hinge
	    • Lunge
	    • Horizontal pull
	    • Vertical pull
	    • Horizontal push
	    • Vertical push

Movements	• Flexibility • Core • Balance • Plyometric • SAQ • Resistance

RECOMMENDATIONS FOR ACUTE TRAINING VARIABLES

	Training Goal (Level of OPT™ Model)	Untrained and Inexperienced	Intermediate	Trained and Experienced
1. Repetitions	Stabilization/muscle endurance	12+	12+	12+
	Strength	8–12	5–10	Depends on performance goal
	Power	3–6	3–6	1–6
2. Sets	Stabilization/muscle endurance	1–2	1–3	1–3
	Strength	1–2	2–5	Depends on performance goal
	Power	1–2	2–3	3
3. Intensity	Stabilization/muscle endurance	Low	Moderate	High
	Strength	50%–70% of estimated 1RM	60%–80% of 1RM	70%–85% of 1RM
	Power	30%–60% of 1RM (velocity)	30%–60% of 1RM (velocity) 60%–70% of 1RM (strength)	30%–60% of 1RM (velocity) 70%–80% of 1RM (strength)
4. Tempo	Stabilization/muscle endurance	Controlled	Moderate	Moderate
	Strength	Moderate	Moderate	Depends on training goal
	Power	Gradually increase the velocity from moderate to fast (1 second or less) as technique improves.	Fast (1 second or less)	Fast (1 second or less)

(continues)

(continued)

	Training Goal (Level of OPT™ Model)	Untrained and Inexperienced	Intermediate	Trained and Experienced
5. Volume	Stabilization/muscle endurance	1–2 sets, 10–15 reps	2–3 sets, 10–15 reps	≥3 sets, 10–15 reps
	Strength	1–2 sets, 10–15 reps	2–3 sets, 8–12 reps	≥3 sets, 6–10 reps
	Power	1–2 sets, 3–6 reps	2–3 sets, 3–6 reps	≥3 sets, 1–6 reps
6. Rest	Stabilization/muscle endurance	As much as needed	30 seconds or less	30 seconds or less
	Strength	1 minute	1 minute	1 minute
	Power	1 minute	1–2 minutes	2–3 minutes
7. Frequency	Stabilization/muscle endurance	2–3 nonconsecutive days	2–3 nonconsecutive days	2–3 nonconsecutive days
	Strength	2–3 days	2–3 days	3–4 days
	Power	2 days	2–3 days	2–3 days
8. Exercise Selection	Stabilization/muscle endurance	Variety of bodyweight and resistance (bands, barbells, dumbbells, kettlebells, etc.)	Variety of bodyweight and resistance (bands, barbells, dumbbells, kettlebells, etc.)	Variety of bodyweight and resistance (bands, barbells, dumbbells, kettlebells, etc.)
	Strength	Single-joint, multi-joint, and total-body; concentric and eccentric	Single-joint, multi-joint, and total-body; concentric and eccentric	Single-joint, multi-joint, and total-body; concentric and eccentric
	Power	Multi-joint and total-body; concentric and eccentric	Multi-joint and total-body; concentric and eccentric	Multi-joint and total-body; concentric and eccentric

CHAPTER 22

TYPES OF FAT

Type of Fat	Role/Health Benefit	Food Sources
Monounsaturated fats	• Heart healthy • Notably high in the Mediterranean diet	• Olives, olive oil • Canola oil • Avocado • Peanuts
Polyunsaturated fats: omega-3 • Eicosapentaenoic acid (EPA) • Docosahexaenoic acid (DHA) • Alpha-linolenic acid (ALA)	• Heart healthy • Lower triglycerides • Associated with improvements in high-density lipoprotein (HDL) cholesterol levels • Reduced inflammation • Associated with improved cognitive function • Associated with a reduced risk of dementia	• Fatty fish (EPA and DHA): salmon, tuna, sardines, mackerel • Walnuts, flaxseed, chia seeds (ALA) • Fortified milk, fortified eggs (DHA) • Dairy from grass-fed cows (DHA, ALA) • Green vegetables (ALA)
Polyunsaturated fats: omega-6	• Essential for normal growth and development	• Vegetable oils, nuts, seeds
Saturated fats	• Exact health benefits remain unclear • General recommendations advise limiting excess saturated fats in the diet	• Animal fats, full-fat dairy, coconut oil, palm oil

(continues)

(continued)

Type of Fat	Role/Health Benefit	Food Sources	
Trans fats	• Artificial/added trans fats increase LDL cholesterol and lower HDL cholesterol. They are also associated with increased inflammation and heart disease (Harvard Medical School, 2015). • Naturally occurring trans fats are less harmful than artificial trans fat		• Artificial/added trans fats are in partially hydrogenated oils and processed foods that contain these oils • Naturally occurring trans fats are found in animal fats and dairy

FOOD FREQUENCY QUESTIONNAIRE

Name _____   **Date** _____

Disclosure: *The following Food Frequency Questionnaire has been adapted from the National Institutes of Health's Diet History Questionnaire III (DHQ III). To simplify this questionnaire and help nutrition coaches remain within their scope of practice, vitamin and mineral supplement questions have been omitted.*

This questionnaire is for informational and nutrition coaching purposes and is not intended to diagnose illness or prescribe nutritional therapy.

Instructions: Answer the following questions to the best of your ability. It is important, for the accuracy of this questionnaire, to answer each question truthfully. Questions are broken into major categories similar to the DHQ III. If a question does not apply to you or you simply do not consume the food or drink in question, leave the associated answer fields blank.

BEVERAGES

Please check the box next to each food/beverage that you ate at least once in the **past 12 months**.		How often did you consume this food/beverage over the **past 12 months**?			What portion size do you usually drink/eat each in one sitting?		
		Rarely	Sometimes	Consistently	Small	Medium	Large
Tomato juice or vegetable juice	☐						
Orange juice or grapefruit juice	☐						
Grape juice	☐						

Please check the box next to each food/beverage that you ate at least once in the **past 12 months**.		How often did you consume this food/beverage over the **past 12 months**?			What portion size do you usually drink/eat each in one sitting?		
		Rarely	Sometimes	Consistently	Small	Medium	Large
Other 100% fruit juices (such as apple)	☐						
Fruit or vegetable smoothies	☐						
Boxed fruit drinks	☐						
Milk as a beverage	☐						
Milkshakes	☐						
Meal replacement or high-protein beverages	☐						
Soda or pop	☐						
Sports drinks	☐						
Energy drinks	☐						
Water	☐						
Vitamin-enhanced water	☐						
Beer	☐						
Wine or wine cooler	☐						
Liquor or mixed drinks	☐						
Coffee (NOT including espresso drinks such as latte, mocha, etc.)	☐						
Espresso drink mixtures (including latte, mocha, cappuccino, etc.)	☐						
Cold or iced tea (caffeinated or decaffeinated)	☐						

FRUITS

Please check the box next to each food/beverage that you ate at least once in the **past 12 months**.		How often did you consume this food/beverage over the **past 12 months**?			What portion size do you usually drink/eat each in one sitting?		
		Rarely	Sometimes	Consistently	Small	Medium	Large
Applesauce	☐						
Apples	☐						
Bananas	☐						
Pineapple	☐						
Pears	☐						
Peaches	☐						
Dried fruit	☐						
Grapes	☐						
Cantaloupe	☐						
Melons (other than cantaloupe)	☐						
Strawberries	☐						
Blueberries	☐						
Oranges, tangerines, clementines	☐						
Grapefruit	☐						
Avocado or guacamole	☐						
Other (not listed above)	☐						

VEGETABLES

Please check the box next to each food/beverage that you ate at least once in the **past 12 months**.		How often did you consume this food/beverage over the **past 12 months**?			What portion size do you usually drink/eat each in one sitting?		
		Rarely	Sometimes	Consistently	Small	Medium	Large
Cooked greens (such as spinach, turnip, collard, mustard, chard, or kale)	☐						
Raw greens (such as spinach, turnip, collard, chard, kale, watercress, seaweed, mustard greens, beet greens, or dandelion greens)	☐						
Coleslaw	☐						
Sauerkraut or cabbage (other than coleslaw)	☐						
Cooked carrots	☐						
Raw carrots	☐						
String beans or green beans	☐						
Peas	☐						
Corn	☐						
Broccoli	☐						
Cauliflower or Brussels sprouts	☐						
Sweet peppers	☐						
Onions	☐						
Garlic	☐						
Mixed vegetables	☐						
Lettuce salads	☐						
Salad dressing on salads	☐						
Mayonnaise on salads	☐						

(continues)

Please check the box next to each food/beverage that you ate at least once in the past 12 months.		How often did you consume this food/beverage over the past 12 months?			What portion size do you usually drink/eat each in one sitting?		
		Rarely	Sometimes	Consistently	Small	Medium	Large
Salsa	☐						
Fresh tomatoes	☐						
Ketchup	☐						
Sweet potatoes or yams	☐						
French fries, home fries, hash browned potatoes, or Tater Tots	☐						
Potato salad	☐						
Baked, boiled, or mashed potatoes	☐						
Cooked dried or canned beans	☐						
Other kinds of vegetables (not listed above)	☐						

SOUPS

Please check the box next to each food/beverage that you ate at least once in the past 12 months.		How often did you consume this food/beverage over the past 12 months?			What portion size do you usually drink/eat each in one sitting?		
		Rarely	Sometimes	Consistently	Small	Medium	Large
Homemade soups	☐						
Canned soups	☐						
Soups (during the winter)	☐						
Soups (during the rest of the year)	☐						
Bean soups	☐						

Please check the box next to each food/beverage that you ate at least once in the **past 12 months**.		How often did you consume this food/beverage over the **past 12 months**?			What portion size do you usually drink/eat each in one sitting?		
		Rarely	Sometimes	Consistently	Small	Medium	Large
Tomato or vegetable soups	☐						
Broth soups with or without noodles and/or rice	☐						
Chili	☐						

RICE, PASTA, PIZZA, TORTILLAS

Please check the box next to each food/beverage that you ate at least once in the **past 12 months**.		How often did you consume this food/beverage over the **past 12 months**?			What portion size do you usually drink/eat each in one sitting?		
		Rarely	Sometimes	Consistently	Small	Medium	Large
Rice or other cooked grains	☐						
Sushi	☐						
Lasagna, stuffed shells, stuffed manicotti, ravioli, or tortellini	☐						
Macaroni and cheese	☐						
Pasta salad or macaroni salad	☐						
Pasta, spaghetti, or other noodles	☐						
Rice or other cooked grains	☐						
Pizza	☐						
Corn or wheat tortillas	☐						
Tacos, tostados	☐						
Burritos, chimichangas	☐						
Enchiladas, quesadillas	☐						

CEREAL, PANCAKES, BREADS

Please check the box next to each food/beverage that you ate at least once in the past 12 months.		How often did you consume this food/beverage over the past 12 months?			What portion size do you usually drink/eat each in one sitting?		
		Rarely	Sometimes	Consistently	Small	Medium	Large
Oatmeal, grits, or other cooked cereals	☐						
Cold cereal	☐						
Pancakes, waffles, or French toast	☐						
Bagels or English muffin	☐						
Breads or rolls (as part of a sandwich)	☐						
Breads or dinner rolls (not as part of a sandwich)	☐						
Cornbread or corn muffins	☐						
Biscuits	☐						
Jam, jelly, or honey (on bagels, muffins, breads, rolls, crackers, etc.)	☐						
Peanut butter or other nut butter	☐						
Hummus	☐						

PROCESSED MEATS

Please check the box next to each food/beverage that you ate at least once in the past 12 months.		How often did you consume this food/beverage over the past 12 months?			What portion size do you usually drink/eat each in one sitting?		
		Rarely	Sometimes	Consistently	Small	Medium	Large
Roast beef or steak (in sandwiches)	☐						
Luncheon or deli-style ham	☐						

Please check the box next to each food/beverage that you ate at least once in the past 12 months.		How often did you consume this food/beverage over the **past 12 months?**			What portion size do you usually drink/eat each in one sitting?		
		Rarely	Sometimes	Consistently	Small	Medium	Large
Turkey or chicken cold cuts	☐						
Bologna	☐						
Other cold cuts or luncheon meats (such as salami, corned beef, pastrami)	☐						
Hot dogs or frankfurters	☐						

MEAT, POULTRY, FISH, AND MEAT SUBSTITUTES

Please check the box next to each food/beverage that you ate at least once in the past 12 months.		How often did you consume this food/beverage over the **past 12 months?**			What portion size do you usually drink/eat each in one sitting?		
		Rarely	Sometimes	Consistently	Small	Medium	Large
Ground chicken or turkey	☐						
Baked, broiled, roasted, stewed, grilled, pan-fried, or fried chicken (including chicken nuggets)	☐						
Chicken in mixed dishes (such as salads, sandwiches, casseroles, stews, or other mixtures)	☐						
Turkey in mixed dishes (such as salads, sandwiches, casseroles, stews, or other mixtures)	☐						
Beef hamburgers or cheeseburger (from a fast-food restaurant)	☐						
Beef hamburgers or cheeseburger (NOT from a fast-food restaurant)	☐						

(continues)

(continued)

Please check the box next to each food/beverage that you ate at least once in the past 12 months.		How often did you consume this food/beverage over the past 12 months?			What portion size do you usually drink/eat each in one sitting?		
		Rarely	Sometimes	Consistently	Small	Medium	Large
Ground beef in mixtures (such as meatballs, casseroles, chili, or meatloaf)	☐						
Beef mixtures (such as beef stew, beef pot pie, beef and noodles, or beef and vegetables)	☐						
Roast beef or pot roast	☐						
Beef steak	☐						
Baked ham or ham steak	☐						
Pork	☐						
Gravy on meat, chicken, potatoes, rice, etc.	☐						
Liver	☐						
Bacon	☐						
Sausage	☐						
Canned tuna or tuna salad	☐						
Fresh tuna, trout, anchovy, mackerel, herring, or sardine	☐						
Salmon	☐						
Fried shellfish (such as crab, lobster, shrimp, or clams)	☐						
Shellfish (such as crab, lobster, or shrimp) that was NOT FRIED	☐						
Fish sticks or other fried fish	☐						
Other fish that was NOT FRIED	☐						

Please check the box next to each food/beverage that you ate at least once in the past 12 months.		How often did you consume this food/beverage over the **past 12 months?**			What portion size do you usually drink/eat each in one sitting?		
		Rarely	Sometimes	Consistently	Small	Medium	Large
Eggs, egg whites	☐						
Tofu, soy burgers, or soy meat substitutes	☐						

CHIPS, PRETZELS, OTHER SNACKS

Please check the box next to each food/beverage that you ate at least once in the **past 12 months.**		How often did you consume this food/beverage over the **past 12 months?**			What portion size do you usually drink/eat each in one sitting?		
		Rarely	Sometimes	Consistently	Small	Medium	Large
Crackers	☐						
Potato chips	☐						
Corn chips or tortilla chips	☐						
Popcorn	☐						
Pretzels	☐						
Whole nuts (including peanuts, almonds, seeds, or other nuts)	☐						
	☐						
High-protein or breakfast bars	☐						
Protein powder	☐						
Granola bars	☐						

YOGURT AND CHEESE

Please check the box next to each food/beverage that you ate at least once in the **past 12 months**.		How often did you consume this food/beverage over the **past 12 months**?			What portion size do you usually drink/eat each in one sitting?		
		Rarely	Sometimes	Consistently	Small	Medium	Large
Yogurt (NOT including frozen yogurt)	☐						
Greek yogurt	☐						
Cottage cheese or ricotta cheese	☐						
Cheese (including low-fat, on cheeseburgers, or in sandwiches or subs)	☐						
Whipped cream	☐						
Nondairy whipped topping	☐						

SWEETS, BAKED GOODS, DESSERTS

Please check the box next to each food/beverage that you ate at least once in the **past 12 months**.		How often did you consume this food/beverage over the **past 12 months**?			What portion size do you usually drink/eat each in one sitting?		
		Rarely	Sometimes	Consistently	Small	Medium	Large
Frozen yogurt, sorbet, or ices	☐						
Ice cream, ice cream bars, or sherbet (including light, low-fat, or fat-free)	☐						
Cake	☐						
Pie	☐						
Cookies	☐						
Brownies	☐						
Doughnuts, sweet rolls, Danish	☐						

Please check the box next to each food/beverage that you ate at least once in the **past 12 months**.		How often did you consume this food/beverage over the **past 12 months**?			What portion size do you usually drink/eat each in one sitting?		
		Rarely	Sometimes	Consistently	Small	Medium	Large
Sweet muffins or dessert breads	☐						
Pudding or custard	☐						
Chocolate bar or chocolate candy	☐						

SPREADS AND DRESSINGS

Please check the box next to each food/beverage that you ate at least once in the **past 12 months**.		How often did you consume this food/beverage over the **past 12 months**?			What portion size do you usually drink/eat each in one sitting?		
		Rarely	Sometimes	Consistently	Small	Medium	Large
Margarine	☐						
Butter	☐						
Mayonnaise or mayonnaise-based dressing	☐						
Salad dressing	☐						

SUMMARY QUESTION

Which of the following foods did you **TOTALLY EXCLUDE** from your diet? **Mark all that apply.**	
☐	Meat (beef, pork, lamb, etc.)
☐	Poultry (chicken, turkey, duck)
☐	Fish and seafood
☐	Eggs
☐	Dairy products (milk, cheese, etc.)

24-HOUR RECALL WORKSHEET

Instructions

Over a 24-hour period, record the foods you consume and when/why you consume them. It is important to be honest when recording what you have eaten over this 24-hour period to help gain an accurate perspective on the types of foods and amounts you consume.

Once you have completed your 24-Hour Recall Worksheet, discuss it with your nutrition coach.

Start Date/Time _____   *End Date/Time* _____

Food Item Description	Serving Size/ Amount/ Portion Description	Time Consumed	Location Consumed and Occasion
Example: Glass of 2% milk	8 ounces	12:37 pm	At home, thirsty

DIET RECORD WORKSHEET

FOOD DESCRIPTION	CALORIES (est.)	PROTEIN (est. grams)	CARBS (est. grams)	FAT (est. grams)
NAME:	**DATE:**		**DAY OF WEEK:**	
Example: 1 cup of 2 % milk	120	8g	11 g	5g

(continues)

(continued)

NAME:	DATE:		DAY OF WEEK:	
FOOD DESCRIPTION	CALORIES (est.)	PROTEIN (est. grams)	CARBS (est. grams)	FAT (est. grams)
TOTAL				
TOTAL WATER INTAKE (OZ.)				
Notes:				

PALEO DIET EXCLUSIONS

Dairy

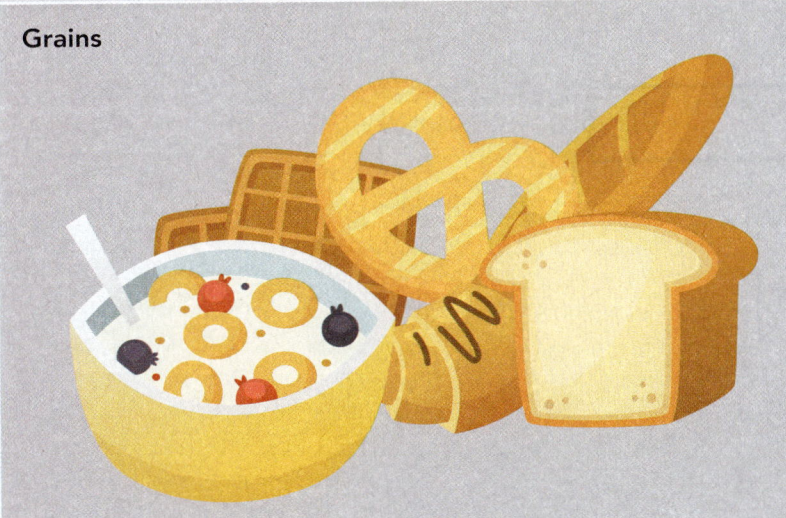

- ✕ Milk
- ✕ Cheese
- ✕ Ice Cream
- ✕ Butter
- ✕ Cream Cheese
- ✕ Evaporated Milk
- ✕ Condensed Milk
- ✕ Yogurt
- ✕ Frozen Yogurt

Grains

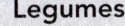

- ✕ Cereal Grains
- ✕ Corn
- ✕ Wheat
- ✕ Pseudocereals: Quinoa, Amaranth, Buckwheat
- ✕ Enriched Flours
- ✕ Pasta
- ✕ Semolina
- ✕ Polenta
- ✕ Grits
- ✕ Oats
- ✕ Barley

Legumes

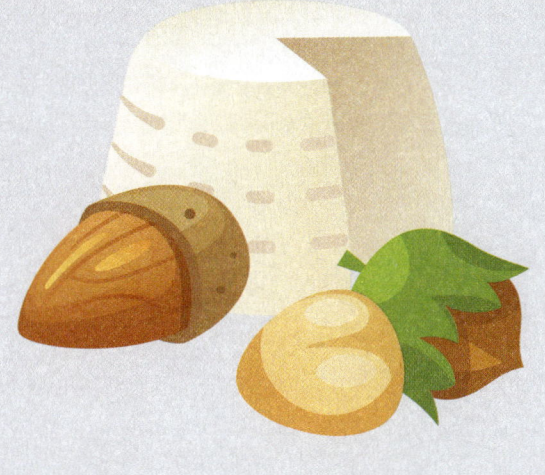

- ✕ Lentils
- ✕ Beans:

  Black Beans, Pinto Beans, Red Beans, Kidney Beans, White Beans, Garbanzo Beans, Black-Eyed Peas, Lima Beans, Adzuki Beans, Mung Beans, Navy Beans, Fava Beans
- ✕ Peas
- ✕ Peanuts and Peanut Products
- ✕ Green Beans
- ✕ String Beans
- ✕ Snap Peas
- ✕ Tofu, Soybeans, and Soy Products

CHAPTER 23

DIETARY SUPPLEMENT USE DECISION TREE

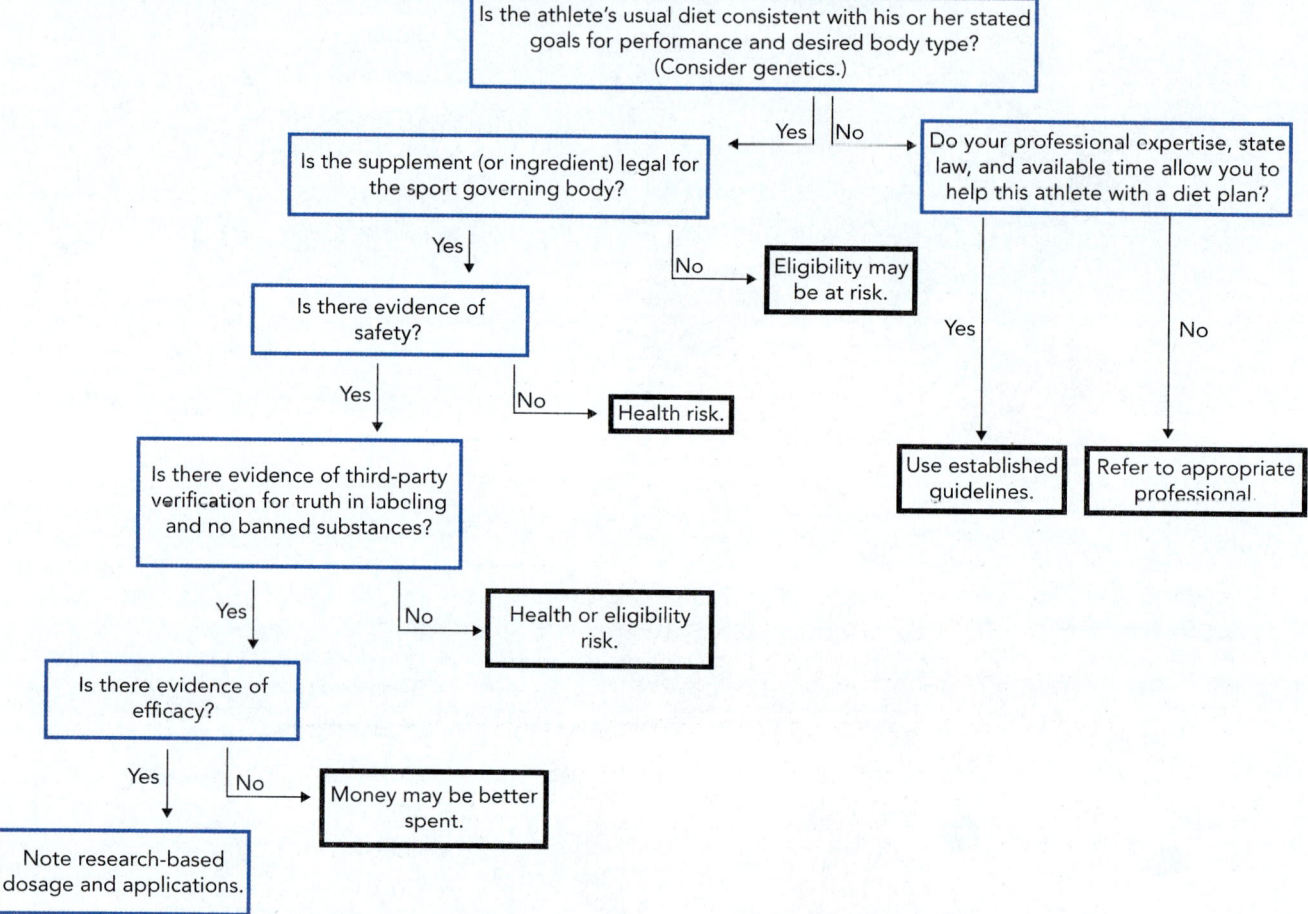

THE ROAD TO CAFFEINE

The ergogenic effect on exercise performance

1 Dose

<3 | 3-6 | >6

All doses might be ergogenic but 1-3 mg/kg in a lower magnitude

Optimal dose depends on:

- Type of sport
- Sport-dependent timing
- Inter-individual responses
- Source of caffeine

>6 mg/kg

No additional benefit vs 3-6 mg/kg

↑ Risk of side effects

6 Safety

>6 mg/kg

- Anxiety
- Insomnia
- Increased blood pressure

5 Ergogenicity

Aerobic Endurance — Small / Moderate / Large

Muscle Endurance — Small / Moderate / Large

Muscle Strength — Small / Moderate / Large

Anaerobic Power — Small / Moderate / Large

2 Mechanism

Adenosine binds to the cell receptor

Adenosine
Caffeine

Hey that's my spot!

Adenosine bound to its receptor causes fatigue

Neuron

Caffeine has affinity for adenosine receptors...

..and inhibits adenosine from binding to its cell receptor

Previous data *suggested*

☕ 3 mg/kg

Caffeine ergogenicity remains up to 20 days of chronic ingestion

Caffeine ergogenicity / Days

Periods of abstinence can maintain sensitivity to lower doses of caffeine and improve ergogenicity, but (as shown) can be used for ~3 weeks without trouble. Athletes may also elect to use a daily undulating pattern where they use it for competition only during the season or only on harder training days during the off-season or pre-season to help maintain low tolerance.

Current data *suggest*

Caffeine ergogenicity / Days

3 Response

Responder

Caffeine intake

Recent research suggests

High-responder

Individualized protocol of caffeine supplementation

Low-responder

Low responders may be slow metabolizers unable to benefit from caffeine supplementation and should reevaluate if they should use caffeine

Non-responder

4 Tolerance

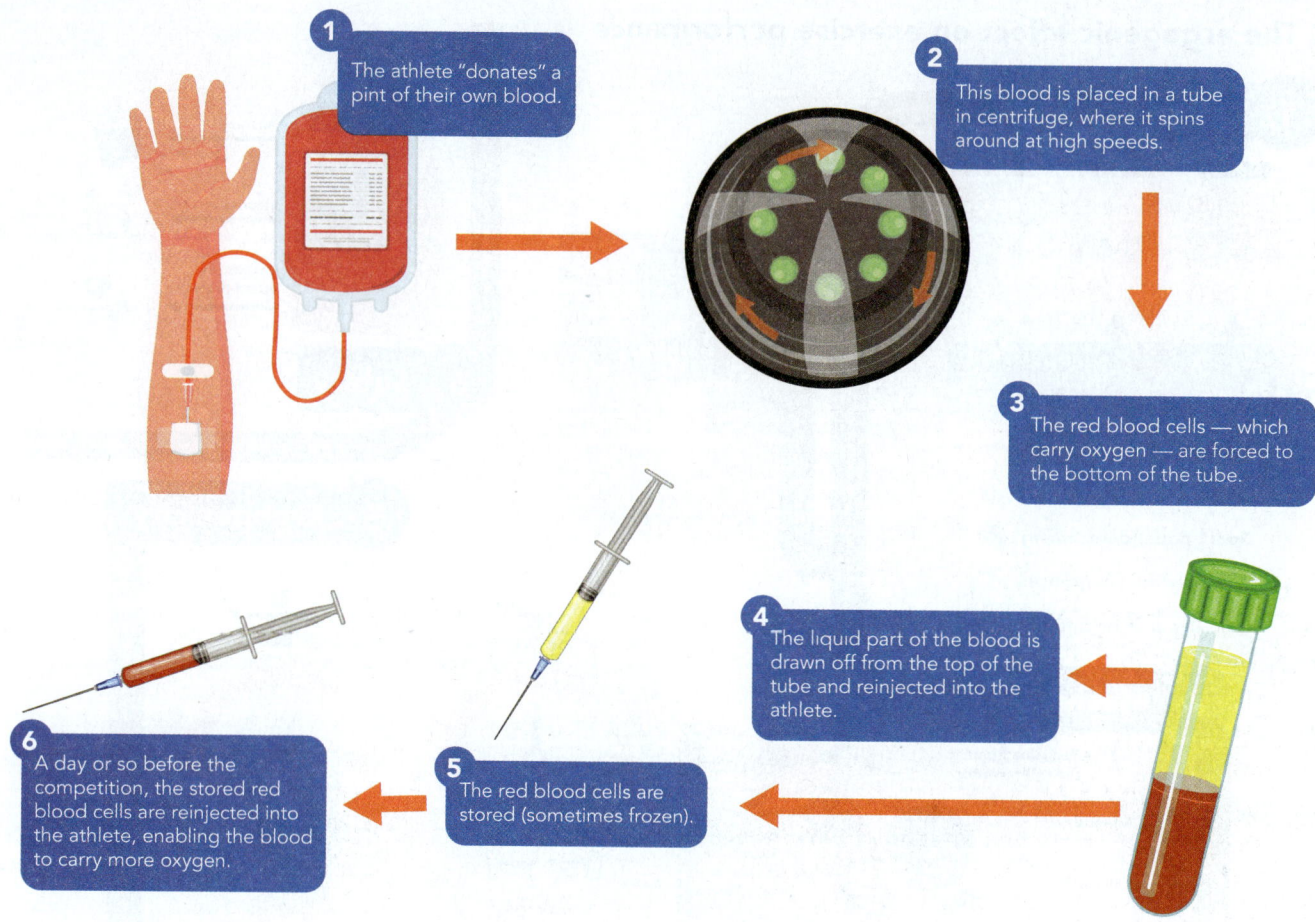

1. The athlete "donates" a pint of their own blood.

2. This blood is placed in a tube in centrifuge, where it spins around at high speeds.

3. The red blood cells — which carry oxygen — are forced to the bottom of the tube.

4. The liquid part of the blood is drawn off from the top of the tube and reinjected into the athlete.

5. The red blood cells are stored (sometimes frozen).

6. A day or so before the competition, the stored red blood cells are reinjected into the athlete, enabling the blood to carry more oxygen.

REFERENCES

Warburton D, Jamnik V, Bredin S, Shephard R, Gledhill N. The 2022 Physical Activity Readiness Questionnaire for Everyone (PAR-Q+) and electronic Physical Activity Readiness Medical Examination (ePARmed-X+). Health & Fitness Journal of Canada 2022;15(1):54-57. https://hfjc.library.ubc.ca/index.php/HFJC/article/view/815

Warburton DER, Gledhill N, Jamnik VK, Bredin SSD, McKenzie DC, Stone J, Charlesworth S, Shephard RJ, on behalf of the PAR-Q+ Collaboration. The Physical Activity Readiness Questionnaire for Everyone (PAR-Q+) and electronic Physical Activity Readiness Medical Examination (ePARmed-X+): Summary of consensus panel recommendations. Health & Fitness Journal of Canada 2011;4:26-37.

GLOSSARY

24-hour dietary recall A method of dietary assessment that involves talking with a client and asking them to recall everything they ate and drank on the previous day.

4-R system A working model of therapeutic rehabilitation that aims to Restore tissue integrity, then Reeducate isolated muscle function, then Recondition whole-body motor sequencing, and finally Return to play.

A

Acceptance and commitment therapy (ACT) A psychological practice that helps individuals develop greater psychological flexibility and well-being by focusing on accepting and having a compassionate attitude toward negative thoughts and emotions and taking committed action toward achieving goals.

Accumulation Similar to traditional periodization; aims to provide general preparation.

Acetylcholine (ACh) A neurotransmitter that helps the action potential cross the synapse into the muscle, which initiates the steps in a muscle contraction.

Achievement motivation theory A person's efforts to master a task, achieve excellence, overcome obstacles, perform better than others, and take pride in exercising talent.

Acid–base balance The balance between intake and production and elimination of hydrogen ions.

Actin The thin, stringlike myofilament that acts along with myosin to produce muscular contraction.

Action potential Nerve impulse that is relayed from the central nervous system, through the peripheral nervous system, and into the muscle across the neuromuscular junction.

Active listening Intently focusing on what is said rather than making judgments or preplanned responses while the athlete is still speaking.

Active rest micro-cycle The primary micro-cycle used during the initial weeks of the preparatory phase.

Active ROM The range of motion achieved with voluntary muscular contractions.

Active stretching A type of stretching that uses agonists and synergists to dynamically move the joint into a range of motion; includes holding the stretched position for 1 to 2 seconds and repeating for 5 to 10 repetitions.

Acute-to-chronic workload ratio (ACWR) A clinical tool used to measure the effects of fatigue (acute workload) on fitness levels (chronic workload).

Adaptation A change by which an organism becomes better matched to its environment.

Adenosine diphosphate (ADP) A high-energy compound occurring in all cells from which adenosine triphosphate is formed.

Adenosine triphosphate (ATP) A high-energy molecule that serves as the main form of energy in the human body; known as the energy currency of the body.

Adolescent growth spurt Period of the lifespan during which a marked increase in growth and puberty occurs.

Adrenaline Also known as epinephrine; a hormone that excites bodily processes, increasing alertness and cell metabolism.

Adverse event Any unfavorable medical occurrence associated with the use of a dietary supplement.

Aerobic tests Tests used to evaluate an athlete's aerobic fitness level and capacity to perform work.

Afferent neurons Sensory neurons that carry signals from sensory stimuli toward the central nervous system.

Agility The ability to change direction or body orientation with rapid and accurate cognitive processing of external and internal information without a substantive loss of movement speed.

Alpha-linolenic acid A short-chain omega-3 fatty acid derived from plants.

Alpha motor neuron A neuron that is one part of a motor unit that arises from the motor cortex in the brain, which sends a specific electrical charge down the central nervous system and out into the periphery to stimulate its associated muscle fibers.

Altered reciprocal inhibition The concept of muscle inhibition caused by a tight agonist, decreasing the neural drive of its functional antagonist.

Amino acid An organic compound that contains a carboxyl group and an amino group and serves as the base unit of all proteins.

Amortization phase The transition from eccentric loading to concentric unloading during the stretch–shortening cycle.

Anabolic Metabolic process that synthesizes smaller molecules into larger units used for building and repairing tissues.

Anabolic androgenic steroid Compound made from testosterone or another hormone that acts upon hormone receptors to produce increases in muscle size or strength.

Anabolism The process of taking smaller pieces, such as individual amino acids, and combining them to make larger structures, such as muscle tissue.

Anaerobic tests Tests that evaluate an athlete's anaerobic fitness and maximally stress the energy systems of the body.

Anaerobic threshold The exercise intensity level at which energy demand is greater than the ability of aerobic metabolism to meet those demands.

Anatomic position The position with the body erect, the arms at the sides, and the palms forward; the position of reference for anatomic nomenclature.

Annual plan The entire training year, which is broken into three distinct phases of periodization: preparation, competition, and transition.

Anterior–posterior axis An imaginary line that passes through a joint from anterior to posterior.

Antioxidants Nutrients that function in the human body to reduce oxidative stress.

Anxiety An emotional state characterized by nervousness, worry, and apprehension, which is associated with activation or arousal of the body.

Arousal The level of psychological and physiological activation that an athlete experiences.

Arthrogenic neuromuscular inhibition (ANI) Inhibition of musculature surrounding a joint after damage to that joint.

Arthrokinematic The description of joint surface movement; consists of three major types—roll, slide, and spin.

Assisted stretching A type of flexibility training in which an individual receives help from a partner, coach, trainer, or physical therapist to perform a stretch more effectively.

Asymmetrical performance assessments Dynamic single-leg movements that challenge the dynamic posture, balance, and neuromuscular control of the lower extremity.

Athleticism The ability to repeatedly perform a range of movements with precision and confidence in a variety of environments, which require competent levels of motor skills, strength, power, speed, agility, balance, coordination, and endurance.

ATP-CP system A rapid-acting energy system that utilizes creatine phosphate to create ATP; also referred to as the ATP-PC or phosphagen system.

Attentional cueing The effort of the coach, trainer, and Sports Performance Coach to direct the attention of the athlete to either an external focus or internal focus to produce improved knowledge of performance or knowledge of results.

Attentional focus The conscious effort of an individual to focus their attention through explicit thoughts so as to execute a motor skill with superior performance.

Autocrine An action in which a hormone or substance acts on the same cell that produced or secreted it.

Autogenic inhibition The process by which neural impulses that sense tension are greater than the impulses that cause muscles to contract, providing an inhibitory effect to the muscle spindles.

Autonomy-supportive style A dialogue-driven approach to communication.

Axis of rotation An imaginary line that runs through a joint, perpendicular to the plane of motion, serving as a pivot point upon which the bones rotate.

#

Ballistic movement A movement that includes a rapid stretching of a muscle, followed immediately by a shortening of the muscle, creating an elastic energy recoil effect, above and beyond the organically produced force of the muscle.

Banned substances Dietary supplements that are prohibited from use in a specific sport or sport league. Banned supplements might not be illegal or banned at all times during the year.

Basal metabolic rate (BMR) The metabolic rate (caloric expenditure) of the body at rest.

Base micro-cycle The first week of formal training.

Base of support The area beneath a person that consists of every point of contact made between the body and the support surface.

Beta-carotene The red-orange pigment found in vegetables and fruits that is converted to vitamin A in the body.

Bi-cycle Annual plan with two peaks or competitive seasons.

Biological age A measurement of a person's age based on various assessments of biological maturity.

Biologically active The form in which a vitamin must be to exert an effect within the body.

Biomotor ability An athletic capacity that forms the basis of physical performance proficiency that can be developed and enhanced by various training methods.

Block periodization Progression of the traditional model with a more targeted and sequential approach; characterized by a focus on one training adaptation for a given time, followed by a large change in acute variables to focus on a different goal.

Blood flow restriction (BFR) The application of a pressurized cuff that restricts the venous return of blood from working muscles; often used in conjunction with light resistance training to stimulate muscle hypertrophy.

Body composition assessments Methods used to measure the proportions of different tissues in the body, such as fat, muscle, and bone.

Borg scale A tool that measures an individual's perception of their physical exertion during activity. It ranges from 6 (no exertion) to 20 (maximal exertion), enabling individuals to subjectively rate their effort, discomfort, and fatigue during exercise.

Bracing A core stabilization technique that contracts the local and global muscles at the same time by stiffening the abdominal wall and pushing the abdomen out externally.

Branched-chain amino acids (BCAA) The three essential amino acids (leucine, isoleucine, and valine) that are abundant in skeletal muscle tissue; named for their branch-like structure.

Broad focus Taking in a large amount of information and processing it quickly, such as an entire field of play.

C

Calorie The amount of energy required to raise the temperature of 1 gram of water by exactly 1°C.

Calories in, calories out (CICO) A way of stating the first law of thermodynamics in the context of human metabolism.

Cardiac output How much blood the heart pumps each minute; a product of heart rate × stroke volume.

Cardiorespiratory fitness The ability of the circulatory and respiratory systems to provide the body with oxygen during activity.

Cardiovascular system The body system that transports blood to tissues of the body; includes the heart, blood vessels, and blood. Also known as the circulatory system.

Carotenoids A class of nutrients that are pigments; they are often yellow, orange, or red.

Catabolic Metabolic process that breaks down molecules into smaller units used for energy.

Catabolism The breakdown of larger structures, such as muscle tissue, into smaller pieces, such as amino acids.

Cell signaling The process of communication between cells by biological messengers to govern cellular function.

Cell swelling An increase in blood flow to the contracting muscle, which results in temporary cell bloating.

Center of gravity The approximate midpoint of the body; although the location may vary between individuals, it is typically located at the midportion of the trunk.

Center of mass (CoM) The point at which the mass or weight (the product of mass and acceleration due to gravity) of the body is evenly distributed.

Central nervous system (CNS) The part of the nervous system consisting of the brain and spinal cord.

Certified dietitian nutritionist (CDN) A registered dietitian who provides safe, effective, evidence-based nutrition services for health, fitness, and athletic performance.

Chemoreceptors Specialized structures that respond to chemical stimuli, such as changes in carbon dioxide, oxygen, and pH levels.

Chronic ankle instability (CAI) A condition characterized by recurrent ankle sprains or a feeling of instability in the ankle joint.

Chronological age The number of years, expressed as a decimal, from the birthdate.

Clean and jerk An Olympic lift involving the lifting of a barbell from a stationary position on the ground to the chest and then directly overhead in multiple phases using a fairly narrow grip.

Closed-loop control system Task-intrinsic feedback and alterations in movement due to the continuous nature of the movement.

Coach A person who is responsible for guiding others from where they are to where they want to be.

Coaching communication loop (CCL) The five-step model used to coach movement within the middle portion of the communication blueprint.

Cognitive age Refers to an individual's cognitive abilities or performance relative to their chronological age, focusing specifically on abilities such as memory, problem-solving skills, understanding, and information processing.

Cognitive anxiety The psychological component of anxiety that involves mental processes such as attention, perception, memory, and reasoning.

Cognitive behavioral orientation The psychophysiological orientation that focuses on an athlete's cognition and thoughts as determinants of their behavior.

Cognitive-general imagery A form of imagery that involves the overall experience of the performance.

Cognitive-specific imagery A form of imagery that involves the specific movements or actions used in a particular skill or task.

Collagen A protein found in connective tissue, muscles, and skin that provides strength and structure; the most abundant protein in the human body.

Compensatory acceleration The maximal intentional acceleration of an external load to develop the internal muscular rate of force development capacity and maximal neuromuscular activation.

Competitive phase The in-season period; the periodization phase in which peak performance is planned to be reached. This phase is generally characterized by decreases in training volume and increases in training intensity.

Complete proteins Foods that contain all nine of the essential amino acids.

Complex training Pairing a resistance training movement with a plyometric movement.

Concentration The ability to exert deliberate mental effort to focus on what is most important in any situation and maintain that focus over time.

Concentric muscle action A muscle action that occurs when a muscle is exerting force greater than the resistive force, resulting in a shortening of the muscle.

Concentric phase The response to the eccentric and amortization phases, in which energy is released and directed toward athletic movement such as jumping or throwing.

Concurrent training Simultaneous use of two or more training modalities for improving more than one biomotor ability, with the aim of improving sports performance at the training session or micro-cycle level.

Conjugate periodization Model of periodization in which blocks of concentrated loading are used to intentionally overreach and promote fatigue in an accumulation block of training.

Constraint Something that eliminates certain possibilities for action.

Constraints-led approach (CLA) A technique for understanding motor skill acquisition and performance that emphasizes the interaction between the individual, the task, and the environment.

Continuous training Training at a constant intensity for a specific period of time.

Contractile element The muscle fibers that are capable of contracting and producing force.

Controlled choice A concept that allows a coach to present choices for coaching cues, and allows the athlete to choose the cue that makes the most sense to them.

Controlling style A monologue-heavy approach to communication.

Contusion Commonly called a bruise; a type of tissue hematoma that results from trauma, causing localized bleeding and skin discoloration.

Coordination The patterning of head, body, and limb movements relative to the patterning of environmental objects and events, regardless of the skill level of the performer.

Core The structures that make up the lumbo-pelvic-hip complex (LPHC), including the lumbar spine, pelvic girdle, abdomen, and hip joint.

Core endurance The ability to control the motion of the spine over a given longer duration.

Core power The ability to control rapid force acceleration and deceleration of the spine.

Core stability The ability of the neuromuscular system to limit unwanted movement of the lumbo-pelvic-hip complex.

Core strength The ability to control the motion of the spine.

Creatine A molecule made from amino acids and used as a dietary supplement to facilitate ATP regeneration for improved training capacity, strength, power, and muscle mass.

Creatine monohydrate The most common, and likely most effective, form of creatine available as a dietary supplement.

Cryotherapy The utilization of cold air or water to cause physiological responses that are intended to improve recovery.

Cue creation A process in which the coach provides the technical error that needs to be corrected and gives the athlete the first opportunity to identify a suitable cue.

Cumulative injury cycle A cycle in which tissue trauma induces inflammation, muscle spasm, adhesions, altered neuromuscular control, and muscle imbalances.

Cutaneous receptors Specialized sensory nerve endings found in the skin that detect and respond to various types of external stimuli.

Cycle training Use of the three main phases of the annual plan to develop the annual training program.

Cytokine Substances including chemokines, interferons, interleukins, lymphokines, and tumor necrosis factors, but generally not hormones or growth factors.

D

Davis's law States that soft tissues (muscle and connective) will remodel along the lines of stress.

Degrees of freedom (DOF) The number of independent directions in which a joint can move.

Dehydration The process of losing body water.

Deliberate play Loosely structured movement activities that are enjoyable, fun, and not goal-oriented.

Deliberate practice Focused, intensive, and high-frequency training approach with the intent of achieving mastery of sport skills, tactics, and physical preparation.

Deload A period of approximately a week utilized to greatly reduce training volume and intensity, which encourages recovery and fitness adaptations.

Derivatives Lifts that emphasize a specific phase found within the two competition Olympic lifts (e.g., snatch pull) and/or are modified versions of them (e.g., hang power clean).

Developmental age Refers to the age at which a child or individual's physical, emotional, social, and cognitive development corresponds to the average levels of others in a specific age group.

Diaphragmatic breathing (DBR) Breathing deeply by allowing the expansion of the abdominal area.

Diet record (food journal) A method of dietary assessment involving real-time tracking of an individual's food on paper, an app, or a computer.

Dietary supplement A product other than tobacco that is intended to supplement the diet that bears or contains one or more of the following dietary ingredients: vitamin; mineral; herb or other botanical; amino acid; dietary supplement that increases the total dietary intake; or a concentrate, metabolite, constituent, extract, or combination of any previously described ingredient.

Dietitian nutritionist (RD/RDN) A health professional with specialized training in the use of diet and nutrition to keep the body healthy as well as addressing disease and engaging in medical nutrition therapy.

Disfacilitation The reduction of excitatory input to specific motor neurons.

Dissociation The ability for one region of the body to perform a task separate from what the rest of the body is doing.

Dissociation exercises Exercises that require the athlete to process separate tasks for different regions of the body, such as running while catching a pass from the side.

Docosahexaenoic acid (DHA) An omega-3 fatty acid derived from animals, usually a marine animal.

Downregulated The process whereby a receptor is not made available for binding with a molecule or hormone.

Drawing-in maneuver A maneuver used to recruit the local core stabilizers by drawing the naval in toward the spine; also referred to as hollowing.

Drive phase Sprint phase that includes the start (first two steps) and acceleration in the first 10 yards; the sprint stride cycle phase in which the foot is in contact with the ground.

Dynamic balance The ability to maintain a stable body position with complete postural control, keeping the center of mass within the base of support when perturbations to the system are present.

Dynamic movement assessments A set of assessments that involve movement with a change in the base of support.

Dynamic stretching A type of stretching that uses the force production of a muscle and the body's momentum to take a joint through the full available range of motion.

E

Early specialization Intensive participation and year-round training in one sport, often prior to the age of 12 or the onset of peak height and weight velocity. Example sports are gymnastics, figure skating, and diving.

Eccentric control balance The ability to effectively maintain the center of mass over a reduced base of support during muscle-lengthening contractions, such as when landing a jump on a single leg.

Eccentric muscle action A muscle action that occurs when a muscle develops tension while lengthening.

Eccentric phase The phase in which muscle spindle activity is increased by pre-stretching the muscle prior to activation.

Efferent neurons Motor neurons that carry signals from the central nervous system toward muscles to create movement.

Effort The internal exertion that muscles produce against an external load.

Effort arm The distance from the effort to the fulcrum.

Eicosapentaenoic acid (EPA) An omega-3 fatty acid derived from animals, usually a marine animal.

Elastic component Noncontractile proteins.

Elasticity The ability of soft tissues to return to resting length after being stretched.

Elastin A protein that provides elasticity to skin, tendons, ligaments, and other structures.

Electronic muscle stimulation (EMS) A type of therapy in which an electrical current is applied to the skin through electrodes and placed on target muscles to help with recovery.

Endocrine system A group of glands that secrete chemical substances (hormones) into the blood to signal cell receptors to respond in a certain manner.

Endogenous Produced or synthesized within an organism.

Endomysium Connective tissue that wraps around individual muscle fibers within a fascicle.

Endurance training Exercise programs designed to optimize oxygen utilization and improve cardiovascular fitness and long duration performances.

Energy In the context of human performance, the power derived from utilizing physical or chemical resources, especially to provide light and heat or to work machines.

Energy balance The relationship between energy intake from food and drink and energy output.

Environmental constraints The external factors in the surrounding environment that can influence an athlete's movement behavior and performance.

Ephedra A plant-sourced alkaloid with metabolism-enhancing effects. It is an illegal supplement in the United States and European Union.

Epimysium Connective tissue surrounding and enclosing an entire skeletal muscle.

Ergogenic aid A dietary supplement that might enhance performance or body composition; also referred to as a performance supplement.

Error management The ability to mitigate the effects of errors and to overcome them.

Essential A nutrient that must be obtained in the diet because the body is incapable of producing the nutrient on its own.

Essential amino acids (EAAs) Amino acids that are necessary for bodily functions but cannot be synthesized by the body and must be obtained in the diet.

Euhydration A state of fluid balance in which fluid loss matches fluid gain.

Excitation–contraction coupling The physiological process of converting an electrical stimulus into a muscle contraction.

Exercise deficit disorder Accumulating less than the recommended 60 minutes of moderate- to vigorous-intensity physical activity per day.

Exercise dose A theoretical quantification of an exercise session, which is a function of both its intensity and its duration.

Exertional rhabdomyolysis A potentially life-threatening metabolic condition caused by extreme physical exertion that causes the cellular breakdown of muscle cell components, resulting in kidney failure.

Exogenous Coming from outside the body.

External feedback Information provided by some external source, such as a coach, video, mirror, or heart rate monitor, to supplement the internal environment.

External focus When an athlete directs attention toward external factors in the environment, focusing on the intention of the movement outcome.

External imagery An imagery practice that involves viewing oneself from a third-person perspective (i.e., an outside vantage point).

Extrinsic motivation The drive that arises from an individual's desire to engage in behavior to obtain external rewards, such as titles, money, praise, or fame.

Extrinsic risk factors Environmental, situational, or circumstantial elements that increase an individual's likelihood of sustaining injury.

F

Fartlek training Speed play; a style of endurance training that uses unstructured intervals to include higher-intensity periods of work within the context of a long-slow distance training stimulus.

Fascia Connective tissue that surrounds muscles and bones.

Fascial slings The interconnected chains of muscles, fascia, and other soft tissues that link the upper and lower extremities together.

Fascicle A bundle of muscle fibers surrounded by perimysium.

Fat-soluble The ability for something to be dissolved in lipids.

Fatty acids (FA) Carboxylic acids that function as the building blocks of fats in the human body.

Feedback The utilization of sensory information and sensorimotor integration to aid in the development of permanent neural representations of motor patterns for efficient movement.

Feed-forward activation When a muscle is automatically activated in anticipation of a movement.

Female athlete triad A medical condition in highly athletic women characterized by low energy availability, menstrual dysfunction, and low bone mineral density.

First law of thermodynamics Within a closed system, energy is neither created nor destroyed.

Fitness–fatigue model A framework in which an individual's performance at any given time is determined by the balance between their level of fitness and their level of fatigue.

FITTE-VP Method of training programming based on manipulating frequency (F), intensity (I), time (T), type (T), enjoyment (E), volume (V), and progression (P).

Flavonoids A class of phytonutrients that are pigments; they are found in plants.

Flexibility The normal extensibility of soft tissues that allows for the full range of motion of a joint.

Fluid balance The relationship between fluid loss and fluid gain.

Food Frequency Questionnaire (FFQ) A survey questionnaire that utilizes a preset list of foods and asks about the frequency of consumption.

Force An influence applied by one object to another, resulting in an acceleration or deceleration of the second object.

Force–couple relationship The synergistic action of multiple muscles working together to produce movement around a joint.

Force–velocity curve A property of skeletal muscle whereby the force in a muscle contraction decreases as the velocity of shortening increases. When this is measured during a complex sport skill, it may be referred to as a force–velocity relationship.

Free nerve endings Unencapsulated sensory nerve endings found in the skin, ligaments, tendons, and joint capsule, which detect temperature and pressure changes, pain, and mechanical stimuli.

Frontal plane An imaginary plane that divides the body into front and back.

Fulcrum The point of pivot or the axis of rotation.

Functional overreaching Intentionally increasing training volume or intensity beyond an athlete's recovery capacity for a short period of time.

Functional strength The ability of the neuromuscular system to contract eccentrically, isometrically, and concentrically in all three planes of motion.

G

General adaptation syndrome (GAS) The human movement system's ability to adapt to stresses placed upon it.

General preparatory phase The early weeks of the preparatory phase, which include more general training and an emphasis on aerobic conditioning.

Gentile's taxonomy A classification of skill progression based on the environment and bodily movement.

Global core stabilizers Muscles spanning over the lumbo-pelvic-hip complex, attaching from the pelvis to the spine and from the pelvis to the femur.

Global muscular system Muscles that are predominately responsible for movement and that consist of more superficial musculature that originates from the pelvis to the rib cage, the lower extremities, or both.

Glucose The simplest form of carbohydrate used by the body for energy.

Glycemic index (GI) A system of scoring foods that is based on the effect the food has on blood sugar levels.

Glycemic load (GL) A measure of how rapidly and how high a food raises blood sugar relative to the actual amount of food consumed.

Glycogen Glucose that is deposited and stored in bodily tissues, such as the liver and muscle cells; the storage form of carbohydrates.

Glycolysis A metabolic process that occurs in a cell's cytosol and converts glucose into pyruvate and adenosine triphosphate.

Goal setting The process of developing a plan to accomplish something.

Goal-setting theory The effects of setting goals on subsequent performance.

Goldilocks effect Finding the "just right" balance in workout intensity and volume to optimize muscle growth and strength gains while minimizing the risk of injury and overtraining.

Golgi tendon organs (GTOs) Specialized sensory receptors located in the musculotendinous junction that are sensitive to changes in tension and the rate of tension change.

Ground contact time (GCT) The time interval during which the foot is in contact with the ground throughout each force application of a stride.

Ground reaction force (GRF) The force applied to the ground by the foot in each phase of the sprint.

Gynecomastia A condition in males characterized by breast tissue growth.

H

Hang Starting position for an Olympic lift that is from a hanging position at the knee, mid-thigh, or hip.

Hang clean Catching derivative of the clean with a starting position at the knee, mid-thigh, or hip and finishing in a full or deep squat position.

Hang power clean Catching derivative of the clean with a starting position at the knee, mid-thigh, or hip and finishing in a half squat position.

Hang power snatch Catching derivative of the snatch with a starting position at the knee, mid-thigh, or hip and finishing in a half squat position.

Hang snatch Catching derivative of the snatch with a starting position at the knee, mid-thigh, or hip and finishing in a full or deep squat position.

Health History questionnaire (HHQ) A questionnaire with lists of questions that pertain to health history and habits, such as exercise history, eating behaviors, and general lifestyle.

Health Insurance Portability and Accountability Act (HIPAA) A federal law that provides privacy and security standards for protected health information.

Heart arrhythmia An irregular heartbeat.

Heart rate reserve (HRR) Difference between HR_{max} or estimated HR_{max} and HR_{rest}: $HRR = HR_{max} - HR_{rest}$.

Heme A type of iron found in animal foods.

Hepcidin A protein that regulates iron levels in the body by slowing iron uptake.

High-intensity interval training (HIIT) Training intensities that range from seconds to minutes; usually multiple repetitions, with rest between each repetition.

Holistic approach Considers the personal, emotional, cultural, academic, athletic, and social identity of the athlete, as well as nutrition, sleep, and recovery, and how these elements influence the athlete's performance.

Homeostasis Any process allowing cells or processes to actively maintain the fairly stable conditions necessary for survival.

Hormesis A characteristic of biological systems that involves the response to stressors in a dose–response manner.

Human movement science An interdisciplinary field that focuses on studying human movement, including the mechanisms that control movement, the factors that influence movement, and the outcomes of movement.

Human movement system (HMS) The muscular, skeletal, and nervous systems; also known as the kinetic chain.

Hyperhydration A state of fluid balance in which fluid gain is greater than fluid loss.

Hypertrophy Enlargement of an organ or tissue; in the context of fitness, the enlargement of skeletal muscle.

Hypermobility Increased movement and functionality of a joint beyond normal range of motion.

Hypohydration A state of fluid balance in which fluid loss is greater than fluid gain.

Hypokinetic A low level of movement throughout the day.

Hyponatremia A state of having lower than normal levels of sodium present in the bloodstream.

I

Imagery A form of simulation in which a person creates a multisensory experience, such as tactile, visual, auditory, or olfactory, through stored memory and information.

Immunodeficiency A weakened immune system.

Incomplete proteins Foods that are missing one or more of the nine essential amino acids.

Individual constraints The unique characteristics of an athlete that influence their movement behavior and performance.

Inflammatory stage A nonspecific response to physical injury that represents the body's attempt to limit the extent of the injury and initiate the tissue repair processes.

Inhibition The suppression or reduction of activity in motor neurons via activation of inhibitory neurons.

Instrument-assisted soft-tissue mobilization (IASTM) Use of specially designed instruments to provide a mobilizing effect to scar tissue and myofascial adhesions.

Integrated Sports Performance Team Analyzes, synthesizes, and harmonizes links between the disciplines to create a coordinated and coherent whole-team approach.

Integrated training A comprehensive training approach that attempts to improve all components necessary for an athlete to perform at the highest level of competition with an injury-risk mitigation focus.

Integrative Neuromuscular Training (INT) A comprehensive training strategy that incorporates general (fundamental movements) and specific (skill-related) strength and conditioning activities designed to enhance health and skill-related fitness.

Interactional view The level of motivation results from the interaction of trait-centered and situation-centered factors.

Intermuscular coordination The ability of the neuromuscular system to allow all muscles to work together with proper activation and timing between them.

Internal feedback Process whereby sensory information is used by the body to reactively monitor movement and the environment.

Internal focus When an athlete focuses on specific body movements or sensations while performing a skill.

Internal imagery An imagery practice that involves viewing oneself from the first-person perspective (i.e., their vantage point).

Inter-personal communication (IC) The coach's capacity to connect with the athlete, build buy-in, and create a motivationally rich environment that the athlete enjoys being a part of.

Intramuscular coordination The ability of the neuromuscular system to allow optimal levels of motor unit recruitment and synchronization within a muscle.

Intramuscular triglycerides A storage form of fatty acids that is found in skeletal muscles.

Intrinsic motivation The drive that arises from an individual's inner desires to achieve specific tasks and fulfill a sense of purpose.

Intrinsic risk factors Individual characteristics or conditions that increase a person's susceptibility to physical harm or injury. These can be physiological, psychological, or related to personal habits and behaviors.

Isometric muscle action When a muscle is exerting a force equal to the force being placed on it, leading to no visible change in the muscle length.

Isotonic muscle contraction A contraction that involves a change in muscle length while maintaining a constant tension or force output.

J

Joint receptors Receptors located in and around the joint capsule that respond to pressure, acceleration, and deceleration of the joint.

Joint translation Joint motion where a bone moves along a linear path without any rotation.

K

Karvonen formula A formula using the heart rate reserve to calculate exercise intensities: Target heart rate = $[(HR_{max} - HR_{rest}) \times \text{exercise intensity}] + HR_{rest}$.

Kilocalorie (kcal) 1,000 calories.

Kinematic characteristics How a body moves in space, including distance, speed, and velocity.

Kinesthetic awareness The awareness of the body's position as it moves through multiple planes of motion.

Kinetic chain checkpoint The five areas of the body that are monitored during movement assessments and exercise: foot/ankle, knees, lumbo-pelvic-hip complex, shoulders, and cervical spine and head.

Knowledge of performance (KP) Information about the quality of movement during an action, skill, or performance.

Knowledge of results (KR) Information used after the completion of a movement to inform individuals about the outcome of their performance.

L

Lactate threshold The amount of lactate in the venous blood, which is typically set at 4 mmol/L of blood and at an exercise intensity below the anaerobic threshold.

Late specialization The identification and participation in one sport, typically after the age of 12 or the initiation of peak height and weight velocity. As they are often preceded by the sampling of many sports or movement activities, team sports are generally characterized as late specialization sports.

Learning-supportive coaching A type of coaching that includes both verbal and nonverbal strategies.

Lengthening reaction When a muscle is lengthened, the cascade of neurological reactions that occur to allow the muscle to be stretched.

Length–tension relationships (LTR) The resting length of a muscle and the tension the muscle can produce at this resting length.

Levers Rigid structures (such as bones) that rotate around a fixed point called a fulcrum in response to the contraction of a muscle.

Licensed nutritionist (LN) A healthcare professional who is licensed to perform nutrition counseling and provide nutrition education.

Linear periodization Model of periodization characterized by an initial high-volume, low-intensity form of training, with decreases in volume and increases in intensity then occurring gradually, usually over a period of months.

Linear speed A scalar quantity (rate) of the distance traveled by the athlete divided by time taken to travel the distance, measured only in magnitude.

Linoleic acid A short-chain omega-6 fatty acid.

Load The external resistance to be moved.

Load arm The distance from the load to the fulcrum.

Loading (nutrition) The practice of using large doses of a supplement to saturate muscle tissues or other body stores prior to resorting to a smaller, maintenance dose.

Load micro-cycle A cycle that follows the base micro-cycle and builds on the volume and intensity.

Local core stabilizers The deepest layer of muscles, which are located closest to the joints of the lumbo-pelvic-hip complex.

Local muscular system Muscles that connect directly to the spine and are predominantly involved in LPHC stabilization.

Long-term athlete development (LTAD) The habitual development of athleticism over time with the goal of improving health, fitness, and physical performance, reducing injury risk, and developing confidence and competence in all youth.

Low energy availability (LEA) A mismatch between energy in and energy out that leaves an inadequate supply of energy for the body to maintain processes that ensure health and wellness. It can occur even if the subject is weight stable.

M

Macro-cycle An annual or seasonal training plan that demonstrates how a training program will progress for the long term, from month to month, to meet the desired goal.

Maturation Progress toward the biologically mature state; varies considerably between individuals in terms of timing (maturity status at a given time) and tempo (maturity progress) especially during adolescence.

Maximal strength The maximal force or torque generated by a muscle or muscles in a single maximum voluntary contraction, which is specific to each type of muscle action.

Maximum oxygen consumption (VO_2 max) The maximal amount of oxygen that the human body utilizes during sustained peak or maximal exercise.

Mechanical specificity The weight and movements required of the body.

Mechanotransduction The process by which cells convert mechanical stimuli or forces, such as pressure, tension, or stretching, into electrochemical signals that elicit specific cellular responses.

Mechanoreceptors Specialized structures that respond to mechanical forces (touch and pressure) within tissues and then transmit signals through sensory nerves.

Medical nutrition therapy (MNT) The diagnosis and treatment of medical conditions, restricted to individuals who have adequate scope of practice for that therapy.

Mediolateral axis An imaginary line that passes through a joint from medial to lateral.

Mental FITness model A model that identifies focus, inspiration, and trust as critical ingredients for conceptualizing and facilitating performance excellence.

Mental skills training (MST) A systematic approach to developing specific mental and psychological skills to enhance performance, increase enjoyment, and achieve greater self-satisfaction.

Mental toughness The ability to cope with stress, pressure, and challenges while maintaining focus and motivation.

Mesocycle A training plan divided into specified monthly cycles or a particular training block within a season.

Metabolic specificity The metabolic route needed to supply energy for a specific exercise accounting for intensity and duration.

Microdosing The programming tactic of introducing shorter, more frequent exercise stimuli to spread out the weekly training load and manage fatigue.

Mindfulness The psychological process of bringing one's attention to the present moment without judgment and accepting attitudes toward current thoughts and feelings.

Mindfulness–acceptance–commitment (MAC) A psychological practice that combines mindfulness-based techniques with acceptance and commitment therapy to help develop greater psychological flexibility and well-being.

Minerals Inorganic substances required in small quantities (usually less than a gram) that must be consumed in the diet because they cannot be manufactured by the body.

Mirroring Reflecting back the relevant words and phrases that the athlete organically shares in their normal day-to-day conversations with the coach.

Mobility The ability of a joint to move through its full range of motion with control and stability; the ability to move freely.

Mobility assessments A set of assessments designed to observe an individual's ability to move through a range of motion at various joints and segments of the body.

Moderate-intensity continuous training (MICT) Continuous training at a medium intensity with the goal of completing a set amount of time.

Moderate-intensity interval training (MIIT) Interval training at a medium intensity with the goal to complete a set number of intervals.

Moment arm The perpendicular distance from the axis of rotation to the line of action.

Momentary failure The brief and acute performance fatigability that limits an individual from performing another repetition with a given load without the assistance of a spotter.

Mono-cycle Annual plan with only one peak or competitive season.

Monounsaturated fat (MUFA) A type of fat that has one carbon without a hydrogen atom and one double bond.

Motivation The direction and intensity of one's effort.

Motor behavior Movement response to internal and external environmental stimuli.

Motor control How the central nervous system integrates internal and external sensory information with previous experiences to produce a motor response.

Motor development Change in skilled motor behavior over time throughout the lifespan.

Motor learning Integration of motor control processes through learning, practice, and experience, leading to a relatively permanent change in the capacity to produce skilled motor behavior.

Motor skill An activity or task that requires voluntary movement of the head, body, and limbs to achieve a specific goal.

Motor unit A motor neuron and the muscle fibers it innervates or activates.

Motor unit recruitment The physiological process by which motor units are activated to produce muscle contraction.

Movement communication (MC) The coach's capacity to use language to generate movement learning.

Movement learning Moving with improved coordination, improved speed, improved strength, and the many other movement-related goals that can be pursued.

Movement system Superficial core muscles that attach the spine and pelvis to the extremities.

Movement velocity A vector quantity of the direction and magnitude of the distance traveled by an athlete divided by the time interval from the start of a movement to completion.

Multidirectional speed (MDS) The ability to propel or move the body at high speed in many directions (e.g., starting, stopping, cutting, feinting, or faking) and to achieve high-speed directional changes rapidly.

Multilateral development Exposure to a variety of fundamental skills to help youth develop general athleticism.

Muscle action spectrum The full range of eccentric, isometric, and concentric muscle contractions required to perform a movement.

Muscle imbalance A condition in which the muscles on each side of a joint have altered length–tension relationships.

Muscle protein breakdown (MPB) The catabolic process of breaking down muscle tissue into individual amino acids.

Muscle protein synthesis (MPS) The anabolic process of making muscle tissue from amino acids.

Muscle spindles Specialized sensory receptors located in muscles that detect changes in muscle length and the rate of length change.

Muscle strain Trauma to the muscle tissue, most commonly occurring at the musculoskeletal junction.

Muscular endurance tests Bodyweight performance tests that evaluate the endurance of a specific muscle group, which is often measured by repeated repetitions within a specific time frame.

Muscular strength tests Tests that evaluate how much muscle force an athlete can produce in

a specific muscle group; often measured as a 1–5 repetition maximum.

Myokine A type of chemical substance released from skeletal muscle upon contraction.

Myosin The thick myofilament that acts along with actin to produce muscular contraction.

N

Narrow focus Taking in specific bits of information, such as a specific area or individual.

Needs analysis Comprehensive written and verbal interview with the athlete to gather more information about their sport, position, and athletic profile.

Negative foot speed The rate at which the foot moves backward as it strikes the ground.

Neural continuum A spectrum of neural involvement in muscular activation, ranging from low to high levels of neural drive.

Neuromuscular control The response (conscious or unconscious) of the muscles within the body to control purposeful movement.

Neuromuscular efficiency The ability of the nervous system to recruit the correct muscles to produce force, reduce force, and dynamically stabilize the body's structure in all three planes of motion.

Neuromuscular efficiency The ability of the nervous system to recruit the correct muscles to produce force, reduce force, and dynamically stabilize the body's structure in all three planes of motion.

Neuromuscular specificity The speed of contraction and exercise selection.

Neuromuscular training continuum Model of exercise progression to optimally develop neuromuscular coordination.

Neurotransmitter A chemical substance used to communicate signals within the nervous system.

Neutralizers The muscles that counteract unwanted actions of other muscles.

Newell's model of constraints Classification of constraints into the categories of individual, task, and environment.

Nociceptors Specialized structures located in the skin and fascial connective tissues that respond to noxious stimuli, such as damage, pain, or perceptions of danger.

Non-essential amino acids Amino acids that the body can manufacture.

Non-exercise activity thermogenesis The energy a body spends moving around during the day that is not from formal, structured exercise.

Non-medical lifestyle-oriented nutrition Education and coaching around lifestyle-based changes that improve the overall nutrition habits of an individual.

Non-rapid eye movement (NREM) sleep A sleep state in which the brain's electrical activity is synchronous; it is measured by an electroencephalograph (EEG) as high-voltage, low-frequency brain activity. This activity reflects neurons that are firing slowly and together.

Nonverbal coaching The aspects of the environment that are influenced by the coach and designed to drive athlete adaptation and learning.

Nutrient density The ratio of high-quality nutrients to calories in food.

O

Omega-3 Polyunsaturated fats; eicosapentaenoic acid (EPA), docosahexaenoic acid (DHA), and alpha-linolenic acid (ALA).

OMNI scale A child-friendly tool used to quantify perceived exertion during physical activity. The scale ranges from 0 to 10 and includes visual cues to help children indicate their perception of the difficulty of a given physical activity, with 0 representing minimal effort and 10 representing maximal effort.

Open-loop control system A control system that does not allow for feedback to alter movement and does not create either immediate change or real-time adjustments.

Orientations The theoretical framework and basis from which sports and performance psychologists obtain information on the mental qualities of an athlete.

Osteokinematic Movement of a limb that is visible.

Osteoporosis A condition of reduced bone mineral density that increases risk of fracture.

Overactive Increased neural facilitation, causing a muscle to be held in a state of chronic contraction.

Overtraining syndrome (OTS) A complex condition marked by an athlete's decrement in performance and increase in fatigue in response to training.

Overuse injury Chronic discomfort or trauma to tissues of the body that occurs as a result of high-volume, repetitive use without adequate opportunity for rest or recovery from training or competition.

Oxidative stress An imbalance between oxidants and antioxidants in the human body.

Oxidative system An energy system that utilizes oxygen and glucose, fatty acids, or amino acids to create ATP; also referred to as the aerobic system or aerobic metabolism.

P

P.A.C.E. sports psychology model A mental fitness model that emphasizes the qualities of perception, activation, concentration, and execution as vital to performance excellence.

Pacinian corpuscles Rapidly adapting, deep receptors found primarily in the skin that respond to deep pressure and high-frequency vibration.

Paracrine The action of a hormone or substance acting locally by diffusing from its source to target cells nearby.

Parallel elastic component (PEC) The passive elastic properties of a muscle that are attributed to the connective tissue elements running parallel to the muscle fibers.

Parasympathetic nervous system (PNS) Subdivision of the autonomic nervous system that works to decrease neural activity and put the body in a more relaxed state.

Passive insufficiency The inability of a biarticular muscle to stretch or lengthen sufficiently across both joints simultaneously. This phenomenon occurs when a muscle reaches its maximum length and can no longer generate effective passive tension.

Passive ROM The range of motion achieved in the absence of muscular contractions, with assistance from a coach or trainer.

Pattern overload Consistently repeating the same pattern of motion over long periods of time, leading to dysfunction or injury.

Pediatric dynapenia The medical term for loss of muscle strength and power that impacts function in children.

Percentage of maximum heart rate (% HR_{max}) Training at an intended percentage of maximum heart rate for a continuous amount of time.

Perceptions The integration of sensory information with past experiences or memories.

Performance anxiety Anxiety experienced in anticipation of or during a performance, such as playing an instrument or participating in a sporting event; also referred to as stage fright.

Performance bandwidth When external feedback like cueing is not provided because the performance falls within an acceptable range of error for the skill.

Performance excellence The consistent on-demand execution of a learned skill.

Perimysium Connective tissue surrounding a muscle fascicle.

Periodization A systematic, planned, and sequential approach to strength and conditioning programming that divides training programs into smaller, progressive stages with the aim of driving physical and metabolic adaptations to improve performance.

Periodized A training program that has been organized into distinct phases or periods with specific goals and characteristics.

Peripheral nervous system (PNS) The part of the nervous

system that connects the rest of the body to the central nervous system.

Perturbation balance training A style of balance training that introduces external instability in a manner that is unpredictable to the athlete, requiring reflexive stabilization of the involved joints.

Phase potentiation The adaptations gained in one training phase enhance adaptations in future training phases, such that the order in which training phases are implemented assumes great importance.

Phosphagen A high-energy molecule that releases energy when its bonds are broken.

Physical Activity Readiness Questionnaire (PAR-Q+) A detailed questionnaire designed to assess an individual's physical readiness to engage in structured exercise.

Physical illiteracy Lack of motor competence and confidence to move well and often.

Physical inactivity triad (PIT) A combination of low levels of physical activity, reduced muscular fitness, and poor movement competency.

Physiological assessments Measurements of the human body or characteristics, including those obtained from smartwatches and other wearable devices.

Physiological system A group of tissues that work together to perform a specific function or set of functions within the body, such as the muscular, skeletal, and nervous systems.

Phytonutrient Plant nutrients believed to benefit human health.

Plasticity The ability of soft tissues to permanently change shape or deform.

Platelet aggregation An accumulation of blood cells prior to a clot.

Plyometrics Exercises that allow individuals to express maximal force in the shortest amount of time.

Plyometric training Exercises that generate quick, powerful movements involving an explosive concentric muscle contraction preceded by an eccentric muscle contraction.

Polyunsaturated fat (PUFA) A type of fat that has two or more carbons without a hydrogen atom and two or more double bonds.

Positive attitude A constructive mindset characterized by optimism, self-confidence, and resilience.

Positive body language The conscious use of nonverbal cues and gestures to communicate confidence, focus, and a winning attitude.

Post-activation potentiation The phenomenon in which acute muscle force generation is increased as a result of the inner contraction of the muscle.

Postural control system The visual, vestibular, and somatosensory peripheral input that is processed by the central nervous system and integrated to create coordinated movement.

Postural control The ability of the body to maintain or change its position in space in a controlled and efficient manner.

Posture The summation of the positions that all joints of the body are in at any given time.

Power The amount of work that can be completed in a fixed amount of time.

Power clean Catching derivative of the clean with a starting position at the floor and finishing in a half squat position.

Power endurance The capacity to maintain mechanical power in a sports skill or task.

Power snatch Catching derivative of the snatch with a starting position at the floor and finishing in a half squat position.

Power tests Tests that evaluate an athlete's ability to explosively exert force in the shortest time.

Preparatory phase The pre-season; the periodization phase that emphasizes the development of the foundational biomotor abilities required for the specific sport to the highest level possible.

Pre-pubertal Relating to or in the period preceding puberty.

Principle of individualization Individuals have unique physical characteristics, fitness levels, goals, and preferences that should be taken into account when designing and implementing training programs.

Principle of interference effect The impairment or blunting of a desired training effect because of the application of a conflicting training stimulus.

Principle of progressive overload Increasing the intensity or volume of exercise programs using a systematic and gradual approach.

Principle of reversibility Benefits of training are not permanent and can be lost if training is discontinued or reduced in frequency, intensity, or duration.

Principle of specificity The adaptive response of specific recruitment of muscles and its associated adaptation to a sport-specific task or training activity. Also known as the SAID (specific adaptation to imposed demands) principle.

Principle of transfer effect Training or practice of one skill can have a positive effect on the performance of another related skill.

Principle of variation Variation in training programs is necessary to stimulate new adaptations.

Proficiency barrier The reduced ability to advance past the fundamental movement stage to the specialized skills phase, due to not attaining a certain level of mastery of fundamental movements; a barrier to later attaining skill mastery of specialized skills, such as those needed for sporting excellence.

Program Design Continuum A comprehensive approach to designing a training program, considering various acute training variables that can be adjusted to meet desired training adaptations.

Progressive relaxation The process of diffusing muscle tension by contracting and subsequently relaxing a group of muscles, bringing awareness to the physical sensations of tension and relaxation.

Proliferative stage The stage of healing in which specialized cells (macrophages) remove dead tissue, dried blood, and other residual factors after physical injury.

Proprioception The body's ability to naturally sense its general orientation and relative position of its parts.

Proprioceptive balance training A type of balance training in which an unstable (yet controllable) exercise environment causes the body to use its internal balance and stabilization mechanisms.

Provitamin A compound that can be converted to a vitamin.

Psychological burnout Condition characterized by emotional and physical exhaustion from excessive physical training and competition. Signs and symptoms include, but are not limited to, fatigue, anxiety, a reduced sense of accomplishment with performance below expectations, and a devalued sense of sport whereby an athlete does not care for the sport anymore.

Psychophysiological orientation The study of behavior during sport to gain insight into an athlete's physiology and brain.

Pulmonary ventilation Breathing; transfer of oxygen from the air through the lungs into the bloodstream.

R

Race pace (RP) Training at a pace that would be maintained during a competitive event.

Range of motion (ROM) The degree to which specific joints or body segments can move; often measured in degrees.

Rapid eye movement (REM) sleep A sleep state in which the brain's electrical activity is dyssynchronous; an electroencephalograph (EEG) shows this as low-voltage, high-frequency activity. This activity reflects brain cells that are very active, firing rapidly at different times.

Rapport building A coach's ongoing process of getting to know an athlete.

Rate coding The speed of the neurological message sent by the brain to the motor units it desires to activate.

Rate of force production Ability of the muscles to exert maximal force output in a minimal amount of time; also known as rate of force development.

Reaction time The interval of time between stimulus detection, pattern recognition, response selection, and initiation of an action.

Reactive neuromuscular training (RNT) A form of training that uses an external load to guide the body toward a weakness, so the body is forced to compensate against the weakness.

Reactive strength The ability to respond to a stimulus (e.g., physical, visual, auditory) with the appropriate amount of strength and control.

Realization The competition and tapering phase/stage of training.

Reciprocal inhibition Contraction of an agonist that causes its antagonist to relax, allowing movement at the joint.

Recovery The adaptive processes to repair, restore, and return the athlete to a normal or supercompensatory state.

Recovery phase Sprint stride cycle phase in which the leg swings from the hip while the foot clears the ground.

Regional interdependence (RI) model A model that proposes problems in one area can lead to compensation patterns and adaptations in other areas, resulting in pain, movement dysfunction, and other symptoms.

Relative age Birth date relative to age group cut-off dates.

Relative age effect A phenomenon in which children born in, or close to, a critical age cut-off period may have an advantage in athletic performance.

Relative energy deficiency in sport (RED-S) syndrome A condition characterized by the interrelationship of low energy availability and menstrual dysfunction, which impair bone structure health. Formerly known as female athlete triad.

Remodeling stage The stage of healing in which the cross-hatched collagen matrix continues to mature and allows the healing of injured tissue.

Repeated-sprint ability (RSA) The ability to execute optimal sprint mechanics in sequential sprints lasting less than or equal to 10 seconds, intermingled with short and infrequent recovery periods.

Repetition maximum (RM) continuum A relationship that describes how the intensity expressed as the percentage of 1RM influences the corresponding number of repetitions that can be performed.

Repetition tempo The speed at which each repetition is performed.

Respiratory system The body system that brings oxygen into the lungs from breathed air while removing carbon dioxide from the lungs to the outside air; includes the airways, lungs, and respiratory muscles. Also known as the pulmonary system.

Response programming A perceptual response involving pattern recognition, response selection, and motor learning of spatial anticipation (i.e., awareness of the sports environment to cognitively organize movements in advance), which is cognitively ingrained in the athlete.

Rest The removal of a training stimulus, activity, or stress.

Rest interval The time taken to recuperate between sets, exercises, or both.

Resting metabolic rate (RMR) The rate of energy expenditure at rest.

Rhythmic breathing Intentionally controlling and regulating breathing patterns to reduce stress and anxiety.

Routine A sequence of relevant thoughts and actions that an athlete systematically engages in before the performance of practice or competition.

Ruffini endings Slow-adapting, encapsulated receptors found in the dermis, subcutaneous tissues, and some connective tissues, which respond to skin stretch.

S

Sagittal plane An imaginary plane that divides the body into left and right.

Sarcomere The structural unit of a myofibril, composed of actin and myosin filaments between two Z-lines.

Saturated fats (SFA) A type of fat that has all of its carbons fully linked with hydrogen atoms.

Scope of practice A term used to describe the skills, actions, procedures, and processes that a qualified individual is permitted to undertake, usually under a professional governing body accreditation and/or law.

Self-confidence The belief that one can successfully perform a task or achieve a goal.

Self-determination theory The belief that one can create and sustain motivation.

Self-myofascial techniques (SMT) Techniques for addressing and breaking up adhesions of the fascia and the surrounding muscle tissues that can be applied and directed by the user; examples include foam rolling and self-massage.

Self-talk The automatic statements and purposeful techniques athletes use to direct sport-related thinking.

Sensations The ability to detect internal and external physical qualities of the environment. Senses include sight, hearing, touch, taste, and smell.

Sensorimotor input Information received from the sensory system (vision, hearing, smell, taste, touch, vestibular, and proprioception).

Series elastic component (SEC) The elastic properties of the tendons and other connective tissues that are located in series, or aligned end-to-end, with the muscle fibers.

Serious adverse event Any adverse event that results in any life-threatening situation, inpatient hospitalization, persistent incapacity of a person's ability to conduct a normal life, a congenital anomaly, reproductive harm, or death.

Session preview The business end of the conversation that outlines what, why, and how.

Session rating of perceived exertion (sRPE) A self-reported outcome measure used to monitor the perceived difficulty of a training session.

Situation-centered view The level of motivation is determined by a given situation.

Size principle Motor unit recruitment occurs from smallest to largest.

Sleep latency The time taken between lying down and falling asleep.

Snatch An Olympic lift involving the lifting of a barbell from a stationary position on the ground to directly overhead in multiple phases using a fairly wide grip.

Social psychoLogical orientation The belief that behavior in sport is determined by a complex interaction between environment and the athlete's personal biological make up.

Somatic anxiety The physiological component of anxiety that involves physical processes such as rapid heartbeat and breathing, sweating, trembling, and stomach discomfort.

Specific preparatory phase The portion of the preparatory phase in which programming shifts toward developing biomotor abilities in a more specific manner required for the athlete's sport—traditionally, shifting to a more anaerobic capacity emphasis using tactics that target repeated sprint ability.

Speed, agility, and quickness (SAQ) tests Tests that evaluate an athlete's ability to move the body as fast as possible in one direction (speed); ability to accelerate, decelerate, stabilize, and quickly change directions with proper posture (agility); and react and change body position with a maximum rate of force production (quickness).

Speed endurance The ability to perform both repetitive short sprints and long sprints greater than 100 yards with minor deceleration due to fatigue.

Speed-strength Moving at high speed with the maximum load possible.

Spiral of engagement Variables within a feedback loop that are positive and continually positively influence the outcome (positive spiral of engagement) or are negative and continually hinder the outcome (negative spiral of engagement).

Sport sampling Participation in two (nonsimultaneous) or more sports over the period of a year.

Sport specialization Intense technical or physical training in a single sport to the exclusion of all other sports.

Sports confidence theory The belief or degree of certainty individuals possess about their ability to be successful in sport.

Sports performance assessments A comprehensive process that involves gathering information and making decisions (e.g., selecting additional tests, designing programs) about an athlete's physiological, physical, and functional abilities.

Sports performance tests A procedure for measuring performance related to a specific skill or ability (e.g., jump height, strength).

Sports psychology The study of performance, mental processes, and well-being of people in sporting settings while considering psychological theory and methods.

Sportsmanship A situation-specific set of behaviors involving concern and respect for rules, opponents, and officials, as well as a positive approach to sporting events.

Stabilization strength The ability of the stabilizing muscles to provide dynamic joint stabilization and postural equilibrium during functional activities.

Standards of practice Standards for providing services consistent with the level of care that another professional with similar education and training would provide. These standards define the criteria that can be used to determine whether quality services have been provided.

State sports confidence (SC state) Situational confidence that wavers and is usually skill-specific.

Static balance The ability to maintain a stable body position with complete postural control, keeping the center of mass within the base of support when minimal movement is present.

Static stretching A type of stretch in which the muscle is passively lengthened to the point of tension and held for a sustained amount of time.

Steady state An exercise intensity at which the oxygen consumption is constant.

Stimulant An agent that increases physiologic or metabolic activity.

Strategic Assessment of Risk and Risk Tolerance (StARRT) A three-step framework that describes when an athlete should be deemed ready to return to participation.

Strength capacity The maximal output of the neuromuscular system; can be classified in different ways such as maximal strength, stabilization, muscle hypertrophy, and power.

Strength reserve The difference between an individual's maximal strength capacity and the strength requirement of the competitive skill or sport movement. A higher strength reserve acts as a buffer between what is needed to play the sport and the strength required to meet unforeseen demands.

Strength-speed Moving relatively heavy loads as fast as possible.

Stretch reflex Neurological signal from the muscle spindle that causes a muscle to contract to prevent excessive lengthening.

Stretch–shortening cycle (SSC) A muscle reflex referred to as the myotatic or stretch reflex, which imparts the ability to store and release elastic energy of the tendons.

Stretch tolerance The ability to experience the physical sensations of stretching to reduce the discomfort felt at the end range of motion.

Stride length The interval of distance completed with each stride, determined by flight time and flight speed.

Stride rate The number of strides accomplished per second, ascertained by ground contact time and flight time.

Stroke volume How much blood the heart pumps each beat.

Subacromial impingement syndrome An inflammatory condition of the shoulder involving tendonitis of the rotator cuff muscles (primarily the supraspinatus muscle) as they pass through the subacromial space below the acromion.

Supercompensation Allowing the body to acclimate to the demands imposed by each exercise to demonstrate improvement and progress.

Superior–inferior axis An imaginary line that passes through a joint from superior to inferior.

Superset Two exercises performed back-to-back in rapid succession with minimal to no rest.

Support phase Sprint stride cycle phase in which the mass of the sprinter is loaded onto or carried by the entire foot.

Sympathetic nervous system (SNS) Subdivision of the autonomic nervous system that works to increase neural activity and put the body in a heightened state of arousal.

Sympatho-adrenergic-adrenal system A physiological connection between the sympathetic nervous system and the adrenal medulla.

Synergistic dominance Compensation by synergists for a weak or inhibited prime mover in an attempt to maintain force production and functional movement patterns.

T

Tabata training A type of HIIT with seven or eight 20-second intervals with 10 seconds of rest between each interval.

Talk test A test used to determine athletes' ability to talk at different exercise intensities.

Tanaka formula A formula used to calculate an estimated maximum heart rate: $HR_{max} = 208 - (0.7 \times age)$.

Task constraints The specific requirements, rules, and goals of a sport or task that influence an athlete's movement behavior and performance.

Tendinopathy Overuse injuries of the tendon characterized by pain, inflammation, tissue structure change, decreased exercise tolerance, and movement dysfunction.

Testosterone A hormone producing secondary male sex characteristics.

Theory of self-efficacy An individual's belief regarding their own capability to produce performances that lead to anticipated outcomes.

Thermic effect of activity The energy that a body spends to engage in formal, structured exercise or sporting events.

Thermic effect of food (TEF) The energy a body spends digesting and absorbing the food it consumes.

Thermoreceptors Sensory organs that respond to changes in temperature, such as heat or cold.

Time-based Olympic sports Events raced against the clock, where the fastest time wins the race; also known as cyclical sports.

Time to exhaustion (TTE) The time remaining before a specific level of work (power or intensity) can no longer be maintained.

Time under tension The number of seconds the muscle is under tension in a single set; calculated by adding the tempo for the speed of movement and multiplying by the number of repetitions.

Tolerable upper limit The greatest quantity of a vitamin or mineral that might be consumed in a day without risk of an adverse health effect.

Tonic reflexes Involuntary, automatic muscle responses to specific sensory stimuli, such as changes in body position or muscle length.

Torque A measure of the amount of force on an object that causes the object to rotate.

Total daily energy expenditure (TDEE) The full sum of all energy expended in a given day by the human body.

Total response time The summation of reaction time and movement time.

Toxicity Accumulation of too much of a vitamin or mineral within the body, resulting in illness or other symptoms.

Training age The number of years or duration of experience that the athlete has participated in systematic (regular, consistent, organized) training.

Trait-centered view The level of motivation is determined by an individual's personal characteristics.

Trait sports confidence (SC trait) Global confidence consistent with an athlete's personality.

Transition phase The off-season; the periodization phase that serves as a rest period for physical and psychological recovery. This phase is generally characterized by the athlete not engaging in formal competitions.

Transition phase (sprinting) Sprint phase in which back-side mechanics transition to front-side mechanics, moving from the acceleration angle to a more upright stance, preparing for top speed.

Transitional movement assessment An assessment that involves movement without a change in the base of support.

Transmutation Sport-specific and skill training that takes advantage of the progress experienced in the accumulation phase.

Transverse plane An imaginary plane that divides the body into top and bottom.

Tri-cycle Annual plan with three peaks or competitive seasons.

Tropomyosin A protein found in muscle fibers that is wound around actin filaments and helps regulate muscle contraction.

Troponin A complex of three proteins found in skeletal and cardiac muscle fibers that regulate muscle contraction.

Type I motor unit An alpha motor neuron that contains only type I slow-twitch muscle fibers.

Type I slow-twitch muscle fiber Muscle fibers that are small in size, generate lower amounts of force, and are more resistant to fatigue.

Type II fast-twitch muscle fiber Muscle fibers that are larger in size, generate higher amounts of force, and are faster to fatigue.

Type II motor unit An alpha motor neuron that contains only type II fast-twitch muscle fibers.

U

Underactive When neural inhibition of a muscle leads to limited neuromuscular recruitment.

Undulating periodization The manipulation of volume and intensities with the training sessions of the week.

Undulation The alternation of higher-intensity resistance training that leads primarily to neural adaptations and lower-intensity resistance training or training that leads to a larger effect on muscle hypertrophy, either between training sessions or between training cycles.

Unidirectional training Use of a single mode of training (i.e., traditional strength training) to improve one biomotor ability during a training session or at the micro-cycle level to enhance sport performance.

Universal athletic position Standing in an approximate one-quarter squat, hips behind the center of gravity, back straight, and feet flat; also referred to as the "ready position."

Unsaturated fats A type of fat that has one or more carbons without a hydrogen atom and at least one double bond.

Upregulated The process whereby a receptor is made available for binding with a molecule or hormone.

V

Valsalva maneuver A process that involves expiring against a closed windpipe, creating additional intra-abdominal pressure and spinal stability.

Vascularization The process of growing blood vessels to improve oxygen and nutrient supply.

Velocity A vector quantity of the direction and magnitude of the distance traveled by an object or athlete divided by the time interval from the start of a movement to completion; the speed at which an object is traveling.

Velocity-based training (VBT) Resistance training approach that focuses on the speed of the lift rather than the weight lifted.

Ventilatory equivalent The amount of ventilation (milliliters per minute, mL/min) divided by how much oxygen is taken in (mL/min).

Ventilatory threshold 1 (VT1) The exercise intensity at which talking becomes challenging; at this point, there is a switch from reliance on mostly aerobic metabolism to a greater reliance on anaerobic metabolism.

Ventilatory threshold 2 (VT2) The exercise intensity at which only single-word speech is possible; the highest exercise intensity at which an athlete can work for a few minutes.

Verbal coaching Spoken communications meant to influence movement learning.

Vestibular system Provides information about the position of the body and head and spatial orientation relative to the surrounding environment; located in the inner ears and assists with balance.

Vitamins Small, organic compounds required in small quantities (usually less than a gram) that must be consumed in the diet because they cannot be manufactured by the body (with some exceptions).

Water-soluble The ability for something to be dissolved in water.

Wet bulb global temperature (WBGT) A measurement of heat stress based on temperature, humidity, and radiant temperature: WBGT = $(0.7 \times T_{wet})$ + $(0.2 \times T_{black\ globe})$ + $(0.1 \times T_{dry})$.

Wolff's law States that bone tissue will adapt to the loads placed upon it along the lines of stress.

Work-to-rest ratio The proportion of sport activity to the proportion of rest, which is used to assign rest intervals that are specific to a sport, sport position, or sporting movement.

YPD Model A framework used in youth training that provides evidence-based guidelines for the appropriate selection of training modes for children and adolescents at different stages of growth and maturation.

Z

Z-disc A protein structure that serves as a boundary between adjacent sarcomeres in muscle fibers.

INDEX

Note: Page numbers followed by *f* and *t* indicate figures and tables, respectively.

flexibility training (*continued*)

  stretching techniques, 371–378

    active, 372–375

    dynamic, 375–378

    static, 371–372, 371*t*

fluid balance, 984

food-first approach, 1011–1012

Food Frequency Questionnaire (FFQ), 989, 990*t*

food journal. *See* diet record (food journal)

foot and ankle injuries, 864–865, 865–867*t*

foot and ankle mobility testing, 247, 247–248*t*

football

  off-season goals and considerations for, 1087*t*

  pre-season goals and considerations for, 1099*t*

  suggested assessments for, 1086*t*

  in-season goals and considerations for, 1107*t*

force-couple relationships, 104, 177–178

force, defined, 174

force-velocity curve, 176–177, 512, 512*f*

force-velocity relationship, 573, 573*f*, 654

4-R system, injury rehabilitation, 1103

free nerve endings, 344–345

frontal plane, 164

fulcrum, 174

functional arm scale for throwers (FAST), 1252–1254*t*, 897

functional overreaching, 717–718

G

GAS. *See* general adaptation syndrome

GCT. *See* ground contact time

general adaptation models, 93–94

general adaptation syndrome (GAS), 94–95

  alarm, 94

  effects on rest and recovery, 720–721

  exhaustion, 95

  periodization, 764, 764*f*

  resistance development, 94–95

generalized exercise instruction, 6–7

general preparatory phase, 766

gentile's taxonomy, 191, 191*t*

GI. *See* glycemic index

global core stabilizers, 396–397, 397*t*

global muscular systems, 179–180

global positioning system (GPS) devices, 700–701

glucose, 680

glycemic index (GI)

and performance, 974

and performance nutrition, 973

vs. glycemic load, 974

glycemic load, 974

glycogen, 680

glycolysis, 680–681

goal setting, 63

goal-setting theory, 58–59

goals, professional and personal, 221

Goldilocks effect, 577

golf

  corrective exercise goals and considerations for, 1114*t*

  pre-practice/play warm-up goals and considerations for, 1119*t*

  strength and conditioning goals and considerations for, 1115*t*

  suggested assessments for, 1112*t*

golgi tendon organs (GTOs), 336, 336*f*

golgi tendon organs, 343, 344*f*, 438, 438, 438*f*

GPS devices. *See* global positioning system devices

greater trochanter pain syndrome (Bursitis), 873*t*

GRF. *See* ground reaction force

grip strength test, 300–301, 301*f*

ground contact time (GCT), 514

ground reaction force (GRF), 506

GTOs. *See* golgi tendon organs

gynecomastia, 1034

H

hamstring muscle strain, 873*t*

handheld myofascial rollers, 367

hang clean, 635

hang position, Olympic lifting, 635, 636*f*

hang power clean, 634, 634*f*

hang power snatch, 634, 634*f*

hang snatch, 635

healing stages, 858–862, 858*f*

  detraining and immobilization characteristics, 862

  inflammatory, 859

  injury rehabilitation, 860–862, 860*f*

  proliferative, 859

  remodeling, 859–860, 859*f*

health-based supplements, 1017

health history questionnaire (HHQ), 209, 211

  demographic information, 211

  injuries and kinetic chain, 211–212

  medical history, 211

  medications, 213, 214*t*

  surgery, 212–213, 213*t*

Health Insurance Portability and Accountability Act (HIPAA), 209

heart arrhythmias, 1019

heart rate monitors, 699–700

  chest strap *vs.* optical sensors, 700

heart rate reserve (HRR), 687–688, 687–688*t*

heart rate variability (HRV), 224–225, 225*f*, 744–745

heme, 1012

hepcidin, 1012

HHQ. *See* health history questionnaire

hierarchy of scientific evidence, 1014, 1014*f*

high-intensity interval training (HIIT), 692–693

high-volume jumping sports, plyometric training, 475

HIIT. *See* high-intensity interval training

HIPAA. *See* Health Insurance Portability and Accountability Act

hip extension prerequisite, for Olympic lifting, 640, 640*f*

hip hinge, Olympic lifting, 635, 636*f*

hip injuries, 872–873, 873–875*t*

HMS. *See* human movement system

hockey

  in-season goals and considerations for, 1133*t*

  off-season goals and considerations for, 1122*t*

  pre-season goals and considerations for, 1129*t*

  suggested assessments for, 1121*t*

holistic approach, 4, 5*f*

holistic athlete development, 5*f*, 8

horizontal jump reference scores for elite male and female athletes, 1212–1213*t*

horizontal (broad) jump test

  double-leg, 308–309, 309*f*

  single-leg, 309–310, 310*f*

hormesis, 983

HRmax. *See* maximum heart rate

HRR. *See* heart rate reserve

HRV. *See* heart rate variability

human movement science

  defined, 162

  language of, 162–163

human movement system (HMS), 211, 7

hydration

  dehydration and hyponatremia symptoms, 986–987

  and evaporative cooling, 985

  hypohydration *vs.* dehydration, 985

  maintaining fluid balance, 984

  monitoring with weight, 985–986

  plan development, 987–988

T

W

Y

Z